**The Maudsley®
Prescribing Guidelines
in Psychiatry**

The Maudsley Guidelines

Other books in the *Maudsley Prescribing Guidelines* series include:

The Maudsley Practice Guidelines for Physical Health Conditions in Psychiatry
David Taylor, Fiona Gaughran, Toby Pillinger

The Maudsley Guidelines on Advanced Prescribing in Psychosis
Paul Morrison, David Taylor, Phillip McGuire

The Maudsley® Prescribing Guidelines in Psychiatry

14th Edition

David M. Taylor, BSc, MSc, PhD, FFRPS, FRPharmS, FRCPEdin, FRCPsychHon

Director of Pharmacy and Pathology, Maudsley Hospital and
Professor of Psychopharmacology, King's College, London, UK

Thomas R. E. Barnes, MBBS, MD, FRCPsych, DSc

Emeritus Professor of Clinical Psychiatry at Imperial College London and
joint head of the Prescribing Observatory for Mental Health at the
Royal College of Psychiatrists' Centre for Quality Improvement, London, UK

Allan H. Young, MB, ChB, MPhil, PhD, FRCP, FRCPsych

Chair of Mood Disorders and Director of the Centre for Affective Disorders in the
Department of Psychological Medicine in the Institute of Psychiatry, Psychology and Neuroscience at King's College,
London, UK

WILEY Blackwell

Registered Office(s)
John Wiley & Sons, Inc., 111 River Street, Hoboken, NJ 07030, USA
John Wiley & Sons Ltd, The Atrium, Southern Gate, Chichester, West Sussex, PO19 8SQ, UK

Editorial Office
The Atrium, Southern Gate, Chichester, West Sussex, PO19 8SQ, UK

For details of our global editorial offices, customer services, and more information about Wiley products visit us at www.wiley.com.

Wiley also publishes its books in a variety of electronic formats and by print-on-demand. Some content that appears in standard print versions of this book may not be available in other formats.

A catalogue record for this book is available from the Library of Congress

Paperback ISBN: 9781119772224; ePDF ISBN: 9781119772248; epub ISBN: 9781119772231

Cover design by Wiley

Set in 10/12pt Sabon by Integra Software Services, Pondicherry, India
Printed and bound by CPI Group (UK) Ltd, Croydon, CR0 4YY

C114213_130521

Contents

Preface

This 14th edition of *The Guidelines* has been written under extraordinary circumstances: the coronavirus pandemic. This global phenomenon has radically altered the lives and working practices of billions of people, and most of us are now familiar, either personally or vicariously, with the experience of the serious physical illness that is associated with COVID-19.

Those working in healthcare have been particularly grievously affected, caring for those made ill by the disease while risking infection themselves. In this environment, the writing of a book has an extremely low priority, if any at all. It is in this context that I give boundless and sincere thanks to all those who have contributed to this edition of *The Guidelines* under such challenging conditions.

Of course, mental health problems have not gone away during the pandemic, and the optimal treatment of mental illness remains a vital imperative. This objective will be all the more critical as we come to deal with the mental health consequences of the pandemic.

This edition of *The Guidelines* has been thoroughly updated to include influential research published since 2017 and all major psychotropic drugs introduced since that time. This edition is also somewhat expanded by the inclusion of new sections on such subjects as the management of agitated delirium, psychotropics at the end of life, intravenous psychotropic formulations, intramuscular clozapine and weekly oral penfluridol. As with previous editions, the 14th edition is written with the intention of having worldwide utility, but it retains its mild emphasis on UK practice.

I would like to pay special tribute to Siobhan Gee for her numerous meticulously prepared contributions on the use of clozapine, Mark Horowitz for his evidence-based and patient-centred guidance on discontinuation of psychotropics, Delia Bishara for her near single-handed production of the chapter on older adults, and Ian Osborne for his contributions on an exceptionally varied range of subjects. Emily Finch deserves particular recognition for organising the writing of the chapter on addictions for the last ten editions of *The Guidelines*. Lastly, I would like to thank my assistant Ivana Clark for managing the production of this edition with patience and an unparalleled attention to detail.

David M. Taylor
London
March 2021

Acknowledgments

The following have contributed to the 14th edition of *The Maudsley® Prescribing Guidelines in Psychiatry*.

Alice Debelle
Andrea Danese
Andrew Wilcock
Annabel Price
Anne Connolly
Bruce Clark
Claire Wilson
Colin Drummond
Daniel Harwood
David Mirfin
Deborah Robson
Delia Bishara
Derek Tracy
Ebenezer Oloyede
Elizabeth Naomi Smith
Emily Finch
Emmert Roberts
Eromona Whiskey
Francis Keaney
Frank Besag
Gabriel Ruane
Georgina Boon
Hubertus Himmerich
Ian Osborne
Irene Guerrini
Iris Rathwell
Ivana Clark
James Stone

Jane Marshall
Janet Treasure
Jemma Theivendran
Jonathan Rogers
Justin Sauer
Kalliopi Vallianatou
Kwame Peprah
Louise Howard
Luke Baker
Luke Jelen
Marinos Kyriakopoulos
Mark Horowitz
Max Henderson
Mike Kelleher
Nicola Funnell
Nicola Kalk
Nilou Nourishad
Oluwakemi Oduniyi
Paramala Santosh
Paul Gringras
Paul Moran
Petrina Douglas-Hall
Sameer Jauhar
Shubhra Mace
Siobhan Gee
Sotiris Posporelis
Stephanie J Lewis
Stephen Barclay

Notes on using *The Maudsley®* *Prescribing Guidelines in Psychiatry*

The main aim of *The Guidelines* is to provide clinicians with practically useful advice on the prescribing of psychotropic agents in both commonly and less commonly encountered clinical situations. The advice contained in this handbook is based on a combination of literature review, clinical experience and expert contribution. We do not claim that this advice is necessarily 'correct' or that it deserves greater prominence than the guidance provided by other professional bodies or special interest groups. We hope, however, to have provided guidance that helps to assure the safe, effective and economic use of medicines in psychiatry. We hope also to have made clear precisely the sources of information used to inform the guidance given. Please note that many of the recommendations provided here go beyond the licensed or labelled indications of many drugs, both in the UK and elsewhere. Note also that, while we have endeavoured to make sure all quoted doses are correct, clinicians should always consult statutory texts before prescribing. Users of *The Guidelines* should also bear in mind that the contents of this handbook are based on information available to us in March 2021. Much of the advice contained here will become out-dated as more research is conducted and published.

No liability is accepted for any injury, loss or damage, however caused.

Notes on inclusion of drugs

The Guidelines are used in many other countries outside the UK. With this in mind, we have included in this edition those drugs in widespread use throughout the Western world in March 2021. These include drugs not marketed in the UK, such as brexpiprazole, desvenlafaxine, pimavanserin and vilazodone, amongst several others. Many older drugs or those not widely available (e.g. levomepromazine, pericyazine, maprotiline, zotepine, oral loxapine, etc.) are either only briefly mentioned or not included on the basis that these drugs are not in widespread use at the time of writing.

Contributors' Conflict of Interest

Most of the contributors to *The Guidelines* have received funding from pharmaceutical manufacturers for research, consultancy or lectures. Readers should be aware that these relationships inevitably colour opinions on such matters as drug selection or preference. We cannot, therefore, guarantee that the guidance provided here is free of indirect influence of the pharmaceutical industry but hope to have mitigated this risk by providing copious literature support for statements made. As regards direct influence, no pharmaceutical company has been allowed to view or comment on any drafts or proofs of *The Guidelines*, and none has made any request for the inclusion or omission of any topic, advice or guidance. To this extent, *The Guidelines* have been written independent of the pharmaceutical industry.

List of abbreviations

AACAP	American Academy of Child and Adolescent Psychiatry	ARB	angiotensin II receptor blocker
		ASD	autism spectrum disorders
ACE	angiotensin-converting enzyme	ASEX	Arizona Sexual Experience Scale
ACh	acetylcholine	AST	aspartate aminotransferase
AChE	acetylcholinesterase	AUDIT	Alcohol Use Disorders
AChE-I	acetylcholinesterase inhibitor		Identification Test
ACR	albumin: creatinine ratio	BAC	blood alcohol concentration
AD	Alzheimer's disease	BAP	British Association for
ADAS-cog	Alzheimer's Disease Assessment		Psychopharmacology
	Scale – cognitive subscale	BBB	blood–brain barrier
ADH	alcohol dehydrogenase	bd	*bis die* (twice a day)
ADHD	attention deficit hyperactivity	BDD	body dysmorphic disorder
	disorder	BDI	Beck Depression Inventory
ADIS	Anxiety Disorders Interview	BDNF	brain-derived neurotrophic
	Schedule		factor
ADL	activities of daily living	BED	binge eating disorder
ADR	adverse drug reaction	BEN	benign ethnic neutropenia
AF	atrial fibrillation	BMI	body mass index
AIDS	acquired immune deficiency	BN	bulimia nervosa
	syndrome	BP	blood pressure
AIMS	Abnormal Involuntary	BPD	borderline personality disorder
	Movement Scale	BPSD	behavioural and psychological
ALP	alkaline phosphatase		symptoms of dementia
ALT	alanine transaminase/	BuChE	butyrylcholinesterase
	aminotransferase	CAM	Confusion Assessment Method
ANC	absolute neutrophil count	CAMS	Childhood Anxiety Multimodal
ANNSERS	Antipsychotic Non-Neurological		Study
	Side-Effects Rating Scale	CATIE	Clinical Antipsychotic Trials of
APA	American Psychological		Intervention Effectiveness
	Association	CBT	cognitive behavioural therapy

CBZ	carbamazepine	DIVA	Diagnostic Interview for
CDRS	Children's Depression Rating		DSM-IV ADHD
	Scale	DLB	dementia with Lewy bodies
CDT	carbohydrate-deficient	DMDD	disruptive mood dysregulation
	transferrin		disorder
CES-D	Centre for Epidemiological	DOAC	direct-acting oral anticoagulant
	Studies Depression scale	DoLS	Deprivation of Liberty
CGAS	Children's Global Assessment		Safeguards
	Scale	DSM	*Diagnostic and Statistical*
CGI	Clinical Global Impression		*Manual of Mental Disorders*
	scales	DVLA	Driver and Vehicle Licensing
CI	confidence interval		Agency
CIBIC-Plus	Clinician's Interview-Based	EAD	early after depolarisation
	Impression of Change	ECG	electrocardiogram
CIGH	clozapine-induced gastrointesti-	ECT	electroconvulsive therapy
	nal hypomotility	EDTA	ethylenediaminetetraacetic acid
CIWA-Ar	Clinical Institute Withdrawal	EEG	electroencephalogram
	Assessment of Alcohol scale	eGFR	estimated glomerular filtration
	revised		rate
CK	creatine kinase	EMDR	eye movement desensitisation
CKD	chronic kidney disease		and reprocessing
CKD-EPI	Chronic Kidney Disease	EOSS	early-onset
	Epidemiology Collaboration		schizophrenia-spectrum
CNS	central nervous system	EPA	eicosapentanoic acid
COMT	catechol-O-methyltransferase	EPS	extrapyramidal symptoms
COPD	chronic obstructive pulmonary	ER	extended release
	disease	ERK	extracellular signal-regulated
COX	cyclo-oxygenase		kinase
CPK	creatinine phosphokinase	ERP	exposure and response
CPP	child–parent psychotherapy		prevention
CPSS	Child PTSD Symptom Scale	ES	effect size
CrCl	creatinine clearance	ESR	erythrocyte sedimentation rate
CREB	cAMP response element-binding	FAST	functional assessment staging
	protein	FBC	full blood count
CRP	C-reactive protein	FDA	Food and Drug Administration
CUtLASS	Cost Utility of the Latest		(USA)
	Antipsychotic Drugs in	FGA	first-generation antipsychotic
	Schizophrenia Study	FPG	fasting plasma glucose
CVA	cerebrovascular accident	FTI	Fatal Toxicity Index
CY-BOCS	Children's Yale-Brown Obsessive	GABA	γ-aminobutyric acid
	Compulsive Scale	GAD	generalised anxiety disorder
CYP	cytochrome P	GASS	Glasgow Antipsychotic
DAI	drug attitude inventory		Side-effect Scale
DESS	Discontinuation–Emergent Signs	GBL	gamma-butyrolactone
	and Symptoms scale	G-CSF	granulocyte colony-stimulating
DEXA	dual-energy X-ray		factor
	absorptiometry	GFR	glomerular filtration rate
DHEA	dehydroepiandrosterone	GGT	γ-glutamyl transferase

GHB	γ-hydroxybutyrate	MASC	Multidimensional Anxiety Scale for Children
GI	gastrointestinal	MCA	Mental Capacity Act
GM-CSF	granulocyte-macrophage colony-stimulating factor	MCI	mild cognitive impairment
GSK3	glycogen synthase kinase 3	MDA	3,4-methylenedioxyam-phetamine
HADS	Hospital Anxiety and Depression Scale	MDMA	3,4-methylenedioxymetham-phetamine
HAMA	Hamilton Anxiety Rating Scale	MDRD	Modification of Diet in Renal Disease
HAND	HIV-associated neurocognitive disorders	MHRA	Medicines and Healthcare Products Regulatory Agency
HD	Huntington's disease	MI	myocardial infarction
HDL	high-density lipoprotein	MMSE	Mini Mental State Examination
HDRS	Hamilton Depression Rating Scale	MR	modified release
HIV	human immunodeficiency virus	MS	mood stabilisers/multiple sclerosis
5-HMT	5-hydroxy-methyl-tolterodine	NAS	neonatal abstinence syndrome
HPA	hypothalamic-pituitary-adrenal	NICE	National Institute for Health and Care Excellence
HR	hazard ratio	NMDA	N-methyl-D-aspartate
IADL	instrumental activities of daily living	NMS	neuroleptic malignant syndrome
ICD	International Classification of Diseases	NNH	number needed to harm
ICH	intracerebral haemorrhage	NNT	number needed to treat
IFG	impaired fasting glucose	nocte	at night
IG	intra-gastric	NPI	neuropsychiatric inventory
IJ	intra-jejunal	NRT	nicotine replacement therapy
IM	intramuscular	NSAID	non-steroidal anti-inflammatory drug
IMCA	independent mental capacity advocate	NVC	neurovascular coupling
IMHP	intramuscular high potency	OCD	obsessive compulsive disorder
INR	international normalised ratio	od	*omni die* (once a day)
IR	immediate release	OD	overdose
IV	intravenous	OGTT	oral glucose tolerance test
IVHP	intravenous high potency	OOWS	Objective Opiate Withdrawal Scale
Kiddie-SADS	Kiddie-Schedule for Affective Disorders and Schizophrenia	OST	opioid substitution treatment
LAI	long-acting injection	PANDAS	Paediatric Autoimmune Neuropsychiatric Disorder Associated with Streptococcus
LD	learning disability		
LDL	low-density lipoprotein	PANS	Paediatric Acute-onset Neuropsychiatric Syndrome
LFTs	liver function tests		
LGIB	lower gastrointestinal bleeding	PANSS	Positive and Negative Syndrome Scale
LSD	lysergic acid diethylamide		
MADRS	Montgomery-Asberg Depression Rating Scale	PBA	pseudobulbar affect
mane	morning	PCP	phencyclidine
MAOI	monoamine oxidase inhibitor	PD	Parkinson's disease
MARS	Medication Adherence Rating Scale		

PDD	pervasive developmental disorders	SCARED	Screen for Child Anxiety and Related Emotional Disorders
PDD-NOS	pervasive developmental disorders not otherwise specified	SCIRS	Severe Cognitive Impairment Rating Scale
P-gp	P-glycoprotein	SCRA	synthetic cannabinoid receptor agonist
PHQ-9	Patient Health Questionnaire-9		
PICU	psychiatric intensive care unit	SGA	second-generation antipsychotics
PLC	pathological laughter and crying		
PLWH	people living with HIV	SIADH	syndrome of inappropriate antidiuretic hormone
PMR	post-mortem redistribution		
po	*per os* (by mouth)	SIB	severe impairment battery
POMH-UK	Prescribing Observatory for Mental Health	SJW	St. John's wort
		SLE	systemic lupus erythematosus
PPH	post-partum haemorrhage	SNRI	serotonin–noradrenaline reuptake inhibitor
PPI	proton pump inhibitor		
prn	*pro re nata* (as required)	SOAD	second opinion appointed doctor
PT	prothrombin time		
PTSD	post-traumatic stress disorder	SPC	summary of product characteristics
PWE	people with epilepsy		
qds	*quarter die sumendum* (four times a day)	SPECT	single photon emission computed tomography
QTc	QT interval adjusted for heart rate	SROM	slow release oral morphine
		SS	steady state
RC	responsible clinician	SSRI	selective serotonin reuptake inhibitor
RCADS	Revised Children's Anxiety and Depression Scale		
		STAR*D	Sequenced Treatment Alternatives to Relieve Depression programme
RCT	randomised controlled trial		
RID	relative infant dose		
RIMA	reversible inhibitor of monoamine oxidase A	STS	selegiline transdermal system
		TADS	Treatment of Adolescents with Depression Study
RLAI	risperidone long-acting injection		
ROMI	Rating of Medication Influences scale	TCA	tricyclic antidepressant
		TD	tardive dyskinesia
RPG	random plasma glucose	tDCS	transcranial direct current stimulation
RR	relative risk		
RRBI	restricted repetitive behaviours and interests	TDP	torsades de pointes
		tds	*ter die sumendum* (three times a day)
RT	rapid tranquillisation		
RTA	road traffic accident	TEAM	Treatment of Early Age Mania
rTMS	repetitive transcranial magnetic stimulation	TF-CBT	trauma-focused cognitive behavioural therapy
RUPP	Research Units on Paediatric Psychopharmacology	TFT	thyroid function test
		THC/CBD	tetrahydrocannabinol/ cannabidiol
RYGB	Roux-en-Y gastric bypass		
SADQ	Severity of Alcohol Dependence Questionnaire	TIA	transient ischaemic attack
		TMS	transcranial magnetic stimulation
SAWS	Short Alcohol Withdrawal Scale		

TORDIA	Treatment of Resistant Depression in Adolescence	VaD	vascular dementia
		VNS	vagal nerve stimulation
TPR	temperature, pulse, respiration	VTE	venous thromboembolism
TRS	treatment-resistant schizophrenia	WBC	white blood cell
		WCC	white cell count
TS	Tourette syndrome	WHO	World Health Organization
U&Es	urea and electrolytes	XL	extended release
UGIB	upper gastrointestinal bleeding	YMRS	Young Mania Rating Scale
UGT	UDP-glucuronosyl transferase	ZA	zuclopenthixol acetate

Part 1

Drug treatment of major psychiatric conditions

Chapter 1

Schizophrenia and related psychoses

ANTIPSYCHOTIC DRUGS

General introduction

Classification of antipsychotics

Before the 1990s, antipsychotics (or major tranquillisers as they were then known) were classified according to their chemistry. The first antipsychotic, chlorpromazine, was a phenothiazine compound – a tricyclic structure incorporating a nitrogen and a sulphur atom. Further phenothiazines were generated and marketed, as were chemically similar thioxanthenes, such as flupentixol. Later entirely different chemical structures were developed according to pharmacological paradigms. These included butyrophenones (haloperidol), diphenylbutylpiperidines (pimozide) and substituted benzamides (sulpiride and amisulpride).

Chemical classification remains useful but is rendered somewhat redundant by the broad range of chemical entities now available and by the absence of any clear structure-activity relationships for newer drugs. The chemistry of some older drugs does relate to their propensity to cause movement disorders. Piperazine phenothiazines (e.g. fluphenazine, trifluoperazine), butyrophenones and thioxanthenes are most likely to cause extrapyramidal effects, while piperidine phenothiazines (e.g. pipotiazine) and benzamides are the least likely. Aliphatic phenothiazines (e.g. chlorpromazine) and diphenylbutylpiperidines (pimozide) are perhaps somewhere in-between.

Relative liability for inducing extrapyramidal symptoms (EPS) was originally the primary factor behind the typical/atypical classification. Clozapine had long been known as an atypical antipsychotic on the basis of its low liability to cause EPS and its failure in animal-based antipsychotic screening tests. Its re-marketing in 1990 signalled the beginning of a series of new medications, all of which were introduced with claims (of varying degrees of accuracy) of 'atypicality'. Of these medications, perhaps only clozapine and, possibly, quetiapine are completely atypical, seemingly having a very low

The Maudsley® Prescribing Guidelines in Psychiatry, Fourteenth Edition. David M. Taylor,
Thomas R. E. Barnes and Allan H. Young.
© 2021 David M. Taylor. Published 2021 by John Wiley & Sons Ltd.

liability for EPS. Others show dose-related effects, although, unlike with typical drugs, therapeutic activity can usually be achieved without EPS. This is possibly the real distinction between typical and atypical drugs: the ease with which a dose can be chosen (within the licensed dosage range), which is effective but does not cause EPS (e.g. compare haloperidol with olanzapine).

The typical/atypical dichotomy does not lend itself well to classification of antipsychotics in the middle ground of EPS liability. Thioridazine was widely described as atypical in the 1980s but is a 'conventional' phenothiazine. Sulpiride was marketed as atypical but is often classified as typical. Risperidone, at its maximum dose of 16mg/day (10mg in the USA), is just about as 'typical' as a drug can be. Alongside these difficulties is the fact that there is nothing either pharmacologically or chemically which clearly binds these so-called atypicals together as a group, save perhaps a general but not universal finding of preference for D2 receptors outside the striatum. Nor are atypicals characterised by improved efficacy over older drugs (clozapine and one or two others excepted) or the absence of hyperprolactinaemia (which is usually worse with risperidone, paliperidone and amisulpride than with typical drugs). Lastly, some more recently introduced agents (e.g. pimavanserin) have antipsychotic activity and do not cause EPS but have almost nothing in common with other atypicals in respect to chemistry, pharmacology or adverse effect profile.

In an attempt to get around some of these problems, typicals and atypicals were reclassified as first- or second-generation antipsychotics (FGA/SGA). All drugs introduced since 1990 are classified as SGAs (i.e. all atypicals), but the new nomenclature dispenses with any connotations regarding atypically, whatever atypicality may mean. However, the FGA/SGA classification remains problematic because neither group is defined by anything other than time of introduction – hardly the most sophisticated pharmacological classification system. Perhaps more importantly, date of introduction is often wildly distant from date of first synthesis. Clozapine is one of the oldest antipsychotics (synthesised in 1959), while olanzapine is hardly in its first flush of youth, having first been patented in 1971. These two drugs are of course SGAs – apparently the most modern of antipsychotics.

In this edition of *The Guidelines*, we conserve the FGA/SGA distinction more because of convention than some scientific basis. Also, we feel that most people know which drugs belong to each group – it thus serves as a useful shorthand. However, it is clearly more sensible to consider the properties of *individual* antipsychotics when choosing drugs to prescribe or in discussions with patients and carers. With this in mind, the use of Neuroscience-based Nomenclature (NbN)[1] – a naming system that reflects pharmacological activity – is strongly recommended.

Choosing an antipsychotic

The NICE guideline for medicines adherence[2] recommends that patients should be as involved as possible in decisions about the choice of medicines that are prescribed for them, and that clinicians should be aware that illness beliefs and beliefs about medicines influence adherence. Consistent with this general advice that covers all of healthcare, the NICE guideline for schizophrenia emphasises the importance of patient choice rather than specifically recommending a class or individual antipsychotic as first-line treatment.[3]

Antipsychotics are effective in both the acute and maintenance treatment of schizo-phrenia and other psychotic disorders. They differ in their pharmacology, pharmacoki-netics, overall efficacy/effectiveness and tolerability, but perhaps more importantly, response and tolerability differ between patients. This variability of individual response means that there is no clear first-line antipsychotic medication that is preferable for all.

Relative efficacy

Following the publication of the independent CATIE[4] and CUtLASS[5] studies, the World Psychiatric Association reviewed the evidence relating to the relative efficacy of 51 FGAs and 11 SGAs and concluded that, if differences in EPS could be minimised (by careful dosing) and anticholinergic use avoided, there was no convincing evidence to support any advantage for SGAs over FGAs.[6] As a class, SGAs may have a lower pro-pensity for EPS and tardive dyskinesia (TD),[7] but this is somewhat offset by a higher propensity to cause metabolic side effects. A meta-analysis of antipsychotic medications for first-episode psychosis[8] found few differences between FGAs and SGAs as groups of drugs but minor advantages for olanzapine and amisulpride individually. A later net-work meta-analysis of first-episode studies found small efficacy advantages for olan-zapine and amisulpride and overall poor performance for haloperidol.[9]

When individual non-clozapine SGAs are compared, initial summary data suggested that olanzapine is marginally more effective than aripiprazole, risperidone, quetiapine and ziprasidone, and that risperidone has a minor advantage over quetiapine and ziprasidone.[10] FGA-controlled trials also suggest an advantage for olanzapine, risperi-done and amisulpride over older drugs.[11,12] A network meta-analysis[13] broadly con-firmed these findings, ranking amisulpride second behind clozapine and olanzapine third. These three drugs were the only ones to show clear efficacy advantages over haloperidol. The magnitude of differences was again small (but potentially substantial enough to be clinically important)[13] and must be weighed against the very different side effect profiles associated with individual antipsychotics. A 2019 network meta-analysis of 32 antipsychotics[14] ranked amisulpride as the most effective drug for positive symp-toms and clozapine as the best for both negative symptoms and overall symptom improvement. Olanzapine and risperidone were also highly ranked for positive symp-tom response. The greatest (beneficial) effect on depressive symptoms was seen with sulpiride, clozapine, amisulpride, olanzapine and the dopamine partial agonists, per-haps reflecting the relative absence of neuroleptic-induced dysphoria common to most FGAs.[15] There was a tendency for more recently introduced drugs to have a lower estimated efficacy – a phenomenon that derives from the substantial increase in placebo response since 1970.[16]

Clozapine is clearly the drug of choice in refractory schizophrenia[17] although, bizarrely, this is not a universal finding,[18] probably because of the nature and quality of many active-comparator trials.[19,20]

Both FGAs and SGAs are associated with a number of adverse effects. These include weight gain, dyslipidaemia, increases in plasma glucose/diabetes,[21,22] hyperprolactinae-mia, hip fracture,[23] sexual dysfunction, EPS including neuroleptic malignant syn-drome,[24] anticholinergic effects, venous thromboembolism (VTE),[25] sedation and postural hypotension. The exact profile is drug-specific (see individual sections on specific adverse effects), although comparative data are not robust[26] (see largescale meta-analyses[13,27] for rankings of some adverse effect risks).

Adverse effects are a common reason for treatment discontinuation,[28] particularly when efficacy is poor.[13] Patients do not always spontaneously report side effects however,[29] and psychiatrists' views of the prevalence and importance of adverse effects differ markedly from patient experience.[30] Systematic enquiry, along with a physical examination and appropriate biochemical tests, is the only way accurately to assess their presence and severity or perceived severity. Patient-completed checklists such as the Glasgow Antipsychotic Side-effect Scale (GASS)[31] can be a useful first step in this process. The clinician-completed Antipsychotic Non-Neurological Side-Effects Rating Scale (ANNSERS) facilitates a more detailed and comprehensive assessment.[32]

Non-adherence to antipsychotic treatment is common, and here the guaranteed medication delivery associated with depot/long-acting injectable antipsychotic preparations is unequivocally advantageous. In comparison with oral antipsychotics, there is strong evidence that depots are associated with a reduced risk of relapse and rehospitalisation.[33–35] The introduction of SGA long-acting injections has to some extent changed the image of depots, which were sometimes perceived as punishments for miscreant patients. Their tolerability advantage probably relates partly to the better definition of their therapeutic dose range, meaning that the optimal dose is more likely to be prescribed (compare aripiprazole, with a licensed dose 300mg or 400mg a month, with flupentixol, which has a licensed dose in the UK of 50mg every four weeks to 400mg a week). The optimal dose of flupentixol is around 40mg every 2 weeks:[27] just 5% of the maximum allowed.

As already mentioned, for patients whose symptoms have not responded sufficiently to adequate, sequential trials of two or more antipsychotic drugs, clozapine is the most effective treatment,[36–38] and its use in these circumstances is recommended by NICE.[3] The biological basis for the superior efficacy of clozapine is uncertain.[39] Olanzapine should probably be one of the two drugs used before clozapine.[10,40] A case might also be made for a trial of amisulpride: it has a uniformly high ranking in meta-analyses, and one trial found continuation with amisulpride to be as effective as switching to olanzapine.[41] This trial also suggested clozapine might be best placed as the second drug used, given that switching provided no benefit over continuing with the first prescribed drug.

This chapter covers the treatment of schizophrenia with antipsychotic drugs, the relative adverse effect profile of these drugs and how adverse effects can be managed.

References

1. Zohar J, et al. A review of the current nomenclature for psychotropic agents and an introduction to the Neuroscience-based Nomenclature. *Eur Neuropsychopharmacol* 2015; 25:2318–2325.
2. National Institute for Clinical Excellence. Medicines adherence: involving patients in decisions about prescribed medicines and supporting adherence. Clinical Guidance [CG76]. 2009 (last checked March 2019); https://www.nice.org.uk/Guidance/CG76.
3. National Institute for Health and Care Excellence. Psychosis and schizophrenia in adults: prevention and management. Clinical Guidance [CG178]. 2014 (last checked March 2019); https://www.nice.org.uk/guidance/cg178.
4. Lieberman JA, et al. Effectiveness of antipsychotic drugs in patients with chronic schizophrenia. *N Engl J Med* 2005; 353:1209–1223.
5. Jones PB, et al. Randomized controlled trial of the effect on Quality of Life of second- vs first-generation antipsychotic drugs in schizophrenia: Cost Utility of the Latest Antipsychotic Drugs in Schizophrenia Study (CUtLASS 1). *Arch Gen Psychiatry* 2006; 63:1079–1087.
6. Tandon R, et al. World Psychiatric Association Pharmacopsychiatry Section statement on comparative effectiveness of antipsychotics in the treatment of schizophrenia. *Schizophr Res* 2008; 100:20–38.
7. Tarsy D, et al. Epidemiology of tardive dyskinesia before and during the era of modern antipsychotic drugs. *Handb Clin Neurol* 2011; 100:601–616.

8. Zhang JP, et al. Efficacy and safety of individual second-generation vs. first-generation antipsychotics in first-episode psychosis: a systematic review and meta-analysis. *Int J Neuro Psychopharmacol* 2013; **16**:1205–1218.

9. Zhu Y, et al. Antipsychotic drugs for the acute treatment of patients with a first episode of schizophrenia: a systematic review with pairwise and network meta-analyses. *Lancet Psychiatry* 2017; **4**:694–705.

10. Leucht S, et al. A meta-analysis of head-to-head comparisons of second-generation antipsychotics in the treatment of schizophrenia. *Am J Psychiatry* 2009; **166**:152–163.

11. Davis JM, et al. A meta-analysis of the efficacy of second-generation antipsychotics. *Arch Gen Psychiatry* 2003; **60**:553–564.

12. Leucht S, et al. Second-generation versus first-generation antipsychotic drugs for schizophrenia: a meta-analysis. *Lancet* 2009; **373**:31–41.

13. Leucht S, et al. Comparative efficacy and tolerability of 15 antipsychotic drugs in schizophrenia: a multiple-treatments meta-analysis. *Lancet* 2013; **382**:951–962.

14. Huhn M, et al. Comparative efficacy and tolerability of 32 oral antipsychotics for the acute treatment of adults with multi-episode schizophrenia: a systematic review and network meta-analysis. *Lancet* 2019; **394**:939–951.

15. Voruganti L, et al. Neuroleptic dysphoria: towards a new synthesis. *Psychopharmacology* 2004; **171**:121–132.

16. Leucht S, et al. Sixty years of placebo-controlled antipsychotic drug trials in acute schizophrenia: systematic review, Bayesian meta-analysis, and meta-regression of efficacy predictors. *Am J Psychiatry* 2017; **174**:927–942.

17. Siskind D, et al. Clozapine v. first- and second-generation antipsychotics in treatment-refractory schizophrenia: systematic review and meta-analysis. *Br J Psychiatry* 2016; **209**:385–392.

18. Samara MT, et al. Efficacy, acceptability, and tolerability of antipsychotics in treatment-resistant schizophrenia: a network meta-analysis. *JAMA Psychiatry* 2016; **73**:199–210.

19. Taylor DM. Clozapine for treatment-resistant schizophrenia: still the gold standard? *CNS Drugs* 2017; **31**:177–180.

20. Kane JM, et al. The role of clozapine in treatment-resistant schizophrenia. *JAMA Psychiatry* 2016; **73**:187–188.

21. Manu P, et al. Prediabetes in patients treated with antipsychotic drugs. *J Clin Psychiatry* 2012; **73**:460–466.

22. Rummel-Kluge C, et al. Head-to-head comparisons of metabolic side effects of second generation antipsychotics in the treatment of schizophrenia: a systematic review and meta-analysis. *Schizophr Res* 2010; **123**:225–233.

23. Sorensen HJ, et al. Schizophrenia, antipsychotics and risk of hip fracture: a population-based analysis. *Eur Neuro Psychopharmacol* 2013; **23**:872–878.

24. Trollor JN, et al. Comparison of neuroleptic malignant syndrome induced by first- and second-generation antipsychotics. *Br J Psychiatry* 2012; **201**:52–56.

25. Masopust J, et al. Risk of venous thromboembolism during treatment with antipsychotic agents. *Psychiatry Clin Neurosci* 2012; **66**:541–552.

26. Pope A, et al. Assessment of adverse effects in clinical studies of antipsychotic medication: survey of methods used. *Br J Psychiatry* 2010; **197**:67–72.

27. Bailey L, et al. Estimating the optimal dose of flupentixol decanoate in the maintenance treatment of schizophrenia-a systematic review of the literature. *Psychopharmacology* 2019; **236**:3081–3092.

28. Falkai P. Limitations of current therapies: why do patients switch therapies? *Eur Neuropsychopharmacol* 2008; **18 Suppl 3**:S135–S139.

29. Yusufi B, et al. Prevalence and nature of side effects during clozapine maintenance treatment and the relationship with clozapine dose and plasma concentration. *Int Clin Psychopharmacol* 2007; **22**:238–243.

30. Day JC, et al. A comparison of patients' and prescribers' beliefs about neuroleptic side-effects: prevalence, distress and causation. *Acta Psychiatr Scand* 1998; **97**:93–97.

31. Waddell L, et al. A new self-rating scale for detecting atypical or second-generation antipsychotic side effects. *J Psychopharmacology* 2008; **22**:238–243.

32. Ohlsen RI, et al. Interrater reliability of the Antipsychotic Non-Neurological Side-Effects Rating Scale measured in patients treated with clozapine. *J Psychopharmacol* 2008; **22**:323–329.

33. Tiihonen J, et al. Effectiveness of antipsychotic treatments in a nationwide cohort of patients in community care after first hospitalisation due to schizophrenia and schizoaffective disorder: observational follow-up study. *BMJ* 2006; **333**:224.

34. Leucht C, et al. Oral versus depot antipsychotic drugs for schizophrenia–a critical systematic review and meta-analysis of randomised long-term trials. *Schizophr Res* 2011; **127**:83–92.

35. Leucht S, et al. Antipsychotic drugs versus placebo for relapse prevention in schizophrenia: a systematic review and meta-analysis. *Lancet* 2012; **379**:2063–2071.

36. Kane J, et al. Clozapine for the treatment-resistant schizophrenic. A double-blind comparison with chlorpromazine. *Arch Gen Psychiatry* 1988; **45**:789–796.

37. McEvoy JP, et al. Effectiveness of clozapine versus olanzapine, quetiapine, and risperidone in patients with chronic schizophrenia who did not respond to prior atypical antipsychotic treatment. *Am J Psychiatry* 2006; **163**:600–610.

38. Lewis SW, et al. Randomized controlled trial of effect of prescription of clozapine versus other second-generation antipsychotic drugs in resistant schizophrenia. *Schizophr Bull* 2006; **32**:715–723.

39. Stone JM, et al. Review: the biological basis of antipsychotic response in schizophrenia. *J Psychopharmacology* 2010; **24**:953–964.

40. Agid O, et al. An algorithm-based approach to first-episode schizophrenia: response rates over 3 prospective antipsychotic trials with a retrospective data analysis. *J Clin Psychiatry* 2011; **72**:1439–1444.

41. Kahn RS, et al. Amisulpride and olanzapine followed by open-label treatment with clozapine in first-episode schizophrenia and schizophreniform disorder (OPTiMiSE): a three-phase switching study. *Lancet Psychiatry* 2018; **5**:797–807.

CHAPTER 1

General principles of prescribing

- The **lowest possible** dose should be used. For each patient, the dose should be titrated to the lowest known to be effective (see the section on minimum effective doses); dose increases should then take place only after one or two weeks of assessment during which the patient is clearly showing poor or no response. (There is gathering evidence that lack of response at 2 weeks is a potent predictor of later poor outcome, unless dose or drug is changed.)

- With regular dosing of **long-acting injections**, plasma levels rise for at least 6–12 weeks after initiation, even without a change in dose (see the section on depot pharmacokinetics in this chapter). Dose increases during this time are therefore difficult to evaluate. The preferred method is to establish efficacy and tolerability of oral medication at a particular dose and then give the equivalent dose of that drug in LAI form. Where this is not possible, the target dose of LAI for an individual should be that established to be optimal in clinical trials (although such data are not always available for older LAIs).

- For the large majority of patients, the use of a **single antipsychotic** (with or without additional mood stabiliser or sedatives) is recommended. Apart from exceptional circumstances (e.g. clozapine augmentation), antipsychotic polypharmacy should generally be avoided because of the increased adverse effect burden and risks associated with QT prolongation and sudden cardiac death (see the section on combined antipsychotics in this chapter).

- **Combinations** of antipsychotics should only be used where response to a single antipsychotic (including clozapine) has been clearly demonstrated to be inadequate. In such cases, the effect of the combination against target symptoms and adverse effects should be carefully evaluated and documented. Where there is no clear benefit, treatment should revert to single antipsychotic therapy.

- In general, **antipsychotics should not be used as 'when necessary' sedatives**. Time-limited prescriptions of benzodiazepines or general sedatives (e.g. promethazine) are recommended (see the section on rapid tranquillisation in this chapter).

- Responses to antipsychotic drug treatment should be **assessed using recognised rating scales** and outcomes documented in patients' records.

- Those receiving antipsychotics should undergo close monitoring of physical health (including blood pressure, pulse, ECG, plasma glucose and plasma lipids) (see appropriate sections in this chapter).

- When withdrawing antipsychotics, reduce the dose slowly in a hyperbolic regimen which minimises the risks of withdrawal symptoms and rebound psychosis.

[*Note*: This section is not referenced. Please see relevant individual sections in this chapter for detailed and referenced guidance.]

Minimum effective doses

Table 1.1 suggests the minimum dose of antipsychotic likely to be effective in first- or multi-episode schizophrenia. Most patients will respond to the dose suggested, although others may require higher doses. Given the variation in individual response, all doses should be considered approximate. Primary references are provided where available, but consensus opinion has also been used. Only oral treatment with commonly used drugs is covered.

Table 1.1 Minimum effective dose/day – antipsychotics

Drug	First episode	Multi-episode
FGAs		
Chlorpromazine[1]	200mg*	300mg
Haloperidol[2–7]	2mg	4mg
Sulpiride[8]	400mg*	800mg
Trifluoperazine[9,10]	10mg*	15mg
SGAs		
Amisulpride[11–16]	300mg*	400mg*
Aripiprazole[7,17–22]	10mg	10mg
Asenapine[7,22,23]	10mg*	10mg
Blonanserin[24]	Not known	8mg
Brexpiprazole[25–27]	2mg*	4mg
Cariprazine[28,29]	1.5mg*	1.5mg
Iloperidone[7,21,22,30]	4mg*	8mg
Lumateperone[31]	Not known	42mg*
Lurasidone[7,32]	40mg HCl/37mg base*	40mg HCl/37mg base
Olanzapine[4,7,33–35]	5mg	7.5mg
Paliperidone[22]	3mg*	3mg
Pimavanserin[36–38]	Not known	34mg**
Quetiapine[39–44]	150mg* (but higher doses often used[45])	300mg
Risperidone[3,7,46–49]	2mg	4mg
Ziprasidone[7,21,50–52]	40mg*	80mg

*Estimate – too few data available
**FDA-approved for Parkinson's disease psychosis; dose in schizophrenia not known

References

1. Dudley K, et al. Chlorpromazine dose for people with schizophrenia. *Cochrane Database Syst Rev* 2017; 4:Cd007778.

2. McGorry PD. Recommended haloperidol and risperidone doses in first-episode psychosis. *J Clin Psychiatry* 1999; 60:794–795.

3. Schooler N, et al. Risperidone and haloperidol in first-episode psychosis: a long-term randomized trial. *Am J Psychiatry* 2005; 162:947–953.

4. Keefe RS, et al. Long-term neurocognitive effects of olanzapine or low-dose haloperidol in first-episode psychosis. *Biol Psychiatry* 2006; 59:97–105.

5. Donnelly L, et al. Haloperidol dose for the acute phase of schizophrenia. *Cochrane Database Syst Rev* 2013; Cd001951.

6. Oosthuizen P, et al. A randomized, controlled comparison of the efficacy and tolerability of low and high doses of haloperidol in the treatment of first-episode psychosis. *Int J Neuropsychopharmacol* 2004; 7:125–131.

7. Leucht S, et al. Dose equivalents for second-generation antipsychotics: the minimum effective dose method. *SchizophrBull* 2014; 40:314–326.

8. Soares BG, et al. Sulpiride for schizophrenia. *Cochrane Database Syst Rev* 2000; CD001162.

9. Armenteros JL, et al. Antipsychotics in early onset schizophrenia: systematic review and meta-analysis. *Eur Child Adolesc Psychiatry* 2006; 15:141–148.

10. Koch K, et al. Trifluoperazine versus placebo for schizophrenia. *Cochrane Database Syst Rev* 2014; Cd010226.

11. Mota NE, et al. Amisulpride for schizophrenia. *Cochrane Database Syst Rev* 2002; CD001357.

12. Puech A, et al. Amisulpride, and atypical antipsychotic, in the treatment of acute episodes of schizophrenia: a dose-ranging study vs. haloperidol. The Amisulpride Study Group. *Acta Psychiatr Scand* 1998; 98:65–72.

13. Moller HJ, et al. Improvement of acute exacerbations of schizophrenia with amisulpride: a comparison with haloperidol. PROD-ASLP Study Group. *Psychopharmacology* 1997; 132:396–401.

14. Sparshatt A, et al. Amisulpride – dose, plasma concentration, occupancy and response: implications for therapeutic drug monitoring. *Acta Psychiatr Scand* 2009; 120:416–428.

15. Buchanan RW, et al. The 2009 schizophrenia PORT psychopharmacological treatment recommendations and summary statements. *SchizophrBull* 2010; 36:71–93.

16. Galletly C, et al. Royal Australian and New Zealand College of Psychiatrists clinical practice guidelines for the management of schizophrenia and related disorders. *Aust N Z J Psychiatry* 2016; 50:410–472.

17. Taylor D. Aripiprazole: a review of its pharmacology and clinical utility. *Int J Clin Pract* 2003; 57:49–54.

18. Cutler AJ, et al. The efficacy and safety of lower doses of aripiprazole for the treatment of patients with acute exacerbation of schizophrenia. *CNS Spectr* 2006; 11:691–702.

19. Mace S, et al. Aripiprazole: dose-response relationship in schizophrenia and schizoaffective disorder. *CNS Drugs* 2008; 23:773–780.

20. Sparshatt A, et al. A systematic review of aripiprazole – dose, plasma concentration, receptor occupancy and response: implications for therapeutic drug monitoring. *J Clin Psychiatry* 2010; 71:1447–1456.

21. Liu CC, et al. Aripiprazole for drug-naive or antipsychotic-short-exposure subjects with ultra-high risk state and first-episode psychosis: an open-label study. *J Clin Psychopharmacol* 2013; 33:18–23.

22. Leucht S, et al. Dose-response meta-analysis of antipsychotic drugs for acute schizophrenia. *Am J Psychiatry* 2020; 177:342–353.

23. Citrome L. Role of sublingual asenapine in treatment of schizophrenia. *Neuropsychiatr Dis Treat* 2011; 7:325–339.

24. Tenjin T, et al. Profile of blonanserin for the treatment of schizophrenia. *Neuropsychiatr Dis Treat* 2013; 9:587–594.

25. Correll CU, et al. Efficacy of brexpiprazole in patients with acute schizophrenia: review of three randomized, double-blind, placebo-controlled studies. *Schizophr Res* 2016; 174:82–92.

26. Malla A, et al. The effect of brexpiprazole in adult outpatients with early-episode schizophrenia: an exploratory study. *Int Clin Psychopharmacol* 2016; 31:307–314.

27. Kane JM, et al. A multicenter, randomized, double-blind, controlled phase 3 trial of fixed-dose brexpiprazole for the treatment of adults with acute schizophrenia. *Schizophr Res* 2015; 164:127–135.

28. Garnock-Jones KP. Cariprazine: a review in schizophrenia. *CNS Drugs* 2017; 31:513–525.

29. Citrome L. Cariprazine for acute and maintenance treatment of adults with schizophrenia: an evidence-based review and place in therapy. *Neuropsychiatr Dis Treat* 2018; 14:2563–2577.

30. Crabtree BL, et al. Iloperidone for the management of adults with schizophrenia. *Clin Ther* 2011; 33:330–345.

31. Correll CU, et al. Efficacy and safety of lumateperone for treatment of schizophrenia: a randomized clinical trial. *JAMA Psychiatry* 2020; 77:349–358.

32. Meltzer HY, et al. Lurasidone in the treatment of schizophrenia: a randomized, double-blind, placebo- and olanzapine-controlled study. *Am J Psychiatry* 2011; 168:957–967.

33. Sanger TM, et al. Olanzapine versus haloperidol treatment in first-episode psychosis. *Am J Psychiatry* 1999; 156:79–87.

34. Kasper S. Risperidone and olanzapine: optimal dosing for efficacy and tolerability in patients with schizophrenia. *Int Clin Psychopharmacol* 1998; 13:253–262.

35. Bishara D, et al. Olanzapine: a systematic review and meta-regression of the relationships between dose, plasma concentration, receptor occupancy, and response. *JClinPsychopharmacol* 2013; 33:329–335.

36. Mathis MV, et al. The US Food and Drug Administration's Perspective on the New Antipsychotic Pimavanserin. *J Clin Psychiatry* 2017; 78:e668–e673.

37. Ballard C, et al. Pimavanserin in Alzheimer's Disease Psychosis: efficacy in patients with more pronounced psychotic symptoms. *J Prev Alzheimers Dis* 2019; 6:27–33.

38. Nasrallah HA, et al. Successful treatment of clozapine-nonresponsive refractory hallucinations and delusions with pimavanserin, a serotonin 5HT-2A receptor inverse agonist. *Schizophr Res* 2019; 208:217–220.

39. Small S, et al. Quetiapine in patients with schizophrenia. A high- and low-dose double-blind comparison with placebo. Seroquel Study Group. *Arch Gen Psychiatry* 1997; 54:549–557.

40. Peuskens J, et al. A comparison of quetiapine and chlorpromazine in the treatment of schizophrenia. *Acta Psychiatr Scand* 1997; 96:265–273.

41. Arvanitis LA, et al. Multiple fixed doses of 'Seroquel' (quetiapine) in patients with acute exacerbation of schizophrenia: a comparison with haloperidol and placebo. *Biol Psychiatry* 1997; 42:233–246.

42. Kopala LC, et al. Treatment of a first episode of psychotic illness with quetiapine: an analysis of 2 year outcomes. *Schizophr Res* 2006; 81:29–39.

43. Sparshatt A, et al. Quetiapine: dose-response relationship in schizophrenia. *CNS Drugs* 2008; 22:49–68.

44. Sparshatt A, et al. Relationship between daily dose, plasma concentrations, dopamine receptor occupancy, and clinical response to quetiapine: a review. *J Clin Psychiatry* 2011; 72:1108–1123.

45. Pagsberg AK, et al. Quetiapine extended release versus aripiprazole in children and adolescents with first-episode psychosis: the multicentre, double-blind, randomised tolerability and efficacy of antipsychotics (TEA) trial. *Lancet Psychiatry* 2017; 4:605–618.

46. Lane HY, et al. Risperidone in acutely exacerbated schizophrenia: dosing strategies and plasma levels. *J Clin Psychiatry* 2000; 61:209–214.

47. Williams R. Optimal dosing with risperidone: updated recommendations. *J Clin Psychiatry* 2001; 62:282–289.

48. Ezewuzie N, et al. Establishing a dose-response relationship for oral risperidone in relapsed schizophrenia. *J Psychopharm* 2006; 20:86–90.

49. Li C, et al. Risperidone dose for schizophrenia. *Cochrane Database Syst Rev* 2009; Cd007474.

50. Bagnall A, et al. Ziprasidone for schizophrenia and severe mental illness. *Cochrane Database Syst Rev* 2000; CD001945.

51. Taylor D. Ziprasidone – an atypical antipsychotic. *Pharm J* 2001; 266:396–401.

52. Joyce AT, et al. Effect of initial ziprasidone dose on length of therapy in schizophrenia. *Schizophr Res* 2006; 83:285–292.

Licensed maximum doses

The following table lists the licensed maximum doses of antipsychotics according to the EMA labelling as of February 2021.

Drug	Maximum dose
FGAs – oral	
Chlorpromazine	1000mg/day
Flupentixol	18mg/day
Haloperidol	20mg/day
Levomepromazine	1200mg/day
Pericyazine	300mg/day
Perphenazine	24mg/day (64mg/day hospitalised patients)
Pimozide	20mg/day
Sulpiride	2400mg/day
Trifluoperazine	20mg/day
Zuclopenthixol	150mg/day
SGAs – oral	
Amisulpride	1200mg/day
Aripiprazole	30mg/day
Asenapine	20mg/day (sublingual)
Cariprazine	6mg/day
Clozapine	900mg/day
Lurasidone	160mg (HCl)/148mg (base)/day
Olanzapine	20mg/day
Paliperidone	12mg/day
Quetiapine	750mg/day schizophrenia (800mg/day for MR preparation) 800mg/day bipolar disorder
Risperidone	16mg/day
Sertindole	24mg/day
Long-acting injections	
Aripiprazole depot	400mg/month
Flupentixol depot	400mg/week
Fluphenazine depot	100mg every 14–35 days
Haloperidol depot	300mg every 4 weeks
Paliperidone depot 1-monthly	150mg/month

Drug	Maximum dose
Paliperidone depot 3-monthly	525mg every 3 months
Pipotiazine depot	200mg every 4 weeks
Risperidone (Janssen)	50mg every 2 weeks
Zuclopenthixol depot	600mg/week

The following table lists the licensed maximum doses of antipsychotics available outside the EU, according to FDA labelling (as of February 2021)

Drug	Maximum dose
SGAs – oral	
Blonanserin*	24mg/day oral[1] (80mg/day patch[2])
Brexpiprazole	4mg/day
Iloperidone	24mg/day
Lumateperone	42mg/day
Molindone	225mg/day
Pimavanserin	34mg/day
RBP-7000 (risperidone 1-monthly)	120mg/month
Ziprasidone	160mg/day

*Available only in China, Japan and South Korea at the time of writing.

References

1. Inoue Y, et al. Safety and effectiveness of oral blonanserin for schizophrenia: a review of Japanese post-marketing surveillances. *J Pharmacol Sci* 2021; **145**:42–51.
2. Nishibe H, et al. Striatal dopamine D2 receptor occupancy induced by daily application of blonanserin transdermal patches: phase 2 study in Japanese patients with schizophrenia. *Int J Neuropsychopharmacol* 2020; **24**:108–117.

Equivalent doses

Knowledge of equivalent dosages is useful when switching between FGAs. Estimates of 'neuroleptic' or 'chlorpromazine' equivalence, in milligrams a day, between these medications are based on clinical experience, expert panel opinion (using various methods) and any dopamine binding studies available.

Table 1.2 provides approximate equivalent doses for FGAs.[1–4] The values given should be seen as a rough guide when switching from one FGA to another and are no substitute for clinical titration of the new medication dose against adverse effects and response.

Equivalent doses of SGAs may be less clinically relevant as these medications tend to have better defined, evidence-based licensed dose ranges. There are several different ways of calculating equivalence based on, for example, defined daily dose,[5] minimum effective dose[6,7] and average dose.[8] These methods give different estimates of equivalence. A very rough guide to equivalent SGA daily dosages is given in the Table 1.3.[3,4,7–9] There is considerable disagreement about exact equivalencies, even amongst the references cited here. Clozapine is not included because this has a distinct initial titration schedule and a high dose-plasma level variability and because it probably has a different mechanism of action.

Comparing potencies of FGAs with SGAs introduces yet more uncertainty with respect to dose equivalence. Very approximately, 100mg chlorpromazine is equivalent to 1.5mg risperidone.[3]

Table 1.2 Equivalent doses of first generation antipsychotics

Drug	Equivalent dose (consensus)	Range of values in literature
Chlorpromazine	100mg/day	Reference
Flupentixol	3mg/day	2–3mg/day
Flupentixol depot	10mg/week	10–20mg/week
Fluphenazine	2mg/day	1–5mg/day
Fluphenazine depot	5mg/week	1–12.5mg/week
Haloperidol	2mg/day	1.5–5mg/day
Haloperidol depot	15mg/week	5–25mg/week
Pericyazine	10mg/day	10mg/day
Perphenazine	10mg/day	5–10mg/day
Pimozide	2mg/day	1.33–2mg/day
Pipotiazine depot	10mg/week	10–12.5mg/week
Sulpiride	200mg/day	133–300mg/day
Trifluoperazine	5mg/day	2.5–5mg/day
Zuclopenthixol	25mg/day	25–60mg/day
Zuclopenthixol depot	100mg/week	40–100mg/week

Table 1.3 Second-generation antipsychotics – approximate equivalent doses[3-10]

Drug	Approximate equivalent dose
Amisulpride	400mg
Aripiprazole	15mg
Asenapine	10mg
Blonanserin	~
Brexpiprazole	2mg
Cariprazine	1.5mg
Clotiapine	100mg
Iloperidone	12mg
Lumateperone	~
Lurasidone	80mg (74mg base)
Melperone	300mg
Molindone	50mg
Olanzapine	10mg
Paliperidone LAI	100mg/month
Pimavanserin	~
Quetiapine	400mg
Risperidone oral	4mg
Risperidone LAI	50mg/2 weeks
Risperidone RBP-7000	120mg/month
Ziprasidone	80mg

~Unknown equivalence at time of writing.

References

1. Foster P. Neuroleptic equivalence. *Pharm J* 1989; **243**:431–432.
2. Atkins M, et al. Chlorpromazine equivalents: a consensus of opinion for both clinical and research implications. *Psychiatric Bull* 1997; **21**:224–226.
3. Patel MX, et al. How to compare doses of different antipsychotics: a systematic review of methods. *Schizophr Res* 2013; **149**:141–148.
4. Gardner DM, et al. International consensus study of antipsychotic dosing. *Am J Psychiatry* 2010; **167**:686–693.
5. Leucht S, et al. Dose equivalents for antipsychotic drugs: the ddd method. *Schizophr Bull* 2016; **42 Suppl 1**:S90–S94.
6. Rothe PH, et al. Dose equivalents for second generation long-acting injectable antipsychotics: the minimum effective dose method. *Schizophr Res* 2018; **193**:23–28.
7. Leucht S, et al. Dose equivalents for second-generation antipsychotics: the minimum effective dose method. *Schizophr Bull* 2014; **40**:314–326.
8. Leucht S, et al. Dose equivalents for second-generation antipsychotic drugs: the classical mean dose method. *Schizophr Bull* 2015; **41**:1397–1402.
9. Woods SW. Chlorpromazine equivalent doses for the newer atypical antipsychotics. *J Clin Psychiatry* 2003; **64**:663–667.
10. Leucht S, et al. Dose-response meta-analysis of antipsychotic drugs for acute schizophrenia. *Am J Psychiatry* 2020; **177**:342–353.

High-dose antipsychotics: prescribing and monitoring

'High dose' antipsychotic medication can result from the prescription of either a single antipsychotic medication at a dose above the recommended maximum or two or more antipsychotic medications concurrently that, when expressed as a percentage of their respective maximum recommended doses and added together, result in a cumulative dose of more than 100%.[1] In clinical practice, antipsychotic polypharmacy and PRN antipsychotic medication are strongly associated with high-dose prescribing.[2,3]

Efficacy

There is no firm evidence that high doses of antipsychotic medication are any more effective than standard doses for schizophrenia. This holds true for the use of antipsychotic medication for rapid tranquillisation, relapse prevention, persistent aggression and the management of acute psychotic episodes.[1] Despite this, in the UK, approximately a quarter to a third of hospitalised patients on antipsychotic medication have been observed to be on a high dose,[2] while the national audit of schizophrenia in 2013, reporting on prescribing practice for over 5,000 predominantly community-based patients, found that, overall, 10% were prescribed a high dose of antipsychotic medication.[4]

Examination of the dose–response effects of a variety of antipsychotic medications has not found any evidence of greater efficacy for doses above accepted licensed ranges.[5,6] Efficacy appears to be optimal at relatively low doses: 4mg/day risperidone;[7] 300mg/day quetiapine,[8] olanzapine 10mg,[9,10] etc. Similarly, treatment with LAI risperidone at a dose of 100mg 2-weekly offers no benefits over 50mg 2-weekly,[11] and 320mg/day ziprasidone[12] is no better than 160mg/day. All currently available antipsychotic medications (with the possible exception of clozapine) exert their antipsychotic effect primarily through antagonism (or partial agonism) at post-synaptic dopamine receptors. There is increasing evidence that in some patients with schizophrenia, refractory symptoms do not seem to be driven through dysfunction of dopamine pathways,[13–16] and so increasing dopamine blockade in such patients is of uncertain value. Just as importantly, the law of mass action dictates that dose increases bring about successively smaller increases in dopamine occupancy once the threshold for efficacy has been reached.[17]

Dold et al.[18] conducted a meta-analysis of RCTs that compared continuation of standard-dose antipsychotic medication with dose escalation in patients whose schizophrenia had proved to be unresponsive to a prospective trial of standard-dose pharmacotherapy with the same antipsychotic medication. In this context, there was no evidence of any benefit associated with the increased dosage. There are a small number of RCTs that have examined the efficacy of high versus standard dosage in patients with a diagnosis of treatment-resistant schizophrenia (TRS).[1] Some demonstrated benefit,[19] but the majority of these studies are old, the number of patients randomised is small and study design is poor by current standards. Some studies used daily doses equivalent to more than 10g chlorpromazine.

In a study of patients with first-episode schizophrenia, increasing the dose of olanzapine up to 30mg/day and the dose of risperidone up to 10mg/day in non-responders to standard doses yielded only a 4% absolute increase in overall response rate; switching to an alternative antipsychotic, including clozapine, was considerably more successful.[20] One small (n = 12) open study of high-dose quetiapine (up to 1400mg/day) found modest benefits in a third of subjects,[21] but other, larger studies of quetiapine have shown no benefit for higher doses.[8,22,23] A further RCT of high-dose olanzapine (up to 45mg/day) versus clozapine for treatment-resistant schizophrenia found similar efficacy for the two treatments, but concluded that, given the small sample size, it would be premature to conclude that they were equivalent.[24] A systematic review of relevant studies comparing olanzapine at above standard dosage with clozapine for TRS concluded that while olanzapine, particularly in higher dosage, might be considered as an alternative to clozapine in TRS, clozapine still had the most robust evidence for efficacy.[25]

The most recent systematic analysis of dose response[26] largely confirmed the observation of a flat or horizontal dose–response curve above a certain dose for all antipsychotics, with the possible exceptions of olanzapine and lurasidone (with these two drugs, there is evidence that doses at the upper end of the licensed range are somewhat more effective than lower doses[10,27]). This systematic review also suggested that doses above which no additional benefit was likely were somewhat higher than those stated above, e.g. risperidone 6.3mg/day; quetiapine 482mg/day. Importantly, however, there was no evidence to support the use of doses of any drug above its licensed does range.

Adverse effects

The majority of side effects associated with antipsychotic treatment are dose-related. These include EPS, sedation, postural hypotension, anticholinergic effects, QTc prolongation and coronary heart disease mortality.[28–31] High-dose antipsychotic treatment is clearly associated with a greater side-effect burden.[12,23,28,32,33] There is some evidence that antipsychotic dose reduction from very high (mean 2253mg chlorpromazine equivalents per day) to high (mean 1315mg chlorpromazine equivalents per day) dose leads to improvements in cognition and negative symptoms.[34]

Recommendations

- The use of high-dose antipsychotic medication should be an exceptional clinical practice and only ever employed when adequate trials of standard treatments, including clozapine, have failed.
- If high-dose antipsychotic medication is prescribed, it should be standard practice to review and document the target symptoms, therapeutic response and side effects, ideally using validated rating scales, so that there is ongoing consideration of the risk-benefit ratio for the patient. Close physical monitoring (including ECG) is essential.

Prescribing high-dose antipsychotic medication

Before using high doses, ensure that:

- Sufficient time has been allowed for response (see section on time to response).
- At least two different antipsychotic medications have been tried sequentially (including, if possible, olanzapine).
- Clozapine has failed or not been tolerated due to agranulocytosis or other serious adverse effect. Most other side-effects can be managed. A small proportion of patients may also decline to take a clozapine regimen.
- Medication adherence is not in doubt (use of blood tests, liquids/dispersible tablets, depot/LAI antipsychotic preparations, etc).
- Adjunctive medications such as antidepressants or mood stabilisers are not indicated.
- Psychological approaches have failed or are not appropriate.

The decision to use high doses should:

- Be made by a senior psychiatrist
- Involve the multidisciplinary team
- Be done, if possible, with a patient's informed consent

Process

- Rule out contraindications (ECG abnormalities, hepatic impairment)
- Consider and minimise any risks posed by concomitant medication (e.g. potential to cause QTc prolongation, electrolyte disturbance or pharmacokinetic interactions via CYP inhibition)
- Document the decision to prescribe high dosage in the clinical notes along with a description of target symptoms. The use of an appropriate rating scale is advised
- Adequate time for response should be allowed after each dosage increment before a further increase is made

Monitoring

- Physical monitoring should be carried out as outlined in the section on monitoring
- All patients on high doses should have regular ECGs (base-line, when steady-state serum levels have been reached after each dosage increment, and then every 6 to 12 months) Additional biochemical/ECG monitoring is advised if drugs that are known to cause electrolyte disturbances or QTc prolongation are subsequently co-prescribed
- Target symptoms should be assessed after 6 weeks and 3 months. If insufficient improvement in these symptoms has occurred, the dose should be decreased to the normal range

References

1. Royal College of Psychiatrists. Consensus statement on high-dose antipsychotic medication. College Report CR190 2014.

2. Paton C, et al. High-dose and combination antipsychotic prescribing in acute adult wards in the UK: the challenges posed by p.r.n. prescribing. *Br J Psychiatry* 2008; **192**:435–439.

3. Roh D, et al. Antipsychotic polypharmacy and high-dose prescription in schizophrenia: a 5-year comparison. *Aust N Z J Psychiatry* 2014; **48**:52–60.

4. Patel MX, et al. Quality of prescribing for schizophrenia: evidence from a national audit in England and Wales. *Eur Neuropsychopharmacol* 2014; **24**:499–509.

5. Davis JM, et al. Dose response and dose equivalence of antipsychotics. *J Clin Psychopharmacol* 2004; **24**:192–208.

6. Gardner DM, et al. International consensus study of antipsychotic dosing. *Am J Psychiatry* 2010; **167**:686–693.

7. Ezewuzie N, et al. Establishing a dose-response relationship for oral risperidone in relapsed schizophrenia. *J Psychopharm* 2006; **20**:86–90.

8. Sparshatt A, et al. Quetiapine: dose-response relationship in schizophrenia. *CNS Drugs* 2008; **22**:49–68.

9. Kinon BJ, et al. Standard and higher dose of olanzapine in patients with schizophrenia or schizoaffective disorder: a randomized, double-blind, fixed-dose study. *J Clin Psychopharmacol* 2008; **28**:392–400.

10. Bishara D, et al. Olanzapine: a systematic review and meta-regression of the relationships between dose, plasma concentration, receptor occupancy, and response. *J Clin Psychopharmacol* 2013; **33**:329–335.

11. Meltzer HY, et al. A six month randomized controlled trial of long acting injectable risperidone 50 and 100 mg in treatment resistant schizophrenia. *Schizophr Res* 2014; **154**:14–22.

12. Goff DC, et al. High-dose oral ziprasidone versus conventional dosing in schizophrenia patients with residual symptoms: the ZEBRAS study. *J Clin Psychopharmacol* 2013; **33**:485–490.

13. Egerton A, et al. Dopamine and glutamate in antipsychotic-responsive compared with antipsychotic-nonresponsive psychosis: a multicenter positron emission tomography and magnetic resonance spectroscopy study (STRATA). *Schizophr Bull* 2020; **47**:505–516.

14. Kapur S, et al. Relationship between dopamine D2 occupancy, clinical response, and side effects: a double-blind PET study of first-episode schizophrenia. *Am J Psychiatry* 2000; **157**:514–520.

15. Demjaha A, et al. Dopamine synthesis capacity in patients with treatment-resistant schizophrenia. *Am J Psychiatry* 2012; **169**:1203–1210.

16. Gillespie AL, et al. Is treatment-resistant schizophrenia categorically distinct from treatment-responsive schizophrenia? A systematic review. *BMC Psychiatry* 2017; **17**:12.

17. Horowitz MA, et al. Tapering Antipsychotic Treatment. *JAMA Psychiatry* 2020; **78**:125–126.

18. Dold M, et al. Dose escalation of antipsychotic drugs in schizophrenia: a meta-analysis of randomized controlled trials. *Schizophr Res* 2015; **166**:187–193.

19. Aubree JC, et al. High and very high dosage antipsychotics: a critical review. *J Clin Psychiatry* 1980; **41**:341–350.

20. Agid O, et al. An algorithm-based approach to first-episode schizophrenia: response rates over 3 prospective antipsychotic trials with a retrospective data analysis. *J Clin Psychiatry* 2011; **72**:1439–1444.

21. Boggs DL, et al. Quetiapine at high doses for the treatment of refractory schizophrenia. *Schizophr Res* 2008; **101**:347–348.

22. Lindenmayer JP, et al. A randomized, double-blind, parallel-group, fixed-dose, clinical trial of quetiapine at 600 versus 1200 mg/d for patients with treatment-resistant schizophrenia or schizoaffective disorder. *J Clin Psychopharmacol* 2011; **31**:160–168.

23. Honer WG, et al. A randomized, double-blind, placebo-controlled study of the safety and tolerability of high-dose quetiapine in patients with persistent symptoms of schizophrenia or schizoaffective disorder. *J Clin Psychiatry* 2012; **73**:13–20.

24. Meltzer HY, et al. A randomized, double-blind comparison of clozapine and high-dose olanzapine in treatment-resistant patients with schizophrenia. *J Clin Psychiatry* 2008; **69**:274–285.

25. Souza JS, et al. Efficacy of olanzapine in comparison with clozapine for treatment-resistant schizophrenia: evidence from a systematic review and meta-analyses. *CNS Spectr* 2013; **18**:82–89.

26. Leucht S, et al. Dose-response meta-analysis of antipsychotic drugs for acute schizophrenia. *Am J Psychiatry* 2020; **177**:342–353.

27. Loebel A, et al. Lurasidone dose escalation in early nonresponding patients with schizophrenia: a randomized, placebo-controlled study. *J Clin Psychiatry* 2016; **77**:1672–1680.

28. Osborn DP, et al. Relative risk of cardiovascular and cancer mortality in people with severe mental illness from the United Kingdom's General Practice Rsearch Database. *Arch Gen Psychiatry* 2007; **64**:242–249.

29. Ray WA, et al. Atypical antipsychotic drugs and the risk of sudden cardiac death. *N Engl J Med* 2009; **360**:225–235.

30. Barbui C, et al. Antipsychotic dose mediates the association between polypharmacy and corrected QT interval. *PLoS One* 2016; **11**:e0148212.

31. Weinmann S, et al. Influence of antipsychotics on mortality in schizophrenia: systematic review. *Schizophr Res* 2009; **113**:1–11.

32. Bollini P, et al. Antipsychotic drugs: is more worse? A meta-analysis of the published randomized control trials. *Psychol Med* 1994; **24**:307–316.

33. Baldessarini RJ, et al. Significance of neuroleptic dose and plasma level in the pharmacological treatment of psychoses. *Arch Gen Psychiatry* 1988; **45**:79–90.

34. Kawai N, et al. High-dose of multiple antipsychotics and cognitive function in schizophrenia: the effect of dose-reduction. *Prog Neuropsychopharmacol Biol Psychiatry* 2006; **30**:1009–1014.

Combined antipsychotics (antipsychotic polypharmacy)

In psychiatric practice, prescriptions for combined antipsychotic medications are common[1–3] and often long term.[4] The medications combined are likely to include LAI antipsychotic preparations,[5,6] quetiapine[7] and FGAs,[8] the last of these perhaps reflecting the frequent use of haloperidol and chlorpromazine as PRN medications.

Poor response to antipsychotic monotherapy

National clinical audits conducted in the UK as part of a Prescribing Observatory for Mental Health (POMH-UK) quality improvement programme[9] found that the most common reasons recorded for prescribing regular, combined antipsychotic medications were a poor response to antipsychotic monotherapy and a period of crossover while switching from one antipsychotic to another. The use of combined antipsychotic medications has been found to be associated with younger patient age, male gender, and increased illness severity, complexity and chronicity, as well as poorer functioning, inpatient status and a diagnosis of schizophrenia.[2,7,10–12] These associations largely reinforce the notion that antipsychotic polypharmacy is used where schizophrenia has proved to be refractory to trials of antipsychotic monotherapy.[10,13–15]

Nonetheless, there is a lack of robust evidence that the efficacy of combined antipsychotic medications is superior to treatment with a single antipsychotic.[16] A meta-analysis of 16 RCTs in schizophrenia, comparing augmentation with a second antipsychotic with continued antipsychotic monotherapy, found that combining antipsychotic medications lacked double-blind/high-quality evidence for overall efficacy.[17] Furthermore, in patients with schizophrenia, the effects of a change back from antipsychotic polypharmacy to monotherapy, even when carefully conducted, are uncertain. While the findings of two randomised studies suggested that the majority of patients may be successfully switched from antipsychotic polypharmacy to monotherapy without loss of symptom control,[18,19] another reported greater increases in symptoms after six months in those participants who had switched to antipsychotic monotherapy,[20] although the expectation is that such exacerbations can be successfully managed.[18]

Long-term antipsychotic treatment

A non-interventional, population-based study in Hungary, sought to compare the effectiveness of antipsychotic monotherapy with the use of combined antipsychotic medications over a one-year observation period. The investigators concluded that while the results provided evidence for the superiority of monotherapy over polypharmacy for SGAs in terms of all-cause treatment discontinuation in schizophrenia, polypharmacy was associated with a lower likelihood of mortality and psychiatric hospitalisations.[21] Similarly, a 20-year, observational study in Finland reported on the risk of rehospitalisation in a cohort of 62,250 hospital-treated patients with schizophrenia. To minimise selection bias, the investigators used within-individual analyses, with each patient used as their own control. The main finding was that antipsychotic combinations, particularly those including clozapine and LAI antipsychotic medications, were associated with a slightly lower risk of psychiatric rehospitalisation than monotherapy.[22] Although the interpretation of such real-world findings is hindered by the issue of confounding by indication,[23] there are perhaps several plausible explanations. It may be that combining antipsychotic medications with different receptor profiles can be more effective and lead to better therapeutic efficacy and/or a lower side-effect burden and therefore better outcomes. It may also be that co-prescribing two antipsychotic medications improves medication adherence in that it increases the likelihood that a patient may use at least one of them.[22] A more complicated and speculative explanation relates to the finding that, in clinical practice, clozapine and LAI antipsychotic preparations appear to be the most effective monotherapies for relapse prevention in schizophrenia.[24] Thus, adding a second antipsychotic medication to clozapine or an LAI antipsychotic medication in an attempt to mitigate metabolic side effects (e.g. by adding aripiprazole) or manage symptoms of agitation, anxiety or sleep disturbance (e.g. by adding olanzapine or quetiapine) might enhance a patient's engagement in their treatment and improve adherence to the effective antipsychotic treatment that has been augmented.

Adverse effects

Evidence for possible harm with combined antipsychotic medications is perhaps more convincing. Clinically significant side effects have been associated with combined antipsychotic medications, which may partly reflect that such a regimen is commonly a high-dose prescription.[8,25] There are reports of an increased prevalence and severity of EPS,[26,27] increased metabolic side effects and diabetes,[20,28,29] sexual dysfunction,[30] an increased risk of hip fracture,[31] paralytic ileus,[32] grand mal seizures,[33] prolonged QTc[34] and arrhythmias.[13] Switching from antipsychotic polypharmacy to monotherapy has been shown to lead to worthwhile improvements in cognitive functioning.[19]

The evidence relating to an increased mortality with a continuing antipsychotic polypharmacy regimen is inconsistent. Two large case–control studies and a database study[35–37] found no increased mortality in patients with schizophrenia receiving antipsychotic polypharmacy, compared with antipsychotic monotherapy. However, a 10-year prospective study of a cohort of 88 patients with schizophrenia reported that receiving more than one antipsychotic medication concurrently was associated with substantially increased mortality.[17,38] These investigators explored the possibility that the use of combined antipsychotic medications might be a proxy for greater severity/increased refractoriness of psychiatric illness but found no association between mortality and any measured index of illness severity, although these measures focussed on negative symptoms and cognitive deficits. Furthermore, analysis of data from a large anonymised mental healthcare database (2007–2014) of 10,945 adult patients with serious mental illness who had been prescribed a single antipsychotic or polypharmacy for six months or more, revealed a weak association between regular, long-term antipsychotic polypharmacy and all-cause mortality and natural causes of death.[39] However, the authors concluded that the evidence for the association was limited, even after controlling for the effect of dose. Another study, involving the follow-up of 99 patients with schizophrenia over a 25-year period, found that those prescribed three antipsychotics simultaneously were twice as likely to die as those who had been prescribed only one.[40] These authors also considered the possibility of indication bias influencing the findings, speculating that combined antipsychotic medication might be more likely to be prescribed for the most severe schizophrenia.

Given the association between combined antipsychotic medication and a greater side-effect burden,[15,41] it follows that it should be standard practice to document in the clinical records the rationale for prescribing combined antipsychotics in individual cases, along with a clear account of the benefits and side effects of an individual trial of the strategy. Medico-legally, this would seem to be prudent although in practice it is rarely done.[42]

The use of combined antipsychotic medications in clinical practice

There are myriad possible antipsychotic medication combinations but very limited data on their relative risk–benefit profiles in relation to overall therapeutic response or target symptom clusters. The clinical disadvantages of antipsychotic polypharmacy include an increased side-effect burden, higher total dosage, increased risk of drug–drug interactions, poorer medication adherence related to the complexity of the treatment, and difficulties in the attribution of any response to one or more of the individual antipsychotic medications prescribed, leading to difficulty in determining the implications for an optimal longer-term regimen.[6]

Despite the limited supportive evidence base, the use of antipsychotic polypharmacy is an established custom and practice in many countries.[43–45] Furthermore, the general consensus across treatment guidelines that the use of combined antipsychotic medication for the treatment of refractory psychotic illness should be considered only after other, evidence-based, pharmacological treatments such as clozapine have been exhausted, is not consistently followed in clinical practice.[6,12,13,46–48] However, it should be noted that a trial of clozapine augmentation with a second antipsychotic medication to enhance efficacy is a potentially supportable practice[49–53] (see the section on clozapine augmentation in this chapter). Other antipsychotic polypharmacy strategies with potentially valid rationales are the addition of aripiprazole to reduce body weight in patients receiving clozapine[54,55] and to normalise prolactin levels in those on haloperidol[56] and risperidone LAI[57] (although not amisulpride[58]). Polypharmacy with aripiprazole in such circumstances may thus represent worthwhile, evidence-based practice, albeit in the absence of regulatory trials demonstrating safety. In many cases, however, using aripiprazole alone might be a more logical choice.

Conclusion

Some of the findings reported above might be considered to challenge the prevailing consensus that prescribing more than one antipsychotic medication is unlikely to improve efficacy and may increase medical morbidity.[59,60] Nevertheless, on the evidence currently available relating to efficacy and the potential for serious adverse effects, the routine use of combined, non-clozapine, antipsychotic medications may be best avoided.

Summary

- There is a lack of robust evidence supporting the efficacy of combined, non-clozapine, antipsychotic medications
- There is substantial evidence supporting the potential for harm and so the use of combined antipsychotic medications, which is commonly a high-dose prescription, should generally be avoided.
- Combined antipsychotic medications are commonly prescribed and this practice seems to be relatively resistant to change
- As a minimum requirement, all patients who are prescribed combined antipsychotic medications should be systematically monitored for side effects (including an ECG) and any beneficial effect on the symptoms of psychotic illness carefully documented.
- Some antipsychotic polypharmacy strategies (e.g. combinations with aripiprazole) show benefits for tolerability but not efficacy.

References

1. Harrington M, et al. The results of a multi-centre audit of the prescribing of antipsychotic drugs for in-patients in the UK. *Psychiatric Bull* 2002; 26:414–418.
2. Gallego JA, et al. Prevalence and correlates of antipsychotic polypharmacy: a systematic review and meta-regression of global and regional trends from the 1970s to 2009. *Schizophr Res* 2012; 138:18–28.
3. Sneider B, et al. Frequency and correlates of antipsychotic polypharmacy among patients with schizophrenia in Denmark: a nation-wide pharmacoepidemiological study. *Eur Neuropsychopharmacol* 2015; 25:1669–1676.
4. Procyshyn RM, et al. Persistent antipsychotic polypharmacy and excessive dosing in the community psychiatric treatment setting: a review of medication profiles in 435 Canadian outpatients. *J Clin Psychiatry* 2010; 71:566–573.
5. Aggarwal NK, et al. Prevalence of concomitant oral antipsychotic drug use among patients treated with long-acting, intramuscular, antipsychotic medications. *J Clin Psychopharmacol* 2012; 32:323–328.
6. Barnes T, et al. Antipsychotic long acting injections: prescribing practice in the UK. *Br J Psychiatry Suppl* 2009; 52:S37–S42.
7. Novick D, et al. Antipsychotic monotherapy and polypharmacy in the treatment of outpatients with schizophrenia in the European Schizophrenia Outpatient Health Outcomes Study. *J Nerv Ment Dis* 2012; 200:637–643.
8. Paton C, et al. High-dose and combination antipsychotic prescribing in acute adult wards in the UK: the challenges posed by p.r.n. prescribing. *Br J Psychiatry* 2008; 192:435–439.
9. Prescribing Observatory for Mental Health. Topic 1g & 3d. Prescribing high dose and combined antipsychotics on adult psychiatric wards. 2017; Prescribing Observatory for Mental Health CCQI1272.
10. Correll CU, et al. Antipsychotic polypharmacy: a comprehensive evaluation of relevant correlates of a long-standing clinical practice. *Psychiatr Clin North Am* 2012; 35:661–681.
11. Baandrup L, et al. Association of antipsychotic polypharmacy with health service cost: a register-based cost analysis. *Eur J Health Econ* 2012; 13:355–363.
12. Kadra G, et al. Predictors of long-term (≥6 months) antipsychotic polypharmacy prescribing in secondary mental healthcare. *Schizophr Res* 2016; 174:106–112.
13. Grech P, et al. Long-term antipsychotic polypharmacy: how does it start, why does it continue? *Ther Adv Psychopharmacol* 2012; 2:5–11.
14. Malandain L, et al. Correlates and predictors of antipsychotic drug polypharmacy in real-life settings: results from a nationwide cohort study. *Schizophr Res* 2018; 192:213–218.
15. Fleischhacker WW, et al. Critical review of antipsychotic polypharmacy in the treatment of schizophrenia. *Int J Neuropsychopharmacol* 2014; 17:1083–1093.
16. Ortiz-Orendain J, et al. Antipsychotic combinations for schizophrenia. *Schizophr Bull* 2018; 44:15–17.
17. Galling B, et al. Antipsychotic augmentation vs. monotherapy in schizophrenia: systematic review, meta-analysis and meta-regression analysis. *World Psychiatry* 2017; 16:77–89.
18. Essock SM, et al. Effectiveness of switching from antipsychotic polypharmacy to monotherapy. *Am J Psychiatry* 2011; 168:702–708.
19. Hori H, et al. Switching to antipsychotic monotherapy can improve attention and processing speed, and social activity in chronic schizophrenia patients. *J Psychiatr Res* 2013; 47:1843–1848.
20. Constantine RJ, et al. The risks and benefits of switching patients with schizophrenia or schizoaffective disorder from two to one antipsychotic medication: a randomized controlled trial. *Schizophr Res* 2015; 166:194–200.
21. Katona L, et al. Real-world effectiveness of antipsychotic monotherapy vs. polypharmacy in schizophrenia: to switch or to combine? A nationwide study in Hungary. *Schizophr Res* 2014; 152:246–254.
22. Tiihonen J, et al. Association of antipsychotic polypharmacy vs monotherapy with psychiatric rehospitalization among adults with schizophrenia. *JAMA Psychiatry* 2019; 76:499–507.
23. Goff DC. Can adjunctive pharmacotherapy reduce hospitalization in schizophrenia?: insights from administrative databases. *JAMA Psychiatry* 2019; 76:468–470.

24. Tiihonen J, et al. Real-world effectiveness of antipsychotic treatments in a nationwide cohort of 29823 patients with schizophrenia. *JAMA Psychiatry* 2017; 74:686–693.

25. López de Torre A, et al. Antipsychotic polypharmacy: a needle in a haystack? *Gen Hosp Psychiatry* 2012; 34:423–432.

26. Carnahan RM, et al. Increased risk of extrapyramidal side-effect treatment associated with atypical antipsychotic polytherapy. *Acta Psychiatr Scand* 2006; 113:135–141.

27. Gomberg RF. Interaction between olanzapine and haloperidol. *J Clin Psychopharmacol* 1999; 19:272–273.

28. Suzuki T, et al. Effectiveness of antipsychotic polypharmacy for patients with treatment refractory schizophrenia: an open-label trial of olanzapine plus risperidone for those who failed to respond to a sequential treatment with olanzapine, quetiapine and risperidone. *Human Psychopharmacology* 2008; 23:455–463.

29. Gallego DW, et al. Safety and tolerability of antipsychotic polypharmacy. *Exp Opin Drug Saf* 2012; 11:527–542.

30. Hashimoto Y, et al. Effects of antipsychotic polypharmacy on side-effects and concurrent use of medications in schizophrenic outpatients. *Psychiatry Clin Neurosci* 2012; 66:405–410.

31. Sorensen HJ, et al. Schizophrenia, antipsychotics and risk of hip fracture: a population-based analysis. *Eur Neuro Psychopharmacol* 2013; 23:872–878.

32. Dome P, et al. Paralytic ileus associated with combined atypical antipsychotic therapy. *Prog Neuropsychopharmacol Biol Psychiatry* 2007; 31:557–560.

33. Hedges DW, et al. New-onset seizure associated with quetiapine and olanzapine. *Ann Pharmacother* 2002; 36:437–439.

34. Beelen AP, et al. Asymptomatic QTc prolongation associated with quetiapine fumarate overdose in a patient being treated with risperidone. *Hum Exp Toxicol* 2001; 20:215–219.

35. Baandrup L, et al. Antipsychotic polypharmacy and risk of death from natural causes in patients with schizophrenia: a population-based nested case-control study. *J Clin Psychiatry* 2010; 71:103–108.

36. Chen Y, et al. Antipsychotics and risk of natural death in patients with schizophrenia. *Neuropsychiatr Dis Treat* 2019; 15:1863–1871.

37. Tiihonen J, et al. Polypharmacy with antipsychotics, antidepressants, or benzodiazepines and mortality in schizophrenia. *Arch Gen Psychiatry* 2012; 69:476–483.

38. Waddington JL, et al. Mortality in schizophrenia. Antipsychotic polypharmacy and absence of adjunctive anticholinergics over the course of a 10-year prospective study. *Br J Psychiatry* 1998; 173:325–329.

39. Kadra G, et al. Long-term antipsychotic polypharmacy prescribing in secondary mental health care and the risk of mortality. *Acta Psychiatr Scand* 2018; 138:123–132.

40. Joukamaa M, et al. Schizophrenia, neuroleptic medication and mortality. *Br J Psychiatry* 2006; 188:122–127.

41. Centorrino F, et al. Multiple versus single antipsychotic agents for hospitalized psychiatric patients: case-control study of risks versus benefits. *Am J Psychiatry* 2004; 161:700–706.

42. Taylor D, et al. Co-prescribing of atypical and typical antipsychotics – prescribing sequence and documented outcome. *Psychiatric Bull* 2002; 26:170–172.

43. Kreyenbuhl J, et al. Adding or switching antipsychotic medications in treatment-refractory schizophrenia. *Psychiatr Serv* 2007; 58:983–990.

44. Nielsen J, et al. Psychiatrists' attitude towards and knowledge of clozapine treatment. *J Psychopharmacology* 2010; 24:965–971.

45. Ascher-Svanum H, et al. Comparison of patients undergoing switching versus augmentation of antipsychotic medications during treatment for schizophrenia. *Neuro Psychiatr Dis Treat* 2012; 8:113–118.

46. Goren JL, et al. Antipsychotic prescribing pathways, polypharmacy, and clozapine use in treatment of schizophrenia. *Psychiatr Serv* 2013; 64:527–533.

47. Howes OD, et al. Adherence to treatment guidelines in clinical practice: study of antipsychotic treatment prior to clozapine initiation. *Br J Psychiatry* 2012; 201:481–485.

48. Thompson JV, et al. Antipsychotic polypharmacy and augmentation strategies prior to clozapine initiation: a historical cohort study of 310 adults with treatment-resistant schizophrenic disorders. *J Psychopharmacology* 2016; 30:436–443.

49. Shiloh R, et al. Sulpiride augmentation in people with schizophrenia partially responsive to clozapine. A double-blind, placebo-controlled study. *Br J Psychiatry* 1997; 171:569–573.

50. Josiassen RC, et al. Clozapine augmented with risperidone in the treatment of schizophrenia: a randomized, double-blind, placebo-controlled trial. *Am J Psychiatry* 2005; 162:130–136.

51. Paton C, et al. Augmentation with a second antipsychotic in patients with schizophrenia who partially respond to clozapine: a meta-analysis. *J Clin Psychopharmacol* 2007; 27:198–204.

52. Barbui C, et al. Does the addition of a second antipsychotic drug improve clozapine treatment? *Schizophr Bull* 2009; 35:458–468.

53. Taylor DM, et al. Augmentation of clozapine with a second antipsychotic – a meta-analysis of randomized, placebo-controlled studies. *Acta Psychiatr Scand* 2009; 119:419–425.

54. Fleischhacker WW, et al. Effects of adjunctive treatment with aripiprazole on body weight and clinical efficacy in schizophrenia patients treated with clozapine: a randomized, double-blind, placebo-controlled trial. *Int J Neuropsychopharmacol* 2010; 13:1115–1125.

55. Cooper SJ, et al. BAP guidelines on the management of weight gain, metabolic disturbances and cardiovascular risk associated with psychosis and antipsychotic drug treatment. *J Psychopharmacology* 2016; 30:717–748.

56. Shim JC, et al. Adjunctive treatment with a dopamine partial agonist, aripiprazole, for antipsychotic-induced hyperprolactinemia: a placebo-controlled trial. *Am J Psychiatry* 2007; 164:1404–1410.

57. Trives MZ, et al. Effect of the addition of aripiprazole on hyperprolactinemia associated with risperidone long-acting injection. *J Clin Psychopharmacol* 2013; 33:538–541.

58. Chen CK, et al. Differential add-on effects of aripiprazole in resolving hyperprolactinemia induced by risperidone in comparison to benzamide antipsychotics. *Prog Neuropsychopharmacol Biol Psychiatry* 2010; 34:1495–1499.

59. Lin SK. Antipsychotic polypharmacy: a dirty little secret or a fashion? *Int J Neuropsychopharmacol* 2020; 23:125–131.

60. Guinart D, et al. Antipsychotic polypharmacy in schizophrenia: why not? *J Clin Psychiatry* 2020; 81:19ac13118.

Antipsychotic prophylaxis

First episode of psychosis

Antipsychotics provide effective protection against relapse, at least in the short to medium term[1] and the introduction of antipsychotics in the 1950s seems to have improved outcomes overall.[2] A meta-analysis of placebo-controlled trials found that 26% of first-episode patients randomised to receive maintenance antipsychotic relapsed after 6–12 months compared with 61% randomised to receive placebo.[3] Although the current consensus is that antipsychotics should be prescribed for 1–2 years after a first episode of schizophrenia,[4,5] one study[6] found that withdrawing antipsychotic treatment in line with this consensus led to a relapse rate of almost 80% after one year medication-free and 98% after 2 years. A 2019 Swedish population study revealed that the longer the treatment with antipsychotics, the lower the risk of hospitalisation (e.g. those with 5 years' treatment had half the hospitalisation rate of those treated for less than 6 months).[7]

Other studies in first-episode schizophrenia confirmed that only a small minority of patients who discontinue remain well 1–2 years later[8-11] (e.g. a small study found 94% of first-episode patients relapsed within 2 years of stopping risperidone long-acting injection, 97% at three years[12]). A 2018 meta-analysis of 8 RCTs was rather more optimistic and found relapse rates averaged 35% (treated) and 61% (discontinued) at 18–24 months.[13]

A 5-year follow-up of a 2-year RCT during which patients received either maintenance antipsychotic treatment or had their antipsychotic dose reduced or discontinued completely found that while there was a clear advantage for maintenance treatment with respect to reducing short-term relapse this advantage was lost in the medium-term. Furthermore, the dose-reduction/discontinuation group were receiving lower doses of antipsychotic drugs at follow-up and had better functional outcomes.[14] There are numerous interpretations of these outcomes, but the most that can be concluded is that dose reduction is a possible option in first-episode psychosis. The study has been heavily criticised[15] and here are certainly other studies showing disastrous outcomes from antipsychotic discontinuation,[16] albeit over shorter periods with fewer subjects. Nonetheless, some patients with first-episode psychosis will not need long-term antipsychotics to stay well – figures as high as 18–30% have been put forward.[17]

There are no reliable patient factors linked to outcome following discontinuation of antipsychotics in first-episode patients (other than cannabis use[18]), and there remains more evidence in favour of continuing antipsychotics than for stopping them.[19] There are indications that very prolonged discontinuation regimens using hyperbolic tapering (see the section of stopping antipsychotics) may offer the best chance of successfully withdrawing from antipsychotic treatment.[20,21]

It should be noted that definitions of relapse usually focus on the severity of positive symptoms, and largely ignore cognitive and negative symptoms: positive symptoms are more likely to lead to hospitalisation while cognitive and negative symptoms (which respond less well, and in some circumstances may even be exacerbated by antipsychotic treatment) have a greater overall impact on quality of life.

With respect to antipsychotic choice, in the context of an RCT, clozapine did not offer any advantage over chlorpromazine in the medium term in first-episode patients with non-refractory illness.[22] But in a large naturalistic study of patients with a first admission for schizophrenia, clozapine and olanzapine fared better with respect to preventing readmission than other oral antipsychotics.[23] In this same study, the use of a long-acting antipsychotic injection seemed to offer advantages over oral antipsychotics despite confounding by indication (depots will have been prescribed to those considered to be poor adherers, oral to those perceived to have good adherence[23]). Later studies show a huge advantage for long-acting risperidone over oral risperidone in first-episode patients[24] and a smaller but substantial benefit for paliperidone LAI over oral antipsychotics in 'recently diagnosed schizophrenia'.[25] In the latest study, amisulpride was shown to give good outcomes and staying on amisulpride after not initially reaching remission was as successful as switching to olanzapine.[26]

In practice, a firm diagnosis of schizophrenia is rarely made after a first episode, and the majority of prescribers and/or patients will have at least attempted to stop antipsychotic treatment within one year.[27] Ideally, patients should have their dose reduced very gradually, and all relevant family members and healthcare staff should be aware of the discontinuation (such a situation is most likely to be achieved by using long-acting injection). It is vital that patients, carers and key-workers are aware of the early signs of relapse and how to access help. Antipsychotics should not be considered the only intervention. Evidence-based psychosocial and psychological interventions are clearly also important.[28]

Multi-episode schizophrenia

The majority of those who have one episode of schizophrenia will go on to have further episodes. Patients with residual symptoms, a greater side effect burden and a less positive attitude to treatment are at greater risk of relapse.[29] With each subsequent episode, the baseline level of functioning deteriorates,[30] and the majority of this decline is seen in the first decade of illness. Suicide risk (10%) is also concentrated in the first decade of illness. Antipsychotic drugs, when taken regularly, protect against relapse in the short, medium and (less certainty) long term.[3,31] Those who receive targeted antipsychotics (i.e. only when symptoms re-emerge) seem to have a worse outcome than those who receive prophylactic antipsychotics,[32,33] and the risk of TD may also be higher. Similarly, low-dose antipsychotics are less effective than standard doses.[34]

Following table summarises the known benefits and harms associated with maintenance antipsychotic treatment as reported in a meta-analysis by Leucht et al. (2012).[3]

Benefits				Harms			
Outcome	Antipsychotic	Placebo	NNT	Adverse effect	Antipsychotic	Placebo	NNH*
Relapse at 7–12 months	27%	64%	3	Movement disorder	16%	9%	17
Re-admission	10%	26%	5	Anticholinergic effects	24%	16%	11
Improvement in mental state	30%	12%	4	Sedation	13%	9%	20
Violent/aggressive behaviour	2%	12%	11	Weight gain	10%	6%	20

NNT = number needed to treat for one patient to benefit; NNH = number treated for one patient to be harmed.
*Likely to be a considerable underestimate as adverse effects are rarely systematically assessed in clinical trials.[35]

Depot preparations may have an advantage over oral in maintenance treatment, most likely because of guaranteed medication delivery (or at least guaranteed awareness of medication delivery). Meta-analyses of clinical trials have shown that the relative and absolute risks of relapse with depot maintenance treatment were 30% and 10% lower, respectively, than with oral treatment.[3,36] Long-acting preparations of antipsychotics may thus be preferred by both prescribers and patients.

Summary

- Relapse rates in patients discontinuing antipsychotics are extremely high.
- Antipsychotics significantly reduce relapse, re-admission and violence/aggression.
- Long-acting depot formulations provide the best protection against relapse.

A large meta-analysis concluded that the risk of relapse with newer antipsychotics is similar to that associated with older drugs.[3] (Note that lack of relapse is not the same as good functioning.[37]) The proportion of multi-episode patients who achieve remission is small and may differ between antipsychotic drugs. The CATIE study reported that only 12% of patients treated with olanzapine achieved remission for at least 6 months, compared with 8% treated with quetiapine and 6% with risperidone.[38] The advantage seen here for olanzapine is consistent with that seen in an acute efficacy network meta-analysis.[39]

Adherence to antipsychotic treatment

Amongst people with schizophrenia, non-adherence with antipsychotic treatment is high. Only 10 days after discharge from hospital up to 25% are partially or non-adherent, rising to 50% at 1 year and 75% at 2 years.[40] Not only does non-adherence increase the risk of relapse, it may also increase the severity of relapse and the duration of hospitalisation.[40] The risk of suicide attempts also increases four-fold[40].

Dose for prophylaxis

Many patients probably receive higher doses than necessary (particularly of the older drugs) when acutely psychotic.[41,42] In the longer term a balance needs to be made between effectiveness and adverse effects. Lower doses of the older drugs (8mg haloperidol/day or equivalent) are, when compared with higher doses, associated with less severe side effects,[43] better subjective state and better community adjustment.[44] Very low doses increase the risk of psychotic relapse.[41,45,46] There are no data to support the use of lower than standard doses of the newer drugs as prophylaxis. Doses that are acutely effective should generally be continued as prophylaxis,[47,48] although an exception to this is prophylaxis after a first episode where very careful dose reduction is probably supportable. There is some recent support for dose reduction in multi-episode schizophrenia,[49] and there are a number of trials in progress at the time of writing.[50–52]

How and when to stop[53]

The decision to stop antipsychotic drugs requires a thorough risk–benefit analysis for each patient. Withdrawal of antipsychotic drugs after long-term treatment should be gradual and closely monitored. The relapse rate in the first 6 months after abrupt withdrawal is double that seen after gradual withdrawal (defined as slow taper down over at least 3 weeks for oral antipsychotics or abrupt withdrawal of depot preparations).[54] One analysis of incidence of relapse after switch to placebo found time to relapse to be very much longer for 3-monthly paliperidone than for 1-monthly and oral.[55] Overall percentage relapse was also reduced. Abrupt withdrawal of oral treatment may also lead to discontinuation symptoms (e.g. headache, nausea, insomnia) in some patients.[56]

The following factors should be considered:[53]

- Is the patient symptom-free, and if so, for how long? Long-standing, non-distressing symptoms which have not previously been responsive to medication may be excluded.
- What is the severity of adverse-effects (EPS, TD, sedation, obesity, etc.)?
- What was the previous pattern of illness? Consider the speed of onset, duration and severity of episodes and any danger posed to self and others.
- Has dosage reduction been attempted before, and, if so, what was the outcome?
- What are the patient's current social circumstances? Is it a period of relative stability, or are stressful life events anticipated?
- What is the social cost of relapse (e.g. is the patient the sole breadwinner for a family)?
- Is the patient/carer able to monitor symptoms, and, if so, will they seek help?

As with first-episode patients, patients, carers and key-workers should be aware of the early signs of relapse and how to access help. Be aware that targeted relapse treatment is much less effective than continuous prophylaxis.[10] Those with a history of aggressive behaviour or serious suicide attempts and those with residual psychotic symptoms should be considered for life-long treatment.

Alternative views

While it is clear that antipsychotics effectively reduce symptom severity and rates of relapse, a minority view is that antipsychotics might also sensitise patients to psychosis. The hypothesis is that relapse on withdrawal can be seen as a type of discontinuation reaction resulting from super-sensitivity of dopamine receptors, although the evidence for this remains uncertain.[57] This phenomenon might explain better outcomes seen in first-episode patients who receive lower doses of antipsychotics, but it also suggests the possibility that the use of antipsychotics might ultimately worsen outcomes. It might also explain the poor outcomes seen with abrupt discontinuation of antipsychotics.[54] This observation in turn leads some to question the validity of long-term studies in which active and successful treatment is abruptly stopped since rebound phenomena and withdrawal reactions may account for at least some of the observed high relapse rates.[58]

The concept of 'super-sensitivity psychosis' was much discussed decades ago[59,60] and has recently seen a resurgence.[57] It is also striking that dopamine antagonists used for non-psychiatric conditions can induce withdrawal psychosis.[61-63] Whilst these theories and observations do not alter recommendations made in this section, they do emphasise the need for using the lowest possible dose of antipsychotic in all patients and the balancing of observed benefit with adverse outcomes including those which might be less clinically obvious (e.g. the possibility of structural brain changes[64]). Clinicians should remain open-minded about the possibility that long-term antipsychotics may worsen, or at least not improve, outcomes in some people with schizophrenia.

References

1. Karson C, et al. Long-term outcomes of antipsychotic treatment in patients with first-episode schizophrenia: a systematic review. *Neuropsychiatr Dis Treat* 2016; **12**:57–67.

2. Taylor M, et al. Are we getting any better at staying better? The long view on relapse and recovery in first episode nonaffective psychosis and schizophrenia. *Ther Adv Psychopharmacol* 2019; **9**:2045125319870033.

3. Leucht S, et al. Antipsychotic drugs versus placebo for relapse prevention in schizophrenia: a systematic review and meta-analysis. *Lancet* 2012; **379**:2063–2071.

4. American Psychiatric Association. Clinical practice guidelines: treatment of patients with schizophrenia. 2019; https://www.psychiatry.org/ psychiatrists/practice/clinical-practice-guidelines.

5. Sheitman BB, et al. The evaluation and treatment of first-episode psychosis. *Schizophr Bull* 1997; **23**:653–661.

6. Gitlin M, et al. Clinical outcome following neuroleptic discontinuation in patients with remitted recent-onset schizophrenia. *Am J Psychiatry* 2001; **158**:1835–1842.

7. Hayes JF, et al. Psychiatric hospitalization following antipsychotic medication cessation in first episode psychosis. *J Psychopharmacology* 2019; **33**:532–534.

8. Wunderink L, et al. Guided discontinuation versus maintenance treatment in remitted first-episode psychosis: relapse rates and functional outcome. *J Clin Psychiatry* 2007; **68**:654–661.

9. Chen EY, et al. Maintenance treatment with quetiapine versus discontinuation after one year of treatment in patients with remitted first episode psychosis: randomised controlled trial. *BMJ* 2010; **341**:c4024.

10. Gaebel W, et al. Relapse prevention in first-episode schizophrenia–maintenance vs intermittent drug treatment with prodrome-based early intervention: results of a randomized controlled trial within the German Research Network on Schizophrenia. *J Clin Psychiatry* 2011; **72**:205–218.

11. Caseiro O, et al. Predicting relapse after a first episode of non-affective psychosis: a three-year follow-up study. *J Psychiatr Res* 2012; **46**:1099–1105.

12. Emsley R, et al. Symptom recurrence following intermittent treatment in first-episode schizophrenia successfully treated for 2 years: a 3-year open-label clinical study. *J Clin Psychiatry* 2012; **73**:e541–e547.

13. Kishi T, et al. Effect of discontinuation v. maintenance of antipsychotic medication on relapse rates in patients with remitted/stable first-episode psychosis: a meta-analysis. *Psychol Med* 2019; **49**:772–779.

14. Wunderink L, et al. Recovery in remitted first-episode psychosis at 7 years of follow-up of an early dose reduction/discontinuation or maintenance treatment strategy: long-term follow-up of a 2-year randomized clinical trial. *JAMA Psychiatry* 2013; **70**:913–920.

15. Correll CU, et al. What is the risk-benefit ratio of long-term antipsychotic treatment in people with schizophrenia? *World Psychiatry* 2018; **17**:149–160.

16. Boonstra G, et al. Antipsychotic prophylaxis is needed after remission from a first psychotic episode in schizophrenia patients: results from an aborted randomised trial. *Int J Psychiatry Clin Pract* 2011; **15**:128–134.

17. Murray RM, et al. Should psychiatrists be more cautious about the long-term prophylactic use of antipsychotics? *Br J Psychiatry* 2016; **209**:361–365.

18. Bowtell M, et al. Rates and predictors of relapse following discontinuation of antipsychotic medication after a first episode of psychosis. *Schizophr Res* 2018; **195**:231–236.

19. Emsley R, et al. How long should antipsychotic treatment be continued after a single episode of schizophrenia? *Curr Opin Psychiatry* 2016; **29**:224–229.

20. Horowitz MA, et al. Tapering antipsychotic treatment. *JAMA Psychiatry* 2020; **78**:125–126.

21. Liu CC, et al. Achieving the lowest effective antipsychotic dose for patients with remitted psychosis: a proposed guided dose-reduction algorithm. *CNS Drugs* 2020; **34**:117–126.

22. Girgis RR, et al. Clozapine v. chlorpromazine in treatment-naive, first-episode schizophrenia: 9-year outcomes of a randomised clinical trial. *Br J Psychiatry* 2011; **199**:281–288.

23. Tiihonen J, et al. A nationwide cohort study of oral and depot antipsychotics after first hospitalization for schizophrenia. *Am J Psychiatry* 2011; **168**:603–609.

24. Subotnik KL, et al. Long-acting injectable risperidone for relapse prevention and control of breakthrough symptoms after a recent first episode of schizophrenia. A randomized clinical trial. *JAMA Psychiatry* 2015; **72**:822–829.

25. Schreiner A, et al. Paliperidone palmitate versus oral antipsychotics in recently diagnosed schizophrenia. *Schizophr Res* 2015; **169**:393–399.

26. Kahn RS, et al. Amisulpride and olanzapine followed by open-label treatment with clozapine in first-episode schizophrenia and schizophreniform disorder (OPTiMiSE): a three-phase switching study. *Lancet Psychiatry* 2018; **5**:797–807.

27. Johnson DAW, et al. Professional attitudes in the UK towards neuroleptic maintenance therapy in schizophrenia. *Psychiatric Bull* 1997; **21**:394–397.

28. National Institute for Health and Care Excellence. Psychosis and schizophrenia in adults: prevention and management. Clinical Guidance [CG178]. 2014 (last checked March 2019); https://www.nice.org.uk/guidance/cg178.

29. Schennach R, et al. Predictors of relapse in the year after hospital discharge among patients with schizophrenia. *Psychiatr Serv* 2012; **63**:87–90.

30. Wyatt RJ. Neuroleptics and the natural course of schizophrenia. *Schizophr Bull* 1991; **17**:325–351.

31. Almerie MQ, et al. Cessation of medication for people with schizophrenia already stable on chlorpromazine. *Schizophr Bull* 2008; **34**:13–14.

32. Jolley AG, et al. Trial of brief intermittent neuroleptic prophylaxis for selected schizophrenic outpatients: clinical and social outcome at two years. *Br Med J* 1990; **301**:837–842.

33. Herz MI, et al. Intermittent vs maintenance medication in schizophrenia. Two-year results. *Arch Gen Psychiatry* 1991; **48**:333–339.

34. Schooler NR, et al. Relapse and rehospitalization during maintenance treatment of schizophrenia. The effects of dose reduction and family treatment. *Arch Gen Psychiatry* 1997; **54**:453–463.

35. Pope A, et al. Assessment of adverse effects in clinical studies of antipsychotic medication: survey of methods used. *Br J Psychiatry* 2010; **197**:67–72.

36. Leucht C, et al. Oral versus depot antipsychotic drugs for schizophrenia–a critical systematic review and meta-analysis of randomised long-term trials. *Schizophr Res* 2011; **127**:83–92.

37. Schooler NR. Relapse prevention and recovery in the treatment of schizophrenia. *J Clin Psychiatry* 2006; **67 Suppl 5**:19–23.

38. Levine SZ, et al. Extent of attaining and maintaining symptom remission by antipsychotic medication in the treatment of chronic schizophrenia: evidence from the CATIE study. *Schizophr Res* 2011; **133**:42–46.

39. Leucht S, et al. Comparative efficacy and tolerability of 15 antipsychotic drugs in schizophrenia: a multiple-treatments meta-analysis. *Lancet* 2013; **382**:951–962.

40. Leucht S, et al. Epidemiology, clinical consequences, and psychosocial treatment of nonadherence in schizophrenia. *J Clin Psychiatry* 2006; **67 Suppl 5**:3–8.

41. Baldessarini RJ, et al. Significance of neuroleptic dose and plasma level in the pharmacological treatment of psychoses. *Arch Gen Psychiatry* 1988; **45**:79–90.

42. Harrington M, et al. The results of a multi-centre audit of the prescribing of antipsychotic drugs for in-patients in the UK. *Psychiatric Bull* 2002; **26**:414–418.

43. Geddes J, et al. Atypical antipsychotics in the treatment of schizophrenia: systematic overview and meta-regression analysis. *Br Med J* 2000; **321**:1371–1376.

44. Hogarty GE, et al. Dose of fluphenazine, familial expressed emotion, and outcome in schizophrenia. Results of a two-year controlled study. *Arch Gen Psychiatry* 1988; **45**:797–805.

45. Marder SR, et al. Low- and conventional-dose maintenance therapy with fluphenazine decanoate. Two-year outcome. *Arch Gen Psychiatry* 1987; **44**:518–521.

46. Uchida H, et al. Low Dose vs Standard Dose of antipsychotics for relapse prevention in schizophrenia: meta-analysis. *Schizophr Bull* 2011; **37**:788–799.

47. Rouillon F, et al. Strategies of treatment with olanzapine in schizophrenic patients during stable phase: results of a pilot study. *Eur Neuropsychopharmacol* 2008; **18**:646–652.

48. Wang CY, et al. Risperidone maintenance treatment in schizophrenia: a randomized, controlled trial. *Am J Psychiatry* 2010; **167**:676–685.

49. Huhn M, et al. Reducing antipsychotic drugs in stable patients with chronic schizophrenia or schizoaffective disorder: a randomized controlled pilot trial. *Eur Arch Psychiatry Clin Neurosci* 2021; **271**:293–302.

50. Stürup AE, et al. TAILOR – tapered discontinuation versus maintenance therapy of antipsychotic medication in patients with newly diagnosed schizophrenia or persistent delusional disorder in remission of psychotic symptoms: study protocol for a randomized clinical trial. *Trials* 2017; **18**:445.

51. Begemann MJH, et al. To continue or not to continue? Antipsychotic medication maintenance versus dose-reduction/discontinuation in first episode psychosis: HAMLETT, a pragmatic multicenter single-blind randomized controlled trial. *Trials* 2020; **21**:147.

52. Moncrieff J, et al. Randomised controlled trial of gradual antipsychotic reduction and discontinuation in people with schizophrenia and related disorders: the RADAR trial (Research into Antipsychotic Discontinuation and Reduction). *BMJ Open* 2019; **9**:e030912.

53. Wyatt RJ. Risks of withdrawing antipsychotic medications. *Arch Gen Psychiatry* 1995; **52**:205–208.

54. Viguera AC, et al. Clinical risk following abrupt and gradual withdrawal of maintenance neuroleptic treatment. *Arch Gen Psychiatry* 1997; **54**:49–55.

55. Weiden PJ, et al. Does half-life matter after antipsychotic discontinuation? A relapse comparison in schizophrenia with 3 different formulations of paliperidone. *J Clin Psychiatry* 2017; **78**:e813–e820.

56. Chouinard G, et al. Withdrawal symptoms after long-term treatment with low-potency neuroleptics. *J Clin Psychiatry* 1984; **45**:500–502.

57. Yin J, et al. Antipsychotic induced dopamine supersensitivity psychosis: a comprehensive review. *Curr Neuropharmacol* 2017; **15**:174–183.

58. Cohen D, et al. Discontinuing psychotropic drugs from participants in randomized controlled trials: a systematic review. *Psychother Psychosom* 2019; **88**:96–104.

59. Chouinard G, et al. Neuroleptic-induced supersensitivity psychosis: clinical and pharmacologic characteristics. *Am J Psychiatry* 1980; **137**:16–21.

60. Kirkpatrick B, et al. The concept of supersensitivity psychosis. *J Nerv Ment Dis* 1992; **180**:265–270.

61. Chaffin DS. Phenothiazine-induced acute psychotic reaction: the 'psychotoxicity' of a drug. *Am J Psychiatry* 1964; **121**:26–32.

62. Lu ML, et al. Metoclopramide-induced supersensitivity psychosis. *Ann Pharmacother* 2002; **36**:1387–1390.

63. Roy-Desruisseaux J, et al. Domperidone-induced tardive dyskinesia and withdrawal psychosis in an elderly woman with dementia. *Ann Pharmacother* 2011; **45**:e51.

64. Huhtaniska S, et al. Long-term antipsychotic use and brain changes in schizophrenia – a systematic review and meta-analysis. *Human Psychopharmacology* 2017; **32**:e2574.

Negative symptoms

Negative symptoms in schizophrenia symptoms represent the absence or diminution of normal behaviours and functions and constitute an important dimension of psychopathology. A subdomain of 'expressive deficits' manifests as a decrease in verbal output or verbal expressiveness and flattened or blunted affect, assessed by diminished facial emotional expression, poor eye contact, decreased spontaneous movement and lack of spontaneity. A second 'avolition/amotivation' subdomain is characterised by a subjective reduction in interests, desires and goals, and a behavioural reduction in purposeful acts, including a lack of self-initiated social interactions.[1,2]

Persistent negative symptoms are held to account for much of the long-term morbidity and poor functional outcome of patients with schizophrenia.[3-6] But the aetiology of negative symptoms is complex, and it is important to determine the most likely cause in any individual case before embarking on a treatment regimen. An important clinical distinction is between primary negative symptoms, which comprise an enduring deficit state, predict a poor prognosis and are stable over time, and secondary negative symptoms, which are consequent upon positive psychotic symptoms, depression or demoralisation, or medication side effects, such as bradykinesia as part of drug-induced parkinsonism.[5,7] Other sources of secondary negative symptoms may include chronic substance/alcohol use, high-dose antipsychotic medication, social deprivation, lack of stimulation and hospitalisation.[8] Secondary negative symptoms may be best tackled by treating the relevant underlying cause. In people with established schizophrenia, negative symptoms are seen to a varying degree in up to three-quarters, with up to 20% having persistent primary negative symptoms.[9,10]

The literature pertaining to the pharmacological treatment of negative symptoms largely consists of sub-analyses of acute efficacy studies, correlational analysis and path analyses.[11] There is often no reliable distinction between primary and secondary negative symptoms or between the two subdomains of expressive deficits and avolition/amotivation, and few studies specifically recruit patients with persistent negative symptoms. While the evidence suggests short-term efficacy for a few interventions, there is no robust evidence for an effective treatment for persistent primary negative symptoms.

In general:

- In first-episode psychosis, the presence of negative symptoms has been related to poor outcome in terms of recovery and level of social functioning.[4,9] There is evidence to suggest that the earlier a psychotic illness is effectively treated, the less likely is the development of negative symptoms over time.[12-14] However, when interpreting such data, it should be borne in mind that an early clinical picture characterised by negative symptoms, being less socially disruptive and more subtle as signs of psychotic illness than positive symptoms, may contribute to delay in presentation to clinical services and thus associated with a longer duration of untreated psychosis. In other words, patients with an inherently poorer prognosis in terms of persistent negative symptoms may be diagnosed and treated later.
- While antipsychotic medication has been shown to improve negative symptoms, this benefit seems to be limited to secondary negative symptoms in acute psychotic episodes.[15] There is no consistent evidence for any superiority of SGAs over FGAs in the

treatment of negative symptoms.[16–20] Similarly, early analyses found no consistent evidence for the superiority of any individual SGA.[21] While a meta-analysis of 38 RCTs found a statistically significant reduction in negative symptoms with SGAs, the effect size did not reach a threshold for 'minimally detectable clinical improvement over time'.[22]

- Nevertheless, a meta-analysis[23] suggests there are robust data suggesting superior efficacy against negative symptoms with certain antipsychotic treatment strategies, such as amisulpride[24–27] and cariprazine,[28,29] and that olanzapine and quetiapine may be more effective than risperidone. Augmentation with aripiprazole may also be effective.[30,31]

- While clozapine remains the only medication with convincing superiority for TRS, whether it has superior efficacy for negative symptoms, at least in the short-term, in such cases remains uncertain.[32–34] One potential confound in studies of clozapine for negative symptoms is that the medication has a low liability for parkinsonian side effects, including bradykinesia, which have a phenomenological overlap with negative symptoms, particularly the subdomain of expressive deficits.

- With respect to non-antipsychotic pharmacological interventions, several drugs that modulate glutamate pathways have been directly tested as adjuncts, but this approach has proved disappointing. Metabotropic glutamate 2/3 (mGlu2/3) receptor agonists have not been found to have any clear effect on negative symptoms over placebo.[35,36] Drugs modulating NMDA receptors in other ways have been tested: for example, there are negative RCTs of glycine,[37] d-serine,[38] modafinil,[39,40] armodafinil,[41] and bitopertin[42,43] augmentation of antipsychotic medication. There is a small preliminary positive RCT of pregnenolone.[44]

- With respect to decreasing glutamate transmission, there are inconsistent meta-analysis findings for lamotrigine augmentation of clozapine[45,46] and one positive[47] and one negative[48] RCT of memantine (the negative study being much larger). There is some suggestion from meta-analyses of relevant studies that adding minocycline, an antibiotic and inflammatory drug, may improve negative symptoms, but the total sample size remains small.[49,50] The BeneMin study was designed to determine whether or not adjunctive minocycline, administered early in the course of schizophrenia, protected against the development of negative symptoms over a year, but the findings did not provide any evidence of clinical benefit with such a strategy.[51]

- With respect to antidepressant augmentation of an antipsychotic for negative symptoms, a Cochrane review concluded that this might be an effective strategy for reducing affective flattening, alogia and avolition,[52] although RCT findings for antidepressant augmentation of antipsychotic medication have found only inconsistent evidence of modest efficacy.[53–56] One meta-analysis of placebo-controlled studies in people with established schizophrenia found that adjunctive antidepressant treatment was associated with a limited reduction in negative symptoms, but only with augmentation of FGAs.[57] Another review of meta-analyses of relevant studies concluded that the evidence suggested a beneficial effect for some SSRIs, such as fluvoxamine, citalopram, and the α2 receptor antagonists mirtazapine and mianserin.[15] Reboxetine may have useful activity.[58]

- Considering glutamate antagonists as adjunctive therapy for negative symptom improvement, there is some limited evidence that topiramate (a noradrenaline reuptake inhibitor) may have some efficacy for symptom reduction in schizophrenia spectrum disorders, including negative symptoms.[59]

- Meta-analyses support the efficacy of augmentation of an antipsychotic with ginkgo biloba[60] and a COX-2 inhibitor (albeit with a small effect size),[61] while small RCTs have demonstrated some benefit for selegiline,[62,63] pramipexole,[64] topical testosterone,[65] ondansetron[66] and granisetron.[67] The findings from studies of repetitive transcranial magnetic stimulation (rTMS) are mixed but promising.[68–70] The evidence for transcranial direct current stimulation (tDCS) as a treatment for negative symptoms is limited and inconclusive.[15,71] A large ($n = 250$) RCT in adults[72] and a smaller RCT in elderly patients[73] each found no benefit for donepezil and there is a further negative RCT of galantamine.[74]

Patients who misuse psychoactive substances experience fewer negative symptoms than patients who do not.[75] But rather than any pharmacological effect, it may be that this association at least partly reflects that those people who develop psychosis in the context of substance use, specifically cannabis, have fewer neurodevelopmental risk factors and thus better cognitive and social function.[76,77]

Summary and recommendations

(Derived from the BAP schizophrenia guideline 2020,[78] Veerman et al. 2017,[8] Aleman et al. 2017[15] and Remington et al. 2016[79])

- There are no well-replicated, large trials, or meta-analyses of trials, with negative symptoms as the primary outcome measure that have yielded convincing evidence for enduring and clinically significant benefit.
- Where some improvement has been demonstrated in clinical trials, this may be limited to secondary negative symptoms.
- Psychotic illness should be identified and treated as early as possible as this may offer some protection against the development of negative symptoms.
- For any given patient, the antipsychotic medication that provides the best balance between overall efficacy and adverse effects should be used at the lowest dose that maintains control of positive symptoms.
- Where negative symptoms persist beyond an acute episode of psychosis:
  - Ensure EPS (specifically bradykinesia) and depression are detected and treated if present, and consider the contribution of the environment to negative symptoms (e.g. institutionalisation, lack of stimulation)
  - There is insufficient evidence at present to support a recommendation for any specific pharmacological treatment for negative symptoms. Nevertheless, a trial of add-on medication for which there is some RCT evidence for efficacy, such as an antidepressant, may be worth considering in some cases, ensuring that the choice of the augmenting agent is based on minimising the potential for compounding side effects through pharmacokinetic or pharmacodynamic drug interactions.

References

1. Messinger JW, et al. Avolition and expressive deficits capture negative symptom phenomenology: implications for DSM-5 and schizophrenia research. *Clin Psychol Rev* 2011; **31**:161–168.

2. Foussias G, et al. Dissecting negative symptoms in schizophrenia: opportunities for translation into new treatments. *J Psychopharmacology* 2015; **29**:116–126.

3. Carpenter WT. The treatment of negative symptoms: pharmacological and methodological issues. *Br J Psychiatry* 1996; **168**:17–22.

4. Galderisi S, et al. Persistent negative symptoms in first episode patients with schizophrenia: results from the European First Episode Schizophrenia Trial. *Eur Neuro PsychoPharmacol* 2013; **23**:196–204.

5. Buchanan RW. Persistent negative symptoms in schizophrenia: an overview. *Schizophr Bull* 2007; **33**:1013–1022.

6. Rabinowitz J, et al. Negative symptoms have greater impact on functioning than positive symptoms in schizophrenia: analysis of CATIE data. *Schizophr Res* 2012; **137**:147–150.

7. Barnes TRE, et al. How to distinguish between the neuroleptic-induced deficit syndrome, depression and disease-related negative symptoms in schizophrenia. *Int Clin Psychopharmacol* 1995; **10 Suppl** 3:115–121.

8. Veerman SRT, et al. Treatment for negative symptoms in schizophrenia: a comprehensive review. *Drugs* 2017; **77**:1423–1459.

9. Rammou A, et al. Negative symptoms in first-episode psychosis: clinical correlates and 1-year follow-up outcomes in London Early Intervention Services. *Early Interv Psychiatry* 2019; **13**:443–452.

10. Bobes J, et al. Prevalence of negative symptoms in outpatients with schizophrenia spectrum disorders treated with antipsychotics in routine clinical practice: findings from the CLAMORS study. *J Clin Psychiatry* 2010; **71**:280–286.

11. Buckley PF, et al. Pharmacological treatment of negative symptoms of schizophrenia: therapeutic opportunity or cul-de-sac? *Acta Psychiatr Scand* 2007; **115**:93–100.

12. Waddington JL, et al. Sequential cross-sectional and 10-year prospective study of severe negative symptoms in relation to duration of initially untreated psychosis in chronic schizophrenia. *Psychol Med* 1995; **25**:849–857.

13. Melle I, et al. Prevention of negative symptom psychopathologies in first-episode schizophrenia: two-year effects of reducing the duration of untreated psychosis. *Arch Gen Psychiatry* 2008; **65**:634–640.

14. Perkins DO, et al. Relationship between duration of untreated psychosis and outcome in first-episode schizophrenia: a critical review and meta-analysis. *Am J Psychiatry* 2005; **162**:1785–1804.

15. Aleman A, et al. Treatment of negative symptoms: where do we stand, and where do we go? *Schizophr Res* 2017; **186**:55–62.

16. Darba J, et al. Efficacy of second-generation-antipsychotics in the treatment of negative symptoms of schizophrenia: a meta-analysis of randomized clinical trials. *Rev Psiquiatr Salud Ment* 2011; **4**:126–143.

17. Leucht S, et al. Second-generation versus first-generation antipsychotic drugs for schizophrenia: a meta-analysis. *Lancet* 2009; **373**:31–41.

18. Erhart SM, et al. Treatment of schizophrenia negative symptoms: future prospects. *Schizophr Bull* 2006; **32**:234–237.

19. Harvey RC, et al. A systematic review and network meta-analysis to assess the relative efficacy of antipsychotics for the treatment of positive and negative symptoms in early-onset schizophrenia. *CNS Drugs* 2016; **30**:27–39.

20. Zhang JP, et al. Efficacy and safety of individual second-generation vs. first-generation antipsychotics in first-episode psychosis: a systematic review and meta-analysis. *Int J Neuro Psychopharmacol* 2013; **16**:1205–1218.

21. Leucht S, et al. A meta-analysis of head-to-head comparisons of second-generation antipsychotics in the treatment of schizophrenia. *Am J Psychiatry* 2009; **166**:152–163.

22. Fusar-Poli P, et al. Treatments of negative symptoms in schizophrenia: meta-analysis of 168 randomized placebo-controlled trials. *Schizophr Bull* 2015; **41**:892–899.

23. Krause M, et al. Antipsychotic drugs for patients with schizophrenia and predominant or prominent negative symptoms: a systematic review and meta-analysis. *Eur Arch Psychiatry Clin Neurosci* 2018; **268**:625–639.

24. Danion JM, et al. Improvement of schizophrenic patients with primary negative symptoms treated with amisulpride. Amisulpride Study Group. *Am J Psychiatry* 1999; **156**:610–616.

25. Speller JC, et al. One-year, low-dose neuroleptic study of in-patients with chronic schizophrenia characterised by persistent negative symptoms. Amisulpride v. haloperidol. *Br J Psychiatry* 1997; **171**:564–568.

26. Leucht S, et al. Amisulpride, an unusual 'atypical' antipsychotic: a meta-analysis of randomized controlled trials. *Am J Psychiatry* 2002; **159**:180–190.

27. Liang Y, et al. Effectiveness of amisulpride in Chinese patients with predominantly negative symptoms of schizophrenia: a subanalysis of the ESCAPE study. *Neuropsychiatr Dis Treat* 2017; **13**:1703–1712.

28. Németh B, et al. Quality-adjusted life year difference in patients with predominant negative symptoms of schizophrenia treated with cariprazine and risperidone. *J Comp Effect Res* 2017; **6**:639–648.

29. Németh G, et al. Cariprazine versus risperidone monotherapy for treatment of predominant negative symptoms in patients with schizophrenia: a randomised, double-blind, controlled trial. *Lancet* 2017; **389**:1103–1113.

30. Zheng W, et al. Efficacy and safety of adjunctive aripiprazole in schizophrenia: meta-analysis of randomized controlled trials. *J Clin Psychopharmacol* 2016; **36**:628–636.

31. Galling B, et al. Antipsychotic augmentation vs. monotherapy in schizophrenia: systematic review, meta-analysis and meta-regression analysis. *World Psychiatry* 2017; **16**:77–89.

32. Siskind D, et al. Clozapine v. first- and second-generation antipsychotics in treatment-refractory schizophrenia: systematic review and meta-analysis. *Br J Psychiatry* 2016; **209**:385–392.

33. Souza JS, et al. Efficacy of olanzapine in comparison with clozapine for treatment-resistant schizophrenia: evidence from a systematic review and meta-analyses. *CNS Spectr* 2013; **18**:82–89.

34. Asenjo Lobos C, et al. Clozapine versus other atypical antipsychotics for schizophrenia. *Cochrane Database Syst Rev* 2010; Cd006633.

35. Adams DH, et al. Pomaglumetad methionil (LY2140023 Monohydrate) and aripiprazole in patients with schizophrenia: a phase 3, multi-center, double-blind comparison. *Schizophr Res Treat* 2014; **2014**:758212.

36. Stauffer VL, et al. Pomaglumetad methionil: no significant difference as an adjunctive treatment for patients with prominent negative symptoms of schizophrenia compared to placebo. *Schizophr Res* 2013; **150**:434–441.

37. Buchanan RW, et al. The Cognitive and Negative Symptoms in Schizophrenia Trial (CONSIST): the efficacy of glutamatergic agents for negative symptoms and cognitive impairments. *Am J Psychiatry* 2007; **164**:1593–1602.

38. Weiser M, et al. A multicenter, add-on randomized controlled trial of low-dose d-serine for negative and cognitive symptoms of schizophrenia. *J Clin Psychiatry* 2012; **73**:e728–e734.

39. Pierre JM, et al. A randomized, double-blind, placebo-controlled trial of modafinil for negative symptoms in schizophrenia. *J Clin Psychiatry* 2007; **68**:705–710.

40. Sabe M, et al. Prodopaminergic drugs for treating the negative symptoms of schizophrenia: systematic review and meta-analysis of randomized controlled trials. *J Clin Psychopharmacol* 2019; **39**:658–664.

41. Kane JM, et al. Adjunctive armodafinil for negative symptoms in adults with schizophrenia: a double-blind, placebo-controlled study. *Schizophr Res* 2012; **135**:116–122.

42. Bugarski-Kirola D, et al. A phase II/III trial of bitopertin monotherapy compared with placebo in patients with an acute exacerbation of schizophrenia – results from the CandleLyte study. *Eur Neuropsychopharmacol* 2014; **24**:1024–1036.

43. Goff DC. Bitopertin: the good news and bad news. *JAMA Psychiatry* 2014; **71**:621–622.

44. Marx CE, et al. Proof-of-concept trial with the neurosteroid pregnenolone targeting cognitive and negative symptoms in schizophrenia. *Neuro Psycho Pharmacology* 2009; **34**:1885–1903.

45. Tiihonen J, et al. The efficacy of lamotrigine in clozapine-resistant schizophrenia: a systematic review and meta-analysis. *Schizophr Res* 2009; **109**:10–14.

46. Veerman SR, et al. Clozapine augmented with glutamate modulators in refractory schizophrenia: a review and metaanalysis. *Pharmacopsychiatry* 2014; **47**:185–194.

47. Rezaei F, et al. Memantine add-on to risperidone for treatment of negative symptoms in patients with stable schizophrenia: randomized, double-blind, placebo-controlled study. *J Clin Psycho Pharmacol* 2013; **33**:336–342.

48. Lieberman JA, et al. A randomized, placebo-controlled study of memantine as adjunctive treatment in patients with schizophrenia. *Neuro Psycho Pharmacology* 2009; **34**:1322–1329.

49. Oya K, et al. Efficacy and tolerability of minocycline augmentation therapy in schizophrenia: a systematic review and meta-analysis of randomized controlled trials. *Human Psycho Pharmacology* 2014; **29**:483–491.

50. Xiang YQ, et al. Adjunctive minocycline for schizophrenia: a meta-analysis of randomized controlled trials. *Eur Neuropsychopharmacol* 2017; **27**:8–18.

51. Deakin B, et al. The benefit of minocycline on negative symptoms of schizophrenia in patients with recent-onset psychosis (BeneMin): a randomised, double-blind, placebo-controlled trial. *Lancet Psychiatry* 2018; **5**:885–894.

52. Rummel C, et al. Antidepressants for the negative symptoms of schizophrenia. *Cochrane Database Syst Rev* 2006; 3:CD005581.

53. Kishi T, et al. Meta-analysis of noradrenergic and specific serotonergic antidepressant use in schizophrenia. *Int J Neuropsychopharmacol* 2014; **17**:343–354.

54. Sepehry AA, et al. Selective serotonin reuptake inhibitor (SSRI) add-on therapy for the negative symptoms of schizophrenia: a meta-analysis. *J Clin Psychiatry* 2007; **68**:604–610.

55. Singh SP, et al. Efficacy of antidepressants in treating the negative symptoms of chronic schizophrenia: meta-analysis. *Br J Psychiatry* 2010; **197**:174–179.

56. Barnes TRE, et al. Antidepressant Controlled Trial For Negative Symptoms In Schizophrenia (ACTIONS): a double-blind, placebo-controlled, randomised clinical trial. *Health Technol Assess* 2016; **20**:1–46.

57. Galling B, et al. Efficacy and safety of antidepressant augmentation of continued antipsychotic treatment in patients with schizophrenia. *Acta Psychiatr Scand* 2018; **137**:187–205.

58. Zheng W, et al. Adjunctive reboxetine for schizophrenia: meta-analysis of randomized double-blind, placebo-controlled trials. *Pharmacopsychiatry* 2020; **53**:5–13.

59. Afshar H, et al. Topiramate add-on treatment in schizophrenia: a randomised, double-blind, placebo-controlled clinical trial. *J Psychopharmacology* 2009; **23**:157–162.

60. Singh V, et al. Review and meta-analysis of usage of ginkgo as an adjunct therapy in chronic schizophrenia. *Int J Neuropsychopharmacol* 2010; **13**:257–271.

61. Sommer IE, et al. Nonsteroidal anti-inflammatory drugs in schizophrenia: ready for practice or a good start? A meta-analysis. *J Clin Psychiatry* 2012; **73**:414–419.

62. Amiri A, et al. Efficacy of selegiline add on therapy to risperidone in the treatment of the negative symptoms of schizophrenia: a double-blind randomized placebo-controlled study. *Human Psychopharmacology* 2008; **23**:79–86.

63. Bodkin JA, et al. Double-blind, placebo-controlled, multicenter trial of selegiline augmentation of antipsychotic medication to treat negative symptoms in outpatients with schizophrenia. *Am J Psychiatry* 2005; **162**:388–390.

64. Kelleher JP, et al. Pilot randomized, controlled trial of pramipexole to augment antipsychotic treatment. *Eur Neuro Psychopharmacol* 2012; **22**:415–418.

65. Ko YH, et al. Short-term testosterone augmentation in male schizophrenics: a randomized, double-blind, placebo-controlled trial. *J Clin Psychopharmacol* 2008; **28**:375–383.

66. Zhang ZJ, et al. Beneficial effects of ondansetron as an adjunct to haloperidol for chronic, treatment-resistant schizophrenia: a double-blind, randomized, placebo-controlled study. *Schizophr Res* 2006; **88**:102–110.

67. Khodaie-Ardakani MR, et al. Granisetron as an add-on to risperidone for treatment of negative symptoms in patients with stable schizophrenia: randomized double-blind placebo-controlled study. *J Psychiatr Res* 2013; **47**:472–478.

68. Shi C, et al. Revisiting the therapeutic effect of rTMS on negative symptoms in schizophrenia: a meta-analysis. *Psychiatry Res* 2014; **215**:505–513.

69. Wobrock T, et al. Left prefrontal high-frequency repetitive transcranial magnetic stimulation for the treatment of schizophrenia with predominant negative symptoms: a sham-controlled, randomized multicenter trial. *Biol Psychiatry* 2015; **77**:979–988.

70. Wang J, et al. Efficacy towards negative symptoms and safety of repetitive transcranial magnetic stimulation treatment for patients with schizophrenia: a systematic review. *Shanghai Arch Psychiatry* 2017; **29**:61–76.

71. Mondino M, et al. Transcranial direct current stimulation for the treatment of refractory symptoms of schizophrenia. Current evidence and future directions. *Curr Pharm Des* 2015; **21**:3373–3383.

72. Keefe RSE, et al. Efficacy and safety of donepezil in patients with schizophrenia or schizoaffective disorder: significant placebo/practice effects in a 12-week, randomized, double-blind, placebo-controlled trial. *Neuro Psycho Pharmacology* 2007; **33**:1217–1228.

73. Mazeh D, et al. Donepezil for negative signs in elderly patients with schizophrenia: an add-on, double-blind, crossover, placebo-controlled study. *Int Psychogeriatr* 2006; **18**:429–436.

74. Conley RR, et al. The effects of galantamine on psychopathology in chronic stable schizophrenia. *Clin Neuropharmacol* 2009; **32**:69–74.

75. Potvin S, et al. A meta-analysis of negative symptoms in dual diagnosis schizophrenia. *Psychol Med* 2006; **36**:431–440.

76. Arndt S, et al. Comorbidity of substance abuse and schizophrenia: the role of pre-morbid adjustment. *Psychol Med* 1992; **22**:379–388.

77. Leeson VC, et al. The effect of cannabis use and cognitive reserve on age at onset and psychosis outcomes in first-episode schizophrenia. *Schizophr Bull* 2012; **38**:873–880.

78. Barnes TRE, et al. Evidence-based guidelines for the pharmacological treatment of schizophrenia: updated recommendations from the British Association for Psychopharmacology. *J Psychopharmacology* 2020; **34**:3–78.

79. Remington G, et al. Treating negative symptoms in schizophrenia: an update. *Curr Treat Options Psychiatry* 2016; **3**:133–150.

Monitoring

The following table summarises suggested monitoring for those receiving antipsychotic medication.[1] Monitoring of people taking antipsychotics is very poor in most countries.[2-5] Guidance given here is strongly recommended to assure safe use of these drugs. More details, references and background are provided in specific sections in this chapter.

Parameter/ test	Suggested frequency	Action to be taken if results outside reference range	Medications with special precautions	Medications for which monitoring is not required
Urea and electrolytes (including creatinine or estimated GFR)	Baseline and yearly as part of a routine physical health check	Investigate all abnormalities detected	Amisulpride and sulpiride renally excreted – consider reducing dose if GFR reduced	None
Full blood count (FBC)[6-11]	Baseline and yearly as part of a routine physical health check and to detect chronic bone marrow suppression (small risk associated with some antipsychotic medications)	Stop suspect medication if neutrophils fall below 1.5 × 10⁹/L Refer to specialist medical care if neutrophils below 0.5 × 10⁹/L. Note high frequency of benign ethnic neutropenia in certain ethnic groups	Clozapine – FBC weekly for 18 weeks, then two-weekly up to one year, then monthly (schedule varies from country to country)	None
Blood lipids[12,13] (cholesterol; triglycerides) Fasting sample, if possible	Baseline, at 3 months then yearly to detect antipsychotic-induced changes, and generally monitor physical health	Offer lifestyle advice. Consider changing antipsychotic medication and/or initiating statin therapy	Clozapine, olanzapine – 3 monthly for first year, then yearly	Some antipsychotic medications (e.g. aripiprazole, lurasidone) not clearly associated with dyslipidaemia, but prevalence is high in this patient group,[14-16] so all patients should be monitored
Weight[12,13,16] (include waist size and BMI, if possible)	Baseline, frequently for three months then yearly to detect antipsychotic-induced changes, and generally monitor physical health	Offer lifestyle advice. Consider changing antipsychotic medication and/or dietary/ pharmacological intervention	Clozapine, olanzapine – frequently for three months then 3 monthly for first year, then yearly	Aripiprazole, ziprasidone, brexpiprazole, cariprazine and lurasidone not clearly associated with weight gain but monitoring recommended nonetheless – obesity prevalence high in this patient group
Plasma glucose (fasting sample, if possible)	Baseline, at 4–6 months, then yearly to detect antipsychotic-induced changes and generally monitor physical health	Offer lifestyle advice. Obtain fasting sample or non-fasting and HbA₁c. Refer to GP or specialist	Clozapine, olanzapine, chlorpromazine – test at baseline, one month, then 4–6 monthly	Some antipsychotic medications not clearly associated with IFG, but prevalence is high in this patient group,[17,18] so all patients should be monitored

(Continued)

Parameter/ test	Suggested frequency	Action to be taken if results outside reference range	Medications with special precautions	Medications for which monitoring is not required
ECG[19,20]	Baseline and when target dose is reached (ECG changes rare in practice[21]) on admission to hospital and before discharge if medication regimen changed.	Discuss with/refer to cardiologist if abnormality detected	Haloperidol, pimozide, sertindole – ECG mandatory; ziprasidone – ECG mandatory in some situations	Risk of sudden cardiac death increased with most antipsychotic medications.[22] Ideally, all patients should be offered an ECG at least yearly
Blood pressure	Baseline; frequently during dose titration and dosage changes to detect antipsychotic-induced changes, and generally monitor physical health	If severe hypotension or hypertension (clozapine) observed, slow rate of titration. Consider switching to another antipsychotic if symptomatic postural hypotension. Treat hypertension in line with NICE guidelines	Clozapine, chlorpromazine and quetiapine most likely to be associated with postural hypotension	Amisulpride, aripiprazole, brexpiprazole, cariprazine, lurasidone, trifluoperazine, sulpiride
Prolactin	Baseline, then at 6 months, then yearly to detect antipsychotic-induced changes	Switch medications if hyperprolactinaemia confirmed and symptomatic. Consider tests of bone mineral density (e.g. DEXA scanning) for those with chronically raised prolactin.	Amisulpride, sulpiride, risperidone and paliperidone particularly associated with hyperprolactinaemia	Asenapine, aripiprazole, brexpiprazole, cariprazine, clozapine, lurasidone, quetiapine, olanzapine (<20mg), and ziprasidone usually do not elevate plasma prolactin, but worth measuring if symptoms arise
Liver function tests (LFTs)[23–25]	Baseline, then yearly as part of a routine physical health check and to detect chronic antipsychotic-induced changes (rare)	Stop suspect medication if LFTs indicate hepatitis (transaminases × 3 normal) or functional damage (PT/albumin change)	Clozapine and chlorpromazine associated with hepatic failure	Amisulpride, sulpiride
Creatinine phospho kinase (CPK)	Baseline, then if NMS suspected	See the section on NMS	NMS more likely with high-potency first-generation antipsychotic medications	None

Other tests: Patients on clozapine may benefit from an **EEG**,[26,27] as this may help determine the need for anticonvulsant treatment (although interpretation is obviously complex). Those on quetiapine should have **thyroid** function tests yearly, although the risk of abnormality is very small.[28,29]

Key: DEXA, dual-energy X-ray absorptiometry; NMS, neuroleptic malignant syndrome; PT, prothrombin time; BMI – body mass index; ECG – electrocardiograph; EEG – electroencephalogram; GFR – glomerular filtration rate; IFG – impaired fasting glucose.

Note: This table is a summary – see individual sections for detail and discussion.

References

1. National Institute for Clinical Excellence. Psychosis and schizophrenia: what monitoring is required? Clinical Knowledge Summaries. 2014 (last revised November 2020); https://cks.nice.org.uk/topics/psychosis-schizophrenia/prescribing-information/monitoring/#:~:text=References-,What%20monitoring%20is%20required%3F,stabilized%20(whichever%20is%20longer).

2. Bulteau S, et al. Advocacy for better metabolic monitoring after antipsychotic initiation: based on data from a French health insurance database. *Exp Opin Drug Saf* 2021; **20**:225–233.

3. Lydon A, et al. Routine screening and rates of metabolic syndrome in patients treated with clozapine and long-acting injectable antipsychotic medications: a cross-sectional study. *Ir J Psychol Med* 2021; **38**:40–48.

4. Poojari PG, et al. Identification of risk factors and metabolic monitoring practices in patients on antipsychotic drugs in South India. *Asian J Psychiatr* 2020; **53**:102186.

5. Perry BI, et al. Prolactin monitoring in the acute psychiatry setting. *Psychiatry Res* 2016; **235**:104–109.

6. Burckart GJ, et al. Neutropenia following acute chlorpromazine ingestion. *Clin Toxicol* 1981; **18**:797–801.

7. Grohmann R, et al. Agranulocytosis and significant leucopenia with neuroleptic drugs: results from the AMUP program. *Psychopharmacology* 1989; **99 Suppl**:S109–S112.

8. Esposito D, et al. Risperidone-induced morning pseudoneutropenia. *Am J Psychiatry* 2005; **162**:397.

9. Montgomery J. Ziprasidone-related agranulocytosis following olanzapine-induced neutropenia. *Gen Hosp Psychiatry* 2006; **28**:83–85.

10. Cowan C, et al. Leukopenia and neutropenia induced by quetiapine. *Prog Neuropsychopharmacol Biol Psychiatry* 2007; **31**:292–294.

11. Buchman N, et al. Olanzapine-induced leukopenia with human leukocyte antigen profiling. *Int Clin Psychopharmacol* 2001; **16**:55–57.

12. Marder SR, et al. Physical health monitoring of patients with schizophrenia. *Am J Psychiatry* 2004; **161**:1334–1349.

13. Fenton WS, et al. Medication-induced weight gain and dyslipidemia in patients with schizophrenia. *Am J Psychiatry* 2006; **163**:1697–1704.

14. Weissman EM, et al. Lipid monitoring in patients with schizophrenia prescribed second-generation antipsychotics. *J Clin Psychiatry* 2006; **67**:1323–1326.

15. Cohn TA, et al. Metabolic monitoring for patients treated with antipsychotic medications. *Can J Psychiatry* 2006; **51**:492–501.

16. Paton C, et al. Obesity, dyslipidaemias and smoking in an inpatient population treated with antipsychotic drugs. *Acta Psychiatr Scand* 2004; **110**:299–305.

17. Taylor D, et al. Undiagnosed impaired fasting glucose and diabetes mellitus amongst inpatients receiving antipsychotic drugs. *J Psychopharmacology* 2005; **19**:182–186.

18. Citrome L, et al. Incidence, prevalence, and surveillance for diabetes in New York State psychiatric hospitals, 1997–2004. *Psychiatr Serv* 2006; **57**:1132–1139.

19. Barnes T, et al. Evidence-based guidelines for the pharmacological treatment of schizophrenia: updated recommendations from the British Association for Psychopharmacology. *J Psychopharmacology* 2020; **34**:3–78.

20. Shah AA, et al. QTc prolongation with antipsychotics: is routine ECG monitoring recommended? *J Psychiatr Pract* 2014; **20**:196–206.

21. Novotny T, et al. Monitoring of QT interval in patients treated with psychotropic drugs. *Int J Cardiol* 2007; **117**:329–332.

22. Ray WA, et al. Atypical antipsychotic drugs and the risk of sudden cardiac death. *N Engl J Med* 2009; **360**:225–235.

23. Hummer M, et al. Hepatotoxicity of clozapine. *J Clin Psychopharmacol* 1997; **17**:314–317.

24. Erdogan A, et al. Management of marked liver enzyme increase during clozapine treatment: a case report and review of the literature. *Int J Psychiatry Med* 2004; **34**:83–89.

25. Regal RE, et al. Phenothiazine-induced cholestatic jaundice. *Clin Pharm* 1987; **6**:787–794.

26. Centorrino F, et al. EEG abnormalities during treatment with typical and atypical antipsychotics. *Am J Psychiatry* 2002; **159**:109–115.

27. Gross A, et al. Clozapine-induced QEEG changes correlate with clinical response in schizophrenic patients: a prospective, longitudinal study. *Pharmacopsychiatry* 2004; **37**:119–122.

28. Twaites BR, et al. The safety of quetiapine: results of a post-marketing surveillance study on 1728 patients in England. *J Psychopharmacology* 2007; **21**:392–399.

29. Kelly DL, et al. Thyroid function in treatment-resistant schizophrenia patients treated with quetiapine, risperidone, or fluphenazine. *J Clin Psychiatry* 2005; **66**:80–84.

Relative adverse effects – a rough guide

Drug	Sedation	Weight gain	Akathisia	Parkinsonism	Anti-cholinergic	Hypotension	Prolactin elevation
Amisulpride*	–	+	+	+	–	–	+++
Aripiprazole	–	–	+	–	–	–	–
Asenapine*	+	+	+	–	–	–	+
Benperidol*	+	+	+	+++	+	+	+++
Brexpiprazole*	–	–	–	–	–	–	–
Cariprazine*	–	–	+	–	–	–	–
Chlorpromazine	+++	++	+	++	++	+++	+++
Clozapine	+++	+++	–	–	+++	+++	–
Flupentixol*	+	++	++	++	++	+	+++
Fluphenazine*	+	+	++	+++	+	+	+++
Haloperidol	+	+	+++	+++	+	+	++
Iloperidone*	–	++	+	+	–	+	–
Lumateperone*	++	–	–	–	–	–	–
Loxapine*	++	+	+	+++	+	++	+++
Lurasidone	+	–	+	+	–	–	–
Olanzapine	++	+++	–	–	+	+	+
Paliperidone	+	++	+	+	+	++	+++
Perphenazine	+	+	++	+++	+	+	+++
Pimavanserin*	-	-	-	-	-	-	-
Pimozide*	+	+	+	+	+	+	+++
Pipothiazine*	++	++	+	++	++	++	+++
Promazine*	+++	++	+	+	++	++	++
Quetiapine	++	++	–	–	+	++	–
Risperidone	+	++	+	+	+	++	+++
Sertindole*	–	+	+	–	–	+++	–
Sulpiride*	–	+	+	+	–	–	+++
Trifluoperazine	+	+	+	+++	+	+	+++
Ziprasidone*	+	–	+	–	–	+	+
Zuclopenthixol*	++	++	++	++	++	+	+++

Key: *Availability varies from country to country; +++ High incidence/severity; ++ Moderate; + Low; – Very low.

Note: The table notes approximate estimates of relative incidence and/or severity, based on clinical experience, manufacturers' literature and published research. This is a very rough guide – see individual sections for more precise and referenced information.

Other adverse effects not mentioned in this table do occur. Please see dedicated sections on other adverse effects included in this book for more information.

Treatment algorithms for schizophrenia

First-episode schizophrenia

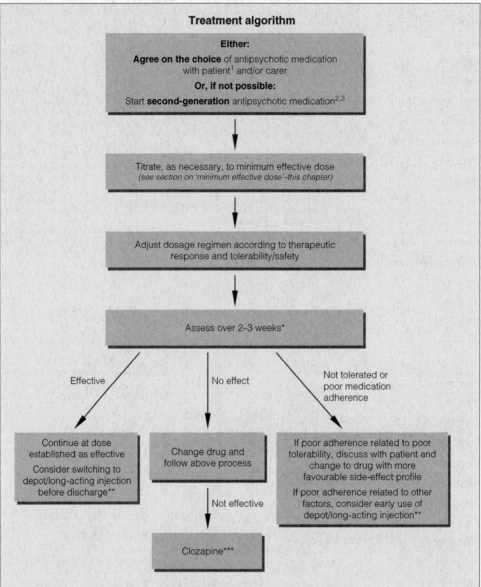

Treatment algorithm

Either:
Agree on the choice of antipsychotic medication with patient[1] and/or carer
Or, if not possible:
Start **second-generation** antipsychotic medication[2,3]

↓

Titrate, as necessary, to minimum effective dose
(see section on 'minimum effective dose'–this chapter)

↓

Adjust dosage regimen according to therapeutic response and tolerability/safety

↓

Assess over 2–3 weeks*

Effective / No effect / Not tolerated or poor medication adherence

Effective:
Continue at dose established as effective
Consider switching to depot/long-acting injection before discharge**

No effect:
Change drug and follow above process

Not effective

↓

Clozapine***

Not tolerated or poor medication adherence:
If poor adherence related to poor tolerability, discuss with patient and change to drug with more favourable side-effect profile
If poor adherence related to other factors, consider early use of depot/long-acting injection**

* Any improvement is likely to be apparent within 2–3 weeks of receiving an effective dose.[4] Most improvement occurs during this period.[5] If <u>no</u> effect by 2–3 weeks, change dose or drug. If some response detected, continue for a total of 10 weeks before abandoning treatment.[6]
** Relapse and readmission rates are vastly reduced by early use of depot/long-acting injections in this patient group.[7–9] First episode patients will accept long-acting injections.[10]
*** Early use of clozapine much more likely than anything else to be successful.[6,11]
Reluctance to use clozapine is associated with poor outcomes.[12]

Relapse or acute exacerbation of schizophrenia

(full adherence to medication confirmed)

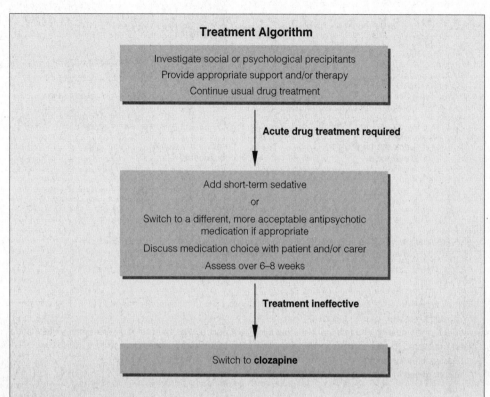

Treatment Algorithm

Investigate social or psychological precipitants
Provide appropriate support and/or therapy
Continue usual drug treatment

Acute drug treatment required

Add short-term sedative

or

Switch to a different, more acceptable antipsychotic
medication if appropriate

Discuss medication choice with patient and/or carer

Assess over 6–8 weeks

Treatment ineffective

Switch to **clozapine**

Notes

- First-generation drugs may be slightly less efficacious than some SGAs.[13,14] FGAs should probably be reserved for second-line use (or not used at all) because of the possibility of poorer outcome compared with SGAs and the higher risk of movement disorder, particularly tardive dyskinesia[15,16]
- Choice should be based largely on comparative adverse effect profile and relative toxicity. Patients seem able to make informed choices based on these factors,[17,18] although in practice they have in the past only very rarely been involved in drug choice.[19] Allowing patients informed choice seems to improve outcomes.[1]
- Where there is prior treatment failure (but not confirmed treatment refractoriness), olanzapine or risperidone may be better options than quetiapine.[20] Olanzapine, because of the wealth of evidence suggesting slight superiority over other antipsychotics, should probably be tried before clozapine unless contra-indicated.[21–24] Note, however, that one RCT[6] found continuing with amisulpride was as effective as switching to olanzapine.
- Before considering clozapine, ensure adherence to prior therapy using depot/LAI formulation or plasma drug level monitoring of oral treatment. Most non-adherence is undetected in practice,[23,25] and apparent treatment resistance may simply be a result of inadequate treatment.[26]
- Time to response is increased, and total response decreased in exacerbation of multi-episode schizophrenia[27]
- Where there is confirmed treatment resistance (failure to respond to adequate trials of at least two antipsychotic medications), evidence supporting the use of clozapine (and only clozapine) is overwhelming[28,29]

CHAPTER 1

Relapse or acute exacerbation of schizophrenia

(adherence doubtful or known to be poor)

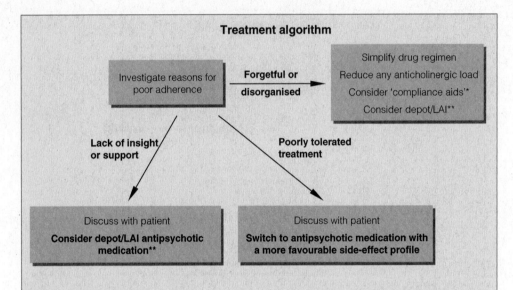

Treatment algorithm

Investigate reasons for poor adherence

Forgetful or disorganised → Simplify drug regimen / Reduce any anticholinergic load / Consider 'compliance aids'* / Consider depot/LAI**

Lack of insight or support

Poorly tolerated treatment

Discuss with patient
Consider depot/LAI antipsychotic medication*

Discuss with patient
Switch to antipsychotic medication with a more favourable side-effect profile

*Compliance aids (e.g. Medidose system in the UK) are not a substitute for patient education. The ultimate aim should be to promote independent living, perhaps with patients filling their own compliance aid, having first been given support and training. Note that such compliance aids are of little use unless the patient is clearly motivated to adhere to prescribed treatment. Note also that some medicines are not suitable for storage in compliance aids.
**Patients generally have positive views of depot medication.[10,30]

References

1. Robinson DG, et al. Psychopharmacological treatment in the RAISE-ETP study: outcomes of a manual and computer decision support system based intervention. *Am J Psychiatry* 2018; **175**:169–179.
2. Zhu Y, et al. Antipsychotic drugs for the acute treatment of patients with a first episode of schizophrenia: a systematic review with pairwise and network meta-analyses. *Lancet Psychiatry* 2017; **4**:694–705.
3. Zhang JP, et al. Efficacy and safety of individual second-generation vs. first-generation antipsychotics in first-episode psychosis: a systematic review and meta-analysis. *Int J Neuropsychopharmacol* 2013; **16**:1205–1218.
4. Leucht S, et al. Early-onset hypothesis of antipsychotic drug action: a hypothesis tested, confirmed and extended. *Biol Psychiatry* 2005; **57**:1543–1549.
5. Agid O, et al. The 'delayed onset' of antipsychotic action–an idea whose time has come and gone. *J Psychiatry Neurosci* 2006; **31**:93–100.
6. Kahn RS, et al. Amisulpride and olanzapine followed by open-label treatment with clozapine in first-episode schizophrenia and schizophreniform disorder (OPTiMiSE): a three-phase switching study. *Lancet Psychiatry* 2018; **5**:797–807.
7. Subotnik KL, et al. Long-acting injectable risperidone for relapse prevention and control of breakthrough symptoms after a recent first episode of schizophrenia. a randomized clinical trial. *JAMA Psychiatry* 2015; **72**:822–829.
8. Schreiner A, et al. Paliperidone palmitate versus oral antipsychotics in recently diagnosed schizophrenia. *Schizophr Res* 2015; **169**:393–399.
9. Alphs L, et al. Treatment effect with paliperidone palmitate compared with oral antipsychotics in patients with recent-onset versus more chronic schizophrenia and a history of criminal justice system involvement. *Early Intervention in Psychiatry* 2018; **12**:55–65.
10. Kane JM, et al. Patients with early-phase schizophrenia will accept treatment with sustained-release medication (Long-Acting Injectable Antipsychotics): results from the recruitment phase of the PRELAPSE trial. *J Clin Psychiatry* 2019; **80**:18m12546.

11. Agid O, et al. An algorithm-based approach to first-episode schizophrenia: response rates over 3 prospective antipsychotic trials with a retrospective data analysis. *J Clin Psychiatry* 2011; 72:1439–1444.

12. Drosos P, et al. One-year outcome and adherence to pharmacological guidelines in first-episode schizophrenia: results from a consecutive cohort study. *J Clin Psychopharmacol* 2020; 40:534–540.

13. Davis JM, et al. A meta-analysis of the efficacy of second-generation antipsychotics. *Arch Gen Psychiatry* 2003; 60:553–564.

14. Leucht S, et al. Second-generation versus first-generation antipsychotic drugs for schizophrenia: a meta-analysis. *Lancet* 2009; 373:31–41.

15. Schooler N, et al. Risperidone and haloperidol in first-episode psychosis: a long-term randomized trial. *Am J Psychiatry* 2005; 162:947–953.

16. Oosthuizen PP, et al. Incidence of tardive dyskinesia in first-episode psychosis patients treated with low-dose haloperidol. *J Clin Psychiatry* 2003; 64:1075–1080.

17. Whiskey E, et al. Evaluation of an antipsychotic information sheet for patients. *Int J Psychiatry Clin Pract* 2005; 9:264–270.

18. Stroup TS, et al. Results of phase 3 of the CATIE schizophrenia trial. *Schizophr Res* 2009; 107:1–12.

19. Olofinjana B, et al. Antipsychotic drugs – information and choice: a patient survey. *Psychiatric Bulletin* 2005; 29:369–371.

20. Stroup TS, et al. Effectiveness of olanzapine, quetiapine, risperidone, and ziprasidone in patients with chronic schizophrenia following discontinuation of a previous atypical antipsychotic. *Am J Psychiatry* 2006; 163:611–622.

21. Haro JM, et al. Remission and relapse in the outpatient care of schizophrenia: three-year results from the Schizophrenia Outpatient Health Outcomes study. *J Clin Psychopharmacol* 2006; 26:571–578.

22. Novick D, et al. Recovery in the outpatient setting: 36-month results from the Schizophrenia Outpatients Health Outcomes (SOHO) study. *Schizophr Res* 2009; 108:223–230.

23. Tiihonen J, et al. Effectiveness of antipsychotic treatments in a nationwide cohort of patients in community care after first hospitalisation due to schizophrenia and schizoaffective disorder: observational follow-up study. *BMJ* 2006; 333:224.

24. Leucht S, et al. A meta-analysis of head-to-head comparisons of second-generation antipsychotics in the treatment of schizophrenia. *Am J Psychiatry* 2009; 166:152–163.

25. Remington G, et al. The use of electronic monitoring (MEMS) to evaluate antipsychotic compliance in outpatients with schizophrenia. *Schizophr Res* 2007; 90:229–237.

26. McCutcheon R, et al. Antipsychotic plasma levels in the assessment of poor treatment response in schizophrenia. *Acta Psychiatr Scand* 2018; 137:39–46.

27. Takeuchi H, et al. Does relapse contribute to treatment resistance? Antipsychotic response in first- vs. second-episode schizophrenia. *Neuropsychopharmacology* 2019; 44:1036–1042.

28. McEvoy JP, et al. Effectiveness of clozapine versus olanzapine, quetiapine, and risperidone in patients with chronic schizophrenia who did not respond to prior atypical antipsychotic treatment. *Am J Psychiatry* 2006; 163:600–610.

29. Lewis SW, et al. Randomized controlled trial of effect of prescription of clozapine versus other second-generation antipsychotic drugs in resistant schizophrenia. *Schizophr Bull* 2006; 32:715–723.

30. Mace S, et al. Positive views on antipsychotic long-acting injections: results of a survey of community patients prescribed antipsychotics. *Ther Adv Psychopharmacol* 2019; 9:2045125319860977.

First-generation antipsychotics – place in therapy

Nomenclature

First-generation ('typical') and second-generation ('atypical') antipsychotic medications are not categorically differentiated, the medications in both groups being heterogeneous in terms of pharmacological and side-effect profiles. First-generation medications were introduced before 1990 and tend to be associated with acute EPS, hyperprolactinaemia and, in the longer term, tardive dyskinesia (TD). There are expectations that such adverse effects are less likely or absent with second-generation antipsychotic medications (introduced after 1990), although in practice most show dose-related EPS, some induce hyperprolactinaemia (often to a greater extent than with FGAs) and all will give rise to TD, albeit at a lower incidence than FGAs. Second-generation medications tend to be associated with metabolic and cardiac complications,[1-3] although this is *not* true of all SGAs and it *is* true of some FGAs. To complicate matters further, it has been suggested that the therapeutic and adverse effects of FGAs can be separated by careful dosing[4] – essentially turning FGAs into SGAs if used in small enough doses (although there is much evidence to the contrary[5-7]).

Given these observations, it seems unwise and unhelpful to consider so-called FGAs and SGAs as distinct groups of drugs. Perhaps the essential difference between the two groups is the size of the therapeutic index in relation to acute EPS. For instance, haloperidol has an extremely narrow range of doses at which it is effective but does not cause extrapyramidal side effects (EPSE) (perhaps 4.0 to 4.5mg/day), whereas olanzapine has a wide range of therapeutic doses (5–40mg/day) at which it does not generally cause EPSE.

The use of Neuroscience-based Nomenclature (NbN)[1,2] (for which there is a free app for iPhone and other devices) obviates the need for classification into an FGA or SGA and describes individual drug by their pharmacological activity. The wider use of NbN will undoubtedly improve understanding of individual drug effects and perhaps forestall future redundant categorisation.

Role of older antipsychotics

FGAs still play an important role in schizophrenia. For example, chlorpromazine and haloperidol are frequent choices for PRN ('when necessary') medication and depot preparations of haloperidol, zuclopenthixol and flupentixol are commonly prescribed. FGAs can offer a valid alternative to SGAs where SGAs are poorly tolerated (usually because of metabolic changes) or where FGAs are preferred by patients themselves. Some FGAs may be less effective than some non-clozapine SGAs (amisulpride, olanzapine and risperidone may be slightly more efficacious[3,4]), but any differences in therapeutic efficacy seem to be modest. Two large pragmatic studies, CATIE[8] and CUtLASS,[5] found few important differences between SGAs and FGAs (mainly perphenazine and sulpiride, respectively).

The main drawbacks of FGAs are, inevitably, acute EPS, hyperprolactinaemia and TD. Hyperprolactinaemia is probably unavoidable in practice (the dose that achieves efficacy is too close to the dose that causes hyperprolactinaemia) and, even when not symptomatic, hyperprolactinaemia may grossly affect hypothalamic function.[6] It is also associated with sexual dysfunction,[7] but be aware that the autonomic effects of some

SGAs may also cause sexual dysfunction.[8] Also, some SGAs (risperidone, paliperidone, amisulpride) increase prolactin to a greater extent than FGAs.[9]

All FGAs are potent dopamine antagonists, which are liable to induce dysphoria.[10] Perhaps as a consequence, some FGAs may produce smaller benefits in quality of life than some SGAs.[11]

TD very probably occurs more frequently with FGAs than SGAs[12–15] (notwithstanding difficulties in defining what is 'atypical'), although there remains some uncertainty[15–17] and the dose of FGA used is a crucial factor. Amongst SGAs, partial agonists may have the lowest risk of TD.[18] Careful observation of patients and the prescribing of the lowest effective dose are essential to help reduce the risk of this serious adverse event.[19,20] Even with these precautions, the risk of TD with some FGAs may be unacceptably high.[21]

A good example of the relative merits of SGAs and a carefully dosed FGA comes from a trial comparing paliperidone palmitate with low-dose haloperidol decanoate.[22] Paliperidone produced more weight gain and prolactin change, but haloperidol was associated with significantly more frequent akathisia and parkinsonism, and, numerically, a higher incidence of TD. Efficacy was identical.

References

1. Blier P, et al. Progress on the neuroscience-based nomenclature (NbN) for psychotropic medications. *Neuropsychopharmacology* 2017; 42:1927–1928.
2. Caraci F, et al. A new nomenclature for classifying psychotropic drugs. *Br J Clin Pharmacol* 2017; 83:1614–1616.
3. Davis JM, et al. A meta-analysis of the efficacy of second-generation antipsychotics. *Arch Gen Psychiatry* 2003; 60:553–564.
4. Leucht S, et al. Second-generation versus first-generation antipsychotic drugs for schizophrenia: a meta-analysis. *Lancet* 2009; 373:31–41.
5. Jones PB, et al. Randomized controlled trial of the effect on quality of life of second- vs first-generation antipsychotic drugs in schizophrenia: Cost Utility of the Latest Antipsychotic Drugs in Schizophrenia Study (CUtLASS 1). *Arch Gen Psychiatry* 2006; 63:1079–1087.
6. Smith S, et al. The effects of antipsychotic-induced hyperprolactinaemia on the hypothalamic-pituitary-gonadal axis. *J Clin Psychopharmacol* 2002; 22:109–114.
7. Smith SM, et al. Sexual dysfunction in patients taking conventional antipsychotic medication. *Br J Psychiatry* 2002; 181:49–55.
8. Aizenberg D, et al. Comparison of sexual dysfunction in male schizophrenic patients maintained on treatment with classical antipsychotics versus clozapine. *J Clin Psychiatry* 2001; 62:541–544.
9. Leucht S, et al. Comparative efficacy and tolerability of 15 antipsychotic drugs in schizophrenia: a multiple-treatments meta-analysis. *Lancet* 2013; 382:951–962.
10. King DJ, et al. Antipsychotic drug-induced dysphoria. *Br J Psychiatry* 1995; 167:480–482.
11. Grunder G, et al. Effects of first-generation antipsychotics versus second-generation antipsychotics on quality of life in schizophrenia: a double-blind, randomised study. *Lancet Psychiatry* 2016; 3:717–729.
12. Tollefson GD, et al. Blind, controlled, long-term study of the comparative incidence of treatment-emergent tardive dyskinesia with olanzapine or haloperidol. *Am J Psychiatry* 1997; 154:1248–1254.
13. Beasley C, et al. Randomised double-blind comparison of the incidence of tardive dyskinesia in patients with schizophrenia during long-term treatment with olanzapine or haloperidol. *Br J Psychiatry* 1999; 174:23–30.
14. Correll CU, et al. Lower risk for tardive dyskinesia associated with second-generation antipsychotics: a systematic review of 1-year studies. *Am J Psychiatry* 2004; 161:414–425.
15. Novick D, et al. Tolerability of outpatient antipsychotic treatment: 36-month results from the European Schizophrenia Outpatient Health Outcomes (SOHO) study. *Eur Neuropsychopharmacol* 2009; 19:542–550.
16. Halliday J, et al. Nithsdale Schizophrenia Surveys 23: movement disorders. 20-year review. *Br J Psychiatry* 2002; 181:422–427.
17. Miller DD, et al. Extrapyramidal side-effects of antipsychotics in a randomised trial. *Br J Psychiatry* 2008; 193:279–288.
18. Carbon M, et al. Tardive dyskinesia prevalence in the period of second-generation antipsychotic use: a meta-analysis. *J Clin Psychiatry* 2017; 78:e264–e278.
19. Jeste DV, et al. Tardive dyskinesia. *Schizophr Bull* 1993; 19:303–315.
20. Cavallaro R, et al. Recognition, avoidance, and management of antipsychotic-induced tardive dyskinesia. *CNS Drugs* 1995; 4:278–293.
21. Oosthuizen P, et al. A randomized, controlled comparison of the efficacy and tolerability of low and high doses of haloperidol in the treatment of first-episode psychosis. *Int J Neuropsychopharmacol* 2004; 7:125–131.
22. McEvoy JP, et al. Effectiveness of paliperidone palmitate vs haloperidol decanoate for maintenance treatment of schizophrenia: a randomized clinical trial. *JAMA* 2014; 311:1978–1987.

NICE guidelines for the treatment of schizophrenia[1]

The 2009 NICE Guidelines[1] differed importantly from previous guidelines. There was no longer an imperative to prescribe an 'atypical' as first-line treatment, and it was recommended only that clozapine be 'offered' (rather than prescribed) after the prior failure of two antipsychotics. These semantic differences pointed respectively towards a disillusionment with SGAs and a recognition of the delay in prescribing clozapine in practice. Much emphasis was placed on involving patients and their carers in prescribing decisions. There is some evidence that this is rarely done[2] but that it can be done.[3] New NICE Guidelines appeared in February 2014 and were reviewed again in March 2019.

NICE Guidelines – a summary

- For people with newly diagnosed schizophrenia, offer oral antipsychotic medication as well as psychological interventions (CBT or family intervention). Provide information and discuss the benefits and side-effect profile of each drug with the service user. The choice of drug should be made by the service user and healthcare professional together, considering:
  - the relative potential of individual antipsychotic drugs to cause extrapyramidal side effects (including akathisia), cardiovascular side effects, metabolic side effects (including weight gain), hormonal side effects (including raised prolactin levels) and other side effects (including unpleasant subjective experiences);
  - the views of the carer where the service user agrees.
- Before starting antipsychotic medication, undertake and record the following baseline investigations:
  - Weight
  - Waist circumference
  - Pulse and blood pressure
  - Fasting blood glucose, HbA_{1C}, blood lipid profile, prolactin
  - Assessment of movement disorders
  - Assessment of nutritional status, diet and level of physical activity
- Before starting antipsychotic medication, offer the person with schizophrenia an electrocardiogram (ECG) if:
  - specified in the SPC
  - a physical examination has identified specific cardiovascular risk (such as diagnosis of high blood pressure)
  - there is personal history of cardiovascular disease, or
  - the service user is being admitted as an inpatient.
- Treatment with antipsychotic medication should be considered an explicit individual therapeutic trial, and the following should be considered:
  - Recording of indications and expected benefits and risks of oral antipsychotic medication, and the expected time for a change in symptoms and appearance of side effects.
  - At the start of treatment, give a dose at the lower end of the licensed range and slowly titrate upwards within the dose range given in the British National Formulary (BNF) or SPC.

- Justify and record reasons for dosages outside the range given in the BNF or SPC.
- Record the rationale for continuing, changing or stopping medication and the effects of such changes.
- Carry out a trial of medication at optimum dosage for 4–6 weeks (although half of this period is probably sufficient if no effect at all is seen).
- Monitor and record the following regularly and systematically throughout treatment, but especially during titration:
  - efficacy, including changes in symptoms and behaviour
  - side effects of treatment, taking into account overlap between certain side effects and clinical features of schizophrenia, for example, the overlap between akathisia and agitation or anxiety
  - adherence
  - weight, weekly for the first 6 weeks, then at 12 weeks, 1 year and annually
  - waist circumference annually
  - pulse and blood pressure at 12 weeks, 1 year and annually
  - fasting blood glucose, HbA_{1C} and blood lipids at 12 weeks, 1 year and annually
  - nutritional status, diet and physical activity.
- Physical monitoring is to be the responsibility of the secondary care team for one year or until the patient is stable.
- Discuss the use of alcohol, tobacco, prescription and non-prescription medication as well as the use of illicit drugs with the service user and carer if appropriate. Discuss their potential interactions with the prescribed therapy and psychological treatments.
- Do not use a loading dose of antipsychotic medication (often referred to as 'rapid neuroleptisation') (Note that this does not apply to loading doses of depot forms of olanzapine and paliperidone).
- Do not routinely initiate regular combined antipsychotic medication, except for short periods (for example, when changing medication).
- If prescribing chlorpromazine, warn of its potential to cause skin photosensitivity. Advise using sunscreen if necessary.
- Consider offering depot/long-acting injectable antipsychotic medication to people with schizophrenia:
  - who would prefer such treatment after an acute episode
  - in patients known to be non-adherent to oral treatment and/or those who prefer this method of administration.
- Offer clozapine to people with schizophrenia whose illness has not responded adequately to treatment despite the sequential use of adequate doses of at least two different antipsychotic drugs alongside psychological therapies. The misuse of illicit substances (including alcohol) and the use of other prescribed medication or physical illness should be excluded. At least one of the drugs should be a non-clozapine second-generation antipsychotic. (See section Treatment Algorithms for schizophrenia – we recommend that one of the drugs should be olanzapine)
- For people with schizophrenia whose illness has not responded adequately to clozapine at an optimised dose, healthcare professionals should establish prior compliance with optimised antipsychotic treatment (including measuring drug levels) and engagement with psychological treatment before adding a second antipsychotic to augment

CHAPTER 1

treatment with clozapine. An adequate trial of such an augmentation may need to be up to 8–10 weeks (some data suggest 6 weeks may be enough[4]). Choose a drug that does not compound the common side effects of clozapine.

References

1. National Institute for Health and Care Excellence. Psychosis and schizophrenia in adults: prevention and management. Clinical Guidance [CG178]. 2014 (last checked March 2019); https://www.nice.org.uk/guidance/cg178.
2. Olofinjana B, et al. Antipsychotic drugs – information and choice: a patient survey. *Psychiatric Bull* 2005;29:369–371.
3. Whiskey E, et al. Evaluation of an antipsychotic information sheet for patients. *Int J Psychiatry Clin Pract* 2005;9:264–270.
4. Taylor D, et al. Augmentation of clozapine with a second antipsychotic. A meta analysis. *Acta Psychiatr Scand* 2012;125:15–24.

Antipsychotic response – to increase the dose, to switch, to add or just wait – what is the right move?

For any clinician actively involved in the care of people with schizophrenia, the single most common clinical dilemma is what to do when treatment with the current antipsychotic medication seems to be suboptimal. This may be for two broad reasons: first, while the symptoms are well controlled the side effects are problematic and, secondly, there is an inadequate therapeutic response. Fortunately, with regard to the first reason, the diversity of the available antipsychotic medications means that it is usually possible to find one that has a side-effect profile that is more appropriate and more tolerable. With regard to the second reason – an inadequate symptom response – what to do next is a more difficult question. If the illness has not shown sufficient improvement despite serial, adequate trials, in terms of dosage, duration and adherence, of two antipsychotic medications, then a trial of clozapine should be considered. However, should the person be reluctant to try clozapine, the clinician has four main choices: to increase the dose of the current medication; to switch to another antipsychotic medication; to add an adjunctive medication, or just to monitor the illness in the hope that changing external factors allow recovery.

When to increase the dose?

While optimal doses of FGAs were always a matter of debate, the recommended doses of the SGAs were generally based on careful and extensive clinical trials. Despite this, the consensus on optimal SGA dosages has changed over time. For example, when risperidone was first launched, it was suggested that optimal titration was from 2mg to 4mg to 6mg or more for all patients. However, subsequently clinical practice moved towards the use of lower doses.[1] On the other hand, when quetiapine was introduced, 300mg was considered the optimal dose. The overall consensus now is towards higher doses,[2] although RCT and other evidence do not support this shift.[2,3] Nonetheless, most clinicians feel comfortable in navigating within the recommended SGA clinical dose ranges. The more critical question is what should be done if the upper limit of the dose range has been reached and, while the individual is tolerating the medication well, there is only limited benefit.

Dose–response observations

Davis and Chen[4] performed a systematic meta-analysis of relevant dose–response data available up to 2004 and concluded that the average dose that produces maximal benefit was 4mg for risperidone, 16mg of olanzapine, 120mg of ziprasidone and 10–15mg of aripiprazole (they could not determine such a dose for quetiapine using their method).[4] More recent trials have tried to compare 'high-dose' with standard dosage. For example, one group[5] studied the dose–response relationship of standard and higher doses of olanzapine in a randomised, double-blind, 8-week, fixed-dose study comparing olanzapine 10mg, 20mg and 40mg. While no additional benefit was found with the higher doses (i.e. 40mg was no better than 10mg), there was clear evidence for an increasing side-effect burden (weight gain and raised plasma prolactin level). Similarly, the initial licensing studies of risperidone compared the usual doses of 2–6mg with higher doses of 8–16mg/day. There was no additional benefit with the higher doses but a clear signal for a greater risk of side effects (EPS and raised plasma prolactin). The findings of these studies are in accord with older studies involving fixed doses of haloperidol,[6] where 8mg/day is clearly the dose above which no additional benefit is seen.[7]

Nonetheless, it is important to keep in mind that these doses are extracted from group evidence where patients are assigned to different doses, which is a different situation from the clinical one where the prescriber considers increasing the dose only in those patients whose illnesses have failed to respond to the initial dosage regimen. Kinon et al.[8] examined patients who failed to respond to the (then) standard dose of fluphenazine (20mg) and tested three strategies: increasing the dose to 80mg, switching to haloperidol or watchful waiting (on the original dose). All three strategies proved to be equivalent in terms of efficacy. These findings provide little supportive evidence at a group level (as opposed to an individual level) for treatment beyond the recommended dose range. Such RCT evidence is corroborated by the clinical practice norms – Hermes and colleagues examined the CATIE data to identify clinical factors that predicted a prescriber's decision to increase the dose and found that decisions for dose change (within the therapeutic ranges) were only weakly associated with clinical measures.[9] More recently, a trial of lurasidone[10] in adult patients with schizophrenia showed that following a lack of response after two weeks on lurasidone 80mg/d, a dose increase to 160mg/d was associated with significant symptom improvement compared with continuing on lurasidone 80mg/d. However, this result may not be generalisable to other antipsychotic medications.

A 2018 Cochrane systematic review of relevant studies concluded that there was no good-quality evidence that for illness not responding to initial antipsychotic treatment, there was any difference between increasing the antipsychotic dose and continuing antipsychotic treatment at the same dose.[11]

Plasma level variations

Group level evidence cannot completely determine individual treatment decisions. There are significant inter-individual variations in plasma drug levels in patients treated with antipsychotic medication. One can often encounter a patient who, when receiving medication at the higher end of the dose range (say 6mg of risperidone or 20mg of olanzapine), would have plasma drug levels that are well below the range expected for 2mg risperidone or 10mg of olanzapine, and these levels may not reach the threshold for response. In such patients, a rational case could be made for increasing the dose, provided the patient is informed, and the side effects are tolerable, to bring the plasma levels to the optimal range for the particular medication. More details on plasma levels and their interpretation are provided in Chapter 11. However, what are the treatment possibilities when a lack of therapeutic response is encountered despite the patient's adherence to their medication regimen, the prescription of a dosage at the top of the recommended range, and apparently sufficient plasma levels?

Treatment choices

There are essentially three options here, a trial of clozapine, switch to another antipsychotic medication or add another (non-clozapine) antipsychotic medication. If the patient meets the criteria for clozapine treatment, this is undoubtedly the preferred option. Yet, in a clinical audit of community (not inpatient) practice in the UK, covering some 5000 patients in 60 different NHS Trusts, it was found that 40% of the patients whose illnesses met the criteria for treatment-resistant schizophrenia had not received clozapine. For the vast majority (85%) of those who had started clozapine, this had been delayed after the failure of two serial trials of antipsychotic medication for much longer than is advised in most guidelines.[12]

Some patients may be averse to the mandatory regular blood testing, the side effects and the regular appointments required as part of the clozapine regimen. In such patients, the options are switching to another antipsychotic medication or to add one. The data on switching are sparse. While almost every clinical trial in patients with established schizophrenia has entailed the patient switching from one antipsychotic medication to another, there are no rigorous studies addressing preferred medication switches (e.g. if risperidone fails – what next? olanzapine, quetiapine, aripiprazole or ziprasidone). If one looks at only the switching trials which have been sponsored by the drug companies – it leads to a rather confusing picture, with the trial results being very closely linked to the sponsors' interest (see Heres S, et al. Why olanzapine beats risperidone, risperidone beats quetiapine, and quetiapine beats olanzapine: an exploratory analysis of head-to-head comparison studies of second-generation antipsychotics[13]).

CATIE, the major US-based publicly funded comparative trial, examined patients who had failed their first SGA and were then randomly assigned to a different second one[14] – patients switched to olanzapine and risperidone did better than those switched to quetiapine and ziprasidone. This greater effectiveness is supported by a meta-analysis that compared a number of SGAs with FGAs and concluded that other than clozapine, only amisulpride, risperidone and olanzapine were superior to FGAs in efficacy;[15] and a meta-analysis comparing SGAs amongst themselves suggested that olanzapine and risperidone (in that order) may be modestly more effective than the others.[16] Nevertheless, if a patient has not yet tried olanzapine or risperidone, it would be a reasonable decision to switch to these medications provided the side-effect balance is favourable. Comparing these two medications – the data are somewhat limited. However, a number of controlled, but open-label studies do show an asymmetrical advantage (i.e. switching to olanzapine being more effective, than to risperidone) – providing some direction, albeit incomplete.[17,18]

The best medication regimen (aside from clozapine) to choose for a patient who fails on olanzapine and risperidone remains unclear. Should one switch to, say, aripiprazole or ziprasidone or even an older FGA, or should another antipsychotic medication be added? Interestingly, studies that have switched patients to aripiprazole for reasons of tolerability (weight gain, etc.) either find no loss of efficacy[19,20] or an improvement in symptom severity after switching.[21,22] The switching method is vitally important, with add-on switching (establishing the dose of aripiprazole before withdrawing the former drug) and cross-tapering giving substantially better outcomes than stop-start.[21]

After 'switching', adding another antipsychotic is probably the most common clinical strategy chosen, as 39–43% of patients in routine care are prescribed more than one antipsychotic.[23] Often, a second antipsychotic is added for additional properties (e.g. quetiapine for sedation or aripiprazole to decrease plasma prolactin – these matters are discussed elsewhere). We are concerned here solely with the use of combined antipsychotic medications to increase efficacy. From a theoretical point of view, since all antipsychotic medications block D_2 receptors (unlike, say, anti-hypertensives which use different mechanisms), there is a limited rationale for addition. Studies of add-ons have often chosen combinations of convenience or based on clinical lore and perhaps the most systematic evidence is available for the addition of a second antipsychotic to clozapine[24,25] – perhaps supported by the rationale that since clozapine has relatively low D_2 occupancy, increasing its D_2 occupancy may yield additional benefits.[26] However, a meta-analysis of RCTs comparing augmentation with a second antipsychotic with continuing antipsychotic monotherapy in schizophrenia[27] found a lack of double-blind/high-quality evidence for efficacy for the combination, in terms of treatment response and symptom improvement. Furthermore, compared with antipsychotic monotherapy, combined antipsychotics seem to be associated with an increased side-effect burden and a greater risk of high-dose prescribing.[28,29]

While augmentation with another antipsychotic medication as a treatment strategy should probably be avoided, under some conditions of acute exacerbation or agitation the prescriber may see this as the only practicable solution. Or quite often the prescriber may inherit the care of a patient on antipsychotic polypharmacy. Most RCT evidence suggests that such a regimen can be safely switched back to antipsychotic monotherapy without symptom exacerbation, at least in the majority of patients,[30–32] although this is not a universal finding.[33] Essock et al.[32] conducted a relatively large trial involving 127 patients with schizophrenia who were stable on antipsychotic polypharmacy. Over a 12-month period, a switch to monotherapy was successful in about two thirds of the patients in whom it was tested. And in those cases where the move to monotherapy resulted in a return of symptoms, the most common recourse was a return to the original polypharmacy; this was achieved without any significant worsening in this group. The advantages for the monotherapy group were exposure to less medication, equivalent symptom severity and some loss of weight.

So when should the prescriber just continue with the current regimen? The evidence reviewed above suggests that no one strategy, such as increasing the dose, switching to another antipsychotic medication or augmentation with a second antipsychotic medication, is the clear winner in all situations. But increasing the dose if plasma drug levels are low, switching to olanzapine or risperidone if these medications have not been tried, or augmentation if there is insufficient response to clozapine, may be beneficial in some cases. Given the limited efficacy of these manoeuvres, perhaps an equally important call by the treating doctor is when to just stay with the current pharmacotherapy and focus on non-pharmacological means: engagement in case management, targeted psychological treatments and vocational rehabilitation as means of enhancing patient well-being. While it may seem a passive option – staying may often do less harm that aimless switching.

Summary

When treatment fails
<ul><li>If the dose of antipsychotic medication has been optimised, consider watchful waiting.</li><li>Consider increasing the antipsychotic dose according to tolerability and plasma levels (little supporting evidence[34,35]).</li><li>If this fails, consider switching to olanzapine or risperidone (if not already used).</li><li>If this fails, use clozapine (supporting evidence very strong).</li><li>If clozapine fails, use time-limited augmentation strategies (supporting evidence variable).</li></ul>

References

1. Ezewuzie N, et al. Establishing a dose-response relationship for oral risperidone in relapsed schizophrenia. *J Psychopharm* 2006;**20**:86–90.
2. Sparshatt A, et al. Quetiapine: dose-response relationship in schizophrenia. *CNS Drugs* 2008;**22**:49–68.
3. Honer WG, et al. A randomized, double-blind, placebo-controlled study of the safety and tolerability of high-dose quetiapine in patients with persistent symptoms of schizophrenia or schizoaffective disorder. *J Clin Psychiatry* 2012;**73**:13–20.
4. Davis JM, et al. Dose response and dose equivalence of antipsychotics. *J Clin Psychopharmacol* 2004;**24**:192–208.
5. Kinon BJ, et al. Standard and higher dose of olanzapine in patients with schizophrenia or schizoaffective disorder: a randomized, double-blind, fixed-dose study. *J Clin Psychopharmacol* 2008;**28**:392–400.
6. Van Putten T, et al. A controlled dose comparison of haloperidol in newly admitted schizophrenic patients. *Arch Gen Psychiatry* 1990;**47**:754–758.
7. Zimbroff DL, et al. Controlled, dose-response study of sertindole and haloperidol in the treatment of schizophrenia. Sertindole Study Group. *Am J Psychiatry* 1997;**154**:782–791.
8. Kinon BJ, et al. Treatment of neuroleptic-resistant schizophrenic relapse. *Psychopharmacol Bull* 1993;**29**:309–314.
9. Hermes E, et al. Predictors of antipsychotic dose changes in the CATIE schizophrenia trial. *Psychiatry Res* 2012;**199**:1–7.
10. Loebel A, et al. Lurasidone dose escalation in early nonresponding patients with schizophrenia: a randomized, placebo-controlled study. *J Clin Psychiatry* 2016;**77**:1672–1680.
11. Samara MT, et al. Increasing antipsychotic dose versus switching antipsychotic for non response in schizophrenia. *Cochrane Database Syst Rev* 2018;**5**:Cd011884.
12. Patel MX, et al. Quality of prescribing for schizophrenia: evidence from a national audit in England and Wales. *Eur Neuropsychopharmacol* 2014;**24**:499–509.
13. Heres S, et al. Why olanzapine beats risperidone, risperidone beats quetiapine, and quetiapine beats olanzapine: an exploratory analysis of head-to-head comparison studies of second-generation antipsychotics. *Am J Psychiatry* 2006;**163**:185–194.
14. Stroup TS, et al. Effectiveness of olanzapine, quetiapine, risperidone, and ziprasidone in patients with chronic schizophrenia following discontinuation of a previous atypical antipsychotic. *Am J Psychiatry* 2006;**163**:611–622.
15. Leucht S, et al. Second-generation versus first-generation antipsychotic drugs for schizophrenia: a meta-analysis. *Lancet* 2009;**373**:31–41.
16. Leucht S, et al. A meta-analysis of head-to-head comparisons of second-generation antipsychotics in the treatment of schizophrenia. *Am J Psychiatry* 2009;**166**:152–163.
17. Hong J, et al. Clinical consequences of switching from olanzapine to risperidone and vice versa in outpatients with schizophrenia: 36-month results from the Worldwide Schizophrenia Outpatients Health Outcomes (W-SOHO) study. *BMC Psychiatry* 2012;**12**:218.
18. Agid O, et al. Antipsychotic response in first-episode schizophrenia: efficacy of high doses and switching. *Eur Neuropsychopharmacol* 2013;**23**:1017–1022.
19. Stroup TS, et al. A randomized trial examining the effectiveness of switching from olanzapine, quetiapine, or risperidone to aripiprazole to reduce metabolic risk: Comparison of Antipsychotics for Metabolic Problems (CAMP). *Am J Psychiatry* 2011;**168**:947–956.
20. Montastruc F, et al. Association of aripiprazole with the risk for psychiatric hospitalization, self-harm, or suicide. *JAMA Psychiatry* 2019;**76**:409–417.
21. Obayashi Y, et al. Switching strategies for antipsychotic monotherapy in schizophrenia: a multi-center cohort study of aripiprazole. *Psychopharmacology* 2020;**237**:167–175.
22. Pae CU, et al. Effectiveness and tolerability of switching to aripiprazole once monthly from antipsychotic polypharmacy and/or other long acting injectable antipsychotics for patients with schizophrenia in routine practice: a retrospective, observation study. *Clin Psychopharmacol Neurosci* 2020;**18**:153–158.
23. Paton C, et al. High-dose and combination antipsychotic prescribing in acute adult wards in the UK: the challenges posed by p.r.n. prescribing. *Br J Psychiatry* 2008;**192**:435–439.
24. Wagner E, et al. Clozapine combination and augmentation strategies in patients with schizophrenia – recommendations from an international expert survey among the Treatment Response and Resistance in Psychosis (TRRIP) Working Group. *Schizophr Bull* 2020; **46**:1459–1470.
25. Taylor DM, et al. Augmentation of clozapine with a second antipsychotic – a meta-analysis of randomized, placebo-controlled studies. *Acta Psychiatr Scand* 2009;**119**:419–425.
26. Kapur S, et al. Increased dopamine D2 receptor occupancy and elevated prolactin level associated with addition of haloperidol to clozapine. *Am J Psychiatry* 2001;**158**:311–314.
27. Galling B, et al. Antipsychotic augmentation vs. monotherapy in schizophrenia: systematic review, meta-analysis and meta-regression analysis. *World Psychiatry* 2017;**16**:77–89.
28. Gallego JA, et al. Safety and tolerability of antipsychotic polypharmacy. *Expert Opinion on Drug Safety* 2012;**11**:527–542.
29. Barnes TRE, et al. Antipsychotic polypharmacy in schizophrenia: benefits and risks. *CNS Drugs* 2011;**25**:383–399.
30. Borlido C, et al. Switching from 2 antipsychotics to 1 antipsychotic in schizophrenia: a randomized, double-blind, placebo-controlled study. *J Clin Psychiatry* 2016;**77**:e14–e20.
31. Hori H, et al. Switching to antipsychotic monotherapy can improve attention and processing speed, and social activity in chronic schizophrenia patients. *J Psychiatr Res* 2013;**47**:1843–1848.
32. Essock SM, et al. Effectiveness of switching from antipsychotic polypharmacy to monotherapy. *Am J Psychiatry* 2011;**168**:702–708.
33. Constantine RJ, et al. The risks and benefits of switching patients with schizophrenia or schizoaffective disorder from two to one antipsychotic medication: a randomized controlled trial. *Schizophr Res* 2015;**166**:194–200.
34. Royal College of Psychiatrists. Consensus statement on high-dose antipsychotic medication. College Report CR190 2014.
35. Barnes TRE, et al. Evidence-based guidelines for the pharmacological treatment of schizophrenia: updated recommendations from the British Association for Psychopharmacology. *J Psychopharmacology* 2020;**34**:3–78.

Acutely disturbed or violent behaviour

Acute behavioural disturbance can occur in the context of psychiatric illness, physical illness, substance abuse or personality disorder. Psychotic symptoms are common and the patient may be aggressive towards others secondary to persecutory delusions or auditory, visual or tactile hallucinations. This section deals with behavioural disturbance in the context of severe mental illness. Excited/agitated delirium caused by illicit substance misuse is dealt with in Chapter 9.

The clinical practice of rapid tranquillisation (RT) is used when appropriate psychological and behavioural approaches have failed to de-escalate acutely disturbed behaviour. It is, essentially, a treatment of last resort. Patients who require RT are often too disturbed to give informed consent and therefore participate in randomised controlled trials (RCTs), but with the use of a number of creative methodologies, the evidence base with respect to the efficacy and tolerability of pharmacological strategies has grown substantially in recent years. A comprehensive and up-to-date consensus guideline has been published[1] and, more recently, a systematic review and meta-analysis.[2]

Oral/inhaled treatment

Several studies supporting the efficacy of oral SGAs have been conducted.[3–6] The level of behavioural disturbance exhibited by the patients in these studies was moderate at most, and all subjects accepted oral treatment (this degree of compliance would be unusual in clinical practice). Patients recruited to these studies received the SGA as antipsychotic monotherapy. The efficacy and safety of adding a second antipsychotic as a 'when necessary' treatment has not been explicitly tested in formal RCTs.

A single-dose RCT showed sublingual asenapine to be more effective than placebo for acute agitation.[7] The efficacy of inhaled loxapine in behavioural disturbance that is moderate in severity is also supported by RCTs[8–10] and case series.[11,12] The use of this preparation requires the co-operation of the patient, and bronchospasm is an established but rare side effect.

Parenteral treatment

Large, placebo-controlled RCTs support the efficacy of IM preparations of olanzapine, ziprasidone and aripiprazole. When considered together, these trials suggested that IM olanzapine is more effective than IM haloperidol which in turn is more effective than IM aripiprazole, which itself is more effective than ziprasidone.[2,13] The level of behavioural disturbance in these studies was moderate at most and differences between treatments small.

A large observational study supports the efficacy and tolerability of IM olanzapine in clinical emergencies (where disturbance was severe).[14] A study comparing IM haloperidol with a combination of IM midazolam and IM haloperidol found the combination more effective than haloperidol alone for controlling agitation in palliative care patients.[15]

Several RCTs have investigated the effectiveness of parenteral medication in 'real-life' acutely disturbed patients. Overall:

- Compared with IV midazolam alone, a combination of IV olanzapine or IV droperidol with IV midazolam was more rapidly effective and resulted in fewer subsequent doses of medication being required.[16]
- IM midazolam 7.5–15mg was more rapidly sedating than a combination of haloperidol 5–10mg and promethazine 50mg (TREC 1).[17]
- Olanzapine 10mg was as effective as a combination of haloperidol 10mg and promethazine 25–50mg in the short term, but the effect did not last as long (TREC 4).[18]
- A combination of haloperidol 5–10mg and promethazine 50mg was more effective and better tolerated than haloperidol 5–10mg alone (6% of patients had an acute dystonic reaction) (TREC 3).[19]
- A combination of haloperidol 10mg and promethazine 25–50mg was more effective than lorazepam 4mg (TREC 2).[20]
- A combination of IM chlorpromazine 100mg, haloperidol 5mg and promethazine 25mg was no better than IM haloperidol 5mg plus promethazine 25mg (TREC Lebanon).[21]
- A combination of IV midazolam and IV droperidol was more rapidly sedating than either IV droperidol or IV olanzapine alone. Fewer patients in the midazolam-droperidol group required additional medication doses to achieve sedation.[22]
- IM olanzapine was more effective than IM aripiprazole in the treatment of agitation in schizophrenia in the short term (at 2 hours), but there was no significant difference between treatments at 24 hours.[23]
- IM midazolam 5mg was faster acting and more effective than olanzapine 10mg, ziprasidone 20mg and both 5 and 10mg haloperidol in a large (n = 737) Emergency Room study.[24]
- In an open-label study, the combination of IM haloperidol and IM lorazepam was found to be similar in efficacy to IM olanzapine.[25]
- IM droperidol and IM haloperidol were equally effective.[26]

Cochrane concluded that haloperidol alone is effective in the management of acute behavioural disturbance but poorly tolerated, and that co-administration of promethazine (but not lorazepam) improves tolerability.[27,28] However, NICE considers the evidence relating to the use of promethazine for this purpose to be inconclusive.[29] When assessing haloperidol plus promethazine, Cochrane concluded that the combination is effective for use in patients who are aggressive due to psychosis, and its use is based on good evidence. The resumption of aggression and need for further injections was more likely with olanzapine than with the haloperidol–promethazine combination. The authors also stated that 'haloperidol used on its own without something to offset its frequent and serious adverse effects does seem difficult to justify'.[30] Cochrane concluded that available data for aripiprazole are rather poor. This evidence suggests that aripiprazole is more effective than placebo and haloperidol alone, but not olanzapine. However, caution is advised when generalising these results to real-world practice.[31]

A systematic review and meta-analysis of IM olanzapine for agitation found IM olanzapine and IM haloperidol to be equally effective, but IM olanzapine was associated with a lower incidence of EPSEs.[32] Cochrane suggests that droperidol is effective and may be used to control people with very disturbed and aggressive behaviours caused by psychosis.[33] Droperidol is seeing a resurgence in use in some countries having become available again (its initial withdrawal was voluntary, so reintroduction is not prohibited).

In a meta-analysis that examined the tolerability of IM antipsychotics when used for the treatment of agitation, the incidence of acute dystonia with haloperidol was reported to be 5%, with SGAs performing considerably better.[34] Acute EPS may adversely affect longer-term compliance.[35] In addition, the formal prescribing information in most countries for haloperidol calls for a pre-treatment ECG[36,37] and recommends that concomitant antipsychotics are not prescribed. The mean increase in QTc after 10mg IM haloperidol can be up to 15ms, but the range is wide.[38]

Note that promethazine may inhibit the metabolism of haloperidol;[39] a pharmacokinetic interaction that is potentially clinically significant given the potential of haloperidol to prolong QTc. While this is unlikely to be problematic if a single dose is administered, repeat dosing may confer risk.

Droperidol is also associated with QT changes (the reason for its past withdrawal). In an observational study set in hospital emergency departments, of the 1009 patients administered parenteral droperidol only 13 patients (1.28%) had an abnormal QT recorded after dose administration. In 7 of these cases another contributory factor was identified. There were no cases of torsades de pointes.[26] In all RT studies of IM droperidol, the overall rate of QT > 500ms was less than 2%.[2]

Intravenous treatment is now rarely used in RT but where benefits are thought to outweigh risks it may be considered as a last resort. A small study comparing high dose IV haloperidol with IV diazepam found both drugs to be effective at 24 hours.[40] Two large observational studies have examined the safety of IV olanzapine when used in the emergency department. The indications for its use varied: agitation being the most common. In one study,[41] in the group treated for agitation ($n = 265$), over a third of patients required an additional sedative dose after the initial IV olanzapine dose. Hypoxia was reported in 17.7% of cases and supplemental oxygen was used in 20.4% cases. Six patients required intubation (two of these because of olanzapine treatment). In the other study,[42] IV olanzapine ($n = 295$) was compared with IM olanzapine ($n = 489$). Additional doses were not required for 81% of patients in the IV group and 84% of patients in the IM group. Respiratory depression was more commonly observed in the group receiving IV olanzapine. Five patients in the IM group and two in the IV group required intubation.

In an acute psychiatric setting, high dose sedation (defined as a dose of more than 10mg of haloperidol, droperidol or midazolam) was not more effective than lower doses but was associated with more adverse effects (hypotension and oxygen desaturation).[43] Consistent with this, a small RCT supports the efficacy of low dose haloperidol, although both efficacy and tolerability were superior when midazolam was co-prescribed.[44] These data broadly support the use of standard doses in clinical emergencies, but the need for further physical restraint after lower doses needs to be considered.

A small observational study supports the effectiveness of buccal midazolam in a PICU setting.[45] Parenteral administration of midazolam, particularly in higher doses, may cause over-sedation accompanied by respiratory depression.[46] Lorazepam IM is an established treatment and TREC 2[20] supports its efficacy, although combining all results from the TREC studies suggests midazolam 7.5–15mg is probably more effective. A Cochrane review of benzodiazepines for psychosis-induced aggression and agitation concluded that most trials were too small to highlight differences in either positive or negative effects and whilst adding a benzodiazepine to another drug may not be clearly advantageous it may lead to unnecessary side effects.[47]

With respect to those who are behaviourally disturbed secondary to acute intoxication with alcohol or illicit drugs, there are fewer data to guide practice. A large observational study of IV sedation in patients intoxicated with alcohol found that combination treatment (most commonly haloperidol 5mg and lorazepam 2mg) was more effective and reduced the need for subsequent sedation than either drug given alone.[48] A case series ($N = 59$) of patients who received modest doses of oral, IM or IV haloperidol to manage behavioural disturbance in the context of PCP consumption, reported that haloperidol was effective and well tolerated (one case each of mild hypotension and mild hypoxia).[49] A section on the treatment of agitated delirium is included in Chapter 9.

Ketamine is widely used for agitation from hospital emergency departments. In a systematic review of 18 studies of ketamine,[50] a mean dose of 315mg IM ketamine achieved adequate sedation in an average of 7.2 minutes. Over 30% of 650 patients were eventually intubated and more than 1% experienced laryngospasm. Ketamine is probably not an option for RT where facilities for intubation are not available.

Overall the current broad consensus is that midazolam and droperidol are the fastest-acting single drug, intramuscular treatments[51] and that haloperidol alone should be avoided and perhaps abandoned completely even in combination.[52] Second-line treatments are combinations of benzodiazepines and antipsychotics and third line would probably now be intravenous benzodiazepines and then ketamine (2–5mg/kg IM), assuming intubation facilities are available.

Practical measures

Plans for the management of individual patients should ideally be made in advance. The aim is to prevent disturbed behaviour and reduce risk of violence. Nursing interventions (de-escalation, time out, seclusion[53]), increased nursing levels, transfer of the patient to a psychiatric intensive care unit (PICU) and pharmacological management are options that may be employed. Care should be taken to avoid combinations and high cumulative doses of antipsychotic drugs. The monitoring of routine physical observations after RT is essential. Note that RT is often viewed as punitive by patients. There is little research into the patient experience of RT.

The aims of RT are threefold:

- To reduce suffering for the patient: psychological or physical (through self-harm or accidents).
- To reduce risk of harm to others by maintaining a safe environment.
- To do no harm (by prescribing safe regimes and monitoring physical health).

Note: Despite the need for rapid and effective treatment, concomitant use of two or more antipsychotics (antipsychotic polypharmacy) should be avoided on the basis of risk associated with QT prolongation (common to almost all antipsychotics). This is a particularly important consideration in RT where the patient's physical state predisposes to cardiac arrhythmia.

Zuclopenthixol acetate

Zuclopenthixol acetate (ZA) is widely used in the UK and elsewhere in Europe and is best known by its trade name Acuphase. Zuclopenthixol itself is a thioxanthene dopamine antagonist first introduced in the early 1960s. ZA is not a rapidly tranquillising agent. Its elimination half-life is around 20 hours. Intramuscular injection of zuclopenthixol base results in rapid absorption and a duration of action of 12–24 hours. By slowing absorption after IM injection, the biological half-life (and so duration of action) becomes dependent on the rate of release from the IM reservoir. This can be achieved by esterification of the zuclopenthixol molecule; the rate of release being broadly proportion to the length of the ester carbon chain. Thus, zuclopenthixol decanoate is slow to act but very long-acting as a result of retarded release after IM injection. Zuclopenthixol acetate (with eight carbon atoms fewer) would be expected to provide relatively prompt release but with an intermediate duration of action. The intention of the manufacturers was that the use of ZA would obviate the need for repeated IM injections in disturbed patients.

An initial pharmacokinetic study of ZA included 19 patients 'in whom calming effect by parenteral neuroleptic was considered necessary'.[54] Zuclopenthixol was detectable in the plasma after 1–2 hours but did not reach peak concentrations until around 36 hours after dosing. At 72 hours, plasma levels were around a third of those at 36 hours. The clinical effect of ZA was not rapid – 10 of 17 patients exhibited minimal or no change in psychotic symptoms at 4 hours. Sedation was evident at 4 hours, but it had effectively abated by 72 hours.

A follow-up study by the same research group[55] examined more closely the clinical effects of ZA in 83 patients. The authors concluded that ZA produced 'pronounced and rapid reduction in psychotic symptoms'. In fact, psychotic symptoms were first assessed only after 24 hours and so a claim of rapid effect is not reasonably supported. Sedative effects were measured after two hours when a statistically significant effect was observed – at baseline mean sedation score was 0.0 (0 = no sign of sedation) and at 2 hours 0.6 (1 = slightly sedated). Maximum sedation was observed at 8 hours (mean score 2.2; 2 = moderately sedated). At 72 hours mean score was 1.1. Dystonia and rigidity were the most commonly reported adverse effects.

Two independently conducted open studies, produced similar results – a slow onset of effect peaking at 24 hours and still being evident at 72 hours.[56,57] The first UK study was reported in 1990.[58] In the trial, a significant reduction in psychosis score was first evident at 8 hours and scores continued to fall until the last measurement at 72 hours. Of 25 patients assessed only 4 showed signs of tranquillisation at 1 hour (19 at 2 hours and 22 at 24 hours).

A comparative trial of ZA[59] examined its effects and those of IM/oral haloperidol and IM/oral zuclopenthixol base (in multiple doses over 6 days). The two non-ester, IM/oral preparations produced a greater degree of sedation at 2 hours than did ZA, but the effect of ZA and zuclopenthixol was more sustained than with haloperidol over 144 hours (although patients received more zuclopenthixol doses). No clear differences between treatments were detected, with the exception of the slow onset of effect of ZA. The number of doses given varied substantially: ZA 1–4; haloperidol 1–26 and zuclopenthixol 1–22. This is the key (and perhaps unique) advantage of ZA – it reduces the need for repeat doses in acute psychosis. Indeed this was the principal finding of the first double-blind study of ZA.[60] Participants were given either ZA or haloperidol IM and assessed over three days. Changes in BPRS and CGI scores were near identical on each daily assessment. However, only 1 of 23 ZA patients required a second injection, whereas 7 of 21 required a repeat dose of haloperidol. Speed of onset was not examined. Similar findings were reported by Thai researchers comparing the same treatments,[61] and in three other studies of moderate size ($n = 44$,[62] $n = 40$,[63] $n = 50$).[64] In each study, the timing of assessments was such that time to onset of effect could not be determined.

A Cochrane review[65] included all of the above comparative studies as well as three further studies[66–68] for which we were unable to obtain full details. The Cochrane authors concluded that all studies were methodically flawed and poorly reported and that ZA did not appear to have a 'rapid onset of action'. They noted that ZA was probably no less effective than other treatments and that its use might 'result in less numerous coercive injections'.

Overall, the utility of ZA in rapid tranquillisation is limited by a somewhat delayed onset of both sedative and antipsychotic actions. Sedation may be apparent in a minority of patients after 2–4 hours, but antipsychotic action is evident only after 8 hours. If ZA is given to a restrained patient, their behaviour on release from restraint is likely to be unchanged and will remain as such for several hours. ZA has a role in reducing the number of restraints for IM injection, but it has no role in rapid tranquillisation.

Guidelines for the use of zuclopenthixol acetate (Acuphase)

Zuclopenthixol acetate (ZA) is not a rapidly tranquillising agent. It should be used only after an acutely psychotic patient has required *repeated* injections of short-acting antipsychotic drugs such as haloperidol or olanzapine, or sedative drugs such as lorazepam. It is perhaps best reserved for those few patients who have a prior history of good response to Acuphase.

ZA should be given only when enough time has elapsed to assess the full response to previously injected drugs: allow 15 minutes after IV injections; 60 minutes after IM.

ZA should never be administered for rapid tranquillisation (onset of effect is too slow) or to a patient who is physically resistant (risk of intravasation and oil embolus) or to neuroleptic-naïve patients (risk of prolonged EPSE).

Rapid tranquillisation summary

In an emergency situation – *Assess if there may be a medical cause.*[69] *Optimise regular prescription. The aim of pharmacological treatment is to calm the patient but not to oversedate. Note: lower doses should be used for children, adolescents and older adults. Patients' levels of consciousness and physical health should be monitored after administration of parenteral medication (see protocol)*

Step Intervention

1 De-escalation, time out, placement, etc., as appropriate

2 Offer oral treatment

If patient is prescribed a regular antipsychotic:

Lorazepam 1–2mg

Promethazine 25–50mg

Monotherapy with **buccal midazolam** may avoid the need for IM treatment. Dose: 10mg *Note that this preparation is unlicensed*

If patient is not already taking a regular oral or depot antipsychotic:

- **Olanzapine** 10mg or
- **Risperidone** 1–2mg or
- **Quetiapine** 50–100mg or
- **Haloperidol** 5mg (best with promethazine 25mg). Note that the EU SPC for haloperidol recommends: A pre-treatment ECG and to avoid concomitant antipsychotics
- **Inhaled loxapine** 10mg Note that use of this preparation requires the co-operation of the patient, and that bronchospasm is a rare side effect (have a salbutamol inhaler to hand).

Repeat after 45–60 minutes, if necessary. Consider combining sedative and antipsychotic treatment.
Go to step 3 if two doses fail or sooner if the patient is placing themselves or others at significant risk.

3 Consider IM treatment

Lorazepam 2mg[ab]	Have flumazenil to hand in case of benzodiazepine-induced respiratory depression.
Promethazine 50mg[c]	IM promethazine is a useful option in a benzodiazepine-tolerant patient.
Olanzapine 10mg[d]	IM olanzapine should NOT be combined with an IM benzodiazepine, particularly if alcohol has been consumed.[70]
Aripiprazole 9.75mg	Less hypotension than olanzapine, but less effective[5,13,71]
Haloperidol 5mg	**Haloperidol should be the last drug considered** ■ The incidence of acute dystonia is high; combine with IM promethazine and ensure IM procyclidine is available ■ Pre-treatment ECG required

Repeat after 30–60 minutes if insufficient effect. Combinations of haloperidol and lorazepam or haloperidol and promethazine may be considered if single drug treatment fails. Drugs must not be mixed in the same syringe. IM olanzapine must never be combined with IM benzodiazepine.

4 Consider **IV treatment**

- **Diazepam** 10mg over at least 2 minutes[be]
- Repeat after 5–10 minutes if insufficient effect (up to 3 times)
- Have flumazenil to hand

5 Seek expert advice[f]

Consider transfer to medical unit for administration of **IM ketamine**

Notes

a. Carefully check administration and dilution instructions, which differ between manufacturers. Many centres use 4mg. An alternative is IM midazolam 5–15mg. 5mg is usually sufficient. The risk of respiratory depression is dose-related with both drugs but generally greater with midazolam.

b. Caution in the very young and elderly and those with pre-existing brain damage or impulse control problems, as disinhibition reactions are more likely.[72]

(Continued)

Rapid tranquillisation summary *(Continued)*

c. Promethazine has a slow onset of action but is often an effective sedative. Dilution is not required before IM injection. May be repeated up to a maximum of 100mg/day. Wait 1–2 hours after injection to assess response. Note that promethazine alone has been reported, albeit very rarely, to cause NMS,[73] although it is an extremely weak dopamine antagonist. Note also the potential pharmacokinetic interaction between promethazine and haloperidol (reduced metabolism of haloperidol), which may confer risk if repeated doses of both are administered.

d. Recommended by NICE only for moderate behavioural disturbance, but data from a large observational study also supports efficacy in clinical emergencies.

e. Use Diazemuls to avoid injection site reactions. Lorazepam can also be given IV. IV therapy may be used instead of IM when a very rapid effect is required. IV therapy also ensures near-immediate delivery of the drug to its site of action and effectively avoids the danger of inadvertent accumulation of slowly absorbed IM doses. IV doses can be repeated after only 5–10 minutes if no effect is observed. Midazolam can also be used IV, but respiratory depression is common.[1]

f. Options at this point are limited, although the wider use of IM ketamine has improved the range of options available. IM amylobarbitone and IM paraldehyde have been used in the past but are used now only extremely rarely and are generally not easy to obtain. IV olanzapine, IV droperidol and IV haloperidol are possible but adverse effects are fairly common. ECT is also an option.

Rapid tranquillisation – physical monitoring

After any parenteral drug administration, monitor as follows:

- **Temperature**
- **Pulse**
- **Blood pressure**
- **Respiratory rate**

Every 15 minutes for 1 hour, and then hourly until the patient is ambulatory. Patients who refuse to have their vital signs monitored or who remain too behaviourally disturbed to be approached should be observed for signs/symptoms of pyrexia, hypoxia, hypotension, over-sedation and general physical well-being.

If the patient is asleep or **unconscious**, the continuous use of pulse oximetry to measure oxygen saturation is desirable. A nurse should remain with the patient until ambulatory.

ECG and haematological monitoring are also strongly recommended when parenteral antipsychotics are given, especially when higher doses are used.[74,75] Hypokalaemia, stress and agitation place the patient at risk of cardiac arrhythmia[76] (see the section on 'QT prolongation'). ECG monitoring is formally recommended for all patients who receive haloperidol.

Remedial measures in rapid tranquillisation

Problem	Remedial measures
Acute dystonia (including oculogyric crises)	Give **procyclidine** 5–10mg IM or IV
Reduced respiratory rate (<10/min) or oxygen saturation (<90%)	Give oxygen, raise legs, ensure patient is not lying face down.
	Give **flumazenil** if benzodiazepine-induced respiratory depression suspected (see protocol)
	If induced by any other sedative agent: **transfer to a medical bed and ventilate mechanically.**

(Continued)

Remedial measures in rapid tranquillisation *(Continued)*	
Irregular or slow (<50/min) **pulse**	**Refer** to specialist medical care immediately.
Fall in blood pressure (>30mmHg orthostatic drop or < 50mmHg diastolic)	**Have patient lie flat**, tilt bed towards head. Monitor closely.
Increased temperature	(risk of NMS and perhaps arrhythmia). Check creatine kinase urgently.

Guidelines for the use of flumazenil	
Indication for use	If, after the administration of lorazepam, midazolam or diazepam, respiratory rate falls below 10/min.
Contraindications	Patients with epilepsy who have been receiving long-term benzodiazepines.
Caution	Dose should be carefully titrated in hepatic impairment.
Dose and route of administration	*Initial*: 200μg *intravenously* over 15 seconds – if required level of consciousness not achieved after 60 seconds, then, *Subsequent dose:* 100μg over 15 seconds.
Time before dose can be repeated	60 seconds.
Maximum dose	1mg in 24 hours (one initial dose and eight subsequent doses).
Side-effects	Patients may become agitated, anxious or fearful on awakening. Seizures may occur in regular benzodiazepine users.
Management	Side-effects usually subside.
Monitoring ▪ **What to monitor?** ▪ **How often?**	 Respiratory rate Continuously until respiratory rate returns to baseline level. Flumazenil has a short half-life (much shorter than diazepam) and respiratory function may recover and then deteriorate again.

Note: If respiratory rate does not return to normal or patient is not alert after initial doses given, assume that sedation is due to some other cause.

References

1. Patel MX, et al. Joint BAP NAPICU evidence-based consensus guidelines for the clinical management of acute disturbance: de-escalation and rapid tranquillisation. *J Psychopharmacology* 2018; 32:601–640.
2. Bak M, et al. The pharmacological management of agitated and aggressive behaviour: a systematic review and meta-analysis. *Eur Psychiatry* 2019; 57:78–100.
3. Currier GW, et al. Acute treatment of psychotic agitation: a randomized comparison of oral treatment with risperidone and lorazepam versus intramuscular treatment with haloperidol and lorazepam. *J Clin Psychiatry* 2004; 65:386–394.
4. Ganesan S, et al. Effectiveness of quetiapine for the management of aggressive psychosis in the emergency psychiatric setting: a naturalistic uncontrolled trial. *Int J Psychiatry Clin Pract* 2005; 9:199–203.
5. Simpson JR, Jr., et al. Impact of orally disintegrating olanzapine on use of intramuscular antipsychotics, seclusion, and restraint in an acute inpatient psychiatric setting. *J Clin Psychopharmacol* 2006; 26:333–335.
6. Hsu WY, et al. Comparison of intramuscular olanzapine, orally disintegrating olanzapine tablets, oral risperidone solution, and intramuscular haloperidol in the management of acute agitation in an acute care psychiatric ward in Taiwan. *J Clin Psychopharmacol* 2010; 30:230–234.
7. Pratts M, et al. A single-dose, randomized, double-blind, placebo-controlled trial of sublingual asenapine for acute agitation. *Acta Psychiatr Scand* 2014; 130:61–68.
8. Lesem MD, et al. Rapid acute treatment of agitation in individuals with schizophrenia: multicentre, randomised, placebo-controlled study of inhaled loxapine. *Br J Psychiatry* 2011; 198:51–58.

9. Kwentus J, et al. Rapid acute treatment of agitation in patients with bipolar I disorder: a multicenter, randomized, placebo-controlled clinical trial with inhaled loxapine. *BipolarDisord* 2012; **14**:31–40.

10. Allen MH, et al. Efficacy and safety of loxapine for inhalation in the treatment of agitation in patients with schizophrenia: a randomized, double-blind, placebo-controlled trial. *J Clin Psychiatry* 2011; **72**:1313–1321.

11. Kahl KG, et al. Inhaled loxapine for acute treatment of agitation in patients with borderline personality disorder: a case series. *J Clin Psychopharmacol* 2015; **35**:741–743.

12. Roncero C, et al. Effectiveness of inhaled loxapine in dual-diagnosis patients: a case series. *Clin Neuropharmacol* 2016; **39**:206–209.

13. Citrome L. Comparison of intramuscular ziprasidone, olanzapine, or aripiprazole for agitation: a quantitative review of efficacy and safety. *J Clin Psychiatry* 2007; **68**:1876–1885.

14. Perrin E, et al. A prospective, observational study of the safety and effectiveness of intramuscular psychotropic treatment in acutely agitated patients with schizophrenia and bipolar mania. *Eur Psychiatry* 2012; **27**:234–239.

15. Ferraz Goncalves JA, et al. Comparison of haloperidol alone and in combination with midazolam for the treatment of acute agitation in an inpatient palliative care service. *J Pain Palliat Care Pharmacother* 2016; **30**:284–288.

16. Chan EW, et al. Intravenous droperidol or olanzapine as an adjunct to midazolam for the acutely agitated patient: a multicenter, randomized, double-blind, placebo-controlled clinical trial. *Ann Emerg Med* 2013; **61**:72–81.

17. TREC Collaborative Group. Rapid tranquillisation for agitated patients in emergency psychiatric rooms: a randomised trial of midazolam versus haloperidol plus promethazine. *BMJ* 2003; **327**:708–713.

18. Raveendran NS, et al. Rapid tranquillisation in psychiatric emergency settings in India: pragmatic randomised controlled trial of intramuscular olanzapine versus intramuscular haloperidol plus promethazine. *BMJ* 2007; **335**:865.

19. Huf G, et al. Rapid tranquillisation in psychiatric emergency settings in Brazil: pragmatic randomised controlled trial of intramuscular haloperidol versus intramuscular haloperidol plus promethazine. *BMJ* 2007; **335**:869.

20. Alexander J, et al. Rapid tranquillisation of violent or agitated patients in a psychiatric emergency setting. Pragmatic randomised trial of intramuscular lorazepam v. haloperidol plus promethazine. *Br J Psychiatry* 2004; **185**:63–69.

21. Dib JE, et al. Rapid tranquillisation in a psychiatric emergency hospital in Lebanon: TREC-Lebanon – a pragmatic randomised controlled trial of intramuscular haloperidol and promethazine v. intramuscular haloperidol, promethazine and chlorpromazine. *Psychol Med* 2021: [Epub ahead of print].

22. Taylor DM, et al. Midazolam-droperidol, droperidol, or olanzapine for acute agitation: a randomized clinical trial. *Ann Emerg Med* 2017; **69**:318–326.e311.

23. Kittipeerachon M, et al. Intramuscular olanzapine versus intramuscular aripiprazole for the treatment of agitation in patients with schizophrenia: a pragmatic double-blind randomized trial. *Schizophr Res* 2016; **176**:231–238.

24. Klein LR, et al. Intramuscular midazolam, olanzapine, ziprasidone, or haloperidol for treating acute agitation in the emergency department. *Ann Emerg Med* 2018; **72**:374–385.

25. Huang CL, et al. Intramuscular olanzapine versus intramuscular haloperidol plus lorazepam for the treatment of acute schizophrenia with agitation: an open-label, randomized controlled trial. *J Formos Med Assoc* 2015; **114**:438–445.

26. Calver L, et al. The safety and effectiveness of droperidol for sedation of acute behavioral disturbance in the emergency department. *Ann Emerg Med* 2015; **66**:230–238.e231.

27. Powney MJ, et al. Haloperidol for psychosis-induced aggression or agitation (rapid tranquillisation). *Cochrane Database Syst Rev* 2012; **11**:CD009377.

28. Ostinelli EG, et al. Haloperidol for psychosis-induced aggression or agitation (rapid tranquillisation). *Cochrane Database Syst Rev* 2017; **7**:Cd009377.

29. National Institute for Health and Clinical Excellence. Violence and aggression: short-term management in mental health, health and community settings. NICE guideline [NG10]. 2015 (last checked December 2019); https://www.nice.org.uk/guidance/NG10.

30. Huf G, et al. Haloperidol plus promethazine for psychosis-induced aggression. *Cochrane Database Syst Rev* 2016; **11**:Cd005146.

31. Ostinelli EG, et al. Aripiprazole (intramuscular) for psychosis-induced aggression or agitation (rapid tranquillisation). *Cochrane Database Syst Rev* 2018; **1**:Cd008074.

32. Kishi T, et al. Intramuscular olanzapine for agitated patients: a systematic review and meta-analysis of randomized controlled trials. *J Psychiatr Res* 2015; **68**:198–209.

33. Khokhar MA, et al. Droperidol for psychosis-induced aggression or agitation. *Cochrane Database Syst Rev* 2016; **12**:Cd002830.

34. Satterthwaite TD, et al. A meta-analysis of the risk of acute extrapyramidal symptoms with intramuscular antipsychotics for the treatment of agitation. *J Clin Psychiatry* 2008; **69**:1869–1879.

35. Van Harten PN, et al. Acute dystonia induced by drug treatment. *Br Med J* 1999; **319**:623–626.

36. Pharmacovigilance Working Party. Public assessment report on neuroleptics and cardiac safety, in particular QT prolongation, cardiac arrhythmias, ventricular tachycardia and torsades de pointes. 2006.

37. Janssen-Cilag Ltd. Summary of product characteristics. haldol decanoate. 2020; https://www.medicines.org.uk/emc/product/968/smpc.

38. Miceli JJ, et al. Effects of high-dose ziprasidone and haloperidol on the QTc interval after intramuscular administration: a randomized, single-blind, parallel-group study in patients with schizophrenia or schizoaffective disorder. *Clin Ther* 2010; **32**:472–491.

39. Suzuki A, et al. Histamine H1-receptor antagonists, promethazine and homochlorcyclizine, increase the steady-state plasma concentrations of haloperidol and reduced haloperidol. *TherDrug Monit* 2003; **25**:192–196.

40. Lerner Y, et al. Acute high-dose parenteral haloperidol treatment of psychosis. *Am J Psychiatry* 1979; **136**:1061–1064.

41. Martel ML, et al. A large retrospective cohort of patients receiving intravenous olanzapine in the emergency department. *Acad Emerg Med* 2016; **23**:29–35.

42. Cole JB, et al. A prospective observational study of patients receiving intravenous and intramuscular olanzapine in the emergency department. *Ann Emerg Med* 2017; **69**:327–336.e322.

43. Calver L, et al. A prospective study of high dose sedation for rapid tranquilisation of acute behavioural disturbance in an acute mental health unit. *BMC Psychiatry* 2013; **13**:225.

44. Mantovani C, et al. Are low doses of antipsychotics effective in the management of psychomotor agitation? A randomized, rated-blind trial of 4 intramuscular interventions. *J Clin Psychopharmacol* 2013; **33**:306–312.

45. Taylor D, et al. Buccal midazolam for rapid tranquillisation. *Int J Psychiatry Clin Pract* 2008; **12**:309–311.

46. Spain D, et al. Safety and effectiveness of high-dose midazolam for severe behavioural disturbance in an emergency department with suspected psychostimulant-affected patients. *Emerg Med Australas* 2008; **20**:112–120.

47. Zaman H, et al. Benzodiazepines for psychosis-induced aggression or agitation. *Cochrane Database Syst Rev* 2017; **12**:Cd003079.

48. Li SF, et al. Safety and efficacy of intravenous combination sedatives in the ED. *Am J Emerg Med* 2013; **31**:1402–1404.

49. MacNeal JJ, et al. Use of haloperidol in PCP-intoxicated individuals. *Clin Toxicol* 2012; **50**:851–853.

50. Mankowitz SL, et al. Ketamine for rapid sedation of agitated patients in the prehospital and emergency department settings: a systematic review and proportional meta-analysis. *J Emerg Med* 2018; **55**:670–681.

51. Kim HK, et al. Safety and efficacy of pharmacologic agents used for rapid tranquilization of emergency department patients with acute agitation or excited delirium. *Exp Opin Drug Saf* 2021; **20**:123–138.

52. Pierre JM. Time to retire haloperidol? For emergency agitation, evidence suggests newer alternatives may be a better choice. *Curr Psychiatry* 2020; **19**:19+.

53. Huf G, et al. Physical restraints versus seclusion room for management of people with acute aggression or agitation due to psychotic illness (TREC-SAVE): a randomized trial. *Psychol Med* 2012; **42**:2265–2273.

54. Amdisen A, et al. Serum concentrations and clinical effect of zuclopenthixol in acutely disturbed, psychotic patients treated with zuclopenthixol acetate in Viscoleo. *Psychopharmacology* 1986; **90**:412–416.

55. Amdisen A, et al. Zuclopenthixol acetate in viscoleo – a new drug formulation. An open Nordic multicentre study of zuclopenthixol acetate in Viscoleo in patients with acute psychoses including mania and exacerbation of chronic psychoses. *Acta Psychiatr Scand* 1987; **75**:99–107.

56. Lowert AC, et al. Acute psychotic disorders treated with 5% zuclopenthixol acetate in 'Viscoleo' ('Cisordinol-Acutard'), a global assessment of the clinical effect: an open multi-centre study. *Pharmatherapeutica* 1989; **5**:380–386.

57. Balant LP, et al. Clinical and pharmacokinetic evaluation of zuclopenthixol acetate in Viscoleo. *Pharmacopsychiatry* 1989; **22**:250–254.

58. Chakravarti SK, et al. Zuclopenthixol acetate (5% in 'Viscoleo'): single-dose treatment for acutely disturbed psychotic patients. *Curr Med Res Opin* 1990; **12**:58–65.

59. Baastrup PC, et al. A controlled Nordic multicentre study of zuclopenthixol acetate in oil solution, haloperidol and zuclopenthixol in the treatment of acute psychosis. *Acta Psychiatr Scand* 1993; **87**:48–58.

60. Chin CN, et al. A double blind comparison of zuclopenthixol acetate with haloperidol in the management of acutely disturbed schizophrenics. *Med J Malaysia* 1998; **53**:365–371.

61. Taymeeyapradit U, et al. Comparative study of the effectiveness of zuclopenthixol acetate and haloperidol in acutely disturbed psychotic patients. *J Med Assoc Thai* 2002; **85**:1301–1308.

62. Brook S, et al. A randomized controlled double blind study of zuclopenthixol acetate compared to haloperidol in acute psychosis. *Human Psychopharmacol Clin Experimental* 1998; **13**:17–20.

63. Chouinard G, et al. A double-blind controlled study of intramuscular zuclopenthixol acetate and liquid oral haloperidol in the treatment of schizophrenic patients with acute exacerbation. *J Clin Psychopharmacol* 1994; **14**:377–384.

64. Al-Haddad MK, et al. Zuclopenthixol versus haloperidol in the initial treatment of schizophrenic psychoses, affective psychoses and paranoid states: a controlled clinical trial. *Arab J Psychiatry* 1996; **7**:44–54.

65. Jayakody K, et al. Zuclopenthixol acetate for acute schizophrenia and similar serious mental illnesses. *Cochrane Database Syst Rev* 2012; **4**:CD000525.

66. Liu P, et al. Observation of clinical effect of clopixol acuphase injection for acute psychosis. *Chin J Pharmacoepidemiology* 1997; **6**:202–204.

67. Ropert R, et al. Where zuclopenthixol acetate stands amid the 'modified release' neuroleptics. Congres de Psychiatrie et de Neurolgie de Langue Francaise, LXXXVIth Session, Chambery, France; June 13–17 1988.

68. Berk M. A controlled double blind study of zuclopenthixol acetate compared with clothiapine in acute psychosis including mania and exacerbation of chronic psychosis. Proceedings of XXth Collegium Internationale Neruo-spychopharmacologicum, Melbourne, Australia; June 23–27 1996.

69. Garriga M, et al. Assessment and management of agitation in psychiatry: expert consensus. *World J Biol Psychiatry* 2016; **17**:86–128.

70. Wilson MP, et al. Potential complications of combining intramuscular olanzapine with benzodiazepines in emergency department patients. *J Emerg Med* 2012; **43**:889–896.

71. Villari V, et al. Oral risperidone, olanzapine and quetiapine versus haloperidol in psychotic agitation. *Prog Neuropsychopharmacol Biol Psychiatry* 2008; **32**:405–413.

72. Paton C. Benzodiazepines and disinhibition: a review. *Psychiatric Bulletin* 2002; **26**:460–462.

73. Chan-Tack KM. Neuroleptic malignant syndrome due to promethazine. *South Med J* 1999; **92**:1017–1018.

74. Appleby L, et al. Sudden unexplained death in psychiatric in-patients. *Br J Psychiatry* 2000; **176**:405–406.

75. Yap YG, et al. Risk of torsades de pointes with non-cardiac drugs. Doctors need to be aware that many drugs can cause QT prolongation. *BMJ* 2000; **320**:1158–1159.

76. Taylor DM. Antipsychotics and QT prolongation. *Acta Psychiatr Scand* 2003; **107**:85–95.

Antipsychotic depots/long-acting injections (LAIs)

Long-acting injectable (LAI) preparations of antipsychotic medication are commonly prescribed in clinical practice, especially in the UK, Australasia and the EU. Observational studies have confirmed that continued treatment is associated with fewer relapses and rehospitalisations compared with oral antipsychotic treatment,[1–5] although there are confounding factors in such studies, such as indication bias.

A Cochrane systematic review of randomised trials comparing maintenance treatment with antipsychotic medication and placebo for people with schizophrenia found LAI antipsychotic medications (in particular, LAI haloperidol and fluphenazine) were more effective than oral antipsychotic medications.[6] However, the authors noted that only head-to-head comparisons of oral and LAI antipsychotic treatment can determine whether the latter are more effective. The findings of such RCTs have generally failed to show a clear superiority for LAI antipsychotic medications,[7–9] although this may be partly related to study design and methodology issues.[2] Specifically, double-blind RCTs are generally relatively short term, and the study samples will tend to be biased towards patients with rather less severe illness, fewer comorbid conditions and better adherence to medication.[10,11] RCTs conducted in a more naturalistic manner may better show the advantages of depots.[12] However, all studies of all types clearly demonstrate that continuous treatment with depots does not confer complete protection against relapse.[13]

LAI antipsychotic medication is recommended where a patient has expressed a preference for such a formulation because of its convenience or where avoidance of covert non-adherence is considered a clinical priority.[14,15] While LAI medication does not ensure adherence, it does assure awareness of adherence, unlike the use of oral medication. Thus, failure to adhere, which may be a sign of relapse or a potential cause, will be signalled by delayed attendance for, or refusal of, an injection, allowing the clinical team to intervene promptly. Another possible advantage for LAI antipsychotic medication is that its use may help clarify whether an unsatisfactory therapeutic response to antipsychotic medication is due to adherence problems or a refractory illness. Many apparently refractory patients are simply non-adherent to oral medication, sometimes completely so.[16] Furthermore, an LAI antipsychotic regimen provides the opportunity for regular scrutiny of a patient's mental state and side effects by the health care professional administering the injection.[17]

The proportion of patients with schizophrenia prescribed LAI antipsychotic medications varies between and across countries suggesting that the use of such medication is influenced by factors beyond the extent of poor adherence. Greater understanding of these factors might allow us to identify possible barriers to the optimal implementation of this treatment.[18–20] A US study found that American first-episode patients were largely willing to accept long-acting treatment.[21] This suggests that low usage of depots in the USA might be largely a result of reluctance on the part of clinicians, rather than patients.

Advice on prescribing LAIs

- **For LAI FGAs, give a test dose**
  Because of its long half-life, any adverse effects that result from the administration of an LAI antipsychotic medication are likely to be long-lived. Therefore, such treatment

should be avoided in patients with a history of serious adverse effects that would warrant immediate discontinuation of the medication, such as neuroleptic malignant syndrome (NMS). For LAI FGAs, a test dose consisting of a small dose of active drug in a small volume of oil serves a dual purpose – it is a test of the patient's sensitivity to EPS and of any sensitivity to the base oil. For LAI SGAs, test doses may not be required (there is a lower propensity to cause EPS and the aqueous base not known to be allergenic), although they could be considered appropriate where a patient is suspected of being non-adherent to oral antipsychotic medication and the LAI preparation will be the first exposure to guaranteed antipsychotic medication delivery. For both LAI FGAs and SGAs, prior treatment with the equivalent oral formulation is preferred to assess efficacy and tolerability, but it is not always necessary from a pharmacokinetic viewpoint. Most SGA depots can be used as sole treatment from the outset, although loading doses are usually necessary (e.g. for paliperidone and aripiprazole).

- **Begin with the lowest therapeutic dose**
There are few data showing clear dose–response effects for FGA LAI antipsychotic medication. There is some information indicating that low doses (within the licensed range) may be at least as effective as higher ones,[22–25] but whether the dosages and frequency of injections for LAI antipsychotic medications achieve the optimal benefit–risk balance seems uncertain.[26–28]

- **Administer at the longest possible licensed interval**
All LAI antipsychotic medications can be safely administered at their licensed dosing intervals, bearing in mind the maximum recommended single dose. There is no evidence to suggest that shortening the dose interval improves efficacy. Moreover, the intramuscular injection site can be a cause of discomfort and pain, so less frequent administration is desirable. Although some patients are reported to deteriorate in the days before their next injection is due, plasma drug concentrations may continue to fall, albeit slowly, for some hours (or even days with some preparations) after each injection. In this context, a patient's apparent recovery soon after the injection is given makes no sense. More importantly, at steady state, trough plasma levels (immediately pre- and post-dose) are usually substantially above the threshold concentration required for therapeutic effect.

- **Adjust doses only after an adequate period of assessment**
Attainment of peak plasma levels, therapeutic effect and steady-state plasma levels are all delayed with LAI antipsychotic medications, compared with oral medications. Doses may be *reduced* if adverse effects occur but should only be increased after careful assessment over at least one month, and preferably longer. Note that with most LAI antipsychotic preparations, at the start of treatment, plasma drug levels increase over several weeks to months without any increase in the dosage. This is due to accumulation: steady state is only achieved after at least 6–8 weeks. Dose increases during this initial period are therefore illogical and impossible to evaluate properly. With continued LAI antipsychotic treatment, the monitoring and recording of therapeutic efficacy, side effects and any impact on physical health are recommended

- **LAIs are not recommended for those who are antipsychotic-naïve**
Tolerability to some LAI antipsychotic medications can be established by using the oral form of the same drug for two weeks before starting. Good examples here are haloperidol, aripiprazole and paliperidone (using oral risperidone).

Table 1.4 Antipsychotic long-acting injections – doses and frequencies[15]

Drug	UK Trade Name	Licences injection site	Test dose (mg)	Dose range (mg/week)	Dosing interval (weeks)	Comments
Aripiprazole	(Abilify Maintena)	Buttock	Not required**	300–400mg monthly	Monthly	Does not increase prolactin; oral loading required
Flupentixol decanoate	(Depixol)	Buttock or thigh	20	50mg every 4 weeks to 400mg a week	2–4	Maximum licensed dose is high relative to other LAIs
Fluphenazine decanoate	(Modecate)	Gluteal region	12.5	12.5mg every 2 weeks to 100mg every 2 weeks	2–5	High EPS
Haloperidol decanoate	(Haldol)	Gluteal region	25*	50–300mg every 4 weeks	4	High EPS
Olanzapine pamoate	(ZypAdhera)	Gluteal	Not required**	150mg every 4 weeks to 300mg every 2 weeks	2–4	Risk of post-injection syndrome
Paliperidone palmitate (monthly)	(Xeplion)	Deltoid or gluteal	Not required**	50–150mg monthly	Monthly	Loading dose required at treatment initiation
Paliperidone palmitate (3-monthly)	(Trevicta)	Deltoid or gluteal	Not required***	175–525mg every 3 months	3 months	
Pipothiazine palmitate	(Piportil)	Gluteal region	25	50–200mg every 4 weeks	4	? Lower incidence of EPS (relative to other FGAs)
Risperidone microspheres	(Risperdal Consta)	Deltoid or gluteal	Not required**	25–50mg every 2 weeks	2	Drug release delayed for 2–3 weeks – oral therapy required
Zuclopenthixol decanote	(Clopixol)	Buttock or thigh	100	200mg every 3 weeks to 600mg a week	2–4	? Slightly better efficacy than LAI FGAs

Notes:

■ The doses mentioned above are for adults. Check formal labelling for appropriate doses in the elderly.

■ After a test dose, wait 4–10 days then titrate to maintenance dose according to response.

■ Avoid using shorter dose intervals than those recommended except in exceptional circumstances (e.g. long interval necessitates high volume (>3–4ml?) injection). Maximum licensed single dose overrides longer intervals and lower volumes. For example, zuclopenthixol 500mg every week is licensed, whereas 1,000mg every two weeks is not (more than the licensed maximum of 600mg is administered). Always check official manufacturer's information.

*Test dose not stated by manufacturer.

**Tolerability and response to the oral preparation should be established before administering the LAI. With respect to paliperidone LAI, oral risperidone can be used for this purpose.

***May not be started until the completion of 4 months' treatment with monthly LAI.

- **Adding an oral antipsychotic medication risks a high-dose prescription**

  The regular prescription of an oral antipsychotic medication in addition to an LAI antipsychotic preparation was once common with FGAs.[17,29] While this may be a possible strategy for the control of breakthrough symptoms and offer greater flexibility in dosage titration, the safety and tolerability of such a combination is uncertain, particularly over the longer term.[30] The co-prescription of an LAI and oral antipsychotic medication may well result in a, possibly inadvertent, high-dose prescription, with an increased side-effect burden and implications for physical health monitoring.[10,17]

Differences between LAIs

None of the individual LAI FGAs has emerged as clearly superior in efficacy, although there is some suggestion of an advantage for zuclopenthixol decanoate in terms of time to discontinuation and hospitalisation, but perhaps at the expense of a greater side-effect burden.[31–33] Cochrane reviews have been completed for pipotiazine palmitate,[34] flupentixol decanoate,[35] zuclopenthixol decanoate,[36] haloperidol decanoate[37] and fluphenazine decanoate.[38]

The LAI SGAs, aripiprazole, paliperidone, risperidone and olanzapine, also have comparable efficacy but vary in their liability for particular adverse effects, such as weight gain, metabolic effects, EPS, and raised plasma prolactin.[39–42] For example, LAI paliperidone is associated with substantial increases in serum prolactin,[41] and LAI olanzapine can cause significant weight gain and is associated with a post-injection delirium/sedation syndrome, assumed to be caused by unintended partial intravascular injection or blood vessel injury.[43,44] Because of the nature of the pharmacokinetic profile of LAI risperidone, administration of an oral antipsychotic medication is required in the three weeks after the first injection (Table 1.4).[45,46] Details on dosing of individual SGAs are given elsewhere in this chapter.

References

1. Tiihonen J, et al. Real-world effectiveness of antipsychotic treatments in a nationwide cohort of 29823 patients with schizophrenia. *JAMA Psychiatry* 2017; **74**:686–693.
2. Kirson NY, et al. Efficacy and effectiveness of depot versus oral antipsychotics in schizophrenia: synthesizing results across different research designs. *J Clin Psychiatry* 2013; **74**:568–575.
3. Marcus SC, et al. Antipsychotic adherence and rehospitalization in schizophrenia patients receiving oral versus long-acting injectable antipsychotics following hospital discharge. *J Manag Care Spec Pharm* 2015; **21**:754–768.
4. Nielsen RE, et al. Second-generation LAI are associated to favorable outcome in a cohort of incident patients diagnosed with schizophrenia. *Schizophr Res* 2018; **202**:234–240.
5. Kishimoto T, et al. Effectiveness of long-acting injectable vs oral antipsychotics in patients with schizophrenia: a meta-analysis of prospective and retrospective cohort studies. *Schizophr Bull* 2018; **44**:603–619.
6. Ceraso A, et al. Maintenance treatment with antipsychotic drugs for schizophrenia. *Cochrane Database Syst Rev* 2020; **8**:Cd008016.
7. Ostuzzi G, et al. Does formulation matter? A systematic review and meta-analysis of oral versus long-acting antipsychotic studies. *Schizophr Res* 2017; **183**:10–21.
8. Kishimoto T, et al. Long-acting injectable vs oral antipsychotics for relapse prevention in schizophrenia: a meta-analysis of randomized trials. *Schizophr Bull* 2014; **40**:192–213.
9. Leucht C, et al. Oral versus depot antipsychotic drugs for schizophrenia–a critical systematic review and meta-analysis of randomised long-term trials. *Schizophr Res* 2011; **127**:83–92.
10. Barnes T, et al. Evidence-based guidelines for the pharmacological treatment of schizophrenia: updated recommendations from the British Association for Psychopharmacology. *J Psychopharmacology* 2020; **34**:3–78.
11. Kane JM, et al. Optimizing treatment choices to improve adherence and outcomes in schizophrenia. *J Clin Psychiatry* 2019; **80**:IN18031AH18031C.

12. Kane JM, et al. Effect of long-acting injectable antipsychotics vs usual care on time to first hospitalization in early-phase schizophrenia: a randomized clinical trial. *JAMA Psychiatry* 2020; 77:1–8.

13. Rubio JM, et al. Psychosis relapse during treatment with long-acting injectable antipsychotics in individuals with schizophrenia-spectrum disorders: an individual participant data meta-analysis. *Lancet Psychiatry* 2020; 7:749–761.

14. National Institute for Health and Care Excellence. Psychosis and schizophrenia in adults: prevention and management. Clinical Guidance [CG178]. 2014 (last checked March 2019); https://www.nice.org.uk/guidance/cg178.

15. Barnes TR. Evidence-based guidelines for the pharmacological treatment of schizophrenia: recommendations from the British Association for Psychopharmacology. *J Psychopharmacology* 2011; 25:567–620.

16. McCutcheon R, et al. Antipsychotic plasma levels in the assessment of poor treatment response in schizophrenia. *Acta Psychiatr Scand* 2018; 137:39–46.

17. Barnes T, et al. Antipsychotic long acting injections: prescribing practice in the UK. *Br J Psychiatry Suppl* 2009; 52:S37–S42.

18. Brissos S, et al. The role of long-acting injectable antipsychotics in schizophrenia: a critical appraisal. *Ther Adv Psychopharmacol* 2014; 4:198–219.

19. Haddad P, et al. Prescribing patterns and determinants of use of antipsychotic long-acting injections: an international perspective, in *Antipsychotic Long-acting Injections* (2nd ed.). Oxford University Press; 2016.

20. Patel MX, et al. Attitudes of European physicians towards the use of long-acting injectable antipsychotics. *BMC Psychiatry* 2020; 20:123.

21. Kane JM, et al. Patients with early-phase schizophrenia will accept treatment with sustained-release medication (Long-Acting Injectable Antipsychotics): results from the recruitment phase of the PRELAPSE trial. *J Clin Psychiatry* 2019; 80.

22. Kane JM, et al. A multidose study of haloperidol decanoate in the maintenance treatment of schizophrenia. *Am J Psychiatry* 2002; 159:554–560.

23. Taylor D. Establishing a dose-response relationship for haloperidol decanoate. *Psychiatric Bulletin* 2005; 29:104–107.

24. McEvoy JP, et al. Effectiveness of paliperidone palmitate vs haloperidol decanoate for maintenance treatment of schizophrenia: a randomized clinical trial. *JAMA* 2014; 311:1978–1987.

25. Bailey L, et al. Estimating the optimal dose of flupentixol decanoate in the maintenance treatment of schizophrenia—a systematic review of the literature. *Psychopharmacology* 2019; 236:3081–3092.

26. Uchida H, et al. Monthly administration of long-acting injectable risperidone and striatal dopamine D2 receptor occupancy for the management of schizophrenia. *J Clin Psychiatry* 2008; 69:1281–1286.

27. Ikai S, et al. Plasma levels and estimated dopamine D(2) receptor occupancy of long-acting injectable risperidone during maintenance treatment of schizophrenia: a 3-year follow-up study. *Psychopharmacology* 2016; 233:4003–4010.

28. Hill AL, et al. Dose-associated changes in safety and efficacy parameters observed in a 24-week maintenance trial of olanzapine long-acting injection in patients with schizophrenia. *BMC Psychiatry* 2011; 11:28.

29. Doshi JA, et al. Concurrent oral antipsychotic drug use among schizophrenia patients initiated on long-acting injectable antipsychotics post-hospital discharge. *J Clin Psychopharmacol* 2015; 35:442–446.

30. Correll CU, et al. Practical considerations for managing breakthrough psychosis and symptomatic worsening in patients with schizophrenia on long-acting injectable antipsychotics. *CNS Spectr* 2018; 24:354–370.

31. Da Silva Freire Coutinho E, et al. Zuclopenthixol decanoate for schizophrenia and other serious mental illnesses. *Cochrane Database Syst Rev* 2006; CD001164.

32. Shajahan P, et al. Comparison of the effectiveness of depot antipsychotics in routine clinical practice. *Psychiatrist* 2010; 34:273–279.

33. Adams CE, et al. Systematic meta-review of depot antipsychotic drugs for people with schizophrenia. *Br J Psychiatry* 2001; 179:290–299.

34. Dinesh M, et al. Depot pipotiazine palmitate and undecylenate for schizophrenia. *Cochrane Database Syst Rev* 2006; CD001720.

35. Mahapatra J, et al. Flupenthixol decanoate (depot) for schizophrenia or other similar psychotic disorders. *Cochrane Database Syst Rev* 2014; 6:CD001470.

36. Coutinho E, et al. Zuclopenthixol decanoate for schizophrenia and other serious mental illnesses. *Cochrane Database Syst Rev* 2000; CD001164.

37. Quraishi S, et al. Depot haloperidol decanoate for schizophrenia. *Cochrane Database Syst Rev* 2000; CD001361.

38. Maayan N, et al. Fluphenazine decanoate (depot) and enanthate for schizophrenia. *Cochrane Database Syst Rev* 2015; Cd000307.

39. Jann MW, et al. Long-acting injectable second-generation antipsychotics: an update and comparison between agents. *CNS Drugs* 2018; 32:241–257.

40. Correll CU, et al. The use of long-acting injectable antipsychotics in schizophrenia: evaluating the evidence. *J Clin Psychiatry* 2016; 77:1–24.

41. Nussbaum AM, et al. Paliperidone palmitate for schizophrenia. *Cochrane Database Syst Rev* 2012; Cd008296.

42. Sampson S, et al. Risperidone (depot) for schizophrenia. *Cochrane Database Syst Rev* 2016; 4:Cd004161.

43. Citrome L. Olanzapine pamoate: a stick in time? *Int J Clin Pract* 2009; 63:140–150.

44. Luedecke D, et al. Post-injection delirium/sedation syndrome in patients treated with olanzapine pamoate: mechanism, incidence, and management. *CNS Drugs* 2015; 29:41–46.

45. Harrison TS, et al. Long-acting risperidone: a review of its use in schizophrenia. *CNS Drugs* 2004; 18:113–132.

46. Knox ED, et al. Clinical review of a long-acting, injectable formulation of risperidone. *Clin Ther* 2004; 26:1994–2002.

Depot/LAI antipsychotics – pharmacokinetics

Drug	UK Trade Name	Time to peak (days)*	Plasma half-life (days)	Time to steady state (weeks)**
Aripiprazole[1]	(Abilify Maintena)	7d	30–46d	~20W
Aripiprazole lauroxil[2–4]	(Aristada (in USA))	44–50d	~54–57d	~16W
Aripiprazole lauroxil nanocrystal[4–6]****	(Aristada Initio (in USA))	4d	~15–18d	
Flupentixol decanoate[7,8]	(Depixol)	4–7d	8–17d	~8–12W
Fluphenazine decanoate[4,9–11]	(Modecate)	8–12d***	7–10d	~8W
Haloperidol decanoate[12,13]	(Haldol)	7d	21d	~14W
Olanzapine pamoate[4,14,15]	(ZypAdhera)	2–3d	30d	~12W
Paliperidone palmitate[4,16] (monthly)	(Xeplion)	13d	25–49d	~20W
Paliperidone palmitate[17,18] (three monthly)	(Trevicta)	25d	Deltoid: 84–95d Gluteal: 118–139d	~52W
Pipotiazine palmitate[19,20]	(Piportil)	7–14d	15d	~9W
RBP-7000[4,21] (risperidone sc monthly)	(Perseris (in USA))	1st peak ~1d 2nd peak ~11d	~8–9d	~8W
Risperidone microspheres[22,23]	(Risperidal Consta)	~30d	4d	~8W
Zuclopenthixol decanoate[7,19,24]	(Clopixol)	4–7d	19d	~12W

*Time to peak is not the same as time to reach therapeutic plasma concentration, but both are dependent on dose. For large (loading) doses, therapeutic activity is often seen before attaining peak levels. For low (test) doses, the initial peak level may be sub-therapeutic.

**Attainment of steady state (SS) follows logarithmic, not linear characteristics: around 90% of SS levels are achieved in three half-lives. Time to attain steady state is independent of dose and dosing frequency (i.e. you can't hurry it up by giving more, more often). Loading doses can be used to produce prompt therapeutic plasma levels but time to SS remains the same.

***Some estimates suggest peak concentrations after only a few hours.[24,25] It is likely that fluphenazine decanoate produces two peaks – one on the day of injection and a second slightly higher peak a week or so later.[12]

****used to initiate treatment with Aristada, IM injection with one 30 mg oral dose of aripiprazole; not designed for repeat dosing.

References

1. Mallikaarjun S, et al. Pharmacokinetics, tolerability and safety of aripiprazole once-monthly in adult schizophrenia: an open-label, parallel-arm, multiple-dose study. *Schizophr Res* 2013; **150**:281–288.
2. Hard ML, et al. Aripiprazole lauroxil: pharmacokinetic profile of this long-acting injectable antipsychotic in persons with schizophrenia. *J Clin Psychopharmacol* 2017; **37**:289–295.
3. Turncliff R, et al. Relative bioavailability and safety of aripiprazole lauroxil, a novel once-monthly, long-acting injectable atypical antipsychotic, following deltoid and gluteal administration in adult subjects with schizophrenia. *Schizophr Res* 2014; **159**:404–410.
4. Correll CU, et al. Pharmacokinetic characteristics of long-acting injectable antipsychotics for schizophrenia: an overview. *CNS Drugs* 2021; **35**:39–59.
5. Alkermes Inc. Highlights of Prescribing Information. ARISTADA INITIO® (aripiprazole lauroxil) extended-release injectable suspension, for intramuscular use. 2020; https://www.aristadahcp.com/downloadables/ARISTADA-INITIO-PI.pdf.

6. Alkermes Inc. ARISTADA INITIO™ (aripiprazole lauroxil) extended-release injectable suspension [product monograph]. 2020; https://www.aristadacaresupport.com/downloadables/ARISTADA-INITIO-ARISTADA-Payer-Hospital-Monograph.pdf.

7. Jann MW, et al. Clinical pharmacokinetics of the depot antipsychotics. *Clin Pharmacokinet* 1985; **10**:315–333.

8. Bailey L, et al. Estimating the optimal dose of flupentixol decanoate in the maintenance treatment of schizophrenia—a systematic review of the literature. *Psychopharmacology* 2019; **236**:3081–3092.

9. Simpson GM, et al. Single-dose pharmacokinetics of fluphenazine after fluphenazine decanoate administration. *J Clin Psychopharmacol* 1990; **10**:417–421.

10. Balant-Gorgia AE, et al. Antipsychotic drugs. Clinical pharmacokinetics of potential candidates for plasma concentration monitoring. *Clin Pharmacokinet* 1987; **13**:65–90.

11. Gitlin MJ, et al. Persistence of fluphenazine in plasma after decanoate withdrawal. *J Clin Psychopharmacol* 1988; **8**:53–56.

12. Wiles DH, et al. Pharmacokinetics of haloperidol and fluphenazine decanoates in chronic schizophrenia. *Psychopharmacology* 1990; **101**:274–281.

13. Nayak RK, et al. The bioavailability and pharmacokinetics of oral and depot intramuscular haloperidol in schizophrenic patients. *J Clin Pharmacol* 1987; **27**:144–150.

14. Heres S, et al. Pharmacokinetics of olanzapine long-acting injection: the clinical perspective. *Int Clin Psychopharmacol* 2014; **29**:299–312.

15. Mitchell M, et al. Single- and multiple-dose pharmacokinetic, safety, and tolerability profiles of olanzapine long-acting injection: an open-label, multicenter, nonrandomized study in patients with schizophrenia. *ClinTher* 2013; **35**:1890–1908.

16. Hoy SM, et al. Intramuscular paliperidone palmitate. *CNS Drugs* 2010; **24**:227–244.

17. Ravenstijn P, et al. Pharmacokinetics, safety, and tolerability of paliperidone palmitate 3-month formulation in patients with schizophrenia: a phase-1, single-dose, randomized, open-label study. *J Clin Pharmacol* 2016; **56**:330–339.

18. Janssen Pharmaceuticals Inc. Highlights of Prescribing Information. INVEGA TRINZA® (paliperidone palmitate) extended-release injectable suspension for intramuscular use. 2019; https://www.janssenlabels.com/package-insert/product-monograph/prescribing-information/INVEGA+TRINZA-pi.pdf.

19. Barnes TR, et al. Long-term depot antipsychotics. A risk-benefit assessment. *Drug Saf* 1994; **10**:464–479.

20. Ogden DA, et al. Determination of pipothiazine in human plasma by reversed-phase high-performance liquid chromatography. *J Pharm Biomed Anal* 1989; **7**:1273–1280.

21. US Food and Drug Administration. Clinical pharmacology and biopharmaceutics review(s). perseris. 2018; https://www.accessdata.fda.gov/drugsatfda_docs/nda/2018/210655Orig1s000ClinPharmR.pdf.

22. Ereshefsky L, et al. Pharmacokinetic profile and clinical efficacy of long-acting risperidone: potential benefits of combining an atypical antipsychotic and a new delivery system. *Drugs RD* 2005; **6**:129–137.

23. Meyer JM. Understanding depot antipsychotics: an illustrated guide to kinetics. *CNS Spectr* 2013; **18 Suppl 1**:58–67.

24. Viala A, et al. Comparative study of the pharmacokinetics of zuclopenthixol decanoate and fluphenazine decanoate. *Psychopharmacology* 1988; **94**:293–297.

25. Soni SD, et al. Plasma levels of fluphenazine decanoate. Effects of site of injection, massage and muscle activity. *Br J Psychiatry* 1988; **153**:382–384.

CHAPTER 1

Management of patients on long-term depots/LAIs

All patients receiving long-term treatment with antipsychotic medication should be seen by their responsible psychiatrist at least once a year (ideally more frequently) in order to review their treatment and progress. A systematic assessment of tolerability and safety should constitute part of this review. The assessment of adverse effects should include EPS (principally parkinsonism, akathisia, and tardive dyskinesia). Assessment of tardive dyskinesia can be recorded by scoring the Abnormal Involuntary Movement Scale (AIMS).[1,2] While some study findings have suggested that LAI antipsychotic medication may be more likely to be associated with tardive dyskinesia than oral antipsychotic medication, this remains uncertain:[3-5] when using the same antipsychotic medication, the risk of tardive dyskinesia does not appear to be different between the LAI and oral formulations.[6,7]

For most people with multi-episode schizophrenia, long-term antipsychotic treatment, even lifelong treatment, may be necessary. Overall, for those with stable illnesses, it has been proposed that the dosage of continuing antipsychotic treatment should be at least 50% of the standard daily dosage, as reduction below this level is associated with a greater risk of relapse.[8] Thus, long-term follow-up is essential when antipsychotic dosage is decreased, particularly to very low doses, as such reduction is associated with a greater risk of treatment failure, hospitalisation and relapse,[9] which may only become evident over the longer term.

However, with the long-term treatment of patients with stable illness with LAI antipsychotic formulations, dose reduction may be considered on the basis that patients often receive supratherapeutic doses. In trials, haloperidol decanoate is optimally effective at 75mg every four weeks,[9,10] paliperidone palmitate at 50mg a month.[11] Doses as low as these are almost unheard of in practice. Furthermore, the threshold level of striatal dopamine D2 receptor occupancy required for relapse prevention may be lower than that for the treatment of an acute episode.[12-14] Nevertheless, for people with schizophrenia, reduction below the standard dosage seems to be clearly associated with a greater risk of relapse, particularly in the longer term. A study comparing fluphenazine decanoate at a low (5mg every two weeks) or standard (25mg every two weeks) dosage found no difference in outcome at one year but a substantial disadvantage for the lower dose at two years (relapse in 69% and 36%, respectively).[15] However, in the same study, the facility to increase the dose when symptoms emerged removed the advantage for the higher dose. Another trial comparing low-dose fluphenazine decanoate (1.25–5mg every two weeks) with standard dosage (12.5 to 50mg every 2 weeks) also found the low-dose to be clearly inferior, with cumulative one-year relapse rates of 56% and 7%, respectively.[16] Similarly, an RCT comparison of four, fixed, monthly doses (25mg, 50mg, 100mg or 200mg) of LAI haloperidol medication over a year[17] found that the standard 200mg dose was associated with the lowest rate of relapse and symptomatic exacerbation (15%), compared with the 100mg (23%) or 50mg (25%) doses (although not statistically significant), but only a minimally increased risk of adverse effects.

There is no simple formula for deciding when or whether to reduce the dose of continuing antipsychotic treatment, and so a risk/benefit analysis must be carried out for every patient. Many patients, it should be noted, prefer to receive LAI antipsychotic preparations.[7,18]

When considering dose reduction, the following prompts may be helpful:

- Is the patient symptom-free and if so for how long? Long-standing, non-distressing symptoms which have not previously been responsive to medication may be excluded.
- How severe, tolerable and disabling are the side effects (EPS including tardive dyskinesia, metabolic side effects including obesity, etc.)? When patients report no or minimal adverse effects, it is usually sensible to continue treatment and monitor closely for signs of tardive dyskinesia.
- What is the previous pattern of illness? Consider the speed of onset, duration and severity of past relapses and any dangers or risks posed to self or others
- Has dosage reduction been attempted before? If so, what was the outcome?
- What are the patient's current social circumstances? Is it a period of relative stability, or should stressful life events be anticipated?
- What is the potential social cost of relapse (e.g. is the patient the sole breadwinner for a family)?
- Is the patient able to monitor his/her own symptoms? If so, will he/she seek appropriate help?

If, after consideration of the above, the decision is taken to reduce the medication dose, the patient's family should be involved and a clear explanation given of what should be done if and when symptoms return or worsen. It would then be reasonable to proceed in the following manner:

- If it has not already been done, any co-prescribed oral antipsychotic medication should be discontinued.
- Where the product labelling allows, the interval between injections should be increased to up to 4 weeks before decreasing the dose given each time.
- The dose should be reduced by no more than a third at any one time. Note: special considerations apply to risperidone Consta LAI.
- Decrements should, if possible, be made no more frequently than every 3 months, preferably every 6 months or more. The slower the rate of withdrawal, the longer the time to relapse.[19]
- Discontinuation of medication should not be seen as the ultimate aim of the above process, although it sometimes results. While an intermittent, targeted (symptom-triggered) treatment approach with antipsychotic medication is not as effective as continuous treatment, it may be preferable to no treatment.[20–22]

If the patient becomes symptomatic, this should be seen not as a failure but rather as an important step in determining the minimum effective dose that the patient requires.

For more discussion, see the section on long-term antipsychotic treatment in this chapter.

References

1. National Institute of Mental Health. *Abnormal Involuntary Movement Scale (AIMS). (U.S. Public Health Service Publication No. MH-9-17).* Washington, DC: US Government Printing Office; 1974.

2. McEvoy JP. How to assess tardive dyskinesia symptom improvement with measurement-based care. *J Clin Psychiatry* 2020; 81:NU19047BR4C.

3. Novick D, et al. Incidence of extrapyramidal symptoms and tardive dyskinesia in schizophrenia: thirty-six-month results from the European schizophrenia outpatient health outcomes study. *J Clin Psychopharmacol* 2010; 30:531–540.

4. Barnes TR, et al. Long-term depot antipsychotics. A risk-benefit assessment. *Drug Saf* 1994; 10:464–479.

5. Baldessarini RJ, et al. Incidence of extrapyramidal syndromes and tardive dyskinesia. *J Clin Psychopharmacol* 2011; 31:382–384; author reply 384–385.

6. Gopal S, et al. Incidence of tardive dyskinesia: a comparison of long-acting injectable and oral paliperidone clinical trial databases. *Int J Clin Pract* 2014; 68:1514–1522.

7. Patel MX, et al. Why aren't depot antipsychotics prescribed more often and what can be done about it? *Adv Psychiatric Treatment* 2005; 11:203–211.

8. Correll CU, et al. What is the risk-benefit ratio of long-term antipsychotic treatment in people with schizophrenia? *World Psychiatry* 2018; 17:149–160.

9. Taylor D. Establishing a dose-response relationship for haloperidol decanoate. *Psychiatric Bulletin* 2005; 29:104–107.

10. McEvoy JP. Effectiveness of paliperidone palmitate vs haloperidol decanoate for maintenance treatment of schizophrenia: a randomized clinical trial. *JAMA* 2014; 311:1978–1987.

11. Rothe PH, et al. Dose equivalents for second generation long-acting injectable antipsychotics: the minimum effective dose method. *Schizophr Res* 2018; 193:23–28.

12. Takeuchi H, et al. Dose reduction of risperidone and olanzapine and estimated dopamine D_2 receptor occupancy in stable patients with schizophrenia: findings from an open-label, randomized, controlled study. *J Clin Psychiatry* 2014; 75:1209–1214.

13. Mizuno Y, et al. Dopamine D2 receptor occupancy with risperidone or olanzapine during maintenance treatment of schizophrenia: a cross-sectional study. *Prog Neuropsychopharmacol Biol Psychiatry* 2012; 37:182–187.

14. Ikai S, et al. A cross-sectional study of plasma risperidone levels with risperidone long-acting injectable: implications for dopamine D2 receptor occupancy during maintenance treatment in schizophrenia. *J Clin Psychiatry* 2012; 73:1147–1152.

15. Marder SR, et al. Low- and conventional-dose maintenance therapy with fluphenazine decanoate. Two-year outcome. *Arch Gen Psychiatry* 1987; 44:518–521.

16. Kane JM, et al. Low-dose neuroleptic treatment of outpatient schizophrenics: i. preliminary results for relapse rates. *Arch Gen Psychiatry* 1983; 40:893–896.

17. Kane JM, et al. A multidose study of haloperidol decanoate in the maintenance treatment of schizophrenia. *Am J Psychiatry* 2002; 159:554–560.

18. Heres S, et al. The attitude of patients towards antipsychotic depot treatment. *Int Clin Psychopharmacol* 2007; 22:275–282.

19. Weiden PJ, et al. Does half-life matter after antipsychotic discontinuation? A relapse comparison in schizophrenia with 3 different formulations of paliperidone. *J Clin Psychiatry* 2017; 78:e813–e820.

20. National Institute for Health and Care Excellence. Psychosis and schizophrenia in adults: prevention and management. Clinical Guidance [CG178]. 2014 (last checked March 2019); https://www.nice.org.uk/guidance/cg178.

21. Barnes T, et al. Evidence-based guidelines for the pharmacological treatment of schizophrenia: updated recommendations from the British Association for Psychopharmacology. *J Psychopharmacology* 2020; 34:3–78.

22. Sampson S, et al. Intermittent drug techniques for schizophrenia. *Cochrane Database Syst Rev* 2013; Cd006196.

Aripiprazole long-acting injection

Abilify brands

Aripiprazole lacks the prolactin-related and metabolic adverse effects of other SGA LAIs and so is a useful alternative to them. Placebo-controlled studies show a good acute and longer term effect in the treatment of schizophrenia.[1] The FDA has also approved Aripiprazole LAI for maintenance monotherapy treatment of bipolar I disorder in adults.[2] Oral aripiprazole 10mg/day for 14 days is recommended initially to establish tolerability and response. One of two regimens may be followed for administering the starting dose of aripiprazole LAI.[3]

One-injection start

On the day of initiation, administer one injection of 400mg aripiprazole LAI and continue treatment with 10mg to 20mg oral aripiprazole per day for 14 consecutive days (28 days in total) to maintain therapeutic aripiprazole concentrations during initiation.

Or

Two-injection start

On the day of initiation, administer two separate injections of 400mg aripiprazole LAI at separate injection sites in two different muscles (separate gluteal, separate deltoid or gluteal and deltoid injection sites) along with one 20mg dose of oral aripiprazole. Oral therapy should not continue after this point.

One month after the day of initiation, begin a regimen of 400mg each month.

After the one-injection + oral starting regimen, peak plasma levels are seen 7 days after the injection and trough levels at four weeks.[4] At steady state, peak plasma levels are up to 50% higher than the first dose peak and trough plasma levels only slightly below the first dose peak.[4] Dose adjustments should take this into account. A population pharmacokinetic modelling study indicated that the two-injection start regimen would produce comparable aripiprazole plasma concentrations to the one injection start method.[5]

A lower dose of 300mg a month can be used in those not tolerating 400mg. A dose of 200mg a month may only be used for those patients receiving particular enzyme inhibiting drugs. The incidence of akathisia, insomnia, nausea and restlessness is similar to that seen with oral aripiprazole[6,7]

There are no formal recommendations for switching to aripiprazole, but we present next recommendations based on our interpretation of available pharmacokinetic data.

Switching to aripiprazole LAI

Switching from	Aripiprazole LAI regimen
Oral antipsychotics	Cross taper antipsychotic with oral aripiprazole* over two weeks
	One-injection start Start aripiprazole LAI, continue aripiprazole oral for another two weeks and then stop
	Two-injection start Start aripiprazole LAI as indicated above after two weeks of oral aripiprazole, then stop oral treatment**.
Depot antipsychotics (not risperidone LAI)	Start oral aripiprazole* on day the last depot injection was due
	One-injection start Start aripiprazole LAI after two weeks and then stop oral aripiprazole two weeks later
	Two-injection start Start aripiprazole LAI as indicated above after two weeks of oral aripiprazole, then stop oral treatment**.
Risperidone LAI	Start oral aripiprazole* 4–6 weeks after the last risperidone injection
	One-injection start Start aripiprazole LAI two weeks later; discontinue oral aripiprazole two weeks after that
	Two-injection start Start aripiprazole LAI as indicated above after two weeks of oral aripiprazole, then stop oral treatment**.

*If prior response and tolerability to aripiprazole are known, pre-injection oral aripiprazole may not be strictly required. However, attainment of effective aripiprazole plasma levels is dependent upon four weeks of oral supplementation for the one-injection start regimen. Similarly, for the two-injection start regimen, the pharmacokinetic modelling study was based on plasma levels from oral aripiprazole being at steady state on the day of initiation.

**If oral aripiprazole cannot be given at all (e.g. patient refusal), always use the two-injection starting regimen. This 800mg dose is likely to afford therapeutic plasma concentrations even in the absence of prior oral treatment.

Other LAI aripiprazole brands

Another long-acting formulation of aripiprazole has been approved by the US Food and Drug Administration (FDA) for the treatment of schizophrenia. It is rarely used outside the United States. Aripiprazole lauroxil is a pro-drug formulated to be administered at monthly, 6-weekly or two-monthly intervals by intramuscular injection into the deltoid or gluteal muscle, depending on the dose.[8,9] It is available as four strengths: 441mg, 662mg, 882mg and 1064mg doses to deliver 300mg, 450mg, 600mg and 724mg of aripiprazole, respectively (see sections on depot pharmacokinetics and new long-acting injections in this chapter). There is also a special initiation formulation (Aristada Initio), which provides effective blood levels within 4 days of injection without oral supplemention.[10]

References

1. Shirley M, et al. Aripiprazole (ABILIFY MAINTENA®): a review of its use as maintenance treatment for adult patients with schizophrenia. *Drugs* 2014; **74**:1097–1110.

2. US Food and Drug Administration. Highlights of Prescribing Information. Abilify Maintena (aripiprazole) for extended-release suspension for intramuscular use. 2020; https://www.accessdata.fda.gov/drugsatfda_docs/label/2020/202971s013lbl.pdf.

3. Otsuka Pharmaceuticals (UK) Ltd. Summary of Product Characteristics. Abilify Maintena 400 mg powder and solvent for prolonged-release suspension for injection. 2020; https://www.medicines.org.uk/emc/product/7965/smpc.

4. Mallikaarjun S, et al. Pharmacokinetics, tolerability and safety of aripiprazole once-monthly in adult schizophrenia: an open-label, parallel-arm, multiple-dose study. *Schizophr Res* 2013; **150**:281–288.

5. Wang Y, et al. The two-injection start of aripiprazole once-monthly provides rapid attainment of therapeutic concentration without the need for 14 day oral Neuropsychopharmacology (ECNP) Congress, 12–15 September 2020, Virtual.

6. Kane JM, et al. Aripiprazole intramuscular depot as maintenance treatment in patients with schizophrenia: a 52-week, multicenter, randomized, double-blind, placebo-controlled study. *J Clin Psychiatry* 2012; **73**:617–624.

7. Potkin SG, et al. Safety and tolerability of once monthly aripiprazole treatment initiation in adults with schizophrenia stabilized on selected atypical oral antipsychotics other than aripiprazole. *Curr Med Res Opin* 2013; **29**:1241–1251.

8. Hard ML, et al. Aripiprazole lauroxil: pharmacokinetic profile of this long-acting injectable antipsychotic in persons with schizophrenia. *J Clin Psychopharmacol* 2017; **37**:289–295.

9. Turncliff R, et al. Relative bioavailability and safety of aripiprazole lauroxil, a novel once-monthly, long-acting injectable atypical antipsychotic, following deltoid and gluteal administration in adult subjects with schizophrenia. *Schizophr Res* 2014; **159**:404–410.

10. Ehret MJ, et al. Aripiprazole Lauroxil NanoCrystal® Dispersion Technology (Aristada Initio®). *Clin Schizophr Relat Psychoses* 2018; **12**:92–96.

Olanzapine long-acting injection

Like all esters, olanzapine pamoate (embonate, in some countries) is very poorly water soluble. An aqueous suspension of olanzapine pamoate, when injected intramuscularly, affords both prompt and sustained release of olanzapine. Peak plasma levels are seen within a week of injection (in most people within 2–4 days[1]), and efficacy can be demonstrated after only three days.[2] Only gluteal injection is licensed; deltoid injection is less effective.[3] Olanzapine LAI is effective when given every four weeks, with two weekly administration only required when the highest dose is prescribed. Half-life is around 30 days.[1] It has not been compared with other long-acting injections in RCTs, but naturalistic data suggest similar effectiveness to paliperidone LAI.[4,5] Loading doses are recommended in some dose regimens (see Table 1.5). Formal labelling/SmPC suggests that patients be given oral olanzapine to assess response and tolerability. This rarely happens in practice but is strongly recommended. Oral supplementation after the first depot injection is not necessary.

Table 1.5 Dosing schedules

Oral olanzapine equivalent	Loading dose	Maintenance dose (given 8 weeks after the first dose)
10mg/day	210mg every 2 weeks or 405mg every 4 weeks	300mg/4 weeks (or 150mg every 2 weeks)
15mg/day	300mg every 2 weeks	405mg/4 weeks (or 210mg every 2 weeks)
20mg/day	None – give 300mg every 2 weeks	300mg every 2 weeks

Switching

Direct switching to olanzapine LAI, ideally following an oral trial, is usually possible. So, when switching from another LAI (but not risperidone), olanzapine oral or LAI can be started on the day the last LAI was due. Likewise, for switching from oral treatment – a direct switch is possible, but prior antipsychotics are probably best reduced slowly after starting olanzapine (either oral or LAI). When switching from risperidone RLAI, olanzapine should be started, we suggest, two weeks after the last injection was due (peak risperidone plasma levels can be expected 4–6 weeks after the last injection).

Post-injection syndrome

Post-injection syndrome occurs when olanzapine pamoate is inadvertently exposed to high blood volumes (probably via accidental intravasation[6]). Olanzapine plasma levels may reach 600mcg/L and delirium and somnolence result.[7] The incidence of post-injection syndrome is less than 0.1% of injections; almost all reactions (86%) occur within one hour of injection.[8] One study suggested an incidence of 0.044% of injections (less than 1 in 2000) with 91% of reactions being apparent within one hour.[9] There are very rare reports of events occurring after three hours, including one case where the reaction occurred 12 hours post injection.[10]

In most countries, olanzapine LAI may only be given in health care facilities under supervision, and patients need to be kept under observation for three hours after the injection is given. Given the tiny number of cases appearing only after two hours, a good case can be made for shortening the observation period to two hours (as is the situation in New Zealand[11] and some other countries). Shorter monitoring periods have been suggested during the COVID-19 pandemic.[12] However, it is worth emphasising that post-injection syndrome may occur at any time, even after multiple uses in the same patient (that is to say, prior safe use of olanzapine LAI does not imply low risk of post-injection syndrome[13]).

In the EU, the exact wording of the SmPC[14] is as follows:

After each injection, patients should be observed in a healthcare facility by appropriately qualified personnel for at least 3 hours for signs and symptoms consistent with olanzapine overdose.

Immediately prior to leaving the healthcare facility, it should be confirmed that the patient is alert, oriented, and absent of any signs and symptoms of overdose. If an overdose is suspected, close medical supervision and monitoring should continue until examination indicates that signs and symptoms have resolved. The 3-hour observation period should be extended as clinically appropriate for patients who exhibit any signs or symptoms consistent with olanzapine overdose.

For the remainder of the day after injection, patients should be advised to be vigilant for signs and symptoms of overdose secondary to post-injection adverse reactions, be able to obtain assistance if needed, and should not drive or operate machinery.

This monitoring requirement has undoubtedly adversely affected the popularity of olanzapine LAI. Interestingly, some patients continue treatment even after an episode of post-injection syndrome.[15]

No patient or medical factor has been identified which might predict post-injection syndrome[7] except that those experiencing the syndrome are more likely to have previously had an injection-site related adverse effect.[16] Male gender and higher doses have also been suggested to be risk factors for post-injection syndrome (the study examined 46 events occurring in 103,505 injections).[9]

References

1. Heres S, et al. Pharmacokinetics of olanzapine long-acting injection: the clinical perspective. *Int Clin Psychopharmacol* 2014; 29:299–312.

2. Lauriello J, et al. An 8-week, double-blind, randomized, placebo-controlled study of olanzapine long-acting injection in acutely ill patients with schizophrenia. *J Clin Psychiatry* 2008; 69:790–799.

3. Mitchell M, et al. Single- and multiple-dose pharmacokinetic, safety, and tolerability profiles of olanzapine long-acting injection: an open-label, multicenter, nonrandomized study in patients with schizophrenia. *Clin Ther* 2013; 35:1890–1908.

4. Denee TR, et al. Treatment continuation and treatment characteristics of four long acting antipsychotic medications (Paliperidone Palmitate, Risperidone Microspheres, Olanzapine Pamoate and Haloperidol Decanoate) in The Netherlands. *Value Health* 2015; 18:A407.

5. Taipale H, et al. Comparative effectiveness of antipsychotic drugs for rehospitalization in schizophrenia-a nationwide study with 20-year follow-up. *Schizophr Bull* 2017; 44:1381–1387.

6. Luedecke D, et al. Post-injection delirium/sedation syndrome in patients treated with olanzapine pamoate: mechanism, incidence, and management. *CNS Drugs* 2015; 29:41–46.

7. McDonnell DP, et al. Post-injection delirium/sedation syndrome in patients with schizophrenia treated with olanzapine long-acting injection, II: investigations of mechanism. *BMC Psychiatry* 2010; 10:45.

8. Bushes CJ, et al. Olanzapine long-acting injection: review of first experiences of post-injection delirium/sedation syndrome in routine clinical practice. *BMC Psychiatry* 2015; 15:65.

9. Meyers KJ, et al. Postinjection delirium/sedation syndrome in patients with schizophrenia receiving olanzapine long-acting injection: results from a large observational study. *B J Psych Open* 2017; 3:186–192.

10. Garg S, et al. Delayed onset postinjection delirium/sedation syndrome associated with olanzapine pamoate: a case report. *J Clin Psychopharmacol* 2019; 39:523–524.

11. Eli Lilly and Company (NZ) Limited. ZYPREXA RELPREVV® (olanzapine pamoate monohydrate). 2019; https://www.medsafe.govt.nz/Consumers/cmi/z/zyprexarelprevvinj.pdf.

12. Siskind D, et al. Monitoring for post-injection delirium/sedation syndrome with long-acting olanzapine during the COVID-19 pandemic. *Aust N Z J Psychiatry* 2020; 54:759–761.

13. Venkatesan V, et al. Postinjection delirium/sedation syndrome after 31st long-acting olanzapine depot injection. *Clin Neuropharmacol* 2019; 42:64–65.

14. Eli Lilly and Company Limited. Summary of Product Characteristics. ZYPADHERA 210 mg powder and solvent for prolonged release suspension for injection. 2020; https://www.medicines.org.uk/emc/product/6429.

15. Anand E, et al. A 6-year open-label study of the efficacy and safety of olanzapine long-acting injection in patients with schizophrenia: a post hoc analysis based on the European label recommendation. *Neuropsychiatr Dis Treat* 2015; 11:1349–1357.

16. Atkins S, et al. A pooled analysis of injection site-related adverse events in patients with schizophrenia treated with olanzapine long-acting injection. *BMC Psychiatry* 2014; 14:7.

Paliperidone palmitate long-acting injection

Paliperidone (9-hydroxyrisperidone) is the major active metabolite of risperidone. Paliperidone palmitate is the ester prodrug of paliperidone available as a monthly and a 3-monthly long-acting injection. The ester is hydrolysed by esterases in the muscle to paliperidone and which is then absorbed into the systemic circulation.[1]

Paliperidone LAI 1-monthly

After the recommended initial loading dose, active paliperidone plasma levels are seen within a few days, and so co-administration of oral paliperidone or risperidone during initiation is not required from a pharmacokinetic viewpoint.[2] Dosing consists of two initiation doses (deltoid) followed by monthly maintenance doses (deltoid or gluteal). After administration of a single IM dose to the deltoid muscle, on average 28% higher peak concentration is observed compared with IM injection to the gluteal muscle.[2] Thus, the two deltoid muscle injections on days 1 and 8 help to quickly attain therapeutic drug concentration (Table 1.6). Improvement in psychotic symptoms has been observed as early as day 4.[2]

Table 1.6 Paliperidone dose and administration information[2]

	Dose	Route
Initiation		
Day 1	150mg IM	Deltoid only
Day 8 (± 4 days)	100mg IM	Deltoid only
Maintenance		
Every month (± 7 days) thereafter	50–150mg IM*	Deltoid or Gluteal**

*The maintenance dose is perhaps best judged by consideration of what might be a suitable dose of oral risperidone and then giving paliperidone palmitate in an equivalent dose (see Table 1.7). Pre-treatment with oral risperidone is helpful in establishing efficacy and tolerability of a given dose.
**Continuation with deltoid injections for the first 6 months may be considered in some patients who switch from higher doses of oral paliperidone or risperidone.[2]

The second initiation dose may be given four days before or after day 8 (after the first initiation dose on day one).[2] The manufacturer recommends that patients may be given maintenance doses up to 7 days before or after the monthly time point.[2] This flexibility should help minimise the number of missed doses. See manufacturer's information for full recommendations regarding missed doses.[2]

Points to note

- No test dose is required for paliperidone palmitate (but patients should (ideally) be currently stabilised on or have previously responded to oral paliperidone or risperidone).
- The median time to maximum plasma concentrations T_{max} is 13 days.[2]
- Patients receiving fewer than 12 injections a year have an increased risk of relapse – correct dosing is critical to the effectiveness of paliperidone monthly.[3,4]

Table 1.7 Approximate dose equivalence[2,5]

Risperidone oral (mg/day) (bioavailability = 70%)[6]	Paliperidone oral (mg/day) (bioavailability = 28%)[7]	Risperidone LAI (Consta) (mg/2 week)	Paliperidone palmitate (mg/monthly) (bioavailability = 100%)[2]
2	4	25	50
3	6	37.5	75
4	9	50	100
6	12	-	150

Paliperidone LAI has been compared with haloperidol depot given in a loading dose schedule matching that of paliperidone.[8] The two formulations were equally effective in preventing relapse, but paliperidone increased prolactin to a greater extent and caused more weight gain. Haloperidol caused more akathisia, more acute movement disorder and there was a trend for a higher incidence of tardive dyskinesia. The average dose of haloperidol was around 75mg a month; a dose rarely used in practice.

There are two studies comparing monthly paliperidone LAI with aripiprazole LAI. The first was a randomised trial that found aripiprazole monthly injection superior in the improvement of quality of life in short term, though the aripiprazole group included more younger patients.[9] The second study compared the two LAIs in patients with psychosis and comorbid substance use disorder (SUD). Improvement in quality of life and reduced substance cravings was seen with both LAIs though aripiprazole fared better. However, there was no clear clinically meaningful superiority for aripiprazole over paliperidone in either of these studies.[10]

Paliperidone LAI 3-monthly

Paliperidone LAI 3-monthly is indicated for patients who are clinically stable on paliperidone LAI 1-monthly (preferably for four months or more) and do not require dose adjustment.[11] It is recommended that the last two doses of the monthly paliperidone remain unchanged before switching to the 3-monthly in order to be certain of the maintenance dose required.[1]

Paliperidone LAI 3-monthly is generally well-tolerated, with a tolerability profile similar to the 1-monthly preparation[12-14] and is non-inferior to paliperidone 1-monthly in terms of relapse rate.[14] In an analysis of predictors for remission, global improvement in the CG I-S during monthly paliperidone increased likelihood of remission after switch to 3-monthly paliperidone.[15]

From a patient's perspective, advantages included less frequent injections and less focus on illness with few disadvantages reported in a qualitative study. The switch did not influence the frequency nor the content of their interaction with health care professionals.[16] Contact with patients should not be reduced because there are fewer antipsychotic administrations.

Table 1.8 Switching to paliperidone palmitate 1-monthly LAI

Switching from	Recommended method of switching	Comments
No treatment	Give the two initiation doses: 150mg IM deltoid on day 1 and 100mg IM deltoid on day 8 Maintenance dose starts 1 month later	The manufacturer recommends a dose of 75mg monthly for the general adult population.[17] This is approximately equivalent to 3mg/day oral risperidone. (see Table 1.7). In practice, the modal dose is 100mg/month[18] Maintenance dose adjustments should be made monthly. However, the full effect of the dose adjustment may not be apparent for several months[2]
Oral paliperidone/ risperidone	Give the two initiation doses followed by the maintenance dose (See Table 1.7 and prescribe equivalent dose)	Oral paliperidone/risperidone supplementation during initiation is not necessary
Oral antipsychotics	Reduce the dose of the oral antipsychotic over 1–2 weeks following the first injection of paliperidone. Give the two initiation doses followed by the maintenance dose	
Depot antipsychotic	Start paliperidone (at the maintenance dose) when the next injection is due. NB. No initiation doses are required	Doses of paliperidone palmitate IM are difficult to predict from the dose of FGA depots. The manufacturer recommends a dose of 75mg monthly for the general adult population but in practice 100mg and 150mg are more often prescribed.[18] If switching from risperidone LAI see Table 1.7 and prescribe equivalent dose Maintenance dose adjustments should be made monthly. However, the full effect of the dose adjustment may not be apparent for several months[2]
Antipsychotic polypharmacy with depot	Start paliperidone (at the maintenance dose) when the next injection is due. NB. No initiation doses are required Reduce the dose of the oral antipsychotic over 1–2 weeks following the first injection of paliperidone	Aim to treat the patient with paliperidone palmitate IM as the sole antipsychotic. The maintenance dose should be governed as far as possible by the total dose of oral and injectable antipsychotic (see dose equivalence table in this chapter)

When initiating paliperidone LAI 3-monthly give the first dose in place of the next scheduled dose of paliperidone LAI 1-monthly (±7 days). The dose of paliperidone LAI 3-monthly should be based on the previous paliperidone LAI 1-monthly dose, see Table 1.9. Dose adjustments should not be necessary but may be made at 3-monthly intervals thereafter, however, the full response to the new dose may not be apparent for several months.[11]

The administration process is important for avoiding incomplete administration of the suspension. This requires shaking vigorously the prefilled syringe with the cap and

CHAPTER 1

a loose wrist, in a vertical motion for at least 15 seconds to ensure an evenly distributed suspension.[11]

Table 1.9 Dosing of paliperidone LAI 3-monthly

Dose of paliperidone LAI 1-monthly	Dose of paliperidone LAI 3-monthly
50mg	175mg
75mg	263mg
100mg	350mg
150mg	525mg

See manufacturer's information for full information in missed doses.

References

1. Lopez A, et al. Role of paliperidone palmitate 3-monthly in the management of schizophrenia: insights from clinical practice. *Neuropsychiatr Dis Treat* 2019; **15**:449–456.
2. Janssen-Cilag Ltd. Summary of Product Characteristics. Xeplion 25 mg, 50 mg, 75 mg, 100 mg, and 150 mg prolonged-release suspension for injection. 2020; https://www.medicines.org.uk/emc/medicine/31329.
3. Pappa S, et al. Partial compliance with long-acting paliperidone palmitate and impact on hospitalization: a 6-year mirror-image study. *Ther Adv Psychopharmacol* 2020; **10**:2045125320924789.
4. Laing E, et al. Relapse and frequency of injection of monthly paliperidone palmitate-A retrospective case-control study. *Eur Psychiatry* 2021; **64**:e11.
5. Russu A, et al. Maintenance dose conversion between oral risperidone and paliperidone palmitate 1 month: practical guidance based on pharmacokinetic simulations. *Int J Clin Pract* 2018; **72**:e13089.
6. Janssen-Cilag Limited. Summary of product characteristics. risperdal 2mg film-coated tablets. 2020; https://www.medicines.org.uk/emc/product/6858/smpc.
7. Janssen-Cilag Limited. Summary of product characteristics. Invega 3 mg prolonged-release tablets. 2020; https://www.medicines.org.uk/emc/product/6816.
8. McEvoy JP, et al. Effectiveness of paliperidone palmitate vs haloperidol decanoate for maintenance treatment of schizophrenia: a randomized clinical trial. *JAMA* 2014; **311**:1978–1987.
9. Naber D, et al. Qualify: a randomized head-to-head study of aripiprazole once-monthly and paliperidone palmitate in the treatment of schizophrenia. *Schizophr Res* 2015; **168**:498–504.
10. Cuomo I, et al. Head-to-head comparison of 1-year aripiprazole long-acting injectable (LAI) versus paliperidone LAI in comorbid psychosis and substance use disorder: impact on clinical status, substance craving, and quality of life. *Neuropsychiatr Dis Treat* 2018; **14**:1645–1656.
11. Janssen-Cilag Limited. Summary of Product Characteristics. TREVICTA 175mg, 263mg, 350mg, 525mg prolonged release suspension for injection. 2021; https://www.medicines.org.uk/emc/medicine/32050.
12. Lamb YN, et al. Paliperidone palmitate intramuscular 3-monthly formulation: a review in schizophrenia. *Drugs* 2016; **76**:1559–1566.
13. Ravenstijn P, et al. Pharmacokinetics, safety, and tolerability of paliperidone palmitate 3-month formulation in patients with schizophrenia: a phase-1, single-dose, randomized, open-label study. *J Clin Pharmacol* 2016; **56**:330–339.
14. Mathews M, et al. Clinical relevance of paliperidone palmitate 3-monthly in treating schizophrenia. *Neuropsychiatr Dis Treat* 2019; **15**:1365–1379.
15. Nash AI, et al. Predictors of achieving remission in schizophrenia patients treated with paliperidone palmitate 3-month formulation. *Neuropsychiatr Dis Treat* 2019; **15**:731–737.
16. Rise MB, et al. Patients' perspectives on three-monthly administration of antipsychotic treatment with paliperidone palmitate – a qualitative interview study. *Nord J Psychiatry* 2020: [Epub ahead of print].
17. Janssen Pharmaceutical Companies. Highlights of Prescribing Information. INVEGA SUSTENNA (paliperidone palmitate) extended-release injectable suspension, for intramuscular use. 2017; http://www.janssenlabels.com/package-insert/product-monograph/prescribing-information/INVEGA+SUSTENNA-pi.pdf.
18. Taylor DM, et al. Paliperidone palmitate: factors predicting continuation with treatment at 2 years. *Eur Neuropsychopharmacol* 2016; **26**:2011–2017.

Risperidone long-acting injection

Risperidone was the first FGA to be made available as a depot, or long-acting, injectable formulation. Doses of 25–50mg every 2 weeks appear to be as effective as oral doses of 2–6mg/day.[1] The long-acting injection also seems to be well tolerated – fewer than 10% of patients experienced EPS, and fewer than 6% withdrew from a long-term trial because of adverse effects.[2] Oral risperidone increases prolactin,[3] as does RLAI,[4] but levels appear to reduce somewhat following a switch from oral to injectable risperidone.[5-7] Rates of tardive dyskinesia are said to be low.[8] There are no direct comparisons with standard depots using randomised controlled designs, but comparisons from observational studies are available and results have been mixed. Switching from FGA depots in stable patients to RLAI has been shown to be less successful than remaining on the FGA depot;[9] in contrast, discontinuation rates were lower with RLAI when compared with FGAs.[10]

Uncertainty remains over the dose–response relationship for RLAI. Studies randomising subjects to different fixed doses of RLAI show no differences in response according to dose.[11] One randomised, fixed-dose yearlong study suggested better outcome for 50mg every two weeks than with 25mg, although no observed difference reached statistical significance.[12] Naturalistic studies indicate doses higher than 25mg/2 weeks are frequently used.[13,14] One study suggested higher doses were associated with better outcome.[15,16]

Plasma levels afforded by 25mg/2 weeks seem to be similar to, or even lower than, levels provided by 2mg/day oral risperidone.[17,18] One study of TDM samples found 9.5% of plasma samples from people apparently receiving risperidone LAI contained no risperidone or 9OH-risperidone.[19] Striatal dopamine D_2 occupancies are low (perhaps subtherapeutic) in people receiving 25mg/2 weeks.[20,21] So, although fixed-dose studies have not revealed clear advantages for doses above 25mg/2 weeks other indicators cast doubt on the assumption that 25mg/2 weeks will be adequate for all or even most patients. While this conundrum remains unresolved the need for careful dose titration becomes of great importance. This is perhaps most efficiently achieved by establishing the required dose of oral risperidone and converting this dose into the equivalent injection dose. Trials have clearly established that switching from 2mg oral to 25mg injection and 4mg oral to 50mg injection is usually successful[2,22,23] (switching from 4mg/day to 25mg/2 week increases the risk of relapse[24]). There remains a question over the equivalent dose for 6mg oral: in theory, patients should be switched to 75mg injection, but this dose showed no advantage over lower doses in clinical trials and is in any case above the licensed maximum dose. Nevertheless, an observational study reported successful outcomes in patients treated with doses in excess of 75mg/2 weeks (range 75–200mg) with continuation rates of 95% after 3 years.[25] Paliperidone palmitate 150mg a month is equivalent to oral risperidone 6mg/day. In fact, for many reasons, paliperidone palmitate (9-hydroxyrisperidone) may be preferred to risperidone injection (as Risperdal Consta): it acts acutely, can be given monthly, does not require cold storage and has a wider, more useful dose range (see the section on paliperidone LAI).

Risperidone long-acting injection differs importantly from other depots, and the following should be noted:

- Risperidone depot is not an esterified form of the parent drug. It contains risperidone coated in polymer to form microspheres. These microspheres have to be suspended in an aqueous base immediately before use.
- The injection must be stored in a fridge (consider the practicalities for community staff).
- It is available in doses of 25mg, 37.5mg and 50mg. The whole vial must be used (because of the nature of the suspension). This means that there is limited flexibility in dosing.
- A test dose is not required or sensible. (Testing tolerability with oral risperidone is desirable but not always practical.)
- It takes 3–4 weeks for the first injection to produce therapeutic plasma levels. Patients must be maintained on a full dose of their previous antipsychotic for at least 3 weeks after the administration of the first risperidone injection. Oral antipsychotic cover is sometimes required for longer (6–8 weeks). If the patient is not already receiving an oral antipsychotic, oral risperidone should be prescribed. (See Table 1.10 for advice on switching from depots.) **Patients who refuse oral treatment and are acutely ill should not be given RLAI because of the long delay in drug release.**
- Risperidone depot must be administered every 2 weeks. The Product Licence does not allow longer intervals between doses. There is little flexibility to negotiate with patients about the frequency of administration, although monthly injections may be effective.[26]
- The most effective way of predicting response to RLAI is to establish dose and response with oral risperidone.
- Risperidone injection is not considered suitable for patients with treatment refractory schizophrenia, although there are studies showing positive effects.[27,28]

For guidance on switching to risperidone long-acting injection, see Table 1.10.

Table 1.10 Switching to risperidone long-acting injection (RLAI)

Switching from	Recommended method of switching	Comments
No treatment (new patient or recently non-compliant)	Start risperidone oral at 2mg/day and titrate to effective dose. If tolerated, prescribe equivalent dose of RLAI Continue with oral risperidone for at least 3 weeks then taper over 1–2 weeks. Be prepared to continue oral risperidone for longer	Use oral risperidone before giving injection to assure good tolerability Those stabilised on 2mg/day start on 25mg/2 weeks Those on higher doses, start on 37.5mg/2 weeks and be prepared to use 50mg/2 weeks (Manufacturer advice may differ from this – our guidance is based on numerous studies of dose-related outcome and on comparative plasma levels)

Table 1.10 (Continued)

Switching from	Recommended method of switching	Comments
Oral risperidone	Prescribe equivalent dose of RLAI	See above
Oral antipsychotics (not risperidone)	**Either:** a. Switch to oral risperidone and titrate to effective dose. If tolerated, prescribe equivalent dose of RLAI	Dose assessment is difficult in those switching from another antipsychotic. Broadly speaking, those on low oral doses should be switched to 25mg/2 weeks
	Continue with oral risperidone for at least 3 weeks then taper over 1–2 weeks. Be prepared to continue oral risperidone for longer	'Low' in this context means towards the lower end of the licensed dose range or around the minimum dose known to be effective
	Or: b. Give RLAI and then slowly discontinue oral antipsychotics after 3–4 weeks. Be prepared to continue oral antipsychotics for longer	Those on higher oral doses should receive 37.5mg or 50mg every two weeks. The continued need for oral antipsychotics after 3–4 weeks may indicate that higher doses of RLAI are required
Depot antipsychotic	Give RLAI one week **before** the last depot injection is given	Dose of RLAI difficult to predict. For those on low doses (see above) start at 25mg/2 weeks and then adjust as necessary
		Start RLAI at 37.5mg/2 weeks in those previously maintained on doses in the middle or upper range of licensed doses. Be prepared to increase to 50mg/2 weeks
Antipsychotic polypharmacy with depot	Give RLAI 1 week before the last depot injection is given Slowly taper oral antipsychotics 3–4 weeks later. Be prepared to continue oral antipsychotics for longer	Aim to treat patient with RLAI as the sole antipsychotic. As before, RLAI dose should be dictated, as far as is possible, by the total dose of oral and injectable antipsychotic

References

1. Chue P, et al. Comparative efficacy and safety of long-acting risperidone and risperidone oral tablets. *Eur Neuropsychopharmacol* 2005; 15:111–117.
2. Fleischhacker WW, et al. Treatment of schizophrenia with long-acting injectable risperidone: a 12-month open-label trial of the first long-acting second-generation antipsychotic. *J Clin Psychiatry* 2003; 64:1250–1257.
3. Kleinberg DL, et al. Prolactin levels and adverse events in patients treated with risperidone. *J Clin Psychopharmacol* 1999; 19:57–61.
4. Fu DJ, et al. Paliperidone palmitate versus oral risperidone and risperidone long-acting injection in patients with recently diagnosed schizophrenia: a tolerability and efficacy comparison. *Int Clin Psychopharmacol* 2014; 29:45–55.
5. Bai YM, et al. A comparative efficacy and safety study of long-acting risperidone injection and risperidone oral tablets among hospitalized patients: 12-week randomized, single-blind study. *Pharmacopsychiatry* 2006; 39:135–141.
6. Bai YM, et al. Pharmacokinetics study for hyperprolactinemia among schizophrenics switched from risperidone to risperidone long-acting injection. *J Clin Psychopharmacol* 2007; 27:306–308.
7. Peng PW, et al. The disparity of pharmacokinetics and prolactin study for risperidone long-acting injection. *J Clin Psychopharmacol* 2008; 28:726–727.
8. Gharabawi GM, et al. An assessment of emergent tardive dyskinesia and existing dyskinesia in patients receiving long-acting, injectable risperidone: results from a long-term study. *Schizophr Res* 2005; 77:129–139.
9. Covell NH, et al. Effectiveness of switching from long-acting injectable fluphenazine or haloperidol decanoate to long-acting injectable risperidone microspheres: an open-label, randomized controlled trial. *J Clin Psychiatry* 2012; 73:669–675.
10. Suzuki H, et al. Comparison of treatment retention between risperidone long-acting injection and first-generation long-acting injections in patients with schizophrenia for 5 years. *J Clin Psychopharmacol* 2016; 36:405–406.

11. Kane JM, et al. Long-acting injectable risperidone: efficacy and safety of the first long-acting atypical antipsychotic. *Am J Psychiatry* 2003; 160:1125–1132.

12. Simpson GM, et al. A 1-year double-blind study of 2 doses of long-acting risperidone in stable patients with schizophrenia or schizoaffective disorder. *J Clin Psychiatry* 2006; 67:1194–1203.

13. Turner M, et al. Long-acting injectable risperidone: safety and efficacy in stable patients switched from conventional depot antipsychotics. *Int Clin Psychopharmacol* 2004; 19:241–249.

14. Taylor DM, et al. Early clinical experience with risperidone long-acting injection: a prospective, 6-month follow-up of 100 patients. *J Clin Psychiatry* 2004; 65:1076–1083.

15. Taylor DM, et al. Prospective 6-month follow-up of patients prescribed risperidone long-acting injection: factors predicting favourable outcome. *Int J Neuropsychopharmacol* 2006; 9:685–694.

16. Taylor DM, et al. Risperidone long-acting injection: a prospective 3-year analysis of its use in clinical practice. *J Clin Psychiatry* 2009; 70:196–200.

17. Nesvag R, et al. Serum concentrations of risperidone and 9-OH risperidone following intramuscular injection of long-acting risperidone compared with oral risperidone medication. *Acta Psychiatr Scand* 2006; 114:21–26.

18. Castberg I, et al. Serum concentrations of risperidone and 9-hydroxyrisperidone after administration of the long-acting injectable form of risperidone: evidence from a routine therapeutic drug monitoring service. *Ther Drug Monit* 2005; 27:103–106.

19. Bowskill SV, et al. Risperidone and total 9-hydroxyrisperidone in relation to prescribed dose and other factors: data from a therapeutic drug monitoring service, 2002–2010. *Ther Drug Monit* 2012; 34:349–355.

20. Gefvert O, et al. Pharmacokinetics and D2 receptor occupancy of long-acting injectable risperidone (Risperdal Consta™) in patients with schizophrenia. *Int J Neuropsychopharmacol* 2005; 8:27–36.

21. Remington G, et al. A PET study evaluating dopamine D2 receptor occupancy for long-acting injectable risperidone. *Am J Psychiatry* 2006; 163:396–401.

22. Lasser RA, et al. Clinical improvement in 336 stable chronically psychotic patients changed from oral to long-acting risperidone: a 12-month open trial. *Int J Neuropsychopharmacol* 2005; 8:427–438.

23. Lauriello J, et al. Long-acting risperidone vs. placebo in the treatment of hospital inpatients with schizophrenia. *Schizophr Res* 2005; 72:249–258.

24. Bai YM, et al. Equivalent switching dose from oral risperidone to risperidone long-acting injection: a 48-week randomized, prospective, single-blind pharmacokinetic study. *J Clin Psychiatry* 2007; 68:1218–1225.

25. Fernandez-Miranda JJ, et al. Effectiveness, good tolerability, and high compliance of doses of risperidone long-acting injectable higher than 75 mg in people with severe schizophrenia: a 3-year follow-up. *J Clin Psychopharmacol* 2015; 35:630–634.

26. Uchida H, et al. Monthly administration of long-acting injectable risperidone and striatal dopamine D2 receptor occupancy for the management of schizophrenia. *J Clin Psychiatry* 2008; 69:1281–1286.

27. Meltzer HY, et al. A six month randomized controlled trial of long acting injectable risperidone 50 and 100mg in treatment resistant schizophrenia. *Schizophr Res* 2014; 154:14–22.

28. Kimura H, et al. Risperidone long-acting injectable in the treatment of treatment-resistant schizophrenia with dopamine supersensitivity psychosis: results of a 2-year prospective study, including an additional 1-year follow-up. *J Psychopharmacology* 2016; 30:795–802.

Risperidone subcutaneous long-acting injection

RBP-7000 or Perseris is a monthly subcutaneous LAI that is available in 90mg and 120mg dosage forms. The lower dose is equivalent to 3mg day oral risperidone and the higher dose 4mg a day.[1]

The injection is acutely effective at both licensed doses, without the need for oral pre-treatment or oral supplementation.[2,3] The 120mg dose was numerically more effective than 90mg at all time points. In the longer term, monthly doses of 120mg are effective in maintaining or improving symptom scale scores.[4] It has clear theoretical advantages over Risperdal Consta, being rapidly active, not requiring oral supplementation and, as a subcutaneous injection, being more acceptable to patients[5] with a low risk of painful injection.[6] One disadvantage is that the injection procedure has several steps and both the complexity of preparation and subcutaneous administration are new to psychiatry.[6] A second potential disadvantage is that doses above the equivalent of 4mg a day may not be given, a fact that may limit clinical utility.[7] (In respect to C_{max}, C_{min} and C_{ave} 3mg/day = 90mg/28 days; and 4mg/day = 120mg/28 days[1,8]). Nonetheless, dopamine receptor occupancies are broadly consistent with clinical efficacy: at steady state, 90mg gives occupancies ranging from approximately 40–80%; 120mg, 60–85%.[9]

Approximate equivalent doses (mg)[10]

Risperidone oral (daily)	Risperdal Consta (2-weekly)	Paliperidone palmitate (monthly)	RBP-7000 (monthly)
2	25	50	Not available*
3	37.5	75	90
4	50	100	120
6	Not available	150	Not available

*Laffont et al.[11] suggest 90mg is equivalent to 25mg/2-weekly Risperdal Consta

References

1. US Food and Drug Administration. Cross-discipline team leader review. RBP-7000 (risperidone-ATRIGEL) 2018; https://www.accessdata.fda.gov/drugsatfda_docs/nda/2018/210655Orig1s000SumR.pdf.

2. Nasser AF, et al. Efficacy, safety, and tolerability of RBP-7000 once-monthly risperidone for the treatment of acute schizophrenia: an 8-week, randomized, double-blind, placebo-controlled, multicenter phase 3 study. *J Clin Psychopharmacol* 2016; **36**:130–140.

3. Le Moigne A, et al. Reanalysis of a phase 3 trial of a monthly extended-release risperidone injection for the treatment of acute schizophrenia. *J Clin Psychopharmacol* 2021; **41**:76–77.

4. Andorn A, et al. Monthly extended-release risperidone (RBP-7000) in the treatment of schizophrenia: results from the phase 3 program. *J Clin Psychopharmacol* 2019; **39**:428–433.

5. Tchobaniouk LV, et al. Once-monthly subcutaneously administered risperidone in the treatment of schizophrenia: patient considerations. *Patient Prefer Adherence* 2019; **13**:2233–2241.

6. Citrome L. Sustained-release risperidone via subcutaneous injection: a systematic review of RBP-7000 (PERSERIS(™)) for the treatment of schizophrenia. *Clin Schizophr Relat Psychoses* 2018; **12**:130–141.

7. Clark I, et al. Newer formulations of risperidone: role in the management of psychotic disorders. *CNS Drugs* 2020; **34**:841–852.

8. US Food and Drug Administration. Clinical pharmacology and biopharmaceutics review(s). Perseris 2018; https://www.accessdata.fda.gov/drugsatfda_docs/nda/2018/210655Orig1s000ClinPharmR.pdf.

9. Laffont CM, et al. Population pharmacokinetics and prediction of dopamine D2 receptor occupancy after multiple doses of RBP-7000, a new sustained-release formulation of risperidone, in schizophrenia patients on stable oral risperidone treatment. *Clin Pharmacokinet* 2014; **53**:533–543.

10. Karas A, et al. Perseris(TM): a new and long-acting, atypical antipsychotic drug-delivery system. *P & T* 2019; **44**:460–466.

11. Laffont CM, et al. Population pharmacokinetic modeling and simulation to guide dose selection for RBP-7000, a new sustained-release formulation of risperidone. *J Clin Pharmacol* 2015; **55**:93–103.

Newer long-acting injectable antipsychotic preparations

The following table provides brief details of some newer LAI antipsychotic formulations.

Drug	Trade name	Formulation	Dosing interval	Site(s) of administration	Dosing information	Pre-mixing required	Pre-treatment with oral therapy essential*	Pre-treatment with oral therapy desirable**	Regulatory status	Additional information
Aripiprazole lauroxil extended-release injectable	Aristada Initio	Nanocrystalline dispersion;[1] LinkeRx technology[2]	Single dose	Intra-muscular injection into the deltoid or gluteal muscle	675mg (IM dispersion = 459mg aripiprazole)[3]	No	Yes – but see additional information	Yes	FDA approved 2018[4]	Aristada initio, together with one 30mg dose of oral aripiprazole, is designed to only be given to initiate treatment with Aristada (see Aripiprazole LAI section in Chapter 1) and should not be used for repeated dosing.[5]
Paliperidone palmitate 6-month formulation	N/A	Micro-crystalline suspension	6-monthly	Intra-muscular injection	700mg/1000mg[6]	No	No	No – patients will already have received long-acting paliperidone	Phase 3 study underway[7]	Designed for patients stabilised on PP1M or PP3M[8]
Risperidone for sub-cutaneous injection (RBP-7000)	Perseris	Suspension, Co-polymer; ATRIGEL technology[3]	1-monthly	Abdominal sub-cutaneous injection only[9]	90mg/120mg	Yes	No[10]	Yes	FDA approved 2018[11]	Does not require loading doses or oral supplementation. Prior tolerability with oral risperidone should be established[9]

(Continued)

Drug	Trade name	Formulation	Dosing interval	Site(s) of administration	Dosing information	Pre-mixing required	Pre-treatment with oral therapy essential*	Pre-treatment with oral therapy desirable**	Regulatory status	Additional information
Risperidone extended release for SC injection (TV-46000)	N/A	Suspension	1- and 2- monthly[12]	Sub-cutaneous injection	2 dose regimens (TV-46000-A & TV-46000-B) being investigated[13]	No[12]	No[13]	Yes[13]	Phase 3 study in progress[13]	Phase 3 results are awaited in 2020[12]
Risperidone	Risperidone ISM or Doria	Suspension[14]	1-monthly[14]	Intra-muscular injection into the gluteal or deltoid muscle[15]	75mg/100mg	Yes	No[16]	Yes	Phase 3 study completed Awaiting EMA approval 2020[17]	Does not require loading doses or oral supplementation/3-day trial of oral risperidone (2mg/day) to check for hypersensitivity in risperidone naïve patients[18]

*LAI tested only in the presence of pre/post-treatment with oral therapy

**Best practice in order to establish efficacy and tolerability

References

1. Krogmann A, et al. Keeping up with the therapeutic advances in schizophrenia: a review of novel and emerging pharmacological entities. *CNS Spectr* 2019; 24:38–69.
2. Alkermes Inc. ARISTADA INITIO™ (aripiprazole lauroxil) extended-release injectable suspension [product monograph]. 2020; https://www.aristadacaresupport.com/downloadables/ARISTADA-INITIO-ARISTADA-Payer-Hospital-Monograph.pdf.
3. Correll CU, et al. Pharmacokinetic characteristics of long-acting injectable antipsychotics for schizophrenia: an overview. *CNS Drugs* 2021; 35:39–59.
4. Pharmaceutical Technology. Alkermes' Aristata Initio approved by FDA for schizophrenia. 2018; https://www.pharmaceutical-technology.com/news/aristada-initio-fda-approval-schizophrenia/:~:text=Alkermes'%20Aristada%20Initio%20approved%20by%20FDA%20for%20schizophrenia.,Aristada%20as%20a%20treatment%20for%20adults%20with%20schizophrenia.
5. U.S. Food & Drug Administration. Drug Approval Package: Aripiprazole lauroxil Nanocrystal Dispersion (AL-NCD). 2019; https://www.accessdata.fda.gov/drugsatfda_docs/nda/2018/209830Orig1s000TOC.cfm.
6. Janssen Research & Development LLC. A study of paliperidone palmitate 6-month formulation. 2020; https://www.centerwatch.com/clinical-trials/listings/160465/schizophrenia-study-paliperidone-palmitate-6-month.
7. ClinicalTrial.gov. A study of paliperidone palmitate 6-month formulation. 2020; https://clinicaltrials.gov/ct2/show/NCT04072575.
8. PRNewswire Press release. Janssen submits paliperidone palmitate 6-month (pp6m) supplemental new drug application to U.S. FDA for treatment of schizophrenia in adults. 2020; https://news.yahoo.com/janssen-submits-paliperidone-palmitate-6-120000670.html?guccounter=1&guce_referrer=aHR0cHM6Ly93d3cuYmluZy5jb20vvc2VhcmNoNoP3E9UGFsaXBlcmlkb25llK1BhbG1pdGF0ZSs2LU1vbnRoRoK0Zvcm11bGF0aW9uJnNyYz1JRS1TZWFyY2hCb3gmRk9STT1JRU5BRTI&guce_referrer_sig=AQAAAEjhHe6O8HxGLi1o0izgasDe15netPJG3l-MUedGGRDHFMtzWa9biyFopIhgzAbCx2sgWOaiFOxF2PLimzGos4vvuSfNDmbS77QWazTi8BXUH9RqzjgWHJsueeTuPPfH-q9OmxpAu-XiwbXTNe1WLVjbFmC7G39qbGtMKyLPH2UDD.
9. Indivior UK Limited. Highlights of prescribing information. Perseris (risperidone) for extended-release injectable suspension for subcutaneous use. 2019; http://www.indivior.com/wp-content/uploads/2018/07/FDA-Label-revised.pdf.
10. Tchobaniouk LV, et al. Once-monthly subcutaneously administered risperidone in the treatment of schizophrenia: patient considerations. *Patient Prefer Adherence* 2019; 13:2233–2241.
11. Indivior. FDA approves PERSERIS (risperidone) for extended-release injectable suspension for the treatment of schizophrenia in adults. 2018; http://indivior.com/wp-content/uploads/2018/07/PERSERIS-Press-Release-FINAL.pdf.
12. Medincell. Building a global pharma leader; through long-acting injectables. January 2019; https://invest.medincell.com/wp-content/uploads/2019/02/19-01-04-JPMprezvdef.pdf.
13. ClinicalTrial.gov. A study to evaluate the safety, tolerability, and effect of risperidone extended-release injectable suspension (TV-46000) for subcutaneous use as maintenance treatment in adult and adolescent patients with schizophrenia. 2020; https://clinicaltrials.gov/ct2/show/NCT03893825.
14. Carabias L, et al. A phase II study to evaluate the pharmacokinetics, safety, and tolerability of risperidone ISM multiple intramuscular injections once every 4 weeks in patients with schizophrenia. *Int Clin Psychopharmacol* 2017; 33:79–87.
15. ClinicalTrial.gov. Study to evaluate the efficacy and safety of risperidone ISM® in patients with acute schizophrenia: open label extension (PRISMA-3_OLE). 2020; https://clinicaltrials.gov/ct2/show/NCT03870880?term=risperidone+ISM&draw=2&rank=1.
16. Llaudo J, et al. Phase I, open-label, randomized, parallel study to evaluate the pharmacokinetics, safety, and tolerability of one intramuscular injection of risperidone ISM at different dose strengths in patients with schizophrenia or schizoaffective disorder (PRISMA-1). *Int Clin Psychopharmacol* 2016; 31:323–331.
17. Rovi. ROVI announces the commencement of the assessment process to obtain marketing authorisation for Doria® in the European Union. 2020; https://www.rovi.es/sites/default/files/Doria%20validation_Press%20release_0.pdf.
18. Correll CU, et al. Efficacy and safety of once-monthly risperidone ISM(®) in schizophrenic patients with an acute exacerbation. *NPJ Schizophr* 2020; 6:37.

Further Reading

Correll CU, et al. Pharmacokinetic characteristics of long-acting injectable antipsychotics for schizophrenia: an overview. *CNS Drugs* 2021; 35:39–59.

Penfluridol weekly

Penfluridol is a diphenylbutylpiperidine FGA, which remains available in some countries such as India and can be imported to other countries. It is similar in efficacy and tolerability to other FGAs.[1]

Penfluridol is unusual in having a very long plasma half-life – at least 60 hours.[2] After oral administration, peak levels are reached within 12 hours and drug can still be detected 168 hours after a single oral dose.[3] Its long duration of action seems to be a result of rapid distribution into fat tissue, which acts as a drug reservoir.[4] This property allows penfluridol to be used as a once-weekly oral therapy for supervised ingestion – an alternative to long-acting injectable antipsychotics.

Several trials have examined the use of once-weekly oral penfluridol, usually in doses ranging from 5mg to 160mg per week.[1] When given in this manner it is at least as effective as depot FGAs[5,6] and is better tolerated overall.[1] Although dose–response relationships remain unclear, a weekly dose of 30mg is adequately effective[7] and a dose of 120mg a day (i.e. a total of 840mg a week) has been used in at least one trial.[8]

Adverse effects include acute EPS, increased prolactin and tardive dyskinesia, as might be expected. It is usually not sedative. Like pimozide (another diphenylbutylpiperidine), penfluridol appears to prolong the QT interval.[9] Penfluridol is a cytotoxic agent which may have anticancer properties.[10]

Summary

- Penfluridol can be given orally once a week.
- Supervised weekly administration is at least as effective as long-acting injections.
- The usual dose is 20–40mg a week.
- Adverse effects are those common to FGAs and include QT prolongation.
- Sedation is minimal.

In practice, penfluridol is usually started at a dose of 20mg, and this dose is increased to a maximum of 40mg after assessment. Steady-state levels are effectively reached after 2–3 weeks. Monitoring includes investigations into renal and hepatic function, changes in cardiometabolic parameter such as lipids, blood glucose, echocardiogram, and general adverse effect screening.

References

1. Soares BG, et al. Penfluridol for schizophrenia. *Cochrane Database Syst Rev* 2006; CD002923.
2. Janssen PA, et al. The pharmacology of penfluridol (R 16341) a new potent and orally long-acting neuroleptic drug. *Eur J Pharmacol* 1970; 11:139–154.
3. Cooper SF, et al. Penfluridol steady-state kinetics in psychiatric patients. *Clin Pharmacol Ther* 1975; 18:325–329.
4. Migdalof BH, et al. Penfluridol: a neuroleptic drug designed for long duration of action. *Drug Metab Rev* 1979; 9:281–299.
5. Iqbal MJ, et al. A long term comparative trial of penfluridol and fluphenazine decanoate in schizophrenic outpatients. *J Clin Psychiatry* 1978; 39:375–379.
6. Quitkin F, et al. Long-acting oral vs injectable antipsychotic drugs in schizophrenics: a one-year double-blind comparison in multiple episode schizophrenics. *Arch Gen Psychiatry* 1978; 35:889–892.
7. Van Praag HM, et al. Controlled trial of penfluridol in acute psychosis. *Br Med J* 1971; 4:710–713.
8. Shopsin B, et al. Penfluridol: an open phase III study in acute newly admitted hospitalized schizophrenic patients. *Psychopharmacology* 1977; 55:157–164.
9. Bhattacharyya R, et al. Resurgence of penfluridol: merits and demerits. *East J Psychiatry* 2015; 18:23–29.
10. Ashraf-Uz-Zaman M, et al. Analogs of penfluridol as chemotherapeutic agents with reduced central nervous system activity. *Bioorg Med Chem Lett* 2018; 28:3652–3657.

Electroconvulsive therapy and psychosis

Evidence from prospective RCTs and retrospective studies suggests that ECT augmentation of antipsychotic medication can have a beneficial effect on persistent positive symptoms in schizophrenia, including medication-resistant schizophrenia.[1-7] However, there is a relative lack of data on long-term effectiveness and efficacy, cognitive deficits, and quality of life.

A Cochrane systematic review[8] assessed randomised controlled clinical trials that had compared ECT with placebo, sham ECT, non-pharmacological interventions, and antipsychotic medication for patients with schizophrenia, schizoaffective disorder or chronic mental disorder. Where ECT was compared with placebo or sham ECT, more people improved in the real ECT group, and there was a suggestion that real ECT resulted in fewer relapses in the short term and a greater likelihood of being discharged from hospital. The review concluded that ECT combined with continuing antipsychotic medication is a valid treatment option for schizophrenia, particularly when rapid global improvement and reduction of symptoms were desired, and where the illness has shown only a limited response to medication alone.

A naturalistic, mirror-image study (2002–2011) compared 2,074 people with schizophrenia on antipsychotic medication who had received ECT while inpatients with control patients prescribed continuing antipsychotic medication.[9] The rate of psychiatric hospitalisation over a one-year post-treatment period decreased in those treated with ECT, but not in the control patients. The effectiveness of ECT was more pronounced among those treated with clozapine or a medium to high antipsychotic dosage.

Treatment-refractory schizophrenia

The benefits and harms of adding ECT to standard care for people with treatment-resistant schizophrenia (TRS) were examined in a Cochrane systematic review.[6] The investigators were able to reach the limited conclusion that the moderate-quality RCT evidence that was available suggested a positive effect for ECT on medium-term clinical response. It was noted that evidence of better quality was required before a stronger conclusion could be made.

Several studies have focussed on ECT augmentation of antipsychotic medication for TRS.[1-3,10,11] For example, in a relatively small sample of patients with TRS characterised by 'dominant negative symptoms', ECT augmentation of a variety of antipsychotic medications produced a significant decrease in symptom severity.[12] A meta-analysis of RCTs[3] in TRS that had examined the efficacy of the combination of ECT and (non-clozapine) antipsychotic medication versus the same antipsychotic medication as monotherapy found that the combination proved to be superior in terms of symptom improvement, study-defined response and remission rate.

ECT augmentation of clozapine may be at least as effective as ECT augmentation of other antipsychotic medications, if not more so.[4,11,13] In a retrospective study[1] assessing the effectiveness and safety of the combination of clozapine and ECT in a sample of patients with TRS, almost two-thirds were responders (defined as a 30% or greater reduction in PANSS total score).[14] Follow-up data on a subsample of these patients, over a mean of 30 months, revealed that the majority had maintained their symptomatic improvement or improved further. Another small retrospective study of ECT augmentation of clozapine reported an acute response (defined as improvement rated on the Clinical Global Impression-Improvement scale[15]) in around three-quarters of the patient sample, and three-quarters of the responders remained out of hospital over a one-year follow-up period.[16]

In a randomised, single-blind study,[2] patients with clozapine-refractory schizophrenia either continued solely on their clozapine treatment or had it augmented with a course of bilateral ECT. After eight weeks, a pre-defined response criterion (which included a 40% or greater reduction in the psychotic symptom subscale of the Brief Psychiatric Rating Scale[17]) was met by half the patients receiving clozapine plus ECT, but none of the group on clozapine alone. When the non-responders from the clozapine-alone group crossed over to an 8-week, open trial of ECT, nearly half met the response criterion.

A systematic review and meta-analysis[18] looking specifically at ECT augmentation of clozapine treatment found a paucity of controlled studies, although the authors acknowledged the methodological challenges of such investigations. They concluded that ECT may be an effective augmentation strategy for schizophrenia that has failed to respond to clozapine monotherapy, but that further research was required to determine the place of such a strategy in any TRS treatment algorithm. A subsequent meta-analysis of RCTs addressing ECT augmentation for clozapine-resistant schizophrenia noted the lack of studies with sham-ECT as a control but reached the conclusion that such a treatment strategy was effective and relatively safe.[19]

Adverse effects

Although ECT augmentation of continuing antipsychotic medication appears to be generally well tolerated, adverse effects such as transient retrograde and anterograde amnesia, headaches and nausea have been reported for a minority of cases,[3,11,12,20] and there are reports of an increase in blood pressure after ECT and prolonged seizures.[1] There is some evidence to suggest that the cognitive side effects may be generally mild and transient.[19,21]

Summary

In summary, the evidence supports ECT augmentation of pharmacotherapy, particularly clozapine, as a potentially efficacious and relatively safe augmentation strategy in TRS,[7,22-24] although further, well-controlled trials are required to establish the benefit–risk balance of such a treatment strategy in both the short and long term.

References

1. Grover S, et al. Effectiveness of electroconvulsive therapy in patients with treatment resistant schizophrenia: a retrospective study. *Psychiatry Res* 2017; 249:349–353.
2. Petrides G, et al. Electroconvulsive therapy augmentation in clozapine-resistant schizophrenia: a prospective, randomized study. *Focus* 2019; 17:76–82.
3. Zheng W, et al. Electroconvulsive therapy added to non-clozapine antipsychotic medication for treatment resistant schizophrenia: meta-analysis of randomized controlled trials. *PLoS One* 2016; 11:e0156510.
4. Kim HS, et al. Effectiveness of electroconvulsive therapy augmentation on clozapine-resistant schizophrenia. *Psychiatry Investig* 2017; 14:58–62.
5. Vuksan Ćusa B, et al. The effects of electroconvulsive therapy augmentation of antipsychotic treatment on cognitive functions in patients with treatment-resistant schizophrenia. *J Ect* 2018; 34:31–34.
6. Sinclair DJM, et al. Electroconvulsive therapy for treatment-resistant schizophrenia. *Schizophr Bull* 2019; 45:730–732.
7. Grover S, et al. ECT in schizophrenia: a review of the evidence. *Acta Neuropsychiatr* 2019; 31:115–127.
8. Tharyan P, et al. Electroconvulsive therapy for schizophrenia. *Cochrane Database Syst Rev* 2005; Cd000076.
9. Lin HT, et al. Impacts of electroconvulsive therapy on 1-year outcomes in patients with schizophrenia: a controlled, population-based mirror-image study. *Schizophr Bull* 2018; 44:798–806.
10. Masoudzadeh A, et al. Comparative study of clozapine, electroshock and the combination of ECT with clozapine in treatment-resistant schizophrenic patients. *Pak J Biol Sci* 2007; 10:4287–4290.
11. Kaster TS, et al. Clinical effectiveness and cognitive impact of electroconvulsive therapy for schizophrenia: a large retrospective study. *J Clin Psychiatry* 2017; 78:e383–e389.
12. Pawełczyk T, et al. Augmentation of antipsychotics with electroconvulsive therapy in treatment-resistant schizophrenia patients with dominant negative symptoms: a pilot study of effectiveness. *Neuropsychobiology* 2014; 70:158–164.
13. Ahmed S, et al. Combined use of electroconvulsive therapy and antipsychotics (both clozapine and non-clozapine) in treatment resistant schizophrenia: a comparative meta-analysis. *Heliyon* 2017; 3:e00429.
14. Kay SR, et al. The positive and negative syndrome scale (PANSS) for schizophrenia. *Schizophr Bull* 1987; 13:261–276.
15. Guy W. ECDEU Assessment Manual for Psychopharmacology, U.S. Department of Health, Education, and Welfare, Public Health Service, Alcohol, Drug Abuse, and Mental Health Administration, National Institute of Mental Health, Psychopharmacology Research Branch, Division of Extramural Research Programs 1976.
16. Lally J, et al. Augmentation of clozapine with ECT: a retrospective case analysis. *Acta Neuropsychiatr* 2021; 33:31–36.
17. Overall JE, et al. The brief psychiatric rating scale. *Psychol Rep* 1962; 10:812.
18. Lally J, et al. Augmentation of clozapine with electroconvulsive therapy in treatment resistant schizophrenia: a systematic review and meta-analysis. *Schizophr Res* 2016; 171:215–224.
19. Wang G, et al. ECT augmentation of clozapine for clozapine-resistant schizophrenia: a meta-analysis of randomized controlled trials. *J Psychiatr Res* 2018; 105:23–32.
20. Zheng W, et al. Memory impairment following electroconvulsive therapy in Chinese patients with schizophrenia: meta-analysis of randomized controlled trials. *Perspect Psychiatr Care* 2018; 54:107–114.
21. Sanghani SN, et al. Electroconvulsive therapy (ECT) in schizophrenia: a review of recent literature. *Curr Opin Psychiatry* 2018; 31:213–222.
22. Zervas IM, et al. Using ECT in schizophrenia: a review from a clinical perspective. *World J Biol Psychiatry* 2012; 13:96–105.
23. Wagner E, et al. Clozapine combination and augmentation strategies in patients with schizophrenia -recommendations from an international expert survey among the Treatment Response and Resistance in Psychosis (TRRIP) Working Group. *Schizophr Bull* 2020; 46:1459–1470.
24. Arumugham SS, et al. Efficacy and safety of combining clozapine with electrical or magnetic brain stimulation in treatment-refractory schizophrenia. *Expert Rev Clin Pharmacol* 2016; 9:1245–1252.

Omega-3 fatty acid (fish oils) in schizophrenia

Fish oils contain the omega-3 fatty acids, eicosapentaenoic acid (EPA) and docosahexaenoic acid (DHA) – also known as polyunsaturated fatty acids or PUFAs. These compounds are thought to be involved in maintaining neuronal membrane structure, in the modulation of membrane proteins and in the production of prostaglandins and leukotrienes.[1] High dietary intake of PUFAs may protect against psychosis,[2] and antipsychotic treatment seems to normalise PUFA deficits.[3] Animal models suggest a protective effect for PUFAs.[4] They have been suggested as treatments for a variety of psychiatric illnesses;[5,6] in schizophrenia, case reports,[7-10] case series[11] and prospective trials originally suggested useful efficacy.[12-16]

Treatment

A meta-analysis of these RCTs[17] concluded that EPA has 'no beneficial effect in established schizophrenia' because the estimate of effect size (0.242) was not statistically significant. Since then, an RCT comprising 71 patients with first-episode schizophrenia given 2.2g EPA + DHA daily for 6 months showed a reduction in symptom severity for patients in the active arm, finding an NNT of 4 to produce a 50% reduction in symptoms measured by PANSS.[18] However, a further RCT of 97 subjects in acute psychosis showed no advantage for EPA 2g daily[19] and a relapse prevention study of EPA 2g + DHA 1g a day failed to demonstrate any value for PUFAs over placebo (relapse rate was 90% with PUFAs, 75% with placebo).[20] The limitations affecting the published data in this area (small sample sizes, heterogeneity of diagnosis and stage of illness, differences in intervention combinations and doses) mean that overall findings remain at best inconclusive.[21,22] Meta-review of published meta-analyses finds no evidence for the use of PUFAs in the treatment of schizophrenia.[23]

On balance, evidence now suggests that EPA (2–3g daily) is unlikely to be a worthwhile option in schizophrenia when added to standard treatment. Set against doubts over efficacy are the facts that fish oils are relatively cheap, well tolerated[24] (mild GI symptoms may occur) and benefit physical health.[1,25-29]

Prevention

A study of 700mg EPA + 480mg DHA in adolescents and young adults at high risk of psychosis showed that such treatment greatly reduced emergence of psychotic symptoms compared with placebo[30] (although a review described this study as 'very low quality evidence'[31]). Since the publication of this single-site study, the large, multi-site NEURAPRO trial[32] gave adult patients at high risk of psychosis 840mg EPA + 560mg DHA for 6 months, and failed to find any evidence of efficacy either for reduction in transition to psychosis, or improvement in symptoms. Cochrane concluded that omega-3 fatty acids 'may' prevent transition to psychosis in the prodromal phase, but that the evidence is of low quality and this conclusion unconfirmed.[33]

Overall

PUFAs are no longer recommended for the treatment of residual symptoms of schizophrenia or for the prevention of transition to psychosis in young people at high risk.[23,34–36] If used, careful assessment of response is important, and fish oils should be withdrawn if no effect is observed after 3 months' treatment, unless required for their beneficial metabolic effects.

Summary recommendations – fish oils (PUFAs)

- Patients at high risk of first-episode psychosis
    - Not recommended. If used, suggest **EPA 700mg/day** (2× Omacor or 6× Maxepa capsules)
- Residual symptoms of multi-episode schizophrenia (added to antipsychotic)
    - Not recommended. If used, suggest dose of **EPA 2g/day** (5× Omacor or 10× Maxepa capsules)

References

1. Fenton WS, et al. Essential fatty acids, lipid membrane abnormalities, and the diagnosis and treatment of schizophrenia. *Biol Psychiatry* 2000; 47:8–21.
2. Hedelin M, et al. Dietary intake of fish, omega-3, omega-6 polyunsaturated fatty acids and vitamin D and the prevalence of psychotic-like symptoms in a cohort of 33,000 women from the general population. *BMC Psychiatry* 2010; 10:38.
3. Sethom MM, et al. Polyunsaturated fatty acids deficits are associated with psychotic state and negative symptoms in patients with schizophrenia. *Prostaglandins Leukot Essent Fatty Acids* 2010; 83:131–136.
4. Zugno AI, et al. Omega-3 prevents behavior response and brain oxidative damage in the ketamine model of schizophrenia. *Neuroscience* 2014; 259:223–231.
5. Freeman MP. Omega-3 fatty acids in psychiatry: a review. *Ann Clin Psychiatry* 2000; 12:159–165.
6. Ross BM, et al. Omega-3 fatty acids as treatments for mental illness: which disorder and which fatty acid? *Lipids Health Dis* 2007; 6:21.
7. Richardson AJ, et al. Red cell and plasma fatty acid changes accompanying symptom remission in a patient with schizophrenia treated with eicosapentaenoic acid. *Eur Neuropsychopharmacol* 2000; 10:189–193.
8. Puri BK, et al. Eicosapentaenoic acid treatment in schizophrenia associated with symptom remission, normalisation of blood fatty acids, reduced neuronal membrane phospholipid turnover and structural brain changes. *Int J Clin Pract* 2000; 54:57–63.
9. Su KP, et al. Omega-3 fatty acids as a psychotherapeutic agent for a pregnant schizophrenic patient. *Eur Neuropsychopharmacol* 2001; 11:295–299.
10. Cuéllar-Barboza AB, et al. Use of omega-3 polyunsaturated fatty acids as augmentation therapy in treatment-resistant schizophrenia. *Prim Care Companion CNS Disord* 2017; 19:16l02040.
11. Sivrioglu EY, et al. The impact of omega-3 fatty acids, vitamins E and C supplementation on treatment outcome and side effects in schizophrenia patients treated with haloperidol: an open-label pilot study. *Prog Neuropsychopharmacol Biol Psychiatry* 2007; 31:1493–1499.
12. Mellor JE, et al. Schizophrenic symptoms and dietary intake of n-3 fatty acids. *Schizophr Res* 1995; 18:85–86.
13. Peet M, et al. Two double-blind placebo-controlled pilot studies of eicosapentaenoic acid in the treatment of schizophrenia. *Schizophr Res* 2001; 49:243–251.
14. Fenton WS, et al. A placebo-controlled trial of omega-3 fatty acid (ethyl eicosapentaenoic acid) supplementation for residual symptoms and cognitive impairment in schizophrenia. *Am J Psychiatry* 2001; 158:2071–2074.
15. Emsley R, et al. Randomized, placebo-controlled study of ethyl-eicosapentaenoic acid as supplemental treatment in schizophrenia. *Am J Psychiatry* 2002; 159:1596–1598.
16. Berger GE, et al. Ethyl-eicosapentaenoic acid in first-episode psychosis: a randomized, placebo-controlled trial. *J Clin Psychiatry* 2007; 68:1867–1875.
17. Fusar-Poli P, et al. Eicosapentaenoic acid interventions in schizophrenia: meta-analysis of randomized, placebo-controlled studies. *J Clin Psychopharmacol* 2012; 32:179–185.
18. Pawelczyk T, et al. A randomized controlled study of the efficacy of six-month supplementation with concentrated fish oil rich in omega-3 polyunsaturated fatty acids in first episode schizophrenia. *J Psychiatr Res* 2016; 73:34–44.
19. Bentsen H, et al. A randomized placebo-controlled trial of an omega-3 fatty acid and vitamins E+C in schizophrenia. *TranslPsychiatry* 2013; 3:e335.

20. Emsley R, et al. A randomized, controlled trial of omega-3 fatty acids plus an antioxidant for relapse prevention after antipsychotic discontinuation in first-episode schizophrenia. *Schizophr Res* 2014; **158**:230–235.

21. Bozzatello P, et al. Polyunsaturated fatty acids: what is their role in treatment of psychiatric disorders? *Int J Molecular Sci* 2019; **20**:5257.

22. Hsu MC, et al. Beneficial effects of omega-3 fatty acid supplementation in schizophrenia: possible mechanisms. *Lipids Health Dis* 2020; **19**:159.

23. Firth J, et al. The efficacy and safety of nutrient supplements in the treatment of mental disorders: a meta-review of meta-analyses of randomized controlled trials. *World Psychiatry* 2019; **18**:308–324.

24. Schlögelhofer M, et al. Polyunsaturated fatty acids in emerging psychosis: a safer alternative? *Early Interv Psychiatry* 2014; **8**:199–208.

25. Scorza FA, et al. Omega-3 fatty acids and sudden cardiac death in schizophrenia: if not a friend, at least a great colleague. *Schizophr Res* 2007; **94**:375–376.

26. Caniato RN, et al. Effect of omega-3 fatty acids on the lipid profile of patients taking clozapine. *Aust N Z J Psychiatry* 2006; **40**:691–697.

27. Emsley R, et al. Safety of the omega-3 fatty acid, eicosapentaenoic acid (EPA) in psychiatric patients: results from a randomized, placebo-controlled trial. *Psychiatry Res* 2008; **161**:284–291.

28. Das UN. Essential fatty acids and their metabolites could function as endogenous HMG-CoA reductase and ACE enzyme inhibitors, anti-arrhythmic, anti-hypertensive, anti-atherosclerotic, anti-inflammatory, cytoprotective, and cardioprotective molecules. *Lipids Health Dis* 2008; **7**:37.

29. Xu F, et al. Effects of omega-3 fatty acids on metabolic syndrome in patients with schizophrenia: a 12-week randomized placebo-controlled trial. *Psychopharmacology* 2019; **236**:1273–1279.

30. Amminger GP, et al. Long-chain omega-3 fatty acids for indicated prevention of psychotic disorders: a randomized, placebo-controlled trial. *Arch Gen Psychiatry* 2010; **67**:146–154.

31. Stafford MR, et al. Early interventions to prevent psychosis: systematic review and meta-analysis. *BMJ* 2013; **346**:f185.

32. McGorry PD, et al. Effect of omega-3 polyunsaturated fatty acids in young people at ultrahigh risk for psychotic disorders: the neurapro randomized clinical trial. *JAMA Psychiatry* 2017; **74**:19–27.

33. Bosnjak Kuharic D, et al. Interventions for prodromal stage of psychosis. *Cochrane Database Syst Rev* 2019; CD012236.

34. Devoe DJ, et al. Attenuated psychotic symptom interventions in youth at risk of psychosis: a systematic review and meta-analysis. *Early Interv Psychiatry* 2019; **13**:3–17.

35. Nasir M, et al. Trim the fat: the role of omega-3 fatty acids in psychopharmacology. *Ther Adv Psychopharmacol* 2019; **9**:2045125319869791.

36. Cho M, et al. Adjunctive use of anti-inflammatory drugs for schizophrenia: a meta-analytic investigation of randomized controlled trials. *Aust N Z J Psychiatry* 2019; **53**:742–759.

Stopping antipsychotics

Antipsychotics are recommended for long-term treatment of schizophrenia because they reduce symptoms and can reduce the risk of relapse.[1] However, antipsychotics have many adverse effects, including metabolic complications, tardive dyskinesia, emotional blunting and brain shrinkage.[2] There is some evidence that reducing or stopping patients' antipsychotics may improve their social functioning (relationships, education or employment, independent living) without worsening their rate of relapse or symptom burden in the medium term,[3] although it might increase their risk of relapse in the short term.[4] There is also evidence that reducing antipsychotic burden may increase cognitive functioning.[5]

Furthermore, the evidence for the relapse prevention properties of antipsychotics relies on discontinuation trials in which antipsychotics were mostly stopped in one day, leading to withdrawal effects that may have elevated the apparent rate of relapse in the discontinuation arm, exaggerating the relapse prevention properties of antipsychotics.[6] Patients often ask to reduce or stop their medication, and in light of the above this may be a reasonable course of action. Cautious de-prescribing should be a component of high-quality prescribing practice.

It should also be noted that more than half of antipsychotic prescriptions in the UK are given to patients without a psychotic or manic disorder and instead are prescribed for insomnia, anxiety, personality disorders and symptoms of dementia,[7] although NICE recommends against medium- or long-term use of antipsychotics in personality disorder,[8] and careful use only in dementia.[9] The principles for de-prescribing outlined below also apply to these patients.

Withdrawal/discontinuation effects of antipsychotics

Stopping or reducing the dose of antipsychotics can cause a variety of symptoms reflecting their various actions (blocking dopamine, histamine, acetylcholine, serotonin and noradrenaline receptors).[10,11] They include autonomic effects (diarrhoea, salivation, sweating), somatic symptoms (headache, nausea, vomiting, anorexia), motor effects (tremulousness, restlessness, dyskinesia) and psychological symptoms (anxiety, irritability, agitation, insomnia and psychotic symptoms) (Figure 1.1).[10,11] Insomnia is probably the most common withdrawal symptom.

Importantly, withdrawal/discontinuation symptoms from antipsychotics can include psychotic symptoms.[11,12] This is suggested by a number of case studies in which people without a psychotic disorder, treated with dopamine antagonists for reasons such as nausea or lactation difficulties, develop psychotic symptoms when these medications are abruptly stopped.[13–15]

In patients with psychotic disorders, relapse often occurs when antipsychotics are withdrawn. This has been widely thought to represent an unmasking of the underlying chronic illness, but the nature of the process of withdrawing antipsychotics may itself be causally related to relapse.[6] This is supported by the marked preponderance of relapses soon after abrupt antipsychotic cessation in patients with schizophrenia in discontinuation trials. In one analysis, 60% of all relapses over four years occurred within three months of drug cessation,[16] the time most likely for withdrawal effects to be evident. It is also supported by evidence that slower tapering can reduce the rate of relapse.[16]

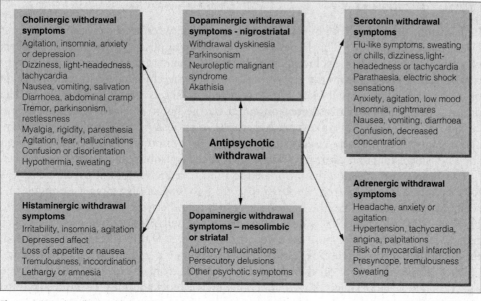

Figure 1.1 Antipsychotic withdrawal symptoms
adapted from Chouinard et al. (2017)[11]

Neurobiology of withdrawal

Withdrawal-associated relapse has been attributed to neural adaptations to long-term antipsychotic treatment (dopaminergic hypersensitivity) that persist after antipsychotic cessation.[17] Indeed, molecular imaging studies in schizophrenia have found increased D2/D3 receptor availability in those subjects who had been exposed to antipsychotic medication but not in antipsychotic-naïve patients.[18] This hypersensitivity to dopamine may render patients more susceptible to psychotic relapse when D2 blockade is diminished by antipsychotic dose reduction.[10,17]

There are converging lines of evidence that suggest that the neuro-adaptive effects of being on antipsychotics can persist for months or years after stopping. Dopaminergic hypersensitivity in animals persists for the equivalent of a human year after treatment is stopped.[19,20] Tardive dyskinesia – attributed to dopaminergic hypersensitivity – can persist for years after antipsychotic medication has been ceased.[21] There is also evidence that patients who have discontinued antipsychotics have increased rates of relapse for three years compared with people maintained on their antipsychotics, after which relapse rates converge,[1] suggesting that adaptations may have resolved by this point.

It follows that the risk of relapse on cessation of antipsychotics might be minimised by more gradual dose tapering because these neuroadaptations would then have time to resolve during the tapering process, and the rate of decline of blockade is more modest. A small analysis found that tapering over three to nine months halves the rate of relapse compared with abrupt discontinuation,[16] while tapering over four weeks showed no difference from abrupt discontinuation.[1]

Pattern of tapering

PET imaging demonstrates a hyperbolic relationship between dose of antipsychotic and D2 receptor occupancy.[22] This hyperbolic relationship applies to other receptor targets of antipsychotics as well (including histaminergic, cholinergic and serotonergic receptors), because it arises from the law of mass action (whereby each additional molecule of a drug has incrementally less effect as receptor targets become saturated).[23] The nature of this relationship is often obscured by the habit of plotting dose–response curves on semi-logarithmic axes.[23] A hyperbolic relationship between dose of antipsychotic and its therapeutic effects (as measured by symptoms scales) has also been shown,[24] suggesting that clinical response mirrors the neurobiological pattern of effects.

This brings into question the rationale for a linear reduction of antipsychotic dose – for example, a reduction from 20 to 15 to 10 to 5 to 0mg of olanzapine. Although this regime appears reasonable, the hyperbolic relationship between dose and effect on D2 blockade dictates that these linear dose decreases will produce increasingly larger reductions of D2 blockade (and the clinical consequences of this) (Figure 1.2A). Indeed, the reduction of dose from 5mg to 0mg will produce a reduction in D2 blockade (52.6%) larger than that produced by the reduction from 40 to 5mg of olanzapine (37.3%). These increasingly large reductions in D2 blockade may be more likely to provoke relapse.

Linear or 'evenly spaced' reductions in D2 blockade require hyperbolically reducing doses of antipsychotic (Figure 1.2B).[25] These hyperbolic reductions are approximated by sequential halving of dose: for example, risperidone doses of 20mg, 10mg, 5mg, 2.5mg, 1.25mg, 0.6mg, 0.3mg, 0mg produce roughly 15 percentage point reductions in D2 blockade. This pattern of reduction may be less likely to provoke relapse because it avoids large increases in dopaminergic signalling. Preliminary support for this notion comes from three studies of gradual antipsychotic reduction: one study achieved a 42% reduction in overall antipsychotic dose in 6 months with no increase in relapse;[26] in

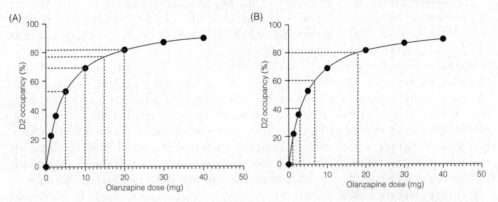

Figure 1.2 (A) Linear dose reductions of risperidone cause increasingly large reductions in D_2 dopaminergic receptor blockade. The relationship between dose of risperidone and D_2 blockade is derived from the line of best fit from meta-analysis of PET studies.[22] (B) Linear reductions of D_2 dopaminergic occupancy (in this case, 20% reductions) correspond to hyperbolically decreasing doses of risperidone. The doses in this case correspond to 6.9mg (80% D_2 occupancy), 2.0mg (60% D_2 occupancy), 0.82mg (40% D_2 occupancy) and 0.30mg (20% D_2 occupancy). Approximations to this regime that correspond to available formulations are given in the text.

another 25–62.5% dose reduction was achieved with three-quarters of patients showing no sign of relapse[27] and 46.0–57.6% dose reduction produced no change in overall PANSS scores between the reduction and maintenance groups.[28]

Exponentially reducing regimes (that is, reducing by a fixed proportion of the most recent dose) will produce roughly linear reductions at all receptor targets of antipsychotics, making it applicable to a wide range of antipsychotic medication. Notably, the study that was able to reduce antipsychotic doses by more than half in some patients with no relapse employed exponentially reducing dose regimens by reducing dose by 25% of the most recent dose every 6 months.[27]

Tapering in practice

All patients should be informed of the risk of withdrawal symptoms on stopping or reducing the dose of any antipsychotic, including insomnia and an increase in psychotic symptoms. Clozapine is associated with the most common and severe withdrawal symptoms, possibly because of its potent anti-cholinergic effects.

Patient should be warned not to stop antipsychotics abruptly, because this is the method thought to be most likely to precipitate a relapse and/or severe withdrawal effects.

When to attempt discontinuation

Longstanding or lifelong antipsychotic treatment is something of a modern-day phenomenon. It the 1960s, discontinuation of antipsychotics was usually attempted after acute response, but abrupt discontinuation often led to relapse (but interestingly, not always[29]). There are currently no evidence-based recommendations for antipsychotic withdrawal, but we suggest that it only be attempted in patients who have been in remission for 6 months (first episode) or one year (multi-episode).

The initial dose reduction could be derived from the patient's previous experience of dose reduction. For many patients the dose could be reduced by approximately 25% of the most recent dose (e.g. for olanzapine this would be a reduction from 20mg to 15mg), although some might require as small a decrease as 10% of their current dose. The patient should then be monitored for three months following this reduction for any withdrawal symptoms or worsening of psychotic symptoms, recalling that these symptoms can be transitory withdrawal effects rather than signs of inevitable relapse, indicating the necessity for reinstatement of their regular dose of medication. If a patient tolerates this reduction with no significant effect on their overall mental state (or perhaps only mild symptoms of insomnia), then further reductions could be made at the same rate (e.g. a reduction of 10–25% of their dose every 3 months). Patients may require increased psychosocial support during this period of withdrawal.

If a patient experiences significant withdrawal symptoms or worsening of psychotic symptoms then an increase back to the original dose (or partway thereof) may be necessary. It should be noted that this does not preclude further attempts at reduction, but these attempts should be delayed till stability is established and should be more gradual than previously attempted (perhaps as small as 5–10% of current dose).

Final doses before complete cessation will need to be very small to prevent a large decrease in D2 blockade. This may need to be as small as 1/80th of the original therapeutic dose (e.g. 0.25mg of olanzapine). Delivery of these small doses will require splitting tablets or using liquid formulations of the medications.

Example reducing regimens are presented in Tables 1.11 and 1.12.

Table 1.11 Reductions of olanzapine dose by 5 percentage points of D2 occupancy at each step

Period	Olanzapine dose (mg)	D2 Occupancy (%)
1	20	81.6
2	14	75
3	10.5	70
4	8.4	65
5	6.8	60
6	5.5	55
7	4.5	50
8	3.7	45
9	3	40
10	2.4	35
11	1.9	30
12	1.5	25
13	1.1	20
14	0.8	15
15	0.5	10
16	0.24	5
17	0	0

Table 1.12 Reductions of olanzapine dose by 2.5 percentage points of D2 occupancy at each step. Larger reductions that are 'evenly spaced' in terms of effect on D2 occupancy could be achieved by following every second or third step of this regimen

Period	Olanzapine dose (mg)	D2 occupancy (%)	Period	Olanzapine dose (mg)	D2 occupancy (%)
1	20	81.6	18	2.7	37.5
2	15.5	77.5	19	2.4	35
3	13.5	75	20	2.2	32.5
4	11.9	72.5	21	1.9	30
5	10.5	70	22	1.7	27.5
6	9.3	67.5	23	1.5	25
7	8.4	65	24	1.3	22.5
8	7.5	62.5	25	1.1	20
9	6.8	60	26	0.95	17.5
10	6.1	57.5	27	0.8	15
11	5.5	55	28	0.65	12.5
12	5	52.5	29	0.5	10
13	4.5	50	30	0.37	7.5
14	4.1	47.5	31	0.24	5
15	3.7	45	32	0.1	2.5
16	3.3	42.5	33	0	0
17	3	40			

Table 1.13 A summary of potential reduction schedules for olanzapine

Reduce olanzapine by 5–10mg every 2–3 months until reaching 20mg per day, *then*

Reduce dose by 2.5–5mg every 2–3 months until reaching 10mg per day, *then*

Reduce dose by 1.25–2.5mg every 2–3 months until reaching 5mg per day, *then*

Reduce dose by 0.6–1.25mg every 2–3 months until reaching 2.5mg per day, *then*

Reduce dose by 0.3–0.6mg every 2–3 months until reaching 1.25mg per day, *then*

Reduce dose by 0.15–0.3mg every 2–3 months until reaching 0.6mg per day, *then*

Reduce dose by 0.07–0.15mg every 2–3 months until olanzapine is **completely stopped**.

This process should take 12–48 months, depending on how the patient tolerates the reductions.

References

1. Leucht S, et al. Antipsychotic drugs versus placebo for relapse prevention in schizophrenia: a systematic review and meta-analysis. *Lancet* 2012; 379:2063–2071.

2. Murray RM, et al. Should psychiatrists be more cautious about the long-term prophylactic use of antipsychotics? *Br J Psychiatry* 2016; 209:361–365.

3. Wunderink L, et al. Recovery in remitted first-episode psychosis at 7 years of follow-up of an early dose reduction/discontinuation or maintenance treatment strategy: long-term follow-up of a 2-year randomized clinical trial. *JAMA Psychiatry* 2013; 70:913–920.

4. Wunderink L, et al. Guided discontinuation versus maintenance treatment in remitted first-episode psychosis: relapse rates and functional outcome. *J Clin Psychiatry* 2007; 68:654–661.

5. Omachi Y, et al. Dose reduction/discontinuation of antipsychotic drugs in psychosis; effect on cognition and functional outcomes. *Frontiers in Psychiatry* 2018; 9:447.

6. Moncrieff J. Antipsychotic Maintenance. Treatment: time to rethink? *PLoS Med* 2015; 12:e1001861.

7. Marston L, et al. Prescribing of antipsychotics in UK primary care: a cohort study. *BMJ Open* 2014; 4:e006135.

8. National Institute for Clinical Excellence. Borderline personality disorder: recognition and management. Clinical Guidance 78 [CG78]. 2009 (Last checked July 2018); https://www.nice.org.uk/guidance/CG78.

9. National Institute for Health and Care Excellence. Dementia: assessment, management and support for people living with dementia and their carers [NG97]. 2018; https://www.nice.org.uk/guidance/ng97.

10. Cerovecki A, et al. Withdrawal symptoms and rebound syndromes associated with switching and discontinuing atypical antipsychotics: theoretical background and practical recommendations. *CNS Drugs* 2013; 27:545–572.

11. Chouinard G, et al. Antipsychotic-induced dopamine supersensitivity psychosis: pharmacology, criteria, and therapy. *Psychother Psychosom* 2017; 86:189–219.

12. Moncrieff J. Does antipsychotic withdrawal provoke psychosis? Review of the literature on rapid onset psychosis (supersensitivity psychosis) and withdrawal-related relapse. *Acta Psychiatr Scand* 2006; 114:3–13.

13. Lu ML, et al. Metoclopramide-induced supersensitivity psychosis. *Ann Pharmacother* 2002; 36:1387–1390.

14. Roy-Desruisseaux J, et al. Domperidone-induced tardive dyskinesia and withdrawal psychosis in an elderly woman with dementia. *Ann Pharmacother* 2011; 45:e51.

15. Seeman P Breast is best but taper domperidone when stopping (e-letter). 2014; https://bjgp.org/content/yes-breast-best-taper-domperidone-when-stopping.

16. Viguera AC, et al. Clinical risk following abrupt and gradual withdrawal of maintenance neuroleptic treatment. *Arch Gen Psychiatry* 1997; 54:49–55.

17. Chouinard G, et al. Atypical antipsychotics: CATIE study, drug-induced movement disorder and resulting iatrogenic psychiatric-like symptoms, supersensitivity rebound psychosis and withdrawal discontinuation syndromes. *Psychother Psychosom* 2008; 77:69–77.

18. Howes OD, et al. The nature of dopamine dysfunction in schizophrenia and what this means for treatment. *Arch Gen Psychiatry* 2012; 69:776–786.

19. Joyce JN. D2 but not D3 receptors are elevated after 9 or 11 months chronic haloperidol treatment: influence of withdrawal period. *Synapse* 2001; 40:137–144.

20. Quinn R. Comparing rat's to human's age: how old is my rat in people years? *Nutrition* 2005; 21:775–777.

21. Marsden CD. Is tardive dyskinesia a unique disorder? *Psychopharmacology Suppl* 1985; 2:64–71.

22. Lako IM, et al. Estimating dopamine D_2 receptor occupancy for doses of 8 antipsychotics: a meta-analysis. *J Clin Psychopharmacol* 2013; 33:675–681.

23. Holford N. Pharmacodynamic principles and the time course of delayed and cumulative drug effects. *Translational and Clinical Pharmacology* 2018; 26:56–59.

24. Leucht S, et al. Dose-response meta-analysis of antipsychotic drugs for acute schizophrenia. *Am J Psychiatry* 2020; 177:342–353.

25. Horowitz MA, et al. Tapering antipsychotic treatment. *JAMA Psychiatry* 2021; 78:125–126.

26. Huhn M, et al. Reducing antipsychotic drugs in stable patients with chronic schizophrenia or schizoaffective disorder: a randomized controlled pilot trial. *Eur Arch Psychiatry Clin Neurosci* 2021; 271:293–302.

27. Liu CC, et al. Achieving the lowest effective antipsychotic dose for patients with remitted psychosis: a proposed guided dose-reduction algorithm. *CNS Drugs* 2020; 34:117–126.

28. Ozawa C, et al. Model-guided antipsychotic dose reduction in schizophrenia: a pilot, single-blind randomized controlled trial. *J Clin Psychopharmacol* 2019; 39:329–335.

29. Prien RF, et al. Relapse in chronic schizophrenics following abrupt withdrawal of tranquillizing medication. *Br J Psychiatry* 1969; 115:679–686.

ANTIPSYCHOTIC ADVERSE EFFECTS

Extrapyramidal symptoms

EPS:

- Tend to be dose-related.
- Appear most likely with high doses of high potency FGAs.
- Are less common with other antipsychotic medications, particularly clozapine, olanzapine, quetiapine and aripiprazole,[1] but once present may be persistent[2] Note that CUtLASS reported no difference in EPS between FGAs and SGAs[3] (although sulpiride was widely used in the FGA group). Vulnerability to EPS may be genetically determined.[4]

Note that similar movement disorder may be seen in never-medicated patients with schizophrenia.[5-7] In one study of such patients at first-episode, 1% had dystonia, 8% parkinsonian symptoms and 11% akathisia.[7] Parkinsonian symptoms and other motor abnormalities in this context may be associated with cognitive impairment[7,8] and poor long-term psychosocial functioning.[9] In a study of never-treated patients with established psychotic illness, 9% exhibited spontaneous dyskinesias and 17% Parkinsonian symptoms.[10] Patients who experience one type of EPS may be more vulnerable to developing others.[11] Substance misuse increases the risk of dystonia, akathisia and TD.[12,13] There is some evidence for an association between alcohol use and akathisia.[14,15]

Table 1.14 Most common extrapyramidal symptoms

	Dystonia (uncontrolled muscular spasm)	Pseudoparkinsonism (bradykinesia, tremor, etc.)	Akathisia (restlessness)[16]	Tardive dyskinesia (abnormal involuntary movements)
Signs and symptoms[17]	Muscle spasm in any part of the body, e.g. ■ Eyes rolling upwards (oculogyric spasm) ■ Head and neck twisted to the side (torticollis) The patient may be unable to swallow or speak clearly. In extreme cases, the back may arch or the jaw dislocate Acute dystonia can be both painful and very frightening	Tremor and/or rigidity Bradykinesia (decreased facial expression, flat monotone voice, slow body movements, inability to initiate movement) Bradyphrenia (slowed thinking) Salivation Pseudoparkinsonism can be mistaken for depression or the negative symptoms of schizophrenia	A subjectively unpleasant state of inner restlessness with a desire or compulsion to move[1] ■ Foot stamping when seated ■ Constantly crossing/uncrossing legs ■ Rocking from foot to foot ■ Constantly pacing up and down Akathisia can be mistaken for psychotic agitation and has been linked with suicidal ideation[18] and aggression towards others[19]	A wide variety of movements can occur,[20] such as: ■ Lip smacking or chewing ■ Tongue protrusion ('fly catching') ■ Choreiform hand movements ('piano playing') ■ Dystonic and choreoathetoid movements of the limbs Severe orofacial movements can lead to difficulty speaking, eating or breathing. Movements are worse when under stress.
Rating scales	No specific scale. Small component of general EPS scales	Simpson–Angus EPS Rating Scale[21]	Barnes Akathisia Rating Scale[22]	Abnormal Involuntary Movement Scale[23] (AIMS)
Prevalence	Approximately 10%,[24] but more common:[25] ■ In young males ■ In those who are antipsychotic-naive ■ With high potency medications (e.g. haloperidol) Dystonic reactions are rare in the elderly	Approximately 20%,[26] but more common in: ■ Elderly females ■ Those with pre-existing neurological damage (head injury, stroke, etc.)	Wide variation but approximately 25%[27] for acute akathisia with FGAs, lower with SGAs The relative liability of individual antipsychotic medications for akathisia is uncertain,[28] but there is consensus that the incidence is lowest for olanzapine, quetiapine and clozapine.[29,30]	5% of patients per year of antipsychotic exposure.[31] More common in respect to:[32] ■ Age ■ Affective illness ■ Schizophrenia ■ Higher doses ■ Acute EPS early in treatment Lower incidence in those on SGAs[33] TD may be associated with neurocognitive deficits.[34]

	Dystonia (uncontrolled muscular spasm)	Pseudoparkinsonism (bradykinesia, tremor, etc.)	Akathisia (restlessness)[16]	Tardive dyskinesia (abnormal involuntary movements)
Time taken to develop	Acute dystonia can occur within hours of starting antipsychotic medication (minutes if the IM or IV route is used). Tardive dystonia occurs after months to years of antipsychotic treatment.	Days to weeks after antipsychotic medication is started or the dose is increased	Acute akathisia occurs within hours to weeks of starting antipsychotic medication or increasing the dose. Akathisia that has persisted for several months or so is called 'chronic akathisia'. Tardive akathisia tends to occur later in treatment and may be exacerbated or provoked by antipsychotic dose reduction or withdrawal.[16]	Months to years The proportion of cases showing reversibility on cessation of antipsychotic medication is unclear and may partly depend on age[20]
Treatment	Anticholinergic drugs given orally, IM or IV depending on the severity of symptoms[20] ■ Remember the patient may be unable to swallow ■ Response to IV administration will be seen within 5 minutes ■ Response to IM administration takes around 20 minutes ■ Tardive dystonia may respond to ECT[35,36] ■ Where severe symptoms do not respond to simpler measures including switching to an antipsychotic with a low propensity for EPS, botulinum toxin may be effective[37,38]	Several options are available depending on the clinical circumstances: ■ Reduce the antipsychotic dose ■ Change to an antipsychotic medication with a lower propensity for pseudoparkinsonism (see section on relative liability of antipsychotic medications for adverse effects) ■ Prescribe an anticholinergic. The majority of patients do not require long-term anticholinergic agents. Use should be reviewed at least every 3 months. Do not prescribe at night (symptoms usually absent during sleep)	■ Reduce the antipsychotic dose ■ Change to an antipsychotic drug with lower propensity for akathisia (see sections on akathisia and relative liability of antipsychotic medications for adverse effects) ■ A reduction in symptoms may be seen with:[39–41] low-dose propranolol, 30–80mg/day, clonazepam (low dose), 5HT$_2$ antagonists such as: cyproheptadine,[36] mirtazapine,[40] trazodone,[42,43] mianserin,[44] and cyproheptadine[36] may help, as may possibly diphenhydramine.[45] All are unlicensed for this indication Anticholinergics are generally unhelpful unless akathisia is part of a general EPS spectrum[46]	■ Stop anticholinergic if prescribed ■ Reduce dose of antipsychotic medication ■ Change to an antipsychotic with lower propensity for TD,[47–50] note that data are conflicting.[51,52] ■ Clozapine is the antipsychotic most likely to be associated with resolution of symptoms.[53,54] Quetiapine may also be useful in this regard.[55] ■ Both valbenazine and deutetrabenazine have a positive risk-benefit balance as add-on treatments[53,56–60] ■ There is also some evidence for tetrabenazine and ginkgo biloba[61] as add-on treatments. For other treatment options[60,62] the review by the American Academy of Neurology[63] and the section on tardive dyskinesia

References

1. Leucht S, et al. Comparative efficacy and tolerability of 15 antipsychotic drugs in schizophrenia: a multiple-treatments meta-analysis. *Lancet* 2013; **382**:951–962.

2. Tenback DE, et al. Incidence and persistence of tardive dyskinesia and extrapyramidal symptoms in schizophrenia. *J Psychopharmacol* 2010; 24:1031–1035.

3. Peluso MJ, et al. Extrapyramidal motor side-effects of first- and second-generation antipsychotic drugs. *Br J Psychiatry* 2012; 200:387–392.

4. Zivkovic M, et al. The association study of polymorphisms in DAT, DRD2, and COMT genes and acute extrapyramidal adverse effects in male schizophrenic patients treated with haloperidol. *J Clin Psychopharmacol* 2013; 33:593–599.

5. Cortese L, et al. Relationship of neuromotor disturbances to psychosis symptoms in first-episode neuroleptic-naive schizophrenia patients. *Schizophr Res* 2005; 75:65–75.

6. Puri BK, et al. Spontaneous dyskinesia in first episode schizophrenia. *J Neurol Neurosurg Psychiatry* 1999; 66:76–78.

7. Rybakowski JK, et al. Extrapyramidal symptoms during treatment of first schizophrenia episode: Results from EUFEST. *Eur Neuropsychopharmacol* 2014; 24:1500–1505.

8. Cuesta MJ, et al. Spontaneous parkinsonism is asociated with cognitive impairment in antipsychotic-naive patients with first-episode psychosis: a 6-month follow-up study. *Schizophr Bull* 2014; 40:1164–1173.

9. Cuesta MJ, et al. Motor abnormalities in first-episode psychosis patients and long-term psychosocial functioning. *Schizophr Res* 2018; 200:97–103.

10. Pappa S, et al. Spontaneous Spontaneous Parkinsonism Is Associated With Cognitive Impairment in Antipsychotic-Naive Patients With First-Episode Psychosis: A 6-Month Follow-up Study. Schizophr Bull; 2014; 40:1164–1173.

11. Kim JH, et al. Prevalence and characteristics of subjective akathisia, objective akathisia, and mixed akathisia in chronic schizophrenic subjects. *Clin Neuropharmacol* 2003; 26:312–316.

12. Potvin S, et al. Increased extrapyramidal symptoms in patients with schizophrenia and a comorbid substance use disorder. *J Neurol Neurosurg Psychiatry* 2006; 77:796–798.

13. Potvin S, et al. Substance abuse is associated with increased extrapyramidal symptoms in schizophrenia: a meta-analysis. *Schizophr Res* 2009; 113:181–188.

14. Hansen LK, et al. Movement disorders in patients with schizophrenia and a history of substance abuse. *Human Psychopharmacology* 2013; 28:192–197.

15. Duke PJ, et al. South Westminster schizophrenia survey. Alcohol use and its relationship to symptoms, tardive dyskinesia and illness onset. *Br J Psychiatry* 1994; **164**:630–636.

16. Barnes TR, et al. Akathisia variants and tardive dyskinesia. *Arch Gen Psychiatry* 1985; 42:874–878.

17. Gervin M, et al. Assessment of drug-related movement disorders in schizophrenia. *Adv Psychiatric Treatment* 2000; 6:332–341.

18. Seemuller F, et al. Akathisia and suicidal ideation in first-episode schizophrenia. *J Clin Psychopharmacol* 2012; 32:694–698.

19. Leong GB, et al. Neuroleptic-induced akathisia and violence: a review. *J Forensic Sci* 2003; 48:187–189.

20. Owens DC. Tardive dyskinesia update: the syndrome. *B J Psych Advances* 2018; 25:57–69.

21. Simpson GM, et al. A rating scale for extrapyramidal side effects. *Acta Psychiatr Scand* 1970; 212:11–19.

22. Barnes TRE. A rating scale for drug-induced akathisia. *Br J Psychiatry* 1989; 154:672–676.

23. Guy W. *ECDEU Assessment Manual for Psychopharmacology*. Washington, DC: US Department of Health, Education, and Welfare; 1976:534–537.

24. American Psychiatric Association. Practice guideline for the treatment of patients with schizophrenia. *Am J Psychiatry* 1997; **154 Suppl** 4:1–63.

25. Van Harten PN, et al. Acute dystonia induced by drug treatment. *Br Med J* 1999; 319:623–626.

26. Bollini P, et al. Antipsychotic drugs: is more worse? A meta-analysis of the published randomized control trials. *Psychol Med* 1994; 24:307–316.

27. Halstead SM, et al. Akathisia: prevalence and associated dysphoria in an in-patient population with chronic schizophrenia. *Br J Psychiatry* 1994; 164:177–183.

28. Martino D, et al. Movement disorders associated with antipsychotic medication in people with schizophrenia: an overview of Cochrane reviews and meta-analysis. *Can J Psychiatry* 2018; 63:706743718777392.

29. Hirose S. The causes of underdiagnosing akathisia. *Schizophr Bull* 2003; 29:547–558.

30. Juncal-Ruiz M, et al. Incidence and risk factors of acute akathisia in 493 individuals with first episode non-affective psychosis: a 6-week randomised study of antipsychotic treatment. *Psychopharmacology* 2017; 234:2563–2570.

31. Caligiuri M. Tardive Dyskinesia: a task force report of the American Psychiatric Association. *Hosp Community Psychiatry* 1993; 44:190.

32. Patterson-Lomba O, et al. Risk assessment and prediction of TD incidence in psychiatric patients taking concomitant antipsychotics: a retrospective data analysis. *BMC Neurol* 2019; 19:174.

33. Widschwendter CG, et al. Antipsychotic-induced tardive dyskinesia: update on epidemiology and management. *Curr Opin Psychiatry* 2019; 32:179–184.

34. Caroff SN, et al. Treatment outcomes of patients with tardive dyskinesia and chronic schizophrenia. *J Clin Psychiatry* 2011; 72:295–303.

35. Yasui-Furukori N, et al. The effects of electroconvulsive therapy on tardive dystonia or dyskinesia induced by psychotropic medication: a retrospective study. *Neuropsychiatr Dis Treat* 2014; 10:1209–1212.

36. Miller CH, et al. Managing antipsychotic-induced acute and chronic akathisia. *Drug Saf* 2000; 22:73–81.

37. Havaki-Kontaxaki BJ, et al. Treatment of severe neuroleptic-induced tardive torticollis. *Ann Gen Hosp Psychiatry* 2003; **2**:9.

38. Hennings JM, et al. Successful treatment of tardive lingual dystonia with botulinum toxin: case report and review of the literature. *Prog Neuropsychopharmacol Biol Psychiatry* 2008; **32**:1167–1171.

39. Pringsheim T, et al. The assessment and treatment of antipsychotic-induced akathisia. *Can J Psychiatry* 2018; **63**:719–729.

40. Poyurovsky M, et al. Efficacy of low-dose mirtazapine in neuroleptic-induced akathisia: a double-blind randomized placebo-controlled pilot study. *J Clin Psychopharmacol* 2003; **23**:305–308.

41. Salem H, et al. Revisiting antipsychotic-induced akathisia: current Issues and prospective challenges. *Curr Neuropharmacol* 2017; **15**:789–798.

42. Stryjer R, et al. Treatment of neuroleptic-induced akathisia with the 5-HT2A antagonist trazodone. *Clin Neuropharmacol* 2003; **26**:137–141.

43. Stryjer R, et al. Trazodone for the treatment of neuroleptic-induced acute akathisia: a placebo-controlled, double-blind, crossover study. *Clin Neuropharmacol* 2010; **33**:219–222.

44. Stryjer R, et al. Mianserin for the rapid improvement of chronic akathisia in a schizophrenia patient. *Eur Psychiatry* 2004; **19**:237–238.

45. Vinson DR. Diphenhydramine in the treatment of akathisia induced by prochlorperazine. *J Emerg Med* 2004; **26**:265–270.

46. Rathbone J, et al. Anticholinergics for neuroleptic-induced acute akathisia. *Cochrane Database Syst Rev* 2006; CD003727.

47. Glazer WM. Expected incidence of tardive dyskinesia associated with atypical antipsychotics. *J Clin Psychiatry* 2000; **61 Suppl 4**:21–26.

48. Kinon BJ, et al. Olanzapine treatment for tardive dyskinesia in schizophrenia patients: a prospective clinical trial with patients randomized to blinded dose reduction periods. *Prog Neuropsychopharmacol Biol Psychiatry* 2004; **28**:985–996.

49. Bai YM, et al. Risperidone for severe tardive dyskinesia: a 12-week randomized, double-blind, placebo-controlled study. *J Clin Psychiatry* 2003; **64**:1342–1348.

50. Tenback DE, et al. Effects of antipsychotic treatment on tardive dyskinesia: a 6-month evaluation of patients from the European Schizophrenia Outpatient Health Outcomes (SOHO) Study. *J Clin Psychiatry* 2005; **66**:1130–1133.

51. Woods SW, et al. Incidence of tardive dyskinesia with atypical versus conventional antipsychotic medications: a prospective cohort study. *J Clin Psychiatry* 2010; **71**:463–474.

52. Pena MS, et al. Tardive dyskinesia and other movement disorders secondary to aripiprazole. *Mov Disord* 2011; **26**:147–152.

53. Stegmayer K, et al. Tardive dyskinesia associated with atypical antipsychotics: prevalence, mechanisms and management strategies. *CNS Drugs* 2018; **32**:135–147.

54. Simpson GM. The treatment of tardive dyskinesia and tardive dystonia. *J Clin Psychiatry* 2000; **61 Suppl 4**:39–44.

55. Peritogiannis V, et al. Can atypical antipsychotics improve tardive dyskinesia associated with other atypical antipsychotics? Case report and brief review of the literature. *J Psychopharmacol* 2010; **24**:1121–1125.

56. Hauser RA, et al. KINECT 3: a phase 3 randomized, double-blind, placebo-controlled trial of valbenazine for tardive dyskinesia. *Am J Psychiatry* 2017; **174**:476–484.

57. Josiassen RC, et al. Long-term safety and tolerability of valbenazine (NBI-98854) in subjects with tardive dyskinesia and a diagnosis of schizophrenia or mood disorder. *Psychopharmacol Bull* 2017; **47**:61–68.

58. Fernandez HH, et al. Randomized controlled trial of deutetrabenazine for tardive dyskinesia: the ARM-TD study. *Neurology* 2017; **88**:2003–2010.

59. Citrome L. Deutetrabenazine for tardive dyskinesia: a systematic review of the efficacy and safety profile for this newly approved novel medication – what is the number needed to treat, number needed to harm and likelihood to be helped or harmed? *Int J Clin Pract* 2017; **71**.

60. Ricciardi L, et al. Treatment recommendations for tardive dyskinesia. *Can J Psychiatry* 2019; **64**:388–399.

61. Zhang WF, et al. Extract of ginkgo biloba treatment for tardive dyskinesia in schizophrenia: a randomized, double-blind, placebo-controlled trial. *J Clin Psychiatry* 2010.

62. Bergman H, et al. Systematic review of interventions for treating or preventing antipsychotic-induced tardive dyskinesia. *Health Technol Assess* 2017; **21**:1–218.

63. Bhidayasiri R, et al. Evidence-based guideline: treatment of tardive syndromes: report of the Guideline Development Subcommittee of the American Academy of Neurology. *Neurology* 2013; **81**:463–469.

CHAPTER 1

Akathisia

Akathisia is a relatively common adverse effect of most antipsychotic medications, although certain SGAs, including some of the recently approved antipsychotic medications, would appear to have a lower liability for the condition.[1,2] In a pooled analysis of three randomised, open-label trials,[3] the incidence of akathisia in FEP was as follows: haloperidol 57%, risperidone 20%, aripiprazole 18%, ziprasidone 17%, olanzapine 4% and quetiapine 3.5%. Lumateperone and pimavanserin are medications available only in some countries: preliminary data suggest that lumateperone may have a low liability for akathisia,[4] and pimavanserin may ameliorate haloperidol-induced akathisia.[5]

The core feature of akathisia is mental unease and dysphoria characterised by a sense of restlessness.[6,7] This is usually accompanied by observable motor restlessness, which, when severe, can cause patients to pace up and down and be unable to stay seated for more than a short time.[6,7] An association between the discomfiting subjective experience of akathisia and suicidal ideation has been postulated[8,9] but remains uncertain.

There is some evidence to suggest that akathisia may be prevented by avoiding high-dose antipsychotic medication, antipsychotic polypharmacy and rapid increase in dosage.[6,10–12] There is limited evidence on the benefit–risk balance for any pharmacological treatment for akathisia, even those most commonly used, such as switching to an antipsychotic medication with a lower liability for the condition, or adding a beta-adrenergic blocker, a 5-HT2A antagonist or anticholinergic agent.[13,14] The following diagram suggests a programme of treatment option for persistent, drug-induced akathisia.

References

1. Demyttenaere K, et al. Medication-induced akathisia with newly approved antipsychotics in patients with a severe mental illness: a systematic review and meta-analysis. *CNS Drugs* 2019; 33:549–566.
2. Chow CL, et al. Akathisia and newer second-generation antipsychotic drugs: a review of current evidence. *Pharmacotherapy* 2020; 40:565–574.
3. Juncal-Ruiz M, et al. Incidence and risk factors of acute akathisia in 493 individuals with first episode non-affective psychosis: a 6-week randomised study of antipsychotic treatment. *Psychopharmacology* 2017; 234:2563–2570.
4. Correll CU, et al. Efficacy and safety of lumateperone for treatment of schizophrenia: a randomized clinical trial. *JAMA Psychiatry* 2020; 77:349–358.
5. Abbas A, et al. Pimavanserin tartrate: a 5-HT2A inverse agonist with potential for treating various neuropsychiatric disorders. *Exp Opin Pharmacother* 2008; 9:3251–3259.
6. Braude WM, et al. Clinical characteristics of akathisia. A systematic investigation of acute psychiatric inpatient admissions. *Br J Psychiatry* 1983; 143:139–150.
7. Barnes TRE. A rating scale for drug-induced akathisia. *Br J Psychiatry* 1989; 154:672–676.
8. Seemuller F, et al. Akathisia and suicidal ideation in first-episode schizophrenia. *J Clin Psychopharmacol* 2012; 32:694–698.
9. Seemuller F, et al. The relationship of akathisia with treatment emergent suicidality among patients with first-episode schizophrenia treated with haloperidol or risperidone. *Pharmacopsychiatry* 2012; 45:292–296.
10. Miller CH, et al. Managing antipsychotic-induced acute and chronic akathisia. *Drug Saf* 2000; 22:73–81.
11. Berardi D, et al. Clinical correlates of akathisia in acute psychiatric inpatients. *Int Clin Psychopharmacol* 2000; 15:215–219.
12. Yoshimura B, et al. Incidence and predictors of acute akathisia in severely ill patients with first-episode schizophrenia treated with aripiprazole or risperidone: secondary analysis of an observational study. *Psychopharmacology* 2019; 236:723–730.
13. Pringsheim T, et al. The assessment and treatment of antipsychotic-induced akathisia. *Can J Psychiatry* 2018; 63:719–729.
14. Stroup TS, et al. Management of common adverse effects of antipsychotic medications. *World Psychiatry* 2018; 17:341–356.
15. Fleischhacker WW, et al. The pharmacologic treatment of neuroleptic-induced akathisia. *J Clin Psychopharmacol* 1990; 10:12–21.
16. Sachdev P. The identification and management of drug-induced akathisia. *CNS Drugs* 1995; 4:28–46.
17. Kumar R, et al. Akathisia and second-generation antipsychotic drugs. *Curr Opin Psychiatry* 2009; 22:293–299.
18. Miller DD, et al. Extrapyramidal side-effects of antipsychotics in a randomised trial. *Br J Psychiatry* 2008; 193:279–288.
19. Rummel-Kluge C, et al. Second-generation antipsychotic drugs and extrapyramidal side effects: a systematic review and meta-analysis of head-to-head comparisons. *Schizophr Bull* 2012; 38:167–177.
20. Kane JM, et al. Akathisia: an updated review focusing on second-generation antipsychotics. *J Clin Psychiatry* 2009; 70:627–643.

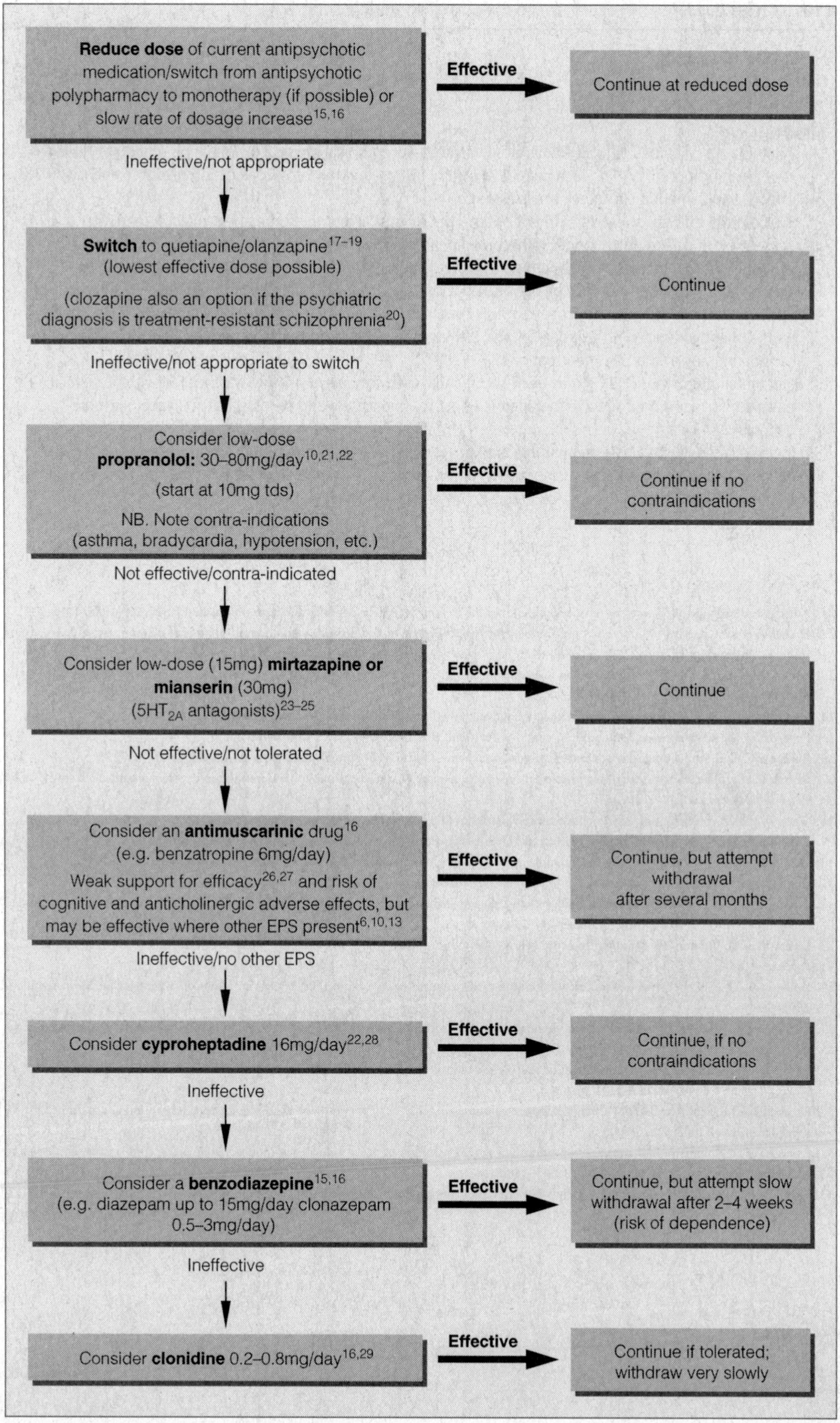

Reduce dose of current antipsychotic medication/switch from antipsychotic polypharmacy to monotherapy (if possible) or slow rate of dosage increase[15,16] — **Effective** → Continue at reduced dose

Ineffective/not appropriate

Switch to quetiapine/olanzapine[17–19] (lowest effective dose possible)

(clozapine also an option if the psychiatric diagnosis is treatment-resistant schizophrenia[20]) — **Effective** → Continue

Ineffective/not appropriate to switch

Consider low-dose **propranolol:** 30–80mg/day[10,21,22]

(start at 10mg tds)

NB. Note contra-indications (asthma, bradycardia, hypotension, etc.) — **Effective** → Continue if no contraindications

Not effective/contra-indicated

Consider low-dose (15mg) **mirtazapine or mianserin** (30mg) ($5HT_{2A}$ antagonists)[23–25] — **Effective** → Continue

Not effective/not tolerated

Consider an **antimuscarinic** drug[16] (e.g. benzatropine 6mg/day)

Weak support for efficacy[26,27] and risk of cognitive and anticholinergic adverse effects, but may be effective where other EPS present[6,10,13] — **Effective** → Continue, but attempt withdrawal after several months

Ineffective/no other EPS

Consider **cyproheptadine** 16mg/day[22,28] — **Effective** → Continue, if no contraindications

Ineffective

Consider a **benzodiazepine**[15,16] (e.g. diazepam up to 15mg/day clonazepam 0.5–3mg/day) — **Effective** → Continue, but attempt slow withdrawal after 2–4 weeks (risk of dependence)

Ineffective

Consider **clonidine** 0.2–0.8mg/day[16,29] — **Effective** → Continue if tolerated; withdraw very slowly

(Continued)

(Continued)

Notes

- Akathisia is sometimes difficult to diagnose with certainty. Clinical physical examination schedules for EPS have been proposed.[30,31] For each patient, a careful history of symptoms, medication response and side effects, and comorbid substance use is essential.
- Evaluate the efficacy of each treatment option over at least 1 month. Some effect may be seen after a few days, but it may take much longer to become apparent in those with chronic akathisia.
- Withdraw previously ineffective akathisia treatments before starting the next option in the algorithm.
- Combinations of treatment may be considered for refractory cases if carefully monitored.
- Other possible treatments for acute akathisia that have been investigated include vitamin B6,[32,33] pregabalin,[34] diphenhydramine,[35] trazodone[23,36] and zolmitriptan.[37,38] Always read the primary literature before considering any of the treatment options.
- Parenteral midazolam (1.5mg) has been successfully used to prevent akathisia associated with IV metoclopramide,[39] suggesting a specific therapeutic effect for midazolam and perhaps benzodiazepines more generally.
- In some cases where agitation/akathisia are known short-lived effects of antipsychotic medication when initiated (e.g. with aripiprazole, cariprazine), prophylactic or rescue benzodiazepines may be prescribed for a limited period. Clinical experience suggests this practice is effective.

21. Adler L, et al. A controlled assessment of propranolol in the treatment of neuroleptic-induced akathisia. *Br J Psychiatry* 1986; **149**:42–45.
22. Fischel T, et al. Cyproheptadine versus propranolol for the treatment of acute neuroleptic-induced akathisia: a comparative double-blind study. *J Clin Psychopharmacol* 2001; **21**:612–615.
23. Laoutidis ZG, et al. 5-HT2A receptor antagonists for the treatment of neuroleptic-induced akathisia: a systematic review and meta-analysis. *Int J Neuropsychopharmacol* 2014; **17**:823–832.
24. Poyurovsky M, et al. Mirtazapine – a multifunctional drug: low dose for akathisia. *CNS Spectr* 2011; **16**:63.
25. Poyurovsky M. Acute antipsychotic-induced akathisia revisited. *Br J Psychiatry* 2010; **196**:89–91.
26. Rathbone J, et al. Anticholinergics for neuroleptic-induced acute akathisia. *Cochrane Database Syst Rev* 2006; CD003727.
27. Baskak B, et al. The effectiveness of intramuscular biperiden in acute akathisia: a double-blind, randomized, placebo-controlled study. *J Clin Psychopharmacol* 2007; **27**:289–294.
28. Weiss D, et al. Cyproheptadine treatment in neuroleptic-induced akathisia. *Br J Psychiatry* 1995; **167**:483–486.
29. Zubenko GS, et al. Use of clonidine in treating neuroleptic-induced akathisia. *Psychiatry Res* 1984; **13**:253–259.
30. Gervin M, et al. Assessment of drug-related movement disorders in schizophrenia. *Adv Psychiatr Treatment* 2000; **6**:332–341.
31. Cunningham Owens DA. *Guide to the extrapyramidal side effects of antipsychotic drugs.* Cambridge University Press; 1999.
32. Miodownik C, et al. Vitamin B6 versus mianserin and placebo in acute neuroleptic-induced akathisia: a randomized, double-blind, controlled study. *Clin Neuropharmacol* 2006; **29**:68–72.
33. Lerner V, et al. Vitamin B6 treatment in acute neuroleptic-induced akathisia: a randomized, double-blind, placebo-controlled study. *J Clin Psychiatry* 2004; **65**:1550–1554.
34. De Berardis D, et al. Reversal of aripiprazole-induced tardive akathisia by addition of pregabalin. *J Neuropsychiatry Clin Neurosci* 2013; **25**:E9–E10.
35. Friedman BW, et al. A randomized trial of diphenhydramine as prophylaxis against metoclopramide-induced akathisia in nauseated emergency department patients. *Ann Emerg Med* 2009; **53**:379–385.
36. Stryjer R, et al. Trazodone for the treatment of neuroleptic-induced acute akathisia: a placebo-controlled, double-blind, crossover study. *Clin Neuropharmacol* 2010; **33**:219–222.
37. Gross-Isseroff R, et al. The 5-HT1D receptor agonist zolmitriptan for neuroleptic-induced akathisia: an open label preliminary study. *Int Clin Psychopharmacol* 2005; **20**:23–25.
38. Avital A, et al. Zolmitriptan compared to propranolol in the treatment of acute neuroleptic-induced akathisia: a comparative double-blind study. *Eur Neuropsychopharmacol* 2009; **19**:476–482.
39. Erdur B, et al. A trial of midazolam vs diphenhydramine in prophylaxis of metoclopramide-induced akathisia. *Am J Emerg Med* 2012; **30**:84–91.

Treatment of tardive dyskinesia

Tardive dyskinesia (TD) is a somewhat less commonly encountered problem now than in previous decades,[1,2] probably because of the introduction and widespread use of SGAs,[3-6] which generally have a lower risk for the condition than FGAs. Treatment of established TD is often unsuccessful, so prevention, early detection and early treatment are essential.[7,8] There is evidence to suggest that TD is associated with greater cognitive impairment,[7,9] more severe psychopathology[10,11] and higher mortality.[12,13]

While SGAs are less likely to cause TD,[14-19] the condition does occur with these medications, with an overall estimated incidence of nearly 4%,[18] although the liability varies across the individual the SGA medications.[20-23] One meta-analysis estimated the yearly risk of TD in those on FGAs to be 3.7–12.5% (depending on the drug) and 1.7–4.8% with SGAs.[24] The risk of developing TD may be related to the extent of D2 receptor occupancy (greater occupancy, higher risk) with a medication.[25] However, data from an extensive meta-analysis of relevant RCTs did not support the notion that the lower risk of TD with SGAs compared with FGAs is related to the use of high dosage of the latter.[24] There is a hint that dopamine partial agonists (or at least aripiprazole) may have the lowest rate of TD.[24] Whether the risk of TD differs between FGA and SGA LAI preparations is unclear,[26] but it might be assumed that lower rates are likely with SGA LAIs.

TD can occur with low doses of haloperidol (and in the absence of prior acute movement disorder[27]) and following the use of other dopamine antagonists such as metoclopramide.[28]

TD has also been observed in never-medicated patients with both first-episode[29,30] and established[31] schizophrenia.

Treatment – first steps

Most authorities recommend the withdrawal of any co-prescribed anticholinergic agents and a reduction in the dose of antipsychotic medication as initial steps in those with early signs of TD[32,33] (although dose reduction can initially worsen TD). Cochrane, however, found little support for dose reduction[34] or anticholinergic withdrawal[35] and the American Academy of Neurology does not recommend dose reduction.[36] Nevertheless, it is common practice to withdraw the antipsychotic medication prescribed when TD is first observed and to substitute another, which is perceived to have a lower liability for the condition. However, the evidence for benefit in switching to any particular SGA is limited.[36] The use of clozapine[32,37] is probably best supported in this regard, but quetiapine, another weak striatal dopamine antagonist, may also be effective,[38-44] and olanzapine[39-42,45,46] and aripiprazole[47] are further potential options. There are a few supporting data for risperidone,[48] but this would not a logical choice in a patient with established TD, given that risperidone is more likely than clozapine, olanzapine and quetiapine to be associated with acute movement disorder.

Treatment – additional agents

Given that there is insufficient evidence to recommend dose reduction as a treatment for TD, and that switching or withdrawing antipsychotic medication is not always effective or advisable, additional agents are often used. A 2020 meta-analysis[49] found clear benefit only for the three licensed VMAT-2 inhibitors, vitamin E, amantadine and vitamin B6 (pyridoxine). Table 1.15 describes the most frequently prescribed add-on drugs for TD.

Table 1.15 First-choice agents (alphabetical order; no preference implied)

Drug	Comments
Amantadine[49–52]	Rarely used but apparently effective at 100–300mg a day
Benzodiazepines[32,33]	Widely used for TD, but Cochrane review considered that the limited evidence for efficacy is inconclusive.[53] Intermittent use may be necessary to avoid tolerance to effects. Most commonly used are clonazepam 1–4mg/day and diazepam 6–25mg/day, with better supporting evidence for the former[36,54]
Deutetrabenazine[8,52,55–57]	Deutetrabenazine (VMAT-2 inhibitor) is also effective as a treatment for TD. Licensed for TD in the USA.[58] Better supporting evidence than for tetrabenazine. Longer half-life than tetrabenazine but still needs to be taken twice a day. Low incidence of psychiatric and neurological effects. Dose is 12–48mg/day
Ginkgo biloba[52,59]	Well tolerated. Cochrane review concluded that while Ginkgo biloba could reduce TD symptoms, the available evidence did not justify its routine use as a treatment.[60] A meta-analysis of three Chinese RCTs showed a good effect with 240mg/day[61]
Pyridoxine[62]	Supported by Cochrane[63] and a meta-analysis.[49] Dose – up to 400mg/day
Tetrabenazine[64,65]	Only licensed treatment for moderate to severe TD in UK. Depression, drowsiness, parkinsonism and akathisia may occur.[54,66] Dose is 25–200mg/day. Reserpine (similar mode of action) also effective but rarely, if ever, used
Valbenazine[8,56,60,67–70]	The evidence supports a favourable benefit-risk ratio for valbenazine (VMAT-2 inhibitor) as a treatment for TD. Licensed for TD in the USA.[71] A dose of 80mg once daily is effective with a benign cardiovascular profile. Low incidence of depression and akathisia
Vitamin E[49,72]	Numerous studies but efficacy remains to be conclusively established. Cochrane suggest that there is evidence only for slowing deterioration of TD.[8,73] Dose is in the range 400–1600 IU/day

Treatment – other possible options

The large number of proposed treatments for TD undoubtedly reflects the somewhat limited effectiveness of standard remedies, at least before the introduction of valbenazine and deutetrabenazine. Table 1.16 lists some of these putative treatments in alphabetical order.

Table 1.16 Other options for the treatment of TD

Drug	Comments
Amino acids[74]	Use is supported by a small randomised, placebo-controlled trial. Low risk of toxicity
Botulinum toxin[75–78]	Case reports of success for localised dyskinesia. Probably now treatment of choice for disabling or distressing focal symptoms
Calcium antagonists[79]	A few published studies but not widely used. Cochrane is dismissive.[80] A meta-analysis found no effect[49]
Donepezil[81–83]	Supported by a single open study and case series. One negative RCT ($n = 12$). Dose is 10mg/day. No clear evidence of efficacy for rivastigmine or galantamine[84]
Fish oils[85,86]	Very limited support for the use of EPA at dose of 2g/day
Fluvoxamine[87]	Three case reports. Dose is 100mg/day. Beware of interactions
Gabapentin[88]	Adds weight to theory that GABAergic mechanisms improve TD. Dose is 900–1200mg/day. Inconclusive data on other GABA agonists[89]
Levetiracetam[90–93]	Three published case studies. One RCT. Dose up to 3000mg/day
Melatonin[94]	Use is supported by a meta-analysis of four trials.[95] Usually well tolerated. Dose is 10mg/day. Some evidence that melatonin receptor genotype determines risk of TD[96]
Naltrexone[97]	May be effective when added to benzodiazepines. Well tolerated. Dose is 200mg/day
Ondansetron[98,99]	Limited evidence but low toxicity. Dose – up to 12mg/day
Propranolol[100–102]	Formerly a relatively widely used treatment. Open-label studies only and a prospective randomized trial is probably warranted. Dose is 40–120mg/day. Beware of contra-indications (asthma, bradycardia, hypotension)
Quercetin[103]	Plant compound which is thought to be an antioxidant. Some promising case reports[103–105]
Sodium oxybate[106]	One case report. Dose was 8g/day
Repetitive transcranial magnetic stimulation (rTMS)[107,108]	RCT data on patients with 'tardive syndromes' suggest the potential for bilateral hemispheric high frequency rTMS to be a feasible treatment where TD is unresponsive to 'first-line' medical treatment[107]
Zolpidem[109]	Three case reports. Dose 10–30mg a day

References

1. Merrill RM, et al. Tardive and spontaneous dyskinesia incidence in the general population. *BMC Psychiatry* 2013; **13**:152.

2. Kane JM, et al. Tardive dyskinesia: prevalence, incidence, and risk factors. *J Clin Psychopharmacol* 1988; **8**:52s–56s.

3. De Leon J. The effect of atypical versus typical antipsychotics on tardive dyskinesia: a naturalistic study. *Eur Arch Psychiatry Clin Neurosci* 2007; **257**:169–172.

4. Halliday J, et al. Nithsdale Schizophrenia Surveys 23: movement disorders. 20-year review. *Br J Psychiatry* 2002; **181**:422–427.

5. Kane JM. Tardive dyskinesia circa 2006. *Am J Psychiatry* 2006; **163**:1316–1318.

6. Eberhard J, et al. Tardive dyskinesia and antipsychotics: a 5-year longitudinal study of frequency, correlates and course. *Int Clin Psychopharmacol* 2006; **21**:35–42.

7. Wu JQ, et al. Tardive dyskinesia is associated with greater cognitive impairment in schizophrenia. *Prog Neuropsychopharmacol Biol Psychiatry* 2013; **46**:71–77.

8. Ricciardi L, et al. Treatment recommendations for tardive dyskinesia. *Can J Psychiatry* 2019; **64**:388–399.

9. Strassnig M, et al. Tardive dyskinesia: motor system impairments, cognition and everyday functioning. *CNS Spectr* 2018; **23**:370–377.

10. Yuen O, et al. Tardive dyskinesia and positive and negative symptoms of schizophrenia. A study using instrumental measures. *Br J Psychiatry* 1996; **168**:702–708.

11. Ascher-Svanum H, et al. Tardive dyskinesia and the 3-year course of schizophrenia: results from a large, prospective, naturalistic study. *J Clin Psychiatry* 2008; **69**:1580–1588.

12. Dean CE, et al. Mortality and tardive dyskinesia: long-term study using the US National Death Index. *Br J Psychiatry* 2009; **194**:360–364.

13. Chong SA, et al. Mortality rates among patients with schizophrenia and tardive dyskinesia. *J Clin Psychopharmacol* 2009; **29**:5–8.

14. Beasley C, et al. Randomised double-blind comparison of the incidence of tardive dyskinesia in patients with schizophrenia during long-term treatment with olanzapine or haloperidol. *Br J Psychiatry* 1999; **174**:23–30.

15. Glazer WM. Expected incidence of tardive dyskinesia associated with atypical antipsychotics. *J Clin Psychiatry* 2000; **61 Suppl 4**:21–26.

16. Correll CU, et al. Lower risk for tardive dyskinesia associated with second-generation antipsychotics: a systematic review of 1-year studies. *Am J Psychiatry* 2004; **161**:414–425.

17. Dolder CR, et al. Incidence of tardive dyskinesia with typical versus atypical antipsychotics in very high risk patients. *Biol Psychiatry* 2003; **53**:1142–1145.

18. Correll CU, et al. Tardive dyskinesia and new antipsychotics. *Curr Opin Psychiatry* 2008; **21**:151–156.

19. Carbon M, et al. Tardive dyskinesia prevalence in the period of second-generation antipsychotic use: a meta-analysis. *J Clin Psychiatry* 2017; **78**:e264–e278.

20. Keck ME, et al. Ziprasidone-related tardive dyskinesia (Letter). *Am J Psychiatry* 2004; **161**:175–176.

21. Maytal G, et al. Aripiprazole-related tardive dyskinesia. *CNS Spectr* 2006; **11**:435–439.

22. Fountoulakis KN, et al. Amisulpride-induced tardive dyskinesia. *Schizophr Res* 2006; **88**:232–234.

23. Sachdev P. Early extrapyramidal side-effects as risk factors for later tardive dyskinesia: a prospective study. *Aust N Z J Psychiatry* 2004; **38**:445–449.

24. Carbon M, et al. Tardive dyskinesia risk with first- and second-generation antipsychotics in comparative randomized controlled trials: a meta-analysis. *World Psychiatry* 2018; **17**:330–340.

25. Yoshida K, et al. Tardive dyskinesia in relation to estimated dopamine D2 receptor occupancy in patients with schizophrenia: analysis of the CATIE data. *Schizophr Res* 2014; **153**:184–188.

26. Saucedo Uribe E, et al. Preliminary efficacy and tolerability profiles of first versus second-generation long-acting injectable antipsychotics in schizophrenia: a systematic review and meta-analysis. *J Psychiatr Res* 2020; **129**:222–233.

27. Oosthuizen PP, et al. Incidence of tardive dyskinesia in first-episode psychosis patients treated with low-dose haloperidol. *J Clin Psychiatry* 2003; **64**:1075–1080.

28. Kenney C, et al. Metoclopramide, an increasingly recognized cause of tardive dyskinesia. *J Clin Pharmacol* 2008; **48**:379–384.

29. Pappa S, et al. Spontaneous movement disorders in antipsychotic-naive patients with first-episode psychoses: a systematic review. *Psychol Med* 2009; **39**:1065–1076.

30. Puri BK, et al. Spontaneous dyskinesia in first episode schizophrenia. *J Neurol Neurosurg Psychiatry* 1999; **66**:76–78.

31. McCreadie RG, et al. Spontaneous dyskinesia and parkinsonism in never-medicated, chronically ill patients with schizophrenia: 18-month follow-up. *Br J Psychiatry* 2002; **181**:135–137.

32. Duncan D, et al. Tardive dyskinesia: how is it prevented and treated? *Psychiatric Bull* 1997; **21**:422–425.

33. Simpson GM. The treatment of tardive dyskinesia and tardive dystonia. *J Clin Psychiatry* 2000; **61 Suppl 4**:39–44.

34. Bergman H, et al. Antipsychotic reduction and/or cessation and antipsychotics as specific treatments for tardive dyskinesia. *Cochrane Database Syst Rev* 2018; **2**:Cd000459.

35. Bergman H, et al. Anticholinergic medication for antipsychotic-induced tardive dyskinesia. *Cochrane Database Syst Rev* 2018; **1**:Cd000204.

36. Bhidayasiri R, et al. Evidence-based guideline: treatment of tardive syndromes: report of the Guideline Development Subcommittee of the American Academy of Neurology. *Neurology* 2013; **81**:463–469.

37. Pardis P, et al. Clozapine and tardive dyskinesia in patients with schizophrenia: a systematic review. *J Psychopharmacology* 2019; **33**:1187–1198.

38. Vesely C, et al. Remission of severe tardive dyskinesia in a schizophrenic patient treated with the atypical antipsychotic substance quetiapine. *Int Clin Psychopharmacol* 2000; **15**:57–60.

39. Alptekin K, et al. Quetiapine-induced improvement of tardive dyskinesia in three patients with schizophrenia. *Int Clin Psychopharmacol* 2002; 17:263–264.

40. Nelson MW, et al. Adjunctive quetiapine decreases symptoms of tardive dyskinesia in a patient taking risperidone. *Clin Neuropharmacol* 2003; 26:297–298.

41. Emsley R, et al. A single-blind, randomized trial comparing quetiapine and haloperidol in the treatment of tardive dyskinesia. *J Clin Psychiatry* 2004; 65:696–701.

42. Bressan RA, et al. Atypical antipsychotic drugs and tardive dyskinesia: relevance of D2 receptor affinity. *J Psychopharmacology* 2004; 18:124–127.

43. Sacchetti E, et al. Quetiapine, clozapine, and olanzapine in the treatment of tardive dyskinesia induced by first-generation antipsychotics: a 124-week case report. *Int Clin Psychopharmacol* 2003; 18:357–359.

44. Gourzis P, et al. Quetiapine in the treatment of focal tardive dystonia induced by other atypical antipsychotics: a report of 2 cases. *Clin Neuropharmacol* 2005; 28:195–196.

45. Soutullo CA, et al. Olanzapine in the treatment of tardive dyskinesia: a report of two cases. *J Clin Psychopharmacol* 1999; 19:100–101.

46. Kinon BJ, et al. Olanzapine treatment for tardive dyskinesia in schizophrenia patients: a prospective clinical trial with patients randomized to blinded dose reduction periods. *Prog Neuropsychopharmacol Biol Psychiatry* 2004; 28:985–996.

47. Chan CH, et al. Switching antipsychotic treatment to aripiprazole in psychotic patients with neuroleptic-induced tardive dyskinesia: a 24-week follow-up study. *Int Clin Psychopharmacol* 2018; 33:155–162.

48. Bai YM, et al. Risperidone for severe tardive dyskinesia: a 12-week randomized, double-blind, placebo-controlled study. *J Clin Psychiatry* 2003; 64:1342–1348.

49. Artukoglu BB, et al. Pharmacologic treatment of tardive dyskinesia: a meta-analysis and systematic review. *J Clin Psychiatry* 2020; 81:19r12798.

50. Angus S, et al. A controlled trial of amantadine hydrochloride and neuroleptics in the treatment of tardive dyskinesia. *J Clin Psychopharmacol* 1997; 17:88–91.

51. Pappa S, et al. Effects of amantadine on tardive dyskinesia: a randomized, double-blind, placebo-controlled study. *Clin Neuropharmacol* 2010; 33:271–275.

52. Bhidayasiri R, et al. Updating the recommendations for treatment of tardive syndromes: a systematic review of new evidence and practical treatment algorithm. *J Neurol Sci* 2018; 389:67–75.

53. Bergman H, et al. Benzodiazepines for antipsychotic-induced tardive dyskinesia. *Cochrane Database Syst Rev* 2018; 1:Cd000205.

54. Rana AQ, et al. New and emerging treatments for symptomatic tardive dyskinesia. *Drug Des Devel Ther* 2013; 7:1329–1340.

55. Cummings MA, et al. Deuterium tetrabenazine for tardive dyskinesia. *Clin Schizophr Relat Psychoses* 2018; 11:214–220.

56. Solmi M, et al. Treatment of tardive dyskinesia with VMAT-2 inhibitors: a systematic review and meta-analysis of randomized controlled trials. *Drug Des Devel Ther* 2018; 12:1215–1238.

57. Claassen DO, et al. Deutetrabenazine for tardive dyskinesia and chorea associated with Huntington's disease: a review of clinical trial data. *Exp Opin Pharmacother* 2019; 20:2209–2221.

58. Citrome L. Deutetrabenazine for tardive dyskinesia: a systematic review of the efficacy and safety profile for this newly approved novel medication – what is the number needed to treat, number needed to harm and likelihood to be helped or harmed? *Int J Clin Pract* 2017; 71:e13030.

59. Zhang WF, et al. Extract of Ginkgo biloba treatment for tardive dyskinesia in schizophrenia: a randomized, double-blind, placebo-controlled trial. *J Clin Psychiatry* 2011; 72:615–621.

60. Soares-Weiser K, et al. Miscellaneous treatments for antipsychotic-induced tardive dyskinesia. *Cochrane Database Syst Rev* 2018; 3:Cd000208.

61. Zheng W, et al. Extract of Ginkgo biloba for tardive dyskinesia: meta-analysis of randomized controlled trials. *Pharmacopsychiatry* 2016; 49:107–111.

62. Lerner V, et al. Vitamin B(6) in the treatment of tardive dyskinesia: a double-blind, placebo-controlled, crossover study. *Am J Psychiatry* 2001; 158:1511–1514.

63. Adelufosi AO, et al. Pyridoxal 5 phosphate for neuroleptic-induced tardive dyskinesia. *Cochrane Database Syst Rev* 2015.

64. Jankovic J, et al. Long-term effects of tetrabenazine in hyperkinetic movement disorders. *Neurology* 1997; 48:358–362.

65. Leung JG, et al. Tetrabenazine for the treatment of tardive dyskinesia. *Ann Pharmacother* 2011; 45:525–531.

66. Kenney C, et al. Long-term tolerability of tetrabenazine in the treatment of hyperkinetic movement disorders. *Mov Disord* 2007; 22:193–197.

67. Hauser RA, et al. KINECT 3: a phase 3 randomized, double-blind, placebo-controlled trial of valbenazine for tardive dyskinesia. *Am J Psychiatry* 2017; 174:476–484.

68. Kane JM, et al. Efficacy of valbenazine (NBI-98854) in treating subjects with tardive dyskinesia and schizophrenia or schizoaffective disorder. *Psychopharmacol Bull* 2017; 47:69–76.

69. Josiassen RC, et al. Long-term safety and tolerability of valbenazine (NBI-98854) in subjects with tardive dyskinesia and a diagnosis of schizophrenia or mood disorder. *Psychopharmacol Bull* 2017; 47:61–68.

70. Lindenmayer JP, et al. A long-term, open-label study of valbenazine for tardive dyskinesia. *CNS Spectr* 2020: [Epub ahead of print].

71. Citrome LL. Medication Options and Clinical Strategies for Treating Tardive Dyskinesia. *J Clin Psychiatry* 2020; 81:TV18059BR18052C.

72. Zhang XY, et al. The effect of vitamin E treatment on tardive dyskinesia and blood superoxide dismutase: a double-blind placebo-controlled trial. *J Clin Psychopharmacol* 2004; 24:83–86.

73. Soares-Weiser K, et al. Vitamin E for antipsychotic-induced tardive dyskinesia. *Cochrane Database Syst Rev* 2018; 1:Cd000209.

74. Richardson MA, et al. Efficacy of the branched-chain amino acids in the treatment of tardive dyskinesia in men. *Am J Psychiatry* 2003; **160**:1117–1124.

75. Tarsy D, et al. An open-label study of botulinum toxin A for treatment of tardive dystonia. *Clin Neuropharmacol* 1997; **20**:90–93.

76. Brashear A, et al. Comparison of treatment of tardive dystonia and idiopathic cervical dystonia with botulinum toxin type A. *Mov Disord* 1998; **13**:158–161.

77. Hennings JM, et al. Successful treatment of tardive lingual dystonia with botulinum toxin: case report and review of the literature. *Prog Neuropsychopharmacol Biol Psychiatry* 2008; **32**:1167–1171.

78. Beckmann YY, et al. Treatment of intractable tardive lingual dyskinesia with botulinum toxin. *J Clin Psychopharmacol* 2011; **31**:250–251.

79. Essali A, et al. Calcium channel blockers for neuroleptic-induced tardive dyskinesia. *Cochrane Database Syst Rev* 2011; Cd000206.

80. Essali A, et al. Calcium channel blockers for antipsychotic-induced tardive dyskinesia. *Cochrane Database Syst Rev* 2018; 3:Cd000206.

81. Caroff SN, et al. Treatment of tardive dyskinesia with donepezil. *J Clin Psychiatry* 2001; **62**:128–129.

82. Bergman J, et al. Beneficial effect of donepezil in the treatment of elderly patients with tardive movement disorders. *J Clin Psychiatry* 2005; **66**:107–110.

83. Ogunmefun A, et al. Effect of donepezil on tardive dyskinesia. *J Clin Psychopharmacol* 2009; **29**:102–104.

84. Tammenmaa-Aho I, et al. Cholinergic medication for antipsychotic-induced tardive dyskinesia. *Cochrane Database Syst Rev* 2018; 3:Cd000207.

85. Emsley R, et al. The effects of eicosapentaenoic acid in tardive dyskinesia: a randomized, placebo-controlled trial. *Schizophr Res* 2006; **84**:112–120.

86. Vaddadi K, et al. Tardive dyskinesia and essential fatty acids. *Int Rev Psychiatry* 2006; **18**:133–143.

87. Albayrak Y, et al. Beneficial effects of sigma-1 agonist fluvoxamine for tardive dyskinesia and tardive akathisia in patients with schizophrenia: report of three cases. *Psychiatry Investig* 2013; **10**:417–420.

88. Hardoy MC, et al. Gabapentin in antipsychotic-induced tardive dyskinesia: results of 1-year follow-up. *J Affect Disord* 2003; **75**:125–130.

89. Alabed S, et al. Gamma-aminobutyric acid agonists for antipsychotic-induced tardive dyskinesia. *Cochrane Database Syst Rev* 2018; 4:Cd000203.

90. McGavin CL, et al. Levetiracetam as a treatment for tardive dyskinesia: a case report. *Neurology* 2003; **61**:419.

91. Meco G, et al. Levetiracetam in tardive dyskinesia. *Clin Neuropharmacol* 2006; **29**:265–268.

92. Woods SW, et al. Effects of levetiracetam on tardive dyskinesia: a randomized, double-blind, placebo-controlled study. *J Clin Psychiatry* 2008; **69**:546–554.

93. Chen PH, et al. Rapid improvement of neuroleptic-induced tardive dyskinesia with levetiracetam in an interictal psychotic patient. *J Clin Psychopharmacol* 2010; **30**:205–207.

94. Shamir E, et al. Melatonin treatment for tardive dyskinesia: a double-blind, placebo-controlled, crossover study. *Arch Gen Psychiatry* 2001; **58**:1049–1052.

95. Sun CH, et al. Adjunctive melatonin for tardive dyskinesia in patients with schizophrenia: a meta-analysis. *Shanghai Arch Psychiatry* 2017; **29**:129–136.

96. Lai IC, et al. Analysis of genetic variations in the human melatonin receptor (MTNR1A, MTNR1B) genes and antipsychotics-induced tardive dyskinesia in schizophrenia. *World J Biol Psychiatry* 2011; **12**:143–148.

97. Wonodi I, et al. Naltrexone treatment of tardive dyskinesia in patients with schizophrenia. *J Clin Psychopharmacol* 2004; **24**:441–445.

98. Sirota P, et al. Use of the selective serotonin 3 receptor antagonist ondansetron in the treatment of neuroleptic-induced tardive dyskinesia. *Am J Psychiatry* 2000; **157**:287–289.

99. Naidu PS, et al. Reversal of neuroleptic-induced orofacial dyskinesia by 5-HT3 receptor antagonists. *Eur J Pharmacol* 2001; **420**:113–117.

100. Perenyi A, et al. Propranolol in the treatment of tardive dyskinesia. *Biol Psychiatry* 1983; **18**:391–394.

101. Pitts FN, Jr. Treatment of tardive dyskinesia with propranolol. *J Clin Psychiatry* 1982; **43**:304.

102. Hatcher-Martin JM, et al. Propranolol therapy for Tardive dyskinesia: a retrospective examination. *Parkinsonism Relat Disord* 2016; **32**:124–126.

103. Naidu PS, et al. Reversal of haloperidol-induced orofacial dyskinesia by quercetin, a bioflavonoid. *Psychopharmacology* 2003; **167**:418–423.

104. Naidu PS, et al. Quercetin, a bioflavonoid, attenuates haloperidol-induced orofacial dyskinesia. *Neuropharmacology* 2003; **44**:1100–1106.

105. Naidu PS, et al. Reversal of reserpine-induced orofacial dyskinesia and cognitive dysfunction by quercetin. *Pharmacology* 2004; **70**:59–67.

106. Berner JE. A case of sodium oxybate treatment of tardive dyskinesia and bipolar disorder. *J Clin Psychiatry* 2008; **69**:862.

107. Khedr EM, et al. Repetitive transcranial magnetic stimulation for treatment of tardive syndromes: double randomized clinical trial. *J Neur Trans* 2019; **126**:183–191.

108. Brambilla P, et al. Transient improvement of tardive dyskinesia induced with rTMS. *Neurology* 2003; **61**:1155.

109. Waln O, et al. Zolpidem improves tardive dyskinesia and akathisia. *Mov Disord* 2013; **28**:1748–1749.

Antipsychotic-induced weight gain

Weight gain, a cardiometabolic risk factor, is a common side effect of antipsychotic medication.[1] The mechanisms underlying antipsychotic-induced weight gain are not well understood,[2] although factors such as $5HT_{2C}$ antagonism, H_1 antagonism, D_2 antagonism, and increased serum leptin (leading to leptin desensitisation)[3-5] are commonly implicated. There is no evidence that these medications exert any direct metabolic effect: weight gain seems to result from increased food intake and, in some cases, reduced energy expenditure.[6,7] The risk of weight gain appears to be related to clinical response[8,9] (although the association may be too small to be clinically important[10]), which may have a genetic basis.[11] Weight gain may be more pronounced in antipsychotic-naïve patients and during the early stages of the treatment of psychotic illness,[12-14] and women may be at greater risk than men.[15,16]

Almost all available antipsychotic medications have been associated with weight gain,[12] although the mean gain in body weight varies substantially between the medications. There is also marked inter-individual variation among those treated, with some losing weight, some gaining no weight and some gaining a great deal of weight. Thus, knowledge of the mean increase in weight reported for a particular medication may not be a helpful predictor of how much weight an individual might gain. Assessment of the relative liability for weight gain of different antipsychotic medications is based largely on short term studies. Notwithstanding these limitations, the results of indirect and direct meta-analyses suggest that these medications can be clustered into three groups based on their relative risk of weight gain[17] (see Table 1.17).

Table 1.17 Antipsychotic-induced weight gain[18-25]

Drug	Risk/extent of weight gain
Clozapine	**High**
Olanzapine	
Chlorpromazine	**Moderate**
Iloperidone	
Sertindole	
Quetiapine	
Risperidone	
Paliperidone	
Amisulpride	**Low**
Asenapine	
Brexpiprazole	
Aripiprazole	
Cariprazine	
Haloperidol	
Lumateperone	
Lurasidone	
Sulpiride	
Trifluoperazine	
Ziprasidone	

See the following section for advice on the management of antipsychotic-induced weight gain.

References

1. Barton BB, et al. Update on weight-gain caused by antipsychotics: a systematic review and meta-analysis. *Exp Opin Drug Saf* 2020; 19:295–314.
2. Correll CU, et al. Antipsychotic drugs and obesity. *Trends Mol Med* 2011; 17:97–107.
3. Nielsen MO, et al. Striatal reward activity and antipsychotic-associated weight change in patients with schizophrenia undergoing initial treatment. *JAMA Psychiatry* 2016; 73:121–128.
4. Ragguett RM, et al. Association between antipsychotic treatment and leptin levels across multiple psychiatric populations: an updated meta-analysis. *Human Psychopharmacology* 2017; 32:e2631.
5. Reynolds GP, et al. Mechanisms underlying metabolic disturbances associated with psychosis and antipsychotic drug treatment. *J Psychopharmacology* 2017; 269881117722987.
6. Benarroch L, et al. Atypical antipsychotics and effects on feeding: from mice to men. *Psychopharmacology* 2016; 233:2629–2653.
7. Cuerda C, et al. The effects of second-generation antipsychotics on food intake, resting energy expenditure and physical activity. *Eur J Clin Nutr* 2014; 68:146–152.
8. Sharma E, et al. Association between antipsychotic-induced metabolic side-effects and clinical improvement: a review on the Evidence for 'metabolic threshold'. *Asian J Psychiatr* 2014; 8:12–21.
9. Garcia-Rizo C. Antipsychotic-induced weight gain and clinical improvement: a psychiatric paradox. *Frontiers in Psychiatry* 2020; 11:560006.
10. Hermes E, et al. The association between weight change and symptom reduction in the CATIE schizophrenia trial. *Schizophr Res* 2011; 128:166–170.
11. Zhang JP, et al. Pharmacogenetic associations of antipsychotic drug-related weight gain: a systematic review and meta-analysis. *Schizophr Bull* 2016; 42:1418–1437.
12. Bak M, et al. Almost all antipsychotics result in weight gain: a meta-analysis. *PLoS One* 2014; 9:e94112.
13. McEvoy JP, et al. Efficacy and tolerability of olanzapine, quetiapine, and risperidone in the treatment of early psychosis: a randomized, double-blind 52-week comparison. *Am J Psychiatry* 2007; 164:1050–1060.
14. Foley DL, et al. Cardiometabolic risk indicators that distinguish adults with psychosis from the general population, by age and gender. *PLoS One* 2013; 8:e82606.
15. Seeman MV. Secondary effects of antipsychotics: women at greater risk than men. *Schizophr Bull* 2009; 35:937–948.
16. Santini I, et al. The metabolic syndrome in an Italian psychiatric sample: a retrospective chart review of inpatients treated with antipsychotics. *Riv Psichiatr* 2016; 51:37–42.
17. Cooper SJ, et al. BAP guidelines on the management of weight gain, metabolic disturbances and cardiovascular risk associated with psychosis and antipsychotic drug treatment. *J Psychopharmacology* 2016; 30:717–748.
18. Rummel-Kluge C, et al. Head-to-head comparisons of metabolic side effects of second generation antipsychotics in the treatment of schizophrenia: a systematic review and meta-analysis. *Schizophr Res* 2010; 123:225–233.
19. Leucht S, et al. Comparative efficacy and tolerability of 15 antipsychotic drugs in schizophrenia: a multiple-treatments meta-analysis. *Lancet* 2013; 382:951–962.
20. Cutler AJ, et al. Long-term safety and tolerability of iloperidone: results from a 25-week, open-label extension trial. *CNSSpectr* 2013; 18:43–54.
21. McEvoy JP, et al. Effectiveness of paliperidone palmitate vs haloperidol decanoate for maintenance treatment of schizophrenia: a randomized clinical trial. *JAMA* 2014; 311:1978–1987.
22. Lao KS, et al. Tolerability and safety profile of cariprazine in treating psychotic disorders, bipolar disorder and major depressive disorder: a systematic review with meta-analysis of randomized controlled trials. *CNS Drugs* 2016; 30:1043–1054.
23. Leucht S, et al. Sixty years of placebo-controlled antipsychotic drug trials in acute schizophrenia: systematic review, Bayesian meta-analysis, and meta-regression of efficacy predictors. *Am J Psychiatry* 2017; 174:927–942.
24. Garay RP, et al. Therapeutic improvements expected in the near future for schizophrenia and schizoaffective disorder: an appraisal of phase III clinical trials of schizophrenia-targeted therapies as found in US and EU clinical trial registries. *Exp Opin Pharmacother* 2016; 17:921–936.
25. Musil R, et al. Weight gain and antipsychotics: a drug safety review. *Exp Opin Drug Saf* 2015; 14:73–96.

Treatment of antipsychotic-induced weight gain

Weight gain is an important adverse effect of nearly all antipsychotic medications with obvious consequences for self-image, morbidity and mortality. Prevention and treatment are therefore matters of some clinical urgency.

Monitoring

Patients starting antipsychotic treatment or changing medication should, as an absolute minimum, be weighed and their weight clearly recorded. Ideally, body mass index (BMI) and waist circumference should also be recorded.[1,2] Early in treatment, monitoring of body weight every week or two is recommended, for at least the first six months.[2,3] Rapid weight gain in early treatment (e.g. an increase of ≥ 5% above baseline after a month of treatment) strongly predicts long-term weight gain and should prompt consideration of preventative or remedial measures.[4-6] With continuing antipsychotic treatment, annual measurement of body weight is recommended as a minimum.[2,3,7]

In clinical practice, the monitoring of body weight and other metabolic side effects in people on continuing antipsychotic medication is inconsistent and limited, falling short of recommended best practice.[8-13]

Treatment and prevention

Most of the relevant literature in this area addresses attempts to reduce body weight gained during treatment with medication, although there are now useful data suggesting that early interventions can prevent or mitigate weight gain.[14,15]

When weight gain occurs, initial options involve switching medications or instituting behavioural programmes (or both). Switching always presents a risk of relapse and treatment discontinuation,[16] but there is fairly strong support for switching to aripiprazole,[17,18] ziprasidone[19-21] or lurasidone[22,23] as a method for reversing weight gain. It is possible that switching to other antipsychotic medications with a low propensity for weight gain can also be beneficial.[2,24,25] Another option is adjunctive aripiprazole: weight loss has been observed when aripiprazole has been added to antipsychotic medications such as clozapine and olanzapine.[15,26]

Stopping antipsychotic treatment altogether can be associated with weight loss,[27,28] but this course of action would not be clinically appropriate for the vast majority of people with multi-episode schizophrenia. Note that, while some switching and augmentation strategies may minimise further weight gain or facilitate weight loss, the overall effect is generally modest and many patients continue to be overweight. Additional lifestyle interventions are often required if BMI is to remain within or move towards the normal range.

A variety of lifestyle interventions has been proposed and evaluated with good results.[2,14,29-32] Interventions vary, but they are mainly 'behavioural lifestyle programmes' aimed at improving diet and increasing physical activity. Meta-analyses of RCTs have shown a robust effect for both prevention and intervention with these non-pharmacological interventions.[14,30]

Pharmacological methods should be considered only where behavioural treatment strategies or switching to a medication with a lower liability for weight gain have failed or where obesity presents a clear, immediate physical risk to the patient. Some drug treatment options for antipsychotic-induced weight gain are listed (in alphabetical order) in Table 1.18. Some treatments recommended in previous editions (e.g., H_2 antagonists) have been removed from this table because evidence no longer supports their use.

Metformin is now probably considered to be the drug of choice for the prevention and treatment of antipsychotic-induced weight gain, although GLP-1 agonists may ultimately prove more effective and better tolerated. Bariatric surgery may have a role in a few of the rare, severe cases where all else has failed;[33] however, the efficacy of bariatric surgery for drug-induced weight gain is not known.[2]

Table 1.18 Drug treatment of antipsychotic-induced weight gain (alphabetical order)

Drug	Comments
Amantadine[34,35] (100–300mg/day)	May attenuate olanzapine-related weight gain. Seems to be well tolerated apart from insomnia and abdominal discomfort. May (theoretically, at least) exacerbate psychosis. Evidence base too limited to recommend[2]
Alpha-lipoic acid[36–38] (1200mg/day)	Supplementation may lead to a small, short-term, weight loss. Limited data for antipsychotic-induced weight gain. Not recommended
Aripiprazole augmentation[15,32,39] (5–15mg/day)	RCTs show beneficial effects on weight loss and possibly other metabolic parameters when used as an adjunct to clozapine or olanzapine. Adjunctive use appears to be safe and unlikely to worsen psychosis. Recommended as a possible option for weight gain associated with clozapine or olanzapine. Not recommended with other antipsychotic medications
Betahistine[40,41] (48mg/day)	May attenuate olanzapine-induced weight gain. Limited data. Not recommended
Bupropion[42,43] (amfebutamone)	Seems to be effective in obesity when combined with calorie-restricted diets. Appears to not exacerbate psychosis symptoms, at least when used for smoking cessation.[44] Few data of its effects on drug-induced weight gain. Not recommended
Bupropion + naltrexone (Contrave/Mysimba)[45]	Combination approved for weight management as an adjunct to diet and exercise. No data in drug-induced weight gain. Not recommended, but should not be ruled out
Fluvoxamine[46–48] (50mg/day)	Earlier conflicting data but one short term RCT shows attenuated clozapine-induced weight gain (possibly related to a higher clozapine to norclozapine ratio). Co-administration markedly increases clozapine levels, requiring extreme caution. Evidence base is too limited to recommend
Liraglutide[49,50] (3mg/day via subcutaneous injection)	GLP-1 agonist that was previously approved for type 2 diabetes and more recently approved as an anti-obesity agent in non-diabetic patients. Dose for weight loss (3mg/day) is higher than the dose used for diabetes (≤1.8mg). Limited data in drug-induced weight gain. One RCT shows significant weight loss in overweight pre-diabetic patients stable on olanzapine or clozapine.[49] Beneficial effects on other metabolic parameters. Well tolerated but can cause GI disturbances. Recommended option in pre-diabetic/diabetic patients and clozapine-induced weight gain. Other GLP-1 agonists are currently only approved for diabetes and have a more limited dose range. Exenatide LA (a once-weekly GLP-1 agonist) may be effective for weight loss in clozapine-treated patients[51] but perhaps not with other antipsychotics[52]

Table 1.18 (Continued)

Drug	Comments
Metformin[2,32,53,54] (500–2000mg/day)	Now a substantial database (in non-diabetic patients) supporting the use of metformin in both reducing and reversing weight gain caused by antipsychotics (mainly olanzapine). Beneficial effects on other metabolic parameters. Some negative studies, but clear and significant effect in meta-analyses. One positive RCT[55] and extension study[56] in children and adolescents with ASD published since then. Ideal for those with weight gain and diabetes or polycystic ovary syndrome. Note that metformin treatment increases the risk of vitamin B_{12} deficiency[57]
Melatonin[58–60] (up to 5mg at night)	One small RCT showing attenuation of olanzapine-induced weight gain. Other studies show negative results. Effect, if any, is small
Methylcellulose (1,500mg ac)	Old-fashioned and rather unpalatable preparation. No data in drug-induced weight gain but once fairly widely used. Also acts as a bulk-forming laxative, so may be suitable for clozapine-related weight gain
Modafinil[61,62] (up to 300mg/day)	Limited positive data and one negative RCT for clozapine-induced weight gain. Not recommended
Naltrexone[63,64] (25–50mg/day)	Some positive results but evidence is limited to two small pilot RCTs. Not recommended
Orlistat[65–70] (120mg tds ac/pc)	Reliable effect in obesity, especially when combined with calorie restriction. Few published data in medication-induced weight gain but widely used in practice with some success. In trials for clozapine or olanzapine-induced weight gain effect was only seen for men.[69,70] When used without calorie restriction in psychiatric patients, the effects are very limited. Failure to adhere to a low-fat diet will result in fatty diarrhoea and possible malabsorption of orally administered medication. Overall, a good choice for clozapine-induced weight gain where it reduces both weight and the incidence of constipation[71]
Reboxetine[15] (4–8mg daily)	Attenuates olanzapine-induced weight gain. Reverses some metabolic changes.[72] Effective when combined with betahistine
Topiramate[32,54,73,74] (Up to 300mg daily)	Reliably reduces weight even when medication-induced. Meta-analyses of RCTs suggest a greater effect for prevention rather than treatment. Problems may arise because of topiramate's propensity for causing sedation, confusion and cognitive impairment. May have antipsychotic properties
Zonisamide[75] (100–600mg/day)	Antiepileptic drug with weight reducing properties. A RCT of 150mg a day showed significant weight reduction in people receiving SGAs. Another RCT (up to 600mg/day) shows attenuated olanzapine-induced weight gain. Sedation, diarrhoea and cognitive impairment are the most common problems. Not recommended

ac, ante cibum (before meals); ASD, autism spectrum disorders. bd, bis in die (twice a day); pc, post cibum (after meals); tds, ter die sumendum (three times a day)

References

1. Marder SR, et al. Physical health monitoring of patients with schizophrenia. *Am J Psychiatry* 2004; **161**:1334–1349.
2. Cooper SJ, et al. BAP guidelines on the management of weight gain, metabolic disturbances and cardiovascular risk associated with psychosis and antipsychotic drug treatment. *J Psychopharmacology* 2016; **30**:717–748.
3. Galletly C, et al. Royal Australian and New Zealand College of Psychiatrists clinical practice guidelines for the management of schizophrenia and related disorders. *Aust N Z J Psychiatry* 2016; **50**:410–472.
4. American Diabetes Association, et al. Consensus Development Conference on antipsychotic drugs and obesity and diabetes. *Diabetes Care* 2004; **27**:596–601.
5. Vandenberghe F, et al. Importance of early weight changes to predict long-term weight gain during psychotropic drug treatment. *J Clin Psychiatry* 2015; **76**:e1417–e1423.
6. Lipkovich I, et al. Early evaluation of patient risk for substantial weight gain during olanzapine treatment for schizophrenia, schizophreniform, or schizoaffective disorder. *BMC Psychiatry* 2008; **8**:78.
7. National Institute for Clinical Excellence. Psychosis and schizophrenia in adults. Quality standard [QS80]. 2015; https://www.nice.org.uk/guidance/qs80.
8. Barnes TR, et al. Screening for the metabolic syndrome in community psychiatric patients prescribed antipsychotics: a quality improvement programme. *Acta Psychiatr Scand* 2008; **118**:26–33.
9. Mitchell AJ, et al. Guideline concordant monitoring of metabolic risk in people treated with antipsychotic medication: systematic review and meta-analysis of screening practices. *Psychol Med* 2012; **42**:125–147.
10. Barnes TR, et al. Screening for the metabolic side effects of antipsychotic medication: findings of a 6-year quality improvement programme in the UK. *BMJ Open* 2015; **5**:e007633.
11. Crawford MJ, et al. Assessment and treatment of physical health problems among people with schizophrenia: national cross-sectional study. *Br J Psychiatry* 2014; **205**:473–477.
12. Hammoudeh S, et al. Risk factors of metabolic syndrome among patients receiving antipsychotics: a retrospective study. *Community Ment Health J* 2020; **56**:760–770.
13. Ward T, et al. Who is responsible for metabolic screening for mental health clients taking antipsychotic medications? *Int J Ment Health Nurs* 2018; **27**:196–203.
14. Bruins J, et al. The effects of lifestyle interventions on (long-term) weight management, cardiometabolic risk and depressive symptoms in people with psychotic disorders: a meta-analysis. *PLoS One* 2014; **9**:e112276.
15. Mizuno Y, et al. Pharmacological strategies to counteract antipsychotic-induced weight gain and metabolic adverse effects in schizophrenia: a systematic review and meta-analysis. *Schizophr Bull* 2014; **40**:1385–1403.
16. Stroup TS, et al. A randomized trial examining the effectiveness of switching from olanzapine, quetiapine, or risperidone to aripiprazole to reduce metabolic risk: comparison of antipsychotics for metabolic problems (CAMP). *Am J Psychiatry* 2011; **168**:947–956.
17. Mukundan A, et al. Antipsychotic switching for people with schizophrenia who have neuroleptic-induced weight or metabolic problems. *Cochrane Database Systematic Rev* 2010; CD006629.
18. Barak Y, et al. Switching to aripiprazole as a strategy for weight reduction: a meta-analysis in patients suffering from schizophrenia. *J Obes* 2011; **2011**:898013.
19. Weiden PJ, et al. Improvement in indices of health status in outpatients with schizophrenia switched to ziprasidone. *J Clin Psychopharmacol* 2003; **23**:595–600.
20. Montes JM, et al. Improvement in antipsychotic-related metabolic disturbances in patients with schizophrenia switched to ziprasidone. *Prog Neuropsychopharmacol Biol Psychiatry* 2007; **31**:383–388.
21. Karayal ON, et al. Switching from quetiapine to ziprasidone: a sixteen-week, open-label, multicenter study evaluating the effectiveness and safety of ziprasidone in outpatient subjects with schizophrenia or schizoaffective disorder. *J Psychiatr Pract* 2011; **17**:100–109.
22. McEvoy JP, et al. Effectiveness of lurasidone in patients with schizophrenia or schizoaffective disorder switched from other antipsychotics: a randomized, 6-week, open-label study. *J Clin Psychiatry* 2013; **74**:170–179.
23. Stahl SM, et al. Effectiveness of lurasidone for patients with schizophrenia following 6 weeks of acute treatment with lurasidone, olanzapine, or placebo: a 6-month, open-label, extension study. *J Clin Psychiatry* 2013; **74**:507–515.
24. Gupta S, et al. Weight decline in patients switching from olanzapine to quetiapine. *Schizophr Res* 2004; **70**:57–62.
25. Ried LD, et al. Weight change after an atypical antipsychotic switch. *Ann Pharmacother* 2003; **37**:1381–1386.
26. Galling B, et al. Antipsychotic augmentation vs. monotherapy in schizophrenia: systematic review, meta-analysis and meta-regression analysis. *World Psychiatry* 2017; **16**:77–89.
27. De Kuijper G, et al. Effects of controlled discontinuation of long-term used antipsychotics on weight and metabolic parameters in individuals with intellectual disability. *J Clin Psychopharmacol* 2013; **33**:520–524.
28. Chen EY, et al. Maintenance treatment with quetiapine versus discontinuation after one year of treatment in patients with remitted first episode psychosis: randomised controlled trial. *BMJ* 2010; **341**:c4024.
29. Werneke U, et al. Behavioural management of antipsychotic-induced weight gain: a review. *Acta Psychiatr Scand* 2003; **108**:252–259.
30. Caemmerer J, et al. Acute and maintenance effects of non-pharmacologic interventions for antipsychotic associated weight gain and metabolic abnormalities: a meta-analytic comparison of randomized controlled trials. *Schizophr Res* 2012; **140**:159–168.
31. Rice J, et al. Integrative management of metabolic syndrome in youth prescribed second-generation antipsychotics. *Med Sci* 2020; **8**:34.
32. Vancampfort D, et al. The impact of pharmacological and non-pharmacological interventions to improve physical health outcomes in people with schizophrenia: a meta-review of meta-analyses of randomized controlled trials. *World Psychiatry* 2019; **18**:53–66.

33. Manu P, et al. Weight gain and obesity in schizophrenia: epidemiology, pathobiology, and management. *Acta Psychiatr Scand* 2015; 132:97–108.

34. Praharaj SK, et al. Amantadine for olanzapine-induced weight gain: a systematic review and meta-analysis of randomized placebo-controlled trials. *Ther Adv Psychopharmacol* 2012; 2:151–156.

35. Zheng W, et al. Amantadine for antipsychotic-related weight gain: meta-analysis of randomized placebo-controlled trials. *J Clin Psychopharmacol* 2017; 37:341–346.

36. Kucukgoncu S, et al. Alpha-lipoic acid (ALA) as a supplementation for weight loss: results from a meta-analysis of randomized controlled trials. *Obes Rev* 2017; 18:594–601.

37. Kim E, et al. A preliminary investigation of alpha-lipoic acid treatment of antipsychotic drug-induced weight gain in patients with schizophrenia. *J Clin Psychopharmacol* 2008; 28:138–146.

38. Ratliff JC, et al. An open-label pilot trial of alpha-lipoic acid for weight loss in patients with schizophrenia without diabetes. *Clin Schizophr Relat Psychoses* 2015; 8:196–200.

39. Zheng W, et al. Efficacy and safety of adjunctive aripiprazole in schizophrenia: meta-analysis of randomized controlled trials. *J Clin Psychopharmacol* 2016; 36:628–636.

40. Barak N, et al. A randomized, double-blind, placebo-controlled pilot study of betahistine to counteract olanzapine-associated weight gain. *J Clin Psychopharmacol* 2016; 36:253–256.

41. Lian J, et al. Ameliorating antipsychotic-induced weight gain by betahistine: mechanisms and clinical implications. *Pharmacol Res* 2016; 106:51–63.

42. Gadde KM, et al. Bupropion for weight loss: an investigation of efficacy and tolerability in overweight and obese women. *Obes Res* 2001; 9:544–551.

43. Jain AK, et al. Bupropion SR vs. placebo for weight loss in obese patients with depressive symptoms. *Obes Res* 2002; 10:1049–1056.

44. Tsoi DT, et al. Interventions for smoking cessation and reduction in individuals with schizophrenia. *Cochrane Database Syst Rev* 2013; 2:CD007253.

45. Greig SL, et al. Naltrexone ER/Bupropion ER: a review in obesity management. *Drugs* 2015; 75:1269–1280.

46. Hinze-Selch D, et al. Effect of coadministration of clozapine and fluvoxamine versus clozapine monotherapy on blood cell counts, plasma levels of cytokines and body weight. *Psychopharmacology* 2000; 149:163–169.

47. Lu ML, et al. Effects of adjunctive fluvoxamine on metabolic parameters and psychopathology in clozapine-treated patients with schizophrenia: a 12-week, randomized, double-blind, placebo-controlled study. *Schizophr Res* 2018; 193:126–133.

48. Lu ML, et al. Adjunctive fluvoxamine inhibits clozapine-related weight gain and metabolic disturbances. *J Clin Psychiatry* 2004; 65:766–771.

49. Larsen JR, et al. Effect of liraglutide treatment on prediabetes and overweight or obesity in clozapine- or olanzapine-treated patients with schizophrenia spectrum disorder: a randomized clinical trial. *JAMA Psychiatry* 2017; 74:719–728.

50. Mayfield K, et al. Glucagon-like peptide-1 agonists combating clozapine-associated obesity and diabetes. *J Psychopharmacology* 2016; 30:227–236.

51. Siskind D, et al. Treatment of clozapine-associated obesity and diabetes with exenatide (CODEX) in adults with schizophrenia: a randomised controlled trial. *Diabetes, Obesity & Metabolism* 2017; 20:1050–1055.

52. Ishoy PL, et al. Effect of GLP-1 receptor agonist treatment on body weight in obese antipsychotic-treated patients with schizophrenia: a randomized, placebo-controlled trial. *Diabetes, Obesity & Metabolism* 2017; 19:162–171.

53. Zheng W, et al. Metformin for weight gain and metabolic abnormalities associated with antipsychotic treatment: meta-analysis of randomized placebo-controlled trials. *J Clin Psychopharmacol* 2015; 35:x499–x509.

54. Wang C, et al. Outcomes and safety of concomitant topiramate or metformin for antipsychotics-induced obesity: a randomized-controlled trial. *Ann General Psychiatry* 2020; 19:68.

55. Anagnostou E, et al. Metformin for treatment of overweight induced by atypical antipsychotic medication in young people with autism spectrum disorder: a randomized clinical trial. *JAMA Psychiatry* 2016; 73:928–937.

56. Handen BL, et al. A randomized, placebo-controlled trial of metformin for the treatment of overweight induced by antipsychotic medication in young people with autism spectrum disorder: open-label extension. *J Am Acad Child Adolesc Psychiatry* 2017; 56:849–856.e846.

57. Chapman LE, et al. Association between metformin and vitamin B12 deficiency in patients with type 2 diabetes: a systematic review and meta-analysis. *Diabetes Metab* 2016; 42:316–327.

58. Agahi M, et al. Effect of melatonin in reducing second-generation antipsychotic metabolic effects: a double blind controlled clinical trial. *Diabetes Metab Syndr* 2017; 12:9–15.

59. Wang HR, et al. The role of melatonin and melatonin agonists in counteracting antipsychotic-induced metabolic side effects: a systematic review. *Int Clin Psychopharmacol* 2016; 31:301–306.

60. Porfirio MC, et al. Can melatonin prevent or improve metabolic side effects during antipsychotic treatments? *Neuropsychiatr Dis Treat* 2017; 13:2167–2174.

61. Henderson DC, et al. Effects of modafinil on weight, glucose and lipid metabolism in clozapine-treated patients with schizophrenia. *Schizophr Res* 2011; 130:53–56.

62. Roerig JL, et al. An exploration of the effect of modafinil on olanzapine associated weight gain in normal human subjects. *Biol Psychiatry* 2009; 65:607–613.

63. Taveira TH, et al. The effect of naltrexone on body fat mass in olanzapine-treated schizophrenic or schizoaffective patients: a randomized double-blind placebo-controlled pilot study. *J Psychopharmacology* 2014; 28:395–400.

64. Tek C, et al. A randomized, double-blind, placebo-controlled pilot study of naltrexone to counteract antipsychotic-associated weight gain: proof of concept. *J Clin Psychopharmacol* 2014; 34:608–612.

65. Sjostrom L, et al. Randomised placebo-controlled trial of orlistat for weight loss and prevention of weight regain in obese patients. European Multicentre Orlistat Study Group. *Lancet* 1998; 352:167–172.

66. Hilger E, et al. The effect of orlistat on plasma levels of psychotropic drugs in patients with long-term psychopharmacotherapy. *J Clin Psychopharmacol* 2002; 22:68–70.

67. Pavlovic ZM. Orlistat in the treatment of clozapine-induced hyperglycemia and weight gain. *Eur Psychiatry* 2005; 20:520.

68. Carpenter LL, et al. A case series describing orlistat use in patients on psychotropic medications. *Med Health R I* 2004; 87:375–377.

69. Joffe G, et al. Orlistat in clozapine- or olanzapine-treated patients with overweight or obesity: a 16-week randomized, double-blind, placebo-controlled trial. *J Clin Psychiatry* 2008; 69:706–711.

70. Tchoukhine E, et al. Orlistat in clozapine- or olanzapine-treated patients with overweight or obesity: a 16-week open-label extension phase and both phases of a randomized controlled trial. *J Clin Psychiatry* 2011; 72:326–330.

71. Chukhin E, et al. In a randomized placebo-controlled add-on study orlistat significantly reduced clozapine-induced constipation. *IntClinPsychopharmacol* 2013; 28:67–70.

72. Amrami-Weizman A, et al. The effect of reboxetine co-administration with olanzapine on metabolic and endocrine profile in schizophrenia patients. *Psychopharmacology* 2013; 230:23–27.

73. Correll CU, et al. Efficacy for psychopathology and body weight and safety of topiramate-antipsychotic cotreatment in patients with schizophrenia spectrum disorders: results from a meta-analysis of randomized controlled trials. *J Clin Psychiatry* 2016; 77:e746–e756.

74. Zheng W, et al. Efficacy and safety of adjunctive topiramate for schizophrenia: a meta-analysis of randomized controlled trials. *Acta Psychiatr Scand* 2016; 134:385–398.

75. Buoli M, et al. The use of zonisamide for the treatment of psychiatric disorders: a systematic review. *Clin Neuropharmacol* 2017; 40:85–92.

Neuroleptic malignant syndrome

Neuroleptic malignant syndrome (NMS) is an acute disorder of thermoregulation and neuromotor control. It is characterised by muscular rigidity, hyperthermia, altered consciousness, and autonomic dysfunction, following exposure to antipsychotic medication, although there is considerable heterogeneity in the clinical presentation.[1-4] Although widely seen as an acute, severe syndrome, NMS may, in many cases, have few overt signs and symptoms, and 'full-blown' NMS may thus represent the extreme of a range of non-malignant related symptoms.[5] Certainly, asymptomatic rises in plasma creatine kinase (CK) are fairly common.[6]

NMS occurs as a rare but potentially serious or even fatal adverse effect of antipsychotics, being medications with dopamine receptor-antagonist properties.[1] Risk factors for developing the condition include being male, dehydration, exhaustion and confusion/agitation.[4,7] Young adult males seem to be particularly at risk while the condition is most likely to be lethal in older people.[4,8]

The incidence and mortality rate of NMS are difficult to establish and probably vary as medication regimens change and recognition of NMS increases. Based on data from a drug safety programme, from 1993 to 2015, the overall incidence was calculated to be 0.16%.[9] A similar study covering the period 2004–2017[10] reported an incidence of 0.11%. High-potency FGAs seem to have the highest incidence, while SGAs and low-potency FGAs have lower incidences.[3,9,11] Nevertheless, most available antipsychotic medications have been reported to be associated with the syndrome,[12-19] including more recently introduced SGAs such as ziprasidone,[20,21] iloperidone,[22] aripiprazole,[23-26] paliperidone[27] (including paliperidone palmitate[28]), asenapine[29] and risperidone injection.[30] Mortality is probably lower with SGAs than with FGAs,[3,31-33] although the clinical picture is essentially similar,[32] except that rigidity and fever may be less common.[3,32] At the time of writing, NMS has yet to be associated with pimavanserin, cariprazine, brexpiprazole or lumateperone.[34]

NMS is also sometimes seen with other medications, such as antidepressants,[35-38] valproate[39,40] phenytoin[41] and lithium.[42] The co-prescription of SSRIs[43] or cholinesterase inhibitors[44,45] with antipsychotic medication may increase the risk of NMS. NMS-type syndromes induced by SGA/SSRI combinations may share their symptoms and pathogenesis with the serotonin syndrome.[46] Benzodiazepines are a recommended treatment for NMS,[47] but an association between their use and NMS has been reported, possibly confounded by diagnosis or explained by the occurrence of NMS-like symptoms during benzodiazepine withdrawal.[11,48,49] NMS is also occasionally seen in people given non-psychotropic dopamine antagonists such as metoclopramide (Table 1.19).[50]

Table 1.19 Neuroleptic malignant syndrome

Signs and symptoms[9,51–53] (presentation varies considerably)[54]	Fever, diaphoresis, rigidity, confusion, fluctuating level of consciousness. Fluctuating blood pressure, tachycardia
	Elevated creatine kinase, leukocytosis, altered liver function tests
Risk factors[8,11,48,52,53,55–57]	High-potency FGAs, recent or rapid dose increase, rapid dose reduction, abrupt withdrawal of anticholinergic agents, antipsychotic polypharmacy
	Psychosis, organic brain disease, alcoholism, Parkinson's disease, hyperthyroidism, psychomotor agitation, mental retardation
	Male gender, younger age
	Agitation, dehydration
Treatments[9,52,58–60] (guideline recommendations for NMS treatment are heterogeneous and based on limited evidence[47])	**In the psychiatric unit:**
	Withdraw antipsychotic medication, monitor temperature, pulse, BP. Consider benzodiazepines if not already prescribed – IM lorazepam has been used[61]
	In the medical/A&E unit:
	Rehydration, bromocriptine + dantrolene, sedation with benzodiazepines, artificial ventilation if required
	L-dopa, apomorphine, and carbamazepine have also been used, among many other drugs. ECT may be effective for NMS, even after pharmacotherapy has failed[62,63]
Restarting antipsychotics[41,52,58,64]	Antipsychotic treatment will be required in most instances and re-challenge is associated with acceptable risk
	Stop antipsychotic medication for at least 5 days, preferably longer. Allow time for symptoms and signs of NMS to resolve completely
	Begin with very small dose and increase very slowly with close monitoring of temperature, pulse and blood pressure. CK monitoring may be used but is controversial.[53,65] Close monitoring of physical and biochemical parameters is effective in reducing progression to 'full-blown' NMS[66,67]
	Consider using an antipsychotic medication structurally unrelated to that previously associated with NMS or a drug with low dopamine affinity (quetiapine or clozapine). Aripiprazole may also be considered,[68] but it has a long plasma half-life and has been linked to an increased risk of NMS[11]
	Avoid depot/LAI antipsychotic preparations (of any kind) and high potency FGAs

References

1. Caroff SN, et al. Neuroleptic malignant syndrome. *Med Clin North Am* 1993; 77:185–202.
2. Gurrera RJ, et al. Thermoregulatory dysfunction in neuroleptic malignant syndrome. *Biol Psychiatry* 1996; 39:207–212.
3. Belvederi Murri M, et al. Second-generation antipsychotics and neuroleptic malignant syndrome: systematic review and case report analysis. *Drugs in R&D* 2015; 15:45–62.
4. Ware MR, et al. Neuroleptic malignant syndrome: diagnosis and management. *Prim Care Companion CNS Disord* 2018; 20.
5. Bristow MF, et al. How 'malignant' is the neuroleptic malignant syndrome? *BMJ* 1993; 307:1223–1224.
6. Meltzer HY, et al. Marked elevations of serum creatine kinase activity associated with antipsychotic drug treatment. *Neuropsychopharmacology* 1996; 15:395–405.
7. Keck PE, Jr., et al. Risk factors for neuroleptic malignant syndrome. A case-control study. *Arch Gen Psychiatry* 1989; 46:914–918.
8. Gurrera RJ. A systematic review of sex and age factors in neuroleptic malignant syndrome diagnosis frequency. *Acta Psychiatr Scand* 2017; 135:398–408.
9. Schneider M, et al. Neuroleptic malignant syndrome: evaluation of drug safety data from the AMSP program during 1993–2015. *Eur Arch Psychiatry Clin Neurosci* 2020; 270:23–33.
10. Lao KSJ, et al. Antipsychotics and risk of neuroleptic malignant syndrome: a population-based cohort and case-crossover study. *CNS Drugs* 2020; 34:1165–1175.
11. Su YP, et al. Retrospective chart review on exposure to psychotropic medications associated with neuroleptic malignant syndrome. *Acta Psychiatr Scand* 2014; 130:52–60.
12. Sing KJ, et al. Neuroleptic malignant syndrome and quetiapine (Letter). *Am J Psychiatry* 2002; 159:149–150.
13. Suh H, et al. Neuroleptic malignant syndrome and low-dose olanzapine (Letter). *Am J Psychiatry* 2003; 160:796.
14. Gallarda T, et al. Neuroleptic malignant syndrome in an 72-year-old-man with Alzheimer's disease: a case report and review of the literature. *Eur Neuropsychopharmacol* 2000; 10 Suppl 3:357.
15. Stanley AK, et al. Possible neuroleptic malignant syndrome with quetiapine. *Br J Psychiatry* 2000; 176:497.
16. Sierra-Biddle D, et al. Neuropletic malignant syndrome and olanzapine. *J Clin Psychopharmacol* 2000; 20:704–705.
17. Hasan S, et al. Novel antipsychotics and the neuroleptic malignant syndrome: a review and critique. *Am J Psychiatry* 1998; 155:1113–1116.
18. Tsai JH, et al. Zotepine-induced catatonia as a precursor in the progression to neuroleptic malignant syndrome. *Pharmacotherapy* 2005; 25:1156–1159.
19. Gortney JS, et al. Neuroleptic malignant syndrome secondary to quetiapine. *Ann Pharmacother* 2009; 43:785–791.
20. Leibold J, et al. Neuroleptic malignant syndrome associated with ziprasidone in an adolescent. *Clin Ther* 2004; 26:1105–1108.
21. Borovicka MC, et al. Ziprasidone- and lithium-induced neuroleptic malignant syndrome. *Ann Pharmacother* 2006; 40:139–142.
22. Guanci N, et al. Atypical neuroleptic malignant syndrome associated with iloperidone administration. *Psychosomatics* 2012; 53:603–605.
23. Spalding S, et al. Aripiprazole and atypical neuroleptic malignant syndrome. *J Am Acad Child Adolesc Psychiatry* 2004; 43:1457–1458.
24. Chakraborty N, et al. Aripiprazole and neuroleptic malignant syndrome. *Int Clin Psychopharmacol* 2004; 19:351–353.
25. Rodriguez OP, et al. A case report of neuroleptic malignant syndrome without fever in a patient given aripiprazole. *J Okla State Med Assoc* 2006; 99:435–438.
26. Srephichit S, et al. Neuroleptic malignant syndrome and aripiprazole in an antipsychotic-naive patient. *J Clin Psychopharmacol* 2006; 26:94–95.
27. Duggal HS. Possible neuroleptic malignant syndrome associated with paliperidone. *J Neuropsychiatry Clin Neurosci* 2007; 19:477–478.
28. Langley-degroot M, et al. Atypical neuroleptic malignant syndrome associated with paliperidone long-acting injection: a case report. *J Clin Psychopharmacol* 2016; 36:277–279.
29. Singh N, et al. Neuroleptic malignant syndrome after exposure to asenapine: a case report. *Prim Care Companion J Clin Psychiatry* 2010; 12:e1.
30. Mall GD, et al. Catatonia and mild neuroleptic malignant syndrome after initiation of long-acting injectable risperidone: case report. *J Clin Psychopharmacol* 2008; 28:572–573.
31. Ananth J, et al. Neuroleptic malignant syndrome and atypical antipsychotic drugs. *J Clin Psychiatry* 2004; 65:464–470.
32. Trollor JN, et al. Comparison of neuroleptic malignant syndrome induced by first- and second-generation antipsychotics. *Br J Psychiatry* 2012; 201:52–56.
33. Nakamura M, et al. Mortality of neuroleptic malignant syndrome induced by typical and atypical antipsychotic drugs: a propensity-matched analysis from the Japanese Diagnosis Procedure Combination database. *J Clin Psychiatry* 2012; 73:427–430.
34. Orsolini L, et al. Up-to-date expert opinion on the safety of recently developed antipsychotics. *Exp Opin Drug Saf* 2020; 19:981–998.
35. Kontaxakis VP, et al. Neuroleptic malignant syndrome after addition of paroxetine to olanzapine. *J Clin Psychopharmacol* 2003; 23:671–672.
36. Young C. A case of neuroleptic malignant syndrome and serotonin disturbance. *J Clin Psychopharmacol* 1997; 17:65–66.
37. June R, et al. Neuroleptic malignant syndrome associated with nortriptyline. *Am J Emerg Med* 1999; 17:736–737.
38. Lu TC, et al. Neuroleptic malignant syndrome after the use of venlafaxine in a patient with generalized anxiety disorder. *J Formos Med Assoc* 2006; 105:90–93.
39. Verma R, et al. An atypical case of neuroleptic malignant syndrome precipitated by valproate. *BMJ Case Rep* 2014; 2014:bcr2013202578.
40. Menon V, et al. Atypical neuroleptic malignant syndrome in a young male precipitated by oral sodium valproate. *Aust N Z J Psychiatry* 2016; 50:1208–1209.

41. Shin HW, et al. Neuroleptic malignant syndrome induced by phenytoin in a patient with drug-induced Parkinsonism. *Neurol Sci* 2014; 35:1641–1643.

42. Gill J, et al. Acute lithium intoxication and neuroleptic malignant syndrome. *Pharmacotherapy* 2003; 23:811–815.

43. Stevens DL. Association between selective serotonin-reuptake inhibitors, second-generation antipsychotics, and neuroleptic malignant syndrome. *Ann Pharmacother* 2008; 42:1290–1297.

44. Stevens DL, et al. Olanzapine-associated neuroleptic malignant syndrome in a patient receiving concomitant rivastigmine therapy. *Pharmacotherapy* 2008; 28:403–405.

45. Warwick TC, et al. Neuroleptic malignant syndrome variant in a patient receiving donepezil and olanzapine. *Nat Clin Pract Neurol* 2008; 4:170–174.

46. Odagaki Y. Atypical neuroleptic malignant syndrome or serotonin toxicity associated with atypical antipsychotics? *Curr Drug Saf* 2009; 4:84–93.

47. Schönfeldt-Lecuona C, et al. Treatment of the neuroleptic malignant syndrome in international therapy guidelines: a comparative analysis. *Pharmacopsychiatry* 2020; 53:51–59.

48. Nielsen RE, et al. Neuroleptic malignant syndrome-an 11-year longitudinal case-control study. *Can J Psychiatry* 2012; 57:512–518.

49. Kishimoto S, et al. Postoperative neuroleptic malignant syndrome-like symptoms improved with intravenous diazepam: a case report. *J Anesth* 2013; 27:768–770.

50. Wittmann O, et al. Neuroleptic malignant syndrome associated with metoclopramide use in a boy: case report and review of the literature. *Am J Ther* 2016; 23:e1246–e1249.

51. Gurrera RJ. Sympathoadrenal hyperactivity and the etiology of neuroleptic malignant syndrome. *Am J Psychiatry* 1999; 156:169–180.

52. Levenson JL. Neuroleptic malignant syndrome. *Am J Psychiatry* 1985; 142:1137–1145.

53. Hermesh H, et al. High serum creatinine kinase level: possible risk factor for neuroleptic malignant syndrome. *J Clin Psychopharmacol* 2002; 22:252–256.

54. Picard LS, et al. Atypical neuroleptic malignant syndrome: diagnostic controversies and considerations. *Pharmacotherapy* 2008; 28:530–535.

55. Viejo LF, et al. Risk factors in neuroleptic malignant syndrome. A case-control study. *Acta Psychiatr Scand* 2003; 107:45–49.

56. Spivak B, et al. Neuroleptic malignant syndrome during abrupt reduction of neuroleptic treatment. *Acta Psychiatr Scand* 1990; 81:168–169.

57. Spivak B, et al. Neuroleptic malignant syndrome associated with abrupt withdrawal of anticholinergic agents. *Int Clin Psychopharmacol* 1996; 11:207–209.

58. Olmsted TR. Neuroleptic malignant syndrome: guidelines for treatment and reinstitution of neuroleptics. *South Med J* 1988; 81:888–891.

59. Lattanzi L, et al. Subcutaneous apomorphine for neuroleptic malignant syndrome. *Am J Psychiatry* 2006; 163:1450–1451.

60. Kuhlwilm L, et al. The neuroleptic malignant syndrome – a systematic case series analysis focusing on therapy regimes and outcome. *Acta Psychiatr Scand* 2020; 142:233–241.

61. Francis A, et al. Is lorazepam a treatment for neuroleptic malignant syndrome? *CNS Spectr* 2000; 5:54–57.

62. BMJ Best Practice. Neuroleptic malignant syndrome. 2020; https://bestpractice.bmj.com/topics/engb/990/pdf/990/Neuroleptic%20malignant%20syndrome.pdf.

63. Morcos N, et al. Electroconvulsive therapy for neuroleptic malignant syndrome: a case series. *J Ect* 2019; 35:225–230.

64. Wells AJ, et al. Neuroleptic rechallenge after neuroleptic malignant syndrome: case report and literature review. *Drug Intell Clin Pharm* 1988; 22:475–480.

65. Klein JP, et al. Massive creatine kinase elevations with quetiapine: report of two cases. *Pharmacopsychiatry* 2006; 39:39–40.

66. Shiloh R, et al. Precautionary measures reduce risk of definite neuroleptic malignant syndrome in newly typical neuroleptic-treated schizophrenia inpatients. *Int Clin Psychopharmacol* 2003; 18:147–149.

67. Hatch CD, et al. Failed challenge with quetiapine after neuroleptic malignant syndrome with conventional antipsychotics. *Pharmacotherapy* 2001; 21:1003–1006.

68. Trutia A, et al. Neuroleptic rechallenge with aripiprazole in a patient with previously documented neuroleptic malignant syndrome. *J Psychiatr Pract* 2008; 14:398–402.

CHAPTER 1

Catatonia

There are two catatonia sub-types, a retarded or stuporous form with decreased psychomotor behaviour and an excited form, characterised by agitation, combativeness, impulsivity and apparently purposeless overactivity.[1,2] The former tends to present as stupor: the key features include mutism, rigidity, marked psychomotor retardation, negativism, posturing, waxy flexibility, and catalepsy. While historically associated with schizophrenia, stupor is also seen in other psychiatric conditions such as depression and, less commonly, mania,[3–8] alcohol[9] or benzodiazepine withdrawal[10] and conversion disorder.[3,4,11–17] If psychiatric stupor is left untreated, physical health complications are unavoidable and develop rapidly. Prompt treatment is crucial to prevent serious complications such as dehydration, venous thrombosis, pulmonary embolism, pneumonia, and ultimately death.[18]

A catatonic syndrome may be produced by a variety of systemic, neurological and toxic conditions, including developmental disorders such as autism, neurodegenerative conditions[19,20] and the following:

- subarachnoid haemorrhages
- basal ganglia disorders
- non-convulsive status epilepticus
- locked-in and akinetic mutism states
- endocrine and metabolic disorders, e.g. Wilson's[21]
- Prader–Willi syndrome
- antiphospholipid syndrome[22]
- autoimmune encephalitis[23]
- systemic lupus erythematosus[24]
- infections (especially CNS infections)
- dementia
- drug withdrawal and toxic drug states, e.g. after abrupt withdrawal of clozapine and withdrawal of zolpidem, benzodiazepines[25] and many non-psychotropic medications, including medicines used in oncology.

The treatment of stupor in the context of catatonia is somewhat dependent on its cause but should usually include benzodiazepines. Benzodiazepines alone are the drugs of choice for stupor occurring in the context of affective and conversion disorders.[5,6,26] It is postulated that benzodiazepines may act by increasing GABAergic transmission or reducing levels of brain-derived neurotrophic factor.[27] There is most clinical experience with lorazepam. Many patients will respond to standard doses (up to 4mg per day), but repeated and higher doses (between 8mg and 24mg per day) may be needed.[28] One small, observational study of patients with catatonic stupor in the context of a mood disorder,[5] either major depressive disorder or bipolar disorder, used a lorazepam-diazepam treatment protocol and reported a response in 10 of the 12 patients with intramuscular lorazepam 2–4mg. In another study using a very similar protocol, relief of symptoms was achieved in 18 out of 21 patients with catatonia caused by general medical conditions or substance misuse.[29] Where benzodiazepines are effective, the benefit is of rapid onset. A test dose of zolpidem (10mg) may predict response to benzodiazepines,[30] and frequent dosing of zolpidem may provide effective treatment.[31,32] IV lorazepam has also been used to predict response.[33]

Catatonia in schizophrenia may be somewhat less likely to respond to benzodiazepines alone, with a response in 40–50%[34] of cases. A double-blind, placebo-controlled, cross-over trial with lorazepam up to 6mg per day demonstrated no effect on chronic catatonic symptoms in patients with established schizophrenia,[35] similar to the poor effect of lorazepam in a non-randomised trial.[36] A Cochrane review[37] searched for RCTs in which people with schizophrenia or other similar SMI had received benzodiazepines or another relevant treatment for catatonia. Only one study was eligible, which involved 17 participants treated with lorazepam or oxazepam: there was no clear difference in effect. The authors noted that no data were available for benzodiazepines compared with either placebo or standard care.

A further complication in schizophrenia is that of differential diagnosis, which includes extrapyramidal side effects and the neuroleptic malignant syndrome (NMS). Debate continues regarding the similarities and differences between catatonic stupor in psychosis and NMS.[38–41] Two terms have been coined – lethal catatonia and malignant catatonia[42] to describe stupor, which is accompanied by autonomic instability or hyperthermia. This potentially fatal condition cannot be distinguished from NMS, either clinically or by laboratory testing, leading to the suggestion that NMS may be a variant form of malignant catatonia.[43] However, NMS can probably be ruled out in the absence of any prior or recent administration of a dopamine antagonist.

The vast majority of evidence published recently as well as over previous decades suggests that prompt ECT remains the most successful treatment for catatonia.[33,36,44–60] ECT-responsive catatonia has been recognised in the context of NMS, delirious mania, self-injurious behaviours in autism, and limbic encephalitis.[41] While it has been suggested that response to ECT may be lower in patients with schizophrenia (or in those who have been treated with antipsychotic medication) than in patients with mood disorders,[61] ECT is still considered the treatment of choice for catatonic schizophrenia that has failed to respond to an adequate trial of benzodiazepines.[62] In malignant catatonia, every effort should be made to maximise the effect of ECT by using liberal stimulus dosing to induce well-generalised seizures.[63] Physical health needs should be prioritised and inpatient medical care obtained when necessary, especially for those showing autonomic instability and those whose dietary intake cannot be managed in psychiatric care.

The use of antipsychotic medication should be carefully considered. Some authors recommend that antipsychotics should be avoided altogether in catatonic patients, although there are case reports of successful treatment with aripiprazole, risperidone, olanzapine, ziprasidone and clozapine.[64–69] There is probably most evidence supporting clozapine and olanzapine. Combination treatment with benzodiazepines can be effective when each fails individually.[70,71]

When considering using antipsychotic medication take into account the history of a patient, their previous diagnosis and previous response to antipsychotic treatment, and the likelihood that non-adherence precipitated stupor. It should be noted that physical health conditions, as in the examples listed earlier in this section, can present with a catatonia-like clinical picture, warranting treatment of the underlying medical condition (e.g. lupus[72]). Antipsychotic medication should be avoided when stupor develops during treatment with antipsychotic medication, if there are clear signs of NMS, and where muscle rigidity is accompanied by autonomic instability. Where NMS can be ruled out, and stupor occurs in the context of non-adherence to antipsychotic treatment, early re-establishment of antipsychotic medication is recommended with consideration of adjunctive benzodiazepines. This may be particularly relevant when catatonic symptoms have occurred following discontinuation of clozapine.[25,73] Catatonia has also been reported after withdrawal of long-term benzodiazepine treatment.[25]

Algorithm for treating catatonic stupor[74]

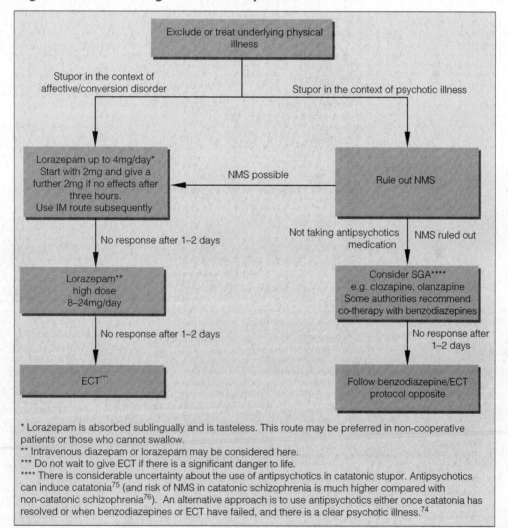

* Lorazepam is absorbed sublingually and is tasteless. This route may be preferred in non-cooperative patients or those who cannot swallow.
** Intravenous diazepam or lorazepam may be considered here.
*** Do not wait to give ECT if there is a significant danger to life.
**** There is considerable uncertainty about the use of antipsychotics in catatonic stupor. Antipsychotics can induce catatonia[75] (and risk of NMS in catatonic schizophrenia is much higher compared with non-catatonic schizophrenia[76]). An alternative approach is to use antipsychotics either once catatonia has resolved or when benzodiazepines or ECT have failed, and there is a clear psychotic illness.[74]

Table 1.20 Medications other than benzodiazepines reported as treatments for catatonia/stupor

Listed in alphabetical order – no ranking or judgement is implied by the order

Antipsychotic medications[64–69,77–80]

- Aripiprazole
- Clozapine
- Olanzapine
- Risperidone
- Ziprasidone

Experimental treatments* [6,7,31,32,53,81–86]

- Amantadine
- Amitriptyline
- Carbamazepine
- Fluoxetine
- Fluvoxamine
- Lithium
- Memantine
- Methylphenidate
- Mirtazapine
- Tramadol
- Valproate
- Zolpidem

*Always read the primary literature before using any of the medications listed in this section.

References

1. Morrison JR. Catatonia. Retarded and excited types. *Arch Gen Psychiatry* 1973; **28**:39–41.
2. Walther S, et al. Structure and neural mechanisms of catatonia. *Lancet Psychiatry* 2019; **6**:610–619.
3. Takacs R, et al. Catatonia in affective disorders. *Curr Psychiatry Rev* 2013; **9**:101–105.
4. Mangas MCC, et al. P-167 – catatonia in bipolar disorder. *Eur Psychiatry* 2012; **27 Suppl 1**:1.
5. Huang YC, et al. Rapid relief of catatonia in mood disorder by lorazepam and diazepam. *Biomed J* 2013; **36**:35–39.
6. Vasudev K, et al. What works for delirious catatonic mania? *BMJ Case Rep* 2010; **2010**.
7. Neuhut R, et al. Resolution of catatonia after treatment with stimulant medication in a patient with bipolar disorder. *Psychosomatics* 2012; **53**:482–484.
8. Ghaffarinejad AR, et al. Periodic catatonia. Challenging diagnosis for psychiatrists. *Neurosciences* 2012; **17**:156–158.
9. Oldham MA, et al. Alcohol and sedative-hypnotic withdrawal catatonia: two case reports, systematic literature review, and suggestion of a potential relationship with alcohol withdrawal delirium. *Psychosomatics* 2016; **57**:246–255.
10. Banerjee D. Etizolam withdrawal catatonia: the first case report. *Asian J Psychiatr* 2018; **37**:32–33.
11. Fink M. Rediscovering catatonia: the biography of a treatable syndrome. *Acta Psychiatr Scand Suppl* 2013; 1–47.
12. Bartolommei N, et al. Catatonia: a critical review and therapeutic recommendation. *J Psychopathology* 2012; **18**:234–246.
13. Lee J. Dissociative catatonia: dissociative-catatonic reactions, clinical presentations and responses to benzodiazepines. *Aust N Z J Psychiatry* 2011; **45**:A42.
14. Suzuki K, et al. Hysteria presenting as a prodrome to catatonic stupor in a depressive patient resolved with electroconvulsive therapy. *J ECT* 2006; **22**:276.
15. Alwaki A, et al. Catatonia: an elusive diagnosis. *Neurology* 2013; **80 Suppl 1**:P05.127.
16. Dhadphale M. Eye gaze diagnostic sign in hysterical stupor. *Lancet* 1980; **2**:374–375.
17. Gomez J. Hysterical stupor and death. *Br J Psychiatry* 1980; **136**:105–106.
18. Petrides G, et al. Synergism of lorazepam and electroconvulsive therapy in the treatment of catatonia. *Biol Psychiatry* 1997; **42**:375–381.
19. Mazzone L, et al. Catatonia in patients with autism: prevalence and management. *CNS Drugs* 2014; **28**:205–215.

20. Dhossche DM, et al. Catatonia in psychiatric illnesses, in SH Fatemi, PJ Clayton, eds. *The medical basis of psychiatry.* Totowa, NJ: Humana Press; 2008:471–486.

21. Shetageri VN, et al. Case report: catatonia as a presenting symptom of Wilsons disease. *Indian J Psychiatry* 2011; 53 **Suppl** 5:S93–S94.

22. Cardinal RN, et al. Psychosis and catatonia as a first presentation of antiphospholipid syndrome. *Br J Psychiatry* 2009; 195:272.

23. Rogers JP, et al. Catatonia and the immune system: a review. *Lancet Psychiatry* 2019; 6:620–630.

24. Pustilnik S, et al. Catatonia as the presenting symptom in systemic lupus erythematosus. *J Psychiatr Pract* 2011; 17:217–221.

25. Lander M, et al. Review of withdrawal catatonia: what does this reveal about clozapine? *Trans Psychiatry* 2018; 8:139.

26. Sienaert P, et al. Adult catatonia: etiopathogenesis, diagnosis and treatment. *Neuropsychiatry* 2013; 3:391–399.

27. Huang TL, et al. Lorazepam reduces the serum brain-derived neurotrophic factor level in schizophrenia patients with catatonia. *Prog Neuropsychopharmacol Biol Psychiatry* 2009; 33:158–159.

28. Fink M, et al. Neuroleptic malignant syndrome is malignant catatonia, warranting treatments efficacious for catatonia. *Prog Neuropsychopharmacol Biol Psychiatry* 2006; 30:1182–1183.

29. Lin CC, et al. The lorazepam and diazepam protocol for catatonia due to general medical condition and substance in liaison psychiatry. *PLoS One* 2017; 12:e0170452.

30. Javelot H, et al. Zolpidem test and catatonia. *J Clin Pharm Ther* 2015; 40:699–701.

31. Bastiampillai T, et al. Treatment refractory chronic catatonia responsive to zolpidem challenge. *Aust N Z J Psychiatry* 2016; 50:98.

32. Peglow S, et al. Treatment of catatonia with zolpidem. *J Neuropsychiatry Clin Neurosci* 2013; 25:E13.

33. Bush G, et al. Catatonia. II: Treatment with lorazepam and electroconvulsive therapy. *Acta Psychiatr Scand* 1996; 93:137–143.

34. Rosebush PI, et al. Catatonia: re-awakening to a forgotten disorder. *Mov Disord* 1999; 14:395–397.

35. Ungvari GS, et al. Lorazepam for chronic catatonia: a randomized, double-blind, placebo-controlled cross-over study. *Psychopharmacology* 1999; 142:393–398.

36. Dutt A, et al. Phenomenology and treatment of Catatonia: a descriptive study from north India. *Indian J Psychiatry* 2011; 53:36–40.

37. Gibson RC, et al. Benzodiazepines for catatonia in people with schizophrenia and other serious mental illnesses. *Cochrane Database Syst Rev* 2008; CD006570.

38. Luchini F, et al. Catatonia and neuroleptic malignant syndrome: two disorders on a same spectrum? Four case reports. *J Nerv Ment Dis* 2013; 201:36–42.

39. Mishima T, et al. [Diazepam-responsive malignant catatonia in a patient with an initial clinical diagnosis of neuroleptic malignant syndrome: a case report]. *Brain Nerve* 2011; 63:503–507.

40. Rodriguez S, et al. Neuroleptic malignant syndrome or catatonia? A case report. *J Crit Care Med* 2020; 6:190–193.

41. Fink M. Expanding the catatonia tent: recognizing electroconvulsive therapy responsive syndromes. *J Ect* 2020: [Epub ahead of print].

42. Mann SC, et al. Catatonia, malignant catatonia, and neuroleptic malignant syndrome. *Curr Psychiatry Rev* 2013; 9:111–119.

43. Taylor MA, et al. Catatonia in psychiatric classification: a home of its own. *Am J Psychiatry* 2003; 160:1233–1241.

44. Cristancho P, et al. Successful use of right unilateral ECT for catatonia: a case series. *J Ect* 2014; 30:69–72.

45. Philbin D, et al. Catatonic schizophrenia: therapeutic challenges and potentially a new role for electroconvulsive therapy? *BMJ Case Rep* 2013; 2013.

46. Takebayashi M. [Electroconvulsive therapy in schizophrenia]. *Nihon Rinsho* 2013; 71:694–700.

47. Oviedo G, et al. Trends in the administration of electroconvulsive therapy for schizophrenia in Colombia: Descriptive study and literature review. *Eur Arch Psychiatry Clin Neurosci* 2013; 263 **Suppl** 1:S98.

48. Pompili M, et al. Indications for electroconvulsive treatment in schizophrenia: a systematic review. *SchizophrRes* 2013; 146:1–9.

49. Ogando Portilla N, et al. Electroconvulsive therapy as an effective treatment in neuroleptic malignant syndrome: purposely a case. *Eur Psychiatry* 2013; 28 **Suppl** 1:1.

50. Unal A, et al. Effective treatment of catatonia by combination of benzodiazepine and electroconvulsive therapy. *J Ect* 2013; 29:206–209.

51. Kaliora SC, et al. The practice of electroconvulsive therapy in Greece. *J ECT* 2013; 29:219–224.

52. Girardi P, et al. Life-saving electroconvulsive therapy in a patient with near-lethal catatonia. *Riv Psichiatr* 2012; 47:535–537.

53. Kumar V, et al. Electroconvulsive therapy in pregnancy. *Indian J Psychiatry* 2011; 53 **Suppl** 5:S100–S101.

54. Weiss M, et al. Treatment of catatonia with electroconvulsive therapy in adolescents. *J Child Adolesc Psychopharmacol* 2012; 22:96–100.

55. Bauer J, et al. Should the term catatonia be explicitly included in the ICD-10 description of acute transient psychotic disorder F23.0? *Nord J Psychiatry* 2012; 66:68–69.

56. Mohammadbeigi H, et al. Electroconvulsive therapy in single manic episodes: a case series. *Afr J Psychiatry* 2011; 14:56–59.

57. Dragasek J. [Utilisation of electroconvulsive therapy in treatment of depression disorders]. *Psychiatrie* 2011; 15:1211–1219.

58. Sienaert P, et al. A clinical review of the treatment of catatonia. *Front Psychiatry* 2014; 5:181.

59. Luchini F, et al. Electroconvulsive therapy in catatonic patients: efficacy and predictors of response. *World J Psychiatry* 2015; 5:182–192.

60. Lloyd JR, et al. Electroconvulsive therapy for patients with catatonia: current perspectives. *Neuropsychiatr Dis Treat* 2020; 16:2191–2208.

61. Van Waarde JA, et al. Electroconvulsive therapy for catatonia: treatment characteristics and outcomes in 27 patients. *J Ect* 2010; 26:248–252.

62. Jain A, et al. Catatonic Schizophrenia. StatPearls. Treasure Island (FL): statPearls Publishing Copyright © 2020, StatPearls Publishing LLC. 2020.

63. Kellner CH, et al. Electroconvulsive therapy for catatonia. *Am J Psychiatry* 2010; 167:1127–1128.

64. Van Den EF, et al. The use of atypical antipsychotics in the treatment of catatonia. *Eur Psychiatry* 2005; 20:422–429.

65. Caroff SN, et al. Movement disorders associated with atypical antipsychotic drugs. *J Clin Psychiatry* 2002; 63 **Suppl** 4:12–19.

66. Guzman CS, et al. Treatment of periodic catatonia with atypical antipsychotic, olanzapine. *Psychiatry Clin Neurosci* 2008; 62:482.

67. Babington PW, et al. Treatment of catatonia with olanzapine and amantadine. *Psychosomatics* 2007; 48:534–536.

68. Bastiampillai T, et al. Catatonia resolution and aripiprazole. *Aust N Z J Psychiatry* 2008; 42:907.

69. Strawn JR, et al. Successful treatment of catatonia with aripiprazole in an adolescent with psychosis. *J Child Adolesc Psychopharmacol* 2007; 17:733–735.

70. Spiegel DR, et al. A case of schizophrenia with catatonia resistant to lorazepam and olanzapine monotherapy but responsive to combination treatment: is it time to consider using select second-generation antipsychotics earlier in the treatment algorithm for this patient type? *Clin Neuropharmacol* 2019; 42:57–59.

71. Cevher Binici N, et al. Response of catatonia to amisulpride and lorazepam in an adolescent with schizophenia. *J Child Adolesc Psychopharmacol* 2018; 28:151–152.

72. Grover S, et al. Catatonia in systemic lupus erythematosus: a case report and review of literature. *Lupus* 2013; 22:634–638.

73. Bilbily J, et al. Catatonia secondary to sudden clozapine withdrawal: a case with three repeated episodes and a literature review. *Case Rep Psychiatry* 2017; 2017:2402731.

74. Rosebush PI, et al. Catatonia and its treatment. *Schizophr Bull* 2010; 36:239–242.

75. Caroff SN, et al. Movement disorders induced by antipsychotic drugs: implications of the CATIE schizophrenia trial. *Neurol Clin* 2011; 29:127–148, viii.

76. Funayama M, et al. Catatonic stupor in schizophrenic disorders and subsequent medical complications and mortality. *Psychosom Med* 2018; 80:370–376.

77. Voros V, et al. [Use of aripiprazole in the treatment of catatonia]. *NeuropsychopharmacolHung* 2010; 12:373–376.

78. Yoshimura B, et al. Is quetiapine suitable for treatment of acute schizophrenia with catatonic stupor? A case series of 39 patients. *Neuropsychiatr Dis Treat* 2013; 9:1565–1571.

79. Todorova K. Olanzapine in the treatment of catatonic stupor – two case reports and discussion. *Eur Neuropsychopharmacol* 2012; **22 Suppl** 2:S326.

80. Prakash O, et al. Catatonia and mania in patient with AIDS: treatment with lorazepam and risperidone. *Gen Hosp Psychiatry* 2012; 34:321–326.

81. Daniels J. Catatonia: clinical aspects and neurobiological correlates. *J Neuropsychiatry Clin Neurosci* 2009; 21:371–380.

82. Obregon DF, et al. Memantine and catatonia: a case report and literature review. *J Psychiatr Pract* 2011; 17:292–299.

83. Hervey WM, et al. Treatment of catatonia with amantadine. *Clin Neuropharmacol* 2012; 35:86–87.

84. Consoli A, et al. Lorazepam, fluoxetine and packing therapy in an adolescent with pervasive developmental disorder and catatonia. *J Physiol Paris* 2010; 104:309–314.

85. Lewis AL, et al. Malignant catatonia in a patient with bipolar disorder, B12 deficiency, and neuroleptic malignant syndrome: one cause or three? *J Psychiatr Pract* 2009; 15:415–422.

86. Padhy SK, et al. The catatonia conundrum: controversies and contradictions. *Asian J Psychiatr* 2014; 7:6–9.

ECG changes – QT prolongation

Introduction

Many psychotropic drugs are associated with ECG changes and some are causally linked to serious ventricular arrhythmia and sudden cardiac death. Specifically, some antipsychotics block cardiac potassium channels and are linked to prolongation of the cardiac QT interval, a risk factor for the ventricular arrhythmia torsade de pointes, which is sometimes fatal.[1]

Case–control studies have suggested that the use of most antipsychotics is associated with an increase in the rate of sudden cardiac death.[2–8] This risk is probably a result of the arrhythmogenic potential of antipsychotics,[9,10] although schizophrenia itself may be associated with QT prolongation.[11] Nonetheless, a study in first-episode patients showed that the use of antipsychotics produced clear prolongation on the QT interval after 2–4 weeks.[12] QT interval is longer in patients with schizophrenia than in controls (e.g. 418ms vs 393ms in one study[13] and in a recent study prolonged QTc was identified in 7.6% of psychiatric in-patients patients who had an ECG.[14]

Overall, risk is probably dose-related and, although the absolute risk is low, it is substantially higher than the, say, risk of fatal agranulocytosis with clozapine.[9] One report of cases gathered by a national database put the risk of TdP at between 0 and 19.2 cases per 100,000 patient-years, depending on the individual antipsychotic and age of patients.[15] The effect of antipsychotic polypharmacy on QT is somewhat uncertain,[16] but the extent of QT prolongation is probably a function of overall dose.[17]

ECG monitoring of drug-induced changes in mental health settings is complicated by a number of factors. Psychiatrists may have limited expertise in ECG interpretation, for example, and still less expertise in manually measuring QT intervals. Even cardiologists show an inter-rater reliability in QT measurement of up to 20ms.[18] Self-reading, computerised ECG devices are now widely available and compensate for some lack of expertise, but different models use different algorithms and different correction formulae.[19] In addition, ECG machines may not be as readily available in all clinical areas as they are in general medicine. Also, there may be insufficient time for ECG determination in many areas (e.g. out-patients). Lastly, ECG determination may be difficult to perform in acutely disturbed, physically uncooperative patients.

ECG monitoring is essential for all patients prescribed antipsychotics. An estimate of QT_C interval should be made on admission to in-patient units (in the UK, this is recommended in the NICE schizophrenia guideline[20]) and yearly thereafter.

QT prolongation

- The cardiac QT interval (usually cited as QTc – QT corrected for heart rate) is a useful, but imprecise indicator of risk of torsade de pointes and of increased cardiac mortality.[21] Different correction factors and methods may give markedly different values.[22]
- The QT interval broadly reflects the duration of cardiac repolarisation. Lengthening of repolarisation duration induces heterogeneity of electrical phasing in different

ventricular structures (a phenomenon known as dispersion), which in turn allows the emergence of early after depolarisations (EADs) which may provoke ventricular extrasystole and torsade de pointes. Measures have been developed (QT dispersion ratio, dispersion transmural repolarisation time) which may better predict arrhythmia.[13]

- There is some controversy over the exact association between QTc and risk of arrhythmia. Very limited evidence suggests that risk is exponentially related to the extent of prolongation beyond normal limits (440ms for men; 470ms for women), although there are well-known exceptions, which appear to disprove this theory[23] (some drugs prolong QT without increasing dispersion). Rather stronger evidence links QTc values over 500ms to a clearly increased risk of arrhythmia.[24] QT intervals of >650ms may be more likely than not to induce torsades.[25] Despite some uncertainties, QTc determination remains an important measure in estimating risk of arrhythmia and sudden death.

- Individual components of the QT interval may have particular importance. The time from the start of the t-wave to t-wave peak has been shown to be an important aspect of QT prolongation associated with sudden cardiac deaths;[26] t-wave peak to end interval may also be predictive of arrhythmia.[13]

- QTc measurements and evaluation are complicated by:
  - difficulty in determining the end of the T wave, particularly where U waves are present (this applies both to manual and self-reading ECG machines).[24]
  - normal physiological variation in QTc interval: QT varies with gender, time of day, food intake, alcohol intake, menstrual cycle, ECG lead, etc.[22,23]
  - variation in the extent of drug-induced prolongation of QTc because of changes in plasma levels. QTc prolongation is most prominent at peak drug plasma levels and least obvious at trough levels.[22,23]

Other ECG changes

Other reported antipsychotic-induced changes include atrial fibrillation, giant P waves, T-wave changes and heart block.[23]

Quantifying risk

Drugs are categorised here according to data available on their effects on the cardiac QTc interval (as reported; mostly using Bazett's correction formula). 'No-effect' drugs are those with which QTc prolongation has not been reported either at therapeutic doses or in overdose. 'Low-effect' drugs are those for which severe QTc prolongation has been reported only following overdose or where only small average increases (<10ms) have been observed at clinical doses. 'Moderate-effect' drugs are those which have been observed to prolong QTc by >10ms on average when given at normal clinical doses or where ECG monitoring is officially recommended in some circumstances. 'High-effect' drugs are those for which extensive average QTc prolongation (usually >20ms at normal clinical doses).

Note that, as outlined above, effect on QTc may not necessarily equate directly to risk of torsade de pointes or sudden death,[27] although this is often assumed. (A good example here is ziprasidone – a drug with a moderate effect on QTc but with minimal evidence of cardiac toxicity[28]). Note also that categorisation is inevitably approximate given the problems associated with QTc measurements. Lastly, keep in mind that differences in the effects of different antipsychotics on the QT interval rarely reach statistical significance, even in meta-analyses (Table 1.21).[29]

Outside these guidelines, readers are directed to the RISQ-PATH study,[30] which provides a scoring system for the prediction of QT prolongation (to above normal ranges) in any patient. RISQ-PATH has a 98% negative predictive value, so allowing a reduction in monitoring in low-risk patients. The RISQ-PATH method uses CredibleMeds categorisation for drug effects on QT – this, too, is recommended.[31]

Table 1.21 Effects of antipsychotics on QTC[13,22,23,32–61].

No effect	Moderate effect
Brexpiprazole*	Amisulpride****
Cariprazine*	Chlorpromazine
Lurasidone	Haloperidol
Lumateperone*	Iloperidone
	Levomepromazine
Low effect	Melperone
Aripiprazole**	Pimavanserin
Asenapine	Quetiapine
Clozapine	Ziprasidone
Flupentixol	
Fluphenazine	**High effect**
Perphenazine	Any intravenous antipsychotic
Prochlorperazine	Pimozide
Olanzapine***	Sertindole
Paliperidone	Any drug or combination of drugs used in doses exceeding
Risperidone	recommended maximum
Sulpiride	
	Unknown effect
	Loxapine
	Pipotiazine
	Trifluoperazine
	Zuclopenthixol

*Limited clinical experience (association with QT prolongation may emerge).
**One case of torsades de pointes (TDP) reported,[62] two cases of QT prolongation[63,64] and an association with TDP found in database study.[65] Healthy volunteer data suggest aripiprazole causes QTc prolongation of around 8ms.[66] Aripiprazole may increase QT dispersion.[67]
***Isolated cases of QTc prolongation[37,68] and has effects on cardiac ion channel, I_{Kr}[69] other data suggest no effect on QT_c.[23,35,36,70]
****TDP common in overdose,[25,71] strong association with TDP in clinical doses.[65]

Aripiprazole remains in the low effect group having previously been firmly placed in 'no effect'. Data are rather contradictory, with most studies showing a decrease in QTc associated with aripiprazole use[52] even in children and adolescents.[72] However, later data[62,63,65,66,73] cast doubt on assumptions of cardiac safety. Interestingly, a 2020 paper analysing reports of events in > 400,000 inpatients over 20 years found aripiprazole had the lowest rate of cardiac events (0.06%) of all antipsychotics.[74]

Lurasidone remains in the 'no effect' group,[52] although one study mentioned in the US labelling[75] reports a QT lengthening of 7.5mg in people receiving 120mg (111mg) a day. Those receiving 600mg (555mg) daily showed a lower change (+4.6ms). These findings are in some contrast with those from studies in patients, which uniformly suggest no or minimal effect.[76–78] This disparity is probably explained by the use of different correction factors and by random change, as often seen in placebo-treated patients[78] and as suggested by the apparent lack of dose-related effect. No cases of QTc > 500ms or TDP have been reported with lurasidone to our knowledge.

Brexpiprazole remains in the 'no effect' group, but be aware that one study of 16 patients found an increase in QTc (Hodges formula) of 10.1ms and an important increase in dispersion transmural repolarisation time.[13] All other data suggest no effect.

Other risk factors

A number of physiological/pathological factors are associated with an increased risk of QT changes and of arrhythmia (Table 1.22) and many non-psychotropic drugs are linked to QT prolongation (Table 1.23).[24] These additional risk factors seem almost always to be present in cases of antipsychotic-induced TDP.[79]

Table 1.22 Physiological risk factors for QTc prolongation and arrhythmia

Cardiac
Long QT syndrome
Bradycardia
Ischaemic heart disease
Myocarditis
Myocardial infarction
Left ventricular hypertrophy

Metabolic
Hypokalaemia
Hypomagnesaemia
Hypocalcaemia

Others
Extreme physical exertion
Stress or shock
Anorexia nervosa
Extremes of age – children and elderly may be more susceptible to QT changes
Female gender

Note: Hypokalaemia-related QTc prolongation is more commonly observed in acute psychotic admissions.[80] Also, be aware that there are a number of physical and genetic factors which may not be discovered on routine examination but which probably predispose patients to arrhythmia.[81,82]

ECG monitoring

Measure QTc in all patients prescribed antipsychotics:

- On admission
- If previous abnormality or known additional risk factor, at annual physical health check

Table 1.23 Non-psychotropics associated with QT prolongation (see Crediblemeds.org for latest information)

Antibiotics	Antiarrhythmics
Erythromycin	Quinidine
Clarithromycin	Disopyramide
Ampicillin	Procainamide
Co-trimoxazole	Sotalol
Pentamidine	Amiodarone
(some four quinolones affect QTc –	Bretylium
see manufacturers' literature)	
Antimalarials	**Others**
Chloroquine	Amantadine
Mefloquine	Cyclosporin
Quinine	Diphenhydramine
	Hydroxyzine
	Methadone
	Nicardipine
	Tamoxifen

Note: β_2 agonists and sympathomimetics may provoke torsade de pointes in patients with prolonged QTc.

Consider measuring QTc within a week of achieving a therapeutic dose of a newly prescribed antipsychotic that is associated with a moderate or high risk of QTc prolongation or of newly prescribed combined antipsychotics (Table 1.24).

Metabolic inhibition

The effect of drugs on the QTc interval is usually plasma level-dependent. Drug interactions are therefore important, especially when metabolic inhibition results in increased plasma levels of the drug affecting QTc. Commonly used metabolic inhibitors include fluvoxamine, fluoxetine, paroxetine and valproate.

Table 1.24 Management of QT prolongation in patients receiving antipsychotic drugs

QTc	Action	Refer to cardiologist
<440ms (men) or <470ms (women)	None unless abnormal T-wave morphology	Consider if in doubt
>440ms (men) or > 470ms (women) but < 500ms	Consider reducing dose or switching to drug of lower effect; repeat ECG	Consider
>500ms	Repeat ECG. Stop suspected causative drug(s) and switch to drug of lower effect	Immediately
Abnormal T-wave morphology	Review treatment. Consider reducing dose or switching to drug of lower effect	Immediately

Other cardiovascular risk factors

The risk of drug-induced arrhythmia and sudden cardiac death with psychotropics is an important consideration. With respect to cardiovascular disease, note that other risk factors such as smoking, obesity and impaired glucose tolerance present a much greater risk to patient morbidity and mortality than the uncertain outcome of QT changes. See relevant sections for discussion of these problems.

Summary

- In the absence of conclusive data, assume all antipsychotics are linked to sudden cardiac death.
- Prescribe the lowest dose possible and avoid polypharmacy/metabolic interactions.
- Perform ECG on admission, and, if previous abnormality or additional risk factor, at yearly check-up.
- Consider measuring QTc within a week of achieving a therapeutic dose of a moderate/high-risk antipsychotic.

References

1. Sicouri S, et al. Mechanisms underlying the actions of antidepressant and antipsychotic drugs that cause sudden cardiac arrest. *Arrhythm Electrophysiol Rev* 2018; 7:199–209.
2. Reilly JG, et al. Thioridazine and sudden unexplained death in psychiatric in-patients. *Br J Psychiatry* 2002; 180:515–522.
3. Murray-Thomas T, et al. Risk of mortality (including sudden cardiac death) and major cardiovascular events in atypical and typical antipsychotic users: a study with the general practice research database. *Cardiovasc Psychiatry Neurol* 2013; 2013:247486.
4. Ray WA, et al. Antipsychotics and the risk of sudden cardiac death. *Arch Gen Psychiatry* 2001; 58:1161–1167.
5. Hennessy S, et al. Cardiac arrest and ventricular arrhythmia in patients taking antipsychotic drugs: cohort study using administrative data. *BMJ* 2002; 325:1070.
6. Straus SM, et al. Antipsychotics and the risk of sudden cardiac death. *Arch Intern Med* 2004; 164:1293–1297.
7. Liperoti R, et al. Conventional and atypical antipsychotics and the risk of hospitalization for ventricular arrhythmias or cardiac arrest. *Arch Intern Med* 2005; 165:696–701.
8. Ray WA, et al. Atypical antipsychotic drugs and the risk of sudden cardiac death. *N Engl J Med* 2009; 360:225–235.
9. Schneeweiss S, et al. Antipsychotic agents and sudden cardiac death–how should we manage the risk? *N Engl J Med* 2009; 360:294–296.
10. Nakagawa S, et al. Antipsychotics and risk of first-time hospitalization for myocardial infarction: a population-based case-control study. *J Intern Med* 2006; 260:451–458.
11. Fujii K, et al. QT is longer in drug-free patients with schizophrenia compared with age-matched healthy subjects. *PLoSOne* 2014; 9:e98555.
12. Zhai D, et al. QTc interval lengthening in first-episode schizophrenia (FES) patients in the earliest stages of antipsychotic treatment. *Schizophr Res* 2017; 179:70–74.
13. Okayasu H, et al. Effects of antipsychotics on arrhythmogenic parameters in schizophrenia patients: beyond corrected QT interval. *Neuropsychiatr Dis Treat* 2021; 17:239–249.
14. Ansermot N, et al. Prevalence of ECG abnormalities and risk factors for QTc interval prolongation in hospitalized psychiatric patients. *Ther Adv Psychopharmacol* 2019; 9:2045125319891386.
15. Danielsson B, et al. Drug use and torsades de pointes cardiac arrhythmias in Sweden: a nationwide register-based cohort study. *BMJ Open* 2020; 10:e034560.
16. Takeuchi H, et al. Antipsychotic polypharmacy and corrected QT interval: a systematic review. *Can J Psychiatry* 2015; 60:215–222.
17. Barbui C, et al. Antipsychotic dose mediates the association between polypharmacy and corrected QT interval. *PLoS One* 2016; 11:e0148212.
18. Goldenberg I, et al. QT interval: how to measure it and what is 'normal'. *J Cardiovasc Electrophysiol* 2006; 17:333–336.
19. Nielsen J, et al. Assessing QT interval prolongation and its associated risks with antipsychotics. *CNS Drugs* 2011; 25:473–490.
20. National Institute for Health and Care Excellence. Psychosis and schizophrenia in adults: prevention and management. Clinical Guidance [CG178]. 2014 (last checked March 2019); https://www.nice.org.uk/guidance/cg178.
21. Malik M, et al. Evaluation of drug-induced QT interval prolongation: implications for drug approval and labelling. *Drug Saf* 2001; 24:323–351.
22. Haddad PM, et al. Antipsychotic-related QTc prolongation, torsade de pointes and sudden death. *Drugs* 2002; 62:1649–1671.
23. Taylor DM. Antipsychotics and QT prolongation. *Acta Psychiatr Scand* 2003; 107:85–95.
24. Botstein P. Is QT interval prolongation harmful? A regulatory perspective. *Am J Cardiol* 1993; 72:50B–52B.
25. Joy JP, et al. Prediction of torsade de pointes from the QT interval: analysis of a case series of amisulpride overdoses. *Clin Pharmacol Ther* 2011; 90:243–245.

26. O'Neal WT, et al. Association between QT-interval components and sudden cardiac death: the ARIC Study (Atherosclerosis Risk in Communities). *Circ Arrhythmia Electrophysiol* 2017; **10**:e005485

27. Witchel HJ, et al. Psychotropic drugs, cardiac arrhythmia, and sudden death. *J Clin Psychopharmacol* 2003; **23**:58–77.

28. Strom BL, et al. Comparative mortality associated with ziprasidone and olanzapine in real-world use among 18,154 patients with schizophrenia: the Ziprasidone Observational Study of Cardiac Outcomes (ZODIAC). *Am J Psychiatry* 2011; **168**:193–201.

29. Chung AK, et al. Effects on prolongation of Bazett's corrected QT interval of seven second-generation antipsychotics in the treatment of schizophrenia: a meta-analysis. *J Psychopharmacology* 2011; **25**:646–666.

30. Vandael E, et al. Development of a risk score for QTc-prolongation: the RISQ-PATH study. *Int J Clin Pharm* 2017; **39**:424–432.

31. CredibleMeds®. CredibleMeds. 2021; https://www.crediblemeds.org.

32. Hui WK, et al. Melperone: electrophysiologic and antiarrhythmic activity in humans. *J Cardiovasc Pharmacol* 1990; **15**:144–149.

33. Glassman AH, et al. Antipsychotic drugs: prolonged QTc interval, torsade de pointes, and sudden death. *Am J Psychiatry* 2001; **158**:1774–1782.

34. Warner B, et al. Investigation of the potential of clozapine to cause torsade de pointes. *Adverse Drug React Toxicol Rev* 2002; **21**:189–203.

35. Harrigan EP, et al. A randomized evaluation of the effects of six antipsychotic agents on QTc, in the absence and presence of metabolic inhibition. *J Clin Psychopharmacol* 2004; **24**:62–69.

36. Lindborg SR, et al. Effects of intramuscular olanzapine vs. haloperidol and placebo on QTc intervals in acutely agitated patients. *Psychiatry Res* 2003; **119**:113–123.

37. Dineen S, et al. QTc prolongation and high-dose olanzapine (Letter). *Psychosomatics* 2003; **44**:174–175.

38. Gupta S, et al. Quetiapine and QTc issues: a case report (Letter). *J Clin Psychiatry* 2003; **64**:612–613.

39. Su KP, et al. A pilot cross-over design study on QTc interval prolongation associated with sulpiride and haloperidol. *Schizophr Res* 2003; **59**:93–94.

40. Chong SA, et al. Prolonged QTc intervals in medicated patients with schizophrenia. *Human Psychopharmacology* 2003; **18**:647–649.

41. Stollberger C, et al. Antipsychotic drugs and QT prolongation. *Int Clin Psychopharmacol* 2005; **20**:243–251.

42. Isbister GK, et al. Amisulpride deliberate self-poisoning causing severe cardiac toxicity including QT prolongation and torsades de pointes. *Med J Aust* 2006; **184**:354–356.

43. Ward DI. Two cases of amisulpride overdose: a cause for prolonged QT syndrome. *Emerg Med Australas* 2005; **17**:274–276.

44. Vieweg WV, et al. Torsade de pointes in a patient with complex medical and psychiatric conditions receiving low-dose quetiapine. *Acta Psychiatr Scand* 2005; **112**:318–322.

45. Huang BH, et al. Sulpiride induced torsade de pointes. *Int J Cardiol* 2007; **118**:e100–e102.

46. Kane JM, et al. Long-term efficacy and safety of iloperidone: results from 3 clinical trials for the treatment of schizophrenia. *J Clin Psychopharmacol* 2008; **28**:S29–S35.

47. Kim MD, et al. Blockade of HERG human K+ channel and IKr of guinea pig cardiomyocytes by prochlorperazine. *Eur J Pharmacol* 2006; **544**:82–90.

48. Meltzer H, et al. Efficacy and tolerability of oral paliperidone extended-release tablets in the treatment of acute schizophrenia: pooled data from three 6-week placebo-controlled studies. *J Clin Psychiatry* 2006; **69**:817–829.

49. Chapel S, et al. Exposure-response analysis in patients with schizophrenia to assess the effect of asenapine on QTc prolongation. *J Clin Pharmacol* 2009; **49**:1297–1308.

50. Ozeki Y, et al. QTc prolongation and antipsychotic medications in a sample of 1017 patients with schizophrenia. *Prog Neuropsychopharmacol Biol Psychiatry* 2010; **34**:401–405.

51. Girardin FR, et al. Drug-induced long QT in adult psychiatric inpatients: the 5-year cross-sectional ECG Screening Outcome in Psychiatry study. *Am J Psychiatry* 2013; **170**:1468–1476.

52. Leucht S, et al. Comparative efficacy and tolerability of 15 antipsychotic drugs in schizophrenia: a multiple-treatments meta-analysis. *Lancet* 2013; **382**:951–962.

53. Grande I, et al. QTc prolongation: is clozapine safe? Study of 82 cases before and after clozapine treatment. *Human Psychopharmacology* 2011; **26**:397–403.

54. Hong HK, et al. Block of hERG K+ channel and prolongation of action potential duration by fluphenazine at submicromolar concentration. *Eur J Pharmacol* 2013; **702**:165–173.

55. Vieweg WV, et al. Risperidone, QTc interval prolongation, and torsade de pointes: a systematic review of case reports. *Psychopharmacology* 2013; **228**:515–524.

56. Suzuki Y, et al. QT prolongation of the antipsychotic risperidone is predominantly related to its 9-hydroxy metabolite paliperidone. *HumPsychopharmacol* 2012; **27**:39–42.

57. Polcwiartek C, et al. The cardiac safety of aripiprazole treatment in patients at high risk for torsade: a systematic review with a meta-analytic approach. *Psychopharmacology* 2015; **232**:3297–3308.

58. Danielsson B, et al. Antidepressants and antipsychotics classified with torsades de pointes arrhythmia risk and mortality in older adults – a Swedish nationwide study. *Br J Clin Pharmacol* 2016; **81**:773–783.

59. Citrome L. Cariprazine in schizophrenia: clinical efficacy, tolerability, and place in therapy. *Adv Ther* 2013; **30**:114–126.

60. Das S, et al. Brexpiprazole: so far so good. *Ther Adv Psychopharmacol* 2016; **6**:39–54.

61. Meyer JM, et al. Lurasidone: a new drug in development for schizophrenia. *Expert Opinion on Investigational Drugs* 2009; **18**:1715–1726.

62. Nelson S, et al. Torsades de pointes after administration of low-dose aripiprazole. *AnnPharmacother* 2013; **47**:e11.

63. Hategan A, et al. Aripiprazole-associated QTc prolongation in a geriatric patient. *J Clin Psychopharmacol* 2014; **34**:766–768.

64. Suzuki Y, et al. Dose-dependent increase in the QTc interval in aripiprazole treatment after risperidone. *Prog Neuropsychopharmacol Biol Psychiatry* 2011; 35:643–644.

65. Raschi E, et al. The contribution of national spontaneous reporting systems to detect signals of torsadogenicity: issues emerging from the ARITMO project. *Drug Saf* 2016; 39:59–68.

66. Belmonte C, et al. Evaluation of the relationship between pharmacokinetics and the safety of aripiprazole and its cardiovascular effects in healthy volunteers. *J Clin Psychopharmacol* 2016; 36:608–614.

67. Germano E, et al. ECG parameters in children and adolescents treated with aripiprazole and risperidone. *Prog Neuropsychopharmacol Biol Psychiatry* 2014; 51:23–27.

68. Su KP, et al. Olanzapine-induced QTc prolongation in a patient with Wolff-Parkinson-White syndrome. *Schizophr Res* 2004; 66:191–192.

69. Morissette P, et al. Olanzapine prolongs cardiac repolarization by blocking the rapid component of the delayed rectifier potassium current. *Journal of Psychopharmacology* 2007; 21:735–741.

70. Bar KJ, et al. Influence of olanzapine on QT variability and complexity measures of heart rate in patients with schizophrenia. *J Clin Psychopharmacol* 2008; 28:694–698.

71. Berling I, et al. Prolonged QT risk assessment in antipsychotic overdose using the qt nomogram. *Ann Emerg Med* 2015; 66:154–164.

72. Jensen KG, et al. Corrected QT changes during antipsychotic treatment of children and adolescents: a systematic review and meta-analysis of clinical trials. *J Am Acad Child Adolesc Psychiatry* 2015; 54:25–36.

73. Karz AJ, et al. Effects of aripiprazole on the QTc: a case report. *J Clin Psychiatry* 2015; 76:1648–1649.

74. Friedrich ME, et al. Cardiovascular adverse reactions during antipsychotic treatment: results of AMSP, a drug surveillance program between 1993 and 2013. *Int J Neuropsychopharmacol* 2020; 23:67–75.

75. Sunovion Pharmaceuticals Inc. Highlights of Prescribing Information: LATUDA (lurasidone hydrochloride) tablets. 2019; http://www.latuda.com/LatudaPrescribingInformation.pdf.

76. Potkin SG, et al. Double-blind comparison of the safety and efficacy of lurasidone and ziprasidone in clinically stable outpatients with schizophrenia or schizoaffective disorder. *Schizophr Res* 2011; 132:101–107.

77. Nakamura M, et al. Lurasidone in the treatment of acute schizophrenia: a double-blind, placebo-controlled trial. *J Clin Psychiatry* 2009; 70:829–836.

78. Meltzer HY, et al. Lurasidone in the treatment of schizophrenia: a randomized, double-blind, placebo- and olanzapine-controlled study. *Am J Psychiatry* 2011; 168:957–967.

79. Hasnain M, et al. Quetiapine, QTc interval prolongation, and torsade de pointes: a review of case reports. *Ther Adv Psychopharmacol* 2014; 4:130–138.

80. Hatta K, et al. Prolonged QT interval in acute psychotic patients. *Psychiatry Res* 2000; 94:279–285.

81. Priori SG, et al. Low penetrance in the long-QT syndrome: clinical impact. *Circulation* 1999; 99:529–533.

82. Frassati D, et al. Hidden cardiac lesions and psychotropic drugs as a possible cause of sudden death in psychiatric patients: a report of 14 cases and review of the literature. *Can J Psychiatry* 2004; 49:100–105.

Effect of antipsychotic medications on plasma lipids

Morbidity and mortality from cardiovascular disease are higher in people with schizophrenia than in the general population.[1] Dyslipidaemia is an established risk factor for cardiovascular disease along with obesity, hypertension, smoking, diabetes and sedentary lifestyle. Specifically, reduced HDL cholesterol and raised triglyceride levels are included in the definition of the metabolic syndrome.[2] The majority of patients with schizophrenia have several of these risk factors and can be considered at 'high risk' of developing cardiovascular disease. Dyslipidaemia is treatable, and intervention is known to reduce morbidity and mortality.[3] Aggressive treatment is particularly important in people with diabetes, the prevalence of which is increased 2- to 3-fold over population norms in people with schizophrenia (see the section on diabetes).

Effect of antipsychotic drugs on lipids

Antipsychotic medications show a marked variation in their effects on total cholesterol, low-density lipoprotein (LDL) cholesterol, high-density lipoprotein (HDL) cholesterol, and triglycerides.[4] Regarding FGAs, phenothiazines are known to be associated with increases in triglycerides and LDL cholesterol and decreases in HDL[5] cholesterol, but the magnitude of these effects is poorly quantified.[6] Haloperidol seems to have minimal effect on lipid profiles.[5] Although there are relatively more data pertaining to some SGAs, they are derived from a variety of sources and are reported in different ways, making it difficult to compare drugs directly. While cholesterol levels can rise, the most profound effect of these drugs seems to be on triglycerides. Raised triglycerides are, in general, associated with obesity and diabetes. From the available data, clozapine and olanzapine[4,7] would seem to have the greatest propensity to increase lipids, while quetiapine and risperidone have a moderate propensity.[8,9] Aripiprazole, lurasidone and ziprasidone appear to have minimal adverse effect on blood lipids[4,7,10-15] and may even modestly reverse dyslipidaemias associated with previous antipsychotics.[14,16,17] For cariprazine and brexpiprazole, the effects on plasma lipids would also appear to be relatively limited.[4,18-21] Iloperidone causes some weight gain but may not have an equivalent impact on cholesterol or triglycerides.[4,22,23] Early RCT data suggest that lumateperone is not associated with any significant effects on plasma cholesterol or triglycerides in the short term, compared with placebo.[24]

Olanzapine

Olanzapine has been shown to increase triglyceride levels by 40% over the short (12 weeks) and medium (16 months) term.[25,26] Levels may continue to rise for up to a year.[27] Up to two-thirds of olanzapine-treated patients have raised triglycerides[28] and just under 10% may develop severe hypertriglyceridaemia.[29] While weight gain with olanzapine is generally associated with both increases in cholesterol[26,30] and triglycerides,[29] severe hypertriglyceridaemia can occur independently of weight gain.[29] In one study, patients treated with olanzapine or risperidone gained a similar amount of weight, but in olanzapine patients serum triglyceride levels increased by four times as much (105mg/dl) as in risperidone patients (32mg/dl).[31] Quetiapine[32] seems to have more modest effects than olanzapine, although the data are conflicting.[33]

A case–control study conducted in the UK found that patients with schizophrenia who were treated with olanzapine were five times more likely to develop hyperlipidaemia than those with no antipsychotic exposure and three times more likely to develop hyperlipidaemia than patients receiving FGAs.[34] Risperidone treatment was not associated with an increased likelihood of hyperlipidaemia compared with no antipsychotic exposure or treatment with an FGA.

Clozapine

Mean triglyceride levels have been shown to double and cholesterol levels to increase by at least 10% after 5 years of treatment with clozapine.[35] Patients treated with clozapine have triglyceride levels that are almost double those of patients who are treated with FGA medications.[36,37] Cholesterol levels are also increased.[7]

Particular care should be taken before prescribing clozapine or olanzapine for patients who are obese, diabetic or known to have pre-existing hyperlipidaemia.[38]

Screening and monitoring

All patients should have their lipids measured at baseline, 3 months after starting treatment with a new antipsychotic medication and then annually. Those prescribed clozapine and olanzapine should ideally have their serum lipids measured every 3 months for the first year of treatment, and then annually. Clinically significant changes in cholesterol are unlikely over the short term, but triglycerides can increase dramatically.[39] In practice, dyslipidaemia is widespread in patients on long-term antipsychotic treatment irrespective of the medication prescribed or of diagnosis.[40–42] Screening for this potentially serious side effect of antipsychotic medication is not yet routine in clinical practice,[43] but is strongly recommended by NICE.[44]

Severe hypertriglyceridemia (fasting level of >5mmol/L) is a risk factor for pancreatitis. Note that antipsychotic-induced dyslipidaemia can occur independent of weight gain.[45]

Clinical management of dyslipidaemia

Patients with raised cholesterol may benefit from dietary advice, lifestyle changes and/or treatment with statins.[46,47] Statins seem to be effective in this patient group, but interactions are possible.[48] The outline of a systematic approach to the diagnosis and management of hypercholesterolaemia is available,[49] based on NICE guidance.[50] Further, risk tables and treatment guidelines can be found in the British National Formulary (BNF). Evidence supports the treatment of cholesterol concentrations as low as 4mmol/l in high-risk patients,[51] and this is the highest level recommended by NICE for secondary prevention of cardiovascular events.[52] NICE makes no recommendations on target levels for primary prevention, but recent advice promotes the use of statins for anyone with a > 10% ten-year risk of cardiovascular disease.[52] Coronary heart disease and stroke risk can be reduced by a third by reducing cholesterol to as low as 3.5mmol/L. When triglycerides alone are raised, diets low in saturated fats, and the taking of fish oil and fibrates are effective treatments,[27,53,54] although there is no proof that mortality is reduced. Such patients should be screened for IGT and diabetes.

If moderate to severe hyperlipidaemia develops during antipsychotic treatment, a switch to another antipsychotic medication less likely to cause this problem should be considered in the first instance. Although not recommended as a strategy in patients with treatment-resistant illness, clozapine-induced hypertriglyceridaemia has been shown to reverse after a switch to risperidone.[55] This may hold true with other switching regimens but data are scarce.[56] Aripiprazole and other D2 partial agonists seem to be the treatments of choice in those with prior antipsychotic-induced dyslipidaemia (lumateperone and ziprasidone are options outside the UK).[17,57] There is evidence to suggest that adjunctive aripiprazole may have beneficial effects on measures of plasma cholesterol and triglycerides when combined with clozapine or olanzapine[16,47,58] and that metformin added to antipsychotic medication may improve total cholesterol and triglyceride levels[47,59] (see the relevant British Association for Psychopharmacology guideline[47] for discussion of the potential risks and benefits of these two strategies).

Summary

Monitoring

Medication	Suggested monitoring schedule
Clozapine Olanzapine	Fasting lipids at baseline then every 3 months for a year, then annually
Other antipsychotic medications	Fasting lipids at baseline, 3 months, and then annually[57]

References

1. Brown S, et al. Causes of the excess mortality of schizophrenia. *Br J Psychiatry* 2000; **177**:212–217.
2. Alberti KG, et al. The metabolic syndrome–a new worldwide definition. *Lancet* 2005; **366**:1059–1062.
3. Durrington P. Dyslipidaemia. *Lancet* 2003; **362**:717–731.
4. Pillinger T, et al. Comparative effects of 18 antipsychotics on metabolic function in patients with schizophrenia, predictors of metabolic dysregulation, and association with psychopathology: a systematic review and network meta-analysis. *Lancet Psychiatry* 2020; **7**:64–77.
5. Sasaki J, et al. Lipids and apolipoproteins in patients treated with major tranquilizers. *Clin Pharmacol Ther* 1985; **37**:684–687.
6. Henkin Y, et al. Secondary dyslipidemia: inadvertent effects of drugs in clinical practice. *JAMA* 1992; **267**:961–968.
7. Chaggar PS, et al. Effect of antipsychotic medications on glucose and lipid levels. *J Clin Pharmacol* 2011; **51**:631–638.
8. Smith RC, et al. Effects of olanzapine and risperidone on lipid metabolism in chronic schizophrenic patients with long-term antipsychotic treatment: a randomized five month study. *Schizophr Res* 2010; **120**:204–209.
9. Perez-Iglesias R, et al. Glucose and lipid disturbances after 1 year of antipsychotic treatment in a drug-naive population. *Schizophr Res* 2009; **107**:115–121.
10. Olfson M, et al. Hyperlipidemia following treatment with antipsychotic medications. *Am J Psychiatry* 2006; **163**:1821–1825.
11. L'Italien GJ, et al. Comparison of metabolic syndrome incidence among schizophrenia patients treated with aripiprazole versus olanzapine or placebo. *J Clin Psychiatry* 2007; **68**:1510–1516.
12. Fenton WS, et al. Medication-induced weight gain and dyslipidemia in patients with schizophrenia. *Am J Psychiatry* 2006; **163**:1697–1704.
13. Meyer JM, et al. Change in metabolic syndrome parameters with antipsychotic treatment in the CATIE Schizophrenia Trial: prospective data from phase 1. *Schizophr Res* 2008; **101**:273–286.
14. Potkin SG, et al. Double-blind comparison of the safety and efficacy of lurasidone and ziprasidone in clinically stable outpatients with schizophrenia or schizoaffective disorder. *Schizophr Res* 2011; **132**:101–107.
15. Correll CU, et al. Long-term safety and effectiveness of lurasidone in schizophrenia: a 22-month, open-label extension study. *CNS Spectr* 2016; **21**:393–402.
16. Fleischhacker WW, et al. Effects of adjunctive treatment with aripiprazole on body weight and clinical efficacy in schizophrenia patients treated with clozapine: a randomized, double-blind, placebo-controlled trial. *Int J Neuropsychopharmacol* 2010; **13**:1115–1125.
17. Chen Y, et al. Comparative effectiveness of switching antipsychotic drug treatment to aripiprazole or ziprasidone for improving metabolic profile and atherogenic dyslipidemia: a 12-month, prospective, open-label study. *J Psychopharmacol* 2012; **26**:1201–1210.
18. Lao KS, et al. Tolerability and safety profile of cariprazine in treating psychotic disorders, bipolar disorder and major depressive disorder: a systematic review with meta-analysis of randomized controlled trials. *CNS Drugs* 2016; **30**:1043–1054.
19. Earley W, et al. Tolerability of cariprazine in the treatment of acute bipolar I mania: a pooled post hoc analysis of 3 phase II/III studies. *J Affect Disord* 2017; **215**:205–212.
20. McEvoy J, et al. Brexpiprazole for the treatment of schizophrenia: a review of this novel serotonin-dopamine activity modulator. *Clin Schizophr Relat Psychoses* 2016; **9**:177–186.
21. Correll CU, et al. Efficacy and safety of brexpiprazole for the treatment of acute schizophrenia: a 6-week randomized, double-blind, placebo-controlled trial. *Am J Psychiatry* 2015; **172**:870–880.
22. Citrome L. Iloperidone: chemistry, pharmacodynamics, pharmacokinetics and metabolism, clinical efficacy, safety and tolerability, regulatory affairs, and an opinion. *Expert Opin Drug Metab Toxicol* 2010; **6**:1551–1564.

23. Cutler AJ, et al. Long-term safety and tolerability of iloperidone: results from a 25-week, open-label extension trial. *CNS Spectr* 2013; **18**:43–54.

24. Correll CU, et al. Efficacy and safety of lumateperone for treatment of schizophrenia: a randomized clinical trial. *JAMA Psychiatry* 2020; **77**:349–358.

25. Sheitman BB, et al. Olanzapine-induced elevation of plasma triglyceride levels. *Am J Psychiatry* 1999; **156**:1471–1472.

26. Osser DN, et al. Olanzapine increases weight and serum triglyceride levels. *J Clin Psychiatry* 1999; **60**:767–770.

27. Meyer JM. Effects of atypical antipsychotics on weight and serum lipid levels. *J Clin Psychiatry* 2001; **62 Suppl 27**:27–34.

28. Melkersson KI, et al. Elevated levels of insulin, leptin, and blood lipids in olanzapine-treated patients with schizophrenia or related psychoses. *J Clin Psychiatry* 2000; **61**:742–749.

29. Meyer JM. Novel antipsychotics and severe hyperlipidemia. *J Clin Psychopharmacol* 2001; **21**:369–374.

30. Kinon BJ, et al. Long-term olanzapine treatment: weight change and weight-related health factors in schizophrenia. *J Clin Psychiatry* 2001; **62**:92–100.

31. Meyer JM. A retrospective comparison of weight, lipid, and glucose changes between risperidone- and olanzapine-treated inpatients: metabolic outcomes after 1 year. *J Clin Psychiatry* 2002; **63**:425–433.

32. Atmaca M, et al. Serum leptin and triglyceride levels in patients on treatment with atypical antipsychotics. *J Clin Psychiatry* 2003; **64**:598–604.

33. De Leon J, et al. A clinical study of the association of antipsychotics with hyperlipidemia. *Schizophr Res* 2007; **92**:95–102.

34. Koro CE, et al. An assessment of the independent effects of olanzapine and risperidone exposure on the risk of hyperlipidemia in schizophrenic patients. *Arch Gen Psychiatry* 2002; **59**:1021–1026.

35. Henderson DC, et al. Clozapine, diabetes mellitus, weight gain, and lipid abnormalities: a five-year naturalistic study. *Am J Psychiatry* 2000; **157**:975–981.

36. Ghaeli P, et al. Serum triglyceride levels in patients treated with clozapine. *Am J Health Syst Pharm* 1996; **53**:2079–2081.

37. Spivak B, et al. Diminished suicidal and aggressive behavior, high plasma norepinephrine levels, and serum triglyceride levels in chronic neuroleptic-resistant schizophrenic patients maintained on clozapine. *Clin Neuropharmacol* 1998; **21**:245–250.

38. Baptista T, et al. Novel antipsychotics and severe hyperlipidemia: comments on the Meyer paper. *J Clin Psychopharmacol* 2002; **22**:536–537.

39. Meyer JM, et al. The effects of antipsychotic therapy on serum lipids: a comprehensive review. *Schizophr Res* 2004; **70**:1–17.

40. Paton C, et al. Obesity, dyslipidaemias and smoking in an inpatient population treated with antipsychotic drugs. *Acta Psychiatr Scand* 2004; **110**:299–305.

41. De Hert M, et al. The METEOR study of diabetes and other metabolic disorders in patients with schizophrenia treated with antipsychotic drugs. I. Methodology. *Int J Methods Psychiatr Res* 2010; **19**:195–210.

42. Jin H, et al. Comparison of longer-term safety and effectiveness of 4 atypical antipsychotics in patients over age 40: a trial using equipoise-stratified randomization. *J Clin Psychiatry* 2013; **74**:10–18.

43. Barnes TR, et al. Screening for the metabolic side effects of antipsychotic medication: findings of a 6-year quality improvement programme in the UK. *BMJ Open* 2015; **5**:e007633.

44. National Institute for Health and Care Excellence. Psychosis and schizophrenia in adults: prevention and management. Clinical Guidance 178 [CG178]. 2014; https://www.nice.org.uk/guidance/cg178.

45. Birkenaes AB, et al. Dyslipidemia independent of body mass in antipsychotic-treated patients under real-life conditions. *J Clin Psychopharmacol* 2008; **28**:132–137.

46. Ojala K, et al. Statins are effective in treating dyslipidemia among psychiatric patients using second-generation antipsychotic agents. *J Psychopharmacol* 2008; **22**:33–38.

47. Cooper SJ, et al. BAP guidelines on the management of weight gain, metabolic disturbances and cardiovascular risk associated with psychosis and antipsychotic drug treatment. *J Psychopharmacol* 2016; **30**:717–748.

48. Tse L, et al. Pharmacological treatment of antipsychotic-induced dyslipidemia and hypertension. *Int Clin Psychopharmacol* 2014; **29**:125–137.

49. Ryan A, et al. Dyslipidaemia and cardiovascular risk. *BMJ* 2018; **360**:k835.

50. Rabar S, et al. Lipid modification and cardiovascular risk assessment for the primary and secondary prevention of cardiovascular disease: summary of updated NICE guidance. *BMJ* 2014; **349**:g4356.

51. Group HPSC. MRC/BHF Heart Protection Study of cholesterol lowering with simvastatin in 20,536 high-risk individuals: a randomised placebo-controlled trial. *Lancet* 2002; **360**:7–22.

52. National Institute for Health and Care Excellence. Cardiovascular disease: risk assessment and reduction, including lipid modification. Clinical guideline [CG181] 2014 (Last updated 2016); https://www.nice.org.uk/Guidance/CG181.

53. Caniato RN, et al. Effect of omega-3 fatty acids on the lipid profile of patients taking clozapine. *Aust N Z J Psychiatry* 2006; **40**:691–697.

54. Freeman MP, et al. Omega-3 fatty acids for atypical antipsychotic-associated hypertriglyceridemia. *Ann Clin Psychiatry* 2015; **27**:197–202.

55. Ghaeli P, et al. Elevated serum triglycerides with clozapine resolved with risperidone in four patients. *Pharmacotherapy* 1999; **19**:1099–1101.

56. Weiden PJ. Switching antipsychotics as a treatment strategy for antipsychotic-induced weight gain and dyslipidemia. *J Clin Psychiatry* 2007; **68 Suppl 4**:34–39.

57. Newcomer JW, et al. A multicenter, randomized, double-blind study of the effects of aripiprazole in overweight subjects with schizophrenia or schizoaffective disorder switched from olanzapine. *J Clin Psychiatry* 2008; **69**:1046–1056.

58. Henderson DC, et al. Aripiprazole added to overweight and obese olanzapine-treated schizophrenia patients. *J Clin Psychopharmacol* 2009; **29**:165–169.

59. Jiang WL, et al. Adjunctive metformin for antipsychotic-induced dyslipidemia: a meta-analysis of randomized, double-blind, placebo-controlled trials. *Trans Psychiatry* 2020; **10**:117.

Diabetes and impaired glucose tolerance

Schizophrenia

Schizophrenia is associated with relatively high rates of insulin resistance and diabetes[1,2] – an observation that predates the discovery and widespread use of antipsychotics.[3-5] Lifestyle interventions (lower weight, more activity) are effective in preventing diabetes[6,7] and should be considered for all people with a diagnosis of schizophrenia.

Antipsychotics

The data relating to diabetes and the use of antipsychotic medication are numerous but less than perfect.[8-12] The main problem is that while incidence and prevalence studies assume full or uniform screening for diabetes, this is unlikely to be occurring in clinical practice.[8] Many studies do not account for other factors affecting the risk of developing diabetes.[11] Small differences between medications are therefore difficult to substantiate but may in any case be ultimately unimportant: risk is probably increased for all those with schizophrenia receiving any antipsychotic medication.

The mechanisms involved in the development of antipsychotic-related diabetes are unclear, but may include $5HT_{2A}/5HT_{2C}$ antagonism, increased plasma lipids, weight gain and leptin resistance.[13] Insulin resistance may occur in the absence of weight gain.[14]

First-generation antipsychotics

Phenothiazine derivatives have long been associated with impaired glucose tolerance and diabetes.[15] Diabetes prevalence was reported to have substantially increased following the introduction and widespread use of FGA drugs.[16] The prevalence of impaired glucose tolerance seems to be higher with the aliphatic phenothiazines than with fluphenazine or haloperidol.[17] Hyperglycaemia has also been reported with other FGAs, such as loxapine,[18] and other data confirm an association with haloperidol.[19] Some studies even suggest that FGAs are no different from SGAs in their propensity to cause diabetes,[20,21] whereas others suggest a modest but statistically significant excess incidence of diabetes with SGAs.[22]

Second-generation antipsychotics

Clozapine

Clozapine is strongly linked to hyperglycaemia, impaired glucose tolerance and diabetic ketoacidosis.[23] The risk of diabetes appears to be higher with clozapine than with other SGAs or FGAs, especially in younger patients,[24-27] although this is not a consistent finding.[28,29]

As many as a third of patients might develop diabetes after 5 years of clozapine treatment.[30] Many cases of diabetes occur in the first 6 months of treatment, some within a month,[31] and some only after many years.[29] Death from ketoacidosis has also been reported.[31] Diabetes associated with clozapine is not necessarily linked to obesity or to family history of diabetes,[23,32] although these factors greatly increase the risk of developing diabetes on clozapine.[33]

Clozapine appears to increase plasma levels of insulin in a clozapine level-dependent fashion.[34,35] It has been shown to be more likely than FGAs to increase plasma glucose and insulin following oral glucose challenge.[36] Testing for diabetes is essential given the high prevalence of diabetes in people receiving clozapine.[37]

Olanzapine

As with clozapine, olanzapine has been strongly linked to impaired glucose tolerance, diabetes and diabetic ketoacidosis.[38] Olanzapine and clozapine appear to directly induce insulin resistance.[39,40] Risk of diabetes has also been reported to be higher with olanzapine than with FGA drugs,[41] again with a particular risk in younger patients.[25] The time course of development of diabetes has not been established but impaired glucose tolerance seems to occur even in the absence of obesity and family history of diabetes.[23,32] Olanzapine is probably more diabetogenic than risperidone.[42-46] Olanzapine is also associated with plasma levels of glucose and insulin higher than those seen with FGAs (after oral glucose load).[36,47]

Risperidone

Risperidone has been linked, mainly in case reports, to impaired glucose tolerance,[48] diabetes[49] and ketoacidosis.[50] The number of reports of such adverse effects is substantially smaller than with either clozapine or olanzapine.[51] At least one study has suggested that changes in fasting glucose are significantly less common with risperidone than with olanzapine,[42] but other studies have detected no difference.[52]

Risperidone seems no more likely than FGA drugs to be associated with diabetes,[25,41,43] although there may be an increased risk in patients under 40 years of age.[25] Risperidone has, however, been observed adversely to affect fasting glucose and plasma glucose (following glucose challenge) compared with the levels seen in healthy volunteers (but not compared with patients taking FGAs).[36]

Quetiapine

Like risperidone, quetiapine has been linked to cases of new-onset diabetes and ketoacidosis.[53-55] Again, the number of reports is much lower than with olanzapine or clozapine. Quetiapine appears to be more likely than FGA medications to be associated with diabetes.[25,56] Two studies showed quetiapine to be equal to olanzapine in the incidence of diabetes.[52,57] The risk with quetiapine may be dose-related, with daily doses of 400mg or more being clearly linked to changes in HbA_{1C}.[58]

Other SGAs

Amisulpride appears not to elevate plasma glucose[59] and seems not to be associated with diabetes.[60] There is one reported case of ketoacidosis occurring in a patient given the closely related medication, sulpiride.[61] Data for aripiprazole[62-65] and ziprasidone[66,67] suggest that neither drug alters glucose homeostasis. Aripiprazole may even reverse diabetes caused by other drugs[68] (although ketoacidosis has been reported with aripiprazole[69-71]). A large case–control study has confirmed that neither amisulpride nor aripiprazole increase the risk of diabetes.[72] These three drugs (amisulpride, aripiprazole and ziprasidone) are recommended for those with a history of or predisposition to diabetes mellitus or as an alternative to other antipsychotics known to be diabetogenic. Data suggest neither lurasidone[73,74] nor asenapine[75,76] has any effect on glucose homeostasis. Likewise, initial data for brexpiprazole[77] and cariprazine[78,79] suggest minimal effects on glucose tolerance. Thus, for patients developing prediabetes or diabetes who are being treated with clozapine, olanzapine or quetiapine, switching to antipsychotic medications with a lower cardiometabolic risk, such as aripiprazole, brexpiprazole, cariprazine, lurasidone or ziprasidone, has been recommended.[80]

Lumateperone appears to have no effect on glucose parameters[81] but clinical experience if limited.

Predicting antipsychotic-related diabetes

The risk of diabetes is increased to a much greater extent in younger adults than in the elderly[82,83] (for whom antipsychotic medication may show no increased risk[84]). First-episode patients seem particularly prone to the development of diabetes, with a variety of antipsychotic medications.[85-87] During treatment, rapid weight gain and a rise in plasma triglycerides seem to be predictive of the development of diabetes.[88]

Monitoring

Diabetes is a growing problem in western society and has a strong association with obesity, (older) age, (lower) educational achievement and certain ethnic groups.[89,90] Diabetes markedly increases cardiovascular mortality, largely as a consequence of atherosclerosis.[91] Likewise, the use of antipsychotic medication also increases cardiovascular mortality.[92-94] Intervention to reduce plasma glucose levels and minimise other risk factors (obesity, hypercholesterolaemia) is therefore essential.[95]

There is no clear consensus on diabetes-monitoring practice for those receiving antipsychotics,[96] and recommendations in formal guidelines vary considerably.[97] Given the previous known parlous state of testing for diabetes in the UK[8,98-100] and elsewhere,[101] arguments over precisely which tests are done and when seem to miss the point. There is an overwhelming need to improve monitoring by any means and so any tests for diabetes are supported – urine glucose and random plasma glucose included.

Ideally, though, all patients should have oral glucose tolerance tests (OGTT) performed as this is the most sensitive method of detection.[102,103] Fasting plasma glucose (FPG) tests are less sensitive but recommended.[104] Any abnormality in FPG should provoke an OGTT. Fasting tests are often difficult to obtain in acutely ill, disorganised patients, so measurement of random plasma glucose or glycosylated haemoglobin (HbA_{1C}) may also be used (fasting not required). HbA_{1C} is now recognised as a useful tool for detecting and monitoring diabetes.[105] Frequency of monitoring should then be determined by physical factors (e.g. weight gain) and known risk factors (e.g. family history of diabetes, lipid abnormalities, smoking status). The absolute minimum is yearly testing for diabetes for all patients. In addition, all patients should be asked to look out for and report signs and symptoms of diabetes (fatigue, candida infection, thirst polyuria).

Treatment of antipsychotic-related diabetes

Switching to an antipsychotic medication with a lower cardiometabolic risk is often effective in reversing changes in glucose tolerance. In this respect, the most compelling evidence is for switching to aripiprazole[106,107] but also to ziprasidone[107] and perhaps lurasidone.[74] Standard antidiabetic treatments are otherwise recommended.[80] Pioglitazone[108] may have particular benefit but note the hepatotoxic potential of this drug. GLP-1 agonists such as liraglutide are increasingly used.[109]

Table 1.25 Recommended monitoring for diabetes in patients receiving antipsychotic drug

Recommended monitoring	Ideally	Minimum
Baseline	OGTT or FPG HbA_{1C} if fasting not possible	Urine glucose (UG) Random plasma glucose (RPG)
Continuation	All drugs: OGTT or FPG + HbA_{1C} at 4–6 months then every 12 months. For clozapine and olanzapine or if other risk factors present: OGTT or FPG after one month, then every 4–6 months. For on-going regular screening, HbA_{1C} is a suitable test. Note that this test is not suitable for detecting short-term change.	UG or RPG every 12 months, with symptom monitoring

FPG, fasting plasma glucose; OGTT, oral glucose tolerance tests; RPG, random plasma glucose

Summary: Antipsychotics – risk of diabetes and impaired glucose tolerance

High risk	Clozapine, olanzapine
Moderate risk	Quetiapine, risperidone, phenothiazines
Low risk	High-potency FGAs (e.g. haloperidol)
Minimal risk	Aripiprazole, amisulpride, asenapine, brexpiprazole, cariprazine, lumateperone, lurasidone, ziprasidone

References

1. Schimmelbusch WH, et al. The positive correlation between insulin resistance and duration of hospitalization in untreated schizophrenia. *Br J Psychiatry* 1971; **118**:429–436.
2. Waitzkin L. A survey for unknown diabetics in a mental hospital. I. Men under age fifty. *Diabetes* 1966; **15**:97–104.
3. Kasanin J. The blood sugar curve in mental disease. II. The schizophrenia (dementia praecox) groups. *Arch Neurol Psychiatry* 1926; **16**:414–419.
4. Braceland FJ, et al. Delayed action of insulin in schizophrenia. *Am J Psychiatry* 1945; **102**:108–110.
5. Kohen D. Diabetes mellitus and schizophrenia: historical perspective. *Br J Psychiatry Suppl* 2004; **47**:S64–S66.
6. Knowler WC, et al. 10-year follow-up of diabetes incidence and weight loss in the Diabetes Prevention Program Outcomes Study. *Lancet* 2009; **374**:1677–1686.

7. Glechner A, et al. Effects of lifestyle changes on adults with prediabetes: a systematic review and meta-analysis. *Prim Care Diabetes* 2018; 12:393–408.

8. Taylor D, et al. Testing for diabetes in hospitalised patients prescribed antipsychotic drugs. *Br J Psychiatry* 2004; 185:152–156.

9. Haddad PM. Antipsychotics and diabetes: review of non-prospective data. *Br J Psychiatry Suppl* 2004; 47:S80–S86.

10. Bushe C, et al. Association between atypical antipsychotic agents and type 2 diabetes: review of prospective clinical data. *Br J Psychiatry* 2004; 184:S87–S93.

11. Gianfrancesco F, et al. The influence of study design on the results of pharmacoepidemiologic studies of diabetes risk with antipsychotic therapy. *Ann Clin Psychiatry* 2006; 18:9–17.

12. Hirigo AT, et al. The magnitude of undiagnosed diabetes and Hypertension among adult psychiatric patients receiving antipsychotic treatment. *Diabetol Metab Syndr* 2020; 12:79.

13. Buchholz S, et al. Atypical antipsychotic-induced diabetes mellitus: an update on epidemiology and postulated mechanisms. *Intern Med J* 2008; 38:602–606.

14. Teff KL, et al. Antipsychotic-induced insulin resistance and postprandial hormonal dysregulation independent of weight gain or psychiatric disease. *Diabetes* 2013; 62:3232–3240.

15. Arneson GA. Phenothiazine derivatives and glucose metabolism. *J Neuropsychiatr* 1964; 5:181.

16. Lindenmayer JP, et al. Hyperglycemia associated with the use of atypical antipsychotics. *J Clin Psychiatry* 2001; 62 Suppl 23:30–38.

17. Keskiner A, et al. Psychotropic drugs, diabetes and chronic mental patients. *Psychosomatics* 1973; 14:176–181.

18. Tollefson G, et al. Nonketotic hyperglycemia associated with loxapine and amoxapine: case report. *J Clin Psychiatry* 1983; 44:347–348.

19. Lindenmayer JP, et al. Changes in glucose and cholesterol levels in patients with schizophrenia treated with typical or atypical antipsychotics. *Am J Psychiatry* 2003; 160:290–296.

20. Carlson C, et al. Diabetes mellitus and antipsychotic treatment in the United Kingdom. *Eur Neuropsychopharmacol* 2006; 16:366–375.

21. Ostbye T, et al. Atypical antipsychotic drugs and diabetes mellitus in a large outpatient population: a retrospective cohort study. *Pharmacoepidemiol Drug Saf* 2005; 14:407–415.

22. Smith M, et al. First- v. second-generation antipsychotics and risk for diabetes in schizophrenia: systematic review and meta-analysis. *Br J Psychiatry* 2008; 192:406–411.

23. Mir S, et al. Atypical antipsychotics and hyperglycaemia. *Int Clin Psychopharmacol* 2001; 16:63–74.

24. Lund BC, et al. Clozapine use in patients with schizophrenia and the risk of diabetes, hyperlipidemia, and hypertension: a claims-based approach. *Arch Gen Psychiatry* 2001; 58:1172–1176.

25. Sernyak MJ, et al. Association of diabetes mellitus with use of atypical neuroleptics in the treatment of schizophrenia. *Am J Psychiatry* 2002; 159:561–566.

26. Gianfrancesco FD, et al. Differential effects of risperidone, olanzapine, clozapine, and conventional antipsychotics on type 2 diabetes: findings from a large health plan database. *J Clin Psychiatry* 2002; 63:920–930.

27. Guo JJ, et al. Risk of diabetes mellitus associated with atypical antipsychotic use among patients with bipolar disorder: a retrospective, population-based, case-control study. *J Clin Psychiatry* 2006; 67:1055–1061.

28. Wang PS, et al. Clozapine use and risk of diabetes mellitus. *J Clin Psychopharmacol* 2002; 22:236–243.

29. Sumiyoshi T, et al. A comparison of incidence of diabetes mellitus between atypical antipsychotic drugs: a survey for clozapine, risperidone, olanzapine, and quetiapine (Letter). *J Clin Psychopharmacol* 2004; 24:345–348.

30. Henderson DC, et al. Clozapine, diabetes mellitus, weight gain, and lipid abnormalities: a five-year naturalistic study. *Am J Psychiatry* 2000; 157:975–981.

31. Koller E, et al. Clozapine-associated diabetes. *Am J Med* 2001; 111:716–723.

32. Sumiyoshi T, et al. The effect of hypertension and obesity on the development of diabetes mellitus in patients treated with atypical antipsychotic drugs (Letter). *J Clin Psychopharmacol* 2004; 24:452–454.

33. Zhang R, et al. The prevalence and clinical-demographic correlates of diabetes mellitus in chronic schizophrenic patients receiving clozapine. *Human Psychopharmacology* 2011; 26:392–396.

34. Melkersson KI, et al. Different influences of classical antipsychotics and clozapine on glucose-insulin homeostasis in patients with schizophrenia or related psychoses. *J Clin Psychiatry* 1999; 60:783–791.

35. Melkersson K. Clozapine and olanzapine, but not conventional antipsychotics, increase insulin release in vitro. *Eur Neuropsychopharmacol* 2004; 14:115–119.

36. Newcomer JW, et al. Abnormalities in glucose regulation during antipsychotic treatment of schizophrenia. *Arch Gen Psychiatry* 2002; 59:337–345.

37. Lamberti JS, et al. Diabetes mellitus among outpatients receiving clozapine: prevalence and clinical-demographic correlates. *J Clin Psychiatry* 2005; 66:900–906.

38. Wirshing DA, et al. Novel antipsychotics and new onset diabetes. *Biol Psychiatry* 1998; 44:778–783.

39. Engl J, et al. Olanzapine impairs glycogen synthesis and insulin signaling in L6 skeletal muscle cells. *Mol Psychiatry* 2005; 10:1089–1096.

40. Vestri HS, et al. Atypical antipsychotic drugs directly impair insulin action in adipocytes: effects on glucose transport, lipogenesis, and antilipolysis. *Neuropsychopharmacology* 2007; 32:765–772.

41. Koro CE, et al. Assessment of independent effect of olanzapine and risperidone on risk of diabetes among patients with schizophrenia: population based nested case-control study. *BMJ* 2002; 325:243.

42. Meyer JM. A retrospective comparison of weight, lipid, and glucose changes between risperidone- and olanzapine-treated inpatients: metabolic outcomes after 1 year. *J Clin Psychiatry* 2002; 63:425–433.

43. Gianfrancesco F, et al. Antipsychotic-induced type 2 diabetes: evidence from a large health plan database. *J Clin Psychopharmacol* 2003; **23**:328–335.

44. Leslie DL, et al. Incidence of newly diagnosed diabetes attributable to atypical antipsychotic medications. *Am J Psychiatry* 2004; **161**:1709–1711.

45. Duncan E, et al. Relative risk of glucose elevation during antipsychotic exposure in a Veterans Administration population. *Int Clin Psychopharmacol* 2007; **22**:1–11.

46. Meyer JM, et al. Change in metabolic syndrome parameters with antipsychotic treatment in the CATIE Schizophrenia Trial: prospective data from phase 1. *Schizophr Res* 2008; **101**:273–286.

47. Ebenbichler CF, et al. Olanzapine induces insulin resistance: results from a prospective study. *J Clin Psychiatry* 2003; **64**:1436–1439.

48. Mallya A, et al. Resolution of hyperglycemia on risperidone discontinuation: a case report. *J Clin Psychiatry* 2002; **63**:453–454.

49. Wirshing DA, et al. Risperidone-associated new-onset diabetes. *Biol Psychiatry* 2001; **50**:148–149.

50. Croarkin PE, et al. Diabetic ketoacidosis associated with risperidone treatment? *Psychosomatics* 2000; **41**:369–370.

51. Koller EA, et al. Risperidone-associated diabetes mellitus: a pharmacovigilance study. *Pharmacotherapy* 2003; **23**:735–744.

52. Lambert BL, et al. Diabetes risk associated with use of olanzapine, quetiapine, and risperidone in veterans health administration patients with schizophrenia. *Am J Epidemiol* 2006; **164**:672–681.

53. Henderson DC. Atypical antipsychotic-induced diabetes mellitus: how strong is the evidence? *CNS Drugs* 2002; **16**:77–89.

54. Koller EA, et al. A survey of reports of quetiapine-associated hyperglycemia and diabetes mellitus. *J Clin Psychiatry* 2004; **65**:857–863.

55. Nanasawa H, et al. Development of diabetes mellitus associated with quetiapine: a case series. *Medicine* 2017; **96**:e5900.

56. Citrome L, et al. Relationship between antipsychotic medication treatment and new cases of diabetes among psychiatric inpatients. *Psychiatr Serv* 2004; **55**:1006–1013.

57. Bushe C, et al. Comparison of metabolic and prolactin variables from a six-month randomised trial of olanzapine and quetiapine in schizophrenia. *J Psychopharmacology* 2010; **24**:1001–1009.

58. Guo Z, et al. A real-world data analysis of dose effect of second-generation antipsychotic therapy on hemoglobin A1C level. *Prog Neuropsychopharmacol Biol Psychiatry* 2011; **35**:1326–1332.

59. Vanelle JM, et al. A double-blind randomised comparative trial of amisulpride versus olanzapine for 2 months in the treatment of subjects with schizophrenia and comorbid depression. *Eur Psychiatry* 2006; **21**:523–530.

60. De Hert MA, et al. Prevalence of the metabolic syndrome in patients with schizophrenia treated with antipsychotic medication. *Schizophr Res* 2006; **83**:87–93.

61. Toprak O, et al. New-onset type II diabetes mellitus, hyperosmolar non-ketotic coma, rhabdomyolysis and acute renal failure in a patient treated with sulpiride. *Nephrol Dial Transplant* 2005; **20**:662–663.

62. Keck PE, Jr., et al. Aripiprazole: a partial dopamine D2 receptor agonist antipsychotic. *Exp Opin Investig Drugs* 2003; **12**:655–662.

63. Pigott TA, et al. Aripiprazole for the prevention of relapse in stabilized patients with chronic schizophrenia: a placebo-controlled 26-week study. *J Clin Psychiatry* 2003; **64**:1048–1056.

64. Van WR, et al. Major changes in glucose metabolism, including new-onset diabetes, within 3 months after initiation of or switch to atypical antipsychotic medication in patients with schizophrenia and schizoaffective disorder. *J Clin Psychiatry* 2008; **69**:472–479.

65. Baker RA, et al. Atypical antipsychotic drugs and diabetes mellitus in the US Food and Drug Administration Adverse Event Database: a Systematic Bayesian Signal Detection Analysis. *Psychopharmacol Bull* 2009; **42**:11–31.

66. Simpson GM, et al. Randomized, controlled, double-blind multicenter comparison of the efficacy and tolerability of ziprasidone and olanzapine in acutely ill inpatients with schizophrenia or schizoaffective disorder. *Am J Psychiatry* 2004; **161**:1837–1847.

67. Sacher J, et al. Effects of olanzapine and ziprasidone on glucose tolerance in healthy volunteers. *Neuropsychopharmacology* 2008; **33**:1633–1641.

68. De Hert M, et al. A case series: evaluation of the metabolic safety of aripiprazole. *Schizophr Bull* 2007; **33**:823–830.

69. Church CO, et al. Diabetic ketoacidosis associated with aripiprazole. *Diabet Med* 2005; **22**:1440–1443.

70. Reddymasu S, et al. Elevated lipase and diabetic ketoacidosis associated with aripiprazole. *J Pancreas* 2006; **7**:303–305.

71. Campanella LM, et al. Severe hyperglycemic hyperosmolar nonketotic coma in a nondiabetic patient receiving aripiprazole. *Ann Emerg Med* 2009; **53**:264–266.

72. Kessing LV, et al. Treatment with antipsychotics and the risk of diabetes in clinical practice. *Br J Psychiatry* 2010; **197**:266–271.

73. McEvoy JP, et al. Effectiveness of lurasidone in patients with schizophrenia or schizoaffective disorder switched from other antipsychotics: a randomized, 6-week, open-label study. *J Clin Psychiatry* 2013; **74**:170–179.

74. Stahl SM, et al. Effectiveness of lurasidone for patients with schizophrenia following 6 weeks of acute treatment with lurasidone, olanzapine, or placebo: a 6-month, open-label, extension study. *J Clin Psychiatry* 2013; **74**:507–515.

75. McIntyre RS, et al. Asenapine for long-term treatment of bipolar disorder: a double-blind 40-week extension study. *J Affect Disord* 2010; **126**:358–365.

76. McIntyre RS, et al. Asenapine versus olanzapine in acute mania: a double-blind extension study. *Bipolar Disorders* 2009; **11**:815–826.

77. Garnock-Jones KP. Brexpiprazole: a review in schizophrenia. *CNS Drugs* 2016; **30**:335–342.

78. Lao KS, et al. Tolerability and safety profile of cariprazine in treating psychotic disorders, bipolar disorder and major depressive disorder: a systematic review with meta-analysis of randomized controlled trials. *CNS Drugs* 2016; **30**:1043–1054.

79. Earley W, et al. Tolerability of cariprazine in the treatment of acute bipolar I mania: a pooled post hoc analysis of 3 phase II/III studies. *J Affect Disord* 2017; **215**:205–212.

80. Cernea S, et al. Pharmacological management of glucose dysregulation in patients treated with second-generation antipsychotics. *Drugs* 2020; **80**:1763–1781.

81. Correll CU, et al. Efficacy and safety of lumateperone for treatment of schizophrenia: a randomized clinical trial. *JAMA Psychiatry* 2020; **77**:349–358.

82. Hammerman A, et al. Antipsychotics and diabetes: an age-related association. *Ann Pharmacother* 2008; **42**:1316–1322.

83. Galling B, et al. Type 2 diabetes mellitus in youth exposed to antipsychotics: a systematic review and meta-analysis. *JAMA Psychiatry* 2016; **73**:247–259.

84. Albert SG, et al. Atypical antipsychotics and the risk of diabetes in an elderly population in long-term care: a retrospective nursing home chart review study. *J Am Med Dir Assoc* 2009; **10**:115–119.

85. De Hert M, et al. Typical and atypical antipsychotics differentially affect long-term incidence rates of the metabolic syndrome in first-episode patients with schizophrenia: a retrospective chart review. *Schizophr Res* 2008; **101**:295–303.

86. Saddichha S, et al. Metabolic syndrome in first episode schizophrenia – a randomized double-blind controlled, short-term prospective study. *Schizophr Res* 2008; **101**:266–272.

87. Saddichha S, et al. Diabetes and schizophrenia – effect of disease or drug? Results from a randomized, double-blind, controlled prospective study in first-episode schizophrenia. *Acta Psychiatr Scand* 2008; **117**:342–347.

88. Reaven GM, et al. In search of moderators and mediators of hyperglycemia with atypical antipsychotic treatment. *J Psychiatr Res* 2009; **43**:997–1002.

89. Mokdad AH, et al. The continuing increase of diabetes in the US. *Diabetes Care* 2001; **24**:412.

90. Mokdad AH, et al. Diabetes trends in the U.S.: 1990–1998. *Diabetes Care* 2000; **23**:1278–1283.

91. Beckman JA, et al. Diabetes and atherosclerosis: epidemiology, pathophysiology, and management. *JAMA* 2002; **287**:2570–2581.

92. Henderson DC, et al. Clozapine, diabetes mellitus, hyperlipidemia, and cardiovascular risks and mortality: results of a 10-year naturalistic study. *J Clin Psychiatry* 2005; **66**:1116–1121.

93. Lamberti JS, et al. Prevalence of the metabolic syndrome among patients receiving clozapine. *Am J Psychiatry* 2006; **163**:1273–1276.

94. Goff DC, et al. A comparison of ten-year cardiac risk estimates in schizophrenia patients from the CATIE study and matched controls. *Schizophr Res* 2005; **80**:45–53.

95. Haupt DW, et al. Hyperglycemia and antipsychotic medications. *J Clin Psychiatry* 2001; **62 Suppl 27**:15–26.

96. Cohn TA, et al. Metabolic monitoring for patients treated with antipsychotic medications. *Can J Psychiatry* 2006; **51**:492–501.

97. De Hert M, et al. Guidelines for screening and monitoring of cardiometabolic risk in schizophrenia: systematic evaluation. *Br J Psychiatry* 2011; **199**:99–105.

98. Barnes TR, et al. Screening for the metabolic syndrome in community psychiatric patients prescribed antipsychotics: a quality improvement programme. *Acta Psychiatr Scand* 2008; **118**:26–33.

99. Barnes TR, et al. Screening for the metabolic side effects of antipsychotic medication: findings of a 6-year quality improvement programme in the UK. *BMJ Open* 2015; **5**:e007633.

100. Crawford MJ, et al. Assessment and treatment of physical health problems among people with schizophrenia: national cross-sectional study. *Br J Psychiatry* 2014; **205**:473–477.

101. Morrato EH, et al. Metabolic screening after the ADA's consensus statement on antipsychotic drugs and diabetes. *Diabetes Care* 2009; **32**:1037–1042.

102. De Hert M, et al. Oral glucose tolerance tests in treated patients with schizophrenia: data to support an adaptation of the proposed guidelines for monitoring of patients on second generation antipsychotics? *Eur Psychiatry* 2006; **21**:224–226.

103. Pillinger T, et al. Impaired glucose homeostasis in first-episode schizophrenia: a systematic review and meta-analysis. *JAMA Psychiatry* 2017; **74**:261–269.

104. Marder SR, et al. Physical health monitoring of patients with schizophrenia. *Am J Psychiatry* 2004; **161**:1334–1349.

105. National Institute for Health and Care Excellence. Type 2 diabetes: the management of type 2 diabetes. Clinical guideline [CG87]. 2009 (Last updated: December 2014); https://www.nice.org.uk/guidance/CG87.

106. Stroup TS, et al. Effects of switching from olanzapine, quetiapine, and risperidone to aripiprazole on 10-year coronary heart disease risk and metabolic syndrome status: results from a randomized controlled trial. *Schizophr Res* 2013; **146**:190–195.

107. Chen Y, et al. Comparative effectiveness of switching antipsychotic drug treatment to aripiprazole or ziprasidone for improving metabolic profile and atherogenic dyslipidemia: a 12-month, prospective, open-label study. *J Psychopharmacol* 2012; **26**:1201–1210.

108. Smith RC, et al. Effects of pioglitazone on metabolic abnormalities, psychopathology, and cognitive function in schizophrenic patients treated with antipsychotic medication: a randomized double-blind study. *SchizophrRes* 2013; **143**:18–24.

109. Larsen JR, et al. Effect of liraglutide treatment on prediabetes and overweight or obesity in clozapine- or olanzapine-treated patients with schizophrenia spectrum disorder: a randomized clinical trial. *JAMA Psychiatry* 2017; **74**:719–728.

Blood pressure changes with antipsychotics

Orthostatic hypotension

Orthostatic hypotension (postural hypotension) is one of the most common cardiovascular adverse effects of antipsychotics and some antidepressants. Orthostatic hypotension generally presents acutely, during the initial dose titration period, but there is evidence to suggest it can also be a chronic problem.[1] Symptoms may include dizziness, light-headedness, asthenia, headache, and visual disturbance. Patients may not be able to communicate the nature of these symptoms effectively and subjective reports of postural dizziness correlate weakly with the magnitude of measured postural hypotension.[2]

Blood pressure monitoring is recommended in suspected cases to confirm orthostatic hypotension (defined as >20mmHg fall in systolic blood pressure or a >10mmHg fall in diastolic blood pressure within 2–5 minutes of standing after a 5-minute period of lying flat[3]). Orthostatic hypotension may result in syncope and falls-related injuries. It has also been associated with an increased risk of coronary heart disease, heart failure and death.[4]

Slow dose titration is a commonly used and often effective strategy to avoid or minimise orthostatic hypotension. However, in some cases orthostasis may be a dose-limiting side effect, preventing optimal treatment. Potential management strategies are shown in Tables 1.26 and 1.27.

Table 1.26 Risk factors for orthostatic hypotension[2]

Treatment factors	■ Intramuscular administration route (as peak levels achieved more rapidly) ■ Rapid dose increases ■ Antipsychotic polypharmacy ■ Drug interactions (e.g. β-blockers and other antihypertensive drugs)
Patient factors	■ Old age (young patients often develop sinus tachycardia with minimal changes in orthostatic blood pressure) ■ Disease states associated with autonomic dysfunction (e.g. Parkinson's disease) ■ Dehydration ■ Cardiovascular disease

Table 1.27 Management of antipsychotic-induced orthostatic hypotension[2]

Minimise the risk of treatment	■ Limit initial doses and titrate slowly according to tolerability (most develop a tolerance to the hypotensive effect) ■ Consider a temporary dose reduction if hypotension develops ■ Avoid antipsychotics that are potent α_1-adrenergic receptor antagonists ■ Reduce peak plasma levels by smaller and more frequent dosing or by using modified-release preparations
Nonpharmacological therapies	■ Advice to patients, e.g. sitting on the edge of the bed for several minutes before attempting to stand in the morning and slowly rising from a seated position, may be helpful ■ Abdominal binders and compression stockings have been recommended in postural hypotension ■ Increasing fluid intake to 1.25–2.5 l/day is advisable for all patients who are not fluid restricted

Table 1.27 (Continued)	
Pharmacological therapies *for patients with a compelling* *indication for treatment where* *alternatives are not suitable (e.g.* *clozapine) and management* *strategies have failed*	■ Sodium chloride supplementation has been used to treat antidepressant-induced orthostatic hypotension ■ Fludrocortisone has been used to treat clozapine-induced orthostatic hypotension where other measures have failed (electrolyte and blood pressure monitoring essential) ■ A single case report describes the use of midodrine (an α1 receptor agonist) for TCA-induced orthostatic hypotension. Of note, midodrine has been linked to acute dystonia when used alongside antipsychotics.[5] Other sympathomimetic drugs have also been used to treat orthostatic hypotension, though there is an absence of evidence in the treatment of psychotropic related cases

Antipsychotics with a high affinity for postsynaptic α_1-adrenergic receptors are most frequently implicated. Among the SGAs, the reported incidence is highest with clozapine (24%), quetiapine (27%) and iloperidone (19.5%) and lowest with lurasidone (<2%) and asenapine (<2%).[2] There are limited quantitative data for FGAs, but low-potency phenothiazines (e.g. chlorpromazine) are considered most likely to cause orthostatic hypotension.[6] All reported frequencies are somewhat dependent on titration schedules used.

Hypertension

There are two ways in which antipsychotic drugs may be associated with the development or worsening of hypertension:

■ **Slow steady rise in blood pressure over time.** This may be linked to weight gain. Being overweight increases the risk of developing hypertension. The magnitude of the effect has been modelled using the Framingham data; for every 30 people who gain 4kg, one will develop hypertension over the next 10 years.[7] Note that this is a very modest weight gain, the majority of patients treated with some antipsychotics gain more than this, increasing further the risk of developing hypertension.

■ **Unpredictable rapid sharp increase in blood pressure on starting a new drug or increasing the dose.** Increases in blood pressure occur shortly after starting, ranging from within hours of the first dose to a month. The information below relates to the pharmacological mechanism behind this and the antipsychotic drugs that are most implicated.

Postural hypotension is commonly associated with antipsychotic drugs that are antagonists at postsynaptic α_1-adrenergic receptors. Some antipsychotics are also antagonists at pre-synaptic α_2-adrenergic receptors; this can lead to increased release of norepinephrine and vasoconstriction. As all antipsychotics that are antagonists at α_2-receptors are also antagonists at α_1 receptors, the end result for any given patient can be difficult to predict, but for a very small number the result can be hypertension. Some antipsychotics are more commonly implicated than others, but individual patient factors are undoubtedly also important.

Receptor binding studies have demonstrated that clozapine, olanzapine and risperidone have the highest affinity for α_2-adrenergic receptors,[8] so it might be predicted that these drugs would be most likely to cause hypertension. Most case reports implicate clozapine,[9–17] with some clearly describing normal blood pressure before clozapine was introduced, a sharp rise during treatment and return to normal when clozapine was discontinued. Blood pressure has also been reported to rise again on re-challenge, and increased plasma catecholamines have been noted in some cases. Case reports also implicate aripiprazole,[18–21] sulpiride,[22,23] risperidone,[24] quetiapine[13] and ziprasidone.[25]

Data available through the UK MHRA yellow card system indicate that clozapine is the antipsychotic drug most associated with hypertension. There are a very small number of reports with aripiprazole, olanzapine, quetiapine and risperidone.[26] The timing of the onset of hypertension in these reports with respect to antipsychotic initiation is unknown, and likely to be variable.

In long-term treatment, hypertension is seen in around 30–40% of patients, regardless of antipsychotic prescribed.[27] A cross-sectional study found an increased risk of hypertension only for perphenazine,[28] a finding not readily explained by its pharmacology.

No antipsychotic is contra-indicated in essential hypertension, but extreme care is needed when clozapine is prescribed. Concomitant treatment with SSRIs may increase risk of hypertension, possibly via inhibition of the metabolism of the antipsychotic.[13] It is also (theoretically) possible that α_2 antagonism may be at least partially responsible for clozapine-induced tachycardia and nausea.[29]

Treatment of antipsychotic-associated hypertension should follow standard protocols. Switching to alternative antipsychotics with a lower cardiometabolic risk should be considered where possible.[30] There is specific evidence for the efficacy of valsartan and telmisartan in antipsychotic-related hypertension.[31]

References

1. Silver H, et al. Postural hypotension in chronically medicated schizophrenics. *J Clin Psychiatry* 1990; 51:459–462.
2. Gugger JJ. Antipsychotic pharmacotherapy and orthostatic hypotension: identification and management. *CNS Drugs* 2011; 25:659–671.
3. Freeman R, et al. Consensus statement on the definition of orthostatic hypotension, neurally mediated syncope and the postural tachycardia syndrome. *Clin Auton Res* 2011; 21:69–72.
4. Ricci F, et al. Cardiovascular morbidity and mortality related to orthostatic hypotension: a meta-analysis of prospective observational studies. *Eur Heart J* 2015; 36:1609–1617.
5. Stroup TS, et al. Management of common adverse effects of antipsychotic medications. *World Psychiatry* 2018; 17:341–356.
6. Casey DE. The relationship of pharmacology to side effects. *J Clin Psychiatry* 1997; **58 Suppl 10**:55–62.
7. Fontaine KR, et al. Estimating the consequences of anti-psychotic induced weight gain on health and mortality rate. *Psychiatry Res* 2001; 101:277–288.
8. Abi-Dargham A, et al. Mechanisms of action of second generation antipsychotic drugs in schizophrenia: insights from brain imaging studies. *Eur Psychiatry* 2005; 20:15–27.
9. Yuen JWY, et al. Clozapine-induced cardiovascular side effects and autonomic dysfunction: a systematic review. *Front Neurosci* 2018; 12:203.
10. Gupta S, et al. Paradoxical hypertension associated with clozapine. *Am J Psychiatry* 1994; 151:148.
11. George TP, et al. Hypertension after initiation of clozapine. *Am J Psychiatry* 1996; 153:1368–1369.
12. Shiwach RS. Treatment of clozapine induced hypertension and possible mechanisms. *Clin Neuropharmacol* 1998; 21:139–140.
13. Coulter D. Atypical antipsychotics may cause hypertension. *Prescriber Update* 2003; 24:4.
14. Li JK, et al. Clozapine: a mimicry of phaeochromocytoma. *Aust N Z J Psychiatry* 1997; 31:889–891.
15. Hoorn EJ, et al. Hypokalemic hypertension related to clozapine: a case report. *J Clin Psychopharmacol* 2014; 34:390–392.
16. Sakalkale A, et al. Pseudophaeochromocytoma: a clinical dilemma in clozapine therapy. *Aust N Z J Psychiatry* 2017; 51 (**Suppl1**).
17. Visscher AJ, et al. Periorbital oedema and treatment-resistant hypertension as rare side effects of clozapine. *Aust N Z J Psychiatry* 2011; 45:1097–1098.
18. Hsiao YL, et al. Aripiprazole augmentation induced hypertension in major depressive disorder: a case report. *Prog Neuropsychopharmacol Biol Psychiatry* 2011; 35:305–306.
19. Yasui-Furukori N, et al. Worsened hypertension control induced by aripiprazole. *Neuropsychiatr Dis Treat* 2013; 9:505–507.
20. Seven H, et al. Aripiprazole-induced asymptomatic hypertension: a case report. *Psychopharmacol Bull* 2017; 47:53–56.

21. Alves BB, et al. Use of atypical antipsychotics and risk of hypertension: a case report and review literature. *SAGE Open Medical Case Reports* 2019; 7:2050313x19841825.

22. Mayer RD, et al. Acute hypertensive episode induced by sulpiride – a case report. *Human Psychopharmacology* 1989; 4:149–150.

23. Corvol P, et al. [Hypertensive episodes initiated by sulpiride (Dogmatil)]. *Ann Med Interne* 1973; 124:647–649.

24. Thomson SR, et al. Risperidone induced hypertension in a young female: a case report. *Adv Sci Lett* 2017; 23:1980–1982.

25. Villanueva N, et al. Probable association between ziprasidone and worsening hypertension. *Pharmacotherapy* 2006; 26:1352–1357.

26. Medicines and Healthcare Products Regulatory Agency. Drug Analysis Profiles (iDAPs) 2021; https://www.gov.uk/drug-analysis-prints.

27. Kelly AC, et al. A naturalistic comparison of the long-term metabolic adverse effects of clozapine versus other antipsychotics for patients with psychotic illnesses. *J Clin Psychopharmacol* 2014; 34:441–445.

28. Boden R, et al. A comparison of cardiovascular risk factors for ten antipsychotic drugs in clinical practice. *Neuropsychiatr Dis Treat* 2013; 9:371–377.

29. Pandharipande P, et al. Alpha-2 agonists: can they modify the outcomes in the postanesthesia care unit? *Curr Drug Targets* 2005; 6:749–754.

30. Whelton PK, et al. 2017 ACC/AHA/AAPA/ABC/ACPM/AGS/APhA/ASH/ASPC/NMA/PCNA guideline for the prevention, detection, evaluation, and management of high blood pressure in adults: a report of the American College of Cardiology/American Heart Association Task Force on Clinical Practice Guidelines. *J Am Coll Cardiol* 2018; 71:e127–e248.

31. Tse L, et al. Pharmacological treatment of antipsychotic-induced dyslipidemia and hypertension. *Int Clin Psychopharmacol* 2014; 29:125–137.

Hyponatraemia in psychosis

Hyponatraemia can occur in the context of:

- **Water intoxication** where water consumption exceeds the maximal renal clearance capacity. Serum and urine osmolality are low. Cross-sectional studies of chronically ill, hospitalised, psychiatric patients have found the prevalence of water intoxication to be 6–17%.[1,2] A longitudinal study found that 10% of severely ill patients with a diagnosis of schizophrenia had episodic hyponatraemia secondary to fluid overload.[3] The primary aetiology is poorly understood. It has been postulated that it may be driven, at least in part, by an extreme compensatory response to the anticholinergic side-effects of some antipsychotic drugs.[4] An alternative theory is that postsynaptic dopamine receptor antagonism results in receptor supersensitivity, increased presynaptic dopamine release, and elevated dopamine in the hypothalamus, driving thirst and polydipsia.[5] The observations that many reported cases occur in patients with long illness histories and treatment with antipsychotics with high D_2 receptor affinity, and that clozapine can improve polydipsia independent of improvement in psychosis, appear to support this suggestion.[5]

- Drug-induced **syndrome of inappropriate antidiuretic hormone (SIADH)** where the kidney retains an excessive quantity of solute-free water. Serum osmolality is low and urine osmolality relatively high. The prevalence of SIADH has been estimated to be as high as 11% in acutely ill psychiatric patients.[6] Risk factors for antidepressant-induced SIADH (increasing age, female gender, medical co-morbidity and polypharmacy) seem to be less relevant in the population of patients treated with antipsychotic drugs.[7] SIADH usually develops in the first few weeks of treatment with the offending drug. Case reports and case series implicate phenothiazines, haloperidol, pimozide, risperidone, paliperidone, quetiapine, olanzapine, aripiprazole, cariprazine and clozapine.[7–26] Systematic review[27] and case–control studies[28,29] suggest a clear increase in the risk of hyponatraemia with antipsychotics. Another review[30] confirmed that drug-induced hyponatraemia is associated with concentrated urine and suggested that an antipsychotic was five times more likely than water intoxication to be the cause of hyponatraemia. Overall, prevalence of antipsychotic-induced hyponatraemia has been estimated at 0.004%[31] and 26.1%[32] of patients. It is assumed the true figure has somewhere between these two extremes. Desmopressin use (for clozapine-induced enuresis) can also result in hyponatraemia.[33] Other drugs, including antidepressants and antiseizure medications (especially carbamazepine[34]), have also been implicated,[35] and the risk may be additive with concomitant prescriptions.[36,37]

- Severe **hyperlipidaemia** and/or **hyperglycaemia** lead to secondary increases in plasma volume and 'pseudohyponatraemia'.[4] Both are more common in people treated with antipsychotic drugs than in the general population and should be excluded as causes.

Mild to moderate hyponatraemia presents as confusion, nausea, headache and lethargy. As the plasma sodium falls, these symptoms become increasingly severe and seizures and coma can develop.

Monitoring of plasma sodium is desirable for all those receiving antipsychotics. Signs of confusion or lethargy should provoke through diagnostic analysis, including plasma sodium determination and urine osmolality (Table 1.28).

Table 1.28 Treatment of hyponatraemia associated with antipsychotic treatment[4,6]

Cause of hyponatraemia	Antipsychotic drugs implicated	Treatment
Water intoxication (serum and urine osmolality low)	Only very speculative evidence to support drugs as a cause. Core part of illness in a minority of patients (e.g. psychotic polydipsia)	■ **Fluid restriction** with careful monitoring of serum sodium, particularly diurnal variation (Na drops as the day progresses). Refer urgently to specialist medical care if Na < 125mmol/l. Note that overly rapid correction of sodium levels can cause irreversible osmotic demyelination syndrome[38] ■ Consider treatment with **clozapine**: shown to increase plasma osmolality into the normal range and increase urine osmolality (not usually reaching the normal range).[39,40] These effects are consistent with reduced fluid intake. This effect is not clearly related to improvements in mental state[41] ■ There are both[7] positive and negative reports for olanzapine[42] and risperidone[43] and one positive case report for quetiapine.[44] Compared with clozapine, the evidence base is weak ■ There is no evidence that either reducing or increasing the dose of an antipsychotic results in improvements in serum sodium in water-intoxicated patients,[45] although there is a suggestion that reducing the number and dose of antipsychotics prescribed may decrease dopamine receptor supersensitivity and drug side effects[5] ■ There are reports of **demeclocycline** use,[46,47] and it is included in some practice guidelines for psychogenic polydipsia.[48] However, it exerts its effect by interfering with ADH and increasing water excretion, which is already at capacity in these patients. Any rationale for its use in the absence of SIADH is therefore debatable (and some cases in the literature may have been complicated by undiagnosed SIADH[49]). A single small RCT showed no benefit[50]
SIADH (serum osmolality low; urine osmolality relatively high)	All antipsychotic drugs	■ If mild, **fluid restriction** with careful monitoring of serum sodium. Refer urgently to specialist medical care if Na < 125mmol/L ■ **Switching to a different antipsychotic drug**. There are insufficient data available to guide choice. Be aware that cross-sensitivity may occur (the individual may be predisposed and the choice of drug relatively less important) ■ Consider **demeclocycline** (see formal prescribing information for details) ■ Lithium may be effective[7] but is a potentially toxic drug – hyponatraemia predisposes to lithium toxicity

More recently introduced drugs such as tolvaptan,[51] a so-called vaptan (non-peptide arginine-vasopressin antagonist – also known as aquaretics because they induce a highly hypotonic diuresis[52]), show promise in the treatment of hyponatraemia of varying aetiology, including that caused by drug-related SIADH and psychogenic polydipsia.[53] Successful use of the carbonic anhydrase inhibitor acetazolamide has also been reported,[54,55] and there are single case reports of irbesartan[56] and propranolol.[57]

Clonidine,[58] enalapril[58] and captopril[59] have also been used with varying success in psychogenic polydipsia.

References

1. De Leon J, et al. Polydipsia and water intoxication in psychiatric patients: a review of the epidemiological literature. *Biol Psychiatry* 1994; 35:408–419.
2. Patel JK. Polydipsia, hyponatremia, and water intoxication among psychiatric patients. *Hosp Community Psychiatry* 1994; 45:1073–1074.
3. De Leon J. Polydipsia–a study in a long-term psychiatric unit. *Eur Arch Psychiatry Clin Neurosci* 2003; 253:37–39.
4. Siegel AJ, et al. Primary and drug-induced disorders of water homeostasis in psychiatric patients: principles of diagnosis and management. *Harv Rev Psychiatry* 1998; 6:190–200.
5. Kirino S, et al. Relationship between polydipsia and antipsychotics: a systematic review of clinical studies and case reports. *Prog Neuropsychopharmacol Biol Psychiatry* 2020; 96:109756.
6. Siegler EL, et al. Risk factors for the development of hyponatremia in psychiatric inpatients. *Arch Intern Med* 1995; 155:953–957.
7. Madhusoodanan S, et al. Hyponatraemia associated with psychotropic medications. A review of the literature and spontaneous reports. *Adv Drug React Toxicol Rev* 2002; 21:17–29.
8. Bachu K, et al. Aripiprazole-induced syndrome of inappropriate antidiuretic hormone secretion (SIADH). *Am J Ther* 2006; 13:370–372.
9. Dudeja SJ, et al. Olanzapine induced hyponatraemia. *Ulster Med J* 2010; 79:104–105.
10. Yam FK, et al. Syndrome of inappropriate antidiuretic hormone associated with aripiprazole. *AmJHealth SystPharm* 2013; 70:2110–2114.
11. Kaur J, et al. Paliperidone inducing concomitantly syndrome of inappropriate antidiuretic hormone, neuroleptic malignant syndrome, and rhabdomyolysis. *Case Reports in Critical Care* 2016; 2016:2587963.
12. Lin MW, et al. Aripiprazole-related hyponatremia and consequent valproic acid-related hyperammonemia in one patient. *Aust N Z J Psychiatry* 2017; 51:296–297.
13. Koufakis T. Quetiapine-Induced Syndrome of Inappropriate Secretion of Antidiuretic Hormone. *Case reports in psychiatry* 2016; 2016:4803132
14. Chen LC, et al. Polydipsia, hyponatremia and rhabdomyolysis in schizophrenia: a case report. *World J Psychiatry* 2014; 4:150–152.
15. Bakhla AK, et al. A suspected case of olanzapine induced hyponatremia. *Indian J Pharmacol* 2014; 46:441–442.
16. Kane JM, et al. Efficacy and safety of cariprazine in acute exacerbation of schizophrenia: results from an international, phase iii clinical trial. *J Clin Psychopharmacol* 2015; 35:367–373.
17. Tibrewal P, et al. Paliperidone-Induced Hyponatremia. *Prim Care Companion CNS Disord* 2017; 19:16l02088.
18. McNally MA, et al. Olanzapine-induced hyponatremia presenting with seizure requiring intensive care unit admission. *Cureus* 2020; 12:e8212.
19. Sachdeva A, et al. Hyponatremia with olanzapine – a suspected association. *Shanghai Arch Psychiatry* 2017; 29:177–179.
20. Kumar PNS, et al. Hyponatremia secondary to SIADH in a schizophrenic patient treated with Quetiapine. *Asian J Psychiatr* 2018; 35:89–90.
21. Mazhar F, et al. Paliperidone-associated hyponatremia: report of a fatal case with analysis of cases reported in the literature and to the US Food and Drug Administration Adverse Event Reporting System. *J Clin Psychopharmacol* 2020; 40:202–205.
22. Chowdhury W, et al. Management of persistent hyponatremia induced by long-acting injectable risperidone therapy. *Cureus* 2018; 10:e2657.
23. Anil SS, et al. A case report of rapid-onset hyponatremia induced by low-dose olanzapine. *J Family Med Primary Care* 2017; 6:878–880.
24. Kang SG, et al. Addendum: low-dose quetiapine-induced syndrome of inappropriate antidiuretic hormone in a patient with traumatic brain syndrome. *Clin Psychopharmacol Neurosci* 2021; 19:179.
25. Aruachán S, et al. Hyponatraemia associated with the use of quetiapine: case report. *Rev Colomb Psiquiatr* 2020; 49:297–300.
26. Zhu X, et al. Rhabdomyolysis and elevated liver enzymes after rapid correction of hyponatremia due to pneumonia and concurrent use of aripiprazole: a case report. *Aust N Z J Psychiatry* 2018; 52:206.
27. Meulendijks D, et al. Antipsychotic-induced hyponatraemia: a systematic review of the published evidence. *Drug Saf* 2010; 33:101–114.
28. Mannesse CK, et al. Hyponatraemia as an adverse drug reaction of antipsychotic drugs: a case-control study in VigiBase. *Drug Saf* 2010; 33:569–578.
29. Falhammar H, et al. Antipsychotics and severe hyponatremia: a Swedish population-based case-control study. *Eur J Intern Med* 2019; 60:71–77.
30. Atsariyasing W, et al. A systematic review of the ability of urine concentration to distinguish antipsychotic- from psychosis-induced hyponatremia. *Psychiatry Res* 2014; 217:129–133.
31. Letmaier M, et al. Hyponatraemia during psychopharmacological treatment: results of a drug surveillance programme. *IntJNeuropsychopharmacol* 2012; 15:739–748.
32. Serrano A, et al. Safety of long-term clozapine administration. Frequency of cardiomyopathy and hyponatraemia: two cross-sectional, naturalistic studies. *Aust N Z J Psychiatry* 2014; 48:183–192.
33. Sarma S, et al. Severe hyponatraemia associated with desmopressin nasal spray to treat clozapine-induced nocturnal enuresis. *Aust N Z J Psychiatry* 2005; 39:949.
34. Yang HJ, et al. Antipsychotic use is a risk factor for hyponatremia in patients with schizophrenia: a 15-year follow-up study. *Psychopharmacology* 2017; 234:869–876.

35. Shepshelovich D, et al. Medication-induced SIADH: distribution and characterization according to medication class. *Br J Clin Pharmacol* 2017; **83**:1801–1807.

36. Yamamoto Y, et al. Prevalence and risk factors for hyponatremia in adult epilepsy patients: large-scale cross-sectional cohort study. *Seizure* 2019; **73**:26–30.

37. Fabrazzo M, et al. The unmasking of hidden severe hyponatremia after long-term combination therapy in exacerbated bipolar patients: a case series. *Int Clin Psychopharmacol* 2019; **34**:206–210.

38. Zaidi AN. Rhabdomyolysis after correction of hyponatremia in psychogenic polydipsia possibly complicated by ziprasidone. *Ann Pharmacother* 2005; **39**:1726–1731.

39. Canuso CM, et al. Clozapine restores water balance in schizophrenic patients with polydipsia-hyponatremia syndrome. *J Neuropsychiatry Clin Neurosci* 1999; **11**:86–90.

40. Fujimoto M, et al. Clozapine improved the syndrome of inappropriate antidiuretic hormone secretion in a patient with treatment-resistant schizophrenia. *Psychiatry Clin Neurosci* 2016; **70**:469.

41. Spears NM, et al. Clozapine treatment in polydipsia and intermittent hyponatremia. *J Clin Psychiatry* 1996; **57**:123–128.

42. Littrell KH, et al. Effects of olanzapine on polydipsia and intermittent hyponatremia. *J Clin Psychiatry* 1997; **58**:549.

43. Kawai N, et al. Risperidone failed to improve polydipsia-hyponatremia of the schizophrenic patients. *Psychiatry Clin Neurosci* 2002; **56**:107–110.

44. Montgomery JH, et al. Adjunctive quetiapine treatment of the polydipsia, intermittent hyponatremia, and psychosis syndrome: a case report. *J Clin Psychiatry* 2003; **64**:339–341.

45. Canuso CM, et al. Does minimizing neuroleptic dosage influence hyponatremia? *Psychiatry Res* 1996; **63**:227–229.

46. Nixon RA, et al. Demeclocycline in the prophylaxis of self-induced water intoxication. *Am J Psychiatry* 1982; **139**:828–830.

47. Vieweg WV, et al. The use of demeclocycline in the treatment of patients with psychosis, intermittent hyponatremia, and polydipsia (PIP syndrome). *Psychiatr Q* 1988; **59**:62–68.

48. Srinivasan S, et al. Psychogenic polydipsia. 2019; https://bestpractice.bmj.com/topics/en-gb/865.

49. Walter-Ryan WG. Water intoxication, demeclocycline, and antidiuretic hormone. *Am J Psychiatry* 1983; **140**:815.

50. Alexander RC, et al. A double blind, placebo-controlled trial of demeclocycline treatment of polydipsia-hyponatremia in chronically psychotic patients. *Biol Psychiatry* 1991; **30**:417–420.

51. Josiassen RC, et al. Tolvaptan: a new tool for the effective treatment of hyponatremia in psychotic disorders. *Expert Opin Pharmacother* 2010; **11**:637–648.

52. Decaux G, et al. Non-peptide arginine-vasopressin antagonists: the vaptans. *Lancet* 2008; **371**:1624–1632.

53. Bhatia MS, et al. Psychogenic polydipsia – management challenges. *Shanghai Arch Psychiatry* 2017; **29**:180–183.

54. Ahmed SE, et al. Acetazolamide: treatment of psychogenic polydipsia. *Cureus* 2017; **9**:e1553.

55. Takagi S, et al. Treatment of psychogenic polydipsia with acetazolamide: a report of 5 cases. *Clin Neuropharmacol* 2011; **34**:5–7.

56. Kruse D, et al. Treatment of psychogenic polydipsia: comparison of risperidone and olanzapine, and the effects of an adjunctive angiotensin-II receptor blocking drug (irbesartan). *Aust N Z J Psychiatry* 2001; **35**:65–68.

57. Shevitz SA, et al. Compulsive water drinking treated with high dose propranolol. *J Nerv Ment Dis* 1980; **168**:246–248.

58. Greendyke RM, et al. Polydipsia in chronic psychiatric patients: therapeutic trials of clonidine and enalapril. *Neuropsychopharmacology* 1998; **18**:272–281.

59. Sebastian CS, et al. Comparison of enalapril and captopril in the management of self-induced water intoxication. *Biol Psychiatry* 1990; **27**:787–790.

Further Reading

Sailer C, et al. Primary polydipsia in the medical and psychiatric patient: characteristics, complications and therapy. *Swiss Med Wkly* 2017; **147**:w14514

Srinivasan S, et al. Psychogenic polydipsia. *BMJ Best Practice* 2019; https://bestpractice.bmj.com/topics/en-gb/865.

Hyperprolactinaemia

Dopamine inhibits prolactin release, and so dopamine antagonists can be expected to increase prolactin plasma levels. The degree of prolactin elevation is probably dose-related,[1] and for most antipsychotic medications the threshold activity (D_2 occupancy) for increased prolactin is very close to that of therapeutic efficacy.[2] Genetic differences may also play a part.[3] Table 1.29 groups individual antipsychotics according to their effect on prolactin concentrations.

Table 1.29 Effects of antipsychotic medication on prolactin concentration[4–11]

Prolactin-sparing (prolactin increase very rare)	Prolactin–elevating (low risk minor changes only)	Prolactin-elevating (high risk; major changes)
Aripiprazole	Lurasidone	Amisulpride
Asenapine	Olanzapine	Paliperidone
Brexpiprazole	Ziprasidone	Risperidone
Cariprazine		Sulpiride
Clozapine		FGAs
Iloperidone		
Lumateperone		
Pimavanserin		
Quetiapine		

Hyperprolactinaemia is often superficially asymptomatic (i.e. the patient does not spontaneously report problems), and there is some evidence that hyperprolactinaemia does not affect subjective quality of life.[12] Nonetheless, persistent elevation of plasma prolactin is associated with suppression of the hypothalamic-pituitary-gonadal axis.[13] Symptoms of this include sexual dysfunction[14] (but note that other pharmacological activities also give rise to sexual dysfunction[15]), menstrual disturbances,[4,16] breast growth and galactorrhoea,[16] and may include delusions of pregnancy.[17] Long-term adverse consequences are reductions in bone mineral density,[18,19] and a possible increase in the risk of breast cancer.[20]

Prolactin can also be raised because of stress, pregnancy and lactation, seizures, renal impairment and other medical conditions,[7,21,22] including prolactinoma. When measuring prolactin, the sample should be taken early in the morning and stress during venepuncture should be minimised.[22]

Contraindications

Prolactin-elevating drugs with high risk should, if possible, be **avoided** in the following patient groups:

- **Patients under 25 years of age (i.e. before peak bone mass)**
- **Patients with osteoporosis**
- **Patients with a history of hormone-dependent breast cancer**
- **Young women**

Management

Treatment of hyperprolactinaemia depends more on symptoms and long-term risk than on the reported plasma prolactin level.

Below, we suggest an algorithm for managing antipsychotic-induced hyperprolactinaemia. If treatment of hyperprolactinaemia is required, switching to an antipsychotic with a lower liability for prolactin elevation is usually the first choice, although switching always carries a risk of destabilising the illness and relapse.[23] An alternative is to add aripiprazole to existing treatment.[24] Aripiprazole lowers prolactin levels in a dose-dependent manner: 3mg/day is effective but 6mg/day more so. Higher doses appear unnecessary.[25] Other strategies to reduce long-term risk to bone mineral density should also be discussed, e.g. stopping smoking, increasing weight-bearing exercise, and ensuring adequate calcium and vitamin D3 intake.[18,26]

For patients who need to remain on a prolactin-elevating antipsychotic medication and who cannot tolerate aripiprazole, dopamine agonists can be effective.[27–29] Amantadine, cabergoline and bromocriptine have all been used, but each has, theoretically at least, the potential to worsen psychosis (although this has not been reported in trials). A herbal remedy – Peony Glycyrrhiza Decoction – has also been shown to improve prolactin-related symptoms,[30,31] but the data are limited. A reduction in prolactin levels was also achieved by taking high daily doses (2.5–3g) of metformin[32] in a study of diabetic women on antipsychotic medication.

Summary of management

First choice	Aripiprazole 5mg a day
Second choice *(in no particular order)*	DA agonists – cabergoline, bromocryptine, amantadine Peony Glycyrrhiza Decoction Metformin 2.5–3g a day

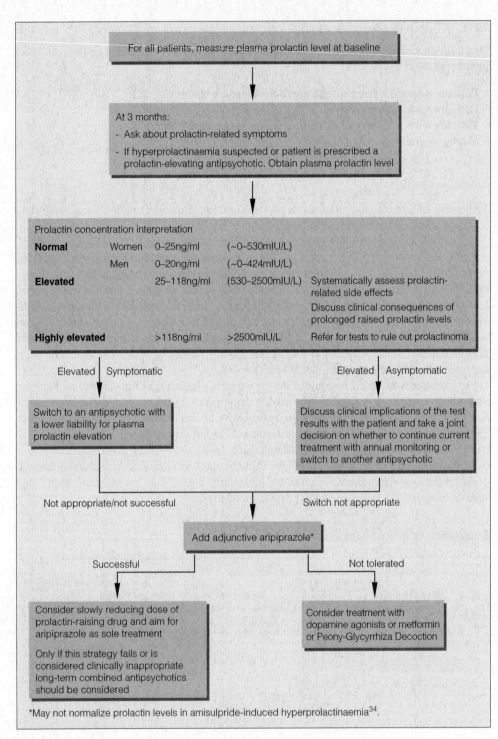

Figure 1.3 Management of antipsychotic-induced hyperprolactinaemia[33].

References

1. Suzuki Y, et al. Differences in plasma prolactin levels in patients with schizophrenia treated on monotherapy with five second-generation antipsychotics. *Schizophr Res* 2013; **145**:116–119.

2. Tsuboi T, et al. Hyperprolactinemia and estimated dopamine D2 receptor occupancy in patients with schizophrenia: analysis of the CATIE data. *Prog Neuropsychopharmacol Biol Psychiatry* 2013; **45**:178–182.

3. Young RM, et al. Prolactin levels in antipsychotic treatment of patients with schizophrenia carrying the DRD2*A1 allele. *Br J Psychiatry* 2004; **185**:147–151.

4. Haddad PM, et al. Antipsychotic-induced hyperprolactinaemia: mechanisms, clinical features and management. *Drugs* 2004; **64**:2291–2314.

5. Holt RI, et al. Antipsychotics and hyperprolactinaemia: mechanisms, consequences and management. *Clin Endocrinol* 2011; **74**:141–147.

6. Leucht S, et al. Comparative efficacy and tolerability of 15 antipsychotic drugs in schizophrenia: a multiple-treatments meta-analysis. *Lancet* 2013; **382**:951–962.

7. Peuskens J, et al. The effects of novel and newly approved antipsychotics on serum prolactin levels: a comprehensive review. *CNS Drugs* 2014; **28**:421–453.

8. Citrome L. Cariprazine: chemistry, pharmacodynamics, pharmacokinetics, and metabolism, clinical efficacy, safety, and tolerability. *Exp Opin Drug Metab Toxicol* 2013; **9**:193–206.

9. Marder SR, et al. Brexpiprazole in patients with schizophrenia: overview of short- and long-term phase 3 controlled studies. *Acta Neuropsychiatr* 2017; **29**:278–290.

10. Vanover KE, et al. Dopamine D(2) receptor occupancy of lumateperone (ITI-007): a positron emission tomography study in patients with schizophrenia. *Neuropsychopharmacology* 2019; **44**:598–605.

11. Yunusa I, et al. Pimavanserin: a novel antipsychotic with potentials to address an unmet need of older adults with dementia-related psychosis. *Front Pharmacol* 2020; **11**:87.

12. Kaneda Y. The impact of prolactin elevation with antipsychotic medications on subjective quality of life in patients with schizophrenia. *Clin Neuropharmacol* 2003; **26**:182–184.

13. Smith S, et al. The effects of antipsychotic-induced hyperprolactinaemia on the hypothalamic-pituitary-gonadal axis. *J Clin Psychopharmacol* 2002; **22**:109–114.

14. De Hert M, et al. Second-generation and newly approved antipsychotics, serum prolactin levels and sexual dysfunctions: a critical literature review. *Exp Opin Drug Saf* 2014; **13**:605–624.

15. Baldwin D, et al. Sexual side-effects of antidepressant and antipsychotic drugs. *Adv Psychiatric Treat* 2003; **9**:202–210.

16. Wieck A, et al. Antipsychotic-induced hyperprolactinaemia in women: pathophysiology, severity and consequences. Selective literature review. *Br J Psychiatry* 2003; **182**:199–204.

17. Ali JA, et al. Delusions of pregnancy associated with increased prolactin concentrations produced by antipsychotic treatment. *Int J Neuropsychopharmacol* 2003; **6**:111–115.

18. De Hert M, et al. Relationship between antipsychotic medication, serum prolactin levels and osteoporosis/osteoporotic fractures in patients with schizophrenia: a critical literature review. *Exp Opin Drug Saf* 2016; **15**:809–823.

19. Tseng PT, et al. Bone mineral density in schizophrenia: an update of current meta-analysis and literature review under guideline of PRISMA. *Medicine* 2015; **94**:e1967.

20. De Hert M, et al. Relationship between prolactin, breast cancer risk, and antipsychotics in patients with schizophrenia: a critical review. *Acta Psychiatr Scand* 2016; **133**:5–22.

21. Holt RI. Medical causes and consequences of hyperprolactinaemia. A context for psychiatrists. *J Psychopharmacology* 2008; **22**:28–37.

22. Melmed S, et al. Diagnosis and treatment of hyperprolactinemia: an Endocrine Society clinical practice guideline. *J Clin Endocrinol Metab* 2011; **96**:273–288.

23. Montejo AL, et al. Multidisciplinary consensus on the therapeutic recommendations for iatrogenic hyperprolactinemia secondary to antipsychotics. *Front Neuroendocrinol* 2017; **45**:25–34.

24. Sá Esteves P, et al. Low doses of adjunctive aripiprazole as treatment for antipsychotic-induced hyperprolactinemia: a literature review. *Eur Psychiatry* 2015; **30 Suppl 1**:393.

25. Yasui-Furukori N, et al. Dose-dependent effects of adjunctive treatment with aripiprazole on hyperprolactinemia induced by risperidone in female patients with schizophrenia. *J Clin Psychopharmacol* 2010; **30**:596–599.

26. Meaney AM, et al. Bone mineral density changes over a year in young females with schizophrenia: relationship to medication and endocrine variables. *Schizophr Res* 2007; **93**:136–143.

27. Hamner MB, et al. Hyperprolactinaemia in antipsychotic-treated patients: guidelines for avoidance and management. *CNS Drugs* 1998; **10**:209–222.

28. Duncan D, et al. Treatment of psychotropic-induced hyperprolactinaemia. *Psychiatric Bulletin* 1995; **19**:755–757.

29. Cavallaro R, et al. Cabergoline treatment of risperidone-induced hyperprolactinemia: a pilot study. *J Clin Psychiatry* 2004; **65**:187–190.

30. Yuan HN, et al. A randomized, crossover comparison of herbal medicine and bromocriptine against risperidone-induced hyperprolactinemia in patients with schizophrenia. *J Clin Psychopharmacol* 2008; **28**:264–370.

31. Man SC, et al. Peony-glycyrrhiza decoction for antipsychotic-related hyperprolactinemia in women with schizophrenia: a randomized controlled trial. *J Clin Psychopharmacol* 2016; **36**:572–579.

32. Krysiak R, et al. The effect of metformin on prolactin levels in patients with drug-induced hyperprolactinemia. *Eur J Intern Med* 2016; **30**:94–98.

33. Walters J, et al. Clinical questions and uncertainty–prolactin measurement in patients with schizophrenia and bipolar disorder. *J Psychopharmacology* 2008; **22**:82–89.

34. Chen CK, et al. Differential add-on effects of aripiprazole in resolving hyperprolactinemia induced by risperidone in comparison to benzamide antipsychotics. *Prog Neuropsychopharmacol Biol Psychiatry* 2010; **34**:1495–1499.

Sexual dysfunction

Primary sexual disorders are common, although reliable normative data are lacking.[1] Physical illness, psychiatric illness, substance misuse and prescribed drug treatment can all cause sexual dysfunction.[2] It has been estimated that 30–82%[3] of people with schizophrenia have problems with sexual dysfunction compared with 30% of the general population,[4] but note that in both groups reported prevalence rates vary depending on the method of data collection (low numbers with spontaneous reports, increasing with confidential questionnaires and further still with direct questioning[2]). In one study of patients with psychosis, 37% spontaneously reported sexual problems, but 46% were found to be experiencing difficulties when directly questioned.[5]

Baseline sexual functioning should be determined if possible (questionnaires may be useful) because sexual function can affect quality of life[6] and compliance with medication (sexual dysfunction is one of the major causes of treatment dropout).[7,8] Complaints of sexual dysfunction may also indicate progression or inadequate treatment of underlying medical or psychiatric conditions.[9,10] Sexual problems may also be caused by drug treatment where intervention may greatly improve quality of life.[11]

The human sexual response

There are four phases of the human sexual response, as detailed in Table 1.30.[2,12,13]

Effects of psychosis

Sexual dysfunction is a well-established phenomenon in first-episode schizophrenia[14,15] and up to 82% of men and 96% of women with established illness report problems, with associated reductions in quality of life.[6] Antipsychotic side effects are not solely

Table 1.30 The human sexual response

Desire	▪ Related to testosterone levels in men ▪ Possibly increased by dopamine and decreased by prolactin ▪ Psychosocial context and conditioning significantly affect desire
Arousal	▪ Influenced by testosterone in men and oestrogen in women ▪ Other potential mechanisms include: central dopamine stimulation, modulation of the cholinergic/adrenergic balance, peripheral α_1 agonism and nitric oxide pathways ▪ Physical pathology such as hypertension or diabetes can have a significant effect
Orgasm	▪ May be related to oxytocin ▪ Inhibition of orgasm may be caused by an increase in serotonin activity and raised prolactin, as well as α_1 blockade
Resolution	▪ Occurs passively after orgasm

Note: Many other hormones and neurotransmitters may interact in a complex way at each phase.

responsible, because prevalence is also high (17 – 70%) in patients who are unmedicated.[16] Men[17] complain of reduced desire, inability to achieve an erection and premature ejaculation, whereas women complain more generally about reduced enjoyment.[17,18] Women with psychosis are known to have reduced fertility.[19] People with psychosis are less able to develop good psychosexual relationships and, for some, treatment with an antipsychotic can improve sexual functioning.[20] Assessment of sexual functioning can clearly be difficult in someone who is psychotic. The Arizona Sexual Experience Scale (ASEX) may be useful in this respect.[21]

Effects of antipsychotic drugs

Sexual dysfunction has been reported as a side-effect of most antipsychotics, and up to 45% of people taking older or conventional antipsychotics experience sexual dysfunction.[22] Individual susceptibility varies and all effects are reversible. Note though that physical illness and drugs other than antipsychotics can cause sexual dysfunction, and many studies do not control for either, making the prevalence of sexual dysfunction with different antipsychotics difficult to compare.[23]

Antipsychotics decrease dopaminergic transmission, which in itself can decrease libido but may also increase prolactin levels via negative feedback. Hyperprolactinaemia has been shown to be associated with sexual dysfunction in several studies,[24] and it has been estimated that prolactin elevation explains 40% of the sexual dysfunction that is associated with antipsychotic medication.[4] Hyperprolactinaemia can also cause amenorrhoea in women and breast enlargement and galactorrhoea in both men and women.[25] Although it has been suggested that the overall propensity of an antipsychotic to cause sexual dysfunction is related to propensity to raise prolactin, i.e. risperidone > haloperidol > olanzapine > quetiapine > aripiprazole,[9,23,26] it should be noted that in the CUtLASS-1 study, FGAs (primarily sulpiride, but also other FGAs known to be associated with prolactin elevation) did not fare any worse than SGAs (70% of patients in this arm were prescribed an antipsychotic not associated with prolactin elevation) with respect to worsening sexual dysfunction. In fact, sexual functioning improved in both arms over the one-year duration of the study.[20] Aripiprazole is relatively free of sexual side effects when used as monotherapy[27] and possibly also in combination with another antipsychotic.[28,29] Cariprazine is a theoretically appropriate alternative (no switching studies are yet available).[30]

Anticholinergic effects can cause disorders of arousal[31] (concomitant anticholinergics may contribute to sexual dysfunction[32]), and drugs that block peripheral α_1 receptors cause particular problems with erection and ejaculation in men.[11] Drugs that are antagonists at both peripheral α_1 receptors and cholinergic receptors can cause priapism.[33] Antipsychotic-induced sedation and weight gain may reduce sexual desire.[33] These principles can be used to predict the sexual side effects of different antipsychotic drugs (see Table 1.31). Bear in mind that switching to an antipsychotic that better controls psychotic symptoms may itself help with sexual dysfunction.

Table 1.31 Sexual adverse effects of antipsychotics

Drug	Type of problem
Aripiprazole	▪ No effect on prolactin or α_1 receptors. No reported adverse effects on sexual function. Improves sexual function in those switched from other antipsychotics.[27,29,34,35] Case reports of aripiprazole-induced hypersexuality have been published[36,37]
Asenapine	▪ Does not appear to significantly affect prolactin levels[38] ▪ No reported cases of sexual dysfunction
Brexpiprazole	▪ Similar mechanism of action to aripiprazole (5-HT$_{1A}$ agonist, 5-HT$_{2A}$ antagonist and partial D$_2$ agonist) ▪ Causes negligible increases in prolactin[39] ▪ No problems with sexual dysfunction reported in clinical trials[40]
Cariprazine	▪ Similar mechanism of action to aripiprazole (5-HT$_{1A}$ agonist, 5-HT$_{2A}$ antagonist and partial D$_2$ agonist) ▪ Not associated with hyperprolactinaemia[41] ▪ No reported cases of sexual dysfunction
Clozapine	▪ Significant α_1 adrenergic blockade and anticholinergic effects.[42] No effect on prolactin[43] ▪ Probably fewer problems than with typical antipsychotics[44]
Haloperidol	▪ Similar problems to the phenothiazines[45] but anticholinergic effects reduced[46] ▪ Prevalence of sexual dysfunction reported to be up to 70%[47]
Lurasidone	▪ Does not appear to significantly affect prolactin levels[48] ▪ No reported cases of sexual dysfunction[49]
Olanzapine	▪ Possibly less sexual dysfunction than drugs such as haloperidol due to relative lack of prolactin-related effects[45] ▪ Priapism reported rarely[50,51] ▪ Prevalence of sexual dysfunction reported to be >50%[47]
Paliperidone	▪ Similar prolactin elevations to risperidone ▪ One small study[52] and one case report[53] showing reduction in sexual dysfunction following switching from risperidone oral or depot to paliperidone depot
Phenothiazines (e.g. chlorpromazine)	▪ Hyperprolactinaemia and anticholinergic effects. Reports of delayed orgasm at lower doses followed by normal orgasm but without ejaculation at higher doses.[18] ▪ Priapism has been reported with thioridazine, risperidone and chlorpromazine (probably due to α_1 blockade)[46,54,55]
Quetiapine	▪ No effect on serum prolactin[56] ▪ Possibly associated with low risk of sexual dysfunction,[57–60] but studies are conflicting[61,62]
Risperidone	▪ Potent elevator of serum prolactin ▪ Less anticholinergic than some other antipsychotics (olanzapine, quetiapine) ▪ Specific peripheral α_1 adrenergic blockade leads to a moderately high reported incidence of ejaculatory problems such as retrograde ejaculation[63,64] ▪ Priapism reported rarely[33] ▪ Prevalence of sexual dysfunction reported to be 60–70%[47]
Sulpiride/ amisulpride	▪ Potent elevators of serum prolactin[22] but note that sulpiride (as the main FGA prescribed in the study) was not associated with greater sexual dysfunction than SGAs (with variable ability to raise prolactin) in the CUtLASS-1 study[20]
Thioxanthenes (e.g. flupentixol)	▪ Arousal problems and anorgasmia[65]

Table 1.31 (*Continued*)

Drug	Type of problem
Lumateperone	▪ Does not appear to affect prolactin[66] ▪ No sexual side effects reported in (short) clinical trials[67]
Pimavanserin	▪ Does not bind to dopamine receptors,[68] therefore has no effect on prolactin ▪ May improve sexual function in patients with depression[69]
Iloperidone	▪ Does not usually affect prolactin[70] ▪ Some reports of sexual dysfunction in adverse event reporting databases,[71] case reports of retrograde ejaculation[72]

Treatment

Before attempting to treat sexual dysfunction, a thorough assessment is essential to determine the most likely cause. Assuming that physical pathology (diabetes, hypertension, cardiovascular disease, etc.) has been excluded or treated (e.g. obesity[73]), the following principles apply.

Spontaneous remission may occasionally occur[33] but may take 6 months to become apparent, if at all,[30] and may be more likely related to a reduction in severity of illness, rather than tolerance to the antipsychotic itself. When symptoms persist, the most obvious first step is to decrease the dose or discontinue the offending drug where appropriate. The next step is to switch to a different drug that is less likely to cause the specific sexual problem experienced (see Table 1.30). Another option is to add 5–10mg aripiprazole – this can normalise prolactin and improve sexual function.[74–77] If this fails or is not practicable, 'antidote' drugs can be tried: for example, cyproheptadine (a $5HT_2$ antagonist at doses of 4–16mg/day) has been used to treat SSRI-induced sexual dysfunction, but sedation is a common side-effect. There is some evidence that mirtazapine (also a $5HT_2$ antagonist as well as an alpha-2 antagonist) may relieve orgasmic dysfunction in FGA-treated patients.[78] Amantadine, bupropion, buspirone, bethanechol and yohimbine have all been used with varying degrees of success but have a number of unwanted side effects and interactions with other drugs. Given that hyperprolactinaemia may contribute to sexual dysfunction, selegiline (enhances dopamine activity) has been tested in an RCT. This was negative.[79] Testosterone patches have been shown to increase libido in women, although be aware that breast cancer risk may be significantly increased (Table 1.32).[80,81]

Table 1.32 Remedial treatments for psychotropic-induced sexual dysfunction

Drug	Pharmacology	Potential treatment for	Side effects
Alprostadil[1,13]	Prostaglandin	Erectile dysfunction	Pain, fibrosis, hypotension, priapism
Amantadine[1,82]	Dopamine agonist	Prolactin-induced reduction in desire and arousal (dopamine increases libido and facilitates ejaculation)	Return of psychotic symptoms, GI effects, nervousness, insomnia, rash
Bethanechol[83]	Cholinergic or cholinergic potentiation of adrenergic neurotransmission	Anticholinergic induced arousal problems and anorgasmia (from TCAs, antipsychotics, etc.)	Nausea and vomiting, colic, bradycardia, blurred vision, sweating
Bromocriptine[11]	Dopamine agonist	Prolactin-induced reduction in desire and arousal	Return of psychotic symptoms, GI effects
Bupropion[84,85]	Noradrenaline and dopamine reuptake inhibitor	SSRI-induced sexual dysfunction (evidence poor)	Concentration problems, reduced sleep, tremor
Buspirone[86]	$5HT_{1a}$ partial agonist	SSRI-induced sexual dysfunction, particularly decreased libido and anorgasmia	Nausea, dizziness, headache
Cyproheptadine[1,86,87]	$5HT_2$ antagonist	Sexual dysfunction caused by increased serotonin transmission (e.g. SSRIs), particularly anorgasmia	Sedation and fatigue. Reversal of the therapeutic effect of antidepressants
Flibanserin (licensed in USA)[88]	$5\text{-}HT_{1A}$ agonist, $5\text{-}HT_{2A}$ antagonist, dopamine antagonist	Lack or loss of sexual desire in premenopausal women. Appears to be safe in women taking antidepressants[89]	Hypotension, syncope, sedation, dizziness, nausea, dry mouth
Sildenafil[13,90–93] tadalafil,[94] lodenafil,[95] vardenafil[96]	Phosphodiesterase inhibitors	Erectile dysfunction of any aetiology. Anorgasmia in women. Effective when prolactin raised	Mild headaches, dizziness, nasal congestion
Yohimbine[1,13,97–99]	Central and peripheral α_2 adrenoceptor antagonist	SSRI-induced sexual dysfunction, particularly erectile dysfunction, decreased libido and anorgasmia (evidence poor)	Anxiety, nausea, fine tremor, increased BP, sweating, fatigue
Pimavanserin[69]	Inverse agonist at $5\text{-}HT_{2A}$ and $5\text{-}HT_{2C}$	Sexual dysfunction in depression with inadequate response to antidepressants. Improvement in sexual function independently of effect on depression unconfirmed.	Peripheral oedema, nausea, confusion
Bremelanotide[100]	Melanocortin receptor agonist	Hypoactive sexual desire in premenopausal women. No published data on use in patients with psychiatric diagnoses.	Flushing, nausea, headache

Note: The use of the drugs listed above should ideally be under the care or supervision of a specialist in sexual dysfunction.

The evidence base supporting the use of 'antidotes' is poor.[33,101] Be aware that generalisability of results from positive trials is limited by small sample sizes, short trial durations, and lack of controlling for confounding factors (age, concurrent medication, antipsychotic switches for reasons other than baseline sexual dysfunction).[101] Comparison of data between studies is further complicated by the use of varying assessment tools to measure outcomes.[102]

Drugs such as sildenafil (Viagra) or alprostadil (Caverject) are effective only in the treatment of erectile dysfunction (they have no effect on libido or central arousal). Psychological approaches used by sexual dysfunction clinics may be difficult for clients with mental health problems to engage in.[11]

References

1. Baldwin DS, et al. Effects of antidepressant drugs on sexual function. *Int J Psychiatry Clin Pract* 1997; **1**:47–58.
2. Pollack MH, et al. Genitourinary and sexual adverse effects of psychotropic medication. *Int J Psychiatry Med* 1992; **22**:305–327.
3. Dumontaud M, et al. Sexual dysfunctions in schizophrenia: beyond antipsychotics. A systematic review. *Prog Neuropsychopharmacol Biol Psychiatry* 2020; **98**:109804.
4. Nunes LV, et al. Strategies for the treatment of antipsychotic-induced sexual dysfunction and/or hyperprolactinemia among patients of the schizophrenia spectrum: a review. *J Sex Marital Ther* 2012; **38**:281–301.
5. Montejo AL, et al. Frequency of sexual dysfunction in patients with a psychotic disorder receiving antipsychotics. *J Sex Med* 2010; **7**:3404–3413.
6. Olfson M, et al. Male sexual dysfunction and quality of life in schizophrenia. *J Clin Psychiatry* 2005; **66**:331–338.
7. Montejo AL, et al. Incidence of sexual dysfunction associated with antidepressant agents: a prospective multicenter study of 1022 outpatients. Spanish Working Group for the Study of Psychotropic-Related Sexual Dysfunction. *J Clin Psychiatry* 2001; **62 Suppl 3**:10–21.
8. Souaiby L, et al. Sexual dysfunction in patients with schizophrenia and schizoaffective disorder and its association with adherence to antipsychotic medication. *J Mental Health* 2020; **29**:623–630.
9. Baggaley M. Sexual dysfunction in schizophrenia: focus on recent evidence. *Human Psychopharmacology* 2008; **23**:201–209.
10. Ucok A, et al. Sexual dysfunction in patients with schizophrenia on antipsychotic medication. *Eur Psychiatry* 2007; **22**:328–333.
11. Segraves RT. Effects of psychotropic drugs on human erection and ejaculation. *Arch Gen Psychiatry* 1989; **46**:275–284.
12. Stahl SM. The psychopharmacology of sex, Part 1: neurotransmitters and the 3 phases of the human sexual response. *J Clin Psychiatry* 2001; **62**:80–81.
13. Garcia-Reboll L, et al. Drugs for the treatment of impotence. *Drugs Aging* 1997; **11**:140–151.
14. Bitter I, et al. Antipsychotic treatment and sexual functioning in first-time neuroleptic-treated schizophrenic patients. *Int Clin Psychopharmacol* 2005; **20**:19–21.
15. Dembler-Stamm T, et al. Sexual dysfunction in unmedicated patients with schizophrenia and in healthy controls. *Pharmacopsychiatry* 2018; **51**:251–256.
16. Vargas-Cáceres S, et al. The impact of psychosis on sexual functioning: a systematic review. *J Sex Med* 2021; S1743-6095(1720) 31126-31127.
17. Macdonald S, et al. Nithsdale schizophrenia surveys 24: sexual dysfunction. Case-control study. *Br J Psychiatry* 2003; **182**:50–56.
18. Smith S. Effects of antipsychotics on sexual and endocrine function in women: implications for clinical practice. *J Clin Psychopharmacol* 2003; **23**:S27–S32.
19. Howard LM, et al. The general fertility rate in women with psychotic disorders. *Am J Psychiatry* 2002; **159**:991–997.
20. Peluso MJ, et al. Non-neurological and metabolic side effects in the Cost Utility of the Latest Antipsychotics in Schizophrenia Randomised Controlled Trial (CUtLASS-1). *SchizophrRes* 2013; **144**:80–86.
21. Byerly MJ, et al. An empirical evaluation of the Arizona sexual experience scale and a simple one-item screening test for assessing antipsychotic-related sexual dysfunction in outpatients with schizophrenia and schizoaffective disorder. *Schizophr Res* 2006; **81**:311–316.
22. Smith SM, et al. Sexual dysfunction in patients taking conventional antipsychotic medication. *Br J Psychiatry* 2002; **181**:49–55.
23. Serretti A, et al. A meta-analysis of sexual dysfunction in psychiatric patients taking antipsychotics. *Int Clin Psychopharmacol* 2011; **26**:130–140.
24. Zhang Y, et al. Prolactin and thyroid stimulating hormone (TSH) levels and sexual dysfunction in patients with schizophrenia treated with conventional antipsychotic medication: a cross-sectional study. *Med Sci Monit* 2018; **24**:9136–9143.
25. Collaborative Working Group on Clinical Trial Evaluations. Adverse effects of the atypical antipsychotics. *J Clin Psychiatry* 1998; **59 Suppl 12**:17–22.
26. Knegtering H, et al. Are sexual side effects of prolactin-raising antipsychotics reducible to serum prolactin? *Psychoneuroendocrinology* 2008; **33**:711–717.
27. Hanssens L, et al. The effect of antipsychotic medication on sexual function and serum prolactin levels in community-treated schizophrenic patients: results from the Schizophrenia Trial of Aripiprazole (STAR) study (NCT00237913). *BMC Psychiatry* 2008; **8**:95.

28. Mir A, et al. Change in sexual dysfunction with aripiprazole: a switching or add-on study. *J Psychopharm* 2008; **22**:244–253.

29. Byerly MJ, et al. Effects of aripiprazole on prolactin levels in subjects with schizophrenia during cross-titration with risperidone or olanzapine: analysis of a randomized, open-label study. *Schizophr Res* 2009; **107**:218–222.

30. Montejo AL, et al. Management strategies for antipsychotic-related sexual dysfunction: a clinical approach. *J Clin Med* 2021; **10**:308.

31. Aldridge SA. Drug-induced sexual dysfunction. *Clin Pharm* 1982; **1**:141–147.

32. Fond G, et al. Sexual dysfunctions are associated with major depression, chronic inflammation and anticholinergic consumption in the real-world schizophrenia FACE-SZ national cohort. *Prog Neuropsychopharmacol Biol Psychiatry* 2019; **94**:109654.

33. Baldwin D, et al. Sexual side-effects of antidepressant and antipsychotic drugs. *Adv Psychiatric Treat* 2003; **9**:202–210.

34. Rykmans V, et al. A comparison of switching strategies from risperidone to aripiprazole in patients with schizophrenia with insufficient efficacy/tolerability on risperidone (cn138–169). *Eur Psychiatry* 2008; **23**:S111–S111.

35. Potkin SG, et al. Reduced sexual dysfunction with aripiprazole once-monthly versus paliperidone palmitate: results from QUALIFY. *Int Clin Psychopharmacol* 2017; **32**:147–154.

36. Chen CY, et al. Improvement of serum prolactin and sexual function after switching to aripiprazole from risperidone in schizophrenia: a case series. *Psychiatry ClinNeurosci* 2011; **65**:95–97.

37. Vrignaud L, et al. [Hypersexuality associated with aripiprazole: a new case and review of the literature]. *Therapie* 2014; **69**:525–527.

38. Ajmal A, et al. Psychotropic-induced hyperprolactinemia: a clinical review. *Psychosomatics* 2014; **55**:29–36.

39. Kane JM, et al. A multicenter, randomized, double-blind, controlled phase 3 trial of fixed-dose brexpiprazole for the treatment of adults with acute schizophrenia. *Schizophr Res* 2015; **164**:127–135.

40. Citrome L. Brexpiprazole for schizophrenia and as adjunct for major depressive disorder: a systematic review of the efficacy and safety profile for this newly approved antipsychotic – what is the number needed to treat, number needed to harm and likelihood to be helped or harmed? *Int J Clin Pract* 2015; **69**:978–997.

41. Nasrallah HA, et al. The safety and tolerability of cariprazine in long-term treatment of schizophrenia: a post hoc pooled analysis. *BMC Psychiatry* 2017; **17**:305.

42. Coward DM. General pharmacology of clozapine. *British J Psychiatry Supp* 1992; **160**:5–11.

43. Meltzer HY, et al. Effect of clozapine on human serum prolactin levels. *Am J Psychiatry* 1979; **136**:1550–1555.

44. Aizenberg D, et al. Comparison of sexual dysfunction in male schizophrenic patients maintained on treatment with classical antipsychotics versus clozapine. *J Clin Psychiatry* 2001; **62**:541–544.

45. Crawford AM, et al. The acute and long-term effect of olanzapine compared with placebo and haloperidol on serum prolactin concentrations. *Schizophr Res* 1997; **26**:41–54.

46. Mitchell JE, et al. Antipsychotic drug therapy and sexual dysfunction in men. *Am J Psychiatry* 1982; **139**:633–637.

47. Serretti A, et al. Sexual side effects of pharmacological treatment of psychiatric diseases. *Clin Pharmacol Ther* 2011; **89**:142–147.

48. Citrome L, et al. Long-term safety and tolerability of lurasidone in schizophrenia: a 12-month, double-blind, active-controlled study. *Int Clin Psychopharmacol* 2012; **27**:165–176.

49. Clayton AH, et al. Safety of flibanserin in women treated with antidepressants: a randomized, placebo-controlled study. *J Sex Med* 2018; **15**:43–51.

50. Dossenbach M, et al. Effects of atypical and typical antipsychotic treatments on sexual function in patients with schizophrenia: 12-month results from the Intercontinental Schizophrenia Outpatient Health Outcomes (IC-SOHO) study. *Eur Psychiatry* 2006; **21**:251–258.

51. Aurobindo Pharma – Milpharm Ltd. Summary of product characteristics. Olanzapine 10 mg tablets. 2020; http://www.medicines.org.uk/emc/medicine/27661/SPC/Olanzapine++10+mg+tablets.

52. Montalvo I, et al. Changes in prolactin levels and sexual function in young psychotic patients after switching from long-acting injectable risperidone to paliperidone palmitate. *Int Clin Psychopharmacol* 2013; **28**:46–49.

53. Shiloh R, et al. Risperidone-induced retrograde ejaculation. *Am J Psychiatry* 2001; **158**:650.

54. Loh C, et al. Risperidone-induced retrograde ejaculation: case report and review of the literature. *Int Clin Psychopharmacol* 2004; **19**:111–112.

55. Thompson JW, Jr., et al. Psychotropic medication and priapism: a comprehensive review. *J Clin Psychiatry* 1990; **51**:430–433.

56. Peuskens J, et al. A comparison of quetiapine and chlorpromazine in the treatment of schizophrenia. *Acta Psychiatr Scand* 1997; **96**:265–273.

57. Bobes J, et al. Frequency of sexual dysfunction and other reproductive side-effects in patients with schizophrenia treated with risperidone, olanzapine, quetiapine, or haloperidol: the results of the EIRE study. *J Sex Marital Ther* 2003; **29**:125–147.

58. Byerly MJ, et al. An open-label trial of quetiapine for antipsychotic-induced sexual dysfunction. *J Sex Marital Ther* 2004; **30**:325–332.

59. Knegtering R, et al. A randomized open-label study of the impact of quetiapine versus risperidone on sexual functioning. *J Clin Psychopharmacol* 2004; **24**:56–61.

60. Montejo Gonzalez AL, et al. A 6-month prospective observational study on the effects of quetiapine on sexual functioning. *J Clin Psychopharmacol* 2005; **25**:533–538.

61. Atmaca M, et al. A new atypical antipsychotic: quetiapine-induced sexual dysfunctions. *Int J Impot Res* 2005; **17**:201–203.

62. Kelly DL, et al. A randomized double-blind 12-week study of quetiapine, risperidone or fluphenazine on sexual functioning in people with schizophrenia. *Psychoneuroendocrinology* 2006; **31**:340–346.

63. Tran PV, et al. Double-blind comparison of olanzapine versus risperidone in the treatment of schizophrenia and other psychotic disorders. *J Clin Psychopharmacol* 1997; **17**:407–418.

64. Raja M. Risperidone-induced absence of ejaculation. *Int Clin Psychopharmacol* 1999; **14**:317–319.

65. Aizenberg D, et al. Sexual dysfunction in male schizophrenic patients. *J Clin Psychiatry* 1995; **56**:137–141.

66. Correll CU, et al. Safety and tolerability of lumateperone 42 mg: an open-label antipsychotic switch study in outpatients with stable schizophrenia. *Schizophr Res* 2021; **228**:198–205.

67. Correll CU, et al. Efficacy and safety of lumateperone for treatment of schizophrenia: a randomized clinical trial. *JAMA Psychiatry* 2020; **77**:349–358.

68. Cruz MP. Pimavanserin (Nuplazid): a treatment for hallucinations and delusions associated with Parkinson's disease. *P & T* 2017; **42**:368–371.

69. Freeman MP, et al. Improvement of sexual functioning during treatment of MDD with adjunctive pimavanserin: a secondary analysis. *Depress Anxiety* 2020; **37**:485–495.

70. Peuskens J, et al. The effects of novel and newly approved antipsychotics on serum prolactin levels: a comprehensive review. *CNS Drugs* 2014; **28**:421–453.

71. Subeesh V, et al. Novel adverse events of iloperidone: a disproportionality analysis in US Food and Drug Administration Adverse Event Reporting System (FAERS) Database. *Current Drug Safety* 2019; **14**:21–26.

72. Freeman SA. Iloperidone-induced retrograde ejaculation. *Int Clin Psychopharmacol* 2013; **28**:156.

73. Theleritis C, et al. Sexual dysfunction and central obesity in patients with first episode psychosis. *Eur Psychiatry* 2017; **42**:1–7.

74. Shim JC, et al. Adjunctive treatment with a dopamine partial agonist, aripiprazole, for antipsychotic-induced hyperprolactinemia: a placebo-controlled trial. *Am J Psychiatry* 2007; **164**:1404–1410.

75. Yasui-Furukori N, et al. Dose-dependent effects of adjunctive treatment with aripiprazole on hyperprolactinemia induced by risperidone in female patients with schizophrenia. *J Clin Psychopharmacol* 2010; **30**:596–599.

76. Trives MZ, et al. Effect of the addition of aripiprazole on hyperprolactinemia associated with risperidone long-acting injection. *J Clin Psychopharmacol* 2013; **33**:538–541.

77. Kelly DL, et al. Adjunct aripiprazole reduces prolactin and prolactin-related adverse effects in premenopausal women with psychosis: results from the DAAMSEL clinical trial. *J Clin Psychopharmacol* 2018; **38**:317–326.

78. Terevnikov V, et al. Add-on mirtazapine improves orgasmic functioning in patients with schizophrenia treated with first-generation antipsychotics. *Nord J Psychiatry* 2017; **71**:77–80.

79. Kodesh A, et al. Selegiline in the treatment of sexual dysfunction in schizophrenic patients maintained on neuroleptics: a pilot study. *Clin Neuropharmacol* 2003; **26**:193–195.

80. Davis SR, et al. Testosterone for low libido in postmenopausal women not taking estrogen. *N Eng J Med* 2008; **359**:2005–2017.

81. Schover LR. Androgen therapy for loss of desire in women: is the benefit worth the breast cancer risk? *FertilSteril* 2008; **90**:129–140.

82. Valevski A, et al. Effect of amantadine on sexual dysfunction in neuroleptic-treated male schizophrenic patients. *Clin Neuropharmacol* 1998; **21**:355–357.

83. Gross MD. Reversal by bethanechol of sexual dysfunction caused by anticholinergic antidepressants. *Am J Psychiatry* 1982; **139**:1193–1194.

84. Masand PS, et al. Sustained-release bupropion for selective serotonin reuptake inhibitor-induced sexual dysfunction: a randomized, double-blind, placebo-controlled, parallel-group study. *Am J Psychiatry* 2001; **158**:805–807.

85. Rezaei O, et al. The effect of bupropion on sexual function in patients with Schizophrenia: a randomized clinical trial. *Eur J Psychiatry* 2017; **32**.

86. Rothschild AJ. Sexual side effects of antidepressants. *J Clin Psychiatry* 2000; **61 Suppl 11**:28–36.

87. Lauerma H. Successful treatment of citalopram-induced anorgasmia by cyproheptadine. *Acta Psychiatr Scand* 1996; **93**:69–70.

88. IBM Watson Health. IBM Micromedex Solutions. 2020; https://www.ibm.com/watson-health/about/micromedex.

89. Clayton AH, et al. Effect of lurasidone on sexual function in major depressive disorder patients with subthreshold hypomanic symptoms (mixed features): results from a placebo-controlled trial. *J Clin Psychiatry* 2018; **79**:18m12132.

90. Nurnberg HG, et al. Sildenafil for women patients with antidepressant-induced sexual dysfunction. *Psychiatr Serv* 1999; **50**:1076–1078.

91. Salerian AJ, et al. Sildenafil for psychotropic-induced sexual dysfunction in 31 women and 61 men. *J Sex Marital Ther* 2000; **26**:133–140.

92. Gopalakrishnan R, et al. Sildenafil in the treatment of antipsychotic-induced erectile dysfunction: a randomized, double-blind, placebo-controlled, flexible-dose, two-way crossover trial. *Am J Psychiatry* 2006; **163**:494–499.

93. Mazzilli R, et al. Erectile dysfunction in patients taking psychotropic drugs and treated with phosphodiesterase-5 inhibitors. *Arch Ital Urol Androl* 2018; **90**:44–48.

94. De Boer MK, et al. Efficacy of tadalafil on erectile dysfunction in male patients using antipsychotics: a double-blind, placebo-controlled, crossover pilot study. *J Clin Psychopharmacol* 2014; **34**:380–382.

95. Nunes LV, et al. Adjunctive treatment with lodenafil carbonate for erectile dysfunction in outpatients with schizophrenia and spectrum: a randomized, double-blind, crossover, placebo-controlled trial. *J Sex Med* 2013; **10**:1136–1145.

96. Mitsonis CI, et al. Vardenafil in the treatment of erectile dysfunction in outpatients with chronic schizophrenia: a flexible-dose, open-label study. *J Clin Psychiatry* 2008; **69**:206–212.

97. Jacobsen FM. Fluoxetine-induced sexual dysfunction and an open trial of yohimbine. *J Clin Psychiatry* 1992; **53**:119–122.

98. Michelson D, et al. Mirtazapine, yohimbine or olanzapine augmentation therapy for serotonin reuptake-associated female sexual dysfunction: a randomized, placebo controlled trial. *J Psychiatr Res* 2002; 36:147–152.

99. Woodrum ST, et al. Management of SSRI-induced sexual dysfunction. *Ann Pharmacother* 1998; 32:1209–1215.

100. Kingsberg SA, et al. Bremelanotide for the treatment of hypoactive sexual desire disorder: two randomized phase 3 trials. *Obstet Gynecol* 2019; 134:899–908.

101. Allen K, et al. Management of antipsychotic-related sexual dysfunction: systematic review. *J Sex Med* 2019; 16:1978–1987.

102. Basson R, et al. Women's sexual dysfunction associated with psychiatric disorders and their treatment. *Womens Health* 2018; 14:1745506518762664.

Further Reading

Clayton AH, et al. Sexual dysfunction due to psychotropic medications. *Psychiatr Clin North Am* 2016; 39:427–463.

Pneumonia

A 2018 meta-analysis of 14 studies reported that antipsychotic use was associated with a near doubling of pneumonia incidence compared with no use.[1] This same analysis found no difference in incidence of pneumonia between FGAs and SGAs and no increase in case fatality rate. A later analysis of spontaneous reporting to the FDA uncovered a signal of greater incidence of reported pneumonia in people prescribed clozapine, olanzapine and multiple antipsychotics (compared with haloperidol).[2] A dose-related increase in risk has been reported for clozapine[3-5] but also for other antipsychotics[6] and for polypharmacy involving FGAs and SGAs[4,5,7] and combinations involving a mood stabiliser[5] have previously been found to be associated with increased risk of pneumonia. In people with bipolar disorder, the risk with combinations involving all three classes of medication was higher than any other combinations.[5]

A study of bipolar patients found that clozapine, olanzapine and haloperidol were linked to increased rates of pneumonia while lithium was protective.[5] Another study suggests amisulpride is not linked to pneumonia.[4] Clozapine re-exposure was associated with a greater risk for (recurrent) pneumonia than the risk of baseline pneumonia with initial clozapine treatment in one study.[3] Schizophrenia itself seems to afford a higher risk of complications (e.g. admission to intensive care) in people diagnosed with pneumonia[8] though neither diagnosis nor age appears to modify the effect of antipsychotic use on pneumonia.[9] Likewise risk of antipsychotic-associated pneumonia was increased in patients with Alzheimer's disease and those without.[10]

Data have emerged recently which to some extent call into question the apparent causal association between antipsychotic use and risk of pneumonia. One study looked at the incidence of pneumonia in over 8000 people before and after starting various antipsychotics and found no change overall (or for any individual antipsychotic). Another analysis, a case-control study, found that duration of antipsychotic use was just one of three factors linked to increased risk of pneumonia (the others being severity of illness and comorbidity index).[11]

In this study, duration of antipsychotic treatment could be considered a proxy for illness duration. It might also be noted, in the time of COVID, that some antipsychotics have demonstrable antiviral activity.[12,13]

The mechanism by which antipsychotics increase the risk of pneumonia is not known. Possibilities include sedation (risk may be highest with drugs that show greatest H_1 antagonism[4,7]), dystonia or dyskinesia, dry mouth causing poor bolus transport and so increasing the risk of aspiration (hypersalivation in the case of clozapine), general poor physical health;[4] or perhaps some ill-defined effect on immune response.[7,14] Nevertheless, the fact that antipsychotics can increase the risk of aspiration pneumonia and not other pneumonia types offers support to this as a plausible (perhaps sole) mechanism.[15] With clozapine, pneumonia may also be secondary to constipation.[16] Clozapine is also fairly strongly associated with antibody deficiency and greater use of antibiotics.[17]

An increased risk of pneumonia should probably be assumed for all patients taking any antipsychotic (but especially clozapine[18]) for any period. All patients should be very carefully monitored for signs of chest infection and effective treatment started promptly. Consideration should be given to using pneumococcal vaccine, although there is no evidence to support its benefit in this group of patients. Extra vigilance is required when re-exposing to clozapine patients with previous history of clozapine-induced pneumonia. Early referral to general medical services should be considered where there is any doubt about the severity or type of chest infection.

Summary

- Assume the use of all antipsychotics increase the risk of pneumonia.
- Monitor all patients for signs of chest infection and treat promptly.

References

1. Dzahini O, et al. Antipsychotic drug use and pneumonia: systematic review and meta-analysis. *J Psychopharmacology* 2018; 32:1167–1181.
2. Cepaityte D, et al. Exploring a safety signal of antipsychotic-associated pneumonia: a pharmacovigilance-pharmacodynamic study. *Schizophr Bull* 2020: [Epub ahead of print].
3. Hung GC, et al. Antipsychotic reexposure and recurrent pneumonia in schizophrenia: a nested case-control study. *J Clin Psychiatry* 2016; 77:60–66.
4. Kuo CJ, et al. Second-generation antipsychotic medications and risk of pneumonia in schizophrenia. *Schizophr Bull* 2013; 39:648–657.
5. Yang SY, et al. Antipsychotic drugs, mood stabilizers, and risk of pneumonia in bipolar disorder: a nationwide case-control study. *J Clin Psychiatry* 2013; 74:e79–e86.
6. Huybrechts KF, et al. Comparative safety of antipsychotic medications in nursing home residents. *J Am Geriatr Soc* 2012; 60:420–429.
7. Trifiro G, et al. Association of community-acquired pneumonia with antipsychotic drug use in elderly patients: a nested case-control study. *Ann Intern Med* 2010; 152:418–440.
8. Chen YH, et al. Poor clinical outcomes among pneumonia patients with schizophrenia. *Schizophr Bull* 2011; 37:1088–1094.
9. Nose M, et al. Antipsychotic drug exposure and risk of pneumonia: a systematic review and meta-analysis of observational studies. *Pharmacoepidemiol Drug Saf* 2015; 24:812–820.
10. Tolppanen AM, et al. Antipsychotic use and risk of hospitalization or death due to pneumonia in persons with and those without Alzheimer disease. *Chest* 2016; 150:1233–1241.
11. Chan HY, et al. Is antipsychotic treatment associated with risk of pneumonia in people with serious mental illness?: the roles of severity of psychiatric symptoms and global functioning. *J Clin Psychopharmacol* 2019; 39:434–440.
12. Plaze M, et al. Repurposing chlorpromazine to treat COVID-19: the reCoVery study. *Encephale* 2020; 46:169–172.
13. Otręba M, et al. Antiviral activity of chlorpromazine, fluphenazine, perphenazine, prochlorperazine, and thioridazine towards RNA-viruses. A review. *Eur J Pharmacol* 2020; 887:173553.
14. Knol W, et al. Antipsychotic drug use and risk of pneumonia in elderly people. *J Am Geriatr Soc* 2008; 56:661–666.
15. Herzig SJ, et al. Antipsychotics and the risk of aspiration pneumonia in individuals hospitalized for nonpsychiatric conditions: a cohort study. *J Am Geriatr Soc* 2017; 65:2580–2586.
16. Galappathie N, et al. Clozapine-associated pneumonia and respiratory arrest secondary to severe constipation. *Med Sci Law* 2014; 54:105–109.
17. Ponsford M, et al. Clozapine is associated with secondary antibody deficiency. *Br J Psychiatry* 2018; 214:1–7.
18. De Leon J, et al. Pneumonia may be more frequent and have more fatal outcomes with clozapine than with other second-generation antipsychotics. *World Psychiatry* 2020; 19:120–121.

Further reading

Schoretsanitis G, et al. An update on the complex relationship between clozapine and pneumonia. *Expert Rev Clin Pharmacol* 2021; 14:145–149.

Switching antipsychotics

Summary of recommendations for switching antipsychotics because of poor tolerability.

Adverse effect	Suggested drugs	Alternatives
Acute EPS[1-8] Dystonia, parkinsonism, bradykinesia	Aripiprazole Brexpiprazole Cariprazine Olanzapine Quetiapine	Clozapine Lurasidone Ziprasidone
Akathisia[2,9,10]	Olanzapine Quetiapine	Clozapine Brexpiprazole
Dyslipidaemia[7,8,11-16]	Amisulpride Aripiprazole§ Lurasidone Ziprasidone	Asenapine Brexpiprazole Cariprazine
Impaired glucose tolerance[7,8,15,17-21]	Amisulpride Aripiprazole§ Lurasidone Ziprasidone	Brexpiprazole Cariprazine Haloperidol
Hyperprolactinaemia[7,8,15,22-28]	Aripiprazole§ Brexpiprazole Cariprazine Lurasidone Quetiapine	Clozapine Olanzapine Ziprasidone
Postural hypotension[8,15,29]	Amisulpride Aripiprazole Brexpiprazole Cariprazine Lurasidone	Haloperidol Sulpiride Trifluoperazine
QT prolongation[27,30-37]	Brexpiprazole Cariprazine Lurasidone Paliperidone	Low dose monotherapy of any drug not formally contra-indicated in QT prolongation (with ECG monitoring)
Sedation[7,8,27]	Amisulpride Aripiprazole Brexpiprazole Cariprazine Risperidone Sulpiride	Haloperidol Trifluoperazine Ziprasidone

(Continued)

(Continued)

Adverse effect	Suggested drugs	Alternatives
Sexual dysfuction[8,38–44]	Aripiprazole Brexpiprazole Cariprazine Lurasidone Quetiapine	Clozapine
Tardive dyskinesia[45–49]	Clozapine	Aripiprazole Olanzapine Quetiapine
Weight gain[16,35,37,50–57]	Amisulpride Aripiprazole§ Brexpiprazole Cariprazine Haloperidol Lurasidone Ziprasidone	Asenapine Haloperidol Trifluoperazine

§There is evidence that both switching to and co-prescription of aripiprazole can be associated with reductions in body weight and plasma prolactin levels, better lipid profiles, and a decrease in plasma glucose levels.[58–61]

Lumateperone and pimavanserin are not listed in the table because of their limited availability. Both drugs cause little or no EPSE or akathisia, have no effect on prolactin or blood pressure and cause minimal weight gain and metabolic disturbance.[62,63] Pimvanserin prolongs QT,[64] whereas lumateperone seems to have no effect on the ECG.[65]

References

1. Stanniland C, et al. Tolerability of atypical antipsychotics. *Drug Saf* 2000; **22**:195–214.
2. Tarsy D, et al. Effects of newer antipsychotics on extrapyramidal function. *CNS Drugs* 2002; **16**:23–45.
3. Caroff SN, et al. Movement disorders associated with atypical antipsychotic drugs. *J Clin Psychiatry* 2002; **63 Suppl 4**:12–19.
4. Lemmens P, et al. A combined analysis of double-blind studies with risperidone vs. placebo and other antipsychotic agents: factors associated with extrapyramidal symptoms. *Acta Psychiatr Scand* 1999; **99**:160–170.
5. Taylor DM. Aripiprazole: a review of its pharmacology and clinical use. *Int J Clin Pract* 2003; **57**:49–54.
6. Meltzer HY, et al. Lurasidone in the treatment of schizophrenia: a randomized, double-blind, placebo- and olanzapine-controlled study. *Am J Psychiatry* 2011; **168**:957–967.
7. Garnock-Jones KP. Cariprazine: a review in schizophrenia. *CNS Drugs* 2017; **31**:513–525.
8. Garnock-Jones KP. Brexpiprazole: a review in schizophrenia. *CNS Drugs* 2016; **30**:335–342.
9. Buckley PF. Efficacy of quetiapine for the treatment of schizophrenia: a combined analysis of three placebo-controlled trials. *Curr Med Res Opin* 2004; **20**:1357–1363.
10. Pringsheim T, et al. The assessment and treatment of antipsychotic-induced akathisia. *Can J Psychiatry* 2018; **63**:719–729.
11. Rettenbacher MA, et al. Early changes of plasma lipids during treatment with atypical antipsychotics. *Int Clin Psychopharmacol* 2006; **21**:369–372.
12. Ball MP, et al. Clozapine-induced hyperlipidemia resolved after switch to aripiprazole therapy. *Ann Pharmacother* 2005; **39**:1570–1572.
13. Chrzanowski WK, et al. Effectiveness of long-term aripiprazole therapy in patients with acutely relapsing or chronic, stable schizophrenia: a 52-week, open-label comparison with olanzapine. *Psychopharmacology* 2006; **189**:259–266.
14. De Hert M, et al. A case series: evaluation of the metabolic safety of aripiprazole. *Schizophr Bull* 2007; **33**:823–830.
15. Citrome L, et al. Long-term safety and tolerability of lurasidone in schizophrenia: a 12-month, double-blind, active-controlled study. *Int Clin Psychopharmacol* 2012; **27**:165–176.
16. Kemp DE, et al. Weight change and metabolic effects of asenapine in patients with schizophrenia and bipolar disorder. *J Clin Psychiatry* 2014; **75**:238–245.

17. Haddad PM. Antipsychotics and diabetes: review of non-prospective data. *Br J Psychiatry Suppl* 2004; 47:S80–S86.

18. Berry S, et al. Improvement of insulin indices after switch from olanzazole to risperidone. *Eur Neuropsychopharmacol* 2002; 12:316.

19. Gianfrancesco FD, et al. Differential effects of risperidone, olanzapine, clozapine, and conventional antipsychotics on type 2 diabetes: findings from a large health plan database. *J Clin Psychiatry* 2002; 63:920–930.

20. Mir S, et al. Atypical antipsychotics and hyperglycaemia. *Int Clin Psychopharmacol* 2001; 16:63–74.

21. Cernea S, et al. Pharmacological management of glucose dysregulation in patients treated with second-generation antipsychotics. *Drugs* 2020; 80:1763–1781.

22. Turrone P, et al. Elevation of prolactin levels by atypical antipsychotics. *Am J Psychiatry* 2002; 159:133–135.

23. David SR, et al. The effects of olanzapine, risperidone, and haloperidol on plasma prolactin levels in patients with schizophrenia. *Clin Ther* 2000; 22:1085–1096.

24. Hamner MB, et al. Hyperprolactinaemia in antipsychotic-treated patients: guidelines for avoidance and management. *CNS Drugs* 1998; 10:209–222.

25. Trives MZ, et al. Effect of the addition of aripiprazole on hyperprolactinemia associated with risperidone long-acting injection. *J Clin Psychopharmacol* 2013; 33:538–541.

26. Suzuki Y, et al. Differences in plasma prolactin levels in patients with schizophrenia treated on monotherapy with five second-generation antipsychotics. *Schizophr Res* 2013; 145:116–119.

27. Leucht S, et al. Comparative efficacy and tolerability of 15 antipsychotic drugs in schizophrenia: a multiple-treatments meta-analysis. *Lancet* 2013; 382:951–962.

28. Keks N, et al. Comparative tolerability of dopamine D2/3 receptor partial agonists for schizophrenia. *CNS Drugs* 2020; 34:473–507.

29. Citrome L. Cariprazine: chemistry, pharmacodynamics, pharmacokinetics, and metabolism, clinical efficacy, safety, and tolerability. *Exp Opin Drug Metab Toxicol* 2013; 9:193–206.

30. Glassman AH, et al. Antipsychotic drugs: prolonged QTc interval, torsade de pointes, and sudden death. *Am J Psychiatry* 2001; 158:1774–1782.

31. Antipsychotics TD. QT prolongation. *Acta Psychiatr Scand* 2003; 107:85–95.

32. Titier K, et al. Atypical antipsychotics: from potassium channels to torsade de pointes and sudden death. *Drug Saf* 2005; 28:35–51.

33. Ray WA, et al. Atypical antipsychotic drugs and the risk of sudden cardiac death. *N Engl J Med* 2009; 360:225–235.

34. Loebel A, et al. Efficacy and safety of lurasidone 80 mg/day and 160 mg/day in the treatment of schizophrenia: a randomized, double-blind, placebo- and active-controlled trial. *Schizophr Res* 2013; 145:101–109.

35. Das S, et al. Brexpiprazole: so far so good. *Ther Adv Psychopharmacol* 2016; 6:39–54.

36. Citrome L. Cariprazine for the treatment of schizophrenia: a review of this dopamine D3-preferring D3/D2 receptor partial agonist. *Clin Schizophr Relat Psychoses* 2016; 10:109–119.

37. Huhn M, et al. Comparative efficacy and tolerability of 32 oral antipsychotics for the acute treatment of adults with multi-episode schizophrenia: a systematic review and network meta-analysis. *Lancet* 2019; 394:939–951.

38. Byerly MJ, et al. An open-label trial of quetiapine for antipsychotic-induced sexual dysfunction. *J Sex Marital Ther* 2004; 30:325–332.

39. Byerly MJ, et al. Sexual dysfunction associated with second-generation antipsychotics in outpatients with schizophrenia or schizoaffective disorder: an empirical evaluation of olanzapine, risperidone, and quetiapine. *Schizophr Res* 2006; 86:244–250.

40. Montejo Gonzalez AL, et al. A 6-month prospective observational study on the effects of quetiapine on sexual functioning. *J Clin Psychopharmacol* 2005; 25:533–538.

41. Dossenbach M, et al. Effects of atypical and typical antipsychotic treatments on sexual function in patients with schizophrenia: 12-month results from the Intercontinental Schizophrenia Outpatient Health Outcomes (IC-SOHO) study. *Eur Psychiatry* 2006; 21:251–258.

42. Kerwin R, et al. A multicentre, randomized, naturalistic, open-label study between aripiprazole and standard of care in the management of community-treated schizophrenic patients Schizophrenia Trial of Aripiprazole: (STAR) study. *Eur Psychiatry* 2007; 22:433–443.

43. Hanssens L, et al. The effect of antipsychotic medication on sexual function and serum prolactin levels in community-treated schizophrenic patients: results from the Schizophrenia Trial of Aripiprazole (STAR) study (NCT00237913). *BMC Psychiatry* 2008; 8:95.

44. Loebel A, et al. Effectiveness of lurasidone vs. quetiapine XR for relapse prevention in schizophrenia: a 12-month, double-blind, noninferiority study. *Schizophr Res* 2013; 147:95–102.

45. Lieberman J, et al. Clozapine pharmacology and tardive dyskinesia. *Psychopharmacology* 1989; 99 Suppl 1:S54–S59.

46. O'Brien J, et al. Marked improvement in tardive dyskinesia following treatment with olanzapine in an elderly subject. *Br J Psychiatry* 1998; 172:186.

47. Sacchetti E, et al. Quetiapine, clozapine, and olanzapine in the treatment of tardive dyskinesia induced by first-generation antipsychotics: a 124-week case report. *Int Clin Psychopharmacol* 2003; 18:357–359.

48. Witschy JK, et al. Improvement in tardive dyskinesia with aripiprazole use. *Can J Psychiatry* 2005; 50:188.

49. Ricciardi L, et al. Treatment recommendations for tardive dyskinesia. *Can J Psychiatry* 2019; 64:388–399.

50. Taylor DM, et al. Atypical antipsychotics and weight gain – a systematic review. *Acta Psychiatr Scand* 2000; 101:416–432.

51. Allison D, et al. Antipsychotic-induced weight gain: a comprehensive research synthesis. *Am J Psychiatry* 1999; 156:1686–1696.

52. Brecher M, et al. The long term effect of quetiapine (Seroquel™) monotherapy on weight in patients with schizophrenia. *Int J Psychiatry Clin Pract* 2000; 4:287–291.

53. Casey DE, et al. Switching patients to aripiprazole from other antipsychotic agents: a multicenter randomized study. *Psychopharmacology* 2003; 166:391–399.

54. Newcomer JW, et al. A multicenter, randomized, double-blind study of the effects of aripiprazole in overweight subjects with schizophrenia or schizoaffective disorder switched from olanzapine. *J Clin Psychiatry* 2008; 69:1046–1056.

CHAPTER 1

55. McEvoy JP, et al. Effectiveness of lurasidone in patients with schizophrenia or schizoaffective disorder switched from other antipsychotics: a randomized, 6-week, open-label study. *J Clin Psychiatry* 2013; **74**:170–179.

56. McEvoy JP, et al. Effectiveness of paliperidone palmitate vs haloperidol decanoate for maintenance treatment of schizophrenia: a randomized clinical trial. *JAMA* 2014; **311**:1978–1987.

57. Nasrallah HA, et al. The safety and tolerability of cariprazine in long-term treatment of schizophrenia: a post hoc pooled analysis. *BMC Psychiatry* 2017; **17**:305.

58. Shim JC, et al. Adjunctive treatment with a dopamine partial agonist, aripiprazole, for antipsychotic-induced hyperprolactinemia: a placebo-controlled trial. *Am J Psychiatry* 2007; **164**:1404–1410.

59. Fleischhacker WW, et al. Weight change on aripiprazole-clozapine combination in schizophrenic patients with weight gain and suboptimal response on clozapine: 16-week double-blind study. *Eur Psychiatry* 2008; **23 Suppl 2**:S114–S115.

60. Henderson DC, et al. Aripiprazole added to overweight and obese olanzapine-treated schizophrenia patients. *J Clin Psychopharmacol* 2009; **29**:165–169.

61. Preda A, et al. A safety evaluation of aripiprazole in the treatment of schizophrenia. *Exp Opin Drug Saf* 2020; **19**:1529–1538.

62. Correll CU, et al. Safety and tolerability of lumateperone 42 mg: an open-label antipsychotic switch study in outpatients with stable schizophrenia. *Schizophr Res* 2021; **228**:198–205.

63. Mathis MV, et al. The US Food and Drug Administration's perspective on the new antipsychotic pimavanserin. *J Clin Psychiatry* 2017; **78**:e668–e673.

64. Cruz MP. Pimavanserin (nuplazid): a treatment for hallucinations and delusions associated with parkinson's disease. *P & T* 2017; **42**:368–371.

65. Greenwood J, et al. Lumateperone: a novel antipsychotic for schizophrenia. *Ann Pharmacother* 2021; **55**:98–104.

Venous thromboembolism

Evidence of an association

Antipsychotic treatment was first linked to an increased risk of thromboembolism in 1965[1] – over a ten-year observation period, 3.1% of 1590 patients developed thromboembolism, of whom 9 (0.6%) died. However, the use of continuing antipsychotic medication is a proxy for severe and enduring mental illness and so observed associations with antipsychotics may reflect inherent pathological processes in the conditions for which they are prescribed. To some extent, the relative contributions to risk of thromboembolism of antipsychotic treatment and the conditions they treat remain to be clearly defined.

In a landmark case–control study of nearly 30,000 patients,[2] an attempt was made to control for age and gender (but not for diagnosed psychiatric conditions). Risk of thromboembolism was greatly increased overall in people prescribed antipsychotics compared with controls (odds ratio (OR) 7.1). The increased risk was driven by the effect of low-potency phenothiazines (thioridazine, chlorpromazine (OR 24.1)) and was seen chiefly in the first few weeks of treatment. Absolute risk of venous thromboembolism was very small – it was seen in only 0.14% of patients. A secondary analysis suggested no association with diagnosis (not all prescribing was for schizophrenia).

A later meta-analysis of seven case-control studies[3] confirmed an increased risk of thromboembolism with low potency drugs (OR 2.91) and suggested lower but significantly increased risks with all types of antipsychotics. Later, a meta-analysis of 17 studies[4] reported a small increased risk of thromboembolism with antipsychotics as a whole (OR 1.54) and with FGAs (OR 1.74) and SGAs (OR 2.07) as individual groups. Risk of thromboembolism clearly decreased with age. The authors suggested that the best that could be said was that antipsychotics probably increased the risk by about 50% but that residual confounding could not be discounted (i.e. other factors may have accounted for the effect seen).

Since this time, several more case–control studies have confirmed both the slightly increased risk of thromboembolism and the small risk overall[5-7] – one study reported a risk for older people taking antipsychotics as 43 per 10,000 patient-years.[7] Other noteworthy findings were a substantially increased association with thromboembolism for prochlorperazine – a drug not always (or even often) prescribed for psychotic disorders,[5] and an increased risk linked to antipsychotic dosage (risk was quadrupled in high-dose patients).[6] An association with prochlorperazine prescribing had previously been suggested by a UK study.[8] These findings add weight to the theory that antipsychotic medication (and not only the conditions they treat) is responsible for the increased hazard of thromboembolism. The highest risk of pathological blood clotting may be in the first 3 months or so of treatment[9,10].

Latest data

Two meta-analyses appeared in early 2021. Their findings are presented in the following table.

Reference	Number of studies included	Relative Risk vs. no use FGAs (OR)	Relative Risk vs. no use SGAs (OR)	Relative Risk vs. no use All anti-psychotics (OR)	Comments
Di et al., 2021[9]	22	1.83 VTE/PE	1.75 VTE 3.79 PE 2.06 VTE/PE	1.53 VTE 3.69 PE 1.60 VTE/PE	Highest risk in younger patients (<60 years). Low potency FGAs highest risk
Liu et al., 2021[10]	28	1.47 VTE/PE	1.62 VTE/PE	1.55 VTE 3.68 PE 2.01 VTE/PE	New users of anti-psychotics had higher risk than continuing patients. Risk slightly elevated with higher doses vs low doses

Mechanisms

Several mechanisms have been suggested to explain the association between antipsychotics and thromboembolism. These proposed mechanisms are outlined in Table 1.33.

Table 1.33 Proposed mechanisms for antipsychotic-associated venous thromboembolism[11-13]

Sedation*
Obesity*
Hyperprolactinaemia*
Elevated phospholipid antibodies
Elevated platelet aggregation**
Elevated plasma homocysteine

*Some evidence that these factors are not the mechanism for antipsychotic-induced thromboembolism.[14]
**In vitro data suggest radically different effects on platelet aggregation for different antipsychotics.[12]

Outcomes

Increased risk of thromboembolism is reflected in numerous published reports of elevated incidence of pulmonary embolism,[15] stroke[16] and myocardial infarction.[17,18]

Summary

Antipsychotics are almost certainly associated with a small but important increased risk of venous thromboembolism and associated hazards of pulmonary embolism, stroke and myocardial infarction. Risk appears to be greatest during the early part of treatment and in younger people, and is probably dose-related.

Practice points

- Monitor closely all patients (but especially younger patients) starting antipsychotic treatment for signs of venous thromboembolism.
  - Calf pain or swelling
  - Sudden breathing difficulties
  - Signs of myocardial infarction (chest pain, nausea, etc.)
  - Signs of stroke (sudden unilateral weakness, etc.)
- Use the lowest therapeutic dose
- Encourage good hydration and physical mobility

References

1. Häfner H, et al. Thromboembolic complications in neuroleptic treatment. *Compr Psychiatry* 1965; 6:25–34.
2. Zornberg GL, et al. Antipsychotic drug use and risk of first-time idiopathic venous thromboembolism: a case-control study. *Lancet* 2000; 356:1219–1223.
3. Zhang R, et al. Antipsychotics and venous thromboembolism risk: a meta-analysis. *Pharmacopsychiatry* 2011; 44:183–188.
4. Barbui C, et al. Antipsychotic drug exposure and risk of venous thromboembolism: a systematic review and meta-analysis of observational studies. *Drug Saf* 2014; 37:79–90.
5. Ishiguro C, et al. Antipsychotic drugs and risk of idiopathic venous thromboembolism: a nested case-control study using the CPRD. *Pharmacoepidemiol Drug Saf* 2014; 23:1168–1175.
6. Wang MT, et al. Use of antipsychotics and risk of venous thromboembolism in postmenopausal women. A population-based nested case-control study. *Thromb Haemost* 2016; 115:1209–1219.
7. Letmaier M, et al. Venous thromboembolism during treatment with antipsychotics: results of a drug surveillance programme. *World J Biol Psychiatry* 2018; 19: 175–186.
8. Parker C, et al. Antipsychotic drugs and risk of venous thromboembolism: nested case-control study. *BMJ* 2010; 341:c4245.
9. Di X, et al. Antipsychotic use and risk of venous thromboembolism: a meta-analysis. *Psychiatry Res* 2021; 296:113691.
10. Liu Y, et al. Current antipsychotic agent use and risk of venous thromboembolism and pulmonary embolism: a systematic review and meta-analysis of observational studies. *Ther Adv Psychopharmacol* 2021; 11:2045125320982720.
11. Hagg S, et al. Risk of venous thromboembolism due to antipsychotic drug therapy. *Exp Opin Drug Saf* 2009; 8:537–547.
12. Dietrich-Muszalska A, et al. The first- and second-generation antipsychotic drugs affect ADP-induced platelet aggregation. *World J Biol Psychiatry* 2010; 11:268–275.
13. Tromeur C, et al. Antipsychotic drugs and venous thromboembolism. *Thromb Res* 2012; 130:S29–S31.
14. Ferraris A, et al. Antipsychotic use among adult outpatients and venous thromboembolic disease: a retrospective cohort study. *J Clin Psychopharmacol* 2017; 37:405–411.
15. Borras L, et al. Pulmonary thromboembolism associated with olanzapine and risperidone. *J Emerg Med* 2008; 35:159–161.
16. Douglas IJ, et al. Exposure to antipsychotics and risk of stroke: self controlled case series study. *BMJ* 2008; 337:a1227.
17. Brauer R, et al. Antipsychotic drugs and risks of myocardial infarction: a self-controlled case series study. *Eur Heart J* 2015; 36:984–992.
18. Huang KL, et al. Myocardial infarction risk and antipsychotics use revisited: a meta-analysis of 10 observational studies. *J Psychopharmacology* 2017; 31:1544–1555.

REFRACTORY SCHIZOPHRENIA AND CLOZAPINE

Clozapine initiation schedule

Clozapine – dosing regimen

Many of the adverse effects of clozapine are dose-dependent and associated with speed of titration. Adverse effects also tend to be more common and severe at the beginning of therapy. Standard maintenance doses may even prove fatal in clozapine-naïve subjects.[1] To minimise these problems it is important to start treatment at a low dose and to increase dosage slowly.

Clozapine should normally be started at a dose of 12.5mg once a day, at night. Blood pressure should be monitored hourly for 6 hours because of the hypotensive effect of clozapine. This monitoring is not usually necessary if the first dose is given at night. On day 2, the dose can be increased to 12.5mg twice daily. If the patient is tolerating clozapine, the dose can be increased by 25–50mg a day, until a dose of 300mg a day is reached. This can usually be achieved in 2–3 weeks. Further dosage increases should be made slowly in increments of 50–100mg each week. A plasma level of 350µg/l should be aimed to ensure an adequate trial, but response may occur at lower plasma level. The *average* (there is substantial variation) dose at which this plasma level is reached varies according to gender and smoking status. The range is approximately 250mg/day (female non-smoker) to 550mg/day (male smoker).[2] The total clozapine dose should be divided (usually twice daily) and, if sedation is a problem, the larger portion of the dose can be given at night.

Table 1.34 is a suggested starting regime for clozapine. This is a cautious regimen – more rapid increases have been used. Slower titration may be necessary where sedation or other dose-related side effects are severe, in the elderly, the very young, those who are physically compromised or those who have poorly tolerated other antipsychotics. If the patient is not tolerating a particular dose, decrease to one that was previously tolerated. If the adverse effect resolves, increase the dose again but at a slower rate.

If, for any reason, a patient misses fewer than 2 days' clozapine, restart at the dose prescribed before the event. Do not administer extra tablets to catch up. If more than 2 days are missed, restart and increase slowly (but at a faster rate than in drug-naïve patients). Please see the section on restarting clozapine.

Table 1.34 Suggested starting regime for clozapine (in-patients)

Day	Morning dose (mg)	Evening dose (mg)
1	–	12.5
2	12.5	12.5
3	25	25
4	25	25
5	25	50
6	25	50
7	50	50
8	50	75
9	75	75
10	75	100
11	100	100
12	100	125
13	125	125[a]
14	125	150
15	150	150
18	150	200[b]
21	200	200
28	200	250[c]

[a]Target dose for female non smokers (250mg/day).
[b]Target dose for male non smokers (350mg/day).
[c]Target dose for female smokers (450mg/day).

References

1. Stanworth D, Hunt NC, Flanagan RJ. Clozapine – a dangerous drug in a clozapine-naive subject. *Forensic Sci Int* 2011; **214**:e23–e5.
2. Rostami-Hodjegan A, Amin AM, Spencer EP, et al. Influence of dose, cigarette smoking, age, sex, and metabolic activity on plasma clozapine concentrations: a predictive model and nomograms to aid clozapine dose adjustment and to assess compliance in individual patients. *J Clin Psychopharmacol* 2004; **24**:70–78.

Intramuscular clozapine

Intramuscular (IM) clozapine is a short-term intervention for patients with a treatment-refractory psychotic disorder who refuse oral medication, with a view to converting to oral clozapine once treatment is established achieved.[1] Although evidence is relatively limited, recent observational data indicate that initiating treatment with IM clozapine does not adversely affect long-term adherence to oral treatment.[1,2] IM clozapine has also been found to be similar to oral clozapine with respect to short-term safety and tolerability.[3] **Importantly, the decision to prescribe IM clozapine should be undertaken on an individual basis and considered as a last resort when all other approaches have failed and only in those who are predicted to respond to clozapine treatment.[1]** This preparation is unlicensed in the UK and many other countries and so adequate precautions should be taken and patient or carer consent obtained.

General recommendations for prescribing intramuscular clozapine in adults are summarised in Table 1.35.

Table 1.35 General recommendations for prescribing IM clozapine

Strength	25mg/ml
Maximum dose*	100mg (4ml) per site
Oral equivalent dose	The oral bioavailability of clozapine is about half that of the IM injection, e.g. 50mg IM injection daily = 100mg tablets/oral solution daily
Site of administration†	The manufacturer states deep intramuscular gluteal injection
Maximum treatment length‡	Before administering each injection, the patient should be offered oral clozapine. Clozapine injection should be used for the shortest duration possible (maximum 2 weeks consecutively)
Dosing frequency	To minimise the number of injections, once daily dosing is preferred
Monitoring	After each administration, patients should be observed every 15 minutes for the first 2 hours to check for excess sedation. Routine clozapine monitoring also applies

*For doses greater than 100mg, the dose may be divided and administered into two sites.
†Case series data report administration via lateral thigh or deltoid — note the injection is painful.[2]
‡Case series data report use of intramuscular clozapine for up to 96 days.[2,3]
Note: If IM benzodiazepines are required leave at least ONE HOUR between administration of IM clozapine and IM benzodiazepines.

References

1. Casetta C, et al. A retrospective study of intramuscular clozapine prescription for treatment initiation and maintenance in treatment-resistant psychosis. *Br J Psychiatry* 2020; **217**:506–513.
2. Henry R, et al. Evaluation of the effectiveness and acceptability of intramuscular clozapine injection: illustrative case series. *B J Psych Bulletin* 2020; **44**:239–243.
3. Schulte PF, et al. Compulsory treatment with clozapine: a retrospective long-term cohort study. *Int J Law Psychiatry* 2007; **30**:539–545.

Optimising clozapine treatment

Using clozapine alone

Target dose	
(Note that dose is best adjusted according to patient tolerability and plasma level)	▪ Average dose in UK is around 450mg/day[1] ▪ Response usually seen in the range 150–900mg/day[2] ▪ Lower doses required in the elderly, females and non-smokers, and in those prescribed certain enzyme inhibitors[3,4] (see clozapine titration schedule)
Plasma levels	▪ Most studies indicate that threshold for response is in the range 350–420µg/l.[5,6] Threshold may be as high as 500µg/l[7] ▪ In male smokers who cannot achieve therapeutic plasma levels, metabolic inhibitors (fluvoxamine[8] or cimetidine[9] for example) can be co-prescribed but extreme caution is required[10] ▪ Importance of norclozapine levels not established but clozapine/norclozapine ratio may aid assessment of recent compliance

Clozapine augmentation

Clozapine 'augmentation' has become common practice because inadequate response to clozapine alone is a frequent clinical event. The evidence base supporting augmentation strategies is growing but remains insufficient to allow the development of any algorithm or schedule of treatment options. In practice, the result of clozapine augmentation is often disappointing and substantial changes in symptom severity are rarely observed. This clinical impression is supported by the equivocal results of many studies, which suggests a small effect size at best. Meta-analyses of antipsychotic augmentation suggest no effect,[11] a small effect in long term studies,[12] a very small effect overall,[13] or small effects in specific symptom domains.[14] It should be noted that few high-quality studies in this area exist – when only large, high-quality studies are included, most meta-analyses report no benefit to pharmacological augmentation.[15] Investigations into dopaminergic activity in refractory schizophrenia suggest there is no overproduction of dopamine.[16,17] Dopamine antagonists are thus unlikely to be effective.

It is recommended that all augmentation attempts are carefully monitored and, if no clear benefit is forthcoming, abandoned after 3–6 months. The addition of another drug to clozapine treatment must be expected to worsen overall adverse effect burden and so continued ineffective treatment is not appropriate. In some cases, the addition of an augmenting agent may reduce the severity of some adverse effects (e.g. weight gain, dyslipidaemia – see below) or allow a reduction in clozapine dose. The addition of aripiprazole to clozapine may be particularly effective in reversing metabolic effects.[18,19] Recently published international consensus guidelines recommend (after optimising plasma levels) tailoring augmentation agent choice to residual symptoms; adding amisulpride or aripiprazole for positive symptoms, antidepressants for negative symptoms, and mood stabilisers for suicidal ideation or aggression.[15]

Table 1.36 shows suggested treatment options (in alphabetical order) where 3–6 months of optimised clozapine alone has provided unsatisfactory benefit.

Table 1.36 Suggested options for augmenting clozapine

Option	Comment
Add amisulpride[20–25] (400–800mg/day)	▪ Some evidence and experience suggest amisulpride augmentation may be worthwhile. Three small RCTs (the largest of which showed no effect), two of which found an increased side effect burden, including cardiac side effects.[26,27] May allow clozapine dose reduction.[28]
Add aripiprazole[18,29–31] (15–30mg/day)	▪ Very limited evidence of therapeutic benefit, although a meta-analysis suggests some effect.[32] Reduces weight and LDL cholesterol.[32] Long-acting injection has been used[33,34]
Add haloperidol[31,35,36] (2–3mg/day)	▪ Modest evidence of benefit
Add lamotrigine[37–39] (25–300mg/day)	▪ May be useful in partial or non-responders. May reduce alcohol consumption.[40] Several equivocal reports;[41–43] some meta-analyses suggest moderate effect size[44] but this is largely influenced by two outlying studies[45]
Add omega-3 triglycerides[46,47] (2–3g EPA daily)	▪ Modest, and somewhat contested evidence to support efficacy in non- or partial responders to antipsychotics, including clozapine
Add risperidone[48,49] (2–6mg/day)	▪ Supported by a randomised, controlled trial but there are also two negative RCTs each with minuscule response rates[50,51] Small number of reports of increases in clozapine plasma levels. Long acting injection also an option;[34,52] paliperidone long-acting injection has also been used[34,53]
Add sulpiride[54] (400mg/day)	▪ May be useful in partial or non-responders. Supported by a single randomised trial in English and three in Chinese.[55] Overall effect modest
Add topiramate[56–60] (50–300mg/day)	▪ Two positive RCTs, two negative. Can worsen psychosis in some.[38,61] Two meta-analyses including hitherto unknown Chinese data[45,62] suggested robust effect on positive and negative symptoms, substantial weight loss but often with psychomotor slowing and attention difficulties
Add sodium valproate[45,63] (400–800mg/day)	▪ Pooled effects from five Chinese RCTs[45] suggest a benefit to positive symptoms, although studies are mostly of poor quality. Cochrane suggests benefit to adding valproate to antipsychotics in general, especially for excitement and aggression[64]
Add ziprasidone[65–68] (80–160mg/day)	▪ Supported by three RCTs.[68,69] Associated with QTc prolongation. Rarely used

Notes

▪ Always consider the use of mood stabilisers and/or antidepressants, especially where mood disturbance is thought to contribute to symptoms[70–72]

▪ Other options include adding **pimozide**, **olanzapine** or **sertindole**. None is recommended: pimozide and sertindole have important cardiac toxicity, and the addition of olanzapine is poorly supported[73] and likely to exacerbate metabolic adverse effects. Studies of pimozide[74,75] and sertindole[76] have shown no effect. One small RCT supports the use of **ginkgo biloba,**[77] another two support the use of **memantine**.[78,79] Another study suggests possible benefit of augmentation with **acetyl-L-carnitine,**[80] and a case study reports good outcome with **thyroxine.**[81] A single RCT describes successful use of **sodium benzoate**.[82] **Minocycline** is probably not effective.[63,83] **Glycine** may be effective for positive symptoms, but studies are of poor quality.[84] A small case series (n = 6) found benefit to adding **pimavanserin**.[85]

References

1. Taylor D, et al. A prescription survey of the use of atypical antipsychotics for hospital inpatients in the United Kingdom. *Int J Psychiatry Clin Pract* 2000; 4:41–46.
2. Murphy B, et al. Maintenance doses for clozapine. *Psychiatric Bull* 1998; 22:12–14.
3. Taylor D. Pharmacokinetic interactions involving clozapine. *Br J Psychiatry* 1997; 171:109–112.
4. Lane HY, et al. Effects of gender and age on plasma levels of clozapine and its metabolites: analyzed by critical statistics. *J Clin Psychiatry* 1999; 60:36–40.
5. Taylor D, et al. The use of clozapine plasma levels in optimising therapy. *Psychiatric Bull* 1995; 19:753–755.
6. Spina E, et al. Relationship between plasma concentrations of clozapine and norclozapine and therapeutic response in patients with schizophrenia resistant to conventional neuroleptics. *Psychopharmacology* 2000; 148:83–89.
7. Perry PJ. Therapeutic drug monitoring of antipsychotics. *Psychopharmacol Bull* 2001; 35:19–29.
8. Polcwiartek C, et al. The clinical potentials of adjunctive fluvoxamine to clozapine treatment: a systematic review. *Psychopharmacology* 2016; 233:741–750.
9. Watras M, et al. A therapeutic interaction between cimetidine and clozapine: case study and review of the literature. *Ther Adv Psychopharmacol* 2013; 3:294–297.
10. Gee S, et al. Optimising treatment of schizophrenia: the role of adjunctive fluvoxamine. *Psychopharmacology* 2016; 233:739–740.
11. Barbui C, et al. Does the addition of a second antipsychotic drug improve clozapine treatment? *Schizophr Bull* 2009; 35:458–468.
12. Paton C, et al. Augmentation with a second antipsychotic in patients with schizophrenia who partially respond to clozapine: a meta-analysis. *J Clin Psychopharmacol* 2007; 27:198–204.
13. Taylor D, et al. Augmentation of clozapine with a second antipsychotic. A meta analysis. *Acta Psychiatr Scand* 2012; 125:15–24.
14. Bartoli F, et al. Adjunctive second-generation antipsychotics for specific symptom domains of schizophrenia resistant to clozapine: a meta-analysis. *J Psychiatr Res* 2019; 108:24–33.
15. Wagner E, et al. Clozapine combination and augmentation strategies in patients with schizophrenia –recommendations from an international expert survey among the Treatment Response and Resistance in Psychosis (TRRIP) working group. *Schizophr Bull* 2020; 46:1459–1470.
16. Demjaha A, et al. Dopamine synthesis capacity in patients with treatment-resistant schizophrenia. *Am J Psychiatry* 2012; 169:1203–1210.
17. Demjaha A, et al. Antipsychotic treatment resistance in schizophrenia associated with elevated glutamate levels but normal dopamine function. *Biol Psychiatry* 2014; 75:e11–e13.
18. Fleischhacker WW, et al. Effects of adjunctive treatment with aripiprazole on body weight and clinical efficacy in schizophrenia patients treated with clozapine: a randomized, double-blind, placebo-controlled trial. *Int J Neuropsychopharmacol* 2010; 13:1115–1125.
19. Correll CU, et al. Selective effects of individual antipsychotic cotreatments on cardiometabolic and hormonal risk status: results from a systematic review and meta-analysis. *Schizophr Bull* 2013; 39 (Suppl 1):S29–S30.
20. Matthiasson P, et al. Relationship between dopamine D2 receptor occupancy and clinical response in amisulpride augmentation of clozapine non-response. *J Psychopharm* 2001; 15:S41.
21. Munro J, et al. Amisulpride augmentation of clozapine: an open non-randomized study in patients with schizophrenia partially responsive to clozapine. *Acta Psychiatr Scand* 2004; 110:292–298.
22. Zink M, et al. Combination of clozapine and amisulpride in treatment-resistant schizophrenia–case reports and review of the literature. *Pharmacopsychiatry* 2004; 37:26–31.
23. Ziegenbein M, et al. Augmentation of clozapine with amisulpride in patients with treatment-resistant schizophrenia: an open clinical study. *German J Psychiatry* 2006; 9:17–21.
24. Kampf P, et al. Augmentation of clozapine with amisulpride: a promising therapeutic approach to refractory schizophrenic symptoms. *Pharmacopsychiatry* 2005; 38:39–40.
25. Assion HJ, et al. Amisulpride augmentation in patients with schizophrenia partially responsive or unresponsive to clozapine. A randomized, double-blind, placebo-controlled trial. *Pharmacopsychiatry* 2008; 41:24–28.
26. Barnes TR, et al. Amisulpride augmentation in clozapine-unresponsive schizophrenia (AMICUS): a double-blind, placebo-controlled, randomised trial of clinical effectiveness and cost-effectiveness. *Health Technol Assess* 2017; 21:1–56.
27. Barnes TRE, et al. Amisulpride augmentation of clozapine for treatment-refractory schizophrenia: a double-blind, placebo-controlled trial. *Ther Adv Psychopharmacol* 2018; 8:185–197.
28. Croissant B, et al. Reduction of side effects by combining clozapine with amisulpride: case report and short review of clozapine-induced hypersalivation-a case report. *Pharmacopsychiatry* 2005; 38:38–39.
29. Chang JS, et al. Aripiprazole augmentation in clozapine-treated patients with refractory schizophrenia: an 8-week, randomized, double-blind, placebo-controlled trial. *J Clin Psychiatry* 2008; 69:720–731.
30. Muscatello MR, et al. Effect of aripiprazole augmentation of clozapine in schizophrenia: a double-blind, placebo-controlled study. *Schizophr Res* 2011; 127:93–99.
31. Cipriani A, et al. Aripiprazole versus haloperidol in combination with clozapine for treatment-resistant schizophrenia: a 12-month, randomized, naturalistic trial. *J Clin Psychopharmacol* 2013; 33:533–537.
32. Srisurapanont M, et al. Efficacy and safety of aripiprazole augmentation of clozapine in schizophrenia: a systematic review and meta-analysis of randomized-controlled trials. *J Psychiatr Res* 2015; 62:38–47.
33. Balcioglu YH, et al. One plus one sometimes equals more than two: long-acting injectable aripiprazole adjunction in clozapine-resistant schizophrenia. *Clin Neuropharmacol* 2020; 43:166–168.
34. Grimminck R, et al. Combination of clozapine with long-acting injectable antipsychotics in treatment-resistant schizophrenia: preliminary evidence from health care utilization indices. *Prim Care Companion CNS Disord* 2020; 22:19m02560.
35. Rajarethinam R, et al. Augmentation of clozapine partial responders with conventional antipsychotics. *Schizophr Res* 2003; 60:97–98.

36. Barbui C, et al. Aripiprazole versus haloperidol in combination with clozapine for treatment-resistant schizophrenia in routine clinical care: a randomized, controlled trial. *J Clin Psychopharmacol* 2011; **31**:266–273.

37. Dursun SM, et al. Clozapine plus lamotrigine in treatment-resistant schizophrenia. *Arch Gen Psychiatry* 1999; **56**:950.

38. Dursun SM, et al. Augmenting antipsychotic treatment with lamotrigine or topiramate in patients with treatment-resistant schizophrenia: a naturalistic case-series outcome study. *J Psychopharm* 2001; **15**:297–301.

39. Tiihonen J, et al. Lamotrigine in treatment-resistant schizophrenia: a randomized placebo-controlled crossover trial. *Biol Psychiatry* 2003; **54**:1241–1248.

40. Kalyoncu A, et al. Use of lamotrigine to augment clozapine in patients with resistant schizophrenia and comorbid alcohol dependence: a potent anti-craving effect? *J Psychopharmacology* 2005; **19**:301–305.

41. Goff DC, et al. Lamotrigine as add-on therapy in schizophrenia: results of 2 placebo-controlled trials. *J Clin Psychopharmacol* 2007; **27**:582–589.

42. Heck AH, et al. Addition of lamotrigine to clozapine in inpatients with chronic psychosis. *J Clin Psychiatry* 2005; **66**:1333.

43. Vayisoglu S, et al. Lamotrigine augmentation in patients with schizophrenia who show partial response to clozapine treatment. *Schizophr Res* 2013; **143**:207–214.

44. Tiihonen J, et al. The efficacy of lamotrigine in clozapine-resistant schizophrenia: a systematic review and meta-analysis. *Schizophr Res* 2009; **109**:10–14.

45. Zheng W, et al. Clozapine augmentation with antiepileptic drugs for treatment-resistant schizophrenia: a meta-analysis of randomized controlled trials. *J Clin Psychiatry* 2017; **78**:e498–e505.

46. Peet M, et al. Double-blind placebo controlled trial of N-3 polyunsaturated fatty acids as an adjunct to neuroleptics. *Schizophr Res* 1998; **29**:160–161.

47. Puri BK, et al. Sustained remission of positive and negative symptoms of schizophrenia following treatment with eicosapentaenoic acid. *Arch Gen Psychiatry* 1998; **55**:188–189.

48. Josiassen RC, et al. Clozapine augmented with risperidone in the treatment of schizophrenia: a randomized, double-blind, placebo-controlled trial. *Am J Psychiatry* 2005; **162**:130–136.

49. Raskin S, et al. Clozapine and risperidone: combination/augmentation treatment of refractory schizophrenia: a preliminary observation. *Acta Psychiatr Scand* 2000; **101**:334–336.

50. Anil Yagcioglu AE, et al. A double-blind controlled study of adjunctive treatment with risperidone in schizophrenic patients partially responsive to clozapine: efficacy and safety. *J Clin Psychiatry* 2005; **66**:63–72.

51. Honer WG, et al. Clozapine alone versus clozapine and risperidone with refractory schizophrenia. *N Engl J Med* 2006; **354**:472–482.

52. Se HK, et al. The combined use of risperidone long-acting injection and clozapine in patients with schizophrenia non-adherent to clozapine: a case series. *J Psychopharmacology* 2010; **24**:981–986.

53. Bioque M, et al. Clozapine and paliperidone palmitate antipsychotic combination in treatment-resistant schizophrenia and other psychotic disorders: a retrospective 6-month mirror-image study. *Eur Psychiatry* 2020; **63**:e71.

54. Shiloh R, et al. Sulpiride augmentation in people with schizophrenia partially responsive to clozapine. A double-blind, placebo-controlled study. *Br J Psychiatry* 1997; **171**:569–573.

55. Wang J, et al. Sulpiride augmentation for schizophrenia. *Schizophr Bull* 2010; **36**:229–230.

56. Tiihonen J, et al. Topiramate add-on in treatment-resistant schizophrenia: a randomized, double-blind, placebo-controlled, crossover trial. *J Clin Psychiatry* 2005; **66**:1012–1015.

57. Afshar H, et al. Topiramate add-on treatment in schizophrenia: a randomised, double-blind, placebo-controlled clinical trial. *J Psychopharmacology* 2009; **23**:157–162.

58. Muscatello MR, et al. Topiramate augmentation of clozapine in schizophrenia: a double-blind, placebo-controlled study. *J Psychopharmacology* 2011; **25**:667–674.

59. Hahn MK, et al. Topiramate augmentation in clozapine-treated patients with schizophrenia: clinical and metabolic effects. *J Clin Psychopharmacol* 2010; **30**:706–710.

60. Behdani F, et al. Effect of topiramate augmentation in chronic schizophrenia: a placebo-controlled trial. *Arch Iran Med* 2011; **14**:270–275.

61. Millson RC, et al. Topiramate for refractory schizophrenia. *Am J Psychiatry* 2002; **159**:675.

62. Zheng W, et al. Efficacy and safety of adjunctive topiramate for schizophrenia: a meta-analysis of randomized controlled trials. *Acta Psychiatr Scand* 2016; **134**:385–398.

63. Siskind DJ, et al. Augmentation strategies for clozapine refractory schizophrenia: a systematic review and meta-analysis. *Aust N Z J Psychiatry* 2018; **52**:751–767.

64. Wang Y, et al. Valproate for schizophrenia. *Cochrane Database Syst Rev* 2016; **11**:Cd004028.

65. Zink M, et al. Combination of ziprasidone and clozapine in treatment-resistant schizophrenia. *Human Psychopharmacology* 2004; **19**:271–273.

66. Ziegenbein M, et al. Clozapine and ziprasidone: a useful combination in patients with treatment-resistant schizophrenia. *J Neuropsychiatry Clin Neurosci* 2006; **18**:246–247.

67. Ziegenbein M, et al. Combination of clozapine and ziprasidone in treatment-resistant schizophrenia: an open clinical study. *Clin Neuropharmacol* 2006; **28**:220–224.

68. Zink M, et al. Efficacy and tolerability of ziprasidone versus risperidone as augmentation in patients partially responsive to clozapine: a randomised controlled clinical trial. *J Psychopharm* 2009; **23**:305–314.

69. Muscatello MR, et al. Augmentation of clozapine with ziprasidone in refractory schizophrenia: a double-blind, placebo-controlled study. *J Clin Psychopharmacol* 2014; **34**:129–133.

70. Citrome L. Schizophrenia and valproate. *Psychopharmacol Bull* 2003; **37 Suppl 2**:74–88.

71. Tranulis C, et al. Somatic augmentation strategies in clozapine resistance–what facts? *Clin Neuropharmacol* 2006; **29**:34–44.

72. Suzuki T, et al. Augmentation of atypical antipsychotics with valproic acid. An open-label study for most difficult patients with schizophrenia. *Human Psychopharmacology* 2009; **24**:628–638.

73. Gupta S, et al. Olanzapine augmentation of clozapine. *Ann Clin Psychiatry* 1998; **10**:113–115.

74. Friedman JI, et al. Pimozide augmentation of clozapine inpatients with schizophrenia and schizoaffective disorder unresponsive to clozapine monotherapy. *Neuropsychopharmacology* 2011; **36**:1289–1295.

75. Gunduz-Bruce H, et al. Efficacy of pimozide augmentation for clozapine partial responders with schizophrenia. *Schizophr Res* 2013; **143**:344–347.

76. Nielsen J, et al. Augmenting clozapine with sertindole: a double-blind, randomized, placebo-controlled study. *J Clin Psychopharmacol* 2012; **32**:173–178.

77. Doruk A, et al. A placebo-controlled study of extract of ginkgo biloba added to clozapine in patients with treatment-resistant schizophrenia. *Int Clin Psychopharmacol* 2008; **23**:223–227.

78. De Lucena D, et al. Improvement of negative and positive symptoms in treatment-refractory schizophrenia: a double-blind, randomized, placebo-controlled trial with memantine as add-on therapy to clozapine. *J Clin Psychiatry* 2009; **70**:1416–1423.

79. Veerman SR, et al. Adjunctive memantine in clozapine-treated refractory schizophrenia: an open-label 1-year extension study. *Psychol Med* 2017; **47**:363–375.

80. Bruno A, et al. Acetyl-L-carnitine augmentation of clozapine in partial-responder schizophrenia: a 12-week, open-label uncontrolled preliminary study. *Clin Neuropharmacol* 2016; **39**:277–280.

81. Seddigh R, et al. Levothyroxine augmentation in clozapine resistant schizophrenia: a case report and review. *Case Rep Psychiatry* 2015; **2015**:678040.

82. Lin CH, et al. Sodium benzoate, a D-Amino acid oxidase inhibitor, added to clozapine for the treatment of schizophrenia: a randomized, double-blind, placebo-controlled trial. *Biol Psychiatry* 2018; **84**:422–432.

83. Kelly DL, et al. Adjunctive minocycline in clozapine-treated schizophrenia patients with persistent symptoms. *J Clin Psychopharmacol* 2015; **35**:374–381.

84. Correll CU, et al. Efficacy of 42 pharmacologic cotreatment strategies added to antipsychotic monotherapy in schizophrenia: systematic overview and quality appraisal of the meta-analytic evidence. *JAMA Psychiatry* 2017; **74**:675–684.

85. Nasrallah HA, et al. Successful treatment of clozapine-nonresponsive refractory hallucinations and delusions with pimavanserin, a serotonin 5HT-2A receptor inverse agonist. *Schizophr Res* 2019; **208**:217–220.

Alternatives to clozapine

Clozapine has the strongest evidence for efficacy for schizophrenia that has proved refractory to adequate trials of standard antipsychotic medication. Where treatment resistance has been established, clozapine treatment should not be delayed or withheld.[1,2] The practice of using successive antipsychotic medications (or the latest) instead of clozapine is widespread but not supported by research. Where clozapine cannot be used (because of toxicity or patient refusal to take the medication or comply with the mandatory monitoring tests), other drugs or drug combinations may be tried (see Table 1.37) but, in practice, outcome is usually disappointing. Long-term data on efficacy and safety/tolerability are generally lacking.

The data that are available do not allow any distinction between treatment regimens to be drawn, particularly choice of antipsychotic medication,[3,4] but it seems wise to use single drugs before trying multiple drug options. Olanzapine is perhaps most often used as antipsychotic monotherapy, usually in dosage above the licensed range. If this fails, then the addition of a second antipsychotic (amisulpride, for example) is a possible next step, although the risk-benefit balance of combined antipsychotic medication regimens remains unclear.[5] A study of antipsychotic drug treatment after clozapine broadly confirms these findings, supporting clozapine reintroduction and olanzapine as the most effective and safest treatment options in those discontinuing clozapine for undefined reasons.[6] Amongst unconventional agents, minocycline and ondansetron have the advantage of low toxicity and good tolerability. A depot/LAI antipsychotic preparation is an option where the avoidance of covert non-adherence is a clinical priority.

Many of the treatments listed below are somewhat experimental and some of the compounds difficult to obtain (e.g. glycine, D-serine, sarcosine, etc.). Before using any of the regimens outlined, readers should consult the primary literature cited. Particular care should be taken to inform patients where prescribing is off-label and to ensure that they understand the potential adverse effects of the more experimental treatments.

Non-clozapine treatment of refractory schizophrenia is an area of active research. Glutamatergic drugs may hold promise (although bitopertin is inactive[7]) as may $5HT_{2A}$ inverse agonists.[8]

Table 1.37 Alternatives to clozapine

Treatment	Comments
Allopurinol 300–600mg/day **(+ antipsychotic)**[9–12]	Increases adenosinergic transmission which may reduce effects of dopamine. Three positive RCTs[9,10,12]
Amisulpride[13] (up to 1200mg/day)	Single, small open study
Antipsychotic polypharmacy	Various antipsychotics in combination have been used. Data are limited, mainly in the form of case reports, open and naturalistic studies
Aripiprazole[14,15] (15–30mg/day)	Single randomized controlled study indicating moderate effect in patients resistant to risperidone or olanzapine (+ others). Higher doses (60mg/day) have been used[16]
Asenapine (+ antipsychotic)[17]	Two case reports

Table 1.37 (*Continued*)

Treatment	Comments
Bexarotene 75mg/day[18] **(+ antipsychotic)**	Retinoid receptor agonist. One RCT (n = 90) in non-refractory but suboptimally treated patients suggest worthwhile effect on positive symptoms
Blonanserin (+ antipsychotic)[19]	Atypical antipsychotic licensed in Japan and Korea. One case series found it to be effective and well tolerated
CBT[20]	Non-drug therapies should always be considered
Celecoxib + risperidone[21] (400mg + 6mg/day)	COX-2 inhibitors modulate immune response and may prevent glutamate-related cell death. One RCT showed useful activity in all main symptom domains. Associated with increased CV mortality
Deep Brain Stimulation (DBS)	Effectiveness of nucleus accumbens (NAcc) and subgenual anterior cingulate cortex (subgenual ACC) targeted DBS demonstrated in 4 of 7 patients with TRS[22]
Donepezil 5–10mg/day **(+ antipsychotic)**[23–25]	Three RCTs, one negative,[24] two positive,[23,25] suggesting a small effect on cognitive and negative symptoms
D-Alanine 100mg/kg/day **(+ antipsychotic)**[26]	Glycine (NMDA) agonist. One positive RCT
D-Serine 30mg/kg/day **(+ olanzapine)**[27]	Glycine (NMDA) agonist. One positive RCT
D-serine up to 3g as monotherapy[28]	Improved negative symptoms in one RCT, but inferior to high dose olanzapine for treatment of positive symptoms
ECT[29]	Open studies suggest moderate effect, as does a retrospective study.[30] Often reserved for last-line treatment in practice but can be successful in the short[31] and long[32] term
Estradiol 100 – 200mcg transdermal/day (+ antipsychotic)[33]	Oestrogens may be psychoprotective and/or antipsychotic. RCT (n = 183) in women of child-bearing age suggested benefits on positive symptoms, especially at higher doses. Note contra-indications include being post-menopausal, history of VTE, stroke, breast cancer, migraine with aura. Unopposed estradiol over long periods increases the risk of endometrial hyperplasia and malignancy – consider consulting an endocrinologist. Evidence in men is lacking
Famotidine 100mg bd + antipsychotic[34]	H_2 antagonist. One short (4 weeks) RCT suggested some benefit in overall PANSS and CGI scores
Ginkgo biloba **(+ antipsychotic)**[6,7]	Possibly effective in combination with haloperidol. Unlikely to give rise to additional adverse effects but clinical experience limited
Lurasidone up to 240mg/day[35] (+ vortioxetine)	One RCT comparing standard with high dose lurasidone produced comparable improvements in TRS when given up to 24 weeks.[36] Appears to be well tolerated, may be effective but no clozapine comparison arm included. The addition of vortioxetine to lurasidone was effective in a small case series[37]
Memantine 20mg/day **(+ antipsychotic)**[38–40]	Memantine is an NMDA antagonist. Two RCTs. The larger of the two (n = 138) was negative. In the smaller (n = 21), memantine improved positive and negative symptoms when added to clozapine. In another study in non-refractory schizophrenia, memantine improved negative symptoms when added to risperidone

(*Continued*)

Table 1.37 (*Continued*)

Treatment	Comments
Mianserin + FGA 30mg/day[32]	5HT$_2$ antagonist. One, small positive RCT
Minocycline 200mg/day **(+ antipsychotic)**[41,42]	May be anti-inflammatory and neuroprotective. One open study (*n* = 22) and one RCT (*n* = 54) suggest good effect on negative and cognitive symptoms. Also one RCT (*n* = 50) of augmentation of clozapine.[43] RCT evidence of neuroprotective effect in early psychosis[44]
Mirtazapine 30mg/day **(+ antipsychotic)**[45–47]	5HT$_2$ antagonist. Two RCTs, one negative,[46] one positive.[45] Effect seems to be mainly on positive symptoms
N-acetylcysteine 2g/day **(+ antipsychotic)**[40]	One RCT suggests small benefits in negative symptoms and rates of akathisia. Another RCT showed benefits in chronic schizophrenia.[48] Case study of successful use of 600mg a day.[49] Large RCT in progress[50]
Olanzapine[51–56] 5–25mg/day	Supported by some well-conducted trials but clinical experience disappointing. Some patients show moderate response
Olanzapine[57–63] 30–60mg/day	Contradictory findings in the literature but possibly effective. High dose olanzapine is not atypical[64] and can be poorly tolerated[65] with gross metabolic changes[63]
Olanzapine + amisulpride[66] (up to 800mg/day)	Small open study suggests benefit
Olanzapine + aripiprazole[67]	Single case report suggests benefit. Probably reduces metabolic toxicity
Olanzapine + glycine[68] (0.8g/kg/day)	Small, double-blind crossover trial suggests clinically relevant improvement in negative symptoms
Olanzapine + lamotrigine[65,69] (up to 400mg/day)	Reports contradictory and rather unconvincing. Reasonable theoretical basis for adding lamotrigine which is usually well tolerated
Olanzapine + risperidone[70] (various doses)	Small study suggests some patients may benefit from combined therapy after sequential failure of each drug alone
Olanzapine + sulpiride[71] (600mg/day)	Some evidence that this combination improves mood symptoms
Omega-3-triglycerides[72,73]	Suggested efficacy but data very limited
Ondansetron 8mg/day **(+ antipsychotic)**	A systematic review of RCTs showed improvements in negative symptoms and general psychopathology. Effect on cognition inconclusive[74]
Paliperidone LAI	Improvement in endocrine and hepatic parameters and lower antipsychotic exposure in a small number of patients switched from clozapine to paliperidone 3 monthly. No data on clinical outcomes[75]

Table 1.37 (Continued)

Treatment	Comments
Pimavanserin (+ antipsychotics)	Clinical improvement with pimavanserin alone or as adjunct to clozapine or other antipsychotics in 10 patients, six of whom had failed to respond to clozapine[76]
Propentofylline + risperidone[77] (900mg + 6mg/day)	One RCT suggests some activity against positive symptoms
Quetiapine[78-81]	Very limited evidence and clinical experience not encouraging. High doses (>1200mg/day) have been used but are no more effective[82]
Quetiapine + amisulpride[83]	Single naturalistic observation of 19 patients suggested useful benefit. Doses averaged 700mg quetiapine and 950mg amisulpride
Quetiapine + haloperidol[84]	Two case reports
Raloxifene 60–120mg/day (+ antipsychotic)[85]	Selective oestrogen receptor modulator; may offer benefits of estradiol without long-term risks. One case report[85] in postmenopausal treatment-resistant schizophrenia. Data in non-treatment resistance are rather conflicting, with two overlapping positive trials[86,87] and one negative trial.[88] One positive RCT in refractory women.[89] Evidence in men is lacking
Riluzole 100mg/day **+ risperidone** up to 6mg/day[90]	Glutamate modulating agent. One RCT demonstrated improvement in negative symptoms
Risperidone[91-93] 4–8mg/day	Doubtful efficacy in true treatment-refractory schizophrenia but some supporting evidence. May also be tried in combination with glycine[68] or lamotrigine[60] or indeed with other atypicals[94]
Risperidone LAI 50/100mg 2/52[95]	One RCT showing good response for both doses in refractory schizophrenia. Plasma levels for 100mg dose similar to 6–8mg/day oral risperidone.
Ritanserin + risperidone (12mg + 6mg/day)[96]	$5HT_{2A/2C}$ antagonist. One RCT suggests small effect on negative symptoms
Sarcosine (2g/day)[97,98] **(+ antipsychotic)**	Enhances glycine action. Supported by two RCTs
Sertindole[99] (12–24mg/day)	One large RCT (conducted in 1996–8 but published in 2011) suggested good effect and equivalence to risperidone. Around half of subjects responded. Another RCT[100] showed no effect at all when added to clozapine. Little experience in practice
Topiramate (300mg/day) **(+ antipsychotic)**[101]	Small effect shown in single RCT. Induces weight loss. Cognitive adverse effects likely
Transcranial magnetic stimulation[102-104]	Conflicting results
Ursodeoxycholic acid[105]	Single case report
Valproate[106]	Doubtful effect but may be useful where there is a clear affective component
Yokukansan (+ antipsychotic)[107]	Japanese herbal medicine, partial agonist at D_2 and $5HT_{1A}$, antagonist at $5HT_{2A}$ and glutamate receptors. Potential small benefit in excitement/hostility symptoms.

(Continued)

Table 1.37 (Continued)

Treatment	Comments
Zotepine 300mg/day[108]	One study showed that some patients do not deteriorate when switched from clozapine.
Ziprasidone 80–160mg/day[109–111]	Two good RCTs. One[111] suggests superior efficacy to chlorpromazine in refractory schizophrenia; the other[109] suggests equivalence to clozapine in subjects with treatment intolerance/resistance. Disappointing results in practice, however. Supratherapeutic doses offer no advantage.[112]

Note: Treatments are listed in alphabetical order: no preference is implied by position in table.

Refractory schizophrenia – alternatives to clozapine: summary

Treatment	Examples	Comments	Strength of evidence
Monotherapy using non-clozapine antipsychotics in standard or high doses	Aripiprazole 15–30mg daily Olanzapine 25–40mg daily	Evidence of efficacy for any antipsychotic other than clozapine in refractory schizophrenia is sparse. Some data suggest efficacy for olanzapine above licensed doses but at the risk of metabolic adverse effects	Very weak ±
Non-clozapine antipsychotic polypharmacy	Amisulpride + olanzapine Quetiapine + amisulpride Aripiprazole + olanzapine	Polypharmacy is common in clinical practice. Evidence from controlled studies limited but open studies and real-world data suggest some effectiveness. Burden of adverse effects is increased	Weak +
Anti-inflammatory agents as adjuncts to antipsychotics	N-acetylcysteine, NSAIDs minocycline, oestrogens, aspirin, omega-3 fatty acids	A heterogeneous group of medicinal agents with inflammatory properties have been tried as adjuncts. Possible benefits in negative and cognitive symptoms but sample sizes have been small	Very weak ±
NMDA receptor modulators as adjuncts	Memantine, glycine, D-serine and sarcosine	Rarely used in clinical practice. May have some benefit in negative symptoms	Very weak ±
Physical treatments	ECT, rTMS, tDCS, DBS	Best evidence for ECT as adjunct to clozapine. Others still largely experimental	Modest ++
Adjunctive antidepressants	Mirtazapine, vortioxetine, SSRIs	Limited data available suggests small benefits in negative and cognitive symptoms	Weak +
Adjunctive antiseizure medications	Lamotrigine, topiramate sodium valproate, carbamazepine	Data difficult to interpret including clozapine and non-clozapine antipsychotics. Modest benefits at best	Weak +
Psychological therapies	CBT	Conflicting findings, effects small	Very weak ±

References

1. Yoshimura B, et al. The critical treatment window of clozapine in treatment-resistant schizophrenia: secondary analysis of an observational study. *Psychiatry Res* 2017; 250:65–70.

2. Howes OD, et al. Adherence to treatment guidelines in clinical practice: study of antipsychotic treatment prior to clozapine initiation. *BrJPsychiatry* 2012; 201:481–485.

3. Molins C, et al. Response to antipsychotic drugs in treatment-resistant schizophrenia: conclusions based on systematic review. *Schizophr Res* 2016; 178:64–67.

4. Samara MT, et al. Efficacy, acceptability, and tolerability of antipsychotics in treatment-resistant schizophrenia: a network meta-analysis. *JAMA Psychiatry* 2016; 73:199–210.

5. Galling B, et al. Antipsychotic augmentation vs. monotherapy in schizophrenia: systematic review, meta-analysis and meta-regression analysis. *World Psychiatry* 2017; 16:77–89.

6. Luykx JJ, et al. In the aftermath of clozapine discontinuation: comparative effectiveness and safety of antipsychotics in patients with schizophrenia who discontinue clozapine. *Br J Psychiatry* 2020; 217:498–505.

7. Bugarski-Kirola D, et al. Efficacy and safety of adjunctive bitopertin versus placebo in patients with suboptimally controlled symptoms of schizophrenia treated with antipsychotics: results from three phase 3, randomised, double-blind, parallel-group, placebo-controlled, multi-centre studies in the SearchLyte clinical trial programme. *Lancet Psychiatry* 2016; 3:1115–1128.

8. Garay RP, et al. Potential serotonergic agents for the treatment of schizophrenia. *Exp Opin Invest Drugs* 2016; 25:159–170.

9. Akhondzadeh S, et al. Beneficial antipsychotic effects of allopurinol as add-on therapy for schizophrenia: a double blind, randomized and placebo controlled trial. *Prog Neuropsychopharmacol Biol Psychiatry* 2005; 29:253–259.

10. Brunstein MG, et al. A clinical trial of adjuvant allopurinol therapy for moderately refractory schizophrenia. *J Clin Psychiatry* 2005; 66:213–219.

11. Buie LW, et al. Allopurinol as adjuvant therapy in poorly responsive or treatment refractory schizophrenia. *Ann Pharmacother* 2006; 40:2200–2204.

12. Dickerson FB, et al. A double-blind trial of adjunctive allopurinol for schizophrenia. *Schizophr Res* 2009; 109:66–69.

13. Kontaxakis VP, et al. Switching to amisulpride monotherapy for treatment-resistant schizophrenia. *Eur Psychiatry* 2006; 21:214–217.

14. Kane JM, et al. Aripiprazole for treatment-resistant schizophrenia: results of a multicenter, randomized, double-blind, comparison study versus perphenazine. *J Clin Psychiatry* 2007; 68:213–223.

15. Hsu WY, et al. Aripiprazole in treatment-refractory schizophrenia. *J Psychiatr Pract* 2009; 15:221–226.

16. Crossman AM, et al. Tolerability of high-dose aripiprazole in treatment-refractory schizophrenic patients. *J Clin Psychiatry* 2006; 67:1158–1159.

17. Smith EN, et al. Asenapine augmentation and treatment-resistant schizophrenia in the high-secure hospital setting. *Ther Adv Psychopharmacol* 2014; 4:193–197.

18. Lerner V, et al. The retinoid X receptor agonist bexarotene relieves positive symptoms of schizophrenia: a 6-week, randomized, double-blind, placebo-controlled multicenter trial. *J Clin Psychiatry* 2013; 74:1224–1232.

19. Tachibana M, et al. Effectiveness of blonanserin for patients with drug treatment-resistant schizophrenia and dopamine supersensitivity: a retrospective analysis. *Asian J Psychiatr* 2016; 24:28–32.

20. Valmaggia LR, et al. Cognitive-behavioural therapy for refractory psychotic symptoms of schizophrenia resistant to atypical antipsychotic medication. Randomised controlled trial. *Br J Psychiatry* 2005; 186:324–330.

21. Akhondzadeh S, et al. Celecoxib as adjunctive therapy in schizophrenia: a double-blind, randomized and placebo-controlled trial. *Schizophr Res* 2007; 90:179–185.

22. Corripio I, et al. Deep brain stimulation in treatment resistant schizophrenia: a pilot randomized cross-over clinical trial. *EBioMedicine* 2020; 51:102568.

23. Lee BJ, et al. A 12-week, double-blind, placebo-controlled trial of donepezil as an adjunct to haloperidol for treating cognitive impairments in patients with chronic schizophrenia. *J Psychopharmacology* 2007; 21:421–427.

24. Keefe RSE, et al. Efficacy and safety of donepezil in patients with schizophrenia or schizoaffective disorder: significant placebo/practice effects in a 12-week, randomized, double-blind, placebo-controlled trial. *Neuropsychopharmacology* 2007; 33:1217–1228.

25. Akhondzadeh S, et al. A 12-week, double-blind, placebo-controlled trial of donepezil adjunctive treatment to risperidone in chronic and stable schizophrenia. *Prog Neuropsychopharmacol Biol Psychiatry* 2008; 32:1810–1815.

26. Tsai GE, et al. D-alanine added to antipsychotics for the treatment of schizophrenia. *Biol Psychiatry* 2006; 59:230–234.

27. Heresco-Levy U, et al. D-serine efficacy as add-on pharmacotherapy to risperidone and olanzapine for treatment-refractory schizophrenia. *Biol Psychiatry* 2005; 57:577–585.

28. Ermilov M, et al. A pilot double-blind comparison of d-serine and high-dose olanzapine in treatment-resistant patients with schizophrenia. *Schizophr Res* 2013; 150:604–605.

29. Zheng W, et al. Electroconvulsive therapy added to non-clozapine antipsychotic medication for treatment resistant schizophrenia: meta-analysis of randomized controlled trials. *PLoS One* 2016; 11:e0156510.

30. Grover S, et al. Effectiveness of electroconvulsive therapy in patients with treatment resistant schizophrenia: a retrospective study. *Psychiatry Res* 2017; 249:349–353.

31. Chanpattana W, et al. Electroconvulsive therapy in treatment-resistant schizophrenia: prediction of response and the nature of symptomatic improvement. *J Ect* 2010; 26:289–298.

32. Ravanic DB, et al. Long-term efficacy of electroconvulsive therapy combined with different antipsychotic drugs in previously resistant schizophrenia. *Psychiatr Danub* 2009; 21:179–186.

33. Kulkarni J, et al. Estradiol for treatment-resistant schizophrenia: a large-scale randomized-controlled trial in women of child-bearing age. *Mol Psychiatry* 2015; 20:695–702.

34. Meskanen K, et al. A randomized clinical trial of histamine 2 receptor antagonism in treatment-resistant schizophrenia. *J Clin Psychopharmacol* 2013; 33:472–478.

35. Meltzer H, et al. W162 – lurasidone is an effective treatment for treatment resistant schizophrenia. *Neuropsychopharmacology* 2015; 40 (Suppl 1):S546.

36. Meltzer HY, et al. Lurasidone improves psychopathology and cognition in treatment-resistant schizophrenia. *J Clin Psychopharmacol* 2020; 40:240–249.

37. Lowe P, et al. When the drugs don't work: treatment-resistant schizophrenia, serotonin and serendipity. *Ther Adv Psychopharmacol* 2018; 8:63–70.

38. Lieberman JA, et al. A randomized, placebo-controlled study of memantine as adjunctive treatment in patients with schizophrenia. *Neuropsychopharmacology* 2009; 34:1322–1329.

39. De Lucena D, et al. Improvement of negative and positive symptoms in treatment-refractory schizophrenia: a double-blind, randomized, placebo-controlled trial with memantine as add-on therapy to clozapine. *J Clin Psychiatry* 2009; 70:1416–1423.

40. Rezaei F, et al. Memantine add-on to risperidone for treatment of negative symptoms in patients with stable schizophrenia: randomized, double-blind, placebo-controlled study. *J Clin Psychopharmacol* 2013; 33:336–342.

41. Levkovitz Y, et al. A double-blind, randomized study of minocycline for the treatment of negative and cognitive symptoms in early-phase schizophrenia. *J Clin Psychiatry* 2010; 71:138–149.

42. Miyaoka T, et al. Minocycline as adjunctive therapy for schizophrenia: an open-label study. *Clin Neuropharmacol* 2008; 31:287–292.

43. Kelly DL, et al. Adjunctive minocycline in clozapine-treated schizophrenia patients with persistent symptoms. *J Clin Psychopharmacol* 2015; 35:374–381.

44. Chaudhry IB, et al. Minocycline benefits negative symptoms in early schizophrenia: a randomised double-blind placebo-controlled clinical trial in patients on standard treatment. *J Psychopharmacol* 2012; 26:1185–1193.

45. Joffe G, et al. Add-on mirtazapine enhances antipsychotic effect of first generation antipsychotics in schizophrenia: a double-blind, randomized, placebo-controlled trial. *Schizophr Res* 2009; 108:245–251.

46. Berk M, et al. Mirtazapine add-on therapy in the treatment of schizophrenia with atypical antipsychotics: a double-blind, randomised, placebo-controlled clinical trial. *Human Psychopharmacology* 2009; 24:233–238.

47. Delle CR, et al. Add-on mirtazapine enhances effects on cognition in schizophrenic patients under stabilized treatment with clozapine. *Exp Clin Psychopharmacol* 2007; 15:563–568.

48. Sepehrmanesh Z, et al. Therapeutic effect of adjunctive N-acetyl cysteine (NAC) on symptoms of chronic schizophrenia: a double-blind, randomized clinical trial. *Prog Neuropsychopharmacol Biol Psychiatry* 2018; 82:289–296.

49. Bulut M, et al. Beneficial effects of N-acetylcysteine in treatment resistant schizophrenia. *World J Biol Psychiatry* 2009; 10:626–628.

50. Rossell SL, et al. N-acetylcysteine (NAC) in schizophrenia resistant to clozapine: a double blind randomised placebo controlled trial targeting negative symptoms. *BMC Psychiatry* 2016; 16:320.

51. Breier A, et al. Comparative efficacy of olanzapine and haloperidol for patients with treatment-resistant schizophrenia. *Biol Psychiatry* 1999; 45:403–411.

52. Conley RR, et al. Olanzapine compared with chlorpromazine in treatment-resistant schizophrenia. *Am J Psychiatry* 1998; 155:914–920.

53. Sanders RD, et al. An open trial of olanzapine in patients with treatment-refractory psychoses. *J Clin Psychopharmacol* 1999; 19:62–66.

54. Taylor D, et al. Olanzapine in practice: a prospective naturalistic study. *Psychiatric Bull* 1999; 23:178–180.

55. Bitter I, et al. Olanzapine versus clozapine in treatment-resistant or treatment-intolerant schizophrenia. *Prog Neuropsychopharmacol Biol Psychiatry* 2004; 28:173–180.

56. Tollefson GD, et al. Double-blind comparison of olanzapine versus clozapine in schizophrenic patients clinically eligible for treatment with clozapine. *Biol Psychiatry* 2001; 49:52–63.

57. Sheitman BB, et al. High-dose olanzapine for treatment-refractory schizophrenia. *Am J Psychiatry* 1997; 154:1626.

58. Fanous A, et al. Schizophrenia and schizoaffective disorder treated with high doses of olanzapine. *J Clin Psychopharmacol* 1999; 19:275–276.

59. Dursun SM, et al. Olanzapine for patients with treatment-resistant schizophrenia: a naturalistic case-series outcome study. *Can J Psychiatry* 1999; 44:701–704.

60. Conley RR, et al. The efficacy of high-dose olanzapine versus clozapine in treatment-resistant schizophrenia: a double-blind crossover study. *J Clin Psychopharmacol* 2003; 23:668–671.

61. Kumra S, et al. Clozapine and 'high-dose' olanzapine in refractory early-onset schizophrenia: a 12-week randomized and double-blind comparison. *Biol Psychiatry* 2008; 63:524–529.

62. Kumra S, et al. Clozapine versus 'high-dose' olanzapine in refractory early-onset schizophrenia: an open-label extension study. *J Child Adolesc Psychopharmacol* 2008; 18:307–316.

63. Meltzer HY, et al. A randomized, double-blind comparison of clozapine and high-dose olanzapine in treatment-resistant patients with schizophrenia. *J Clin Psychiatry* 2008; 69:274–285.

64. Bronson BD, et al. Adverse effects of high-dose olanzapine in treatment-refractory schizophrenia. *J Clin Psychopharmacol* 2000; 20:382–384.

65. Kelly DL, et al. Adverse effects and laboratory parameters of high-dose olanzapine vs. clozapine in treatment-resistant schizophrenia. *Ann Clin Psychiatry* 2003; **15**:181–186.

66. Zink M, et al. Combination of amisulpride and olanzapine in treatment-resistant schizophrenic psychoses. *Eur Psychiatry* 2004; **19**:56–58.

67. Duggal HS. Aripirazole-olanzapine combination for treatment of schizophrenia. *Can J Psychiatry* 2004; **49**:151.

68. Heresco-Levy U, et al. High-dose glycine added to olanzapine and risperidone for the treatment of schizophrenia. *Biol Psychiatry* 2004; **55**:165–171.

69. Dursun SM, et al. Augmenting antipsychotic treatment with lamotrigine or topiramate in patients with treatment-resistant schizophrenia: a naturalistic case-series outcome study. *J Psychopharm* 2001; **15**:297–301.

70. Suzuki T, et al. Effectiveness of antipsychotic polypharmacy for patients with treatment refractory schizophrenia: an open-label trial of olan-zapine plus risperidone for those who failed to respond to a sequential treatment with olanzapine, quetiapine and risperidone. *Human Psychopharmacology* 2008; **23**:455–463.

71. Kotler M, et al. Sulpiride augmentation of olanzapine in the management of treatment-resistant chronic schizophrenia: evidence for improve-ment of mood symptomatology. *Int Clin Psychopharmacol* 2004; **19**:23–26.

72. Mellor JE, et al. Omega-3 fatty acid supplementation in schizophrenic patients. *Human Psychopharmacology* 1996; **11**:39–46.

73. Puri BK, et al. Sustained remission of positive and negative symptoms of schizophrenia following treatment with eicosapentaenoic acid. *Arch Gen Psychiatry* 1998; **55**:188–189.

74. Zheng W, et al. Adjunctive ondansetron for schizophrenia: a systematic review and meta-analysis of randomized controlled trials. *J Psychiatr Res* 2019; **113**:27–33.

75. Martínez-Andrés JA, et al. Switching from clozapine to paliperidone palmitate-3-monthly improved obesity, hyperglycemia and dyslipidemia lowering antipsychotic dose equivalents in a treatment-resistant schizophrenia cohort. *Int Clin Psychopharmacol* 2020; **35**:163–169.

76. Nasrallah HA, et al. Successful treatment of clozapine-nonresponsive refractory hallucinations and delusions with pimavanserin, a serotonin 5HT-2A receptor inverse agonist. *Schizophr Res* 2019; **208**:217–220.

77. Salimi S, et al. A placebo controlled study of the propentofylline added to risperidone in chronic schizophrenia. *Prog Neuropsychopharmacol Biol Psychiatry* 2008; **32**:726–732.

78. Reznik I, et al. Long-term efficacy and safety of quetiapine in treatment-refractory schizophrenia: a case report. *Int J Psychiatry Clin Pract* 2000; **4**:77–80.

79. De Nayer A, et al. Efficacy and tolerability of quetiapine in patients with schizophrenia switched from other antipsychotics. *Int J Psychiatry Clin Pract* 2003; **7**:59–66.

80. Larmo I, et al. Efficacy and tolerability of quetiapine in patients with schizophrenia who switched from haloperidol, olanzapine or risperi-done. *Human Psychopharmacology* 2005; **20**:573–581.

81. Boggs DL, et al. Quetiapine at high doses for the treatment of refractory schizophrenia. *Schizophr Res* 2008; **101**:347–348.

82. Lindenmayer JP, et al. A randomized, double-blind, parallel-group, fixed-dose, clinical trial of quetiapine at 600 versus 1200 mg/d for patients with treatment-resistant schizophrenia or schizoaffective disorder. *J Clin Psychopharmacol* 2011; **31**:160–168.

83. Quintero J, et al. The effectiveness of the combination therapy of amisulpride and quetiapine for managing treatment-resistant schizophrenia: a naturalistic study. *J Clin Psychopharmacol* 2011; **31**:240–242.

84. Aziz MA, et al. Remission of positive and negative symptoms in refractory schizophrenia with a combination of haloperidol and quetiapine: two case studies. *J Psychiatr Pract* 2006; **12**:332–336.

85. Tharoor H, et al. Raloxifene trial in postmenopausal woman with treatment-resistant schizophrenia. *Arch Women's Mental Health* 2015; **18**:741–742.

86. Usall J, et al. Raloxifene as an adjunctive treatment for postmenopausal women with schizophrenia: a 24-week double-blind, randomized, parallel, placebo-controlled trial. *Schizophr Bull* 2016; **42**:309–317.

87. Usall J, et al. Raloxifene as an adjunctive treatment for postmenopausal women with schizophrenia: a double-blind, randomized, placebo-controlled trial. *J Clin Psychiatry* 2011; **72**:1552–1557.

88. Weiser M, et al. Raloxifene plus antipsychotics versus placebo plus antipsychotics in severely ill decompensated postmenopausal women with schizophrenia or schizoaffective disorder: a randomized controlled trial. *J Clin Psychiatry* 2017; **78**:e758–e765.

89. Kulkarni J, et al. Effect of adjunctive raloxifene therapy on severity of refractory schizophrenia in women: a randomized clinical trial. *JAMA Psychiatry* 2016; **73**:947–954.

90. Farokhnia M, et al. A double-blind, placebo controlled, randomized trial of riluzole as an adjunct to risperidone for treatment of negative symptoms in patients with chronic schizophrenia. *Psychopharmacology* 2014; **231**:533–542.

91. Breier AF, et al. Clozapine and risperidone in chronic schizophrenia: effects on symptoms, parkinsonian side effects, and neuroendocrine response. *Am J Psychiatry* 1999; **156**:294–298.

92. Bondolfi G, et al. Risperidone versus clozapine in treatment-resistant chronic schizophrenia: a randomized double-blind study. The Risperidone Study Group. *Am J Psychiatry* 1998; **155**:499–504.

93. Conley RR, et al. Risperidone, quetiapine, and fluphenazine in the treatment of patients with therapy-refractory schizophrenia. *Clin Neuropharmacol* 2005; **28**:163–168.

94. Lerner V, et al. Combination of 'atypical' antipsychotic medication in the management of treatment-resistant schizophrenia and schizoaffec-tive disorder. *Prog Neuropsychopharmacol Biol Psychiatry* 2004; **28**:89–98.

95. Meltzer HY, et al. A six month randomized controlled trial of long acting injectable risperidone 50 and 100mg in treatment resistant schizo-phrenia. *Schizophr Res* 2014; **154**:14–22.

96. Akhondzadeh S, et al. Effect of ritanserin, a 5HT2A/2C antagonist, on negative symptoms of schizophrenia: a double-blind randomized placebo-controlled study. *Prog Neuropsychopharmacol Biol Psychiatry* 2008; **32**:1879–1883.

97. Lane HY, et al. Sarcosine or D-serine add-on treatment for acute exacerbation of schizophrenia: a randomized, double-blind, placebo-controlled study. *Arch Gen Psychiatry* 2005; **62**:1196–1204.

98. Tsai G, et al. Glycine transporter I inhibitor, N-methylglycine (sarcosine), added to antipsychotics for the treatment of schizophrenia. *Biol Psychiatry* 2004; **55**:452–456.

99. Kane JM, et al. A double-blind, randomized study comparing the efficacy and safety of sertindole and risperidone in patients with treatment-resistant schizophrenia. *J Clin Psychiatry* 2011; **72**:194–204.

100. Nielsen J, et al. Augmenting clozapine with sertindole: a double-blind, randomized, placebo-controlled study. *J Clin Psychopharmacol* 2012; **32**:173–178.

101. Tiihonen J, et al. Topiramate add-on in treatment-resistant schizophrenia: a randomized, double-blind, placebo-controlled, crossover trial. *J Clin Psychiatry* 2005; **66**:1012–1015.

102. Franck N, et al. Left temporoparietal transcranial magnetic stimulation in treatment-resistant schizophrenia with verbal hallucinations. *Psychiatry Res* 2003; **120**:107–109.

103. Fitzgerald PB, et al. A double-blind sham-controlled trial of repetitive transcranial magnetic stimulation in the treatment of refractory auditory hallucinations. *J Clin Psychopharmacol* 2005; **25**:358–362.

104. Tuppurainen H, et al. Repetitive navigated αTMS in treatment-resistant schizophrenia. *Brain Stimulation* 2017; **10**:397–398.

105. Khosravi M. Ursodeoxycholic acid augmentation in treatment-refractory schizophrenia: a case report. *J Med Case Rep* 2020; **14**:137.

106. Basan A, et al. Valproate as an adjunct to antipsychotics for schizophrenia: a systematic review of randomized trials. *Schizophr Res* 2004; **70**:33–37.

107. Miyaoka T, et al. Efficacy and safety of yokukansan in treatment-resistant schizophrenia: a randomized, multicenter, double-blind, placebo-controlled trial. *Evid Based Complement Alternat Med* 2015; **2015**:201592.

108. Lin CC, et al. Switching from clozapine to zotepine in patients with schizophrenia: a 12-week prospective, randomized, rater blind, and parallel study. *J Clin Psychopharmacol* 2013; **33**:211–214.

109. Sacchetti E, et al. Ziprasidone vs clozapine in schizophrenia patients refractory to multiple antipsychotic treatments: the MOZART study. *Schizophr Res* 2009; **110**:80–89.

110. Loebel AD, et al. Ziprasidone in treatment-resistant schizophrenia: a 52-week, open-label continuation study. *J Clin Psychiatry* 2007; **68**:1333–1338.

111. Kane JM, et al. Efficacy and tolerability of ziprasidone in patients with treatment-resistant schizophrenia. *Int Clin Psychopharmacol* 2006; **21**:21–28.

112. Goff DC, et al. High-dose oral ziprasidone versus conventional dosing in schizophrenia patients with residual symptoms: the ZEBRAS study. *J Clin Psychopharmacol* 2013; **33**:485–490.

Re-starting clozapine after a break in treatment

Patients prescribed clozapine should be advised to contact their prescriber if they stop taking the medication. This is partly because, if clozapine treatment is stopped abruptly, there is a need to monitor for symptoms of cholinergic rebound, such as nausea, vomiting, diarrhoea, sweating and headache,[1,2] as well as the possible emergence of dystonias, dyskinesias and catatonic symptoms.[3–6] Furthermore, if clozapine treatment is missed for more than 48 hours, re-titration from a 12.5mg dose is required.[7,8]

Depending on tolerability, it may be feasible to re-titrate the dose to a therapeutic level more rapidly than is recommended for initial treatment. While there is some evidence to suggest that faster titrations may be safe in those patients naïve to clozapine[2] and those re-starting it,[3] there is the risk that titration schedules that are too rapid will lead to unnecessary drug discontinuation because of side-effects. More cautious dosage titration will be appropriate for certain patients, such as those who are elderly, people with Parkinson's disease, and outpatients starting clozapine who are uncertain about the potential benefits of the medication.[9,10]

Re-starting clozapine after gaps of various lengths should take account of the need to regain antipsychotic activity with clozapine while ensuring safety during titration. A key element is flexibility: the dosage schedule prescribed for a patient will depend upon how previous dosages were tolerated. Examples of slow, fast and ultra-fast titration schedules are available,[8] but it is probably best to individualise titration according to patient tolerability. In broad terms, this means starting with 12.5mg and increasing to 25mg for the next dose if the initial dose causes no adverse problems with, for example, sedation, heart rate or blood pressure. If the 25mg dose is well tolerated then 50mg can be given for the next dose, and so on. Twice daily dosing probably allows an optimum rate of titration, but some centres use three times daily dosing. Accumulation effects are more likely with the latter schedule. Where a given dose in the titration schedule is not tolerated, the next dose should usually be delayed and not increased (possibly decreased).

It is usually better to prescribe a series of single 'stat' doses one at a time rather than to write up a complete schedule of doses which might then have to be changed.

References

1. Shiovitz TM, et al. Cholinergic rebound and rapid onset psychosis following abrupt clozapine withdrawal. *Schizophr Bull* 1996; **22**:591–595.
2. Galova A, et al. A case report of cholinergic rebound syndrome following abrupt low-dose clozapine discontinuation in a patient with type I bipolar affective disorder. *BMC Psychiatry* 2019; **19**:73.
3. Ahmed S, et al. Clozapine withdrawal-emergent dystonias and dyskinesias: a case series. *J Clin Psychiatry* 1998; **59**:472–477.
4. Shrivastava M, et al. Relapse of tardive dyskinesia due to reduction in clozapine dose. *Indian J Pharmacol* 2009; **41**:201–202.
5. Boazak M, et al. Catatonia due to clozapine withdrawal: a case report and literature review. *Psychosomatics* 2019; **60**:421–427.
6. Lander M, et al. Review of withdrawal catatonia: what does this reveal about clozapine? *Trans Psychiatry* 2018; **8**:139.
7. Mylan Products Ltd. Clozaril 25mg and 100mg tablets. 2020; https://www.medicines.org.uk/emc/medicine/32564.
8. Rubio JM, et al. How and when to use clozapine. *Acta Psychiatr Scand* 2020; **141**:178–189.
9. Gee SH, et al. Patient attitudes to clozapine initiation. *Int Clin Psychopharmacol* 2017; **32**:337–342.
10. Schulte PF, et al. Comment on 'effectiveness and safety of rapid clozapine titration in schizophrenia'. *Acta Psychiatr Scand* 2014; **130**:69–70.

Guidelines for the initiation of clozapine for patients based in the community

Contra-indications to community initiation

- History of seizures, significant cardiac disease, unstable diabetes, paralytic ileus, blood dyscrasia, neuroleptic malignant syndrome or other disorder that increases the risk of serious side-effects (initiation with close monitoring in hospital may still be possible)
- Previous severe side effects on titration of clozapine or other antipsychotics
- Unreliable or chaotic life-style that may affect adherence to the medication or the monitoring regimen
- Significant abuse of alcohol or other drugs likely to increase the risk of side-effects (e.g. cocaine)

Suitability for community initiation (answers should all be yes)

- Is the patient likely to be adherent with oral medication and to monitoring requirements?
- Has the patient understood the need for regular physical monitoring and blood tests?
- Has the patient understood the possible side-effects and what to do about them (particularly the rare but serious ones)?
- Is the patient readily contactable (e.g. in the event of a result that needs follow-up)?
- Is it possible for the patient to be seen every day during the early titration phase?
- Is the patient able to collect medication every week or can medication be delivered to their home?
- Is the patient likely to be able to seek help out-of-hours if they experience potentially serious side-effects (e.g. indicators of myocarditis or infection such as fever, malaise, chest pain)?

Initial work-up

To screen for risk factors and provide a baseline:

- Physical examination, FBC (see below), LFTs, urea and electrolytes (U&Es), lipids, glucose/HbA1c. Consider troponin, C-reactive protein (CRP), beta-natriuretic peptide, erythrocyte sedimentation rate (ESR) (as baseline for further tests)
- ECG- particularly to screen for evidence of past MI or ventricular abnormality
- Echocardiogram if clinically indicated

Mandatory blood monitoring and registration

- Register with the relevant monitoring service.
- Perform baseline blood tests (white cell count (WCC) and differential count) before starting clozapine.
- Further blood testing continues weekly for the first 18 weeks and then every 2 weeks for the remainder of the year. After that, the blood monitoring is usually done monthly.
- Inform the patient's GP.

Dosing

Starting clozapine in the community requires a slow and flexible titration schedule. Prior antipsychotics should be slowly discontinued during the titration phase (depots can usually be stopped at the start of titration). Clozapine can cause marked postural hypotension. The initially monitoring is partly aimed at detecting and managing this.

There are two basic methods for starting clozapine in the community. One is to give the first dose in the morning in clinic and then monitor the patient for at least three hours. If the dose is well tolerated, the patient is then allowed home with a dose to take before going to bed. This dosing schedule is described in Table 1.38. This is a very cautious schedule: most patients will tolerate faster titration. The second method involves giving the patient the first dose to take immediately before bed, so avoiding the need for close physical monitoring immediately after administration. Subsequent doses and monitoring is as for the first method. All initiations should take place early in the week (e.g. on a Monday) so that adequate staffing and monitoring are assured.

Table 1.38 Suggested titration regime for initiation of clozapine in the community (note that much faster titrations can be undertaken in many patients where tolerability allows)

Day	Day of the week	Morning dose (mg)	Evening dose (mg)	Monitoring	Percentage dose of previous antipsychotic
1	Monday	6.25	6.25	A	100
2	Tuesday	6.25	6.25	A	
3	Wednesday	6.25	6.25	A	
4	Thursday	6.25	12.5	A, B, FBC	
5	Friday	12.5	12.5	A Check results from day 4. Remind patient of out-of-hours arrangements for weekend	
6	Saturday	12.5	12.5	No routine monitoring unless clinically indicated	
7	Sunday	12.5	12.5	No routine monitoring unless clinically indicated	
8	Monday	12.5	25	A	75*
9	Tuesday	12.5	25	A	
10	Wednesday	25	25	A	
11	Thursday	25	37.5	A, B, FBC	
12	Friday	25	37.5	A Check results from day 1. Remind patient of out-of-hours arrangements for week-end	
13	Saturday	25	37.5	No routine monitoring unless clinically indicated	

(Continued)

Table 1.38 (*Continued*)

Day	Day of the week	Morning dose (mg)	Evening dose (mg)	Monitoring	Percentage dose of previous antipsychotic
14	Sunday	25	37.5	No routine monitoring unless clinically indicated	
15	Monday	37.5	37.5	A	50*
16	Tuesday	37.5	37.5	Not seen unless problems	
17	Wednesday	37.5	50	A	
18	Thursday	37.5	50	Not seen unless problems	
19	Friday	50	50	A, B, FBC	
20	Saturday	50	50	No routine monitoring unless clinically indicated	
21	Sunday	50	50	No routine monitoring unless clinically indicated	
22	Monday	50	75	A	25*
23	Tuesday	50	75	Not seen unless problems	
24	Wednesday	75	75	A	
25	Thursday	75	75	Not seen unless problems	
26	Friday	75	100	A, B, FBC	
27	Saturday	75	100	No routine monitoring unless clinically indicated	
28	Sunday	75	100	No routine monitoring unless clinically indicated	

Further increments should be 25–50mg/day (generally 25mg/day) until target dose is reached (use plasma levels). Beware sudden increase in plasma levels due to saturation of first-pass metabolism (watch for increase in sedation/other side-effects).

Note:
A. Pulse, postural BP, temperature should be taken before the dose and, ideally, between 30 minutes and 6 hours after the dose. Enquire about side effects.
B. Mental state, weight, review and actively manage side-effects (e.g. behavioural advice, slow clozapine titration or reduce dose of other antipsychotic, start adjunctive treatments- see the section on clozapine side-effects). Consider troponin, CRP, beta-natriuretic peptide.
* May need to be adjusted depending on side effects and mental state.

Adverse effects

Sedation, hypersalivation and hypotension are common at the start of treatment. These effects can usually be managed (see the section on common adverse effects) but require particular attention in community titration. Consider regular systematic assessment of side effects using a recognised scale such as the Glasgow Antipsychotic Side-effects Scale for Clozapine GASS-C.

The formal carer (usually the Community Psychiatric Nurse) should inform the prescriber if:

- **temperature rises above 38°C** (this is very common and is not a good reason, on its own, for stopping clozapine)
- **pulse is > 100bpm** (also common and not, on its own a reason for stopping, but may sometimes be linked to myocarditis)
- **postural drop of >30mmHg**
- **patient is clearly over-sedated**
- **any signs of constipation**
- **flu-like symptoms (malaise, fatigue, etc.)**
- **chest pain, dyspnoea, tachypnoea**
- **any other adverse effect that is intolerable**
- **changes in smoking habit**

A doctor should see the patient at least once a week for the first month to assess mental and physical state.

Recommended additional monitoring

Baseline	1 month	3 months	4–6 months	12 months
Weight/BMI/waist	Weight/BMI/weight	Weight/BMI/waist	Weight/BMI/waist	Weight/BMI/waist
Plasma glucose and lipids	Plasma glucose and lipids		Plasma glucose and lipids	Plasma glucose and lipids
Liver function tests (LFTs)			LFTs	

Consider monitoring plasma troponin, beta-natriuretic peptide and c-reactive protein weekly in the first six weeks of treatment, particularly where there is any suspicion of myocarditis (see the section on myocarditis).

Switching from other antipsychotics

- The switching regime will be largely dependent on the patient's mental state
- Consider potential additive side-effects of antipsychotics (e.g. hypotension, sedation, effect on QTc interval)
- Consider drug interactions (e.g. some SSRIs may increase clozapine levels)
- All depots, sertindole, pimozide and ziprasidone should be stopped before clozapine is started
- Other antipsychotics and clozapine may be cross-tapered with varying degrees of caution. ECG monitoring is prudent when clozapine is co-prescribed with other drugs known to affect QT interval

Serious cardiac adverse effects

Patients should be closely observed for signs or symptoms of myocarditis, particularly during the first 2 months and advised to inform staff if they experience these, and to seek out-of-hours review if necessary. These include persistent tachycardia (although commonly benign), palpitations, shortness of breath, fever, arrhythmia, symptoms mimicking myocardial infarction, chest pain and other unexplained symptoms of heart failure. See section on Clozapine: serious haematological and cardiovascular adverse effects in this chapter.

CLOZAPINE ADVERSE EFFECTS

Clozapine: common adverse effects

Adverse effect	Time course	Action
Sedation	First few months. May persist, but usually wears off to some extent.	Give smaller dose in the morning. Give evening dose earlier if morning waking is troublesome. Reduce dose if possible. Case reports of successful use of psychostimulants (methylphenidate[1]) and betahistine[2] but long-term data are lacking. Modafinil does not appear to be effective[3]
Hypersalivation	First few months. Usually persists, but sometimes wears off. Often very troublesome at night	Give hyoscine 300mcg sucked and swallowed up to three times a day. Many other options – see the section on hypersalivation. Note anticholinergics worsen constipation and cognition
Constipation	First 4 months are the highest risk.[4] Usually persists and so requires continuous monitoring/ treatment	Advise patients of the risks before starting, screen regularly, ensure adequate fibre, fluid and exercise. Stimulant laxatives (senna) are first-line treatments, adding emollients (docusate) and/or osmotics (macrogols) if needed.[5] Bulk-forming laxatives should usually be avoided as the underlying cause is gastric hypomotility. Stop other medicines that may be contributing and reduce clozapine dose if possible. Effective treatment or prevention of constipation is essential as death may result.[4,6–9] See the section of clozapine-induced constipation
Hypotension	First 4 weeks	Advise patient to take time when standing up. Reduce dose or slow down rate of increase. Increase fluid intake to 2l daily.[10] If severe, consider moclobemide and Bovril,[11] fludrocortisone, desmopressin or abdominal binders.[10] Over longer term, weight gain may lead to hypertension
Hypertension[12]	First 4 weeks, sometimes longer	Monitor closely and increase dose as slowly as is necessary. Hypotensive therapy is sometimes necessary[13]
Tachycardia	First 4 weeks, but sometimes persists	Very common in early stages of treatment but usually benign. May be dose-related.[14] Tachycardia, if persistent at rest and associated with fever, hypotension or chest pain, may indicate myocarditis[15,16] (see the section on cardiovascular side effects). Referral to a cardiologist is advised. Clozapine should be stopped if tachycardia occurs in the context of chest pain or heart failure. Benign sinus tachycardia can be treated with bisoprolol[17] or atenolol,[18] although evidence base is poor.[19,20] Ivabradine may be used if hypotension or contra-indications limit the use of beta blockers.[21] Note that prolonged tachycardia can itself precipitate cardiomyopathy[22] or other cardiovascular consequences[10]

(Continued)

Adverse effect	Time course	Action
Weight gain	Usually during the first year of treatment, but may continue	Dietary counselling is essential. Advice may be more effective if given before weight gain occurs. Weight gain is common and often profound (4.5kg in the first 10 weeks[23]). Many treatments available – see the section on treating weight gain
Fever[24]	First 4 weeks	Clozapine induces inflammatory response (increased C-Reactive Protein, interleukin-6[25] and eosinophils).[25–27] Give paracetamol but check FBC for neutropenia. Reduce rate of dose titration.[28] This fever is not usually related to blood dyscrasias[29] but beware myocarditis, NMS, pneumonia and other rarer types of inflammatory organ damage (see the section on uncommon side effects)
Seizures[30]	May occur at any time[31]	Related to dose, plasma level and rapid dose escalation.[32] Consider prophylactic, topiramate, lamotrigine, gabapentin or valproate* if on high dose (≥500mg/day) or with high plasma level (≥500mcg/L). Some suggest risk of seizures below 1300mcg/L (about 1 in 20 people) is not enough to support primary prophylaxis.[33] After a seizure: withhold clozapine for one day; restart at half previous dose; give antiseizure medication**. EEG abnormalities are common in those on clozapine[34,35]
Nausea	First 6 weeks	May give anti-emetic. Avoid prochlorperazine and metoclopramide if previous EPS. Avoid domperidone if underlying cardiac risk or QTc prolongation. Ondansetron is a good choice, but it may worsen constipation. One case of nausea and vomiting being the only presenting symptoms of myocarditis[36]
Nocturnal enuresis	May occur at any time	Try reducing the dose or manipulating dose schedule to avoid periods of deep sedation. Avoid fluids before bedtime. Consider scheduled night-time toileting. May resolve spontaneously,[37] but may persist for months or years.[38] Seems to affect 1 in 5 people on clozapine.[39] In severe cases, desmopressin nasal spray (10–20mcg nocte) is usually effective[40] but is not without risk: hyponatraemia may result.[41] Anticholinergic agents may be effective[42] but support for this approach is weak and constipation and sedation may worsen. Ephedrine,[43] pseudoephedrine[44] and aripiprazole[45,46] have also been used

(Continued)

Adverse effect	Time course	Action
Gastro-oesophageal reflux disease[47,48]	Any time	Proton pump inhibitors often prescribed but some are CYP1A2 inducers, and possibly increase risk of neutropenia and agranulocytosis.[49,50] Reasons for GORD association unclear – clozapine is an H_2 antagonist[51]
Myoclonus[32,52–54]	During dose titration or plasma level increases	May precede full tonic-clonic seizure. Reduce dose. Antiepileptics may help, and will reduce the likelihood of progression to seizures. Valproate is first choice, lamotrigine may worsen some types of myoclonus
Pneumonia[55–62]	Usually early in treatment, but may be any time	May result from saliva aspiration (this may be why pneumonia sometimes appears to be dose related[63,64]), and very rarely from constipation.[65] Pneumonia is a common cause of death in people on clozapine.[56] Infections in general may be more common in those on clozapine[66] and use of antibiotics is also increased.[67] Note that respiratory infections may give rise to elevated clozapine levels.[68–71] (Possibly an artefact: smoking usually ceases during an infection but may be due to inflammation causing reduction in CYP1A2 activity[72,73]). Clozapine is often successfully continued after the pneumonia has resolved, but recurrence may be more likely[74–76]

*Usual dose is 1000–2000mg/day. Plasma levels may be useful as a rough guide to dosing – aim for 50–100mg/l. Use of modified-release preparation (Epilim Chrono) may aid compliance: can be given once-daily and may be better tolerated.
**Use valproate if schizoaffective; lamotrigine if female of child-bearing age, poor response to clozapine or continued negative symptoms; topiramate if weight loss required (but beware cognitive adverse effects); gabapentin if other antiseizure medications are poorly tolerated.[32]

References

1. Sarfati D, et al. Methylphenidate as treatment for clozapine-induced sedation in patients with treatment-resistant schizophrenia. *Clin Schizophr Relat Psychoses* 2018: [Epub ahead of print].
2. Poyurovsky M, et al. Beneficial effect of betahistine, a structural analog of histamine, in clozapine-related sedation. *Clin Neuropharmacol* 2019; 42:145.
3. Freudenreich O, et al. Modafinil for clozapine-treated schizophrenia patients: a double-blind, placebo-controlled pilot trial. *J Clin Psychiatry* 2009; 70:1674–1680.
4. Palmer SE, et al. Life-threatening clozapine-induced gastrointestinal hypomotility: an analysis of 102 cases. *J Clin Psychiatry* 2008; 69:759–768.
5. Taylor D, et al. *The Maudsley Practice Guidelines for Physical Health Conditions in Psychiatry*. United Kingdom Wiley – Blackwell; 2020.
6. Townsend G, et al. Case report: rapidly fatal bowel ischaemia on clozapine treatment. *BMC Psychiatry* 2006; 6:43.
7. Rege S, et al. Life-threatening constipation associated with clozapine. *Aust Psychiatry* 2008; 16:216–219.
8. Leung JS, et al. Rapidly fatal clozapine-induced intestinal obstruction without prior warning signs. *Aust N Z J Psychiatry* 2008; 42:1073–1074.
9. Flanagan RJ, et al. Gastrointestinal hypomotility: an under-recognised life-threatening adverse effect of clozapine. *Forensic Sci Int* 2011; 206:e31–e36.
10. Ronaldson KJ. Cardiovascular disease in clozapine-treated patients: evidence, mechanisms and management. *CNS Drugs* 2017; 31:777–795.
11. Taylor D, et al. Clozapine-induced hypotension treated with moclobemide and Bovril. *Br J Psychiatry* 1995; 167:409–410.
12. Gonsai NH, et al. Effects of dopamine receptor antagonist antipsychotic therapy on blood pressure. *J Clin Pharm Ther* 2017; 43:1–7.
13. Henderson DC, et al. Clozapine and hypertension: a chart review of 82 patients. *J Clin Psychiatry* 2004; 65:686–689.

14. Nilsson BM, et al. Tachycardia in patients treated with clozapine versus antipsychotic long-acting injections. *Int Clin Psychopharmacol* 2017; 32:219–224.

15. Medicines CoSo. Clozapine and cardiac safety: updated advice for prescribers. *Curr Prob Pharmacovigilance* 2002; 28:8.

16. Hagg S, et al. Myocarditis related to clozapine treatment. *J Clin Psychopharmacol* 2001; 21:382–388.

17. Nilsson BM, et al. Persistent tachycardia in clozapine treated patients: a 24-hour ambulatory electrocardiogram study. *Schizophr Res* 2018; 199:403–406.

18. Stryjer R, et al. Beta-adrenergic antagonists for the treatment of clozapine-induced sinus tachycardia: a retrospective study. *Clin Neuropharmacol* 2009; 32:290–292.

19. Lally J, et al. Pharmacological interventions for clozapine-induced sinus tachycardia. *Cochrane Database Syst Rev* 2016; Cd011566.

20. Yuen JWY, et al. Clozapine-induced cardiovascular side effects and autonomic dysfunction: a systematic review. *Front Neurosci* 2018; 12:203.

21. Lally J, et al. Ivabradine, a novel treatment for clozapine-induced sinus tachycardia: a case series. *Ther Adv Psychopharmacol* 2014; 4:117–122.

22. Shinbane JS, et al. Tachycardia-induced cardiomyopathy: a review of animal models and clinical studies. *J Am Coll Cardiol* 1997; 29:709–715.

23. Allison D, et al. Antipsychotic-induced weight gain: a comprehensive research synthesis. *Am J Psychiatry* 1999; 156:1686–1696.

24. Verdoux H, et al. Clinical determinants of fever in clozapine users and implications for treatment management: a narrative review. *Schizophr Res* 2019; 211:1–9.

25. Hung YP, et al. Role of cytokine changes in clozapine-induced fever: a cohort prospective study. *Psychiatry Clin Neurosci* 2017; 71:395–402.

26. Kohen I, et al. Increases in C-reactive protein may predict recurrence of clozapine-induced fever. *Ann Pharmacother* 2009; 43:143–146.

27. Kluge M, et al. Effects of clozapine and olanzapine on cytokine systems are closely linked to weight gain and drug-induced fever. *Psychoneuroendocrinology* 2009; 34:118–128.

28. Chung JP, et al. The incidence and characteristics of clozapine – induced fever in a local psychiatric unit in Hong Kong. *Can J Psychiatry* 2008; 53:857–862.

29. Tham JC, et al. Clozapine-induced fevers and 1-year clozapine discontinuation rate. *J Clin Psychiatry* 2002; 63:880–884.

30. Grover S, et al. Association of clozapine with seizures: a brief report involving 222 patients prescribed clozapine. *East Asian Arch Psychiatry* 2015; 25:73–78.

31. Pacia SV, et al. Clozapine-related seizures: experience with 5,629 patients. *Neurology* 1994; 44:2247–2249.

32. Varma S, et al. Clozapine-related EEG changes and seizures: dose and plasma-level relationships. *Ther Adv Psychopharmacol* 2011; 1:47–66.

33. Caetano D. Use of anticonvulsants as prophylaxis for seizures in patients on clozapine. *Australas Psychiatry* 2014; 22:78–83.

34. Centorrino F, et al. EEG abnormalities during treatment with typical and atypical antipsychotics. *Am J Psychiatry* 2002; 159:109–115.

35. Jackson A, et al. EEG changes in patients on antipsychotic therapy: a systematic review. *Epilepsy Behav* 2019; 95:1–9.

36. Van Der Horst MZ, et al. Isolated nausea and vomiting as the cardinal presenting symptoms of clozapine-induced myocarditis: a case report. *BMC Psychiatry* 2020; 20:568.

37. Warner JP, et al. Clozapine and urinary incontinence. *Int Clin Psychopharmacol* 1994; 9:207–209.

38. Jeong SH, et al. A 2-year prospective follow-up study of lower urinary tract symptoms in patients treated with clozapine. *J Clin Psychopharmacol* 2008; 28:618–624.

39. Harrison-Woolrych M, et al. Nocturnal enuresis in patients taking clozapine, risperidone, olanzapine and quetiapine: comparative cohort study. *Br J Psychiatry* 2011; 199:140–144.

40. Steingard S. Use of desmopressin to treat clozapine-induced nocturnal enuresis. *J Clin Psychiatry* 1994; 55:315–316.

41. Sarma S, et al. Severe hyponatraemia associated with desmopressin nasal spray to treat clozapine-induced nocturnal enuresis. *Aust N Z J Psychiatry* 2005; 39:949.

42. Praharaj SK, et al. Amitriptyline for clozapine-induced nocturnal enuresis and sialorrhoea. *Br J Clin Pharmacol* 2007; 63:128–129.

43. Fuller MA, et al. Clozapine-induced urinary incontinence: incidence and treatment with ephedrine. *J Clin Psychiatry* 1996; 57:514–518.

44. Hanes A, et al. Pseudoephedrine for the treatment of clozapine-induced incontinence. *Innov Clin Neurosci* 2013; 10:33–35.

45. Palaniappan P. Aripiprazole as a treatment option for clozapine-induced enuresis. *Indian J Pharmacol* 2015; 47:574–575.

46. Lee MJ, et al. Use of aripiprazole in clozapine induced enuresis: report of two cases. *J Korean Med Sci* 2010; 25:333–335.

47. Taylor D, et al. Use of antacid medication in patients receiving clozapine: a comparison with other second-generation antipsychotics. *J Clin Psychopharmacol* 2010; 30:460–461.

48. Van Veggel M, et al. Clozapine and gastro-oesophageal reflux disease (GORD) – an investigation of temporal association. *Acta Psychiatr Scand* 2013; 127:69–77.

49. Wicinski M, et al. Potential mechanisms of hematological adverse drug reactions in patients receiving clozapine in combination with proton pump inhibitors. *J Psychiatr Pract* 2017; 23:114–120.

50. Shuman MD, et al. Exploring the potential effect of polypharmacy on the hematologic profiles of clozapine patients. *J Psychiatr Pract* 2014; 20:50–58.

51. Humbert-Claude M, et al. Involvement of histamine receptors in the atypical antipsychotic profile of clozapine: a reassessment in vitro and in vivo. *Psychopharmacology* 2011; 220:225–241.

52. Osborne IJ, et al. Clozapine-induced myoclonus: a case report and review of the literature. *Ther Adv Psychopharmacol* 2015; 5:351–356.

53. Praharaj SK, et al. Clozapine-induced myoclonus: a case study and brief review. *Prog Neuropsychopharmacol Biol Psychiatry* 2010; 34:242–243.

54. Sajatovic M, et al. Clozapine-induced myoclonus and generalized seizures. *Biol Psychiatry* 1996; 39:367–370.

55. Hinkes R, et al. Aspiration pneumonia possibly secondary to clozapine-induced sialorrhea. *J Clin Psychopharmacol* 1996; 16:462–463.

56. Taylor DM, et al. Reasons for discontinuing clozapine: matched, case-control comparison with risperidone long-acting injection. *Br J Psychiatry* 2009; 194:165–167.

57. Stoecker ZR, et al. Clozapine usage increases the incidence of pneumonia compared with risperidone and the general population: a retrospective comparison of clozapine, risperidone, and the general population in a single hospital over 25 months. *Int Clin Psychopharmacol* 2017; 32:155–160.

58. Kaplan J, et al. Clozapine-associated aspiration pneumonia: case series and review of the literature. *Psychosomatics* 2017; 58:199–203.

59. Gurrera RJ, et al. Aspiration pneumonia: an underappreciated risk of clozapine treatment. *J Clin Psychopharmacol* 2016; 36:174–176.

60. Aldridge G, et al. Clozapine-induced pneumonitis. *Aust N Z J Psychiatry* 2013; 47:1215–1216.

61. Saenger RC, et al. Aspiration pneumonia due to clozapine-induced sialorrhea. *Clin Schizophr Relat Psychoses* 2016; 9:170–172.

62. Patel SS, et al. Physical complications in early clozapine treatment: a case report and implications for safe monitoring. *Ther Adv Psychopharmacol* 2011; 1:25–29.

63. Trigoboff E, et al. Sialorrhea and aspiration pneumonia: a case study. *Innov Clin Neurosci* 2013; 10:20–27.

64. Kuo CJ, et al. Second-generation antipsychotic medications and risk of pneumonia in schizophrenia. *SchizophrBull* 2013; 39:648–657.

65. Galappathie N, et al. Clozapine-associated pneumonia and respiratory arrest secondary to severe constipation. *MedSciLaw* 2014; 54:105–109.

66. Landry P, et al. Increased use of antibiotics in clozapine-treated patients. *Int Clin Psychopharmacol* 2003; 18:297–298.

67. Nielsen J, et al. Increased use of antibiotics in patients treated with clozapine. *Eur Neuropsychopharmacol* 2009; 19:483–486.

68. Raaska K, et al. Bacterial pneumonia can increase serum concentration of clozapine. *Eur J Clin Pharmacol* 2002; 58:321–322.

69. De Leon J, et al. Serious respiratory infections can increase clozapine levels and contribute to side effects: a case report. *Prog Neuropsychopharmacol Biol Psychiatry* 2003; 27:1059–1063.

70. Ruan CJ, et al. Pneumonia can cause clozapine intoxication: a case report. *Psychosomatics* 2017; 58:652–656.

71. Leung JG, et al. Necrotizing pneumonia in the setting of elevated clozapine levels. *J Clin Psychopharmacol* 2016; 36:176–178.

72. De Leon J, et al. A rational use of clozapine based on adverse drug reactions, pharmacokinetics, and clinical pharmacopsychology. *Psychother Psychosom* 2020; 89:200–214.

73. Clark SR, et al. Elevated clozapine levels associated with infection: a systematic review. *Schizophr Res* 2018; 192:50–56.

74. Hung GC, et al. Antipsychotic reexposure and recurrent pneumonia in schizophrenia: a nested case-control study. *J Clin Psychiatry* 2016; 77:60–66.

75. Galappathie N, et al. Clozapine re-trial in a patient with repeated life threatening pneumonias. *Acta Biomed* 2014; 85:175–179.

76. Schmidinger S, et al. Pulmonary embolism and aspiration pneumonia after reexposure to clozapine: pulmonary adverse effects of clozapine. *J Clin Psychopharmacol* 2014; 34:385–387.

Clozapine: uncommon or unusual adverse effects

Adverse effect	Time course	Comment
Agranulocytosis/ neutropenia (delayed)[1–4]	Usually first 3 months but may occur at any time	Occasional reports of apparent clozapine-related blood dyscrasia even after 1 year of treatment. Risk may be elevated for up to 9 years.[5] It is possible that clozapine is not the causative agent in some cases.[6,7] See section on haematological adverse effects
Colitis/gastrointestinal necrosis[8–15]	Usually within the first month but may be any time[16]	Growing body of case reports. Any severe or chronic diarrhoea should prompt specialist referral as there is a substantial risk of death. Anticholinergic use probably increases risk of colitis and necrosis[17]
Delirium[18–20]	Any time	Reported to be fairly common (8–10%[18,21]) but rarely seen in practice if dose is titrated slowly and plasma level determinations are used. Older age and medical comorbidity increase the risk of delirium. Ensure common causes of delirium are treated (see the section on delirium)
Eosinophilia[22–24]	First weeks[25,26]	Reasonably common but significance unclear. Some suggestion that eosinophilia predicts neutropenia but this is disputed. Usually benign but investigate for signs of inflammatory organ damage[27] (myocarditis,[28] interstitial nephritis,[26,29] interstitial lung disease, hepatitis, pancreatitis[30]). May be associated with colitis and related symptoms.[15,31] Six case reports of DRESS syndrome.[32] Successful rechallenge in the absence of organ inflammation is possible.[33] Concomitant antidepressants may increase risk[34,35]
Heat stroke[36,37]	Any time	Two cases reported, both occurred during a heatwave. May be mistaken for NMS (CK was elevated in both cases)
Hepatic failure/enzyme abnormalities[38–44]	First few months	Benign changes in LFTs are common (up to 50% of patients) but worth monitoring because of the very small risk of fulminant hepatic failure.[45] Rash may be associated with clozapine-related hepatitis.[46] See section on hepatic impairment
Hypothermia[47]	Any time	A few case reports and events in pharmacovigilance databases. Can be fatal
Interstitial nephritis[29,48–56]	Usually first three weeks, possibly up to three months[26,57]	A handful of reports implicating clozapine. Immune-mediated. May occur after only a few doses. Symptoms include fever, tachycardia, nausea, vomiting, diarrhoea, raised creatinine, urinary difficulties and eosinophilia. The classic nephritis-associated rash may not be present.[26] There are no cases of successful rechallenge[26]
Interstitial lung disease	Usually first few months, possibly later in treatment	Six case reports.[58] May be caused by aspiration or an immune reaction. Symptoms are non-specific: shortness of breath, fever, cough, fatigue. Pneumonitis has also been reported[59]
Ocular effects	Any time	Single case report of ocular pigmentation,[60] five of periorbital oedema.[61] Clozapine may cause dry eye syndrome[62]

(Continued)

(Continued)

Adverse effect	Time course	Comment
Pancreatitis[63–70]	Usually first six weeks, possibly later in treatment[71]	Several reports of asymptomatic and symptomatic pancreatitis. Symptoms include fever, abdominal pain and distension, nausea and vomiting, raised CRP and raised lipase and/or amylase. Sodium valproate may increase the risk.[26] Majority of attempts to rechallenge fail[66,72–74] but one successful case is reported[75]
Parotid gland swelling[76–82]	Usually first few weeks, but may occur later[83]	Several case reports. Unclear mechanism, possibly immunological or thickening of saliva leading to calcium precipitation. Can be recurrent. May resolve spontaneously.[84] Treatment of hypersalivation with terazosin in combination with benzatropine may be helpful
Pericarditis and pericardial effusion[85–93]	Any time	Several reports in the literature. Symptoms include fatigue, chest pain, dyspnoea and tachycardia, but may be asymptomatic.[94] Signs include raised inflammatory markers (specifically trop I) and pro-BNP levels.[95] Use echocardiogram to confirm/rule out effusion. Successful rechallenge possible[96,97]
Stuttering[98–106]	Any time	Case reports. May be a result of EPS or epileptiform activity. Check plasma levels, consider dose reduction and/or antiseizure drugs – may be a warning sign for impending generalised seizures[107]
Thrombocytopenia[108–111]	First 3 months	Few data but apparently fairly common (incidence over 1 year of 3[112]–8%[113]). Probably transient and clinically unimportant, but persistent in some cases[114,115] and recurrent on rechallenge in others.[116] Thrombocytosis also reported[117]
Skin reactions[118]	Any time	Presence of skin diseases in general is higher in those with schizophrenia.[119] Four reports of vasculitis[120–123] in which patients developed confluent erythematous rash on lower limbs. One report of Stevens-Johnson syndrome,[124] two reports of pityriasis rosea,[125,126] one report of a papular rash,[127] one report of exanthematic pustulosis[128] and one fatal case of Sweet's syndrome.[129] Skin rash is commonly reported in DRESS syndrome[32]
Thromboembolism[130–134]	Any time[135]	Weight increase and sedation may contribute to risk. Mechanism may be increased platelet aggregation via $5HT_{2A}$ receptor activation.[136] Clozapine increases risk of pulmonary thromboembolism by 28 times compared with the general population.[137] The risk may be dose-related.[138] Threshold for prophylactic antithrombotic treatment where additional risk factors are present (surgery, immobility) should be low. Continuation of therapy after embolism may be possible[139] but consult haematologist as without prophylactic antithrombotic treatment recurrence is likely[140,141]

References

1. Thompson A, et al. Late onset neutropenia with clozapine. *Can J Psychiatry* 2004; **49**:647–648.

2. Bhanji NH, et al. Late-onset agranulocytosis in a patient with schizophrenia after 17 months of clozapine treatment. *J Clin Psychopharmacol* 2003; **23**:522–523.

3. Sedky K, et al. Clozapine-induced agranulocytosis after 11 years of treatment (Letter). *Am J Psychiatry* 2005; **162**:814.

4. De Araujo CF, et al. Delayed-onset severe neutropenia associated with clozapine with successful rechallenge at lower dose. *J Clin Psychopharmacol* 2021; **41**:77–79.

5. Kang BJ, et al. Long-term patient monitoring for clozapine-induced agranulocytosis and neutropenia in Korea: when is it safe to discontinue CPMS? *Human Psychopharmacology* 2006; **21**:387–391.

6. Panesar N, et al. Late onset neutropenia with clozapine. *Aust N Z J Psychiatry* 2011; **45**:684.

7. Tourian L, et al. Late-onset agranulocytosis in a patient treated with clozapine and lamotrigine. *J Clin Psychopharmacol* 2011; **31**:665–667.

8. Hawe R, et al. Response to clozapine-induced microscopic colitis: a case report and review of the literature. *J Clin Psychopharmacol* 2008; **28**:454–455.

9. Shah V, et al. Clozapine-induced ischaemic colitis. *BMJ Case Rep* 2013; **2013**:bcr2012007933.

10. Linsley KR, et al. Clozapine-associated colitis: case report and review of the literature. *J Clin Psychopharmacol* 2012; **32**:564–566.

11. Baptista T. A fatal case of ischemic colitis during clozapine administration. *Rev Bras Psiquiatr* 2014; **36**:358.

12. Rodriguez-Sosa JT, et al. Apropos of a case: relationship of ischemic colitis with clozapine. *Actas Esp Psiquiatr* 2014; **42**:325–326.

13. Osterman MT, et al. Clozapine-induced acute gastrointestinal necrosis: a case report. *J Med Case Rep* 2017; **11**:270.

14. Holz K, et al. Clozapine associated with microscopic colitis in the setting of biopsy-proven celiac disease. *J Clin Psychopharmacol* 2018; **38**:150–152.

15. Rask SM, et al. Clozapine-related diarrhea and colitis: report of 4 cases. *J Clin Psychopharmacol* 2020; **40**:293–296.

16. Verdoux H, et al. Clinical determinants of fever in clozapine users and implications for treatment management: a narrative review. *Schizophr Res* 2019; **211**:1–9.

17. Peyriere H, et al. Antipsychotics-induced ischaemic colitis and gastrointestinal necrosis: a review of the French pharmacovigilance database. *Pharmacoepidemiol Drug Saf* 2009; **18**:948–955.

18. Centorrino F, et al. Delirium during clozapine treatment: incidence and associated risk factors. *Pharmacopsychiatry* 2003; **36**:156–160.

19. Shankar BR. Clozapine-induced delirium. *J Neuropsychiatry Clin Neurosci* 2008; **20**:239–240.

20. Khanra S, et al. An unusual case of delirium after restarting clozapine. *Clin Psychopharmacol Neurosci* 2016; **14**:107–108.

21. Gaertner HJ, et al. Side effects of clozapine. *Psychopharmacology* 1989; **99 Suppl**:S97–S100.

22. Hummer M, et al. Does eosinophilia predict clozapine induced neutropenia? *Psychopharmacology* 1996; **124**:201–204.

23. Ames D, et al. Predictive value of eosinophilia for neutropenia during clozapine treatment. *J Clin Psychiatry* 1996; **57**:579–581.

24. Wysokinski A, et al. Rapidly developing and self-limiting eosinophilia associated with clozapine. *Psychiatry Clin Neurosci* 2015; **69**:122.

25. Aneja J, et al. Eosinophilia induced by clozapine: a report of two cases and review of the literature. *J Family Med Primary Care* 2015; **4**:127–129.

26. Lally J, et al. Hepatitis, interstitial nephritis, and pancreatitis in association with clozapine treatment: a systematic review of case series and reports. *J Clin Psychopharmacol* 2018; **38**:520–527.

27. Marchel D, et al. Multiorgan eosinophilic infiltration after initiation of clozapine therapy: a case report. *BMC Res Notes* 2017; **10**:316.

28. Chatterton R. Eosinophilia after commencement of clozapine treatment. *AustNZJPsychiatry* 1997; **31**:874–876.

29. Chan SY, et al. Clozapine-induced acute interstitial nephritis. *Hong Kong Med J* 2015; **21**:372–374.

30. Lally J, et al. Rechallenge following clozapine-associated eosinophilia: a case report and literature review. *J Clin Psychopharmacol* 2019; **39**:504–506.

31. Linsley KR, et al. Clozapine-induced eosinophilic colitis (letter). *Am J Psychiatry* 2005; **162**:1386–1387.

32. De Filippis R, et al. Clozapine-related drug reaction with eosinophilia and systemic symptoms (DRESS) syndrome: a systematic review. *Expert Rev Clin Pharmacol* 2020; **13**:875–883.

33. McArdle PA, et al. Successful rechallenge with clozapine after treatment associated eosinophilia. *Aust Psychiatry* 2016; **24**:365–367.

34. Fabrazzo M, et al. Clozapine versus other antipsychotics during the first 18 weeks of treatment: a retrospective study on risk factor increase of blood dyscrasias. *Psychiatry Res* 2017; **256**:275–282.

35. Sanader B, et al. Clozapine-induced DRESS syndrome: a case series from the AMSP multicenter drug safety surveillance project. *Pharmacopsychiatry* 2019; **52**:156–159.

36. Kerwin RW, et al. Heat stroke in schizophrenia during clozapine treatment: rapid recognition and management. *J Psychopharmacology* 2004; **18**:121–123.

37. Hoffmann MS, et al. Heat stroke during long-term clozapine treatment: should we be concerned about hot weather? *Trends in Psychiatry and Psychotherapy* 2016; **38**:56–59.

38. Erdogan A, et al. Management of marked liver enzyme increase during clozapine treatment: a case report and review of the literature. *Int J Psychiatry Med* 2004; **34**:83–89.

39. Macfarlane B, et al. Fatal acute fulminant liver failure due to clozapine: a case report and review of clozapine-induced hepatotoxicity. *Gastroenterology* 1997; **112**:1707–1709.

40. Chang A, et al. Clozapine-induced fatal fulminant hepatic failure: a case report. *Can J Gastroenterol* 2009; **23**:376–378.

41. Chaplin AC, et al. Re: recent case report of clozapine-induced acute hepatic failure. *Can J Gastroenterol* 2010; **24**:739–740.

42. Wu Chou AI, et al. Hepatotoxicity induced by clozapine: a case report and review of literature. *Neuropsychiatr Dis Treat* 2014; **10**:1585–1587.

43. Kane JP, et al. Clozapine-induced liver injury and pleural effusion. *Mental Illness* 2014; **6**:5403.

44. Douros A, et al. Drug-induced liver injury: results from the hospital-based Berlin Case-Control Surveillance Study. *Br J Clin Pharmacol* 2015; **79**:988–999.

45. Tucker P. Liver toxicity with clozapine. *Aust N Z J Psychiatry* 2013; **47**:975–976.

46. Fong SY, et al. Clozapine-induced toxic hepatitis with skin rash. *J Psychopharmacol* 2005; **19**:107.

47. Burk BG, et al. A case report of acute hypothermia during initial inpatient clozapine titration with review of current literature on clozapine-induced temperature dysregulations. *BMC Psychiatry* 2020; **20**:290.

48. Hunter R, et al. Clozapine-induced interstitial nephritis – a rare but important complication: a case report. *J Med Case Rep* 2009; **3**:8574.

49. Elias TJ, et al. Clozapine-induced acute interstitial nephritis. *Lancet* 1999; **354**:1180–1181.

50. Parekh R, et al. Clozapine induced tubulointerstitial nephritis in a patient with paranoid schizophrenia. *BMJ Case Rep* 2014; bcr2013203502.

51. An NY, et al. A case of clozapine induced acute renal failure. *Psychiatry Investig* 2013; 10:92–94.

52. Kanofsky JD, et al. A case of acute renal failure in a patient recently treated with clozapine and a review of previously reported cases. *Prim Care Companion CNS Disord* 2011; 13:PCC.10br01091.

53. Au AF, et al. Clozapine-induced acute interstitial nephritis. *Am J Psychiatry* 2004; 161:1501.

54. Southall KE. A case of interstitial nephritis on clozapine. *Aust N Z J Psychiatry* 2000; 34:697–698.

55. Fraser D, et al. An unexpected and serious complication of treatment with the atypical antipsychotic drug clozapine. *Clin Nephrol* 2000; 54:78–80.

56. McLoughlin C, et al. Clozapine-induced interstitial nephritis in a patient with schizoaffective disorder in the forensic setting: a case report and review of the literature. *Ir J Psychol Med* 2019; [Epub ahead of print].

57. Mohan T, et al. Clozapine-induced nephritis and monitoring implications. *Aust N Z J Psychiatry* 2013; 47:586–587.

58. Can KC, et al. A very rare adverse effect of clozapine, clozapine-induced interstitial lung disease: case report and literature review. *Noro Psikiyatri Arsivi* 2019; 56:313–315.

59. Torrico T, et al. Clozapine-induced pneumonitis: a case report. *Frontiers in Psychiatry* 2020; 11:572102.

60. Borovik AM, et al. Ocular pigmentation associated with clozapine. *Med J Aust* 2009; 190:210–211.

61. Huttlin EA, et al. Periorbital edema associated with clozapine and gabapentins: a case report. *J Clin Psychopharmacol* 2020; 40:198–199.

62. Ceylan E, et al. The ocular surface side effects of an anti-psychotic drug, clozapine. *Cutan Ocul Toxicol* 2016; 35:62–66.

63. Bergemann N, et al. Asymptomatic pancreatitis associated with clozapine. *Pharmacopsychiatry* 1999; 32:78–80.

64. Raja M, et al. A case of clozapine-associated pancreatitis. *Open Neuropsychopharmacol J* 2011; 4:5–7.

65. Bayard JM, et al. Case report: acute pancreatitis induced by Clozapine. *Acta Gastroenterol Belg* 2005; 68:92–94.

66. Sani G, et al. Development of asymptomatic pancreatitis with paradoxically high serum clozapine levels in a patient with schizophrenia and the CYP1A2*1F/1F genotype. *J Clin Psychopharmacol* 2010; 30:737–739.

67. Wehmeier PM, et al. Pancreatitis followed by pericardial effusion in an adolescent treated with clozapine. *J Clin Psychopharmacol* 2003; 23:102–103.

68. Garlipp P, et al. The development of a clinical syndrome of asymptomatic pancreatitis and eosinophilia after treatment with clozapine in schizophrenia: implications for clinical care, recognition and management. *J Psychopharmacology* 2002; 16:399–400.

69. Gatto EM, et al. Clozapine and pancreatitis. *Clin Neuropharmacol* 1998; 21:203.

70. Martin A. Acute pancreatitis associated with clozapine use. *Am J Psychiatry* 1992; 149:714.

71. Cerulli TR. Clozapine-associated pancreatitis. *Harv Rev Psychiatry* 1999; 7:61–63.

72. Huang YJ, et al. Recurrent pancreatitis without eosinophilia on clozapine rechallenge. *Prog Neuropsychopharmacol Biol Psychiatry* 2009; 33:1561–1562.

73. Chengappa KN, et al. Recurrent pancreatitis on clozapine re-challenge. *J Psychopharmacology* 1995; 9:381–382.

74. Frankenburg FR, et al. Eosinophilia, clozapine, and pancreatitis. *Lancet* 1992; 340:251.

75. DeRemer CE, et al. Clozapine drug-induced pancreatitis of intermediate latency of onset confirmed by de-challenge and re-challenge. *Int J Clin Pharmacol Ther* 2019; 57:37–40.

76. Immadisetty V, et al. A successful treatment strategy for clozapine-induced parotid swelling: a clinical case and systematic review. *TherAdvPsychopharmacol* 2012; 2:235–239.

77. Gouzien C, et al. [Clozapine-induced parotitis: a case study]. *Encephale* 2014; 40:81–85.

78. Saguem BN, et al. Eosinophilia and parotitis occurring early in clozapine treatment. *Int J Clin Pharm* 2015; 37:992–995.

79. Vohra A. Clozapine- induced recurrent and transient parotid gland swelling. *African Journal of Psychiatry* 2013; 16:236, 238.

80. Acosta-Armas AJ. Two cases of parotid gland swelling in patients taking clozapine. *Hosp Med* 2001; 62:704–705.

81. Patkar AA, et al. Parotid gland swelling with clozapine. *J Clin Psychiatry* 1996; 57:488.

82. Kathirvel N, et al. Recurrent transient parotid gland swelling with clozapine therapy. *Ir J Psychol Med* 2014; 25:69–70.

83. Brodkin ES, et al. Treatment of clozapine-induced parotid gland swelling. *Am J Psychiatry* 1996; 153:445.

84. Vasile JS, et al. Clozapine and the development of salivary gland swelling: a case study. *J Clin Psychiatry* 1995; 56:511–513.

85. Raju P, et al. Pericardial effusion in patients with schizophrenia: are they on clozapine? *Emerg Med J* 2008; 25:383–384.

86. Dauner DG, et al. Clozapine-induced pericardial effusion. *J Clin Psychopharmacol* 2008; 28:455–456.

87. Markovic J, et al. Clozapine-induced pericarditis. *Afr J Psychiatry* 2011; 14:236–238.

88. Bhatti MA, et al. Clozapine-induced pericarditis, pericardial tamponade, polyserositis, and rash. *J Clin Psychiatry* 2005; 66:1490–1491.

89. Boot E, et al. Pericardial and bilateral pleural effusion associated with clozapine treatment. *Eur Psychiatry* 2004; 19:65.

90. Murko A, et al. Clozapine and pericarditis with pericardial effusion. *Am J Psychiatry* 2002; 159:494.

91. Imon Paul MD, et al. Clozapine induced pericarditis. *Clin Schizophr Relat Psychoses* 2014; 4;1–6

92. Bath AS, et al. Pericardial effusion: rare adverse effect of clozapine. *Cureus* 2019; 11:e4890.

93. Johal HK, et al. Clozapine-induced pericarditis: an ethical dilemma. *BMJ Case Rep* 2019; 12:e229872.

94. Prisco V, et al. Brain natriuretic peptide as a biomarker of asymptomatic clozapine-related heart dysfunction: a criterion for a more cautious administration. *Clin Schizophr Relat Psychoses* 2016; 12:185–188.

95. Prisco V, et al. Brain natriuretic peptide as a biomarker of asymptomatic clozapine-related heart dysfunction: a criterion for a more cautious administration. *Clin Schizophr Relat Psychoses* 2019; 12:185–188.

96. Crews MP, et al. Clozapine rechallenge following clozapine-induced pericarditis. *J Clin Psychiatry* 2010; 71:959–961.

97. Sarathy K, et al. A successful re-trial after clozapine myopericarditis. *J R Coll Physicians Edinb* 2017; 47:146–147.

98. Kumar T, et al. Dose dependent stuttering with clozapine: a case report. *Asian J Psychiatr* 2013; 6:178–179.

99. Grover S, et al. Clozapine-induced stuttering: a case report and analysis of similar case reports in the literature. *Gen Hosp Psychiatry* 2012; 34:703–703.

100. Murphy R, et al. Clozapine-induced stuttering: an estimate of prevalence in the west of Ireland. *Ther Adv Psychopharmacol* 2015; 5:232–236.

101. Rachamallu V, et al. Clozapine-induced microseizures, orofacial dyskinesia, and speech dysfluency in an adolescent with treatment resistant early onset schizophrenia on concurrent lithium therapy. *Case Rep Psychiatry* 2017: 7359095

102. Bar KJ, et al. Olanzapine- and clozapine-induced stuttering. A case series. *Pharmacopsychiatry* 2004; 37:131–134.

103. Chochol MD, et al. Clozapine-associated myoclonus and stuttering secondary to smoking cessation and drug interaction: a case report. *J Clin Psychopharmacol* 2019; 39:275–277.

104. Gica S, et al. Clozapine-associated stuttering: a case report. *Am J Ther* 2020; 27:e624–e627.

105. Das S, et al. Clozapine-induced weight loss and stuttering in a patient with schizophrenia. *Indian J Psychol Med* 2018; 40:385–387.

106. Nagendrappa S, et al. 'I stopped hearing voices, started to stutter' – a case of clozapine-induced stuttering. *Indian J Psychol Med* 2019; 41:97–98.

107. Duggal HS, et al. Clozapine-induced stuttering and seizures. *Am J Psychiatry* 2002; 159:315.

108. Jagadheesan K, et al. Clozapine-induced thrombocytopenia: a pilot study. *Hong Kong J Psychiatry* 2003; 13:12–15.

109. Mihaljevic-Peles A, et al. Thrombocytopenia associated with clozapine and fluphenazine. *Nord J Psychiatry* 2001; 55:449–450.

110. Rudolf J, et al. Clozapine-induced agranulocytosis and thrombopenia in a patient with dopaminergic psychosis. *J Neur Trans* 1997; 104:1305–1311.

111. Assion HJ, et al. Lymphocytopenia and thrombocytopenia during treatment with risperidone or clozapine. *Pharmacopsychiatry* 1996; 29:227–228.

112. Lee J, et al. The effect of clozapine on hematological indices: a 1-year follow-up study. *J Clin Psychopharmacol* 2015; 35:510–516.

113. Grover S, et al. Haematological side effects associated with clozapine: a retrospective study from India. *Asian J Psychiatr* 2020; 48:101906.

114. Kate N, et al. Clozapine associated thrombocytopenia. *J Pharmacol Pharmacother* 2013; 4:149–151.

115. Gonzales MF, et al. Evidence for immune etiology in clozapine-induced thrombocytopenia of 40 months' duration: a case report. *CNS Spectr* 2000; 5:17–18.

116. Hauseux PA, et al. Clozapine rechallenge after thrombocytopenia: a case report. *Schizophr Res* 2020; 222:477–479.

117. Hampson ME. Clozapine-induced thrombocytosis. *Br J Psychiatry* 2000; 176:400.

118. Warnock JK, et al. Adverse cutaneous reactions to antipsychotics. *Am J Clin Dermatol* 2002; 3:629–636.

119. Wu BY, et al. Prevalence and associated factors of comorbid skin diseases in patients with schizophrenia: a clinical survey and national health database study. *Gen Hosp Psychiatry* 2014; 36:415–421.

120. Voulgari C, et al. Clozapine-induced late agranulocytosis and severe neutropenia complicated with streptococcus pneumonia, venous thromboembolism, and allergic vasculitis in treatment-resistant female psychosis. *Case Rep Med* 2015. http://dx.doi.org/10.1155/2015/703218.

121. Penaskovic K, et al. Clozapine-induced allergic vasculitis (letter). *Am J Psychiatry* 2005; 162:1543–1542.

122. Mukherjee S, et al. Leukocytoclastic vasculitis secondary to clozapine. *Indian J Psychiatry* 2019; 61:94–96.

123. Fujimoto S, et al. Clozapine-induced antineutrophil cytoplasmic antibody-associated vasculitis: a case report. *Mod Rheumatol Case Rep* 2020; 4:70–73.

124. Wu MK, et al. The severe complication of Stevens-Johnson syndrome induced by long-term clozapine treatment in a male schizophrenia patient: a case report. *Neuropsychiatr Dis Treat* 2015; 11:1039–1041.

125. Lai YW, et al. Pityriasis rosea-like eruption associated with clozapine: a case report. *Gen Hosp Psychiatry* 2012; 34:703.e705–707.

126. Bhatia MS, et al. Clozapine induced pityriasiform eruption. *Indian J Dermatol* 1997; 42:245–246.

127. Stanislav SW, et al. Papular rash and bilateral pleural effusion associated with clozapine. *Ann Pharmacother* 1999; 33:1008–1009.

128. Bosonnet S, et al. [Acute generalized exanthematic pustulosis after intake of clozapine (leponex) First case]. *Ann Dermatol Venereol* 1997; 124:547–548.

129. Kleinen JM, et al. [Clozapine-induced agranulocytosis and Sweet's syndrome in a 74-year-old female patient A Case Study]. *Tijdschrift Voor Psychiatrie* 2008; 50:119–123.

130. Chate S, et al. Pulmonary thromboembolism associated with clozapine. *J Neuropsychiatry Clin Neurosci* 2013; 25:E3–6.

131. Srinivasaraju R, et al. Clozapine-associated cerebral venous thrombosis. *J Clin Psychopharmacol* 2010; 30:335–336.

132. Werring D, et al. Cerebral venous sinus thrombosis may be associated with clozapine. *J Neuropsychiatry Clin Neurosci* 2009; 21:343–345.

133. Paciullo CA. Evaluating the association between clozapine and venous thromboembolism. *Am J Health Syst Pharm* 2008; 65:1825–1829.

134. Yang TY, et al. Massive pulmonary embolism in a young patient on clozapine therapy. *J Emerg Med* 2004; 27:27–29.

135. Gami RK, et al. Pulmonary embolism and clozapine use: a case report and literature review. *Psychosomatics* 2017; 58:203–208.

136. Hagg S, et al. Risk of venous thromboembolism due to antipsychotic drug therapy. *Exp Opin Drug Saf* 2009; 8:537–547.

137. De Fazio P, et al. Rare and very rare adverse effects of clozapine. *Neuropsychiatr Dis Treat* 2015; 11:1995–2003.

138. Sarvaiya N, et al. Clozapine-associated pulmonary embolism: a high-mortality, dose-independent and early-onset adverse effect. *Am J Ther* 2018; 25:e434–e438.

139. Goh JG, et al. A case report of clozapine continuation after pulmonary embolism in the context of other risk factors for thromboembolism. *Aust N Z J Psychiatry* 2016; 50:1205–1206.

140. Munoli RN, et al. Clozapine-induced recurrent pulmonary thromboembolism. *J Neuropsychiatry Clin Neurosci* 2013; 25:E50–E51.

141. Selten JP, et al. Clozapine and venous thromboembolism: further evidence. *J Clin Psychiatry* 2003; 64:609.

Clozapine: serious haematological and cardiovascular adverse effects

Agranulocytosis, thromboembolism, cardiomyopathy and myocarditis

Clozapine is a somewhat toxic drug, but it may reduce overall mortality in schizophrenia,[1] largely because of a reduction in the rate of suicide.[2-4] Clozapine can cause serious, life-threatening adverse effects, of which **agranulocytosis** is the best known, and which is seen in 0.4% of clozapine patients.[5] The incidence of death related to agranulocytosis following clozapine prescription is 0.013%, with a case fatality rate of 2.1%.[6] Risk is clearly well managed by the approved clozapine monitoring systems and the incidence of severe neutropenia declines to negligible levels after the first year of treatment.[6] Successful rechallenge after clozapine-associated neutropenia may be possible,[7] but not after agranulocytosis.[8] Most neutropenia occurring in the context of clozapine treatment is coincidental to the use of clozapine.[9]

Thromboembolism

A possible association between clozapine and **thromboembolism** has been suggested.[10] Initially, Walker *et al.*[2] uncovered a risk of fatal pulmonary embolism of 1 in 4500 – about 20 times the risk in the population as a whole. Following a case report of non-fatal pulmonary embolism possibly related to clozapine,[11] data from the Swedish authorities were published.[12] Twelve cases of venous thromboembolism were described, of which five were fatal. The risk of thromboembolism was estimated to be 1 in 2000 to 1 in 6000 patients treated. Thromboembolism may be related to clozapine's observed effects on antiphospholipid antibodies[13] and platelet aggregation.[14] It seems most likely to occur in the first 6 months of treatment[15] but can occur at any time. The risk may be independent of dose,[15] but some studies suggest a correlation with higher doses.[16] Other antipsychotics are also strongly linked to thromboembolism, although clozapine may present the highest risk.[16,17]

With all drugs, the causes of thromboembolism are probably multifactorial.[18] Sedation may lead to a reduction in movement and consequent venous stasis. Obesity, hyperprolactinaemia and smoking are additional independent risk factors for thromboembolism.[19,20] Encouraging exercise and ensuring good hydration are essential precautionary measures.[21]

Myocarditis and cardiomyopathy

Clozapine is associated with **myocarditis** and **cardiomyopathy**. Myocarditis is a hypersensitivity response to clozapine, resulting in inflammation of the myocardium. Some debate surrounds the prevalence of myocarditis, with several Australian studies finding it to occur in around 3% of patients.[22-24] Studies conducted elsewhere[25-27] have suggested much a lower incidence of 1% or less. The reason for such variation in reported incidence is unclear; some authors propose that a lack of robust monitoring leads to missed diagnoses in those countries reporting lower incidences.[28] Meta-analysis suggests an event rate of less than 1% – 7 per 1000 patients.[29] Myocarditis is potentially fatal (case fatality rate of 12.7%[29]), and is most likely to occur in the first 6–8 weeks of starting clozapine treatment (median 3 weeks),[30] but may occur at any time.

Cardiomyopathy is usually diagnosed from echocardiography to establish left ventricular dilatation (resulting in a reduced ejection fraction) and/or hypertrophy. It may develop following myocarditis (if clozapine is not stopped), but other causative factors may include persistent tachycardia, obesity, diabetes, and previous personal or familial cardiac events.[28] Most incidence data originate from Australia, and range from 0.02% to 5%.[24,31] Meta-analysis suggests an event rate of 6 per 1000 patients, with a case fatality rate of 7.8%.[29] Cardiomyopathy may occur later in treatment than myocarditis (median 9 months),[30] but as with myocarditis it may occur at any time.

Despite uncertainty over incidence, patients should be closely monitored for signs of myocarditis, especially in the first few months of treatment.[32] Symptoms include hypotension, tachycardia, fever, flu-like symptoms, fatigue, dyspnoea (with increased respiratory rate) and chest pain.[33] Signs include ECG changes (ST depression), enlarged heart on radiography/echo and eosinophilia. Many of these symptoms occur in patients on clozapine not developing myocarditis[34] and conversely, their absence does not rule out myocarditis.[35] Nonetheless, signs of heart failure should provoke immediate cessation of clozapine and referral to a cardiologist. Rechallenge has been successfully completed[8,36–41] (the use of beta blockers, ACE inhibitors and mineralocorticoid receptor antagonists may help[42–44]), but recurrence is also possible.[45–48] Use of echocardiography, measurement of CRP and troponin are essential in cases of rechallenge.[49–51] Effective treatment of comorbid metabolic syndrome and diabetes may also help.[29]

Autopsy findings suggest that fatal myocarditis can occur in the absence of clear cardiac symptoms, although tachycardia and fever are usually present.[52] A group from Melbourne, Australia, has put forward a monitoring programme which is said to detect 100% of symptomatic cases of myocarditis[53] using measurement of troponin I or T and C-reactive protein (See Table 1.39). Echocardiography at baseline, six months and yearly thereafter is routine practice in Australia, although the benefit of this monitoring in the absence of other symptoms has been questioned.[54] Baseline echocardiography may at least be useful to establish a comparator if concerns arise later, especially in those with known cardiac disease, structural abnormalities, or other cardiac risk factors.[55] The absence of resources to provide monitoring beyond routine blood tests (including CRP and troponin) and ECG should not be a barrier to prescribing for most patients.[27]

Factors that may increase the risk of developing myocarditis include rapid dose increases, concurrent use of sodium valproate, and older age (31% increased risk for each additional decade).[56] Other psychotropics, including lithium, risperidone, haloperidol, chlorpromazine and fluphenazine have also been associated with myocarditis.[57] It is probably preferable to avoid concomitant use of other medicines that may contribute to the risk, but this may be practically difficult. Any pre-existing cardiac disorder, previous cardiac event, use of illicit drugs[23] or family history of cardiac disease should provoke extra caution.

Cardiomyopathy should be suspected in any patient showing signs of heart failure, which should provoke immediate cessation of clozapine and referral. Presentation of cardiomyopathy varies somewhat[58,59] and is often asymptomatic in the early stages,[24] so any reported symptoms of palpitations, chest pain, syncope, sweating, decreased exercise capacity or breathing difficulties should be closely investigated. Successful rechallenge with rigorous cardiac monitoring (including ECHO) and instigation of disease-modifying cardiac medications may be possible.[44,60,61]

Note also that, despite an overall reduction in mortality, younger patients may have an increased risk of sudden death,[62] perhaps because of clozapine-induced ECG changes.[63] The overall picture remains very unclear but caution is required. There may, of course, be similar problems with other antipsychotics.[57,64,65]

Summary

- Overall mortality is lower for those on clozapine than in schizophrenia as a whole.
- Risk of fatal agranulocytosis is less than 1 in 8000 during standard monitoring.
- Risk of fatal pulmonary embolism is estimated to be around 1 in 4500 patients treated.
- Risk of fatal myocarditis or cardiomyopathy may be as high as 1 in 1000 patients.
- Careful monitoring is essential during clozapine treatment, particularly during the first 3 months (see box).

Table 1.39 Suggested monitoring for myocarditis[52,53,66,67]

Baseline	Pulse, blood pressure, temperature, respiratory rate
	Full blood count (FBC)
	C-reactive protein (CRP)
	Troponin
	Echocardiography (if available)
	Electrocardiogram (ECG)
Daily, if possible	Pulse, blood pressure, temperature, respiratory rate
	Ask about: chest pain, fever, cough, shortness of breath, exercise capacity
On days 7, 14, 21, and 28	CRP
	Troponin
	FBC
	ECG if possible
If CRP > 100mg/L or troponin > twice upper limit of normal	Stop clozapine; repeat echo
If fever + tachycardia + raised CRP or troponin (but not as above)	Daily CRP and troponin measures

References

1. Vermeulen JM, et al. Clozapine and long-term mortality risk in patients with schizophrenia: a systematic review and meta-analysis of studies lasting 1.1–12.5 years. *Schizophr Bull* 2019; **45**:315–329.

2. Walker AM, et al. Mortality in current and former users of clozapine. *Epidemiology* 1997; **8**:671–677.

3. Van Der Zalm Y, et al. Clozapine and mortality: a comparison with other antipsychotics in a nationwide Danish cohort study. *Acta Psychiatr Scand* 2020: [Epub ahead of print].

4. Munro J, et al. Active monitoring of 12760 clozapine recipients in the UK and Ireland. *Br J Psychiatry* 1999; **175**:576–580.

5. Li XH, et al. The prevalence of agranulocytosis and related death in clozapine-treated patients: a comprehensive meta-analysis of observational studies. *Psychol Med* 2020; **50**:583–594.

6. Myles N, et al. Meta-analysis examining the epidemiology of clozapine-associated neutropenia. *Acta Psychiatr Scand* 2018; **138**:101–109.

7. Prokopez CR, et al. Clozapine rechallenge after neutropenia or leucopenia. *J Clin Psychopharmacol* 2016; **36**:377–380.

8. Manu P, et al. Clozapine rechallenge after major adverse effects: clinical guidelines based on 259 cases. *Am J Ther* 2018; **25**:e218–e223.

9. Oloyede E, et al. There is life after the UK clozapine central non-rechallenge database. *Schizophr Bull* 2021: sbab006 [Epub ahead of print].

10. Paciullo CA. Evaluating the association between clozapine and venous thromboembolism. *Am J Health Syst Pharm* 2008; **65**:1825–1829.

11. Lacika S, et al. Pulmonary embolus possibly associated with clozapine treatment (Letter). *Can J Psychiatry* 1999; **44**:396–397.

12. Hagg S, et al. Association of venous thromboembolism and clozapine. *Lancet* 2000; **355**:1155–1156.

13. Davis S, et al. Antiphospholipid antibodies associated with clozapine treatment. *Am J Hematol* 1994; **46**:166–167.

14. Axelsson S, et al. In vitro effects of antipsychotics on human platelet adhesion and aggregation and plasma coagulation. *Clin Exp Pharmacol Physiol* 2007; **34**:775–780.

15. Sarvaiya N, et al. Clozapine-associated pulmonary embolism: a high-mortality, dose-independent and early-onset adverse effect. *Am J Ther* 2018; **25**:e434–e438.

16. Allenet B, et al. Antipsychotic drugs and risk of pulmonary embolism. *PharmacoepidemiolDrug Saf* 2012; **21**:42–48.

17. Dai L, et al. The association and influencing factors between antipsychotics exposure and the risk of VTE and PE: a systematic review and meta-analysis. *Curr Drug Targets* 2020; **21**:930–942.

18. Lacut K. Association between antipsychotic drugs, antidepressant drugs, and venous thromboembolism. *Clin Adv Hematol Oncol* 2008; **6**:887–890.

19. Masopust J, et al. Risk of venous thromboembolism during treatment with antipsychotic agents. *Psychiatry Clin Neurosci* 2012; **66**:541–552.

20. Jonsson AK, et al. Venous thromboembolism in recipients of antipsychotics: incidence, mechanisms and management. *CNS Drugs* 2012; **26**:649–662.

21. Maly R, et al. Assessment of risk of venous thromboembolism and its possible prevention in psychiatric patients. *Psychiatry Clin Neurosci* 2008; **62**:3–8.

22. Ronaldson KJ. Cardiovascular disease in clozapine-treated patients: evidence, mechanisms and management. *CNS Drugs* 2017; **31**:777–795.

23. Khan AA, et al. Clozapine and incidence of myocarditis and sudden death – long term Australian experience. *Int J Cardiol* 2017; **238**:136–139.

24. Youssef DL, et al. Incidence and risk factors for clozapine-induced myocarditis and cardiomyopathy at a regional mental health service in Australia. *Austr Psychiatry* 2016; **24**:176–180.

25. Cohen D, et al. Beyond white blood cell monitoring: screening in the initial phase of clozapine therapy. *J Clin Psychiatry* 2012; **73**:1307–1312.

26. Kilian JG, et al. Myocarditis and cardiomyopathy associated with clozapine. *Lancet* 1999; **354**:1841–1845.

27. Freudenreich O. Clozapine-induced myocarditis: prescribe safely but do prescribe. *Acta Psychiatr Scand* 2015; **132**:240–241.

28. Ronaldson KJ, et al. Clozapine-induced myocarditis, a widely overlooked adverse reaction. *Acta Psychiatr Scand* 2015; **132**:231–240.

29. Siskind D, et al. Systematic review and meta-analysis of rates of clozapine-associated myocarditis and cardiomyopathy. *Aust N Z J Psychiatry* 2020; **54**:467–481.

30. La Grenade L, et al. Myocarditis and cardiomyopathy associated with clozapine use in the United States (Letter). *N Engl J Med* 2001; **345**:224–225.

31. Curto M, et al. Systematic review of clozapine cardiotoxicity. *Current Psychiatry Reports* 2016; **18**:68.

32. Marder SR, et al. Physical health monitoring of patients with schizophrenia. *Am J Psychiatry* 2004; **161**:1334–1349.

33. Annamraju S, et al. Early recognition of clozapine-induced myocarditis. *J Clin Psychopharmacol* 2007; **27**:479–483.

34. Wehmeier PM, et al. Chart review for potential features of myocarditis, pericarditis, and cardiomyopathy in children and adolescents treated with clozapine. *J Child Adolesc Psychopharmacol* 2004; **14**:267–271.

35. McNeil JJ, et al. Clozapine-induced myocarditis: characterisation using case-control design. *Eur Heart J* 2013; **34 (Suppl 1)**:688.

36. Reinders J, et al. Clozapine-related myocarditis and cardiomyopathy in an Australian metropolitan psychiatric service. *Aust N Z J Psychiatry* 2004; **38**:915–922.

37. Bellissima BL, et al. A systematic review of clozapine-induced myocarditis. *Int J Cardiol* 2018; **259**:122–129.

38. Nguyen B, et al. Successful clozapine re-challenge following myocarditis. *Austr Psychiatry* 2017; **25**:385–386.

39. Otsuka Y, et al. Clozapine-induced myocarditis: follow-up for 3.5 years after successful retrial. *J Gen Fam Med* 2019; **20**:114–117.

40. Noël MC, et al. Clozapine-related myocarditis and rechallenge: a case series and clinical review. *J Clin Psychopharmacol* 2019; **39**:380–385.

41. Hosseini SA, et al. Successful clozapine re-challenge after suspected clozapine-induced myocarditis. *Am J Case Rep* 2020; 21:e926507.

42. Rostagno C, et al. Beta-blocker and angiotensin-converting enzyme inhibitor may limit certain cardiac adverse effects of clozapine. *Gen Hosp Psychiatry* 2008; 30:280–283.

43. Floreani J, et al. Successful re-challenge with clozapine following development of clozapine-induced cardiomyopathy. *Aust N Z J Psychiatry* 2008; 42:747–748.

44. Patel RK, et al. Clozapine and cardiotoxicity – a guide for psychiatrists written by cardiologists. *Psychiatry Res* 2019; 282:112491.

45. Roh S, et al. Cardiomyopathy associated with clozapine. *Exp Clin Psychopharmacol* 2006; 14:94–98.

46. Masopust J, et al. Repeated occurrence of clozapine-induced myocarditis in a patient with schizoaffective disorder and comorbid Parkinson's disease. *Neuro Endocrinol Lett* 2009; 30:19–21.

47. Ronaldson KJ, et al. Observations from 8 cases of clozapine rechallenge after development of myocarditis. *JClinPsychiatry* 2012; 73:252–254.

48. Nielsen J, et al. Termination of clozapine treatment due to medical reasons: when is it warranted and how can it be avoided? *J Clin Psychiatry* 2013; 74:603–613; quiz 613.

49. Hassan I, et al. Monitoring in clozapine rechallenge after myocarditis. *Austr Psychiatry* 2011; 19:370–371.

50. Bray A, et al. Successful clozapine rechallenge after acute myocarditis. *Aust N Z J Psychiatry* 2011; 45:90.

51. Rosenfeld AJ, et al. Successful clozapine retrial after suspected myocarditis. *Am J Psychiatry* 2010; 167:350–351.

52. Ronaldson KJ, et al. Clinical course and analysis of ten fatal cases of clozapine-induced myocarditis and comparison with 66 surviving cases. *Schizophr Res* 2011; 128:161–165.

53. Ronaldson KJ, et al. A new monitoring protocol for clozapine-induced myocarditis based on an analysis of 75 cases and 94 controls. *Aust N Z J Psychiatry* 2011; 45:458–465.

54. Robinson G, et al. Echocardiography and clozapine: is current clinical practice inhibiting use of a potentially life-transforming therapy? *Aust Fam Physician* 2017; 46:169–170.

55. Knoph KN, et al. Clozapine-induced cardiomyopathy and myocarditis monitoring: a systematic review. *Schizophr Res* 2018; 199:17–30.

56. Ronaldson KJ, et al. Rapid clozapine dose titration and concomitant sodium valproate increase the risk of myocarditis with clozapine: a case-control study. *Schizophr Res* 2012; 141:173–178.

57. Coulter DM, et al. Antipsychotic drugs and heart muscle disorder in international pharmacovigilance: data mining study. *BMJ* 2001; 322:1207–1209.

58. Pastor CA, et al. Masked clozapine-induced cardiomyopathy. *J Am Board Fam Med* 2008; 21:70–74.

59. Sagar R, et al. Clozapine-induced cardiomyopathy presenting as panic attacks. *J Psychiatr Pract* 2008; 14:182–185.

60. Nederlof M, et al. Clozapine re-exposure after dilated cardiomyopathy. *BMJ Case Rep* 2017; 2017:bcr2017219652.

61. Alawami M, et al. A systematic review of clozapine induced cardiomyopathy. *Int J Cardiol* 2014; 176:315–320.

62. Modai I, et al. Sudden death in patients receiving clozapine treatment: a preliminary investigation. *J Clin Psychopharmacol* 2000; 20:325–327.

63. Kang UG, et al. Electrocardiographic abnormalities in patients treated with clozapine. *J Clin Psychiatry* 2000; 61:441–446.

64. Thomassen R, et al. Antipsychotic drugs and venous thromboembolism (Letter). *Lancet* 2000; 356:252.

65. Hagg S, et al. Antipsychotic-induced venous thromboembolism: a review of the evidence. *CNS Drugs* 2002; 16:765–776.

66. Ronaldson KJ, et al. Diagnostic characteristics of clozapine-induced myocarditis identified by an analysis of 38 cases and 47 controls. *J Clin Psychiatry* 2010; 71:976–981.

67. Yuen JWY, et al. Clozapine-induced cardiovascular side effects and autonomic dysfunction: a systematic review. *Front Neurosci* 2018; 12:203.

Clozapine-induced hypersalivation

Clozapine is well known to be causally associated with hypersalivation (sialorrhoea)[1] with excess salivary pooling in the mouth and drooling, particularly at night. The problem tends to occur in the early stages of treatment and is probably dose-related. Hypersalivation has been found to be more common in those prescribed standard doses of clozapine rather than low dosage[2] and to be associated with elevated plasma clozapine concentrations.[3] Clinical observation suggests that hypersalivation reduces somewhat in severity over time (usually several months) but may persist. Clozapine-induced hypersalivation is socially embarrassing, has a negative impact on quality of life[1] and, given that it has been implicated as a contributory factor in the development of aspiration pneumonia, could be potentially life-threatening.[4-7] So treatment is a matter of some urgency.

The pharmacological basis of clozapine-related hypersalivation remains unclear.[8] Suggested mechanisms include muscarinic M_4 agonism, adrenergic α_2 antagonism, and inhibition of the swallowing reflex.[9,10] The last of these is supported by trials which suggest that saliva production is not increased in clozapine-treated patients,[11,12] although at least one study has observed marked increases in salivary flow in the first three weeks of treatment.[13]

Whatever the mechanism, medications that reduce saliva production might be expected to diminish the severity of clozapine-induced sialorrhoea. However, there are no medications licensed for this condition, and many of the relevant published studies have limitations that preclude any confident treatment recommendations.[14] The evidence, such as it is, tends to favour anti-muscarinic agents, such as propantheline and diphenhydramine.[15,16] Use of antimuscarinic agents should take account of the risk of compounding clozapine's liability for serious, potentially life-threatening, gastrointestinal hypomotility.[17,18] Table 1.40 describes putative pharmacological treatments that have been examined. Non-drug treatments may be used if appropriate – these include chewing gum during the day, elevating pillows and placing a towel on the pillow to prevent soaking.[8]

Table 1.40 Clozapine-related hypersalivation – summary

Treatment	Comments
Amisulpride 100–400mg/day[16,19,20]	Supported by a positive RCT compared with placebo, one other in which it was compared with moclobemide and numerous case studies.[21-25] May allow dose reduction of clozapine
Amitriptyline 25–100mg/day[26-28]	Limited literature support. Adverse effects may be troublesome. Worsens constipation
Atropine given sublingually[29-33] or as solution (1mg/10ml) used as a mouthwash	Limited literature support and benefit-risk uncertain. Rarely used. Problems with administration have been reported[34]

(Continued)

CHAPTER 1

Table 1.40 (*Continued*)

Treatment	Comments
Benzhexol (trihexyphenidyl) 5–15mg/day[35]	Small, open study suggests useful activity. Used in some centres but may impair cognitive function. Lower doses (2mg) may be effective[36]
Benzatropine 2mg/day + **terazosin** 2mg/day[37]	Combination shown to be better than either drug alone. Terazosin is an α_1 antagonist so it may cause hypotension.
Botulinum toxin[38–41] (Botox) Bilateral parotid gland injections (150 IU into each gland)	Effective in treating sialorrhoea associated with neurological disorders. Six cases of successful treatment of clozapine-related hypersalivation in the literature
Bupropion 100–150mg/day[42]	Single case report. May lower seizure threshold
Chlorphenamine[16]	Antihistamine and relatively weak antimuscarinic. One high-quality study
Clonidine 0.1–0.2mg patch weekly or 0.1mg orally at night[43,44]	α_2 partial agonist. Limited literature support. May exacerbate psychosis, depression and cause hypotension
Diphenhydramine[15,16]	Antihistamine and potent antimuscarinic. Few high-quality studies
Glycopyrrolate 0.5mg to 4mg BD[45–49]	One RCT showed glycopyrrolate to be more effective than biperiden without worsening cognitive function while another found significant clinical improvement of 'nocturnal sialorrhoea' with 2mg a day compared with placebo
Guanfacine 1mg daily[50]	α_2 agonist. Single case report. May cause hypotension
Hyoscine 0.3mg tablet sucked or chewed up to 3 times daily or 1.5mg/72 hours patch[51–54]	Peripheral and central anticholinergic. Very widely used but only one double-blind RCT. May cause cognitive impairment, drowsiness and worsen constipation
Ipratropium Nasal spray (0.03% or 0.06%) – given sublingually up to 2 sprays three times a day of the 0.06% or intranasally, 1 spray into each nostril daily of the 0.03%[55,56]	Limited literature support. The only placebo-controlled RCT conducted was negative[57]
Lofexidine 0.2mg twice daily[58]	α_2 agonist. Very few data. May exacerbate psychosis, depression and cause hypotension
Metoclopramide Starting dose of 10mg a day[16,59,60]	Double-blind, placebo-controlled trial found metoclopramide was associated with a significant reduction in nocturnal hypersalivation and drooling.
Moclobemide 150–300mg/day[45]	Effective in 9 of 14 patients treated in one open study. Appears to be as effective as amisulpride (see above)
N-Acetylcysteine[61]	An antioxidant that also modulates glutamatergic, neurotrophic and inflammatory pathways. Small case series reported with significant decrease in sialorrhea.

CHAPTER 1

Table 1.40 *(Continued)*

Treatment	Comments
Oxybutynin 5mg up to twice daily[62]	Single case report
Pirenzepine 50–150mg/day[63–65]	Selective M_1, M_4 antagonist. Extensive clinical experience suggests efficacy in some but only randomised trial suggested no effect. Still widely used. Does not have a UK licence for any indication. May cause constipation.
Propantheline 7.5mg at night[15,16]	Peripheral anticholinergic. No central effects. Two RCTs (one positive). May worsen constipation
Quetiapine[51]	May reduce hypersalivation by allowing lower doses of clozapine to be used
Sulpiride 150–300mg/day[5,16,66,67]	Supported by one, small positive RCT and a Cochrane Review of clozapine augmentation with sulpiride (at higher sulpiride doses). May allow dose reduction of clozapine

References

1. Man WH, et al. Reporting patterns of sialorrhea comparing users of clozapine to users of other antipsychotics: a disproportionality analysis using vigibase. *J Clin Psychopharmacol* 2020; 40:283–286.
2. Subramanian S, et al. Clozapine dose for schizophrenia. *Cochrane Database Syst Rev* 2017; 6:Cd009555.
3. Schoretsanitis G, et al. Elevated clozapine concentrations in clozapine-treated patients with hypersalivation. *Clin Pharmacokinet* 2021; 60:329–335.
4. Hinkes R, et al. Aspiration pneumonia possibly secondary to clozapine-induced sialorrhea. *J Clin Psychopharmacol* 1996; 16:462–463.
5. Saenger RC, et al. Aspiration pneumonia due to clozapine-induced sialorrhea. *Clin Schizophr Relat Psychoses* 2016; 9:170–172.
6. Gurrera RJ, et al. Aspiration pneumonia: an underappreciated risk of clozapine treatment. *J Clin Psychopharmacol* 2016; 36:174–176.
7. Kaplan J, et al. Clozapine-associated aspiration pneumonia: case series and review of the literature. *Psychosomatics* 2017; 58:199–203.
8. Praharaj SK, et al. Clozapine-induced sialorrhea: pathophysiology and management strategies. *Psychopharmacology* 2006; 185:265–273.
9. Davydov L, et al. Clozapine-induced hypersalivation. *Ann Pharmacother* 2000; 34:662–665.
10. Rogers DP, et al. Therapeutic options in the treatment of clozapine-induced sialorrhea. *Pharmacotherapy* 2000; 20:1092–1095.
11. Rabinowitz T, et al. The effect of clozapine on saliva flow rate: a pilot study. *Biol Psychiatry* 1996; 40:1132–1134.
12. Ben Aryeh H, et al. Salivary flow-rate and composition in schizophrenic patients on clozapine: subjective reports and laboratory data. *Biol Psychiatry* 1996; 39:946–949.
13. Praharaj SK, et al. Salivary flow rate in patients with schizophrenia on clozapine. *Clin Neuropharmacol* 2010; 33:176–178.
14. Sockalingam S, et al. Review: insufficient evidence to guide use of drugs for clozapine induced hypersalivation. *Evid Based Ment Health* 2009; 12:12.
15. Syed R, et al. Pharmacological interventions for clozapine-induced hypersalivation. *Cochrane Database Syst Rev* 2008; Cd005579.
16. Chen SY, et al. Treatment strategies for clozapine-induced sialorrhea: a systematic review and meta-analysis. *CNS Drugs* 2019; 33:225–238.
17. Palmer SE, et al. Life-threatening clozapine-induced gastrointestinal hypomotility: an analysis of 102 cases. *J Clin Psychiatry* 2008; 69:759–768.
18. West S, et al. Clozapine induced gastrointestinal hypomotility: a potentially life threatening adverse event. A review of the literature. *Gen Hosp Psychiatry* 2017; 46:32–37.
19. Kreinin A, et al. Amisulpride treatment of clozapine-induced hypersalivation in schizophrenia patients: a randomized, double-blind, placebo-controlled cross-over study. *Int Clin Psychopharmacol* 2006; 21:99–103.
20. Kreinin A, et al. Amisulpride versus moclobemide in treatment of clozapine-induced hypersalivation. *World J Biol Psychiatry* 2010; 12:620–626.

21. Praharaj SK, et al. Amisulpride treatment for clozapine-induced sialorrhea. *J Clin Psychopharmacol* 2009; **29**:189–190.

22. Aggarwal A, et al. Amisulpride for clozapine induced sialorrhea. *Psychopharmacol Bull* 2009; **42**:69–71.

23. Croissant B, et al. Reduction of side effects by combining clozapine with amisulpride: case report and short review of clozapine-induced hypersalivation-a case report. *Pharmacopsychiatry* 2005; **38**:38–39.

24. Praharaj SK, et al. Amisulpride improved debilitating clozapine-induced sialorrhea. *Am J Ther* 2011; **18**:e84–e85.

25. Kulkarni RR. Low-dose amisulpride for debilitating clozapine-induced sialorrhea: case series and review of literature. *Indian J Psychol Med* 2015; **37**:446–448.

26. Copp P, et al. Amitriptyline in clozapine-induced sialorrhoea. *Br J Psychiatry* 1991; **159**:166.

27. Praharaj SK, et al. Amitriptyline for clozapine-induced nocturnal enuresis and sialorrhoea. *Br J Clin Pharmacol* 2007; **63**:128–129.

28. Sinha S, et al. Very low dose amitriptyline for clozapine-associated sialorrhea. *Curr Drug Saf* 2016; **11**:262–263.

29. Antonello C, et al. Clozapine and sialorrhea: a new intervention for this bothersome and potentially dangerous side effect. *J Psychiatry Neurosci* 1999; **24**:250.

30. Mustafa FA, et al. Sublingual atropine for the treatment of severe and hyoscine-resistant clozapine-induced sialorrhea. *Afr J Psychiatry* 2013; **16**:242.

31. Matos Santana TE, et al. Sublingual atropine in the treatment of clozapine-induced sialorrhea. *Schizophr Res* 2017; **182**:144–145.

32. Mubaslat O, et al. The effect of sublingual atropine sulfate on clozapine-induced hypersalivation: a multicentre, randomised placebo-controlled trial. *Psychopharmacology* 2020; **237**:2905–2915.

33. Van Der Poorten T, et al. The sublingual use of atropine in the treatment of clozapine-induced sialorrhea: a systematic review. *Clin Case Rep* 2019; **7**:2108–2113.

34. Leung JG, et al. Potential problems surrounding the use of sublingually administered ophthalmic atropine for sialorrhea. *Schizophr Res* 2017; **185**:202–203.

35. Spivak B, et al. Trihexyphenidyl treatment of clozapine-induced hypersalivation. *Int Clin Psychopharmacol* 1997; **12**:213–215.

36. Praharaj SK, et al. Complete resolution of clozapine-induced sialorrhea with low dose trihexyphenidyl. *Psychopharmacol Bull* 2010; **43**:73–75.

37. Reinstein M, et al. Comparative efficacy and tolerability of benzatropine and terazosin in the treatment of hypersalivation secondary to clozapine. *Clin Drug Investig* 1999; **17**:97–102.

38. Kahl KG, et al. Botulinum toxin as an effective treatment of clozapine-induced hypersalivation. *Psychopharmacology* 2004; **173**:229–230.

39. Steinlechner S, et al. Botulinum toxin B as an effective and safe treatment for neuroleptic-induced sialorrhea. *Psychopharmacology* 2010; **207**:593–597.

40. Kahl KG, et al. [Pharmacological strategies for clozapine-induced hypersalivation: treatment with botulinum toxin B in one patient and review of the literature]. *Nervenarzt* 2005; **76**:205–208.

41. Verma R, et al. Botulinum toxin: a novel therapy for clozapine-induced sialorrhoea. *Psychopharmacology* 2018; **235**:369–371.

42. Stern RG, et al. Clozapine-induced sialorrhea alleviated by bupropion–a case report. *Prog Neuropsychopharmacol Biol Psychiatry* 2009; **33**:1578–1580.

43. Grabowski J. Clonidine treatment of clozapine-induced hypersalivation. *J Clin Psychopharmacol* 1992; **12**:69–70.

44. Praharaj SK, et al. Is clonidine useful for treatment of clozapine-induced sialorrhea? *Journal of Psychopharmacology* 2005; **19**:426–428.

45. Duggal HS. Glycopyrrolate for clozapine-induced sialorrhea. *Prog Neuropsychopharmacol Biol Psychiatry* 2007; **31**:1546–1547.

46. Robb AS, et al. Glycopyrrolate for treatment of clozapine-induced sialorrhea in three adolescents. *J Child Adolesc Psychopharmacol* 2008; **18**:99–107.

47. Liang CS, et al. Comparison of the efficacy and impact on cognition of glycopyrrolate and biperiden for clozapine-induced sialorrhea in schizophrenic patients: a randomized, double-blind, crossover study. *Schizophr Res* 2010; **119**:138–144.

48. Man WH, et al. The effect of glycopyrrolate on nocturnal sialorrhea in patients using clozapine: a randomized, crossover, double-blind, placebo-controlled trial. *J Clin Psychopharmacol* 2017; **37**:155–161.

49. Praharaj SK, et al. Low-dose glycopyrrolate for clozapine-associated sialorrhea. *J Clin Psychopharmacol* 2014; **34**:392.

50. Webber MA, et al. Guanfacine treatment of clozapine-induced sialorrhea. *J Clin Psychopharmacol* 2004; **24**:675–676.

51. McKane JP, et al. Hyoscine patches in clozapine-induced hypersalivation. *Psychiatric Bulletin* 2001; **25**:277.

52. Gaftanyuk O, et al. Scolpolamine patch for clozapine-induced sialorrhea. *Psychiatr Serv* 2004; **55**:318.

53. Segev A, et al. Hyoscine for clozapine-induced hypersalivation: a double-blind, randomized, placebo-controlled cross-over trial. *Int Clin Psychopharmacol* 2019; **34**:101–107.

54. Takeuchi I, et al. Effect of scopolamine butylbromide on clozapine-induced hypersalivation in schizophrenic patients: a case series. *Clin Psychopharmacol Neurosci* 2015; **13**:109–112.

55. Calderon J, et al. Potential use of ipatropium bromide for the treatment of clozapine-induced hypersalivation: a preliminary report. *Int Clin Psychopharmacol* 2000; **15**:49–52.

56. Freudenreich O, et al. Clozapine-induced sialorrhea treated with sublingual ipratropium spray: a case series. *J Clin Psychopharmacol* 2004; **24**:98–100.

57. Sockalingam S, et al. Treatment of clozapine-induced hypersalivation with ipratropium bromide: a randomized, double-blind, placebo-controlled crossover study. *J Clin Psychiatry* 2009; **70**:1114–1119.

58. Corrigan FM, et al. Clozapine-induced hypersalivation and the alpha 2 adrenoceptor. *Br J Psychiatry* 1995; **167**:412.

59. Kreinin A, et al. Double-blind, randomized, placebo-controlled trial of metoclopramide for hypersalivation associated with clozapine. *J Clin Psychopharmacol* 2016; **36**:200–205.

60. Hallahan B. Metoclopramide may be effective for clozapine-induced hypersalivation. *Evid Based Ment Health* 2016; **19**:124.

61. Uzun Ö, et al. Effect of N-acetylcysteine on clozapine-induced sialorrhea in schizophrenic patients: a case series. *Int Clin Psychopharmacol* 2020; **35**:229–231.

62. Leung JG, et al. Immediate-release oxybutynin for the treatment of clozapine-induced sialorrhea. *Ann Pharmacother* 2011; **45**:e45.

63. Fritze J, et al. Pirenzepine for clozapine-induced hypersalivation. *Lancet* 1995; **346**:1034.

64. Bai YM, et al. Therapeutic effect of pirenzepine for clozapine-induced hypersalivation: a randomized, double-blind, placebo-controlled, cross-over study. *J Clin Psychopharmacol* 2001; **21**:608–611.

65. Schneider B, et al. Reduction of clozapine-induced hypersalivation by pirenzepine is safe. *Pharmacopsychiatry* 2004; **37**:43–45.

66. Kreinin A, et al. Sulpiride addition for the treatment of clozapine-induced hypersalivation: preliminary study. *Isr J Psychiatry Relat Sci* 2005; **42**:61–63.

67. Wang J, et al. Sulpiride augmentation for schizophrenia. *Cochrane Database Syst Rev* 2010; CD008125.

Clozapine-induced gastrointestinal hypomotility (CIGH)

Constipation is a common adverse effect of clozapine treatment with a prevalence of more than 30%, three times that is seen with other antipsychotics.[1] The mechanism of action is not completely understood but is thought to be a combination of the drug's anticholinergic[2,3] and antihistaminergic properties,[4] which are further complicated by antagonism at 5-HT3 receptors.[2,3,5] In addition, clozapine-induced sedation can result in a sedentary lifestyle,[4] which is itself a risk factor for constipation. Clozapine causes constipation by slowing transit time through the gut. Mean transit times are four times longer than normal and 80% of clozapine patients show reduced transit time.[6]

Clozapine-induced constipation is much more common than blood dyscrasias, and mortality rates are also higher.[4] When constipation is severe, the case fatality rate is around 20–30%.[4,7,8] The most recent (and largest) study[9] found an incidence of 37/10,000 cases of severe hypomotility and 7/10,000 constipation-related death. Case fatality was 18%. Enhanced monitoring of CIGH is clearly needed to reduce the likelihood of constipation-related fatality.

A gastrointestinal history and abdominal examination is recommended prior to starting treatment and if the patient is constipated, clozapine should not be initiated until this has resolved.[8] CIGH is most severe during the first four months of treatment,[8] but may occur at any time. Adopting the Rome III criteria[10] at routine FBCs might be a successful strategy to combat preventable deaths due to CIGH, although even this does not guarantee identification of hypomotility.[11]

Opinions differ on the relationship between clozapine dose and constipation, and between clozapine plasma level and constipation.[8,12,13] However, deaths that have occurred as a result of CIGH had higher than average daily doses (mean 535mg/day).[8,14] At the time of death, median duration of clozapine treatment is 2.5 years.[9] Older age, male sex and higher daily doses have been proposed as possible risk factors for death based on case series review (Table 1.41).[14]

Table 1.41 Risk factors for developing clozapine-induced constipation[8,15–18]

Increasing age
Female sex
Anticholinergic medication
Higher clozapine dose/plasma level (consider the effect of interacting drugs or stopping smoking)
Hypercalcaemia
Gastrointestinal disease
Obesity
Diaphoresis
Low fibre diet
Poor bowel habit
Dehydration (exacerbated by hypersalivation)
Diabetes
Hypothyroidism
Parkinson's disease
Multiple sclerosis

Prevention and simple management of CIGH

A slow clozapine titration may reduce the risk of developing constipation, with dose increments not exceeding 25mg/day or 100mg/week.[19] Increasing dietary fibre intake to at least 20–25g per day can increase stool weight and but can decrease gut transit time[18,20] (fibre decreases or increases transit time depending on the initial transit time[21]). If fibre intake is increased it is important that adequate fluid intake (1.5–2L/day) is also maintained to avoid intestinal obstruction.[8,18,22] Daily food and fluid charts would be ideal to monitor fibre and fluid intake especially during the titration phase of clozapine. Regular exercise (150 minutes/week)[23] in addition to a high fibre diet and increased fluid intake also assist in the prevention of CIGH.[24,25]

Active monitoring of patients, including direct questioning, is essential. Patients often do not self-report even life-threatening constipation.[8] Use of stool charts daily for the first 4 weeks, and weekly or monthly thereafter is recommended. If there is a change from usual baseline bowel habit or fewer than three bowel movements (BM) per week[10] an abdominal examination is indicated.[8] Where this excludes intestinal obstruction, both a stimulant and stool-softening laxative should be started, as suggested by the Porirua Protocol[26] (e.g. senna 15mg nocte and docusate 100mg three times daily[8,26,27]). Bulk forming laxatives are not usually effective in slow-transit constipation[2,28] and therefore should be avoided. There is some evidence that lactulose and polyethylene glycol (e.g. Movicol) are effective[2,29] and could be considered in addition to the stimulant and softener combination.[26] Most people with CIGH will need a stimulant laxative such as senna or bisacodyl. These should not be withheld on the basis that long-term use of stimulants is usually proscribed.

Choice of laxative should also be guided by the patient's previous response to certain agents in association with consideration of the required speed of action.[30] It would not be appropriate, for example, to start lactulose treatment (which takes up to 72 hours of regular use to work[31]) for someone in need of urgent treatment. Stimulant laxatives are usually the fastest acting (6–10 hours). Laxative doses should be increased every 48 hours until resolution of symptoms (usual maximum dose of senna is 30mg, docusate 500mg). Glycerin suppositories (2x4g) can be used and are usually effective within 30 minutes, but there are no data on their use in CIGH. It fact, it should be noted that published data supporting laxative choice for antipsychotic-related constipation are sparse and of poor quality.[11]

Management of suspected acute CIGH

Signs and symptoms that warrant immediate medical attention are abdominal pain, distension, vomiting, overflow diarrhoea, absent bowel sounds, acute abdomen, feculent vomitus and symptoms of sepsis.[7,8,19,32–39] There have been case reports of fatalities occurring only hours after first symptoms present,[40] and this emphasises the urgency for prompt assessment and management (including cessation of clozapine). There should therefore be a low threshold for referral to a gastroenterologist and/or A&E when conservative management fails or constipation is severe and acute.[8,41]

Clozapine re-challenge following severe constipation

Some patients have been successfully re-challenged following severe cases of CIGH, however, this process does not come without risk. Prophylactic measures should therefore be used for those with a history of CIGH or who are deemed high risk of developing CIGH. Minimise the use of other constipating drugs and ensure other modifiable risk factors are addressed (fibre and fluid intake, exercise). Where conventional laxatives have not been tried in regular and adequate doses, this should be done. However, when this approach has previously failed, a number of more experimental options are available. Prescribers must familiarise themselves with the literature (at the very least by reading the SPC) before using any of these treatments and involvement of gastrointestinal specialists is encouraged.

The prostaglandin E1 analogue **lubiprostone** was licensed in the UK (it was discontinued in 2018 for commercial reasons) for the treatment of chronic idiopathic constipation and associated symptoms in adults, when response to diet and other non-pharmacological measures (e.g. educational measures, physical activity) are inappropriate.[42] The recommended dose for the previously licensed indication is 24 micrograms twice daily for a maximum of 2 weeks duration.[42] Lubiprostone has been reported to be effective in obviating the need for other laxatives in a clozapine re-challenge following a severe case of CIGH,[43] and is used in some centres for this indication.[43]

Orlistat, a drug used to aid weight loss, is also known to have a laxative effect particularly when a high-fat diet is consumed. It was reported as being successfully used for three patients with severe constipation associated with opioid use (hypomotility-induced constipation).[44] A small, randomised placebo-controlled study of orlistat for clozapine-induced constipation found a statistically significant favourable difference at study endpoint (week 16) for the prevalence of constipation, diarrhoea, and normal stools for orlistat compared with placebo,[45] although 47 of the 54 participants required conventional laxatives. Note also that orlistat is known to reduce the absorption of some drugs from the GI tract. It is therefore important to monitor plasma clozapine levels if starting treatment with orlistat. Orlistat may be particularly difficult to use outside clinical study settings as without adherence to a strict low fat diet, gastric side effects can be unpleasant (specifically, oily rectal leakage).

Bethanechol, a cholinergic agonist, has been described as being effective in reducing the amount of laxatives and enemas required to maintain regular bowel movements for a patient diagnosed with clozapine-related CIGH.[46] Bethanechol, in this case, was used at a dose of 10mg TDS. It should only ever be initiated after other options have failed and in consultation with a gastroenterologist.[46]

Prucalopride is a 5HT4 agonist which increases gut motility, and is licensed for chronic constipation where laxatives have failed to provide adequate relief. Case reports of successful use for clozapine-induced constipation have been described,[47,48] and superior efficacy to lactulose for this indication was demonstrated in an open-label study.[49]

Linaclotide (licensed in the UK for constipation in irritable bowel syndrome) and **plecanatide** (available in the US for chronic idiopathic constipation) are oral guanylate cyclase C agonists. Neither has any published data to date supporting use in antipsychotic-induced constipation.

References

1. Shirazi A, et al. Prevalence and predictors of clozapine-associated constipation: a systematic review and meta-analysis. *Int J Molecular Sci* 2016; 17:863.
2. Hibbard KR, et al. Fatalities associated with clozapine-related constipation and bowel obstruction: a literature review and two case reports. *Psychosomatics* 2009; 50:416–419.
3. Rege S, et al. Life-threatening constipation associated with clozapine. *Austr Psychiatry* 2008; 16:216–219.

4. De Hert M, et al. Second-generation antipsychotics and constipation: a review of the literature. *Eur Psychiatry* 2011; 26:34–44.

5. Meltzer HY, et al. Effects of antipsychotic drugs on serotonin receptors. *Pharmacol Rev* 1991; 43:587–604.

6. Every-Palmer S, et al. Clozapine-treated patients have marked gastrointestinal hypomotility, the probable basis of life-threatening gastrointestinal complications: a cross sectional study. *E Bio Med* 2016; 5:125–134.

7. Cohen D, et al. Beyond white blood cell monitoring: screening in the initial phase of clozapine therapy. *J Clin Psychiatry* 2012; 73:1307–1312.

8. Palmer SE, et al. Life-threatening clozapine-induced gastrointestinal hypomotility: an analysis of 102 cases. *J Clin Psychiatry* 2008; 69:759–768.

9. Every-Palmer S, et al. Clozapine-induced gastrointestinal hypomotility: a 22-year bi-national pharmacovigilance study of serious or fatal 'slow gut' reactions, and comparison with international drug safety advice. *CNS Drugs* 2017; 31:699–709.

10. Rome Foundation. Rome IV disorders and criteria. 2020; https://theromefoundation.org.

11. Every-Palmer S, et al. Pharmacological treatment for antipsychotic-related constipation. *Cochrane Database Syst Rev* 2017; 1:Cd011128.

12. Chengappa KN, et al. Anticholinergic differences among patients receiving standard clinical doses of olanzapine or clozapine. *J Clin Psychopharmacol* 2000; 20:311–316.

13. Vella-Brincat J, et al. Clozapine-induced gastrointestinal hypomotility. *Austr Psychiatry* 2011; 19:450–451.

14. West S, et al. Clozapine induced gastrointestinal hypomotility: a potentially life threatening adverse event. A review of the literature. *Gen Hosp Psychiatry* 2017; 46:32–37.

15. Nielsen J, et al. Termination of clozapine treatment due to medical reasons: when is it warranted and how can it be avoided? *J Clin Psychiatry* 2013; 74:603–613; quiz 613.

16. Nielsen J, et al. Risk factors for ileus in patients with schizophrenia. *Schizophr Bull* 2012; 38:592–598.

17. Longmore M, et al. *Oxford handbook of clinical medicine*. Oxford, UK: OUP Oxford; 2010.

18. ZTAS. Zaponex fact sheet – constipation. 2013; https://dokumen.tips/documents/zaponex-fact-sheet-constipation-ztascom-aj-van-beelen-phd-december-2013-m.html.

19. Hayes G, et al. Clozapine-induced constipation. *Am J Psychiatry* 1995; 152:298.

20. Muller-Lissner SA. Effect of wheat bran on weight of stool and gastrointestinal transit time: a meta analysis *Br Med J (Clin Res Ed)* 1988; 296:615–617.

21. Harvey RF, et al. Effects of increased dietary fibre on intestinal transit. *Lancet* 1973; 1:1278–1280.

22. National Prescribing Centre. The management of constipation. *MedRec Bulletin* 2011; 21:1–8.

23. NHS. Exercise: physical activity guidelines for adults aged 19 to 64. 2019; https://www.nhs.uk/live-well/exercise.

24. Fitzsimons J, et al. A review of clozapine safety. *Expert Opinion on Drug Safety* 2005; 4:731–744.

25. Young CR, et al. Management of the adverse effects of clozapine. *Schizophr Bull* 1998; 24:381–390.

26. Every-Palmer S, et al. The porirua protocol in the treatment of clozapine-induced gastrointestinal hypomotility and constipation: a pre- and post-treatment study. *CNS Drugs* 2017; 31:75–85.

27. Swegle JM, et al. Management of common opioid-induced adverse effects. *Am Fam Physician* 2006; 74:1347–1354.

28. Voderholzer WA, et al. Clinical response to dietary fiber treatment of chronic constipation. *Am J Gastroenterol* 1997; 92:95–98.

29. Brandt LJ, et al. Systematic review on the management of chronic constipation in North America. *Am J Gastroenterol* 2005; 100 Suppl 1:S5–S21.

30. Bleakley S, et al. *Clozapine handbook*. Warwickshire, UK: Lloyd-Reinhold Communications LLP; 2013.

31. Intrapharm Laboratories Limited. Summary of Product Characteristics. Lactulose 10 g/15 ml oral solution sachets. 2017; https://www.medicines.org.uk/emc/medicine/25597.

32. Leong QM, et al. Necrotising colitis related to clozapine? A rare but life threatening side effect. *World J Emerg Surg* 2007; 2:21.

33. Shammi CM, et al. Clozapine-induced necrotizing colitis. *J Clin Psychopharmacol* 1997; 17:230–232.

34. Rondla S, et al. A case of clozapine-induced paralytic ileus. *Emerg Med J* 2007; 24:e12.

35. Levin TT, et al. Death from clozapine-induced constipation: case report and literature review. *Psychosomatics* 2002; 43:71–73.

36. Townsend G, et al. Case report: rapidly fatal bowel ischaemia on clozapine treatment. *BMC Psychiatry* 2006; 6:43.

37. Karmacharya R, et al. Clozapine-induced eosinophilic colitis. *Am J Psychiatry* 2005; 162:1386–1387.

38. Erickson B, et al. Clozapine-associated postoperative ileus: case report and review of the literature. *Arch Gen Psychiatry* 1995; 52:508–509.

39. Schwartz BJ, et al. A case report of clozapine-induced gastric outlet obstruction. *Am J Psychiatry* 1993; 150:1563.

40. Drew L, et al. Clozapine and constipation: a serious issue. *Aust N Z J Psychiatry* 1997; 31:149.

41. Ikai S, et al. Reintroduction of clozapine after perforation of the large intestine–a case report and review of the literature. *Ann Pharmacother* 2013; 47:e31.

42. National Institute for Clinical Excellence. Final appraisal determination – lubiprostone for treating chronic idiopathic constipation. 2014; https://www.nice.org.uk/guidance/ta318/documents/constipation-chronic-idiopathic-lubiprostone-final-appraisal-determination-document2.

43. Meyer JM, et al. Lubiprostone for treatment-resistant constipation associated with clozapine use. *Acta Psychiatr Scand* 2014; 130:71–72.

44. Guarino AH. Treatment of intractable constipation with orlistat: a report of three cases *Pain Med* 2005; 6:327–328.

45. Chukhin E, et al. In a randomized placebo-controlled add-on study orlistat significantly reduced clozapine-induced constipation. *Int Clin Psychopharmacol* 2013; 28:67–70.

46. Poetter CE, et al. Treatment of clozapine-induced constipation with bethanechol. *J Clin Psychopharmacol* 2013; 33:713–714.

47. Thomas N, et al. Prucalopride in clozapine-induced constipation. *Aust N Z J Psychiatry* 2018; 52:804.

48. Hui H. Prucalopride for the treatment of clozapine induced constipation: a case report *JOJ Case Studies* 2018; 6:555683.

49. Damodaran I, et al. An open-label, head to head comparison study between prucalopride and lactulose for clozapine induced constipation in patients with treatment resistant schizophrenia. *Healthcare* 2020; 8:533.

Clozapine, neutropenia and lithium

Risk of clozapine-induced neutropenia and agranulocytosis

Around 2.7% of patients treated with clozapine develop neutropenia. Of these, half do so within the first 18 weeks of treatment and three-quarters by the end of the first year.[1] Risk factors include being Afro-Caribbean, younger age and having a low baseline white cell count (WCC).[1] Risk is not dose-related. The mechanism of clozapine-induced neutropenia/agranulocytosis is unclear; both immune-mediated and direct cytotoxic effects may be important. Furthermore, the mechanism may differ between individuals and also between mild and severe forms of marrow suppression.[2] One third of patients who stop clozapine because they have developed neutropenia or agranulocytosis will develop a blood dyscrasia on rechallenge. Where the index dyscrasia was agranulocytosis, the second blood dyscrasia is inevitable and invariably occurs more rapidly and is more severe and lasts longer.[3] This is not necessarily the case where the index dyscrasia was neutropenia.[4]

Confusion arises because of the various possible reasons for a low neutrophil count in people taking clozapine. A single low count might just be a coincidental finding of no clinical relevance, as is common with all drugs. Several low counts (consecutive or intermittent) might be seen in people with benign ethnic neutropenia (BEN – see below) or as a result of clozapine-associated bone marrow suppression (especially if consecutive and progressively falling). Full-blown agranulocytosis can probably always be interpreted as being the result of severe bone marrow suppression caused by clozapine. The pattern of the results can be important. In non-BEN patients agranulocytosis is generally preceded by normal neutrophil counts which are then followed by a precipitous fall in neutrophils (usually over a week or less)[5,6] and a prolonged period of counts near to zero (assuming that it has not been treated).

Neutrophil counts that do not follow this characteristic pattern are difficult to interpret. An Icelandic study found no difference in the risk of severe neutropenia between clozapine and non-clozapine antipsychotics, suggesting that many cases of neutropenia during clozapine treatment are probably not caused by clozapine.[7] Indeed, a meta-analysis comparing the risk of neutropenia between clozapine and other antipsychotics found that clozapine did not have a stronger association with neutropenia than other antipsychotic medications.[8]

The prevalence of agranulocytosis during clozapine treatment is (0.4%),[9] lower than previously thought and risk of death resulting from this is 0.05%: a rare event. Over 80% of cases of agranulocytosis develop within the first 18 weeks of treatment.[1] The Netherlands Clozapine Collaboration Group[10] consider the risk of agranulocytosis so low that a mentally competent patient may stop routine haematological monitoring after 6 months of treatment. The group still nevertheless recommend low frequency testing, for example, four times a year if routine monitoring is stopped.

Risk factors for agranulocytosis include increasing age and Asian race.[1] Some patients may be genetically predisposed.[11] Although the timescale and individual risk factors for the development of agranulocytosis are different from those associated with neutropenia/coincidental low neutrophil counts, it is difficult to be certain in any given patient that neutropenia is not a precursor to agranulocytosis.

Haematological monitoring is mandatory to mitigate the haematological risk. However, worldwide, there are marked variations in the recommendations for monitoring frequency and the threshold for clozapine cessation,[12] reflecting, perhaps, the weak evidence on which they are based. In October 2015, the US Food and Drugs Administration (FDA) introduced changes to the clozapine monitoring system making only the absolute neutrophil count (ANC) mandatory and effectively lowering the threshold for cessation of clozapine treatment.[13] It is recommended that treatment with clozapine be stopped when neutrophils fall below 1000/mm³ (compared with UK recommendations for cessation if ANC < 1500/mm³). The new FDA regulations will undoubtedly improve clozapine use in the USA and may have implications internationally.

There is evidence that clozapine is grossly underutilised worldwide, with very wide variation in prescribing frequency from one country to another.[14] This may be explained at least in part by the stringent blood monitoring requirements. The worldwide outbreak of COVID-19 in 2020 prompted a re-evaluation of clozapine haematological monitoring with a group proposing a reduction from monthly to three-monthly for patients who have received clozapine for more than one year without a history of neutropenia.[15] When considering that the development of agranulocytosis occurs over a week or less, the value of monthly monitoring is clearly questionable, especially in patients for whom the overall risk of agranulocytosis is near to zero.

Benign ethnic neutropenia

Benign ethnic neutropenia (BEN) is a widely recognised, hereditary condition in which the neutrophil count is relatively low. People of African or Middle Eastern descent have a higher prevalence. BEN is characterised by low WCCs which may frequently fall below the lower limit of normal. This pattern may be observed before, during and after the use of clozapine and very probably accounts for a proportion of observed or apparent clozapine-associated neutropenias and treatment cessation. Many countries allow registration of BEN status whereby different (lower) limits are set for neutrophil counts in these patients. While true clozapine-induced neutropenia can occur in the context of BEN, the current evidence suggests that BEN does not pose an increased risk of dyscrasias during clozapine treatment.[16,17]

Concurrent medications

Different classes of medicines associated with haematological adverse effects are co-prescribed with clozapine. These include other antipsychotics, antiseizure medications such as sodium valproate and carbamazepine, antibacterials, gastrointestinal agents such as proton-pump inhibitors. Many patients develop neutropenia on clozapine but not all are clozapine-related or even pathological. The possible contributory role of these agents should always be considered and these agents discontinued if clozapine rechallenge is attempted.[18]

Management options

Before treatment initiation, it is important to evaluate baseline haematological values. If a patient is suspected of having BEN, there should be a referral to a haematologist for confirmation should be undertaken.[19]

Distinguishing between true clozapine toxicity and neutropenia unrelated to clozapine is not possible with certainty but some factors are important. Consultation with a haematologist is advisable regarding BEN and to exclude any other co-prescribed medication that may be responsible. The use of iatrogenic agents to elevate WCC in patients with clear prior clozapine-induced neutropenia (i.e. certainty that clozapine was the cause) is not recommended. Lithium or other medicines should only be used to elevate WCC where it is strongly felt that prior neutropenic episodes were unrelated to clozapine. Patients who have had a previous episode of agranulocytosis that is attributable to clozapine should not be re-challenged.

Lithium

Lithium increases the neutrophil count and total WCC both acutely and chronically. The magnitude of this effect is poorly quantified, but a mean neutrophil count of 11.9 × 10^9/L has been reported in lithium-treated patients and a mean rise in neutrophil count of 2 × 10^9/L was seen in clozapine-treated patients after the addition of lithium. This effect does not seem to be clearly dose-related, although a minimum lithium serum level of 0.4mmol/L may be required. The mechanism is not completely understood.[20]

Lithium has been used to increase the WCC in patients who have developed neutropenia whilst taking clozapine, allowing clozapine treatment to continue. Several case reports in adults[21-25] and in children[26,27] have been published. Almost all patients had serum lithium levels of > 0.6mmol/L. In a case series ($n = 25$) of patients who had stopped clozapine because of a blood dyscrasia and were rechallenged in the presence of lithium, only one developed a subsequent dyscrasia.[28] If considering lithium, discuss with the medical advisor at the relevant monitoring service to determine the optimum pharmacological strategy for the particular patient.

Lithium does not seem to protect against true clozapine-induced agranulocytosis: One case of fatal agranulocytosis has occurred with this combination[25] and a second case of agranulocytosis has been reported where the bone marrow was resistant to treatment with granulocyte colony stimulating factor (G-CSF).[29]

Granulocyte-colony stimulating factor (G-CSF)

The use of G-CSF to facilitate uninterrupted clozapine therapy in patients with previous neutropenia is a strategy that is attracting increasing interest, but is somewhat controversial. There are both successful[30-32] and unsuccessful[32,33] case reports of patients receiving regular long-term G-CSF to enable clozapine therapy. As well as the commonly reported side effects of bone pain[34] and neutrophil dysplasia,[35] the administration of G-CSF in the face of a low or declining neutrophil count may mask an impending neutropenia or agranulocytosis, leading to dire consequences. The long term safety of G-CSF has not been determined; bone density and spleen size should probably be monitored.

'When required' G-CSF, to be administered if neutrophils drop below a defined threshold, may allow rechallenge with clozapine of patients in whom lithium is

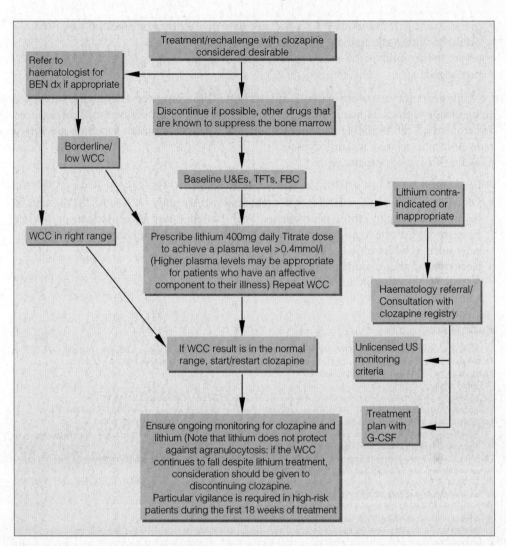

Figure 1.4 The use of lithium with clozapine

insufficient to prevent 'dipping' of WCC below the normal range. Again, this strategy risks masking a severe neutropenia or agranulocytosis. It is also likely to be practically difficult to manage outside a specialist unit, as frequent blood testing (twice to three times a week) is required, as well as immediate access to medical review and the G-CSF itself.

Consultation with a haematologist and discussion with the medical adviser at the clozapine monitoring service is essential before considering the use of G-CSF. A patient's individual clinical circumstances should be considered. In particular, patients should be considered to be very high risk for rechallenge with clozapine if the first episode of dyscrasia fulfilled any of the following criteria, all of which suggest that the low counts are clozapine related:

- inconsistent with previous WCCs (i.e. not part of a pattern of repeated low WCCs)
- occurred within the first 18 weeks of treatment
- severe (neutrophils $< 0.5 \times 10^9/1$) or
- prolonged.

While granulocyte-colony stimulating factor has been reported as allowing successful re-challenge with clozapine in some people with previous episodes of clozapine-induced neutropenia,[36] the available evidence excludes this course of action for someone with a true clozapine-related agranulocytosis.[37]

Management of patients with:

- Low initial WCC ($<4 \times 10^9/L$) or neutrophils ($<2.5 \times 10^9/L$)
- Leucopenia (WCC $< 3 \times 10^9/L$) or neutropenia (neutrophils $< 1.5 \times 10^9/L$) thought to be linked to benign ethnic neutropenia. Such patients may be of African or Middle Eastern descent, have no history of susceptibility to infection and have morphologically normal white blood cells[38]
- Recurrent 'amber' results during clozapine treatment
- A 'red' result probably unrelated to clozapine

References

1. Munro J, et al. Active monitoring of 12760 clozapine recipients in the UK and Ireland. *Br J Psychiatry* 1999; 175:576–580.
2. Whiskey E, et al. Restarting clozapine after neutropenia: evaluating the possibilities and practicalities. *CNS Drugs* 2007; 21:25–35.
3. Dunk LR, et al. Rechallenge with clozapine following leucopenia or neutropenia during previous therapy. *Br J Psychiatry* 2006; 188:255–263.
4. Prokopez CR, et al. Clozapine rechallenge after neutropenia or leucopenia. *J Clin Psychopharmacol* 2016; 36:377–380.
5. Almaghrebi AH. Safety of a clozapine trial following quetiapine-induced leukopenia: a case report. *Curr Drug Saf* 2019; 14:80–83.
6. Patel NC, et al. Sudden late onset of clozapine-induced agranulocytosis. *Ann Pharmacother* 2002; 36:1012–1015.
7. Ingimarsson O, et al. Neutropenia and agranulocytosis during treatment of schizophrenia with clozapine versus other antipsychotics: an observational study in Iceland. *BMC Psychiatry* 2016; 16:441.
8. Myles N, et al. A meta-analysis of controlled studies comparing the association between clozapine and other antipsychotic medications and the development of neutropenia. *Aust N Z J Psychiatry* 2019; 53:403–412.
9. Li XH, et al. The prevalence of agranulocytosis and related death in clozapine-treated patients: a comprehensive meta-analysis of observational studies. *Psychol Med* 2020; 50:583–594.
10. Netherlands Clozapine Collaboration Group. Guideline for the use of Clozapine version 05-02-2013. 2013; https://www.clozapinepluswerkgroep.nl/wp-content/uploads/2013/07/Guideline-for-the-use-of-Clozapine-2013.pdf.
11. Dettling M, et al. Further evidence of human leukocyte antigen-encoded susceptibility to clozapine-induced agranulocytosis independent of ancestry. *Pharmacogenetics* 2001; 11:135–141.
12. Nielsen J, et al. Worldwide differences in regulations of clozapine use. *CNS Drugs* 2016; 30:149–161.
13. FDA. FDA Drug Safety Communication: FDA modifies monitoring for neutropenia associated with schizophrenia medicine clozapine; approves new shared REMS program for all clozapine medicines. 2016; https://www.fda.gov/Drugs/DrugSafety/ucm461853.htm.
14. Bachmann CJ, et al. International trends in clozapine use: a study in 17 countries. *Acta Psychiatr Scand* 2017; 136:37–51.
15. Siskind D, et al. Consensus statement on the use of clozapine during the COVID-19 pandemic. *J Psychiatry Neurosci* 2020; 45:222–223.
16. Manu P, et al. Benign ethnic neutropenia and clozapine use: a systematic review of the evidence and treatment recommendations. *J Clin Psychiatry* 2016; 77:e909–916.
17. Richardson CM, et al. Evaluation of the safety of clozapine use in patients with benign neutropenia. *J Clin Psychiatry* 2016; 77:e1454–e1459.
18. Shuman MD, et al. Exploring the potential effect of polypharmacy on the hematologic profiles of clozapine patients. *J Psychiatr Pract* 2014; 20:50–58.
19. Whiskey E, et al. The importance of the recognition of benign ethnic neutropenia in black patients during treatment with clozapine: case reports and database study. *J Psychopharmacology* 2011; 25:842–845.
20. Paton C, et al. Managing clozapine-induced neutropenia with lithium. *Psychiatric Bull* 2005; 29:186–188.
21. Adityanjee A. Modification of clozapine-induced leukopenia and neutropenia with lithium carbonate. *Am J Psychiatry* 1995; 152:648–649.
22. Silverstone PH. Prevention of clozapine-induced neutropenia by pretreatment with lithium. *J Clin Psychopharmacol* 1998; 18:86–88.

23. Boshes RA, et al. Initiation of clozapine therapy in a patient with preexisting leukopenia: a discussion of the rationale of current treatment options. *Ann Clin Psychiatry* 2001; **13**:233–237.

24. Papetti F, et al. Treatment of clozapine-induced granulocytopenia with lithium (two observations). *Encephale* 2004; **30**:578–582.

25. Kutscher EC, et al. Clozapine-induced leukopenia successfully treated with lithium. *Am J Health Syst Pharm* 2007; **64**:2027–2031.

26. Sporn A, et al. Clozapine-induced neutropenia in children: management with lithium carbonate. *J Child Adolesc Psychopharmacol* 2003; **13**:401–404.

27. Mattai A, et al. Adjunctive use of lithium carbonate for the management of neutropenia in clozapine-treated children. *Human Psychopharmacology* 2009; **24**:584–589.

28. Kanaan RA, et al. Lithium and clozapine rechallenge: a restrospective case analysis. *J Clin Psychiatry* 2006; **67**:756–760.

29. Valevski A, et al. Clozapine-lithium combined treatment and agranulocytosis. *Int Clin Psychopharmacol* 1993; **8**:63–65.

30. Spencer BW, et al. Granulocyte colony stimulating factor (G-CSF) can allow treatment with clozapine in a patient with severe benign ethnic neutropaenia (BEN): a case report. *J Psychopharmacol* 2012; **26**:1280–1282.

31. Hagg S, et al. Long-term combination treatment with clozapine and filgrastim in patients with clozapine-induced agranulocytosis. *Int Clin Psychopharmacol* 2003; **18**:173–174.

32. Joffe G, et al. Add-on filgrastim during clozapine rechallenge in patients with a history of clozapine-related granulocytopenia/agranulocytosis. *Am J Psychiatry* 2009; **166**:236.

33. Mathewson KA, et al. Clozapine and granulocyte colony-stimulating factor: potential for long-term combination treatment for clozapine-induced neutropenia. *J Clin Psychopharmacol* 2007; **27**:714–715.

34. Puhalla S, et al. Hematopoietic growth factors: personalization of risks and benefits. *Mol Oncol* 2012; **6**:237–241.

35. Bain BJ, et al. Neutrophil dysplasia induced by granulocyte colony-stimulating factor. *Am J Hematol* 2010; **85**:354.

36. Myles N, et al. Use of granulocyte-colony stimulating factor to prevent recurrent clozapine-induced neutropenia on drug rechallenge: a systematic review of the literature and clinical recommendations. *Aust N Z J Psychiatry* 2017; 4867417720516.

37. Lally J, et al. The use of granulocyte colony-stimulating factor in clozapine rechallenge: a systematic review. *J Clin Psychopharmacol* 2017; **37**:600–604.

38. Hsieh MM, et al. Prevalence of neutropenia in the U.S. population: age, sex, smoking status, and ethnic differences. *Ann Intern Med* 2007; **146**:486–492.

Clozapine and chemotherapy

The use of clozapine with agents which cause neutropenia is formally contraindicated. Most chemotherapy treatments cause significant bone marrow suppression. When the white blood cell count drops below 3.0×10^9/L clozapine is usually discontinued; this is an important safety precaution outlined in the formal licence/labelling. For many regimens it can be predicted that chemotherapy will reduce the white blood cell count below this level, irrespective of the use of clozapine.

Where possible, clozapine should be discontinued before chemotherapy. However, this will place most patients at high risk of relapse or deterioration, which may then affect their capacity to consent to chemotherapy. This poses a therapeutic dilemma in patients prescribed clozapine and requiring chemotherapy. In practice, many patients, perhaps even a majority, continue clozapine during chemotherapy.

There are a number of case reports supporting continuing clozapine during chemotherapy,[1-18] but interpretation of this literature should take account of possible publication bias.[2] Before initiating chemotherapy for a patient receiving clozapine, it is essential to put in place a treatment plan that is agreed with all relevant healthcare staff involved and, of course, the patient and family members/carers; this will include the oncologist/physician, psychiatrist, pharmacist and the clozapine monitoring service. Plans should be made in advance for the action that should be taken when the white blood count drops below the normally accepted minimum. This plan should cover the frequency of haematological monitoring, increased vigilance regarding the clinical consequences of neutropenia/agranulocytosis, if and when clozapine should be stopped, and the place of medication such as lithium and granulocyte-colony stimulating factor (G-CSF)[19,20] to try and support the maintenance of normal neutrophil counts.

In the UK, the clozapine monitoring service will normally ask the psychiatrist to sign an 'unlicensed use' form and will request additional blood monitoring. Complications appear to be rare but there is one case report of neutropenia persisting for 6 months after doxorubicin, radiotherapy and clozapine.[8] G-CSF has been used to treat agranulocytosis associated with chemotherapy and clozapine in combination.[9,10,21] Risks of life-threatening blood dyscrasia are probably lowest in those who have received clozapine for longer than a year, in whom clozapine-induced neutropenia would be highly unusual.

Summary

- If possible, clozapine should be discontinued before starting chemotherapy. However, for most patients, withdrawal is not possible or sensible.
- The risk of relapse or deterioration of the psychotic illness must be considered before discontinuing clozapine.
- If the patient's mental state deteriorates, they may retract their consent for chemotherapy.
- When clozapine treatment is continued during chemotherapy, a collaborative approach between the oncologist, psychiatrist, pharmacy, patient and clozapine monitoring service is strongly recommended.

References

1. Wesson ML, et al. Continuing clozapine despite neutropenia. *Br J Psychiatry* 1996; **168**:217–220.
2. Cunningham NT, et al. Continuation of clozapine during chemotherapy: a case report and review of literature. *Psychosomatics* 2014; **55**:673–679.
3. Bareggi C, et al. Clozapine and full-dose concomitant chemoradiation therapy in a schizophrenic patient with nasopharyngeal cancer. *Tumori* 2002; **88**:59–60.
4. Avnon M, et al. Clozapine, cancer, and schizophrenia. *Am J Psychiatry* 1993; **150**:1562–1563.
5. Hundertmark J, et al. Reintroduction of clozapine after diagnosis of lymphoma. *Br J Psychiatry* 2001; **178**:576.
6. McKenna RC, et al. Clozapine and chemotherapy. *Hosp Community Psychiatry* 1994; **45**:831.
7. Haut FA. Clozapine and chemotherapy. *J Drug Devolop Clin Pract* 1995; **7**:237–239.
8. Rosenstock J. Clozapine therapy during cancer treatment. *Am J Psychiatry* 2004; **161**:175.
9. Lee SY, et al. Combined antitumor chemotherapy in a refractory schizophrenic receiving clozapine. *J Korean Neuropsychiatr Assoc* 2000; **39**:234–239.
10. Usta NG, et al. Clozapine treatment of refractory schizophrenia during essential chemotherapy: a case study and mini review of a clinical dilemma. *Ther Adv Psychopharmacol* 2014; **4**:276–281.
11. Rosenberg I, et al. Restarting clozapine treatment during ablation chemotherapy and stem cell transplant for Hodgkin's lymphoma. *Am J Psychiatry* 2007; **164**:1438–1439.
12. Goulet K, et al. Case report: clozapine given in the context of chemotherapy for lung cancer. *Psychooncology* 2008; **17**:512–516.
13. Frieri T, et al. Maintaining clozapine treatment during chemotherapy for non-Hodgkin's lymphoma. *Prog Neuropsychopharmacol Biol Psychiatry* 2008; **32**:1611–1612.
14. Sankaranarayanan A, et al. Clozapine, cancer chemotherapy and neutropenia – dilemmas in management. *PsychiatrDanub* 2013; **25**:419–422.
15. De Berardis D, et al. Safety and efficacy of combined clozapine-azathioprine treatment in a case of resistant schizophrenia associated with Behcet's disease: a 2-year follow-up. *GenHospPsychiatry* 2013; **35**:213–211.
16. Deodhar JK, et al. Clozapine and cancer treatment: adding to the experience and evidence. *Indian J Psychiatry* 2014; **56**:191–193.
17. Monga V, et al. Clozapine and concomitant chemotherapy in a patient with schizophrenia and new onset esophageal cancer. *Psychooncology* 2015; **24**:971–972.
18. Overbeeke MR, et al. Successful clozapine continuation during chemotherapy for the treatment of malignancy: a case report. *Int J Clin Pharm* 2016; **38**:199–202.
19. Whiskey E, et al. Restarting clozapine after neutropenia: evaluating the possibilities and practicalities. *CNS Drugs* 2007; **21**:25–35.
20. Silva E, et al. Clozapine rechallenge and initiation despite neutropenia- a practical, step-by-step guide. *BMC Psychiatry* 2020; **20**:279.
21. Kolli V, et al. Treating chemotherapy induced agranulocytosis with granulocyte colony-stimulating factors in a patient on clozapine. *Psychooncology* 2013; **22**:1674–1675.

Clozapine-genetic testing for clozapine treatment

A great number of studies have sought to detect genetic predictors of clozapine outcomes, both therapeutic and adverse. Generally, only small effects have been uncovered and clinical utility is limited unless genetic variant effects are mathematically combined. Sensitivity (the likelihood of accurately predicting a specific outcome) is usually low but specificity (the likelihood of excluding that outcome) is often very high. Numerical values for these categories can be combined with population incidence data to generate positive predictive value (PPV – the % of people who will experience the outcome when predicted) and negative predictive value (NPV – the % of people who will not experience that outcome when it is not predicted).

Response

Three variants have been reliably shown to predict therapeutic outcome with clozapine[1]

HTR2A rs6313C	CC carriers less likely to respond than <u>T carriers</u> CC 146/272 response, CT/TT 366/596 response (54% vs 62%)
HTR2A rs6314	<u>C allele</u> more likely to respond than T allele C allele response 685/1215, T allele 55/127 (56% vs 43%)
HTR3A rs1062613	C allele less likely to respond than <u>T allele</u> C allele response 528/841, T allele 134/185 (63% vs 72%)

Agranulocytosis

Four genetic variants are reliably associated with altered risk of agranulocytosis. Some variants are found only in certain ethnic groups.

HLA-DQB1	Sequence variant 6672 G > C (REC 21 G) confers 1,175% higher risk of agranulocytosis than general population. Sensitivity 21.5%, specificity 98.4%.[2] Positive predictive value 5.1%, negative predictive value 99.7%
HLA-DQB1	DQB1*0502 allele associated with agranulocytosis in 5/7 studies (eg. Dettling et al,[3] Yunis et al[4]). Effect size variable.
HLA-B*59:01	Presence of allele highly predictive of agranulocytosis but is rare in East Asian populations and almost absent in Caucasians. Sensitivity 31.8%, specificity 95.3%[5] PPV 6.4%, NPV 99.3%
HLA DQB1/HLA-B	Single amino acid changes HLA DQB1 126Q and HLA-B 158 T Associated with increased risk of agranulocytosis. Overall 39 of 95 cases had one or both alleles; 175 of 206 controls had neither allele. Sensitivity 41.0%, specificity 85.0%[6,7] (36% and 89% figures given elsewhere[8]). PPV/NPV not given but can be calculated

The HLA-DQB1 variants and the HLA-B variants are in linkage disequilibrium (LD)[8] and are likely to convey the same association signal. Variants in LD are inherited together

Benign ethnic neutropenia

ACKR1 rs2814778   CC genotype at rs2814778 (Duffy Null Status) is considered to be the cause of BEN[9]

Metabolism

Clozapine is largely metabolised by CYP1A2 and, to a lesser extent, CYP3A4/5. CYP2D6 plays almost no role. Metabolic rate is usually classified as poor (PM), intermediate (IM) or extensive (EM) and each is associated with a particular genetic variant. Genetic analysis can therefore allow an estimate of the target dose of clozapine for an individual.

Cytochrome p4501A2   PM/IM/EM status as normally defined by analysis of e.g. CYP1A2*1 F/1 C/1A/1K[10]

Cytochrome p4503A4   PM/IM/EM status

CYP3A4 is a minor route of clozapine metabolism but metaboliser status affects blood concentration.[11]

Cytochrome p4503A5   PM/IM/EM status

CYP3A5 PM status associated with elevated clozapine blood levels[12]

Other non-CYP genetic associations have also been demonstrated.

NFIB rs28379954 *T > C*   CT carriers have much lower blood concentrations than TT carriers in both smokers and non-smokers[13]

Also the **rs2472297** genotype independently predicts clozapine plasm levels.[14] Levels are highest in C/C carriers and lowest in T/T carriers (C/T somewhere in between). This single nucleotide polymorphism is located bewteen genes coding for CYP1A1 and CYP1A2 on chromosome 15.

Other adverse effects

Genetic predictors of myocarditis[15] and weight gain[16] have also been found but associations are probably too weak to allow clinical application.[10]

References

1. Gressier F, et al. Pharmacogenetics of clozapine response and induced weight gain: a comprehensive review and meta-analysis. *Eur Neuropsychopharmacol* 2016; **26**:163–185.

2. Athanasiou MC, et al. Candidate gene analysis identifies a polymorphism in HLA-DQB1 associated with clozapine-induced agranulocytosis. *J Clin Psychiatry* 2011; **72**:458–463.

3. Dettling M, et al. Genetic determinants of clozapine-induced agranulocytosis: recent results of HLA subtyping in a non-jewish caucasian sample. *Arch Gen Psychiatry* 2001; **58**:93–94.

4. Yunis JJ, et al. HLA associations in clozapine-induced agranulocytosis. *Blood* 1995; **86**:1177–1183.

5. Saito T, et al. Pharmacogenomic study of clozapine-induced agranulocytosis/granulocytopenia in a Japanese population. *Biol Psychiatry* 2016; **80**:636–642.

6. Girardin FR, et al. Cost-effectiveness of HLA-DQB1/HLA-B pharmacogenetic-guided treatment and blood monitoring in US patients taking clozapine. *Pharmacogenomics J* 2019; **19**:211–218.

7. Goldstein JI, et al. Clozapine-induced agranulocytosis is associated with rare HLA-DQB1 and HLA-B alleles. *Nat Commun* 2014; **5**:4757.

8. Legge SE, et al. Genetics of clozapine-associated neutropenia: recent advances, challenges and future perspective. *Pharmacogenomics* 2019; **20**:279–290.

9. Charles BA, et al. Analyses of genome wide association data, cytokines, and gene expression in African-Americans with benign ethnic neutropenia. *PLoS One* 2018; **13**:e0194400.

10. Thorn CF, et al. PharmGKB summary: clozapine pathway, pharmacokinetics. *Pharmacogenet Genomics* 2018; **28**:214–222.

11. Tóth K, et al. Potential role of patients' CYP3A-status in clozapine pharmacokinetics. *Int J Neuropsychopharmacol* 2017; **20**:529–537.

12. John AP, et al. Unusually high serum levels of clozapine associated with genetic polymorphism of CYP3A enzymes. *Asian J Psychiatr* 2020; **57**:102126.

13. Smith RL, et al. Identification of a novel polymorphism associated with reduced clozapine concentration in schizophrenia patients-a genome-wide association study adjusting for smoking habits. *Trans Psychiatry* 2020; **10**:198.

14. Pardiñas AF, et al. Pharmacogenomic variants and drug interactions identified through the genetic analysis of clozapine metabolism. *Am J Psychiatry* 2019; **176**:477–486.

15. Lacaze P, et al. Genetic associations with clozapine-induced myocarditis in patients with schizophrenia. *Translational Psychiatry* 2020; **10**:37.

16. Li N, et al. Progress in genetic polymorphisms related to lipid disturbances induced by atypical antipsychotic drugs. *Front Pharmacol* 2020; **10**:1669.

Bipolar disorder

Lithium

Mechanism of action

Lithium is the third element of the periodic table, in the same column as hydrogen and sodium. Potentially implicated in a wide range of biological processes and with a multiplicity of other effects, it has proven very difficult to ascertain the key mechanism(s) of action of lithium in regulating mood and behaviour. For example, there is some older evidence that people with bipolar illness have higher intracellular concentrations of sodium and calcium than controls and that lithium can reduce these. Interestingly, calcium-related genes have been implicated by genetic studies in bipolar disorder (BD).[1] Glycogen synthase kinase 3 (GSK3), cAMP response element-binding protein (CREB) and Na(+)/K(+) ATPase-related mechanisms may be important for lithium's effects. For a review of lithium's potential mechanism(s) of action, see Alda.[2] Lithium may have neuroprotective effects that preserve the function of neurones and neuronal circuits.[3] Lithium also promotes the creation of new neurones (neurogenesis) in the hippocampus, which is potentially important for learning, memory and stress responses.[4] Although the older literature pertaining to the possible neuroprotective effect of lithium consisted largely on either in vitro or animal studies, a meta-analysis suggests that lithium may prevent transition to dementia.[5] Notably, however, both reversible and irreversible neurotoxicities related to lithium are recognised as adverse effects.[6,7] Lithium is present in low levels in the environment (e.g. in drinking water), and environmental lithium has been reported to be inversely related to suicide and dementia at population levels.[8,9]

Clinical indications

Acute treatment of mania

Lithium is effective for the treatment of mania, at a plasma level of 0.8–1.0mmol/L.[10] If a faster action is needed, an adjunctive or single-agent antipsychotic with an evidence base for treating mania is recommended.[10] It can be difficult to achieve therapeutic

The Maudsley® Prescribing Guidelines in Psychiatry, Fourteenth Edition. David M. Taylor, Thomas R. E. Barnes and Allan H. Young.
© 2021 David M. Taylor. Published 2021 by John Wiley & Sons Ltd.

plasma lithium levels rapidly, and monitoring may be problematic if the patient is unco-operative. Treatment may be most successful in those without psychotic symptoms or evidence of rapid cycling.[11]

Treatment of acute mania in patients already on long-term lithium

BAP guidelines[10] suggest that in the event of relapse, an urgent plasma lithium level should be obtained to indicate the level of compliance with lithium therapy and inform possible dose adjustment. If lithium level measurement indicates non-compliance, the reason should be ascertained. If the lithium level is confirmed to be optimal, but the control of mania is inadequate, then adding a dopamine antagonist, dopamine partial agonist or valproate is recommended.[10]

Bipolar depression

Lithium is widely used in bipolar depression but evidence supporting robust efficacy is lacking.[12,13] Evidence for prevention of depressive episodes is more compelling.

Maintenance treatment of bipolar disorder

Aim for the highest tolerable lithium plasma level in the range of 0.6–0.8mmol/L[10,14] with the option to reduce it to 0.40–0.60mmol/L in case of good response but poor tolerance or to increase it to 0.80–1.00mmol/L in case of insufficient response and good tolerance. The aim of treatment is complete remission of both manic and depressive episodes.[15] Lithium may be the best performing medicine for BD in practice: Hayes et al.[16] prospectively analysed the progress of 5089 bipolar patients prescribed mono-therapy maintenance treatment: lithium ($n = 1505$), olanzapine ($n = 1366$), valproate ($n = 1173$) and quetiapine ($n = 1075$). It was found that monotherapy failure in 75% of each cohort occurred by 2.05 years for lithium monotherapy, 1.13 years for olanzap-ine monotherapy, 0.98 years for valproate monotherapy and 0.76 years for quetiapine monotherapy.[16]

Augmentation of antidepressants in unipolar depression

Approximately 30–50% of patients fail to respond to trials of first- or second-line anti-depressants, and outcomes from 'treatment-resistant depression' are poor.[17] Evidence-based guidelines for treating depressive orders with antidepressants, e.g. Cleare et al.,[18] suggest that either lithium or quetiapine are agents of first choice for augmenting the existing antidepressant and that lithium augmentation of selective serotonin reuptake inhibitors (SSRIs) or venlafaxine is most effective at a lithium plasma level of 0.6–1.0mmol/L. To help determine which, if either, is the better of these two augment-ing agents over a follow-up period of 1 year, a head-to-head, parallel group, open-label, multi-site randomised pragmatic trial of lithium versus quetiapine augmentation in treatment-resistant depression is underway and should report in 2021.[19] Clinical pre-dictors associated with a better outcome in lithium augmentation for treatment-resistant depression include more severe depressive symptomatology, psychomotor retardation, significant weight loss, a family history of major depression and a personal experience of more than three episodes.[20] Of course, compliance with lithium augmentation should also be added to this list.

Prophylaxis of unipolar depression

The use of lithium for long-term treatment of unipolar depression has recently been reviewed.[21] Cipriani et al. (2006)[22] analysed eight randomised controlled trials (RCTs) (*n* = 475), and found lithium was significantly superior to antidepressants in preventing relapses that required hospitalisation with a relative risk of 0.34. Abou-Saleh et al. (2017)[23] proposed lithium prophylaxis in unipolar depression if a patient has suffered two depressive episodes in 5 years; or after one episode if the episode is severe and there is a strong suicide risk; with indefinite treatment if there is adherence and adverse events are not problematic, particularly if a bipolar background is suspected.

Other uses of lithium

Lithium is also used to treat aggressive and self-mutilating behaviour, and recent studies have confirmed benefits[24] to both prevent and treat steroid-induced psychosis[25] and to raise the white blood cell (WBC) count in patients receiving clozapine.[26]

Lithium and suicide

It is estimated that 15% of people with BD eventually take their own life.[27] A meta-analysis of clinical trials concluded that lithium reduced the risk of both attempted and completed suicide by 80% in patients with bipolar illness,[28] and large database studies have shown that lithium-treated patients are less likely to complete suicide than patients treated with other mood-stabilising drugs.[29]

In patients with unipolar depression, lithium also seems to protect against suicide although the mechanism of this protective effect is unknown.[28] As noted earlier, environmental lithium has been reported to be inversely related to suicide at a population levels.[8]

Plasma levels

The minimum effective plasma level for prophylaxis is 0.4mmol/L, with the optimal range being 0.6–0.8mmol/L.[30] Levels above 0.75mmol/L offer additional protection only against manic symptoms,[31] so the target range for prophylaxis is effectively 0.6–0.8mmol/L.[14] Changes in plasma levels seem to worsen the risk of relapse.[31] The optimal plasma level range in patients who have unipolar depression is less clear and much research remains to be done in this area.[21]

Children and adolescents may require higher plasma levels than adults to ensure that an adequate concentration of lithium is present in the central nervous system (CNS).[32]

Lithium is rapidly absorbed from the gastrointestinal tract but has a long distribution phase. Blood samples for plasma lithium level estimations should be taken 10–14 (ideally 12) hours post dose in patients who are prescribed a single daily dose of a prolonged release preparation at bedtime.[10]

Formulations

There is no clinically significant difference in the pharmacokinetics of the two most widely prescribed brands of lithium in the UK: Priadel and Camcolit. The UK manufacturers of Priadel attempted to withdraw the formulation but this is currently under review.[33] Other preparations should not be assumed to be bioequivalent and should be prescribed by brand.

- Each of the lithium carbonate 400mg tablets contains 10.8mmol/lithium.
- Lithium citrate liquid is available in two strengths and should be administered twice daily:
  - 5.4mmol/5mL is equivalent to 200mg lithium carbonate.
  - 10.8mmol/5mL is equivalent to 400mg lithium carbonate.

Lack of clarity over which liquid preparation is intended when prescribing can lead to the patient receiving a sub-therapeutic or toxic dose.

Adverse effects

Most side effects are dose and plasma level related. These include mild gastrointestinal upset, fine tremor, polyuria and polydipsia. Polyuria may occur more frequently with twice daily dosing.[34,35] Propranolol can be useful in lithium-induced tremor. Some skin conditions such as psoriasis and acne can be aggravated by lithium therapy. Lithium can also cause a metallic taste in the mouth, ankle oedema and weight gain.

Lithium can cause a reduction in urinary concentrating capacity – nephrogenic diabetes insipidus – hence the occurrence of thirst and polyuria. This effect is usually reversible in the short to medium term but renal effects may be irreversible after long-term treatment (>15 years).[36] Lithium treatment can also lead to a reduction in the glomerular filtration rate (GFR) although the magnitude of the risk is uncertain.[36] Lithium levels of >0.8mmol/L are associated with a higher risk of renal toxicity, and prolonged lithium treatment requires regular monitoring of kidney function.[37]

In the longer term, lithium increases the risk of hypothyroidism;[38] in middle-aged women, the risk may be up to 20%.[39] A case has been made for testing thyroid autoantibodies in this group before starting lithium (to better estimate risk) and for measuring thyroid function tests (TFTs) more frequently in the first year of treatment.[40] Hypothyroidism is easily treated with thyroxine. TFTs usually return to normal when lithium is discontinued. Lithium also more rarely increases the risk of hyperthyroidism and hyperparathyroidism, and some recommend that calcium levels should be monitored in patients on long-term treatment.[41,42] Clinical consequences of chronically increased serum calcium include renal stones, osteoporosis, dyspepsia, hypertension and renal impairment. For a review of the toxicity profile of lithium, see McKnight et al.[41]

Lithium toxicity

Toxic effects reliably occur at levels >1.5mmol/L and usually consist of gastrointestinal effects (increasing anorexia, nausea and diarrhoea) and CNS effects (muscle weakness, drowsiness, confusion, ataxia, course tremor and muscle twitching).[43] Above 2mmol/L, increased disorientation and seizures usually occur, which can progress to coma, and ultimately death. In the presence of more severe symptoms, osmotic or forced alkaline diuresis should be used (note NEVER thiazide or loop diuretics). Above 3mmol/L peritoneal or haemodialysis is often used. These plasma levels are only a guide, and individuals vary in their susceptibility to symptoms of toxicity. Neurotoxicity at normal plasma levels has also been described as brain lithium levels may not be reflected in the plasma.[44,45]

Most *risk factors for toxicity* involve changes in sodium levels or the way the body handles sodium; for example, low salt diets, dehydration, drug interactions (see summary table) and some uncommon physical illnesses such as Addison's disease.

Information relating to the symptoms of toxicity and the common risk factors should always be given to patients when treatment with lithium is initiated.[46] This information should be repeated at appropriate intervals to make sure that it is clearly understood.

Pre-treatment tests

Before prescribing lithium, renal, thyroid and cardiac functions should be checked. As a minimum, estimated eGFR[47] and TFTs should be checked. An electrocardiogram (ECG) is also recommended in patients who have risk factors for, or existing cardiovascular disease. A baseline measure of weight is also desirable.

Lithium is a putative human teratogen. Women of child-bearing age should be advised to use a reliable form of contraception. See section 'Psychotropics and pregnancy' (Chapter 7).

On-treatment monitoring[10]

BAP guidelines recommend that before lithium is prescribed, baseline eGFR, thyroid function and calcium should be checked. Plasma lithium, eGFR and TFTs should be checked every 6 months. More frequent tests may be required in those who are prescribed interacting drugs, elderly or have established chronic kidney disease. A patient safety alert related to the importance of biochemical monitoring in patients prescribed that lithium has been issued by the National Patient Safety Agency.[48] Weight (or body mass index (BMI)) should also be monitored. Lithium monitoring in clinical practice in the UK is known to be suboptimal,[49] although there has been a modest improvement over time.[50] The use of automated reminder systems has been shown to improve monitoring rates.[51]

Discontinuation

Intermittent treatment with lithium may worsen the natural course of bipolar illness. A much greater than expected incidence of manic relapse is seen in the first few months after abruptly discontinuing lithium,[52] even in patients who have been symptom free for as long as 5 years.[53] This has led to recommendations that lithium treatment should not be started unless there is a clear intention to continue it for at least 3 years.[54] This advice has obvious implications for initiating lithium treatment against a patient's will (or in a patient known to be non-compliant with medication) during a period of acute illness.

The risk of relapse *may* be reduced by decreasing the dose gradually over a period of at least a month,[55] and avoiding decremental plasma level reductions of >0.2mmol/L.[31]

In contrast with these recommendations, a naturalistic study found that, in patients who had been in remission for at least 2 years and had discontinued lithium very slowly, the recurrence rate was at least 3 times greater than in patients who continued lithium; significant survival differences persisted for many years. Patients maintained on high lithium levels prior to discontinuation were particularly prone to relapse.[56]

A large US study based on prescription records found that half of those prescribed lithium took almost all of their prescribed doses, a quarter took between 50% and 80%, and the remaining quarter took less than 50%; in addition, a third of patients took lithium for less than 6 months in total.[57] A large audit found that one in ten patients prescribed long-term lithium treatment had a plasma level below the therapeutic range.[58] It is clear that suboptimal adherence limits the effectiveness of lithium in clinical practice. A database study suggested the extent to which lithium taken was directly related to the risk of suicide (more prescriptions = lower suicide rate).[59]

Less convincing data support the emergence of depressive symptoms in bipolar patients after lithium discontinuation.[52] There are few data relating to patients with unipolar depression.

Table 2.1 Lithium – prescribing and monitoring

Indications	Mania, hypomania, prophylaxis of bipolar affective disorder and recurrent depression. Reduces aggression and suicidality.
Pre-lithium workup	eGFR and TFTs. ECG recommended in patients who have risk factors for, or existing cardiovascular disease. Baseline measure of weight desirable.
Prescribing	Start at 400mg at night (200mg in the elderly). Plasma level after 7 days, then 7 days after every dose change until the desired level is reached (0.4mmol/L may be effective in unipolar depression, 0.6–1.0mmol/L in bipolar illness and slightly higher levels in difficult-to-treat mania). Blood should be taken 12 hours after the last dose. Take care when prescribing liquid preparations to clearly specify the strength required.
Monitoring	Plasma lithium every 6 months (more frequent monitoring is necessary in those prescribed interacting drugs, the elderly and those with established renal impairment or other relevant physical illness). eGFR and TFTs every 6 months. Weight (or BMI) should also be monitored.
Stopping	Reduce slowly over at least 1 month and preferably 3 months. Avoid reductions in plasma levels of >0.2mmol/L.

Interactions with other drugs[60–62]

Because of lithium's relatively narrow therapeutic index, pharmacokinetic interactions with other drugs can precipitate lithium toxicity. Most clinically significant interactions are with drugs that alter renal sodium handling.

ACE inhibitors

Angiotensin-converting enzyme (ACE) inhibitors can (1) reduce thirst leading to mild dehydration and (2) increase renal sodium loss leading to increased Na re-absorption by the kidney, resulting in an increase in lithium plasma levels. The magnitude of this effect is variable: from no increase to a four-fold increase. The full effect can take several weeks to develop. The risk seems to be increased in patients with heart failure, dehydration and renal impairment (presumably because of changes in fluid balance/handling). In the elderly, ACE inhibitors increase seven-fold the risk of hospitalisation due to lithium toxicity. ACE inhibitors can also precipitate renal failure, so, if co-prescribed with lithium, more frequent monitoring of eGFR and plasma lithium is required.

The following drugs are ACE inhibitors: captopril, cilazapril, enalapril, fosinopril, imidapril, lisinopril, moexipril, perindopril, quinapril, ramipril and trandolapril.

Care is also required with **angiotensin II receptor antagonists:** candesartan, eprosartan, irbesartan, losartan, olmesartan, telmisartan and valsartan.

Diuretics

Diuretics can reduce the renal clearance of lithium, the magnitude of this effect being greater with thiazide than loop diuretics. Lithium levels usually rise within 10 days of a *thiazide diuretic* being prescribed; the magnitude of the rise is unpredictable and can vary from an increase of 25–400%.

The following drugs are thiazide (or related) diuretics: bendroflumethiazide, chlorthalidone, cyclopenthiazide, indapamide, metolazone and xipamide.

Although there are case reports of lithium toxicity induced by *loop diuretics*, many patients receive this combination of drugs without apparent problems. The risk of an interaction seems to be greatest in the first month after the loop diuretic has been prescribed, and extra lithium plasma level monitoring during this time is recommended if these drugs are co-prescribed. Loop diuretics can increase sodium loss and subsequent re-absorption by the kidney. Patients taking loop diuretics may also have been advised to restrict their salt intake; this may contribute to the risk of lithium toxicity in these individuals.

The following drugs are loop diuretics: bumetanide, furosemide and torasemide.

Non-steroidal anti-inflammatory drugs (NSAIDs)

NSAIDs inhibit the synthesis of renal prostaglandins, thereby reducing renal blood flow and possibly increasing renal re-absorption of sodium and therefore lithium. The magnitude of the rise is unpredictable for any given patient; case reports vary from increases of around 10% to over 400%. The onset of effect also seems to be variable: from a few days to several months. Risk appears to be increased in those patients who have impaired renal function, renal artery stenosis or heart failure and who are dehydrated or on a low salt diet. There are a number of case reports of an interaction between lithium and COX-2 inhibitors. NSAIDs do not appear to diminish the therapeutic effects of lithium[63] as has previously been reported.

NSAIDs (or COX-2 inhibitors) can be combined with lithium but (1) they should be prescribed regularly *not* PRN and (2) more frequent plasma lithium monitoring is essential.

Some NSAIDs can be purchased without a prescription, so it is particularly important that patients are aware of the potential for interaction.

CHAPTER 2

The following drugs are NSAIDs or COX-2 inhibitors: aceclofenac, acemetacin, celecoxib, dexibuprofen, dexketoprofen, diclofenac, diflunisal, etodolac, etoricoxib, fenbufen, fenoprofen, flurbiprofen, ibuprofen, indometacin, ketoprofen, lumiracoxib, mefenamic acid, meloxicam, nabumetone, naproxen, piroxicam, sulindac, tenoxicam and tiaprofenic acid.

Carbamazepine

There are rare reports of neurotoxicity when carbamazepine is combined with lithium. Most are old and in the context of treatment involving high plasma lithium levels. It is of note though that carbamazepine can cause hyponatraemia, which may in turn lead to lithium retention and toxicity. Similarly, rare reports of CNS toxicity implicate *SSRIs*, another group of drugs that can cause hyponatraemia.

Table 2.2 Lithium – clinically relevant drug interactions

Drug group	Magnitude of effect	Timescale of effect	Additional information
ACE inhibitors	▪ Unpredictable ▪ Up to fourfold increases in [Li]	Develops over several weeks	▪ Sevenfold increased risk of hospitalisation for lithium toxicity in the elderly ▪ **Angiotensin II receptor antagonists** may be associated with similar risk.
Thiazide diuretics	▪ Unpredictable ▪ Up to fourfold increases in [Li]	Usually apparent in first 10 days	▪ Loop diuretics are safer ▪ Any effect will be apparent in the first month
NSAIDs	▪ Unpredictable ▪ From 10% to more than fourfold increases in [Li]	Variable; few days to several months	▪ NSAIDs are widely used on a PRN basis ▪ Can be bought without a prescription

[Li], lithium concentration, prn, pro re nata (as required).

References

1. Bray NJ, et al. The genetics of neuropsychiatric disorders. *Brain Neurosci Adv* 2019; 2:2398212818799271.
2. Alda M. Lithium in the treatment of bipolar disorder: pharmacology and pharmacogenetics. *Mol Psychiatry* 2015; 20:661–670.
3. Jope RS, et al. Lithium to the rescue. 2016; http://dana.org/Cerebrum/2016/Lithium_to_the_Rescue.
4. Hanson ND, et al. Lithium, but not fluoxetine or the corticotropin-releasing factor receptor 1 receptor antagonist R121919, increases cell proliferation in the adult dentate gyrus. *J Pharmacol Exp Ther* 2011; 337:180–186.
5. Matsunaga S, et al. Lithium as a treatment for Alzheimer's disease: a systematic review and meta-analysis. *J Alzheimer's Dis* 2015; 48:403–410.
6. Netto I, et al. Reversible lithium neurotoxicity: review of the literature. *Prim Care Companion CNS Disord* 2012; **14**. PCC.11r01197.
7. Adityanjee, et al. The syndrome of irreversible lithium-effectuated neurotoxicity. *Clin Neuropharmacol* 2005; 28:38–49.
8. Memon A, et al. Association between naturally occurring lithium in drinking water and suicide rates: systematic review and meta-analysis of ecological studies. *Br J Psychiatry* 2020; 1–12. 217:667-678.
9. Kessing LV, et al. Association of lithium in drinking water with the incidence of dementia. *JAMA Psychiatry* 2017; 74:1005–1010.
10. Goodwin GM, et al. Evidence-based guidelines for treating bipolar disorder: revised third edition recommendations from the British Association for Psychopharmacology. *J Psychopharmacol* 2016; 30:495–553.
11. Hui TP, et al. A systematic review and meta-analysis of clinical predictors of lithium response in bipolar disorder. *Acta Psychiatr Scand* 2019; 140:94–115.
12. Bahji A, et al. Comparative efficacy and tolerability of pharmacological treatments for the treatment of acute bipolar depression: a systematic review and network meta-analysis. *J Affect Disord* 2020; 269:154–184.
13. Taylor DM, et al. Comparative efficacy and acceptability of drug treatments for bipolar depression: a multiple-treatments meta-analysis. *Acta Psychiatr Scand* 2014; 130:452–469.

14. Nolen WA, et al. What is the optimal serum level for lithium in the maintenance treatment of bipolar disorder? A systematic review and recommendations from the ISBD/IGSLI Task Force on treatment with lithium. *Bipolar Disord* 2019; **21**:394–409.

15. Severus E, et al. Lithium for prevention of mood episodes in bipolar disorders: systematic review and meta-analysis. *Int J Bipolar Disord* 2014; **2**:15.

16. Hayes JF, et al. Lithium vs. valproate vs. olanzapine vs. quetiapine as maintenance monotherapy for bipolar disorder: a population-based UK cohort study using electronic health records. *World Psychiatry* 2016; **15**:53–58.

17. Dunner DL, et al. Prospective, long-term, multicenter study of the naturalistic outcomes of patients with treatment-resistant depression. *J Clin Psychiatry* 2006; **67**:688–695.

18. Cleare A, et al. Evidence-based guidelines for treating depressive disorders with antidepressants: A revision of the 2008 British Association for Psychopharmacology guidelines. *J Psychopharmacol* 2015; **29**:459–525.

19. Marwood L, et al. Study protocol for a randomised pragmatic trial comparing the clinical and cost effectiveness of lithium and quetiapine augmentation in treatment resistant depression (the LQD study). *BMC Psychiatry* 2017; **17**:231.

20. Bauer M, et al. Role of lithium augmentation in the management of major depressive disorder. *CNS Drugs* 2014; **28**:331–342.

21. Young AH. Lithium for long-term treatment of unipolar depression. *Lancet Psychiatry* 2017; **4**:511–512.

22. Cipriani A, et al. Lithium versus antidepressants in the long-term treatment of unipolar affective disorder. *Cochrane Database Syst Rev* 2006; CD003492.

23. Abou-Saleh MT, et al. Lithium in the episode and suicide prophylaxis and in augmenting strategies in patients with unipolar depression. *Int J Bipolar Disord* 2017; **5**:11.

24. Correll CU, et al. Biological treatment of acute agitation or aggression with schizophrenia or bipolar disorder in the inpatient setting. *Ann Clin Psychiatry* 2017; **29**:92–107.

25. Sirois F. Steroid psychosis: a review. *Gen Hosp Psychiatry* 2003; **25**:27–33.

26. Aydin M, et al. Continuing clozapine treatment with lithium in schizophrenic patients with neutropenia or leukopenia: brief review of literature with case reports. *Ther Adv Psychopharmacol* 2016; **6**:33–38.

27. Harris EC, et al. Excess mortality of mental disorder. *Br J Psychiatry* 1998; **173**:11–53.

28. Cipriani A, et al. Lithium in the prevention of suicide in mood disorders: updated systematic review and meta-analysis. *BMJ* 2013; **346**:f3646.

29. Hayes JF, et al. Self-harm, unintentional injury, and suicide in bipolar disorder during maintenance mood stabilizer treatment: a UK population-based electronic health records study. *JAMA Psychiatry* 2016; **73**:630–637.

30. Nolen WA, et al. The association of the effect of lithium in the maintenance treatment of bipolar disorder with lithium plasma levels: a post hoc analysis of a double-blind study comparing switching to lithium or placebo in patients who responded to quetiapine (Trial 144). *Bipolar Disord* 2013; **15**:100–109.

31. Severus WE, et al. What is the optimal serum lithium level in the long-term treatment of bipolar disorder–a review? *Bipolar Disord* 2008; **10**:231–237.

32. Moore CM, et al. Brain-to-serum lithium ratio and age: an in vivo magnetic resonance spectroscopy study. *Am J Psychiatry* 2002; **159**:1240–1242.

33. Gov.UK Guidance. CMA to investigate the supply of bipolar drug. Press release. 2020; https://www.gov.uk/government/news/cma-to-investigate-the-supply-of-bipolar-drug.

34. Bowen RC, et al. Less frequent lithium administration and lower urine volume. *Am J Psychiatry* 1991; **148**:189–192.

35. Ljubicic D, et al. Lithium treatments: single and multiple daily dosing. *Can J Psychiatry* 2008; **53**:323–331.

36. Gong R, et al. What we need to know about the effect of lithium on the kidney. *Am J Physiol Renal Physiol* 2016; **311**:F1168–F1171.

37. Aiff H, et al. Effects of 10 to 30 years of lithium treatment on kidney function. *J Psychopharmacol* 2015; **29**:608–614.

38. Frye MA, et al. Depressive relapse during lithium treatment associated with increased serum thyroid-stimulating hormone: results from two placebo-controlled bipolar I maintenance studies. *Acta Psychiatr Scand* 2009; **120**:10–13.

39. Johnston AM, et al. Lithium-associated clinical hypothyroidism. Prevalence and risk factors. *Br J Psychiatry* 1999; **175**:336–339.

40. Livingstone C, et al. Lithium: a review of its metabolic adverse effects. *J Psychopharmacol* 2006; **20**:347–355.

41. McKnight RF, et al. Lithium toxicity profile: a systematic review and meta-analysis. *Lancet* 2012; **379**:721–728.

42. Czarnywojtek A, et al. Effect of lithium carbonate on the function of the thyroid gland: mechanism of action and clinical implications. *J Physiol Pharmacol* 2020; **71**: [Epub ahead of print].

43. Ott M, et al. Lithium intoxication: incidence, clinical course and renal function – a population-based retrospective cohort study. *J Psychopharmacol* 2016; **30**:1008–1019.

44. Bell AJ, et al. Lithium neurotoxicity at normal therapeutic levels. *Br J Psychiatry* 1993; **162**:689–692.

45. Smith FE, et al. 3D (7)Li magnetic resonance imaging of brain lithium distribution in bipolar disorder. *Mol Psychiatry* 2018; **23**:2184–2191.

46. Gerrett D, et al. Prescribing and monitoring lithium therapy: summary of a safety report from the National Patient Safety Agency. *BMJ* 2010; **341**:c6258.

47. Morriss R, et al. Lithium and eGFR: a new routinely available tool for the prevention of chronic kidney disease. *Br J Psychiatry* 2008; **193**:93–95.

48. National Patient Safety Agency. Safer lithium therapy. NPSA/2009/PSA005. 2009 (Last updated August 2018); https://www.sps.nhs.uk/articles/npsa-alert-safer-lithium-therapy-2009.

49. Collins N, et al. Standards of lithium monitoring in mental health trusts in the UK. *BMC Psychiatry* 2010; **10**:80.

50. Paton C, et al. Monitoring lithium therapy: the impact of a quality improvement programme in the UK. *Bipolar Disord* 2013; **15**:865–875.

51. Kirkham E, et al. Impact of active monitoring on lithium management in Norfolk. *Ther Adv Psychopharmacol* 2013; **3**:260–265.

CHAPTER 2

52. Cavanagh J, et al. Relapse into mania or depression following lithium discontinuation: a 7-year follow-up. *Acta Psychiatr Scand* 2004; **109**:91–95.

53. Yazici O, et al. Controlled lithium discontinuation in bipolar patients with good response to long-term lithium prophylaxis. *J Affect Disord* 2004; **80**:269–271.

54. Goodwin GM. Recurrence of mania after lithium withdrawal. Implications for the use of lithium in the treatment of bipolar affective disorder. *Br J Psychiatry* 1994; **164**:149–152.

55. Baldessarini RJ, et al. Effects of the rate of discontinuing lithium maintenance treatment in bipolar disorders. *J Clin Psychiatry* 1996; **57**:441–448.

56. Biel MG, et al. Continuation versus discontinuation of lithium in recurrent bipolar illness: a naturalistic study. *Bipolar Disord* 2007; **9**:435–442.

57. Sajatovic M, et al. Treatment adherence with lithium and anticonvulsant medications among patients with bipolar disorder. *Psychiatr Serv* 2007; **58**:855–863.

58. Paton C, et al. Lithium in bipolar and other affective disorders: prescribing practice in the UK. *J Psychopharmacol* 2010; **24**:1739–1746.

59. Kessing LV, et al. Suicide risk in patients treated with lithium. *Arch Gen Psychiatry* 2005; **62**:860–866.

60. Medicines Complete. Stockley's drug interactions. 2020; https://www.medicinescomplete.com.

61. Juurlink DN, et al. Drug-induced lithium toxicity in the elderly: a population-based study. *J Am Geriatr Soc* 2004; **52**:794–798.

62. Finley PR. Drug interactions with lithium: an update. *Clin Pharmacokinet* 2016; **55**:925–941.

63. Kohler-Forsberg O, et al. Nonsteroidal anti-inflammatory drugs (NSAIDs) and paracetamol do not affect 6-month mood-stabilizing treatment outcome among 482 patients with bipolar disorder. *Depress Anxiety* 2017; **34**:281–290.

Valproate

Mechanism of action[1]

Valproate is a simple branched-chain fatty acid. Its mechanism of action is complex and not fully understood. Valproate inhibits the catabolism of γ-aminobutyric acid (GABA), reduces the turnover of arachidonic acid, activates the extracellular signal-regulated kinase (ERK) pathway and thus alters synaptic plasticity, interferes with intracellular, signalling promotes BDNF expression and reduces levels of protein kinase C. Recent research has focused on the ability of valproate to alter the expression of multiple genes that are involved in transcription regulation, cytoskeletal modifications and ion homeostasis. Other mechanisms that have been proposed include depletion of inositol, and indirect effects on non-GABA pathways through inhibition of voltage-gated sodium channels.

There is a growing literature relating to the potential use of valproate as an adjunctive treatment in several types of cancer; the relevant mechanism of action being inhibition of histone deacetylase,[2-4] a property that may also confer some effects on neuroplasticity.[5]

Formulations

Valproate is available in the UK in three forms: sodium valproate, valproic acid (licensed for the treatment of epilepsy) and semi-sodium valproate (licensed for the treatment of acute mania). Both semi-sodium and sodium valproate are metabolised to valproic acid, which is responsible for the pharmacological activity of all three preparations.[6] Clinical studies of the treatment of affective disorders variably use sodium valproate, semi-sodium valproate, 'valproate' or valproic acid. The great majority has used semi-sodium valproate.

In the US, valproic acid is widely used in the treatment of bipolar illness,[7] and in the UK sodium valproate is widely used. It is important to remember that doses of sodium valproate and semi-sodium valproate are not equivalent; a slightly higher (approximately 10%) dose is required if sodium valproate is used to allow for the extra sodium content.

It is unclear if there is any difference in efficacy between valproic acid, valproate semi-sodium and sodium valproate. A large US quasi-experimental study found that inpatients who initially received the semi-sodium preparation had a hospital stay that was a third longer than patients who initially received valproic acid.[8] Note that sodium valproate controlled release (Epilim Chrono[9]) can be administered as a once daily dose, whereas other sodium and semi-sodium valproate preparations require at least twice daily administration.

Indications

Randomised controlled trials (RCTs) have shown valproate to be effective in the treatment of **mania**,[10,11] with a response rate of 50% and a number needed to treat (NNT) of 2–4,[12] although large negative studies do exist.[13] One RCT found lithium to be more effective overall than valproate[11] but a large (n = 300) randomised open trial of 12 weeks duration found lithium and valproate to be equally effective in the treatment of acute mania.[14] Valproate may be effective in patients who have failed to respond to lithium; in a small placebo-controlled RCT (n = 36) in patients who had failed to respond to or could not tolerate lithium, the median decrease in the Young Mania Rating Scale scores was 54% in the valproate group and 5% in the placebo group.[15] It may be less effective than olanzapine, both as monotherapy[16] **and** as an adjunctive treatment to lithium[12] in acute mania. A network meta-analysis reported that valproate was less effective but better tolerated than lithium.[17]

A meta-analysis of four small RCTs concluded that valproate is effective in **bipolar depression** with a small to medium effect size.[18] A 2020 meta-analysis placed divalproex 5th out of 21 treatments for bipolar depression.[19]

Although open-label studies suggest that valproate is effective in the **prophylaxis** of bipolar affective disorder,[20] RCT data are limited.[21,22] Bowden et al.[23] found no difference between lithium, valproate and placebo in the primary outcome measure, time to any mood episode, although valproate was superior to lithium and placebo on some secondary outcome measures. This study can be criticised for including patients who were 'not ill enough' and for not lasting 'long enough' (1 year). In another RCT,[21] which lasted for 47 weeks, there was no difference in relapse rates between valproate and olanzapine. The study had no placebo arm and the attrition rate was high, so is difficult to interpret. A post hoc analysis of data from this study found that patients with rapid cycling illness had a better very early response to valproate than to olanzapine but that this advantage was not maintained.[22] Outcomes with respect to manic symptoms for those who did not have a rapid cycling illness were better at 1 year with olanzapine than valproate. In a further 20 months' RCT of lithium versus valproate in patients with rapid cycling illness, both the relapse and attrition rate were high, and no difference in efficacy between valproate and lithium was apparent.[24] More recently, the BALANCE study found lithium to be numerically superior to valproate, and the combination of lithium and valproate to be statistically superior to valproate alone.[25] Aripiprazole in combination with valproate is superior to valproate alone.[26]

The National Institute for Health and Clinical Excellence (NICE) recommends valproate as a first-line option for the treatment of acute episodes of mania, in combination with an antidepressant for the treatment of acute episodes of depression, and for prophylaxis,[27] but importantly NOT in women of child-bearing potential.[27,28] Cochrane conclude that the evidence supporting the use of valproate as prophylaxis is limited,[29] yet use for this indication has substantially increased in recent years.[30] Indeed, in the US, valproate use in BD has risen at the expense of lithium use, despite the latter drug's recommendation as the first-line drug.[31]

Valproate is sometimes used to treat aggressive behaviours of variable aetiology.[32] One **very** small RCT (n = 16) failed to detect any advantage for risperidone augmented with valproate over risperidone alone in reducing hostility in patients with schizophrenia.[33] A mirror-image study found that, in patients with schizophrenia or BD in a secure setting, valproate decreased agitation.[34]

There is a small positive placebo-controlled RCT of valproate in generalised anxiety disorder.[35]

Plasma levels

The pharmacokinetics of valproate are complex, following a three-compartmental model and showing protein-binding saturation. Plasma level monitoring is supposedly of more limited use than with lithium or carbamazepine.[36] There may be a linear association between valproate serum levels and response in acute mania, with serum levels <55mg/L being no more effective than placebo and levels >94mg/L being associated with the most robust response,[37] although these data are weak.[36] Note that this is the top of the reference range (for epilepsy) that is quoted on laboratory forms. Optimal serum levels during the maintenance phase are unknown, but are likely to be at least 50mg/L.[38] Achieving therapeutic plasma levels rapidly using a loading dose regimen is generally well tolerated. Plasma levels can also be used to detect non-compliance or toxicity.

Adverse effects

Valproate can cause both gastric irritation and hyperammonaemia,[39] both of which can lead to nausea. Lethargy and confusion can occasionally occur with starting doses above 750mg/day. Weight gain can be significant,[40] particularly when valproate is used in combination with clozapine. Valproate causes dose-related tremor in up to a quarter of patients.[41] In the majority of these patients, it is intention/postural tremor that is problematic, but a very small proportion develop parkinsonism associated with cognitive decline; these symptoms are reversible when valproate is discontinued.[42]

Hair loss (with curly regrowth) and peripheral oedema can occur, as can thrombocytopenia, leucopenia, red cell hypoplasia and pancreatitis.[43] Valproate can cause hyperandrogenism in women[44] and has been linked with the development of polycystic ovaries; the evidence supporting this association is conflicting. Valproate is a major human teratogen (see section 'Pregnancy', Chapter 7). Valproate may very rarely cause fulminant hepatic failure. Young children receiving multiple antiseizure medications are most at risk. Any patient with raised liver function tests (LFTs; common in early treatment[45]) should be evaluated clinically and other markers of hepatic function such as albumin and clotting time should be checked.

Many side effects of valproate are dose related (peak plasma-level related) and an increase in frequency and severity when the plasma level is >100mg/L. The once daily Chrono form of sodium valproate does not produce as high peak plasma levels as the conventional formulation, and so may be better tolerated.

Valproate and other antiseizure medications have been associated with an increased risk of suicidal behaviour,[46] but this finding is not consistent across studies.[47] Patients with depression[48] or who take another antiseizure medication that increases the risk of developing depression may be a subgroup at greater risk.[49]

Note that valproate is eliminated mainly through the kidneys, partly in the form of ketone bodies, and may give a false positive urine test for ketones.

Pre-treatment tests

Baseline full blood count (FBC), LFTs and weight or BMI are recommended by NICE.

On-treatment monitoring

NICE recommends that FBC and LFTs should be repeated after 6 months, and that Body Mass Index (BMI) should be monitored. Valproate SPCs recommend more frequent LFTs during the first 6 months with albumin and clotting measured if enzyme levels are abnormal.

Discontinuation

It is unknown if abrupt discontinuation of valproate worsens the natural course of bipolar illness in the same way that discontinuation of lithium does. A small naturalistic retrospective study suggests that it might.[50] Until further data are available, if valproate is to be discontinued, it should be done slowly over at least a month.

Use in women of child-bearing age

Valproate is an established human teratogen. NICE recommends that alternative antiseizure medications are preferred in women with epilepsy[51] and that valproate should not be used to treat bipolar illness in women of child-bearing age.[27] The Medicines and Healthcare products Regulatory Agency (MHRA) published the valproate toolkit, providing a set of resources for patients, GPs, pharmacists and specialists.[52]

The toolkit and the SPCs for sodium valproate and semi-sodium valproate[9,53] state that:

- these drugs should not be initiated in women of child-bearing potential without specialist advice (from a neurologist or a psychiatrist)
- women who are trying to conceive and require valproate should be prescribed prophylactic folate.

Women who have mania are likely to be sexually disinhibited **when unwell**. The risk of unplanned pregnancy is likely to be above population norms (where 50% of pregnancies are unplanned).

The teratogenic potential of valproate is not widely appreciated and many women of child-bearing age are not advised of the need for contraception or prophylactic folate.[54,55] Valproate may also cause impaired cognitive function in children exposed to valproate in utero.[56] See section 'Pregnancy'. Most now agree that valproate should not be used in women under 50 years of age, and an outright prohibition of its use in these patients is being considered in some countries.

Interactions with other drugs

Valproate is highly protein bound and can be displaced by other protein bound drugs such as aspirin, leading to toxicity. Aspirin also inhibits the metabolism of valproate: a dose of at least 300mg aspirin is required.[57] Other, less strongly protein bound drugs such as warfarin can be displaced by valproate, leading to higher free levels and toxicity.

Valproate is hepatically metabolised; drugs that inhibit CYP enzymes can increase valproate levels (e.g. erythromycin, fluoxetine and cimetidine). Valproate can increase the plasma levels of some drugs by inhibition of glucuronidation. Examples include tricyclic antidepressant (TCAs; particularly clomipramine[58]), lamotrigine,[59] quetiapine,[60] warfarin[61] and phenobarbital. Valproate may also significantly lower plasma olanzapine concentrations; the mechanism is unknown.[62]

Pharmacodynamic interactions also occur. The anticonvulsant effect of valproate is antagonised by drugs that lower the seizure threshold (e.g. antipsychotics). Weight gain can be exacerbated by other drugs such as clozapine and olanzapine.

CHAPTER 2

Table 2.3 Valproate – prescribing and monitoring

Indications	Mania, hypomania, bipolar depression and prophylaxis of bipolar affective disorder. May reduce aggression in a range of psychiatric disorders (data weak).
	Note that sodium valproate is licensed only for epilepsy and semi-sodium valproate only for acute mania.
Pre-valproate workup	FBC and LFTs. Baseline measure of weight desirable
Prescribing	Titrate dose upwards against response and side effects. Loading doses can be used and are generally well tolerated.
	Note that CR sodium valproate (Epilim Chrono⁹) can be given once daily. All other formulations must be administered at least twice daily.
	Plasma levels can be used to assure adequate dosing and treatment compliance. Blood should be taken immediately before the next dose.
Monitoring	FBC and LFTs if clinically indicated
	Weight (or BMI)
Stopping	Reduce slowly over at least 1 month

References

1. Rosenberg G. The mechanisms of action of valproate in neuropsychiatric disorders: can we see the forest for the trees? *Cell Mol Life Sci* 2007; 64:2090–2103.
2. Kuendgen A, et al. Valproic acid for the treatment of myeloid malignancies. *Cancer* 2007; 110:943–954.
3. Atmaca A, et al. Valproic acid (VPA) in patients with refractory advanced cancer: a dose escalating phase I clinical trial. *Br J Cancer* 2007; 97:177–182.
4. Hallas J, et al. Cancer risk in long-term users of valproate: a population-based case-control study. *Cancer Epidemiol Biomarkers Prev* 2009; 18:1714–1719.
5. Gervain J, et al. Valproate reopens critical-period learning of absolute pitch. *Front Syst Neurosci* 2013; 7:1–11.
6. Fisher C, et al. Sodium valproate or valproate semisodium: is there a difference in the treatment of bipolar disorder? *Psychiatric Bull* 2003; 27:446–448.
7. Iqbal SU, et al. Divalproex sodium vs. valproic acid: drug utilization patterns, persistence rates and predictors of hospitalization among VA patients diagnosed with bipolar disorder. *J Clin Pharm Ther* 2007; 32:625–632.
8. Wassef AA, et al. Lower effectiveness of divalproex versus valproic acid in a prospective, quasi-experimental clinical trial involving 9,260 psychiatric admissions. *Am J Psychiatry* 2005; 162:330–339.
9. Sanofi. Summary of product characteristics. Epilim Chrono 500mg. 2020; https://www.medicines.org.uk/emc/medicine/6779.
10. Bowden CL, et al. Efficacy of divalproex vs lithium and placebo in the treatment of mania. The Depakote Mania Study Group. *JAMA* 1994; 271:918–924.

11. Freeman TW, et al. A double-blind comparison of valproate and lithium in the treatment of acute mania. *Am J Psychiatry* 1992; **149**:108–111.

12. Nasrallah HA, et al. Carbamazepine and valproate for the treatment of bipolar disorder: a review of the literature. *J Affect Disord* 2006; **95**:69–78.

13. Hirschfeld RM, et al. A randomized, placebo-controlled, multicenter study of divalproex sodium extended-release in the acute treatment of mania. *J Clin Psychiatry* 2010; **71**:426–432.

14. Bowden C, et al. A 12-week, open, randomized trial comparing sodium valproate to lithium in patients with bipolar I disorder suffering from a manic episode. *Int Clin Psychopharmacol* 2008; **23**:254–262.

15. Pope HG, Jr., et al. Valproate in the treatment of acute mania. A placebo-controlled study. *Arch Gen Psychiatry* 1991; **48**:62–68.

16. Novick D, et al. Translation of randomised controlled trial findings into clinical practice: comparison of olanzapine and valproate in the EMBLEM study. *Pharmacopsychiatry* 2009; **42**:145–152.

17. Cipriani A, et al. Comparative efficacy and acceptability of antimanic drugs in acute mania: a multiple-treatments meta-analysis. *Lancet* 2011; **378**:1306–1315.

18. Smith LA, et al. Valproate for the treatment of acute bipolar depression: systematic review and meta-analysis. *J Affect Disord* 2010; **122**:1–9.

19. Bahji A, et al. Comparative efficacy and tolerability of pharmacological treatments for the treatment of acute bipolar depression: A systematic review and network meta-analysis. *J Affect Disord* 2020; **269**:154–184.

20. Calabrese JR, et al. Spectrum of efficacy of valproate in 55 patients with rapid-cycling bipolar disorder. *Am J Psychiatry* 1990; **147**:431–434.

21. Tohen M, et al. Olanzapine versus divalproex sodium for the treatment of acute mania and maintenance of remission: a 47-week study. *Am J Psychiatry* 2003; **160**:1263–1271.

22. Suppes T, et al. Rapid versus non-rapid cycling as a predictor of response to olanzapine and divalproex sodium for bipolar mania and maintenance of remission: post hoc analyses of 47-week data. *J Affect Disord* 2005; **89**:69–77.

23. Bowden CL, et al. A randomized, placebo-controlled 12-month trial of divalproex and lithium in treatment of outpatients with bipolar I disorder. Divalproex Maintenance Study Group. *Arch Gen Psychiatry* 2000; **57**:481–489.

24. Calabrese JR, et al. A 20-month, double-blind, maintenance trial of lithium versus divalproex in rapid-cycling bipolar disorder. *Am J Psychiatry* 2005; **162**:2152–2161.

25. Geddes JR, et al. Lithium plus valproate combination therapy versus monotherapy for relapse prevention in bipolar I disorder (BALANCE): a randomised open-label trial. *Lancet* 2010; **375**:385–395.

26. Marcus R, et al. Efficacy of aripiprazole adjunctive to lithium or valproate in the long-term treatment of patients with bipolar I disorder with an inadequate response to lithium or valproate monotherapy: a multicenter, double-blind, randomized study. *Bipolar Disord* 2011; **13**:133–144.

27. National Institute for Health and Care Excellence. Bipolar disorder: assessment and management. Clinical Guidance [CG198]. 2014 (Last updated February 2020); https://www.nice.org.uk/guidance/cg185.

28. National Institute for Health and Care Excellence. Antenatal and postnatal mental health: clinical management and service guidance. Clinical Guidance [CG192]. 2014 (Last updated: February 2020); https://www.nice.org.uk/guidance/cg192.

29. Cipriani A, et al. Valproic acid, valproate and divalproex in the maintenance treatment of bipolar disorder. *Cochrane Database Syst Rev* 2013; **10**:CD003196.

30. Hayes J, et al. Prescribing trends in bipolar disorder: cohort study in the United Kingdom THIN primary care database 1995–2009. *PLoSOne* 2011; **6**:e28725.

31. Lin Y, et al. Trends in prescriptions of lithium and other medications for patients with bipolar disorder in office-based practices in the United States: 1996–2015. *J Affect Disord* 2020; **276**:883–889.

32. Lindenmayer JP, et al. Use of sodium valproate in violent and aggressive behaviors: a critical review. *J Clin Psychiatry* 2000; **61**:123–128.

33. Citrome L, et al. Risperidone alone versus risperidone plus valproate in the treatment of patients with schizophrenia and hostility. *Int Clin Psychopharmacol* 2007; **22**:356–362.

34. Gobbi G, et al. Efficacy of topiramate, valproate, and their combination on aggression/agitation behavior in patients with psychosis. *J Clin Psychopharmacol* 2006; **26**:467–473.

35. Aliyev NA, et al. Valproate (depakine-chrono) in the acute treatment of outpatients with generalized anxiety disorder without psychiatric comorbidity: randomized, double-blind placebo-controlled study. *Eur Psychiatry* 2008; **23**:109–114.

36. Haymond J, et al. Does valproic acid warrant therapeutic drug monitoring in bipolar affective disorder? *Ther Drug Monit* 2010; **32**:19–29.

37. Allen MH, et al. Linear relationship of valproate serum concentration to response and optimal serum levels for acute mania. *Am J Psychiatry* 2006; **163**:272–275.

38. Taylor D, et al. Doses of carbamazepine and valproate in bipolar affective disorder. *Psychiatric Bull* 1997; **21**:221–223.

39. Segura-Bruna N, et al. Valproate-induced hyperammonemic encephalopathy. *Acta Neurol Scand* 2006; **114**:1–7.

40. El-Khatib F, et al. Valproate, weight gain and carbohydrate craving: a gender study. *Seizure* 2007; **16**:226–232.

41. Zadikoff C, et al. Movement disorders in patients taking anticonvulsants. *J Neurol Neurosurg Psychiatry* 2007; **78**:147–151.

42. Ristic AJ, et al. The frequency of reversible parkinsonism and cognitive decline associated with valproate treatment: a study of 364 patients with different types of epilepsy. *Epilepsia* 2006; **47**:2183–2185.

43. Gerstner T, et al. Valproic acid-induced pancreatitis: 16 new cases and a review of the literature. *J Gastroenterol* 2007; **42**:39–48.

44. Joffe H, et al. Valproate is associated with new-onset oligoamenorrhea with hyperandrogenism in women with bipolar disorder. *Biol Psychiatry* 2006; **59**:1078–1086.

45. Bjornsson E. Hepatotoxicity associated with antiepileptic drugs. *Acta Neurol Scand* 2008; **118**:281–290.

46. Patorno E, et al. Anticonvulsant medications and the risk of suicide, attempted suicide, or violent death. *JAMA* 2010; **303**:1401–1409.

47. Gibbons RD, et al. Relationship between antiepileptic drugs and suicide attempts in patients with bipolar disorder. *Arch Gen Psychiatry* 2009; **66**:1354–1360.

48. Arana A, et al. Suicide-related events in patients treated with antiepileptic drugs. *N Engl J Med* 2010; **363**:542–551.

49. Andersohn F, et al. Use of antiepileptic drugs in epilepsy and the risk of self-harm or suicidal behavior. *Neurology* 2010; **75**:335–340.

50. Franks MA, et al. Bouncing back: is the bipolar rebound phenomenon peculiar to lithium? A retrospective naturalistic study. *J Psychopharmacol* 2008; **22**:452–456.

51. National Institute for Health and Clinical Excellence. The epilepsies: the diagnosis and management of the epilepsies in adults and children in primary and secondary care. Clinical Guidance 137. 2012 (Last updated February 2016); https://www.nice.org.uk/guidance/cg137.

52. GOV.UK Guidance. Valproate use by women and girls. 2020; https://www.gov.uk/guidance/valproate-use-by-women-and-girls.

53. Sanofi. Summary of product characteristics. Depakote 250mg tablets. 2020; https://www.medicines.org.uk/emc/medicine/25929.

54. James L, et al. Informing patients of the teratogenic potential of mood stabilising drugs; a case notes review of the practice of psychiatrists. *J Psychopharmacol* 2007; **21**:815–819.

55. James L, et al. Mood stabilizers and teratogenicity – prescribing practice and awareness amongst practising psychiatrists. *J Mental Health* 2009; **18**:137–143.

56. Meador KJ, et al. Cognitive function at 3 years of age after fetal exposure to antiepileptic drugs. *N Engl J Med* 2009; **360**:1597–1605.

57. Sandson NB, et al. An interaction between aspirin and valproate: the relevance of plasma protein displacement drug-drug interactions. *Am J Psychiatry* 2006; **163**:1891–1896.

58. Fehr C, et al. Increase in serum clomipramine concentrations caused by valproate. *J Clin Psychopharmacol* 2000; **20**:493–494.

59. Morris RG, et al. Clinical study of lamotrigine and valproic acid in patients with epilepsy: using a drug interaction to advantage? *Ther Drug Monit* 2000; **22**:656–660.

60. Aichhorn W, et al. Influence of age, gender, body weight and valproate comedication on quetiapine plasma concentrations. *Int Clin Psychopharmacol* 2006; **21**:81–85.

61. Gunes A, et al. Inhibitory effect of valproic acid on cytochrome P450 2C9 activity in epilepsy patients. *Basic Clin Pharmacol Toxicol* 2007; **100**:383–386.

62. Bergemann N, et al. Valproate lowers plasma concentration of olanzapine. *J Clin Psychopharmacol* 2006; **26**:432–434.

CHAPTER 2

Carbamazepine

Mechanism of action[1]

Carbamazepine blocks voltage-dependent sodium channels thus inhibiting repetitive neuronal firing. It reduces glutamate release and decreases the turnover of dopamine and nor adrenaline. Carbamazepine has a similar molecular structure to TCAs.

As well as blocking voltage-dependent sodium channels, oxcarbazepine (a structural derivative of carbamazepine) also increases potassium conductance and modulates high-voltage activated calcium channels.

Formulations

Carbamazepine is available as a liquid, chewable, immediate-release and controlled-release tablets. Conventional formulations generally have to be administered two to three times daily. The controlled release preparation can be given once or twice daily, and the reduced fluctuation in serum levels usually leads to improved tolerability. This preparation has a lower bioavailability and an increase in dose of 10–15% may be required.

Indications

Carbamazepine is primarily used as an antiseizure medication in the treatment of grand mal and focal seizures. It is also used in the treatment of trigeminal neuralgia and, in the UK, is licensed for the treatment of bipolar illness in patients who do not respond to lithium.

With respect to the treatment of *mania*, two placebo-controlled randomised studies have found the extended release formulation of carbamazepine to be effective; in both studies, the response rate in the carbamazepine arm was twice that in the placebo arm.[2,3] Carbamazepine was not particularly well tolerated; the incidence of dizziness, somnolence and nausea was high. Another study found carbamazepine alone to be as effective as carbamazepine plus olanzapine.[4] NICE does not recommend carbamazepine as a first-line treatment for mania.[5] A Cochrane review concluded that there were insufficient trials of adequate methodological quality on oxcarbazepine in the acute treatment of BD to inform about on its efficacy and acceptability.[6]

Open studies suggest that carbamazepine monotherapy has some efficacy in *bipolar depression*;[7] note that the evidence base supporting other strategies is stronger (see section 'Bipolar depression'). Carbamazepine may also be useful in *unipolar depression* either alone[8] or as an augmentation strategy.[9]

Carbamazepine is generally considered to be less effective than lithium in the *prophylaxis* of bipolar illness;[10] several published studies report a low response rate and high drop-out rate. A meta-analysis ($n = 464$) failed to find a significant difference in efficacy between lithium and carbamazepine, but those who received carbamazepine were more likely to drop out of treatment because of side effects.[11] Lithium is considered to be superior to carbamazepine in reducing suicidal behaviour,[12] although data are not consistent[13] and carbamazepine may have anti-suicidal properties.[14] NICE considers carbamazepine to be a third-line prophylactic agent,[5] and data emerging since this guidance support this positioning.[15] Three small studies suggest that the related oxcarbazepine may have some prophylactic efficacy when used in combination with other mood-stabilising drugs.[16-18]

There are data supporting the use of carbamazepine in the management of alcohol withdrawal symptoms,[19] although the high doses required initially are often poorly tolerated. Cochrane does not consider the evidence strong enough to support the use of carbamazepine for this indication.[20] Carbamazepine has also been used to manage aggressive behaviour in patients with schizophrenia;[21] the quality of data is weak and the mode of action unknown. There are a number of case reports and open case series that report on the use of carbamazepine in various psychiatric illnesses such as panic disorder, borderline personality disorder and episodic dyscontrol syndrome.

Plasma levels

When carbamazepine is used as an antiseizure medication, the therapeutic range is generally considered to be 4–12mg/L, although the supporting evidence is not strong. In patients with affective illness, a dose of at least 600mg/day and a plasma level of at least 7mg/L may be required,[22] although this is not a consistent finding.[4,8,23] Levels above 12mg/L are associated with a higher side effect burden.

Carbamazepine serum levels vary markedly within a dosage interval. It is therefore important to sample at a point in time where levels are likely to be reproducible for any given individual. The most appropriate way of monitoring is to take a trough level before the first dose of the day.

Carbamazepine is a hepatic enzyme inducer that induces its own metabolism as well as that of other drugs including some antipsychotics. An initial plasma half-life of around 30 hours is reduced to around 12 hours on chronic dosing. For this reason, plasma levels should be checked 2–4 weeks after an increase in dose to ensure that the desired level is still being obtained.

Most published clinical trials that demonstrate the efficacy of carbamazepine as a mood stabiliser use doses that are significantly higher (800–1200mg/day) than those commonly prescribed in the UK clinical practice.[24]

Adverse effects[1]

The main side effects associated with carbamazepine therapy are dizziness, diplopia, drowsiness, ataxia, nausea and headaches. They can sometimes be avoided by starting with a low dose and increasing slowly. Avoiding high peak blood levels by splitting the dose throughout the day or using a controlled release formulation may also help. Dry mouth, oedema and hyponatraemia are also common. Sexual dysfunction can occur, probably mediated through reduced testosterone levels.[25] Around 3% of patients treated with carbamazepine develop a generalised erythematous rash. Serious exfoliative dermatological reactions can rarely occur; vulnerability is genetically determined,[26] and genetic testing of people of Han Chinese or Thai origin is recommended before carbamazepine is prescribed. Carbamazepine is a known human teratogen (see Chapter 7).

Carbamazepine commonly causes a chronic low white blood cell (WBC) count. One patient in 20,000 develops agranulocytosis and/or aplastic anaemia.[27] Raised alkaline phosphatase (ALP) and gamma-glutamyl transferase (GGT) are common (a GGT of

2–3 times normal is rarely a cause for concern[28]). A delayed multi-organ hypersensitivity reaction rarely occurs, mainly manifesting itself as various skin reactions, a low WBC count and abnormal LFTs. Fatalities have been reported.[28,29] There is no clear timescale for these events.

Some antiseizure medications have been associated with an increased risk of suicidal behaviour. Carbamazepine has not been implicated, either in general[30,31] or more specifically in those with bipolar illness.[32]

Pre-treatment tests

Baseline urea and electrolytes (U&Es) FBC and LFTs are recommended by NICE. A baseline measure of weight is also desirable.

On-treatment monitoring

NICE recommends that U&Es, FBC and LFTs should be repeated after 6 months, and that weight (or BMI) should also be monitored.

Discontinuation

It is not known if abrupt discontinuation of carbamazepine worsens the natural course of bipolar illness in the same way that abrupt cessation of lithium does. In one small case series ($n = 6$), one patient developed depression within a month of discontinuation,[33] while in another small case series ($n = 4$), three patients had a recurrence of their mood disorder within 3 months.[34] Until further data are available, if carbamazepine is to be discontinued, it should be done slowly (over at least a month).

Use in women of child-bearing age

Carbamazepine is an established human teratogen (see Chapter 7).

Women who have mania are likely to be sexually disinhibited. The risk of unplanned pregnancy is likely to be above population norms (where 50% of pregnancies are unplanned). If carbamazepine cannot be avoided, adequate contraception should be ensured (note the interaction between carbamazepine and oral contraceptives outlined below) and prophylactic folate prescribed.

Interactions with other drugs[35–38]

Carbamazepine is a potent inducer of hepatic cytochrome enzymes and is metabolised by CYP3A4. Plasma levels of most **antidepressants**, most **antipsychotics, benzodiazepines, warfarin, zolpidem,** some **cholinesterase inhibitors, methadone, thyroxine, theophylline, oestrogens** and **other steroids** may be reduced by carbamazepine, resulting in treatment failure. Patients requiring contraception should either receive a preparation containing not less than 50µg oestrogen or use a non-hormonal method. Drugs that inhibit CYP3A4 will increase carbamazepine plasma levels and may precipitate toxicity. Examples include **fluconazole, cimetidine, diltiazem, verapamil, erythromycin** and some **SSRIs.**

Pharmacodynamic interactions also occur. The anticonvulsant activity of carbamazepine is reduced by drugs that lower the seizure threshold (e.g. antipsychotics and antidepressants), the potential for carbamazepine to cause neutropenia may be increased by other drugs that have the potential to depress the bone marrow (e.g. clozapine), and the risk of hyponatraemia may be increased by other drugs that have the potential to deplete sodium (e.g. diuretics). Neurotoxicity has been reported when carbamazepine is used in combination with lithium. This is rare. For a full review of carbamazepine interactions, see chapter 17 of *Applied Clinical Pharmacokinetics of Psychopharmacological Agents*.[39]

As carbamazepine is structurally similar to TCAs, in theory it should not be given within 14 days of discontinuing a monoamine oxidase inhibitor (MAOI).

Table 2.4 Carbamazepine – prescribing and monitoring

Indications	Mania (not first line), bipolar depression (evidence weak), unipolar depression (evidence weak) and prophylaxis of bipolar disorder (third line after antipsychotics and valproate). Alcohol withdrawal (may be poorly tolerated)
	Carbamazepine is licensed for the treatment of bipolar illness in patients who do not respond to lithium
Pre-carbamazepine workup	U&Es, FBC and LFTs. Baseline measure of weight desirable
Prescribing	Titrate dose upwards against response and side effects; start with 100–200mg bd and aim for 400mg bd (some patients will require higher doses)
	Note that the modified release formulation (Tegretol Retard) can be given once to twice daily, is associated with less severe fluctuations in serum levels and is generally better tolerated
	Plasma levels can be used to assure adequate dosing and treatment compliance. Blood should be taken immediately before the next dose. Carbamazepine induces its own metabolism; serum levels (if used) should be re-checked a month after an increase in dose
Monitoring	U&Es, FBC and LFTs if clinically indicated
	Weight (or BMI)
Stopping	Reduce slowly over at least 1 month

bd, bis in die (twice a day)

References

1. Novartis Pharmaceuticals UK Limited. Summary of product characteristics. Tegretol tablets 100mg, 200mg, 400mg. 2020; https://www.medicines.org.uk/emc/medicine/1328.
2. Weisler RH, et al. A multicenter, randomized, double-blind, placebo-controlled trial of extended-release carbamazepine capsules as monotherapy for bipolar disorder patients with manic or mixed episodes. *J Clin Psychiatry* 2004; 65:478–484.
3. Weisler RH, et al. Extended-release carbamazepine capsules as monotherapy for acute mania in bipolar disorder: a multicenter, randomized, double-blind, placebo-controlled trial. *J Clin Psychiatry* 2005; 66:323–330.
4. Tohen M, et al. Olanzapine plus carbamazepine v. carbamazepine alone in treating manic episodes. *Br J Psychiatry* 2008; 192:135–143.
5. National Institute for Health and Care Excellence. Bipolar disorder: assessment and management. Clinical Guidance 185 [CG185]. 2014 (Last updated February 2020); https://www.nice.org.uk/guidance/cg185.
6. Vasudev A, et al. Oxcarbazepine for acute affective episodes in bipolar disorder. *Cochrane Database Syst Rev* 2011; Cd004857.
7. Dilsaver SC, et al. Treatment of bipolar depression with carbamazepine: results of an open study. *Biol Psychiatry* 1996; 40:935–937.
8. Zhang ZJ, et al. The effectiveness of carbamazepine in unipolar depression: a double-blind, randomized, placebo-controlled study. *J Affect Disord* 2008; 109:91–97.

9. Kramlinger KG, et al. The addition of lithium to carbamazepine. Antidepressant efficacy in treatment-resistant depression. *Arch Gen Psychiatry* 1989; 46:794–800.

10. Nasrallah HA, et al. Carbamazepine and valproate for the treatment of bipolar disorder: a review of the literature. *J Affect Disord* 2006; 95:69–78.

11. Ceron-Litvoc D, et al. Comparison of carbamazepine and lithium in treatment of bipolar disorder: a systematic review of randomized controlled trials. *Human Psychopharmacol* 2009; 24:19–28.

12. Kleindienst N, et al. Differential efficacy of lithium and carbamazepine in the prophylaxis of bipolar disorder: results of the MAP study. *Neuropsychobiology* 2000; 42 Suppl 1:2–10.

13. Yerevanian BI, et al. Bipolar pharmacotherapy and suicidal behavior. Part I: lithium, divalproex and carbamazepine. *J Affect Disord* 2007; 103:5–11.

14. Tsai CJ, et al. The rapid suicide protection of mood stabilizers on patients with bipolar disorder: a nationwide observational cohort study in Taiwan. *J Affect Disord* 2016; 196:71–77.

15. Peselow ED, et al. Prophylactic efficacy of lithium, valproic acid, and carbamazepine in the maintenance phase of bipolar disorder: a naturalistic study. *Int Clin Psychopharmacol* 2016; 31:218–223.

16. Vieta E, et al. A double-blind, randomized, placebo-controlled prophylaxis trial of oxcarbazepine as adjunctive treatment to lithium in the long-term treatment of bipolar I and II disorder. *Int J Neuropsychopharmacol* 2008; 11:445–452.

17. Conway CR, et al. An open-label trial of adjunctive oxcarbazepine for bipolar disorder. *J Clin Psychopharmacol* 2006; 26:95–97.

18. Juruena MF, et al. Bipolar I and II disorder residual symptoms: oxcarbazepine and carbamazepine as add-on treatment to lithium in a double-blind, randomized trial. *Prog Neuropsychopharmacol Biol Psychiatry* 2009; 33:94–99.

19. Malcolm R, et al. The effects of carbamazepine and lorazepam on single versus multiple previous alcohol withdrawals in an outpatient randomized trial. *J Gen Intern Med* 2002; 17:349–355.

20. Minozzi S, et al. Anticonvulsants for alcohol withdrawal. *Cochrane Database Syst Rev* 2010; CD005064.

21. Brieden T, et al. Psychopharmacological treatment of aggression in schizophrenic patients. *Pharmacopsychiatry* 2002; 35:83–89.

22. Taylor D, et al. Doses of carbamazepine and valproate in bipolar affective disorder. *Psychiatric Bull* 1997; 21:221–223.

23. Simhandl C, et al. The comparative efficacy of carbamazepine low and high serum level and lithium carbonate in the prophylaxis of affective disorders. *J Affect Disord* 1993; 28:221–231.

24. Taylor DM, et al. Prescribing and monitoring of carbamazepine and valproate – a case note review. *Psychiatric Bull* 2000; 24:174–177.

25. Lossius MI, et al. Reversible effects of antiepileptic drugs on reproductive endocrine function in men and women with epilepsy–a prospective randomized double-blind withdrawal study. *Epilepsia* 2007; 48:1875–1882.

26. Hung SI, et al. Genetic susceptibility to carbamazepine-induced cutaneous adverse drug reactions. *Pharmacogenet Genomics* 2006; 16:297–306.

27. Kaufman DW, et al. Drugs in the aetiology of agranulocytosis and aplastic anaemia. *Eur J Haematol Suppl* 1996; 60:23–30.

28. Bjornsson E. Hepatotoxicity associated with antiepileptic drugs. *Acta Neurol Scand* 2008; 118:281–290.

29. Ganeva M, et al. Carbamazepine-induced drug reaction with eosinophilia and systemic symptoms (DRESS) syndrome: report of four cases and brief review. *Int J Dermatol* 2008; 47:853–860.

30. Patorno E, et al. Anticonvulsant medications and the risk of suicide, attempted suicide, or violent death. *JAMA* 2010; 303:1401–1409.

31. Andersohn F, et al. Use of antiepileptic drugs in epilepsy and the risk of self-harm or suicidal behavior. *Neurology* 2010; 75:335–340.

32. Gibbons RD, et al. Relationship between antiepileptic drugs and suicide attempts in patients with bipolar disorder. *Arch Gen Psychiatry* 2009; 66:1354–1360.

33. Macritchie KA, et al. Does 'rebound mania' occur after stopping carbamazepine? A pilot study. *J Psychopharmacol* 2000; 14:266–268.

34. Franks MA, et al. Bouncing back: is the bipolar rebound phenomenon peculiar to lithium? A retrospective naturalistic study. *J Psychopharmacol* 2008; 22:452–456.

35. Spina E, et al. Clinical significance of pharmacokinetic interactions between antiepileptic and psychotropic drugs. *Epilepsia* 2002; 43 Suppl 2:37–44.

36. Patsalos PN, et al. The importance of drug interactions in epilepsy therapy. *Epilepsia* 2002; 43:365–385.

37. Crawford P. Interactions between antiepileptic drugs and hormonal contraception. *CNS Drugs* 2002; 16:263–272.

38. Citrome L, et al. Pharmacokinetics of aripiprazole and concomitant carbamazepine. *J Clin Psychopharmacol* 2007; 27:279–283.

39. Taylor D, et al. Clinically significant interactions with mood stabilisers, inM Jann, S Penzak, L Cohen, eds. Applied clinical pharmacokinetics and pharmacodynamics of psychopharmacological agents. Switzerland: ADIS 2016; 423–449.

Antipsychotics in bipolar disorder

Antipsychotic drugs do not only have 'antipsychotic' actions, with individual antipsychotics variously possessing sedative, anxiolytic, antimanic, mood-stabilising and antidepressant properties. Some antipsychotics (quetiapine and olanzapine) show all of these activities.[1]

Antipsychotics have been used in acute and maintenance treatment of BD since the 1960s, with evidence to suggest effectiveness at both poles of the illness, as well as mixed states.

Antipsychotics licensed by the Food and Drug Administration (FDA) for use in BD include aripiprazole (mania, mixed episodes, maintenance treatment), asenapine (mania, mixed states), cariprazine (depression), lurasidone (depression), olanzapine (mania, mixed episodes, maintenance), olanzapine and fluoxetine (depression), quetiapine (mania, maintenance, depression), risperidone (mania, mixed episodes) and ziprasidone (mania, maintenance). Risperidone long-acting injection (LAI) has been approved for monotherapy or adjunctive maintenance, and aripiprazole depot for monotherapy maintenance treatment. European Union (EU) labelling is similar except that olanzapine/fluoxetine in combination is not licensed for any indication, and no second-generation antipsychotic (SGA) LAI has a licence for maintenance.

First-generation antipsychotics

First-generation antipsychotics (FGAs) have long been used in mania, and several studies support their use in the acute phase of illness, with superiority over placebo and comparable effects to lithium.[2,3] Their effectiveness is enhanced by combination with lithium.[4,5] In the longer term (maintenance) treatment of BD, FGAs are widely used (presumably for prophylaxis)[6] but robust supporting data are absent.[7] The observation that FGAs are associated with both depression and tardive dyskinesia in BD militates against their long-term use.[7-9] The use of FGA depots is common in practice but poorly supported and seems to be associated with a high risk of depression[10] (see section 'Antipsychotic long-acting injections in bipolar disorder'). SGAs are less likely to cause depression than treatment with haloperidol.[11]

Second-generation antipsychotics

Mania

Network meta-analyses indicate superiority of antipsychotics over placebo in mania, but no statistical superiority to other compounds, such as lithium.[12] The order determined was: risperidone, haloperidol, cariprazine, olanzapine, aripiprazole, quetiapine, paliperidone, asenapine and ziprasidone, in terms of response rate. It should also be noted that response rate was similar to lithium and antiseizure medications.[13]

Adjunctive treatment with antipsychotics is more effective than monotherapy with mood stabiliser medication at 1 and 3 weeks, and augmentation with mood stabiliser medication is more effective than antipsychotics monotherapy at 3 weeks. The combination is associated with more side effects, especially somnolence.[14] Interpretation of outcomes is made difficult by trials including patients whose mania occurred in the context of failed mood stabiliser treatment.

Although mechanism is difficult to discern, converging evidence suggests antimanic effects of antipsychotics are related to their effects on the dopamine system.[15,16]

Depression

In acute treatment of bipolar depression, antipsychotics that are found to be effective include cariprazine, lurasidone, olanzapine (+/- fluoxetine) and quetiapine.[13,17] In terms of mechanism, this does not appear to be a dopamine-mediated effect, as aripiprazole and other dopamine-blocking antipsychotics do not show efficacy in acute bipolar depression.[17]

Maintenance

It is striking that compounds which appear to have efficacy in the acute phase of BD, whether that be mania or depression, seem to exert effects in maintenance treatment, i.e. prophylaxis.[18] This is borne out by a network meta-analysis of maintenance treatments in BD, which included aripiprazole, olanzapine, paliperidone, quetiapine and risperidone LAI, all of which, with the exception of aripiprazole and paliperidone, showed effects against relapse.[19] It should be noted that this analysis did not include more recent trials of aripiprazole (see further).[19]

Specific antipsychotics

Aripiprazole

Aripiprazole is effective in acute treatment of mania both alone[20-22] as an add-on agent[23] and in long-term prophylaxis.[24,25] No difference is seen when directly compared with lithium or haloperidol although one small RCT suggested that lithium was more effective in mania.[26] In trials in mania, it is associated with nausea and movement disorder (mainly akathisia).[27] Aripiprazole LAI is also effective for prophylaxis in bipolar 1 disorder with the effect predominantly on prevention of manic episodes.[28]

Asenapine

Asenapine is given by the sublingual route and is effective in mania.[29,30] Efficacy seems to be maintained in the longer term,[31] RCT evidence showing efficacy in preventing depression and manic episodes, in people with bipolar 1 disorder.[32] Asenapine is unlikely to cause weight gain and metabolic disturbance[33] than other antipsychotics.

Cariprazine

Cariprazine is efficacious for treating mania as well as depression symptoms in people with mania with mixed features,[34] and has a low propensity for weight gain.[33]

Clozapine

The earliest observational study of antipsychotics for maintenance treatment in BD examined clozapine in people attending a service for resistant mood disorders.[35] There is evidence from 15 trials to suggest improvements in treatment-resistant BD (where two treatments have failed, despite adequate dose and duration), in depression, mania, rapid cycling states and psychotic symptoms.[36]

Lurasidone

Lurasidone is licensed by the FDA as monotherapy and adjunctive treatment to lithium and divalproex for acute treatment of bipolar depression, on the basis of RCTs of monotherapy versus placebo[37] and as adjunct to lithium or valproate.[38] Main side effects include nausea and akathisia, with minimal effects on weight and metabolic parameters.[33]

Olanzapine

Olanzapine is effective in mania.[39,40] As with other FGAs, olanzapine is most effective when used in combination with a mood stabiliser in acute mania and for symptomatic (though not syndromal) relapse prevention[41,42] (although in one study, olanzapine + carbamazepine was no better than carbamazepine alone[43]). Data suggest that olanzapine may offer benefits in longer term treatment.[44,45] It may be more effective than lithium.[46,47] Olanzapine is of course associated with significant metabolic effects, including weight gain.

Quetiapine

Data relating to quetiapine[48–50] suggest robust efficacy in all aspects of BD, including prevention of bipolar depression.[51] It has low propensity for EPSEs, though significant effects on weight and metabolic parameters.

Risperidone

Risperidone has shown efficacy in mania,[52] particularly in combination with a mood stabiliser.[53,54] Risperidone LAI is also effective[55] (note though that the pharmacokinetics of this formulation generally render it an unsuitable choice for the acute treatment of mania). The long-acting version is used as prophylaxis (an unlicensed use in most countries). It is effective as prophylaxis against mania in the longer term.[18] Paliperidone can be assumed to have similar effects.

Other antipsychotics

There are few data for amisulpride[56] and rather more for ziprasidone,[57] which is widely used for mania in the US. Iloperidone may be effective in mixed episodes[58] but data are insufficient to support its use.

References

1. ECNP. Neuroscience based nomenclature, 2nd edition. 2017; http://www.nbn2.com.
2. Cipriani A, et al. Comparative efficacy and acceptability of antimanic drugs in acute mania: a multiple-treatments meta-analysis. *Lancet* 2011; 378:1306–1315.
3. Goodwin GM, et al. Evidence-based guidelines for treating bipolar disorder: revised third edition recommendations from the British Association for Psychopharmacology. *J Psychopharmacol* 2016; 30:495–553.
4. Chou JC, et al. Acute mania: haloperidol dose and augmentation with lithium or lorazepam. *J Clin Psychopharmacol* 1999; 19:500–505.
5. Small JG, et al. A placebo-controlled study of lithium combined with neuroleptics in chronic schizophrenic patients. *Am J Psychiatry* 1975; 132:1315–1317.
6. Soares JC, et al. Adjunctive antipsychotic use in bipolar patients: an open 6-month prospective study following an acute episode. *J Affect Disord* 1999; 56:1–8.
7. Keck PE, Jr., et al. Anticonvulsants and antipsychotics in the treatment of bipolar disorder. *J Clin Psychiatry* 1998; 59 Suppl 6:74–81.
8. Tohen M, et al. Antipsychotic agents and bipolar disorder. *J Clin Psychiatry* 1998; 59 Suppl 1:38–48.
9. Zarate CA, Jr., et al. Double-blind comparison of the continued use of antipsychotic treatment versus its discontinuation in remitted manic patients. *Am J Psychiatry* 2004; 161:169–171.
10. Gigante AD, et al. Long-acting injectable antipsychotics for the maintenance treatment of bipolar disorder. *CNS Drugs* 2012; 26:403–420.
11. Goikolea JM, et al. Lower rate of depressive switch following antimanic treatment with second-generation antipsychotics versus haloperidol. *J Affect Disord* 2013; 144:191–198.
12. Yildiz A, et al. A network meta-analysis on comparative efficacy and all-cause discontinuation of antimanic treatments in acute bipolar mania. *Psychol Med* 2015; 45:299–317.
13. Baldessarini RJ, et al. Pharmacological treatment of adult bipolar disorder. *Mol Psychiatry* 2019; 24:198–217.
14. Ogawa Y, et al. Mood stabilizers and antipsychotics for acute mania: a systematic review and meta-analysis of combination/augmentation therapy versus monotherapy. *CNS Drugs* 2014; 28:989–1003.
15. Ashok AH, et al. The dopamine hypothesis of bipolar affective disorder: the state of the art and implications for treatment. *Mol Psychiatry* 2017; 22:666–679.
16. Jauhar S, et al. A test of the transdiagnostic dopamine hypothesis of psychosis using positron emission tomographic imaging in bipolar affective disorder and schizophrenia. *JAMA Psychiatry* 2017; 74:1206–1213.
17. Taylor DM, et al. Comparative efficacy and acceptability of drug treatments for bipolar depression: a multiple-treatments meta-analysis. *Acta Psychiatr Scand* 2014; 130:452–469.
18. Taylor MJ. Bipolar treatment efficacy. *Lancet Psychiatry* 2014; 1:418.
19. Miura T, et al. Comparative efficacy and tolerability of pharmacological treatments in the maintenance treatment of bipolar disorder: a systematic review and network meta-analysis. *Lancet Psychiatry* 2014; 1:351–359.
20. Sachs G, et al. Aripiprazole in the treatment of acute manic or mixed episodes in patients with bipolar I disorder: a 3-week placebo-controlled study. *J Psychopharmacol* 2006; 20:536–546.
21. Keck PE, et al. Aripiprazole monotherapy in the treatment of acute bipolar I mania: a randomized, double-blind, placebo- and lithium-controlled study. *J Affect Disord* 2009; 112:36–49.
22. Young AH, et al. Aripiprazole monotherapy in acute mania: 12-week randomised placebo- and haloperidol-controlled study. *Brit J Psychiatry* 2009; 194:40–48.
23. Vieta E, et al. Efficacy of adjunctive aripiprazole to either valproate or lithium in bipolar mania patients partially nonresponsive to valproate/lithium monotherapy: a placebo-controlled study. *Am J Psychiatry* 2008; 165:1316–1325.
24. Keck PE, Jr., et al. Aripiprazole monotherapy for maintenance therapy in bipolar I disorder: a 100-week, double-blind study versus placebo. *J Clin Psychiatry* 2007; 68:1480–1491.
25. Vieta E, et al. Assessment of safety, tolerability and effectiveness of adjunctive aripiprazole to lithium/valproate in bipolar mania: a 46-week, open-label extension following a 6-week double-blind study. *Curr Med Res Opin* 2010; 26:1485–1496.
26. Shafti SS. Aripiprazole versus lithium in management of acute mania: a randomized clinical trial. *East Asian Arch Psychiatry* 2018; 28:80–84.
27. Brown R, et al. Aripiprazole alone or in combination for acute mania. *Cochrane Database Syst Rev* 2013; Cd005000.
28. Calabrese JR, et al. Efficacy and safety of aripiprazole once-monthly in the maintenance treatment of bipolar I disorder: a double-blind, placebo-controlled, 52-week randomized withdrawal study. *J Clin Psychiatry* 2017; 78:324–331.
29. McIntyre RS, et al. Asenapine in the treatment of acute mania in bipolar I disorder: a randomized, double-blind, placebo-controlled trial. *J Affect Disord* 2010; 122:27–38.
30. McIntyre RS, et al. Asenapine versus olanzapine in acute mania: a double-blind extension study. *Bipolar Disord* 2009; 11:815–826.
31. McIntyre RS, et al. Asenapine for long-term treatment of bipolar disorder: a double-blind 40-week extension study. *J Affect Disord* 2010; 126:358–365.
32. Szegedi A, et al. Randomized, double-blind, placebo-controlled trial of asenapine maintenance therapy in adults with an acute manic or mixed episode associated with bipolar I disorder. *Am J Psychiatry* 2018; 175:71–79.
33. Pillinger T, et al. Comparative effects of 18 antipsychotics on metabolic function in patients with schizophrenia, predictors of metabolic dysregulation, and association with psychopathology: a systematic review and network meta-analysis. *Lancet Psychiatry* 2020; 7:64–77.
34. McIntyre RS, et al. Cariprazine for the treatment of bipolar mania with mixed features: a post hoc pooled analysis of 3 trials. *J Affect Disord* 2019; 257:600–606.

CHAPTER 2

35. Zarate CA, Jr., et al. Clozapine in severe mood disorders. *J Clin Psychiatry* 1995; 56:411–417.

36. Li XB, et al. Clozapine for treatment-resistant bipolar disorder: a systematic review. *Bipolar Disord* 2015; 17:235–247.

37. Loebel A, et al. Lurasidone monotherapy in the treatment of bipolar I depression: a randomized, double-blind, placebo-controlled study. *Am J Psychiatry* 2014; 171:160–168.

38. Loebel A, et al. Lurasidone as adjunctive therapy with lithium or valproate for the treatment of bipolar I depression: a randomized, double-blind, placebo-controlled study. *Am J Psychiatry* 2014; 171:169–177.

39. Tohen M, et al. Olanzapine versus placebo in the treatment of acute mania. Olanzapine HGEH Study Group. *Am J Psychiatry* 1999; 156:702–709.

40. Tohen M, et al. Efficacy of olanzapine in acute bipolar mania: a double-blind, placebo-controlled study. The Olanzipine HGGW Study Group. *Arch Gen Psychiatry* 2000; 57:841–849.

41. Tohen M, et al. Efficacy of olanzapine in combination with valproate or lithium in the treatment of mania in patients partially nonresponsive to valproate or lithium monotherapy. *Arch Gen Psychiatry* 2002; 59:62–69.

42. Tohen M, et al. Relapse prevention in bipolar I disorder: 18-month comparison of olanzapine plus mood stabiliser v. mood stabiliser alone. *Br J Psychiatry* 2004; 184:337–345.

43. Tohen M, et al. Olanzapine plus carbamazepine v. carbamazepine alone in treating manic episodes. *Br J Psychiatry* 2008; 192:135–143.

44. Sanger TM, et al. Long-term olanzapine therapy in the treatment of bipolar I disorder: an open-label continuation phase study. *J Clin Psychiatry* 2001; 62:273–281.

45. Vieta E, et al. Olanzapine as long-term adjunctive therapy in treatment-resistant bipolar disorder. *J Clin Psychopharmacol* 2001; 21:469–473.

46. Tohen M, et al. Olanzapine versus lithium in the maintenance treatment of bipolar disorder: a 12-month, randomized, double-blind, controlled clinical trial. *Am J Psychiatry* 2005; 162:1281–1290.

47. McKnight RF, et al. Lithium for acute mania. *Cochrane Database Syst Rev* 2019; 6:Cd004048.

48. Ghaemi SN, et al. The use of quetiapine for treatment-resistant bipolar disorder: a case series. *Ann Clin Psychiatry* 1999; 11:137–140.

49. Sachs G, et al. Quetiapine with lithium or divalproex for the treatment of bipolar mania: a randomized, double-blind, placebo-controlled study. *Bipolar Disorders* 2004; 6:213–223.

50. Altamura AC, et al. Efficacy and tolerability of quetiapine in the treatment of bipolar disorder: preliminary evidence from a 12-month open label study. *J Affect Disord* 2003; 76:267–271.

51. Young AH, et al. A randomised, placebo-controlled 52-week trial of continued quetiapine treatment in recently depressed patients with bipolar I and bipolar II disorder. *World J Biol Psychiatry* 2014; 15:96–112.

52. Segal J, et al. Risperidone compared with both lithium and haloperidol in mania: a double-blind randomized controlled trial. *Clin Neuropharmacol* 1998; 21:176–180.

53. Sachs GS, et al. Combination of a mood stabilizer with risperidone or haloperidol for treatment of acute mania: a double-blind, placebo-controlled comparison of efficacy and safety. *Am J Psychiatry* 2002; 159:1146–1154.

54. Vieta E, et al. Risperidone in the treatment of mania: efficacy and safety results from a large, multicentre, open study in Spain. *J Affect Disord* 2002; 72:15–19.

55. Quiroz JA, et al. Risperidone long-acting injectable monotherapy in the maintenance treatment of bipolar I disorder. *Biol Psychiatry* 2010; 68:156–162.

56. Vieta E, et al. An open-label study of amisulpride in the treatment of mania. *J Clin Psychiatry* 2005; 66:575–578.

57. Vieta E, et al. Ziprasidone in the treatment of acute mania: a 12-week, placebo-controlled, haloperidol-referenced study. *J Psychopharm* 2010; 24:547–558.

58. Singh V, et al. An open trial of iloperidone for mixed episodes in bipolar disorder. *J Clin Psychopharmacol* 2017; 37:615–619.

CHAPTER 2

Antipsychotic long-acting injections in bipolar disorder

LAIs are widely used in BD although none is formally licensed in the UK for this indication (Abilify Maintena is approved by the FDA in the US[1]). Support for their use is rather limited: there have been dozens of open-label trials or case series published, but few included more than a handful of subjects.[2-4] Retrospective cohort studies and population level studies do, nonetheless, offer some support for the use of LAIs (mainly SGAs) in bipolar maintenance.[2] There have also been seven RCTs, only five of which were sufficiently powered to produce interpretable results (the remaining two trials included only 30 subjects in total[5,6]). These five RCTs represent the highest level of evidence for LAIs in BD. Their details are set out in Table 2.5.

Few firm conclusions can be drawn from the controlled trials outlined in the table. Risperidone LAI is clearly effective either as the sole treatment or as an adjunct but provides protection only against manic, hypomanic and mixed-manic episodes and neither decreases nor increases the risk of depressive relapse. Risperidone LAI may be less effective than oral olanzapine. It might be tentatively assumed that paliperidone LAI has similar effects to risperidone LAI. Oral paliperidone prevents manic relapse in BD[7] and case reports describe good outcomes with the LAI form.[8] Aripiprazole LAI also protects against manic relapse and does not appear to affect the risk of depression.

Table 2.5 Randomised controlled trials of long-acting injections in bipolar disorder

Study	N	LAI	Comparator	Duration	Outcome
Ahlfors et al. 1981[9]	33 (19/14)	Flupentixol decanoate	Lithium	18 months	Neither treatment improved main outcome (number of mood episodes)
MacFadden et al.[10]*	124 (65/59)	Risperidone (adjunct)	Placebo (adjunct)	12 months	Risperidone LAI reduced rate of relapse compared with placebo (relative risk 2.3)
Quiroz et al.[11]*	303 (154/149)	Risperidone monotherapy	Placebo monotherapy	24 months	Overall relapse rate was 30% with risperidone, 56% with placebo. Risperidone did not protect against depressive relapse
Vieta et al.[12]*	398 (132/135/131)	Risperidone monotherapy	Placebo or oral olanzapine monotherapy	18 months	Recurrence of any mood episode: oral olanzapine 23.8%; risperidone LAI 38.9%; placebo 56.4%. Olanzapine and risperidone reduced the risk of elevated mood episode but only olanzapine reduced the risk of depression
Calabrese et al.[13]*	266 (133/133)	Aripiprazole monotherapy	Placebo monotherapy	12 months	Relapse to any mood episode 26.5% with aripiprazole; 51.1% with placebo. No clear effect on recurrence of depression. An open follow-on study of this RCT (that also included patients newly prescribed aripiprazole) showed somewhat better levels of protection: 87–98% of participants remained well over 12 months.[14]

*Trial sponsored by the manufacturer.

Data for FGAs in BD are scarce and generally of low quality (open trials, case series and retrospective analyses). In these studies, FGA LAIs seem to reduce the risk of relapse compared with prior treatments. The largest (open) study[9] (*n* = 85) (note: reference 9 reports the results of two studies) suggested flupentixol decanoate (20mg every 2–3 weeks) reduced the risk of elevated mood episodes. Other reports describe similar effects for other FGA LAIs. An RCT conducted with flupentixol LAI[9] showed no effect and no superiority over lithium.

Taking into account this single RCT and all of the small and uncontrolled observations, there is very little evidence to support the often-repeated lore that flupentixol LAI increases the risk of manic relapse, and haloperidol LAI and fluphenazine LAI increase the risk of depressive relapse (or at least that FGAs provoke depression). It is notable that authors of systematic reviews[15,16] repeat this view, which seems to be based on the observed increase in depressive episodes in the open study conducted by Ahlfors et al.[9] In fact, this increase occurred only in subjects whose lithium treatment had been stopped immediately before the study began. Nonetheless, oral haloperidol, when used for mania, is more likely than oral SGAs to cause a switch to depression,[17] so some caution is clearly required.

There are no controlled comparisons of FGA and SGA LAIs.[2–4] A Taiwanese retrospective cohort study[18] uncovered a higher risk of depressive episode recurrence and a higher likelihood of hospitalisation in those prescribed FGA LAIs (50% were prescribed flupentixol, 25% haloperidol and 25% others) compared with those prescribed risperidone LAI. The hazard ratio for readmission was 1.20 (95% CI: 1.04–1.38) – risperidone incident rate 0.42; FGAs 0.51. Of particular note was the substantial rate of treatment discontinuation. At 1 year, only 7.2% of those initially prescribed risperidone and 2.2% of those initiated on FGA LAIs remained on the original treatment.

Conclusions

- Support for the use of FGA LAIs in bipolar is weak.
- Very limited evidence suggests that FGA LAIs may be effective in reducing recurrence of mania/hypomania but they do not prevent recurrence of depression and may increase the risk.
- Risperidone LAI and aripiprazole LAI are robustly associated with a reduced risk of recurrence of episodes of mania/hypomania compared with placebo.
- There is no evidence to suggest that SGAs increase the risk of depression.
- Risperidone LAI and aripiprazole LAI have no effect on the risk of depressive recurrence.
- There is no evidence to support the benefit of LAIs over oral antipsychotic treatment in bipolar maintenance.
- As with other conditions, the use of LAIs offers the advantage of transparency with respect to compliance: the LAI injection is either given or it is not.

CHAPTER 2

References

1. MDedge Psychiatry. Abilify Maintena OK'd by FDA for adults with bipolar I disorder. 2017; https://www.mdedge.com/psychiatry/article/143846/bipolar-disorder/abilify-maintena-okd-fda-adults-bipolar-i-disorder?sso=true.

2. Keramatian K, et al. Long-acting injectable second-generation/atypical antipsychotics for the management of bipolar disorder: a systematic review. *CNS Drugs* 2019; 33:431–456.

3. Pacchiarotti I, et al. Long-acting injectable antipsychotics (LAIs) for maintenance treatment of bipolar and schizoaffective disorders: a systematic review. *Eur Neuropsychopharmacol* 2019; 29:457–470.

4. Prajapati AR, et al. Second-generation antipsychotic long-acting injections in bipolar disorder: systematic review and meta-analysis. *Bipolar Disorders* 2018; 20:687–696.

5. Esparon J, et al. Comparison of the prophylactic action of flupenthixol with placebo in lithium treated manic-depressive patients. *Br J Psychiatry* 1986; 148:723–725.

6. Yatham L, et al. Randomised trial of oral vs. injectable antipsychotics in bipolar disorder. *Presented at the 6th International Conference on Bipolar Disorder: June 16–18 2005*, Pittsburgh, PA; 2005.

7. Berwaerts J, et al. A randomized, placebo- and active-controlled study of paliperidone extended-release as maintenance treatment in patients with bipolar I disorder after an acute manic or mixed episode. *J Affect Disord* 2012; 138:247–258.

8. Buoli M, et al. Paliperidone palmitate depot in the long-term treatment of psychotic bipolar disorder: a case series. *Clin Neuropharmacol* 2015; 38:209–211.

9. Ahlfors UG, et al. Flupenthixol decanoate in recurrent manic-depressive illness. A comparison with lithium. *Acta Psychiatr Scand* 1981; 64:226–237.

10. Macfadden W, et al. A randomized, double-blind, placebo-controlled study of maintenance treatment with adjunctive risperidone long-acting therapy in patients with bipolar I disorder who relapse frequently. *Bipolar Disord* 2009; 11:827–839.

11. Quiroz JA, et al. Risperidone long-acting injectable monotherapy in the maintenance treatment of bipolar I disorder. *Biol Psychiatry* 2010; 68:156–162.

12. Vieta E, et al. A randomized, double-blind, placebo-controlled trial to assess prevention of mood episodes with risperidone long-acting injectable in patients with bipolar I disorder. *Eur Neuropsychopharmacol* 2012; 22:825–835.

13. Calabrese JR, et al. Efficacy and safety of aripiprazole once-monthly in the maintenance treatment of bipolar I disorder: a double-blind, placebo-controlled, 52-week randomized withdrawal study. *J Clin Psychiatry* 2017; 78:324–331.

14. Calabrese JR, et al. Aripiprazole once-monthly as maintenance treatment for bipolar I disorder: a 52-week, multicenter, open-label study. *Int J Bipolar Disord* 2018; 6:14.

15. Bond DJ, et al. Depot antipsychotic medications in bipolar disorder: a review of the literature. *Acta Psychiatr Scand Suppl* 2007; 116:3–16.

16. Gigante AD, et al. Long-acting injectable antipsychotics for the maintenance treatment of bipolar disorder. *CNS Drugs* 2012; 26:403–420.

17. Goikolea JM, et al. Lower rate of depressive switch following antimanic treatment with second-generation antipsychotics versus haloperidol. *J Affect Disord* 2013; 144:191–198.

18. Wu CS, et al. Comparative effectiveness of long-acting injectable risperidone vs. long-acting injectable first-generation antipsychotics in bipolar disorder. *J Affect Disord* 2016; 197:189–195.

Physical monitoring for people with bipolar disorder[1,2]

Test or measurement	Monitoring of all patients		Additional monitoring of specific drugs			
	Initial health check	Annual check-up	Antipsychotics	Lithium	Valproate	Carbamazepine
Thyroid function	Yes	Yes		At start and every 6 months; more often if evidence of change		
Liver function tests (LFTs)	Yes	Yes			Every 3 months for the first year then annually	Monthly for the first 3 months then annually
Renal function (eGFR)	Yes	Yes		At start and every 6 months; more often if there is evidence of deterioration or the patient starts taking interacting drugs		
Electrolytes, urea and creatinine (EUC)	Yes	Yes		At start and then every 3–6 months (include serum calcium)		Monthly for the first 3 months then annually
Full blood count (FBC)	Yes	Yes		Only if clinically indicated	Every 3 months for the first year then annually	Monthly for the first 3 months then annually
Blood (plasma) glucose	Yes	Yes, as part of a routine physical health check	At start and then every 4–6 months (and at 1 month if taking olanzapine); more often if evidence of elevated levels			
Lipid profile	Yes	Yes, as part of a routine physical health check	At start and at 3 months; more often initially if evidence of elevated levels			
Blood pressure and pulse	Yes	Yes, as part of a routine physical health check	During dosage titration if antipsychotic prescribed is associated with postural hypotension			

(Continued)

(Continued)

Prolactin	Children and adolescents only	At start and if symptoms of raised prolactin develop. Raised prolactin unlikely with quetiapine or aripiprazole. Very occasionally seen with olanzapine and asenapine. Very common with risperidone and FGAs			
ECG	If indicated by cardiovascular disease or risk factors	At start if there are risk factors for or existing cardiovascular disease (or haloperidol is prescribed). If relevant abnormalities are detected, as a minimum recheck after each dose increase.	At start if risk factors for or existing cardiovascular disease. If relevant abnormalities are detected, as a minimum recheck after each dose increase.		At start if risk factors for or existing cardiovascular disease. If relevant abnormalities are detected, as a minimum recheck after each dose increase.
Waist circumference and/or BMI	Yes	Yes, as part of a routine physical health check.	Monthly for the first 3 months then annually	At start, and then every 6 months	Every 3 months for the first year then annually	At start and when needed if the patient gains weight rapidly
Plasma levels of drug			At least 3–4 days after initiation and 3–4 days after every dose change until levels stable, then **every 3 months** in the first year, then every 6 months for most patients (see NICE²)	Titrate by effect and tolerability. Do not routinely measure unless there is evidence of lack of effectiveness, poor adherence or toxicity	Two weeks after initiation and two weeks after dose change. Thereafter, do not routinely measure unless there is evidence of lack of effectiveness, poor adherence or toxicity

For patients on **lamotrigine**, do an annual health check, but no special monitoring tests are needed although blood levels may indicate if high doses might be considered.

References

1. Ng F, et al. The International Society for Bipolar Disorders (ISBD) consensus guidelines for the safety monitoring of bipolar disorder treatments. *Bipolar Disord* 2009; 11:559–595.
2. National Institute for Health and Care Excellence. Bipolar disorder: assessment and management. Clinical Guidance [CG185]. 2014 (Last updated February 2020); https://www.nice.org.uk/guidance/cg185.

Treatment of acute mania or hypomania

Drug treatment is the mainstay of therapy for mania and hypomania. Both antipsychotics and mood stabilisers are effective (although the nomenclature here is unhelpful – most, possibly all, antipsychotics are antimanic and most mood stabilisers reduce psychotic symptoms in mania). Sedative and anxiolytic drugs (e.g. benzodiazepines) may add to the effects of these drugs.

Drug choice is made difficult by the small number of direct comparisons and so no drug can be recommended over another on efficacy grounds. However, a multiple treatments meta-analysis[1] (which allows indirect comparison) suggested that olanzapine, risperidone, haloperidol and quetiapine had the best combination of efficacy and acceptability. Cochrane suggests olanzapine is more effective than both lithium[2] and valproate[3] when used as monotherapy. Olanzapine may also be more effective than asenapine.[4]

The benefit of antipsychotic–mood stabiliser combinations (compared with mood stabiliser alone) is established for those relapsing while on mood stabilisers but less clear for those presenting on no treatment.[5–9] The most recent international guidelines

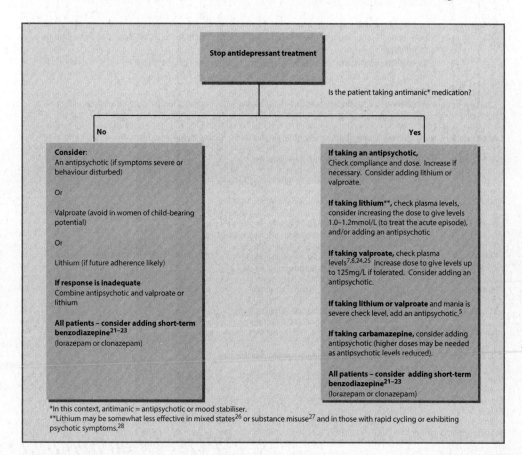

Figure 2.1 Treatment of acute mania or hypomania[5–20]

available[29] suggest combination treatments 'tend to work faster' and that '20% more patients will respond to combination therapy' (compared with monotherapy). Conversely, guidelines from Australia and New Zealand suggest trying an antipsychotic first and only adding a mood stabiliser 'if monotherapy does not suffice'.[30] In practice, there is often a strong tendency to use combination therapy from the outset.

The diagram outlines a treatment strategy for mania and hypomania. These recommendations are based on the UK NICE guidelines,[6] BAP guidelines[31] and individual references cited. Where an antipsychotic is recommended, choose from those licensed for mania/BD, that is, most conventional drugs including aripiprazole, asenapine, olanzapine, risperidone and quetiapine. Suggested doses and alternative treatments are outlined in the tables that follow.

Table 2.6 Drug treatment of mania - suggested doses

Drug	Dose
Lithium	400mg/day, increasing every 3–4 days according to plasma levels. At least one study has used 800mg as a starting dose[32]
Valproate	As **semi-sodium** – 250mg three times daily increasing according to tolerability and plasma levels. Slow release semi-sodium valproate may also be effective (at 15–30mg/kg)[33] but there is one failed study[34] As **sodium valproate** slow release – 500mg/day increasing as above Higher, 'loading doses' have been used, both oral[35–37] and intravenous (IV).[38,39] Dose is 20–30mg/kg/day A review of 13 studies suggested 'IV valproate as a loading therapy is an efficacious, safe and well-tolerated treatment'[40]
Aripiprazole	15mg/day increasing up to 30mg/day as required.[41] Doses lower than 15mg may not be effective[42]
Asenapine	5mg bd increasing to 10mg bd as required
Cariprazine	3mg/day increasing up to 12mg a day as required[43]
Olanzapine	10mg/day increasing to 15mg or 20mg as required
Risperidone	2mg or 3mg/day increased to 6mg/day as required The use of paliperidone in mania is not well supported[44]
Quetiapine	**IR** – 100mg/day increasing to 800mg as required. Higher starting doses have been used[45] **XL** – 300/day increasing to 600mg/day on day 2
Haloperidol	5–10mg/day increasing to 15mg if required
Lorazepam[22,23]	Up to 4mg/day (some centres use higher doses)
Clonzapam[21,23]	Up to 8mg/day

bd, bis die (twice a day), IR, immediate release, XL, extended release

Table 2.7 Mania – other possible treatments
Alphabetical order – no preference implied by order in the table. Consult specialist and primary literature before using any treatment listed.

Treatment	Comments
Allopurinol (300–600mg/day)	A meta-analysis of five studies of adjunct allopurinol found an effect size of just less than 0.3[46]
Celecoxib (400mg/day)[47]	Small RCT (n = 46) suggests benefit when used as adjunct to valproate
Clozapine[48–50]	Established treatment option for refractory mania/bipolar disorder. Rapid titration has been reported[51]
Ebselen[52]	Inhibits inositol monophosphatase (similar to lithium). Preliminary evidence of benefit
Gabapentin[53–55] (up to 2.4g/day)	Probably only effective by virtue of an anxiolytic effect. Rarely used. Possibly useful as prophylaxis[56]
Levetiracetam[57,58] (up to 4000mg/day)	Possibly effective but controlled studies required. One case of levetiracetam causing mania[59]
Memantine[60] (10–30mg/day)	Conflicting evidence[61–63]
Melatonin 6mg/day[64]	Preliminary evidence of benefit as an adjunct to standard treatment. One small negative study[65]
Oxcarbazepine[66–72] (around 300–3000mg/day)	Probably effective acutely and as prophylaxis although one controlled study conducted (in youths) was negative[73]
Phenytoin[74] (300–400mg/day)	Rarely used. Limited data Complex kinetics with narrow therapeutic range
Ritanserin[75] (10mg/day)	Supported by a single RCT. Well tolerated. May protect against extrapyramidal symptoms (EPS)
Tamoxifen[76] (20–140mg/day)	Possibly effective. Five small RCTs. Dose–response relationship is unclear. Good evidence for efficacy as adjunct and as monotherapy, with large effect size
Topiramate[77] (up to 300mg/day)	Probably not effective. Less effective than lithium.[2]
Tryptophan depletion[78]	Supported by a small RCT
Ziprasidone[79–81]	Supported by three RCTs. Widely used outside the UK

References

1. Cipriani A, et al. Comparative efficacy and acceptability of antimanic drugs in acute mania: a multiple-treatments meta-analysis. *Lancet* 2011; **378**:1306–1315.
2. McKnight RF, et al. Lithium for acute mania. *Cochrane Database Syst Rev* 2019; **6**:Cd004048.
3. Jochim J, et al. Valproate for acute mania. *Cochrane Database Syst Rev* 2019; **10**:Cd004052.
4. Mahajan V, et al. Efficacy and safety of asenapine versus olanzapine in combination with divalproex for acute mania: a randomized controlled trial. *J Clin Psychopharmacol* 2019; **39**:305–311.
5. Smith LA, et al. Acute bipolar mania: a systematic review and meta-analysis of co-therapy vs. monotherapy. *Acta Psychiatr Scand* 2007; **115**:12–20.

6. National Institute for Health and Care Excellence. Bipolar disorder: assessment and management. Clinical Guidance [CG185]. 2014 (Last updated February 2020); https://www.nice.org.uk/guidance/cg185.

7. Goodwin GM. Evidence-based guidelines for treating bipolar disorder: revised second edition–recommendations from the British Association for Psychopharmacology. *J Psychopharmacol* 2009; 23:346–388.

8. American Psychiatric Association. Guideline watch: practice guideline for the treatment of patients with bipolar disorder, 2nd edition. Washington, DC: American Psychiatric Association; 2005. doi:10.1176/appi.books.9780890423363.148430.

9. Sachs GS. Decision tree for the treatment of bipolar disorder. *J Clin Psychiatry* 2003; 64 Suppl 8:35–40.

10. Tohen M, et al. A 12-week, double-blind comparison of olanzapine vs haloperidol in the treatment of acute mania. *Arch Gen Psychiatry* 2003; 60:1218–1226.

11. Baldessarini RJ, et al. Olanzapine versus placebo in acute mania treatment responses in subgroups. *J Clin Psychopharmacol* 2003; 23:370–376.

12. Sachs G, et al. Quetiapine with lithium or divalproex for the treatment of bipolar mania: a randomized, double-blind, placebo-controlled study. *Bipolar Disord* 2004; 6:213–223.

13. Yatham LN, et al. Quetiapine versus placebo in combination with lithium or divalproex for the treatment of bipolar mania. *J Clin Psychopharmacol* 2004; 24:599–606.

14. Yatham LN, et al. Risperidone plus lithium versus risperidone plus valproate in acute and continuation treatment of mania. *Int Clin Psychopharmacol* 2004; 19:103–109.

15. Bowden CL, et al. Risperidone in combination with mood stabilizers: a 10-week continuation phase study in bipolar I disorder. *J Clin Psychiatry* 2004; 65:707–714.

16. Hirschfeld RM, et al. Rapid antimanic effect of risperidone monotherapy: a 3-week multicenter, double-blind, placebo-controlled trial. *Am J Psychiatry* 2004; 161:1057–1065.

17. Bowden CL, et al. A randomized, double-blind, placebo-controlled efficacy and safety study of quetiapine or lithium as monotherapy for mania in bipolar disorder. *J Clin Psychiatry* 2005; 66:111–121.

18. Khanna S, et al. Risperidone in the treatment of acute mania: double-blind, placebo-controlled study. *Br J Psychiatry* 2005; 187:229–234.

19. Young RC, et al. GERI-BD: a randomized double-blind controlled trial of lithium and divalproex in the treatment of mania in older patients with bipolar disorder. *Am J Psychiatry* 2017; 174:1086–1093.

20. Conus P, et al. Olanzapine or chlorpromazine plus lithium in first episode psychotic mania: an 8-week randomised controlled trial. *Eur Psychiatry* 2015; 30:975–982.

21. Sachs GS, et al. Adjunctive clonazepam for maintenance treatment of bipolar affective disorder. *J Clin Psychopharmacol* 1990; 10:42–47.

22. Modell JG, et al. Inpatient clinical trial of lorazepam for the management of manic agitation. *J Clin Psychopharmacol* 1985; 5:109–113.

23. Curtin F, et al. Clonazepam and lorazepam in acute mania: a Bayesian meta-analysis. *J Affect Disord* 2004; 78:201–208.

24. Taylor D, et al. Doses of carbamazepine and valproate in bipolar affective disorder. *Psychiatric Bull* 1997; 21:221–223.

25. Allen MH, et al. Linear relationship of valproate serum concentration to response and optimal serum levels for acute mania. *Am J Psychiatry* 2006; 163:272–275.

26. Swann AC, et al. Lithium treatment of mania: clinical characteristics, specificity of symptom change, and outcome. *Psychiatry Res* 1986; 18:127–141.

27. Goldberg JF, et al. A history of substance abuse complicates remission from acute mania in bipolar disorder. *J Clin Psychiatry* 1999; 60:733–740.

28. Hui TP, et al. A systematic review and meta-analysis of clinical predictors of lithium response in bipolar disorder. *Acta Psychiatr Scand* 2019; 140:94–115.

29. Yatham LN, et al. Canadian Network for Mood and Anxiety Treatments (CANMAT) and International Society for Bipolar Disorders (ISBD) 2018 guidelines for the management of patients with bipolar disorder. *Bipolar Disord* 2018; 20:97–170.

30. Malhi GS, et al. The 2020 Royal Australian and New Zealand College of Psychiatrists Clinical Practice Guidelines for mood disorders: bipolar disorder summary. *Bipolar Disord* 2020. 22:805–821.

31. Goodwin GM, et al. Evidence-based guidelines for treating bipolar disorder: revised third edition recommendations from the British Association for Psychopharmacology. *J Psychopharmacol* 2016; 30:495–553.

32. Bowden CL, et al. Efficacy of valproate versus lithium in mania or mixed mania: a randomized, open 12-week trial. *Int Clin Psychopharmacol* 2010; 25:60–67.

33. McElroy SL, et al. Randomized, double-blind, placebo-controlled study of divalproex extended release loading monotherapy in ambulatory bipolar spectrum disorder patients with moderate-to-severe hypomania or mild mania. *J Clin Psychiatry* 2010; 71:557–565.

34. Hirschfeld RM, et al. A randomized, placebo-controlled, multicenter study of divalproex sodium extended-release in the acute treatment of mania. *J Clin Psychiatry* 2010; 71:426–432.

35. McElroy SL, et al. A randomized comparison of divalproex oral loading versus haloperidol in the initial treatment of acute psychotic mania. *J Clin Psychiatry* 1996; 57:142–146.

36. Hirschfeld RM, et al. Safety and tolerability of oral loading divalproex sodium in acutely manic bipolar patients. *J Clin Psychiatry* 1999; 60:815–818.

37. Hirschfeld RM, et al. The safety and early efficacy of oral-loaded divalproex versus standard-titration divalproex, lithium, olanzapine, and placebo in the treatment of acute mania associated with bipolar disorder. *J Clin Psychiatry* 2003; 64:841–846.

38. Jagadheesan K, et al. Acute antimanic efficacy and safety of intravenous valproate loading therapy: an open-label study. *Neuropsychobiology* 2003; 47:90–93.

39. Sekhar S, et al. Efficacy of sodium valproate and haloperidol in the management of acute mania: a randomized open-label comparative study. *J Clin Pharmacol* 2010; 50:688–692.

40. Fontana E, et al. Intravenous valproate in the treatment of acute manic episode in bipolar disorder: a review. *J Affect Disord* 2020; 260:738–743.

41. Li DJ, et al. Efficacy, safety and tolerability of aripiprazole in bipolar disorder: an updated systematic review and meta-analysis of randomized controlled trials. *Prog Neuropsychopharmacol Biol Psychiatry* 2017; 79:289–301.

42. Romeo B, et al. Meta-analysis and review of dopamine agonists in acute episodes of mood disorder: efficacy and safety. *J Psychopharmacol* 2018; 32:385–396.

43. Vieta E, et al. Effect of cariprazine across the symptoms of mania in bipolar I disorder: analyses of pooled data from phase II/III trials. *Eur Neuropsychopharmacol* 2015; 25:1882–1891.

44. Chang HY, et al. The efficacy and tolerability of paliperidone in mania of bipolar disorder: a preliminary meta-analysis. *Exp Clin Psychopharmacol* 2017; 25:422–433.

45. Pajonk FG, et al. Rapid dose titration of quetiapine for the treatment of acute schizophrenia and acute mania: a case series. *J Psychopharmacol* 2006; 20:119–124.

46. Chen AT, et al. Allopurinol augmentation in acute mania: a meta-analysis of placebo-controlled trials. *J Affect Disord* 2018; 226:245–250.

47. Arabzadeh S, et al. Celecoxib adjunctive therapy for acute bipolar mania: a randomized, double-blind, placebo-controlled trial. *Bipolar Disord* 2015; 17:606–614.

48. Mahmood T, et al. Clozapine in the management of bipolar and schizoaffective manic episodes resistant to standard treatment. *Aust N Z J Psychiatry* 1997; 31:424–426.

49. Green AI, et al. Clozapine in the treatment of refractory psychotic mania. *Am J Psychiatry* 2000; 157:982–986.

50. Ifteni P, et al. Switching bipolar disorder patients treated with clozapine to another antipsychotic medication: a mirror image study. *Neuropsychiatr Dis Treat* 2017; 13:201–204.

51. Aksoy Poyraz C, et al. Effectiveness of ultra-rapid dose titration of clozapine for treatment-resistant bipolar mania: case series. *Ther Adv Psychopharmacol* 2015; 5:237–242.

52. Sharpley AL, et al. A phase 2a randomised, double-blind, placebo-controlled, parallel-group, add-on clinical trial of ebselen (SPI-1005) as a novel treatment for mania or hypomania. *Psychopharmacology (Berl)* 2020; 237:3773–3782.

53. Macdonald KJ, et al. Newer antiepileptic drugs in bipolar disorder: rationale for use and role in therapy. *CNS Drugs* 2002; 16:549–562.

54. Cabras PL, et al. Clinical experience with gabapentin in patients with bipolar or schizoaffective disorder: results of an open-label study. *J Clin Psychiatry* 1999; 60:245–248.

55. Pande AC, et al. Gabapentin in bipolar disorder: a placebo-controlled trial of adjunctive therapy. Gabapentin Bipolar Disorder Study Group. *Bipolar Disord* 2000; 2 (3 Pt 2):249–255.

56. Vieta E, et al. A double-blind, randomized, placebo-controlled, prophylaxis study of adjunctive gabapentin for bipolar disorder. *J Clin Psychiatry* 2006; 67:473–477.

57. Grunze H, et al. Levetiracetam in the treatment of acute mania: an open add-on study with an on-off-on design. *J Clin Psychiatry* 2003; 64:781–784.

58. Goldberg JF, et al. Levetiracetam for acute mania (Letter). *Am J Psychiatry* 2002; 159:148.

59. Park EM, et al. Acute mania associated with levetiracetam treatment. *Psychosomatics* 2014; 55:98–100.

60. Koukopoulos A, et al. Antimanic and mood-stabilizing effect of memantine as an augmenting agent in treatment-resistant bipolar disorder. *Bipolar Disord* 2010; 12:348–349.

61. Veronese N, et al. Acetylcholinesterase inhibitors and memantine in bipolar disorder: a systematic review and best evidence synthesis of the efficacy and safety for multiple disease dimensions. *J Affect Disord* 2016; 197:268–280.

62. Serra G, et al. Three-year, naturalistic, mirror-image assessment of adding memantine to the treatment of 30 treatment-resistant patients with bipolar disorder. *J Clin Psychiatry* 2015; 76:e91–e97.

63. Omranifard V, et al. Evaluation of the effect of memantine supplementation in the treatment of acute phase of mania in bipolar disorder of elderly patients: a double-blind randomized controlled trial. *Adv Biomed Res* 2018; 7:148.

64. Moghaddam HS, et al. Efficacy of melatonin as an adjunct in the treatment of acute mania: a double-blind and placebo-controlled trial. *Int Clin Psychopharmacol* 2020; 35:81–88.

65. Quested DJ, et al. Melatonin in acute mania investigation (MIAMI-UK). A randomized controlled trial of add-on melatonin in bipolar disorder. *Bipolar Disord* 2021; 23:176–185

66. Benedetti A, et al. Oxcarbazepine as add-on treatment in patients with bipolar manic, mixed or depressive episode. *J Affect Disord* 2004; 79:273–277.

67. Lande RG. Oxcarbazepine: efficacy, safety, and tolerability in the treatment of mania. *Int J Psychiatry Clin Pract* 2004; 8:37–40.

68. Ghaemi SN, et al. Oxcarbazepine treatment of bipolar disorder. *J Clin Psychiatry* 2003; 64:943–945.

69. Pratoomsri W, et al. Oxcarbazepine in the treatment of bipolar disorder: a review. *Can J Psychiatry* 2006; 51:540–545.

70. Juruena MF, et al. Bipolar I and II disorder residual symptoms: oxcarbazepine and carbamazepine as add-on treatment to lithium in a double-blind, randomized trial. *Prog Neuropsychopharmacol Biol Psychiatry* 2009; 33:94–99.

71. Suppes T, et al. Comparison of two anticonvulsants in a randomized, single-blind treatment of hypomanic symptoms in patients with bipolar disorder. *Aust N Z J Psychiatry* 2007; 41:397–402.

72. Vieta E, et al. A double-blind, randomized, placebo-controlled prophylaxis trial of oxcarbazepine as adjunctive treatment to lithium in the long-term treatment of bipolar I and II disorder. *Int J Neuropsychopharmacol* 2008; 11:445–452.

CHAPTER 2

73. Wagner KD, et al. A double-blind, randomized, placebo-controlled trial of oxcarbazepine in the treatment of bipolar disorder in children and adolescents. *Am J Psychiatry* 2006; **163**:1179–1186.

74. Mishory A, et al. Phenytoin as an antimanic anticonvulsant: a controlled study. *Am J Psychiatry* 2000; **157**:463–465.

75. Akhondzadeh S, et al. Ritanserin as an adjunct to lithium and haloperidol for the treatment of medication-naive patients with acute mania: a double blind and placebo controlled trial. *BMC Psychiatry* 2003; **3**:7.

76. Palacios J, et al. Tamoxifen for bipolar disorder: systematic review and meta-analysis. *J Psychopharmacol* 2019; **33**:177–184.

77. Pigott K, et al. Topiramate for acute affective episodes in bipolar disorder in adults. *Cochrane Database Syst Rev* 2016.

78. Applebaum J, et al. Rapid tryptophan depletion as a treatment for acute mania: a double-blind, pilot-controlled study. *Bipolar Disord* 2007; **9**:884–887.

79. Keck PE, Jr., et al. Ziprasidone in the treatment of acute bipolar mania: a three-week, placebo-controlled, double-blind, randomized trial. *Am J Psychiatry* 2003; **160**:741–748.

80. Potkin SG, et al. Ziprasidone in acute bipolar mania: a 21-day randomized, double-blind, placebo-controlled replication trial. *J Clin Psychopharmacol* 2005; **25**:301–310.

81. Vieta E, et al. Ziprasidone in the treatment of acute mania: a 12-week, placebo-controlled, haloperidol-referenced study. *J Psychopharm* 2010; **24**:547–558.

Rapid cycling bipolar affective disorder

Rapid cycling is usually defined as BD in which four or more episodes of (hypo)mania or depression (or four clear switches in polarity) occur in a 12-month period. It is generally held to be less responsive to drug treatment than non-rapid cycling bipolar illness[1,2] and entails considerable depressive morbidity and suicide risk.[3] Important clinical differences between bipolar patients with and without a rapid cycling include more depressive morbidity, higher incidence of anxiety disorders, addiction, bulimia and borderline personality disorder, as well as atypical features during depression and symptoms such as irritability, risky behaviour, impulsivity and agitation. Rapid cycling patients have poorer functioning than patients without, more obesity, and have to be treated with more drugs.[4] Drug doses tend to be somewhat higher in rapid cycling than in other bipolar patients.[5]

Table 2.8 outlines a treatment strategy for rapid cycling based on rather limited data and very few direct comparisons of drugs.[6,7] This strategy is broadly in line with the findings of published systematic reviews.[7,8] NICE concluded in 2016 that there is no evidence to support rapid cycling illness being managed any differently from that with a more conventional course.[9] There is no formal first choice agent or combination – prescribing depends partly on what treatments have already been used in an attempt to

Table 2.8 Recommended treatment strategy for rapid-cycling bipolar disorder

Step	Suggested treatment
Step 1	**Withdraw antidepressants** in all patients[10–14] (some controversial evidence supports continuation of SSRIs[15,16])
Step 2	**Evaluate possible precipitants** (e.g. alcohol, thyroid dysfunction (including antithyroid antibodies[17]), external stressors)[2]
Step 3	**Optimise mood stabiliser treatment**[18–21] (using plasma levels), and **Consider combining mood stabilisers**, e.g. lithium + valproate; lithium + lamotrigine, valproate + carbamazepine or go to Step 4
Step 4	**Consider other (usually adjunct) treatment options**: (alphabetical order; preferred treatment options in bold) **Aripiprazole**[22,23] (15–30mg/day) Clozapine[24] (usual doses) Lamotrigine[25–27] (up to 225mg/day) Levetiracetam[28] (up to 2000mg/day) Nimodipine[29,30] (180mg/day) **Olanzapine**[18] (usual doses) **Quetiapine**[31–34] (300–600mg/day) Risperidone[35–37] (up to 6mg/day) Thyroxine[38–40] (150–400µg/day) Topiramate[41] (up to 300mg/day)

Choice of drug is determined by patient factors – few comparative efficacy data to guide choice at the time of writing. **Quetiapine** *probably has best supporting data[31–33] but there is no evidence of superiority over aripiprazole or olanzapine. Supporting data for levetiracetam, nimodipine, thyroxine and topiramate are rather limited.*

Clozapine *has a clear role in treatment-resistant bipolar disorder,[42] a definition that might include rapid cycling in which it shows acute and long-term efficacy.[24,43]*

prevent or treat mood episodes. Evidence suggests that lithium is less likely to be effective in rapid cycling than in non-rapid cycling,[44] a finding supported by psychiatrists' experiences.[45]

In practice, response to treatment is sometimes idiosyncratic: individuals may show significant response only to one or two drugs. Spontaneous or treatment-related remissions occur in around a third of rapid cyclers[46] and rapid cycling may come and go in many patients.[47]

References

1. Calabrese JR, et al. Current research on rapid cycling bipolar disorder and its treatment. *J Affect Disord* 2001; 67:241–255.
2. Kupka RW, et al. Rapid and non-rapid cycling bipolar disorder: a meta-analysis of clinical studies. *J Clin Psychiatry* 2003; 64:1483–1494.
3. Coryell W, et al. The long-term course of rapid-cycling bipolar disorder. *Arch Gen Psychiatry* 2003; 60:914–920.
4. Furio M, et al. Characterization of rapid cycling bipolar patients presenting with major depressive episode within the BRIDGE-II-MIX study. *Bipolar Disord* 2020. [Epub ahead of print].
5. Yasui-Furukori N, et al. Factors Associated with Doses of Mood Stabilizers in Real-world Outpatients with Bipolar Disorder. *Clin Psychopharmacol Neurosci* 2020; 18:599–606.
6. Tondo L, et al. Rapid-cycling bipolar disorder: effects of long-term treatments. *Acta Psychiatr Scand* 2003; 108:4–14.
7. Fountoulakis KN, et al. A systematic review of the evidence on the treatment of rapid cycling bipolar disorder. *Bipolar Disord* 2013; 15:115–137.
8. Fountoulakis KN, et al. The international college of neuro-psychopharmacology (CINP) treatment guidelines for bipolar disorder in adults (CINP-BD-2017), Part 2: review, grading of the evidence, and a Precise Algorithm. *Int J Neuropsychopharmacol* 2017; 20:121–179.
9. National Institute for Health and Care Excellence. Bipolar disorder: assessment and management. Clinical Guidance [CG185]. 2014 (Last updated February 2020); https://www.nice.org.uk/guidance/cg185.
10. Wehr TA, et al. Can antidepressants cause mania and worsen the course of affective illness? *Am J Psychiatry* 1987; 144:1403–1411.
11. Altshuler LL, et al. Antidepressant-induced mania and cycle acceleration: a controversy revisited. *Am J Psychiatry* 1995; 152:1130–1138.
12. Ghaemi SN, et al. Antidepressant discontinuation in bipolar depression: a Systematic Treatment Enhancement Program for Bipolar Disorder (STEP-BD) randomized clinical trial of long-term effectiveness and safety. *J Clin Psychiatry* 2010; 71:372–380.
13. Ghaemi SN. Treatment of rapid-cycling bipolar disorder: are antidepressants mood destabilizers? *Am J Psychiatry* 2008; 165:300–302.
14. El-Mallakh RS, et al. Antidepressants worsen rapid-cycling course in bipolar depression: a STEP-BD randomized clinical trial. *J Affect Disord* 2015; 184:318–321.
15. Amsterdam JD, et al. Efficacy and mood conversion rate during long-term fluoxetine v. lithium monotherapy in rapid- and non-rapid-cycling bipolar II disorder. *Br J Psychiatry* 2013; 202:301–306.
16. Amsterdam JD, et al. Effectiveness and mood conversion rate of short-term fluoxetine monotherapy in patients with rapid cycling bipolar II depression versus patients with nonrapid cycling bipolar II depression. *J Clin Psychopharmacol* 2013; 33:420–424.
17. Gan Z, et al. Rapid cycling bipolar disorder is associated with antithyroid antibodies, instead of thyroid dysfunction. *BMC Psychiatry* 2019; 19:378.
18. Sanger TM, et al. Olanzapine in the acute treatment of bipolar I disorder with a history of rapid cycling. *J Affect Disord* 2003; 73:155–161.
19. Kemp DE, et al. A 6-month, double-blind, maintenance trial of lithium monotherapy versus the combination of lithium and divalproex for rapid-cycling bipolar disorder and Co-occurring substance abuse or dependence. *J Clin Psychiatry* 2009; 70:113–121.
20. da Rocha FF, et al. Addition of lamotrigine to valproic acid: a successful outcome in a case of rapid-cycling bipolar affective disorder. *Prog Neuropsychopharmacol Biol Psychiatry* 2007; 31:1548–1549.
21. Woo YS, et al. Lamotrigine added to valproate successfully treated a case of ultra-rapid cycling bipolar disorder. *Psychiatry Clin Neurosci* 2007; 61:130–131.
22. Suppes T, et al. Efficacy and safety of aripiprazole in subpopulations with acute manic or mixed episodes of bipolar I disorder. *J Affect Disord* 2008; 107:145–154.
23. Muzina DJ, et al. Aripiprazole monotherapy in patients with rapid-cycling bipolar I disorder: an analysis from a long-term, double-blind, placebo-controlled study. *Int J Clin Pract* 2008; 62:679–687.
24. Calabrese JR, et al. Clozapine prophylaxis in rapid cycling bipolar disorder. *J Clin Psychopharmacol* 1991; 11:396–397.
25. Fatemi SH, et al. Lamotrigine in rapid-cycling bipolar disorder. *J Clin Psychiatry* 1997; 58:522–527.
26. Calabrese JR, et al. A double-blind, placebo-controlled, prophylaxis study of lamotrigine in rapid-cycling bipolar disorder. Lamictal 614 Study Group. *J Clin Psychiatry* 2000; 61:841–850.
27. Wang Z, et al. Lamotrigine adjunctive therapy to lithium and divalproex in depressed patients with rapid cycling bipolar disorder and a recent substance use disorder: a 12-week, double-blind, placebo-controlled pilot study. *Psychopharmacol Bull* 2010; 43:5–21.
28. Braunig P, et al. Levetiracetam in the treatment of rapid cycling bipolar disorder. *J Psychopharmacol* 2003; 17:239–241.
29. Goodnick PJ. Nimodipine treatment of rapid cycling bipolar disorder. *J Clin Psychiatry* 1995; 56:330.

30. Pazzaglia PJ, et al. Preliminary controlled trial of nimodipine in ultra-rapid cycling affective dysregulation. *Psychiatry Res* 1993; **49**:257–272.

31. Goldberg JF, et al. Effectiveness of quetiapine in rapid cycling bipolar disorder: a preliminary study. *J Affect Disord* 2008; **105**:305–310.

32. Vieta E, et al. Quetiapine monotherapy in the treatment of patients with bipolar I or II depression and a rapid-cycling disease course: a randomized, double-blind, placebo-controlled study. *Bipolar Disord* 2007; **9**:413–425.

33. Langosch JM, et al. Efficacy of quetiapine monotherapy in rapid-cycling bipolar disorder in comparison with sodium valproate. *J Clin Psychopharmacol* 2008; **28**:555–560.

34. Vieta E, et al. Quetiapine in the treatment of rapid cycling bipolar disorder. *Bipolar Disord* 2002; **4**:335–340.

35. Jacobsen FM. Risperidone in the treatment of affective illness and obsessive-compulsive disorder. *J Clin Psychiatry* 1995; **56**:423–429.

36. Bobo WV, et al. A randomized open comparison of long-acting injectable risperidone and treatment as usual for prevention of relapse, rehospitalization, and urgent care referral in community-treated patients with rapid cycling bipolar disorder. *Clin Neuropharmacol* 2011; **34**:224–233.

37. Vieta E, et al. Treatment of refractory rapid cycling bipolar disorder with risperidone. *J Clin Psychopharmacol* 1998; **18**:172–174.

38. Extein IL. High doses of levothyroxine for refractory rapid cycling. *Am J Psychiatry* 2000; **157**:1704–1705.

39. Walshaw PD, et al. Adjunctive thyroid hormone treatment in rapid cycling bipolar disorder: a double-blind placebo-controlled trial of levothyroxine (L-T(4)) and triiodothyronine (T(3)). *Bipolar Disord* 2018; **20**:594–603.

40. Qureshi MM, et al. The chimera of circular insanity and the labours of Thyreoidea. *Bipolar Disord* 2019; **21**:794–796.

41. Chen CK, et al. Combination treatment of clozapine and topiramate in resistant rapid-cycling bipolar disorder. *Clin Neuropharmacol* 2005; **28**:136–138.

42. Delgado A, et al. Clozapine in bipolar disorder: a systematic review and meta-analysis. *J Psychiatr Res* 2020; **125**:21–27.

43. Kılınçel O, et al. The role of clozapine as a mood regulator in the treatment of rapid cycling bipolar affective disorder. *Turk J Psychiatry* 2019; **30**:268–271.

44. Hui TP, et al. A systematic review and meta-analysis of clinical predictors of lithium response in bipolar disorder. *Acta Psychiatr Scand* 2019; **140**:94–115.

45. Montlahuc C, et al. Response to lithium in patients with bipolar disorder: what are psychiatrists' experiences and practices compared to literature review? *Pharmacopsychiatry* 2019; **52**:70–77.

46. Koukopoulos A, et al. Duration and stability of the rapid-cycling course: a long-term personal follow-up of 109 patients. *J Affect Disord* 2003; **73**:75–85.

47. Carvalho AF, et al. Rapid cycling in bipolar disorder: a systematic review. *J Clin Psychiatry* 2014; **75**:e578–e586.

CHAPTER 2

Bipolar depression

Bipolar depression shares the same diagnostic criteria for a major depressive episode in major depressive disorder but episodes may differ in severity, time course, liability to recurrence and response to drug treatment. Episodes of bipolar depression are, compared with unipolar depression, more rapid in onset, more frequent, more severe, shorter and more likely to involve delusions and reverse neuro-vegetative symptoms such as hyperphagia and hypersomnia.[1-3] Around 15% of people with bipolar depression commit suicide,[4] a statistic that reflects the severity and frequency of depressive episodes. Bipolar depression affords greater socio-economic burden than either mania or unipolar major depression[5] and comprises the majority of symptomatic illness in bipolar affective disorder with respect to time.[6,7]

The drug treatment of bipolar depression is somewhat controversial for two reasons. First, there are few well-conducted RCTs specifically in bipolar depression, and second, the condition entails consideration of the long-term outcome rather than only the discrete depressive episode response.[8] We have some knowledge of the therapeutic effects of drugs in bipolar depressive episodes but more limited awareness of the therapeutic or deleterious effects of drugs in the longer term.

In the UK, NICE recommends the initial use of fluoxetine combined with olanzapine or quetiapine on its own (assuming an antipsychotic is not already prescribed).[9] Lamotrigine is considered to be a second-line treatment. BAP guidelines[10] have lamotrigine as a first-line option, albeit with the caveat that a mood stabiliser or antipsychotic will be needed to protect against mania in the longer term. Lurasidone is also a first-line option in the BAP guidelines.

More recent consensus guidelines are broadly but not precisely in agreement. The Canadian Network for Mood and Anxiety Treatments (CANMAT)/International Society for Bipolar Disorders (ISBD) guidelines recommend quetiapine, lurasidone (with or without a mood stabiliser), lamotrigine and lithium as first-line treatments.[11] The 2020 RANZCP guidelines suggest lithium, lamotrigine and valproate (in that order) as first-line agents, and quetiapine, lurasidone and cariprazine (again, in that order) as second-line treatments.[12]

Tables 2.9–2.11 give some broad guidance on treatment options in bipolar depression.

Meta-analysis in bipolar depression

Meta-analytic studies in bipolar depression are constrained by the variety of methods used to assess efficacy. This means that many scientifically robust studies cannot be included in some meta-analyses because their parameters (outcomes, duration, etc.) are not shared with other studies and so cannot be compared with them. Early lithium studies are an important example – their short duration and cross-over design precludes their inclusion in meta-analysis. BAP guidelines are somewhat dismissive (perhaps correctly) of network meta-analyses because outcome is heavily influenced by inclusion criteria and because findings often contradict direct comparisons.[10]

A meta-analysis of five trials (906 participants) revealed that antidepressants were no better than placebo with respect to response or remission, although results approached

Table 2.9 Established treatments (listed in alphabetical order)

Drug/regime	Comments
Lamotrigine[1,13–19]	Lamotrigine appears to be effective both as a treatment for bipolar depression and as prophylaxis against further episodes. It does not induce switching or rapid cycling. It is as effective as citalopram and causes less weight gain than lithium. Overall, the effect of lamotrigine is difficult to be clear about with numerous equivocal trials[20,21] that perhaps failed to allow for the time taken for full titration of the drug. It may be useful as an adjunct to lithium[22] or as an alternative to it in pregnancy.[23] A later trial[24] suggests robust efficacy when combined with quetiapine. There is a small antimanic effect of lamotrigine.[25]
	Treatment is somewhat complicated by the small risk of rash, which is associated with speed of dose titration. The necessity for titration may limit clinical utility.
	A further complication is the question of dose: 50mg/day has efficacy, but 200mg/day is probably better. In the US, doses of up to 1200mg/day have been used (mean around 250mg/day). Plasma concentrations (only the range for anticonvulsant effects is known) may guide the need for higher doses.
Lithium[1,13,26–28]	Lithium is probably effective in treating bipolar depression but supporting data are methodologically questionable.[29] There is some evidence that lithium prevents depressive relapse but its effects on manic relapse are considered more robust. Fairly strong support for lithium in reducing suicidality in bipolar disorder[30,31]
Lurasidone	Three RCTs show good effect for lurasidone either alone[32] or as an adjunct to mood stabilisers.[33,34] A further RCT reported good outcome in bipolar depression with sub-syndromal hypomanic symptoms.[35] Pooled analysis suggests response is dose related.[36] A network meta-analysis suggests that lurasidone is more effective than aripiprazole and ziprasidone but not quetiapine or olanzapine.[37]
Mood stabiliser + antidepressant[38–44]	Antidepressants are still widely used in bipolar depression, particularly for breakthrough episodes occurring in those on mood stabilisers. They have been assumed to be effective, although there is a risk of cycle acceleration and/or switching. Studies suggest that mood stabilisers alone are just as effective as mood stabilisers–antidepressant combination although sub-analysis suggested higher doses of antidepressants may be effective.[45–47] Tricyclics and MAOIs are usually best avoided. SSRIs are generally recommended if an antidepressant is to be prescribed. Venlafaxine and bupropion (amfebutamone) have also been used. Venlafaxine may be more likely to induce a switch to mania.[48,49]
	Continuing antidepressant treatment after resolution of symptoms may protect against depressive relapse,[50,51] although only in the absence of a mood stabiliser.[52] At the time of writing, there is no consensus on whether or not to continue antidepressants long term.[53] The most recent findings suggest that switch rates are no higher than with sertraline alone than with lithium + sertraline.[54]
	Some guidelines recommend the use of antidepressant in bipolar II depression,[11] and there is evidence that sertraline does not increase switch rates in these patients.[54]

(Continued)

Drug/regime	Comments
Olanzapine ± fluoxetine[13,29,55–58]	This combination (Symbyax®) is more effective than both placebo and olanzapine alone in treating bipolar depression. The dose is 6mg/day and 25mg/day or 12mg/day and 50mg/day (so presumably 5/20mg and 10/40mg are effective). May be more effective than lamotrigine. Reasonable evidence of prophylactic effect. Recommended as first-line treatment by NICE.[9]
	Olanzapine alone is effective when compared with placebo,[59] but the combination with fluoxetine is more effective. (This is possibly the strongest evidence for a beneficial effect for an antidepressant in bipolar depression.)
Quetiapine[60–64]	Five large RCTs have demonstrated clear efficacy for doses of 300mg and 600mg daily (as monotherapy) in bipolar I and bipolar II depression. A later study in Chinese patients demonstrated the efficacy of 300mg/day[65] in bipolar I depression. May be superior to both lithium and paroxetine.
	Quetiapine also prevents relapse into depression and mania[66,67] and so is one of the treatments of choice in bipolar depression. It appears not to be associated with switching to mania.
Valproate[1,13,68–72]	Limited evidence of efficacy as monotherapy but recommended in some guidelines. Several very small RCTs but many negative, however, meta-analyses do support antidepressant efficacy.[71] Probably protects against depressive relapse but database is small.

Table 2.10 Alternative treatments – refer to primary literature before using

Drug/regime	Comments
Antidepressants[73–81]	'Unopposed' antidepressants (i.e. without mood stabiliser protection) are generally to be avoided in bipolar depression because of the risk of switching and inducing rapid cycling. There is also evidence that they are relatively less effective (perhaps not effective at all) in bipolar depression than in unipolar depression although dose may be critical.[47] Short-term use of fluoxetine, venlafaxine and moclobemide seems reasonably effective and safe even as monotherapy. A meta-analysis suggested a large effect size for tranylcypromine in the absence of any risk of switching.[82] Overall, however, unopposed antidepressant treatment should be avoided, especially in bipolar I disorder.[53]
Cariprazine[83]	One RCT suggests that cariprazine at 1.5mg/day is effective in bipolar I depression. A second, larger study showed 1.5mg/day and 3mg/day to be effective.[84] The most recent study[84] found benefit for 1.5mg/day but not 3mg/day.
Ketamine[85–88]	IV dose of 0.5mg/kg is effective in refractory bipolar depression. Very high response rate. Dissociative symptoms common but brief. Now accepted as standard treatment for refractory bipolar depression.[89,90] IV racemate is possibly more effective than intranasal esketamine.[91] Switching to mania is a potential problem[92] although probably a remote risk.
Pramipexole[93,94]	Two small placebo-controlled trials suggest useful efficacy in bipolar depression. Effective dose averages around 1.7mg/day. Both studies used pramipexole as an adjunct to the existing mood stabiliser treatment. Neither study detected an increased risk of switching to mania/hypomania (a theoretical consideration) but data are insufficient to exclude this possibility. A meta-analysis of studies showed a robust effect on response but not remission.[95]

Table 2.11 Other possible treatments – seek specialist advice before using

Drug/regime	Comments
Aripiprazole[96–99]	Limited support from open studies as add-on treatment. RCT negative. Possibly not effective.[95]
Carbamazepine[1,13,100]	Occasionally recommended but database is poor and effect modest. May have useful activity when added to other mood stabilisers.
Gabapentin[1,101,102]	Open studies suggest modest effect when added to mood stabilisers or antipsychotics. Doses average around 1750mg/day. Anxiolytic effect may account for apparent effect in bipolar depression
Inositol[103]	Small, randomised, pilot study suggests that 12g/day inositol is effective in bipolar depression
Mifepristone[104,105]	Some evidence of mood-elevating properties in bipolar depression although this was not replicated in a larger trial. Improved cognitive function in both trials. Dose used was 600mg/day.
Modafinil[106]	Meta-analysis of five studies of modafinil/armodafinil suggests robust benefit on response and remission with good tolerability and no evidence of increased risk of switching.
Omega-3 fatty acids[107,108]	One positive RCT (1g/2g a day) and one negative (6g a day)

CHAPTER 2

statistical significance.[98] Another analysis of trials not involving antidepressants[109] (7307 participants) found a statistical advantage over placebo for olanzapine + fluoxetine, valproate, quetiapine, lurasidone, olanzapine, aripiprazole and carbamazepine (in order of effect size, highest first).

A 2014 network meta-analysis of 29 studies included 8331 subjects.[110] Overall olanzapine + fluoxetine, lurasidone, olanzapine, valproate, SSRIs and quetiapine were ranked highest in terms of effect size and response with olanzapine + fluoxetine ranked first for both. The most recent network meta-analysis included 11,448 participants in 50 studies.[111] Drugs found to be more effective than placebo were olanzapine + fluoxetine, olanzapine, valproate, cariprazine, lamotrigine, lurasidone and quetiapine. Interestingly, imipramine and fluoxetine were also more effective than placebo (but with wide confidence intervals).

Summary of drug choice

The combination of olanzapine + fluoxetine is probably the most effective treatment available for bipolar depression but its use is constrained by the well known adverse effect profile of olanzapine. SSRIs other than fluoxetine may be effective but should probably be avoided unless clear individual benefit is obvious.[53] Alternative first-line choices are quetiapine, olanzapine, lurasidone, lamotrigine and valproate. These drugs differ substantially in adverse effect profile, tolerability and cost, each of which needs to be considered when prescribing for an individual. Lithium is also effective but supporting evidence is relatively weak. Second-line drugs include ketamine and, increasingly, modafinil. Aripiprazole, risperidone, ziprasidone, tricyclics (with the exception of imipramine) and MAOIs (with the exception of tranylcypromine) are probably not effective and should not be used routinely.[110]

References

1. Malhi GS, et al. Bipolar depression: management options. *CNS Drugs* 2003; **17**:9–25.
2. Perlis RH, et al. Clinical features of bipolar depression versus major depressive disorder in large multicenter trials. *Am J Psychiatry* 2006; **163**:225–231.
3. Mitchell PB, et al. Comparison of depressive episodes in bipolar disorder and in major depressive disorder within bipolar disorder pedigrees. *Br J Psychiatry* 2011; **199**:303–309.
4. Haddad P, et al. Pharmacological management of bipolar depression. *Acta Psychiatr Scand* 2002; **105**:401–403.
5. Hirschfeld RM. Bipolar depression: the real challenge. *Eur Neuropsychopharmacol* 2004; **14 Suppl 2**:S83–S88.
6. Judd LL, et al. The long-term natural history of the weekly symptomatic status of bipolar I disorder. *Arch Gen Psychiatry* 2002; **59**:530–537.
7. Judd LL, et al. A prospective investigation of the natural history of the long-term weekly symptomatic status of bipolar II disorder. *Arch Gen Psychiatry* 2003; **60**:261–269.
8. Baldassano CF, et al. Rethinking the treatment paradigm for bipolar depression: the importance of long-term management. *CNS Spectr* 2004; **9**:11–18.
9. National Institute for Health and Care Excellence. Bipolar disorder: assessment and management. Clinical Guidance [CG185]. 2014 (Last updated February 2020); https://www.nice.org.uk/guidance/cg185.
10. Goodwin GM, et al. Evidence-based guidelines for treating bipolar disorder: revised third edition recommendations from the British Association for Psychopharmacology. *J Psychopharmacol* 2016; **30**:495–553.
11. Yatham LN, et al. Canadian network for mood and anxiety treatments (CANMAT) and International Society for Bipolar Disorders (ISBD) 2018 guidelines for the management of patients with bipolar disorder. *Bipolar Disord* 2018; **20**:97–170.
12. Malhi GS, et al. The 2020 Royal Australian and New Zealand College of Psychiatrists Clinical Practice Guidelines for mood disorders: bipolar disorder summary. *Bipolar Disord* 2020; **22**:805–821.
13. Yatham LN, et al. Bipolar depression: criteria for treatment selection, definition of refractoriness, and treatment options. *Bipolar Disord* 2003; **5**:85–97.
14. Calabrese JR, et al. A double-blind placebo-controlled study of lamotrigine monotherapy in outpatients with bipolar I depression. Lamictal 602 Study Group. *J Clin Psychiatry* 1999; **60**:79–88.
15. Bowden CL, et al. Lamotrigine in the treatment of bipolar depression. *Eur Neuropsychopharmacol* 1999; **9 Suppl 4**:S113–S117.
16. Marangell LB, et al. Lamotrigine treatment of bipolar disorder: data from the first 500 patients in STEP-BD. *Bipolar Disord* 2004; **6**:139–143.
17. Schaffer A, et al. Randomized, double-blind pilot trial comparing lamotrigine versus citalopram for the treatment of bipolar depression. *J Affect Disord* 2006; **96**:95–99.
18. Bowden CL, et al. Impact of lamotrigine and lithium on weight in obese and nonobese patients with bipolar I disorder. *Am J Psychiatry* 2006; **163**:1199–1201.
19. Suppes T, et al. A single blind comparison of lithium and lamotrigine for the treatment of bipolar II depression. *J Affect Disord* 2008; **111**:334–343.
20. Geddes JR, et al. Lamotrigine for treatment of bipolar depression: independent meta-analysis and meta-regression of individual patient data from five randomised trials. *Br J Psychiatry* 2009; **194**:4–9.
21. Calabrese JR, et al. Lamotrigine in the acute treatment of bipolar depression: results of five double-blind, placebo-controlled clinical trials. *Bipolar Disord* 2008; **10**:323–333.
22. van der Loos ML, et al. Efficacy and safety of lamotrigine as add-on treatment to lithium in bipolar depression: a multicenter, double-blind, placebo-controlled trial. *J Clin Psychiatry* 2009; **70**:223–231.
23. Newport DJ, et al. Lamotrigine in bipolar disorder: efficacy during pregnancy. *Bipolar Disord* 2008; **10**:432–436.
24. Geddes JR, et al. Comparative evaluation of quetiapine plus lamotrigine combination versus quetiapine monotherapy (and folic acid versus placebo) in bipolar depression (CEQUEL): a 2 x 2 factorial randomised trial. *Lancet Psychiatry* 2016; **3**:31–39.
25. Goodwin GM, et al. A pooled analysis of 2 placebo-controlled 18-month trials of lamotrigine and lithium maintenance in bipolar I disorder. *J Clin Psychiatry* 2004; **65**:432–441.
26. Geddes JR, et al. Long-term lithium therapy for bipolar disorder: systematic review and meta-analysis of randomized controlled trials. *Am J Psychiatry* 2004; **161**:217–222.
27. Calabrese JR, et al. A placebo-controlled 18-month trial of lamotrigine and lithium maintenance treatment in recently depressed patients with bipolar I disorder. *J Clin Psychiatry* 2003; **64**:1013–1024.
28. Prien RF, et al. Lithium carbonate and imipramine in prevention of affective episodes. A comparison in recurrent affective illness. *Arch Gen Psychiatry* 1973; **29**:420–425.
29. Grunze H, et al. The world federation of societies of biological psychiatry (WFSBP) guidelines for the biological treatment of bipolar disorders: update 2010 on the treatment of acute bipolar depression. *World J Biol Psychiatry* 2010; **11**:81–109.
30. Goodwin FK, et al. Suicide risk in bipolar disorder during treatment with lithium and divalproex. *JAMA* 2003; **290**:1467–1473.
31. Kessing LV, et al. Suicide risk in patients treated with lithium. *Arch Gen Psychiatry* 2005; **62**:860–866.
32. Loebel A, et al. Lurasidone monotherapy in the treatment of bipolar I depression: a randomized, double-blind, placebo-controlled study. *Am J Psychiatry* 2014; **171**:160–168.
33. Loebel A, et al. Lurasidone as adjunctive therapy with lithium or valproate for the treatment of bipolar I depression: a randomized, double-blind, placebo-controlled study. *Am J Psychiatry* 2014; **171**:169–177.

34. Suppes T, et al. Lurasidone adjunctive with lithium or valproate for bipolar depression: a placebo-controlled trial utilizing prospective and retrospective enrolment cohorts. *J Psychiatr Res* 2016; **78**:86–93.

35. Suppes T, et al. Lurasidone for the treatment of major depressive disorder with mixed features: a randomized, double-blind, placebo-controlled study. *Am J Psychiatry* 2016; **173**:400–407.

36. Chapel S, et al. Lurasidone dose response in bipolar depression: a population dose-response analysis. *Clin Ther* 2016; **38**:4–15.

37. Ostacher M, et al. Lurasidone compared to other atypical antipsychotic monotherapies for bipolar depression: A systematic review and network meta-analysis. *World J Biol Psychiatry* 2018; **19**:586–601.

38. Calabrese JR, et al. International consensus group on bipolar i depression treatment guidelines. *J Clin Psychiatry* 2004; **65**:571–579.

39. Nemeroff CB, et al. Double-blind, placebo-controlled comparison of imipramine and paroxetine in the treatment of bipolar depression. *Am J Psychiatry* 2001; **158**:906–912.

40. Vieta E, et al. A randomized trial comparing paroxetine and venlafaxine in the treatment of bipolar depressed patients taking mood stabilizers. *J Clin Psychiatry* 2002; **63**:508–512.

41. Young LT, et al. Double-blind comparison of addition of a second mood stabilizer versus an antidepressant to an initial mood stabilizer for treatment of patients with bipolar depression. *Am J Psychiatry* 2000; **157**:124–126.

42. Fawcett JA. Lithium combinations in acute and maintenance treatment of unipolar and bipolar depression. *J Clin Psychiatry* 2003; **64 Suppl 5**:32–37.

43. Altshuler L, et al. The impact of antidepressant discontinuation versus antidepressant continuation on 1-year risk for relapse of bipolar depression: a retrospective chart review. *J Clin Psychiatry* 2001; **62**:612–616.

44. Erfurth A, et al. Bupropion as add-on strategy in difficult-to-treat bipolar depressive patients. *Neuropsychobiology* 2002; **45 Suppl 1**:33–36.

45. Sachs GS, et al. Effectiveness of adjunctive antidepressant treatment for bipolar depression. *N Engl J Med* 2007; **356**:1711–1722.

46. Goldberg JF, et al. Adjunctive antidepressant use and symptomatic recovery among bipolar depressed patients with concomitant manic symptoms: findings from the STEP-BD. *Am J Psychiatry* 2007; **164**:1348–1355.

47. Tada M, et al. Antidepressant dose and treatment response in bipolar depression: reanalysis of the Systematic Treatment Enhancement Program for Bipolar Disorder (STEP-BD) data. *J Psychiatr Res* 2015; **68**:151–156.

48. Post RM, et al. Mood switch in bipolar depression: comparison of adjunctive venlafaxine, bupropion and sertraline. *Br J Psychiatry* 2006; **189**:124–131.

49. Leverich GS, et al. Risk of switch in mood polarity to hypomania or mania in patients with bipolar depression during acute and continuation trials of venlafaxine, sertraline, and bupropion as adjuncts to mood stabilizers. *Am J Psychiatry* 2006; **163**:232–239.

50. Salvi V, et al. The use of antidepressants in bipolar disorder. *J Clin Psychiatry* 2008; **69**:1307–1318.

51. Altshuler LL, et al. Impact of antidepressant continuation after acute positive or partial treatment response for bipolar depression: a blinded, randomized study. *J Clin Psychiatry* 2009; **70**:450–457.

52. Ghaemi SN, et al. Long-term antidepressant treatment in bipolar disorder: meta-analyses of benefits and risks. *Acta Psychiatr Scand* 2008; **118**:347–356.

53. Pacchiarotti I, et al. The International Society for Bipolar Disorders (ISBD) task force report on antidepressant use in bipolar disorders. *Am J Psychiatry* 2013; **170**:1249–1262.

54. Altshuler LL, et al. Switch rates during acute treatment for bipolar II depression with lithium, sertraline, or the two combined: a randomized double-blind comparison. *Am J Psychiatry* 2017; **174**:266–276.

55. Tohen M, et al. Efficacy of olanzapine and olanzapine-fluoxetine combination in the treatment of bipolar I depression. *Arch Gen Psychiatry* 2003; **60**:1079–1088.

56. Brown EB, et al. A 7-week, randomized, double-blind trial of olanzapine/fluoxetine combination versus lamotrigine in the treatment of bipolar I depression. *J Clin Psychiatry* 2006; **67**:1025–1033.

57. Corya SA, et al. A 24-week open-label extension study of olanzapine-fluoxetine combination and olanzapine monotherapy in the treatment of bipolar depression. *J Clin Psychiatry* 2006; **67**:798–806.

58. Dube S, et al. Onset of antidepressant effect of olanzapine and olanzapine/fluoxetine combination in bipolar depression. *Bipolar Disord* 2007; **9**:618–627.

59. Tohen M, et al. Randomised, double-blind, placebo-controlled study of olanzapine in patients with bipolar I depression. *Br J Psychiatry* 2012; **201**:376–382.

60. Calabrese JR, et al. A randomized, double-blind, placebo-controlled trial of quetiapine in the treatment of bipolar I or II depression. *Am J Psychiatry* 2005; **162**:1351–1360.

61. Thase ME, et al. Efficacy of quetiapine monotherapy in bipolar I and II depression: a double-blind, placebo-controlled study (the BOLDER II study). *J Clin Psychopharmacol* 2006; **26**:600–609.

62. Suppes T, et al. Effectiveness of the extended release formulation of quetiapine as monotherapy for the treatment of acute bipolar depression. *J Affect Disord* 2010; **121**:106–115.

63. Young AH, et al. A double-blind, placebo-controlled study of quetiapine and lithium monotherapy in adults in the acute phase of bipolar depression (EMBOLDEN I). *J Clin Psychiatry* 2010; **71**:150–162.

64. McElroy SL, et al. A double-blind, placebo-controlled study of quetiapine and paroxetine as monotherapy in adults with bipolar depression (EMBOLDEN II). *J Clin Psychiatry* 2010; **71**:163–174.

65. Li H, et al. Efficacy and safety of quetiapine extended release monotherapy in bipolar depression: a multi-center, randomized, double-blind, placebo-controlled trial. *Psychopharmacology (Berl)* 2016; **233**:1289–1297.

CHAPTER 2

66. Vieta E, et al. Efficacy and safety of quetiapine in combination with lithium or divalproex for maintenance of patients with bipolar I disorder (international trial 126). *J Affect Disord* 2008; 109:251–263.

67. Suppes T, et al. Maintenance treatment for patients with bipolar I disorder: results from a North American study of quetiapine in combination with lithium or divalproex (trial 127). *Am J Psychiatry* 2009; 166:476–488.

68. Goodwin GM. Evidence-based guidelines for treating bipolar disorder: revised second edition–recommendations from the British Association for Psychopharmacology. *J Psychopharmacol* 2009; 23:346–388.

69. Davis LL, et al. Divalproex in the treatment of bipolar depression: a placebo-controlled study. *J Affect Disord* 2005; 85:259–266.

70. Ghaemi SN, et al. Divalproex in the treatment of acute bipolar depression: a preliminary double-blind, randomized, placebo-controlled pilot study. *J Clin Psychiatry* 2007; 68:1840–1844.

71. Smith LA, et al. Valproate for the treatment of acute bipolar depression: systematic review and meta-analysis. *J Affect Disord* 2010; 122:1–9.

72. Muzina DJ, et al. Acute efficacy of divalproex sodium versus placebo in mood stabilizer-naive bipolar I or II depression: a double-blind, randomized, placebo-controlled trial. *J Clin Psychiatry* 2011; 72:813–819.

73. Amsterdam JD, et al. Short-term fluoxetine monotherapy for bipolar type II or bipolar NOS major depression – low manic switch rate. *Bipolar Disord* 2004; 6:75–81.

74. Amsterdam JD, et al. Efficacy and safety of fluoxetine in treating bipolar II major depressive episode. *J Clin Psychopharmacol* 1998; 18:435–440.

75. Amsterdam J. Efficacy and safety of venlafaxine in the treatment of bipolar II major depressive episode. *J Clin Psychopharmacol* 1998; 18:414–417.

76. Amsterdam JD, et al. Venlafaxine monotherapy in women with bipolar II and unipolar major depression. *J Affect Disord* 2000; 59:225–229.

77. Silverstone T. Moclobemide vs. imipramine in bipolar depression: a multicentre double-blind clinical trial. *Acta Psychiatr Scand* 2001; 104:104–109.

78. Ghaemi SN, et al. Antidepressant treatment in bipolar versus unipolar depression. *Am J Psychiatry* 2004; 161:163–165.

79. Post RM, et al. A re-evaluation of the role of antidepressants in the treatment of bipolar depression: data from the Stanley Foundation Bipolar Network. *Bipolar Disord* 2003; 5:396–406.

80. Amsterdam JD, et al. Comparison of fluoxetine, olanzapine, and combined fluoxetine plus olanzapine initial therapy of bipolar type I and type II major depression–lack of manic induction. *J Affect Disord* 2005; 87:121–130.

81. Amsterdam JD, et al. Fluoxetine monotherapy of bipolar type II and bipolar NOS major depression: a double-blind, placebo-substitution, continuation study. *Int Clin Psychopharmacol* 2005; 20:257–264.

82. Heijnen WT, et al. Efficacy of tranylcypromine in bipolar depression: a systematic review. *J Clin Psychopharmacol* 2015; 35:700–705.

83. Durgam S, et al. An 8-week randomized, double-blind, placebo-controlled evaluation of the safety and efficacy of cariprazine in patients with bipolar I depression. *Am J Psychiatry* 2016; 173:271–281.

84. Earley W, et al. Cariprazine treatment of bipolar depression: a randomized double-blind placebo-controlled phase 3 study. *Am J Psychiatry* 2019; 176:439–448.

85. Diazgranados N, et al. A randomized add-on trial of an N-methyl-D-aspartate antagonist in treatment-resistant bipolar depression. *Arch Gen Psychiatry* 2010; 67:793–802.

86. Shahani R, et al. Ketamine-associated ulcerative cystitis: a new clinical entity. *Urology* 2007; 69:810–812.

87. Zarate CA, Jr., et al. Replication of ketamine's antidepressant efficacy in bipolar depression: a randomized controlled add-on trial. *Biol Psychiatry* 2012; 71:939–946.

88. Permoda-Osip A, et al. Single ketamine infusion and neurocognitive performance in bipolar depression. *Pharmacopsychiatry* 2015; 48:78–79.

89. Jha MK, et al. Psychopharmacology and experimental therapeutics for bipolar depression. *Focus (American Psychiatric Publishing)* 2019; 17:232–237.

90. Włodarczyk A, et al. Safety and tolerability of ketamine use in treatment-resistant bipolar depression patients with regard to central nervous system symptomatology: literature review and analysis. *Medicina (Kaunas)* 2020; 56:67.

91. Bahji A, et al. Comparative efficacy of racemic ketamine and esketamine for depression: a systematic review and meta-analysis. *J Affect Disord* 2021; 278:542–555.

92. Alison McInnes L, et al. Possible affective switch associated with intravenous ketamine treatment in a patient with bipolar I disorder. *Biol Psychiatry* 2016; 79:e71–e72.

93. Goldberg JF, et al. Preliminary randomized, double-blind, placebo-controlled trial of pramipexole added to mood stabilizers for treatment-resistant bipolar depression. *Am J Psychiatry* 2004; 161:564–566.

94. Zarate CA, Jr., et al. Pramipexole for bipolar II depression: a placebo-controlled proof of concept study. *Biol Psychiatry* 2004; 56:54–60.

95. Romeo B, et al. Meta-analysis and review of dopamine agonists in acute episodes of mood disorder: efficacy and safety. *J Psychopharmacol* 2018; 32:385–396.

96. Ketter TA, et al. Adjunctive aripiprazole in treatment-resistant bipolar depression. *Ann Clin Psychiatry* 2006; 18:169–172.

97. Mazza M, et al. Beneficial acute antidepressant effects of aripiprazole as an adjunctive treatment or monotherapy in bipolar patients unresponsive to mood stabilizers: results from a 16-week open-label trial. *Expert Opin Pharmacother* 2008; 9:3145–3149.

98. Sidor MM, et al. Antidepressants for the acute treatment of bipolar depression: a systematic review and meta-analysis. *J Clin Psychiatry* 2011; 72:156–167.

99. Cruz N, et al. Efficacy of modern antipsychotics in placebo-controlled trials in bipolar depression: a meta-analysis. *Int J Neuropsychopharmacol* 2010; **13**:5–14.

100. Dilsaver SC, et al. Treatment of bipolar depression with carbamazepine: results of an open study. *Biol Psychiatry* 1996; **40**:935–937.

101. Wang PW, et al. Gabapentin augmentation therapy in bipolar depression. *Bipolar Disorders* 2002; **4**:296–301.

102. Ashton H, et al. GABA-ergic drugs: exit stage left, enter stage right. *J Psychopharmacol* 2003; **17**:174–178.

103. Chengappa KN, et al. Inositol as an add-on treatment for bipolar depression. *Bipolar Disord* 2000; **2**:47–55.

104. Young AH, et al. Improvements in neurocognitive function and mood following adjunctive treatment with mifepristone (RU-486) in bipolar disorder. *Neuropsychopharmacology* 2004; **29**:1538–1545.

105. Watson S, et al. A randomized trial to examine the effect of mifepristone on neuropsychological performance and mood in patients with bipolar depression. *Biol Psychiatry* 2012; **72**:943–949.

106. Nunez NA, et al. Efficacy and tolerability of adjunctive modafinil/armodafinil in bipolar depression: a meta-analysis of randomized controlled trials. *Bipolar Disord* 2020; **22**:109–120.

107. Frangou S, et al. Efficacy of ethyl-eicosapentaenoic acid in bipolar depression: randomised double-blind placebo-controlled study. *Br J Psychiatry* 2006; **188**:46–50.

108. Keck PE, Jr., et al. Double-blind, randomized, placebo-controlled trials of ethyl-eicosapentanoate in the treatment of bipolar depression and rapid cycling bipolar disorder. *Biol Psychiatry* 2006; **60**:1020–1022.

109. Selle V, et al. Treatments for acute bipolar depression: meta-analyses of placebo-controlled, monotherapy trials of anticonvulsants, lithium and antipsychotics. *Pharmacopsychiatry* 2014; **47**:43–52.

110. Taylor DM, et al. Comparative efficacy and acceptability of drug treatments for bipolar depression: a multiple-treatments meta-analysis. *Acta Psychiatr Scand* 2014; **130**:452–469.

111. Bahji A, et al. Comparative efficacy and tolerability of pharmacological treatments for the treatment of acute bipolar depression: a systematic review and network meta-analysis. *J Affect Disord* 2020; **269**:154–184.

CHAPTER 2

Prophylaxis in bipolar disorder

There is general agreement that successful drug regimens used in acute episodes should be continued as prophylaxis. To a large extent, therefore, the choice of maintenance treatment for individual patients is dictated by the efficacy and tolerability of acute treatment. Possible exceptions include the consideration of withdrawing antipsychotic treatment from a mood stabiliser combination after an episode of mania (recommended by some authorities[1]) and the withdrawal of antidepressants after the successful treatment of an acute episode of bipolar depression, assuming a mood stabiliser is continued (recommended by most authorities, at least implicitly[2]). There is some evidence that withdrawing antipsychotics from combination regimens with lithium or valproate worsens the risk of relapse.[3]

Residual mood symptoms after an acute episode are a strong predictor of recurrence.[4,5] With respect to monotherapy, most evidence supports the efficacy of lithium[6–10] in preventing episodes of mania and depression.[11] Carbamazepine is somewhat less effective,[10,12] and the long-term efficacy of valproate is uncertain,[8,9,13–15] although it too may protect against relapse both into depression and mania.[10,16] Lithium has the advantage of a proven anti-suicidal effect[17–20] but perhaps, relative to other mood stabilisers, the disadvantage of a worsened outcome following abrupt discontinuation[21–24] (although the effect of abrupt discontinuation of other drugs may be similar[24]). Early use of lithium might increase the likelihood of efficacy.[25]

The independent BALANCE study found that valproate as monotherapy was relatively less effective than lithium or the combination of lithium and valproate,[14] casting doubt on its use as a first-line single treatment. Also, a large observational study has shown that lithium is much more effective than valproate in preventing relapse to any condition and in preventing rehospitalisation.[26] Given this and the fact that valproate is not licensed for prophylaxis, it should be considered a second-line treatment.

Conventional antipsychotics have traditionally been used and are perceived to be effective although the objective evidence base is rather weak.[27,28] FGA depots probably protect against mania but may worsen depression[29] (see section 'Antipsychotic long acting injections in bipolar disorder'). Evidence supports the efficacy of many SGAs particularly olanzapine,[9,30] quetiapine,[31] aripiprazole[32] and risperidone.[33] Most studies examine combinations with mood stabilisers and there are few supportive monotherapy trials: only olanzapine, quetiapine and risperidone monotherapy could be shown to out-perform placebo in a 2017 review.[34]

Olanzapine, quetiapine and aripiprazole are licensed for prophylaxis and appear to protect against both mania and depression.[34] Asenapine may also be effective,[35] as may ziprasidone.[36] There is little to choose between individual SGAs.[34]

All antipsychotic + mood stabiliser combinations were more effective than mood stabiliser alone in a 2020 meta-analysis of 41 studies and 9821 participants.[37] Aripiprazole + valproate was numerically the best maintenance treatment (risk of relapse to any episode) in this analysis. A contemporary meta-analysis of 14 monotherapy studies found that monotherapy with aripiprazole, olanzapine, lurasidone, risperidone or quetiapine was more effective than placebo over 6 months or longer.[38]

Long-acting aripiprazole has been shown to delay the time to, and reduced the rate of recurrence of, manic episodes and was generally safe and well tolerated.[39] The use of risperidone LAI is well supported by RCTs[40] and naturalistic studies[41] (see section 'Antipsychotic long acting injections in bipolar disorder').

> **NICE recommendations[30]**
>
> - When planning long-term pharmacological interventions to prevent relapse, take into account drugs that have been effective during episodes of mania or bipolar depression. Discuss with the person whether they prefer to continue this treatment or switch to lithium, and explain that lithium is the most effective long-term treatment for BD.
> - Offer lithium as a first-line, long-term pharmacological treatment for BD and: if lithium is insufficiently effective, consider adding valproate; if lithium is poorly tolerated, consider valproate or olanzapine instead, or if it has been effective during an episode of mania or bipolar depression, quetiapine.
> - Do not offer valproate to women of child-bearing potential.
> - Discuss with the person the possible benefits and risks of each drug for them.
> - The secondary care team should maintain responsibility for monitoring the efficacy and tolerability of antipsychotic medication until the person's condition has stabilised.
> - Before stopping medication, discuss with the person how to recognise early signs of relapse and what to do if symptoms recur.
> - If stopping medication, do so gradually and monitor for signs of relapse.
> - Continue monitoring symptoms, mood and mental state for 2 years after stopping medication. This may be undertaken in primary care.

Optimising lithium treatment[42]

For adults with BD, the standard lithium serum level should be 0.60–0.80mmol/L with the option to reduce it to 0.40–0.60mmol/L in case of good response but poor tolerance or to increase it to 0.80–1.00mmol/L in case of insufficient response and good tolerance. For children and adolescents no consensus exists, but the majority of the International Society for Bipolar Disorders (ISBD)/ International Study Group on Lithium (IGSLI) Task Force endorsed the same recommendation. For the elderly, a more conservative approach may be adopted: usually 0.40–0.60mmol/L, with the option to go to maximally 0.70 or 0.80mmol/L at 65–79 years and to maximally 0.70mmol/L over 80 years.

Combination treatment

A significant proportion of patients with bipolar illness fail to be treated adequately with a single mood stabiliser,[14] so combinations of mood stabilisers[43,44] or a mood stabiliser and an antipsychotic[44,45] are commonly used.[46] Also, there is evidence that where combination treatments are effective in mania or depression, then continuation with the same combination provides optimal prophylaxis.[31,45] The use of polypharmacy needs to be balanced against the likely increased side-effect burden. Combinations of olanzapine, risperidone, quetiapine or haloperidol with lithium or valproate are recommended by NICE[30] and BAP guidelines.[10] Alternative antipsychotics (e.g. aripiprazole) are also options in combinations with lithium or valproate, particularly if these have been found to be effective during the treatment of an acute episode of mania or depression[31,47] Carbamazepine is considered to be third line. Lamotrigine may be useful in bipolar II disorder[30] but seems only to significantly prevent recurrence of depression.[48] Lurasidone may have broadly similar long-term efficacy, both as monotherapy and when combined with a mood stabiliser.[49,50]

Extrapolation of currently available data suggests that lithium plus an SGA is probably the polypharmacy regimen of choice. There are naturalistic data to support combinations of three treatments; in one study,[51] the two best treatments were lithium + valproate + quetiapine followed by lithium + valproate + olanzapine. Monotherapy with antipsychotics can be considered where mood stabilisers are poorly tolerated or where adherence cannot be.[52]

A meta-analysis of long-term antidepressant treatment found that continued treatment was more likely to induce a switch to mania than prevent a depressive episode.[53] The Systematic Treatment Enhancement Program for Bipolar Disorder (STEP-BD) found no significant benefit for continuing (compared with discontinuing) an antidepressant and worse outcomes in those with rapid cycling illness.[54] There is thus essentially no strong support for long-term use of antidepressants in bipolar illness although some bipolar patients may relapse into depression when antidepressants are discontinued.[24]

Substance misuse increases the risk of switching into mania.[55]

Summary table

Prophylaxis in bipolar disorder

First line: lithium monotherapy
Second line: olanzapine, aripiprazole, risperidone or quetiapine in combination with *valproate or lithium
Third line: alternative antipsychotic (lurasidone, asenapine, ziprasidone) or alternative mood stabiliser (carbamazepine, lamotrigine) in combination
Fourth line: antipsychotic with two mood stabilisers

- Always maintain successful acute treatment regimens (e.g. mood stabiliser + antipsychotic) as prophylaxis
- Avoid long-term antidepressants if possible

*Not in women of child-bearing potential.

References

1. Malhi GS, et al. The 2020 Royal Australian and New Zealand College of Psychiatrists Clinical Practice Guidelines for mood disorders: bipolar disorder summary. *Bipolar Disord* 2020; **22**:805–821.

2. Yatham LN, et al. Canadian network for mood and anxiety treatments (CANMAT) and International Society for Bipolar Disorders (ISBD) 2018 guidelines for the management of patients with bipolar disorder. *Bipolar Disord* 2018; **20**:97–170.

3. Kang MG, et al. Lithium vs valproate in the maintenance treatment of bipolar I disorder: a post- hoc analysis of a randomized double-blind placebo-controlled trial. *Aust N Z J Psychiatry* 2020; **54**:298–307.

4. Solomon DA, et al. Longitudinal course of bipolar I disorder: duration of mood episodes. *Arch Gen Psychiatry* 2010; **67**:339–347.

5. Perlis RH, et al. Predictors of recurrence in bipolar disorder: primary outcomes from the Systematic Treatment Enhancement Program for Bipolar Disorder (STEP-BD). *Am J Psychiatry* 2006; **163**:217–224.

6. Young AH, et al. Lithium in mood disorders: increasing evidence base, declining use? *Brit J Psychiatry* 2007; **191**:474–476.

7. Biel MG, et al. Continuation versus discontinuation of lithium in recurrent bipolar illness: a naturalistic study. *Bipolar Disord* 2007; **9**:435–442.

8. Bowden CL, et al. A randomized, placebo-controlled 12-month trial of divalproex and lithium in treatment of outpatients with bipolar I disorder. Divalproex Maintenance Study Group. *Arch Gen Psychiatry* 2000; **57**:481–489.

9. Tohen M, et al. Olanzapine versus divalproex sodium for the treatment of acute mania and maintenance of remission: a 47-week study. *Am J Psychiatry* 2003; **160**:1263–1271.

10. Goodwin GM, et al. Evidence-based guidelines for treating bipolar disorder: revised third edition recommendations from the British Association for Psychopharmacology. *J Psychopharmacol* 2016; **30**:495–553.

11. Sani G, et al. Treatment of bipolar disorder in a lifetime perspective: is lithium still the best choice? *Clin Drug Investig* 2017; **37**:713–727.

12. Hartong EG, et al. Prophylactic efficacy of lithium versus carbamazepine in treatment-naive bipolar patients. *J Clin Psychiatry* 2003; **64**:144–151.

13. Cipriani A, et al. Valproic acid, valproate and divalproex in the maintenance treatment of bipolar disorder. *Cochrane Database Syst Rev* 2013; 10:CD003196.

14. Geddes JR, et al. Lithium plus valproate combination therapy versus monotherapy for relapse prevention in bipolar I disorder (BALANCE): a randomised open-label trial. *Lancet* 2010; 375:385–395.

15. Kemp DE, et al. A 6-month, double-blind, maintenance trial of lithium monotherapy versus the combination of lithium and divalproex for rapid-cycling bipolar disorder and Co-occurring substance abuse or dependence. *J Clin Psychiatry* 2009; 70:113–121.

16. Smith LA, et al. Effectiveness of mood stabilizers and antipsychotics in the maintenance phase of bipolar disorder: a systematic review of randomized controlled trials. *Bipolar Disorders* 2007; 9:394–412.

17. Cipriani A, et al. Lithium in the prevention of suicidal behavior and all-cause mortality in patients with mood disorders: a systematic review of randomized trials. *Am J Psychiatry* 2005; 162:1805–1819.

18. Kessing LV, et al. Suicide risk in patients treated with lithium. *Arch Gen Psychiatry* 2005; 62:860–866.

19. Young AH, et al. Lithium in maintenance therapy for bipolar disorder. *J Psychopharmacol* 2006; 20:17–22.

20. Song J, et al. Suicidal behavior during lithium and valproate treatment: a within-individual 8-year prospective study of 50,000 patients with bipolar disorder. *Am J Psychiatry* 2017; 174:795–802.

21. Mander AJ, et al. Rapid recurrence of mania following abrupt discontinuation of lithium. *Lancet* 1988; 2:15–17.

22. Faedda GL, et al. Outcome after rapid vs gradual discontinuation of lithium treatment in bipolar disorders. *Arch Gen Psychiatry* 1993; 50:448–455.

23. Macritchie KA, et al. Does 'rebound mania' occur after stopping carbamazepine? A pilot study. *J Psychopharmacol* 2000; 14:266–268.

24. Franks MA, et al. Bouncing back: is the bipolar rebound phenomenon peculiar to lithium? A retrospective naturalistic study. *J Psychopharmacol* 2008; 22:452–456.

25. Kessing LV, et al. Starting lithium prophylaxis early v. late in bipolar disorder. *Br J Psychiatry* 2014; 205:214–20.

26. Kessing LV, et al. Valproate v. lithium in the treatment of bipolar disorder in clinical practice: observational nationwide register-based cohort study. *Brit J Psychiatry* 2011; 199:57–63.

27. Gao K, et al. Typical and atypical antipsychotics in bipolar depression. *J Clin Psychiatry* 2005; 66:1376–1385.

28. Hellewell JS. A review of the evidence for the use of antipsychotics in the maintenance treatment of bipolar disorders. *J Psychopharmacol* 2006; 20:39–45.

29. Gigante AD, et al. Long-acting injectable antipsychotics for the maintenance treatment of bipolar disorder. *CNS Drugs* 2012; 26:403–420.

30. National Institute for Health and Care Excellence. Bipolar disorder: assessment and management. Clinical Guidance [CG185]. 2014 (Last updated February 2020); https://www.nice.org.uk/guidance/cg185.

31. Vieta E, et al. Efficacy and safety of quetiapine in combination with lithium or divalproex for maintenance of patients with bipolar I disorder (international trial 126). *J Affect Disord* 2008; 109:251–263.

32. McIntyre RS. Aripiprazole for the maintenance treatment of bipolar I disorder: A review. *Clin Ther* 2010; 32 Suppl 1:S32–S38.

33. Ghaemi SN, et al. Long-term risperidone treatment in bipolar disorder: 6-month follow up. *Int Clin Psychopharmacol* 1997; 12:333–338.

34. Lindstrom L, et al. Maintenance therapy with second generation antipsychotics for bipolar disorder – A systematic review and meta-analysis. *J Affect Disord* 2017; 213:138–150.

35. Szegedi A, et al. Randomized, double-blind, placebo-controlled trial of asenapine maintenance therapy in adults with an acute manic or mixed episode associated with bipolar I disorder. *Am J Psychiatry* 2017; 175:71–79.

36. Bowden CL, et al. Efficacy of valproate versus lithium in mania or mixed mania: a randomized, open 12-week trial. *Int Clin Psychopharmacol* 2010; 25:60–67.

37. Kishi T, et al. Mood stabilizers and/or antipsychotics for bipolar disorder in the maintenance phase: a systematic review and network meta-analysis of randomized controlled trials. *Mol Psychiatry* 2020. [Epub ahead of print].

38. Escudero MAG, et al. Second generation antipsychotics monotherapy as maintenance treatment for bipolar disorder: a systematic review of long-term studies. *Psychiatr Q* 2020; 91:1047–1060.

39. Calabrese JR, et al. Efficacy and safety of aripiprazole once-monthly in the maintenance treatment of bipolar i disorder: a double-blind, placebo-controlled, 52-week randomized withdrawal study. *J Clin Psychiatry* 2017; 78:324–331.

40. Kishi T, et al. Long-acting injectable antipsychotics for prevention of relapse in bipolar disorder: a systematic review and meta-analyses of randomized controlled trials. *Int J Neuropsychopharmacol* 2016; 19.

41. Hsieh MH, et al. Bipolar patients treated with long-acting injectable risperidone in Taiwan: A 1-year mirror-image study using a national claims database. *J Affect Disord* 2017; 218:327–334.

42. Nolen WA, et al. What is the optimal serum level for lithium in the maintenance treatment of bipolar disorder? A systematic review and recommendations from the ISBD/IGSLI Task Force on treatment with lithium. *Bipolar Disord* 2019; 21:394–409.

43. Freeman MP, et al. Mood stabilizer combinations: a review of safety and efficacy. *Am J Psychiatry* 1998; 155:12–21.

44. Muzina DJ, et al. Maintenance therapies in bipolar disorder: focus on randomized controlled trials. *Aust N Z J Psychiatry* 2005; 39:652–661.

45. Tohen M, et al. Relapse prevention in bipolar I disorder: 18-month comparison of olanzapine plus mood stabiliser v. mood stabiliser alone. *Br J Psychiatry* 2004; 184:337–345.

46. Paton C, et al. Lithium in bipolar and other affective disorders: prescribing practice in the UK. *J Psychopharmacol* 2010; 24:1739–1746.

47. Marcus R, et al. Efficacy of aripiprazole adjunctive to lithium or valproate in the long-term treatment of patients with bipolar I disorder with an inadequate response to lithium or valproate monotherapy: a multicenter, double-blind, randomized study. *Bipolar Disord* 2011; 13:133–144.

CHAPTER 2

48. Bowden CL, et al. A placebo-controlled 18-month trial of lamotrigine and lithium maintenance treatment in recently manic or hypomanic patients with bipolar I disorder. *Arch Gen Psychiatry* 2003; 60:392–400.

49. Pikalov A, et al. Long-term use of lurasidone in patients with bipolar disorder: safety and effectiveness over 2 years of treatment. *Int J Bipolar Disord* 2017; 5:9.

50. Calabrese JR, et al. Lurasidone in combination with lithium or valproate for the maintenance treatment of bipolar I disorder. *Eur Neuropsychopharmacol* 2017; 27:865–876.

51. Wingård L, et al. Monotherapy vs. combination therapy for post mania maintenance treatment: a population based cohort study. *Eur Neuropsychopharmacol* 2019; 29:691–700.

52. Jauhar S, et al. Controversies in bipolar disorder; role of second-generation antipsychotic for maintenance therapy. *Int J Bipolar Disord* 2019; 7:10.

53. Ghaemi SN, et al. Long-term antidepressant treatment in bipolar disorder: meta-analyses of benefits and risks. *Acta Psychiatr Scand* 2008; 118:347–356.

54. Ghaemi SN, et al. Antidepressant discontinuation in bipolar depression: a Systematic Treatment Enhancement Program for Bipolar Disorder (STEP-BD) randomized clinical trial of long-term effectiveness and safety. *J Clin Psychiatry* 2010; 71:372–380.

55. Ostacher MJ, et al. Impact of substance use disorders on recovery from episodes of depression in bipolar disorder patients: prospective data from the Systematic Treatment Enhancement Program for Bipolar Disorder (STEP-BD). *Am J Psychiatry* 2010; 167:289–297.

Stopping lithium and mood stabilisers

Rationale for stopping

Patients may ask to stop lithium and other mood stabilisers because of the range of adverse effects experienced. In one cohort, 54% of patients discontinued lithium most because of tolerability problems, including diarrhoea (13%), tremor (11%), polyuria/polydipsia/diabetes insipidus (9%), creatinine increase (9%) and weight gain (7%).[1] Alternatively, although lithium and mood stabilisers are useful in controlling acute symptoms and preventing relapse, a clinician may judge that the balance of risks and benefits have shifted over time (e.g. adverse physical effects accumulate, alternative coping strategies developed) such that dose reduction or stopping may be considered. Other patients may be prescribed mood stabilisers for conditions such as personality disorders, for which there is a lack of evidence. Stopping should be done in a manner that minimises the risk of withdrawal effects and relapse (the two key risks).

Withdrawal effects from lithium and other mood stabilisers

Discontinuation of lithium can cause withdrawal effects, including both physical and psychological symptoms (see Table 2.12). These withdrawal effects include mood episodes (depression, but more commonly, mania) and are sometimes called 'rebound' effects.[2,3] The risk of relapse in the period following abrupt cessation greatly exceeds the rate of relapse in the untreated disorder.[2] For example, a review of studies of lithium discontinuation in people with BD found that the untreated disorder had a mean cycle length (the average time between episodes) of 11.6 months, whereas the time to a new episode following lithium discontinuation was 1.7 months.[2] This represents a seven-fold increase in the rate of relapse and suggests that manic and depressive symptoms that occur immediately following lithium withdrawal are largely because of lithium withdrawal.

Rebound effects have been variously thought to be due to the development of dopaminergic hypersensitivity,[4] changes in neuronal membranes, cell transport function or other neurotransmitter systems during lithium treatment.[5] Other mood stabilisers have also been associated with a 'withdrawal' syndrome.[6]

Table 2.12 Withdrawal effects from lithium[3,7,8]

Physical	Psychological
■ Tremor	■ Anxiety
■ Polyuria	■ Nervousness
■ Muscular weakness	■ Irritability
■ Polydipsia	■ Alertness
■ Dryness of mouth	■ Sleep disturbances
	■ Elated mood/mania
	■ Depressed mood

Evidence for long-term treatment

Although lithium is accepted as the first-line choice for prophylaxis in BD,[9] older evidence for long-term treatment with lithium and other mood stabilisers was derived from discontinuation studies where patients established on these medications are randomised to either continue or cease treatment.[10,11] In these studies, lithium is sometimes stopped abruptly. As mentioned, abrupt stopping of lithium is likely to produce withdrawal effects, which can include precipitating mood episodes.[2] Indeed, in one study abruptly stopping lithium in patients with apparent unipolar depression produced manic episodes in 13%.[12]

There is evidence that abrupt cessation of other mood stabilisers can also precipitate mood episodes.[3] Patients who are discontinued from these medications rapidly demonstrate relapse rates that are greater than the untreated disorder, suggesting that withdrawal effects may inflate the apparent rate and extent of relapse.[2,13] Few maintenance studies extend beyond a 2-year follow-up period, but significant naturalistic data (over longer periods) strongly supports longer term use of lithium.[14]

Duration of tapering

Abrupt discontinuation (1–14 days) is far more dangerous than 'gradual' (14–30 days) tapering.[15–17] Time to relapse is decreased, and proportion of patients relapsed at the end of study is greatly increased. These robust and reproducible findings support a recommendation that lithium should not be stopped abruptly unless a serious adverse effect occurs, and that withdrawal should normally take place over at least a month and preferably longer if practicable.

There are few studies examining the optimal rate or duration of tapering lithium. However, the finding that 50% of relapses occur in the first 3 months after lithium is stopped but then lessen over time,[2] suggests that this period might be required for underlying adaptations to lithium to resolve and suggests that tapering over 3 months may be beneficial. One study which discontinued lithium over 2–5 months found higher relapse rates in those patients compared to those who stayed on lithium.[18] This might suggest that tapering should be even slower than the 4-week to 3-month period suggested by NICE.[19]

Such long withdrawal schedules are not unusual in different areas of medicine: antiepileptic drugs (AEDs) are tapered over between 1 month and 4 years in non-psychiatric conditions, with relapse rates increased in the first 6 months before converging with patients continuing with AEDs.[6]

Practice guide to tapering

- Patients should be told that there is the possibility of rebound effects, and that there may be an increased risk of affective relapse from stopping lithium or mood stabilisers more quickly. These effects will be reduced if these medications are reduced in a more gradual fashion.
- There is no clear evidence on how to taper (or for how long), but following principles from other psychotropic medications, an initial reduction of 10–25% of the current

dose should be offered, with withdrawal symptoms (Table 2.12) and symptoms monitored for 2–4 weeks to ensure stability.

- Further reductions should be titrated against the tolerability of this dose decrease. Reductions should probably be made according to an exponentially reducing pattern, whereby each reduction is calculated as a fixed proportion (e.g. 10–25%) of the *most recent* dose (effectively becoming smaller and smaller as the total dose becomes lower) each month or so, or until stability is assured.
- Occasionally, the final dose before completely stopping may be very small, because small doses have relatively large effects on target receptors. To achieve small doses, liquid preparations (lithium) or tablet cutters (valproate and carbamazepine) will be required.
- As the process of reducing lithium or mood stabilisers might be destabilising, it may be wise to pursue other strategies during the tapering period.[20] Ongoing monitoring may be necessary for a number of months after complete cessation to ensure stability.
- If withdrawal symptoms or symptoms of relapse emerge at any point, pausing the reduction, a small increase in dose or returning to a previously effective dose are all possible responses. Difficulty reducing medication does not preclude a further attempt at reduction, but might indicate the need for a more gradual reduction regimen.
- Other modalities for people with BD, including family therapy, interpersonal therapy, cognitive behavioural therapy, psychoeducation and social rhythm therapy, may be considered as well as more individualised, idiosyncratic medication strategies.[21-23]

References

1. Öhlund L, et al. Correction to: reasons for lithium discontinuation in men and women with bipolar disorder: a retrospective cohort study. *BMC Psychiatry* 2018; **18:**322.
2. Suppes T, et al. Risk of recurrence following discontinuation of lithium treatment in bipolar disorder. *Arch Gen Psychiatry* 1991; **48:**1082–1088.
3. Franks MA, et al. Bouncing back: is the bipolar rebound phenomenon peculiar to lithium? A retrospective naturalistic study. *J Psychopharmacol* 2008; **22:**452–456.
4. Ferrie L, et al. Effect of chronic lithium and withdrawal from chronic lithium on presynaptic dopamine function in the rat. *J Psychopharmacol* 2005; **19:**229–234.
5. Balon R, et al. Lithium discontinuation: withdrawal or relapse? *Compr Psychiatry* 1988; **29:**330–334.
6. Vernachio K, et al. A review of withdraw strategies for discontinuing antiepileptic therapy in epilepsy and pain management. *Pharm Pharmacol Int J* 2015; **3:**232–235.
7. Baastrup PC, et al. Prophylactic lithium: double blind discontinuation in manic-depressive and recurrent-depressive disorders. *Lancet* 1970; **2:**326–330.
8. Klein E, et al. Discontinuation of lithium treatment in remitted bipolar patients: relationship between clinical outcome and changes in sleep-wake cycles. *J Nerv Ment Dis* 1991; **179:**499–501.
9. Nolen WA, et al. What is the optimal serum level for lithium in the maintenance treatment of bipolar disorder? A systematic review and recommendations from the ISBD/IGSLI Task Force on treatment with lithium. *Bipolar Disord* 2019; **21:**394–409.
10. Geddes JR, et al. Long-term lithium therapy for bipolar disorder: systematic review and meta-analysis of randomized controlled trials. *Am J Psychiatry* 2004; **161:**217–222.
11. Moncrieff J. Lithium: evidence reconsidered. *Br J Psychiatry* 1997; **171:**113–119
12. Faedda GL, et al. Lithium discontinuation: uncovering latent bipolar disorder? *Am J Psychiatry* 2001; **158:**1337–1339.
13. Goodwin GM. Recurrence of mania after lithium withdrawal. Implications for the use of lithium in the treatment of bipolar affective disorder. *Br J Psychiatry* 1994; **164:**149–152.
14. Kessing LV, et al. Effectiveness of maintenance therapy of lithium vs other mood stabilizers in monotherapy and in combinations: a systematic review of evidence from observational studies. *Bipolar Disord* 2018; **20:**419–431
15. Faedda GL, et al. Outcome after rapid vs gradual discontinuation of lithium treatment in bipolar disorders. *Arch Gen Psychiatry* 1993; **50:**448–455.

16. Baldessarini RJ, et al. Illness risk following rapid versus gradual discontinuation of antidepressants. *Am J Psychiatry* 2010; 167:934–941.

17. Baldessarini RJ, et al. Effects of the rate of discontinuing lithium maintenance treatment in bipolar disorders. *J Clin Psychiatry* 1996; 57:441–448.

18. Biel MG, et al. Continuation versus discontinuation of lithium in recurrent bipolar illness: a naturalistic study. *Bipolar Disord* 2007; 9:435–442.

19. National Institute for Health and Care Excellence. Bipolar disorder: assessment and management. Clinical Guidance [CG185]. 2014 (Last updated February 2020); https://www.nice.org.uk/guidance/cg185.

20. Guy A, et al. Guidance for psychological therapists: enabling conversations with clients taking or withdrawing from prescribed psychiatric drugs. London: APPG for Prescribed Drug Dependence; 2019.

21. Reinares M, et al. Psychosocial interventions in bipolar disorder: what, for whom, and when. *J Affect Disord* 2014; 156:46–55.

22. Cappleman R, et al. Managing bipolar moods without medication: a qualitative investigation. *J Affect Disord* 2015; 174:241–249.

23. Miklowitz DJ. Adjunctive psychotherapy for bipolar disorder: state of the evidence. *Am J Psychiatry* 2008; 165:1408–1419.

Chapter 3

Depression and anxiety disorders

Introduction to Depression

Depression is widely recognised as a major public health problem around the world. The mainstay of treatment is the prescription of antidepressants, although psychological treatments have a place as first-line alternative to antidepressants in milder forms of depression.[1] Other methods of treating depression (VNS,[2] rTMS,[3] etc.) are also used but are not widely available.

The basic principles of prescribing are described here, along with a summary of NICE guidance.

Table 3.1 Basic principles of prescribing in depression

- Discuss with the patient choice of drug and utility/availability of other, non-pharmacological treatments.
- Discuss with the patient likely outcomes, such as gradual relief from depressive symptoms over several weeks.
- Prescribe a dose of antidepressant (after titration, if necessary) that is likely to be effective.
- For a single episode, continue treatment for at least 6–9 months after resolution of symptoms (multiple episodes may require longer).
- Withdraw antidepressants very gradually; always inform patients of the risk and nature of discontinuation symptoms.

Official guidance on the treatment of depression

NICE guidelines[1] – a summary

- Antidepressants are not recommended as a first-line treatment in recent onset, mild depression – active monitoring, individual guided self-help, CBT or exercise are preferred.

The Maudsley® Prescribing Guidelines in Psychiatry, Fourteenth Edition. David M. Taylor, Thomas R. E. Barnes and Allan H. Young.
© 2021 David M. Taylor. Published 2021 by John Wiley & Sons Ltd.

- Antidepressants are recommended for the treatment of moderate to severe depression and for dysthymia.
- When an antidepressant is prescribed, a generic SSRI is recommended.
- All patients should be informed about the withdrawal (discontinuation) effects of antidepressants.
- For treatment-resistant depression, recommended strategies include augmentation with lithium or an antipsychotic or the addition of a second antidepressant (see sections on treatment resistant depression in this chapter).
- Patients with two prior episodes and functional impairment should be treated for at least 2 years.
- The use of ECT is supported in severe and treatment-resistant depression.

At the time of writing, the new NICE Guidelines are available only in draft form.[4] Basic principles appear to be the same as in the earlier guideline, but important differences are proposed for drug choice after first treatment failure (see Drug Treatment in Depression section in this chapter). The final guideline is to be published in 2021/2022.

This chapter concentrates on the use of antidepressants and offers advice on drug choice, dosing, switching strategies and sequencing of treatments. The near exclusion of other non-drug treatment modalities does not imply any lack of confidence in their efficacy but simply reflects the need (in a prescribing guideline) to concentrate on medicines-related subjects.

References

1. National Institute for Clinical Excellence. Depression: the treatment and management of depression in adults. Clinical Guidance [CG90]. 2009 (last reviewed December 2013); https://www.nice.org.uk/guidance/cg90.
2. George MS, et al. Vagus nerve stimulation for the treatment of depression and other neuropsychiatric disorders. *Expert Rev Neurother* 2007; 7:63–74.
3. Loo CK, et al. A review of the efficacy of transcranial magnetic stimulation (TMS) treatment for depression, and current and future strategies to optimize efficacy. *J Affect Disord* 2005; 88:255–267.
4. National Institute for Health and Care Excellence. Depression in adults: treatment and management – full guideline (Draft for Consultation). 2017; https://www.nice.org.uk/guidance/GID-CGWAVE0725/documents/draft-guideline.

Antidepressants – general overview

Effectiveness

A 2018 comprehensive review found that all antidepressants were more efficacious than placebo in adults with major depressive disorder,[1] and a further review found equal benefit from antidepressant treatments for mild, moderate or severe major depression.[2]

Antidepressants are normally recommended as first-line treatment in patients whose depression is of at least moderate severity, with psychological treatments being used for milder forms. Of the moderate-severe patient group, approximately 20% will recover with no treatment at all, 30% will respond to placebo and 50% will respond to antidepressant drug treatment.[3] This gives a number needed to treat (NNT) of 3 for antidepressant over true no-treatment control and an NNT of 5 for antidepressant over placebo. Note though that response in clinical trials is generally defined as a 50% reduction in depression rating scale scores, a somewhat arbitrary dichotomy, and that change measured using continuous scales tends to show a relatively small mean difference between active treatment and placebo (which itself is an effective treatment for depression).

Drug-placebo differences may have diminished over time largely because of methodological changes.[4] It is possible that rating scales obscure the effects of antidepressants to some extent. Hieronymus et al.[5] undertook patient-level post-hoc analyses of 18 industry-sponsored placebo-controlled trials of paroxetine, citalopram, sertraline or fluoxetine, including in total 6669 adults with major depression, with the aim being to assess what the outcome would have been if the single item 'depressed mood' (rated 0–4) had been used as the measure of efficacy. While 18 out of 32 comparisons (56%) failed to separate active drug from placebo at week 6 with respect to reduction in Hamilton Depression Rating Scale (HDRS)-17 total score, only 3 out of 32 comparisons (9%) were negative when depressed mood was used as the sole effect parameter. As noted earlier, even when whole depression scales are used, a recent network meta-analysis showed robust superiority for antidepressants over placebo, with amitriptyline being the most efficacious.[1]

The 2019 PANDA trial results support the prescription of selective serotonin reuptake inhibitor (SSRI) antidepressants in a wider group of participants than previously thought, including those with mild to moderate symptoms who do not meet diagnostic criteria for depression or generalised anxiety disorder.[6]

Onset of Action

It is widely held that antidepressants do not exert their effects for 2–4 weeks. This is a myth. All antidepressants show a pattern of response where the rate of improvement is highest during weeks 1–2 and lowest during weeks 4–6. Statistical separation from placebo is seen at 2–4 weeks in single trials (hence the idea of a lag effect) but after only 1–2 weeks in (statistically more powerful) meta-analyses.[7,8] Thus, where large numbers of patients are treated and detailed rating scales are used, an antidepressant effect is statistically evident at 1 week. In clinical practice using simple observations, an antidepressant effect in an individual is usually seen by 2 weeks.[9] It follows that in individuals where *no* antidepressant effect is evident after 3–4 weeks' treatment, a change in dose or drug should be considered. It is important, however, to be clear about what constitutes 'no effect'. Different patterns of response have been identified,[10] and in some individuals response is slow to emerge. However, in those ultimately responsive to treatment, all will very probably have begun to show at least minor improvement at 4 weeks. Thus, those showing no discernible improvement at this time will very probably never respond to the prescribed drug at that dose. In contrast, those showing small improvements at 4 weeks (that is, improvement not meeting criteria for 'response') may well go on to respond fully.[11] A 'mega-analysis'[12] has shown that if antidepressant (citalopram, paroxetine or sertraline specifically) trials are examined with regards to the effects on depressed mood alone (rather than the total Hamilton Depression Rating Scale score), then both a rapid effect and a dose-response relationship are evident.

Choice of antidepressant and relative side effects

Selective serotonin re-uptake inhibitors (*SSRIs*) are well tolerated compared with the older tricyclic antidepressants (TCAs) and mono-amine oxidase inhibitors (MAOIs), and are generally recommended as *first-line* pharmacological treatment for depression.[13] There is a suggestion from network meta-analyses[1,14] that some antidepressants may be more effective overall than others, but this has not been consistently demonstrated in head-to-head studies and should therefore be treated with caution. Side effect profiles of antidepressants do differ. For example, paroxetine has been associated with more weight gain and a higher incidence of sexual dysfunction, and sertraline with a higher incidence of diarrhoea than other SSRIs.[15] Dual re-uptake inhibitors such as venlafaxine and duloxetine tend to be tolerated less well than SSRIs but better than TCAs. With all drugs there is marked inter-individual variation in tolerability which is not easily predicted by knowledge of a drug's likely adverse effects. A flexible approach is usually required to find the right drug for a particular patient.

As well as *headache* and *GI symptoms*, SSRIs as a class are associated with a range of other side effects, including *sexual dysfunction* (see the relevant section in this chapter), *hyponatraemia* (see the section on hyponatraemia) and *GI bleeds* (see SSRIs and bleeding). TCAs have a number of *adverse cardiovascular effects* (hypotension, tachycardia and QTc prolongation), and are particularly *toxic in overdose*[16] (see section on Psychotropic drugs in overdose in Chapter 13). The now rarely used *MAOIs* have the potential to interact with tyramine-containing foods to cause *hypertensive crisis and much more commonly cause hypotension*. All antidepressant drugs can cause *discontinuation symptoms*, with short half-life drugs probably being most problematic in this respect (see section on Stopping antidepressants). See the following pages for a summary of the clinically relevant side effects of available antidepressant drugs.

Drug interactions

Some *SSRIs* are potent *inhibitors* of individual or multiple *hepatic cytochrome P450 (CYP)* pathways and the magnitude of these effects is dose-related. A number of clinically significant drug interactions can therefore be predicted. For example, fluvoxamine is a potent inhibitor of CYP1A2, which can result in increased theophylline serum levels, fluoxetine is a potent inhibitor of CYP2D6, which can result in increased seizure risk with clozapine, and paroxetine is a potent inhibitor of CYP2D6, which can result in treatment failure with tamoxifen (a pro-drug) leading to increased mortality.[17]

Antidepressants can also cause pharmacodynamic interactions. For example, the cardiotoxicity of TCAs may be exacerbated by drugs such as diuretics that can cause electrolyte disturbances. A summary of clinically relevant drug interactions with antidepressants can be found later in this chapter.

Potential *pharmacokinetic* and *pharmacodynamic* interactions between antidepressants have to be considered when *switching* from one antidepressant to another (see section on Switching antidepressants in this chapter).

Suicidality

Antidepressant treatment has been associated with an increased risk of suicidal thoughts and acts, particularly in adolescents and young adults,[18–21] leading to the recommendation that patients should be warned of this potential adverse effect during the early weeks of treatment and know how to seek help if required. Suicide and self-harm rates tend to be higher when antidepressants are started or stopped, so the same care over risk assessment should be carried out when treatment is stopped as when it is started.[22] Furthermore, switching antidepressants may be a marker of increased risk of suicidal behaviours in those who initiate antidepressant treatment aged 75 years and over.[23]

All antidepressants have been implicated,[24] including those that are marketed for an indication other than depression (e.g. atomoxetine). It should be noted that (1) although the relative risk may be elevated above placebo rates in some patient groups, the absolute risk remains very small; (2) the most effective way to prevent suicidal thoughts and acts is to treat depression;[25–27] and (3) antidepressant drugs are the most effective treatment currently available.[3,28] For the most part, suicidality is greatly reduced by the use of antidepressants.[29–31] Note, however, that those who experience treatment-emergent or worsening suicidal ideation with one antidepressant may be more likely to have a similar experience with subsequent treatments.[32] Some recent data suggests that an increasing proportion of young women who later committed suicide had in the last few years been treated with antidepressants prior to and at the time of the suicide.[33] At the time of writing, there is no clear consensus on the potential dangers of antidepressants except that young people are most at risk.[34]

Toxicity in overdose varies both between and within groups of antidepressants.[35] See section on 'Psychotropics in overdose' in Chapter 13.

Duration of treatment

Antidepressants relieve the symptoms of depression but do not treat the underlying cause. A reasonable amount of evidence suggests that they should be taken for 6–9 months after recovery from a single episode (presumably to cover the duration of an untreated episode). In those patients who have had multiple episodes, there is evidence of benefit from maintenance treatment for at least 2 years, but no upper duration of treatment has been identified (see section on 'Antidepressant prophylaxis' in this chapter). There are little data on which to base recommendations about the duration of treatment of augmentation regimens. A minority view is that antidepressants worsen outcome in the long term.[36]

Next step treatments

Approximately a third of patients do not respond to the first antidepressant that is prescribed. Options in this group include dose escalation, switching to a different drug and a number of augmentation strategies. The lessons from STAR*D are that a small proportion of non-responders will respond with each treatment change, but that effect sizes are modest, and there is no clear difference in effectiveness between strategies. (See sections on treatment-resistant depression in this chapter.)

Use of antidepressants in anxiety spectrum disorders

Antidepressants are first-line treatments in a number of anxiety spectrum disorders. (See section on Anxiety spectrum disorders in this chapter.)

References

1. Cipriani A, et al. Comparative efficacy and acceptability of 21 antidepressant drugs for the acute treatment of adults with major depressive disorder: a systematic review and network meta-analysis. *Lancet* 2018; 391:1357–1366.

2. Furukawa TA, et al. Initial severity of major depression and efficacy of new generation antidepressants: individual participant data meta-analysis. *Acta Psychiatr Scand* 2018; 137:450–458.

3. Anderson IM, et al. Evidence-based guidelines for treating depressive disorders with antidepressants: a revision of the 2000 British Association for Psychopharmacology guidelines. *J Psychopharmacology* 2008; 22:343–396.

4. Khan A, et al. Why has the antidepressant-placebo difference in antidepressant clinical trials diminished over the past three decades? *CNS Neurosci Ther* 2010; 16:217–226.

5. Hieronymus F, et al. Consistent superiority of selective serotonin reuptake inhibitors over placebo in reducing depressed mood in patients with major depression. *Mol Psychiatry* 2016; 21:523–530.

6. Lewis G, et al. The clinical effectiveness of sertraline in primary care and the role of depression severity and duration (PANDA): a pragmatic, double-blind, placebo-controlled randomised trial. *Lancet Psychiatry* 2019; 6:903–914.

7. Taylor MJ, et al. Early onset of selective serotonin reuptake inhibitor antidepressant action: systematic review and meta-analysis. *Arch Gen Psychiatry* 2006; 63:1217–1223.

8. Papakostas GI, et al. A meta-analysis of early sustained response rates between antidepressants and placebo for the treatment of major depressive disorder. *J Clin Psychopharmacol* 2006; 26:56–60.

9. Szegedi A, et al. Early improvement in the first 2 weeks as a predictor of treatment outcome in patients with major depressive disorder: a meta-analysis including 6562 patients. *J Clin Psychiatry* 2009; 70:344–353.

10. Uher R, et al. Early and delayed onset of response to antidepressants in individual trajectories of change during treatment of major depression: a secondary analysis of data from the Genome-Based Therapeutic Drugs for Depression (GENDEP) study. *J Clin Psychiatry* 2011; 72:1478–1484.

11. Posternak MA, et al. Response rates to fluoxetine in subjects who initially show no improvement. *J Clin Psychiatry* 2011; 72:949–954.

12. Hieronymus F, et al. A mega-analysis of fixed-dose trials reveals dose-dependency and a rapid onset of action for the antidepressant effect of three selective serotonin reuptake inhibitors. *Trans Psychiatry* 2016; 6:e834.

13. National Institute for Health and Care Excellence. Depression in adults: recognition and management. Clinical guideline [CG90]. 2009 (last updated: December 2013); https://www.nice.org.uk/Guidance/cg90.

14. Cipriani A, et al. Comparative efficacy and acceptability of 12 new-generation antidepressants: a multiple-treatments meta-analysis. *Lancet* 2009; 373:746–758.

15. Gartlehner G, et al. Comparative benefits and harms of second-generation antidepressants: background paper for the American College of Physicians. *Ann Intern Med* 2008; 149:734–750.

16. Flanagan RJ. Fatal toxicity of drugs used in psychiatry. *Human Psychopharmacology* 2008; 23 Suppl 1:43–51.

17. Kelly CM, et al. Selective serotonin reuptake inhibitors and breast cancer mortality in women receiving tamoxifen: a population based cohort study. *BMJ* 2010; 340:c693.

18. Stone M, et al. Risk of suicidality in clinical trials of antidepressants in adults: analysis of proprietary data submitted to US Food and Drug Administration. *BMJ* 2009; 339:b2880.

19. Carpenter DJ, et al. Meta-analysis of efficacy and treatment-emergent suicidality in adults by psychiatric indication and age subgroup following initiation of paroxetine therapy: a complete set of randomized placebo-controlled trials. *J Clin Psychiatry* 2011; **72**:1503–1514.

20. Barbui C, et al. Selective serotonin reuptake inhibitors and risk of suicide: a systematic review of observational studies. *CMAJ* 2009; **180**:291–297.

21. Umetsu R, et al. Association between selective serotonin reuptake inhibitor therapy and suicidality: analysis of U.S. Food and drug administration adverse event reporting system data. *Biol Pharm Bull* 2015; **38**:1689–1699.

22. Coupland C, et al. Antidepressant use and risk of suicide and attempted suicide or self harm in people aged 20 to 64: cohort study using a primary care database. *BMJ* 2015; **350**:h517.

23. Hedna K, et al. Antidepressants and suicidal behaviour in late life: a prospective population-based study of use patterns in new users aged 75 and above. *Eur J Clin Pharmacol* 2018; **74**:201–208.

24. Schneeweiss S, et al. Variation in the risk of suicide attempts and completed suicides by antidepressant agent in adults: a propensity score-adjusted analysis of 9 years' data. *Arch Gen Psychiatry* 2010; **67**:497–506.

25. Isacsson G, et al. The increased use of antidepressants has contributed to the worldwide reduction in suicide rates. *Br J Psychiatry* 2010; **196**:429–433.

26. Gibbons RD, et al. Suicidal thoughts and behavior with antidepressant treatment: reanalysis of the randomized placebo-controlled studies of fluoxetine and venlafaxine. *Arch Gen Psychiatry* 2012; **69**:580–587.

27. Lu CY, et al. Changes in antidepressant use by young people and suicidal behavior after FDA warnings and media coverage: quasi-experimental study. *BMJ* 2014; **348**:g3596.

28. Isacsson G, et al. Antidepressant medication prevents suicide in depression. *Acta Psychiatr Scand* 2010; **122**:454–460.

29. Simon GE, et al. Suicide risk during antidepressant treatment. *Am J Psychiatry* 2006; **163**:41–47.

30. Mulder RT, et al. Antidepressant treatment is associated with a reduction in suicidal ideation and suicide attempts. *Acta Psychiatr Scand* 2008; **118**:116–122.

31. Tondo L, et al. Suicidal status during antidepressant treatment in 789 Sardinian patients with major affective disorder. *Acta Psychiatr Scand* 2008; **118**:106–115.

32. Perlis RH, et al. Do suicidal thoughts or behaviors recur during a second antidepressant treatment trial? *J Clin Psychiatry* 2012; **73**:1439–1442.

33. Larsson J. Antidepressants and suicide among young women in Sweden 1999–2013. *Int J Risk Saf Med* 2017; **29**:101–106.

34. Spielmans GI, et al. Duty to warn: antidepressant black box suicidality warning is empirically justified. *Front Psychiatry* 2020; **11**:18.

35. Hawton K, et al. Toxicity of antidepressants: rates of suicide relative to prescribing and non-fatal overdose. *Br J Psychiatry* 2010; **196**:354–358.

36. Fava GA. May antidepressant drugs worsen the conditions they are supposed to treat? The clinical foundations of the oppositional model of tolerance. *Ther Adv Psychopharmacol* 2020; [Epub ahead of print].

CHAPTER 3

Recognised minimum effective doses of antidepressants

The recommended minimum effective doses of antidepressants are summarised in Table 3.2.

Table 3.2 The recommended minimum effective doses of antidepressants

Antidepressant	Dose
Tricyclics	Unclear; at least 75–100mg/day,[1] possibly 125mg/day[2]
Lofepramine	140mg/day[3]
SSRIs	
Citalopram	20mg/day[4]
Escitalopram	10mg/day[5]
Fluoxetine	20mg/day[6]
Fluvoxamine	50mg/day[7]
Paroxetine	20mg/day[8]
Sertraline	50mg/day[9]
Others	
Agomelatine	25mg/day[10]
Bupropion	150mg/day[11]
Desvenlafaxine	50mg/day[12]
Duloxetine	60mg/day[13,14]
Levomilnacipran	40mg/day[15]
Mirtazapine	30mg/day (15mg?[16])
Moclobemide	300mg/[17]
Reboxetine	8mg/day[18]
Trazodone	150mg/day[19]
Venlafaxine	75mg/day[20]
Vilazodone	20mg/day[15]
Vortioxetine	10mg/day[15]

References

1. Furukawa TA, et al. Meta-analysis of effects and side effects of low dosage tricyclic antidepressants in depression: systematic review. *BMJ* 2002; **325**:991.

2. Donoghue J, et al. Suboptimal use of antidepressants in the treatment of depression. *CNS Drugs* 2000; **13**:365–368.

3. Lancaster SG, et al. Lofepramine. A review of its pharmacodynamic and pharmacokinetic properties, and therapeutic efficacy in depressive illness. *Drugs* 1989; **37**:123–140.

4. Montgomery SA, et al. The optimal dosing regimen for citalopram – a meta-analysis of nine placebo-controlled studies. *Int Clin Psychopharmacol* 1994; **9 Suppl 1**:35–40.

5. Burke WJ, et al. Fixed-dose trial of the single isomer SSRI escitalopram in depressed outpatients. *J Clin Psychiatry* 2002; **63**:331–336.

6. Altamura AC, et al. The evidence for 20mg a day of fluoxetine as the optimal dose in the treatment of depression. *Br J Psychiatry Suppl* 1988; 109–112.

7. Walczak DD, et al. The oral dose-effect relationship for fluvoxamine: a fixed-dose comparison against placebo in depressed outpatients. *Ann Clin Psychiatry* 1996; **8**:139–151.

8. Dunner DL, et al. Optimal dose regimen for paroxetine. *J Clin Psychiatry* 1992; **53 Suppl**:21–26.

9. Moon CAL, et al. A double-blind comparison of sertraline and clomipramine in the treatment of major depressive disorder and associative anxiety in general practice. *J Psychopharm* 1994; **8**:171–176.

10. Loo H, et al. Determination of the dose of agomelatine, a melatoninergic agonist and selective 5-HT(2C) antagonist, in the treatment of major depressive disorder: a placebo-controlled dose range study. *Int Clin Psychopharmacol* 2002; **17**:239–247.

11. Hewett K, et al. Eight-week, placebo-controlled, double-blind comparison of the antidepressant efficacy and tolerability of bupropion XR and venlafaxine XR. *J Psychopharmacology* 2009; **23**:531–538.

12. Kornstein SG, et al. The effect of desvenlafaxine 50 mg/day on a subpopulation of anxious/depressed patients: a pooled analysis of seven randomized, placebo-controlled studies. *Human Psychopharmacology* 2014; **29**:492–501.

13. Goldstein DJ, et al. Duloxetine in the treatment of depression: a double-blind placebo-controlled comparison with paroxetine. *J Clin Psychopharmacol* 2004; **24**:389–399.

14. Detke MJ, et al. Duloxetine, 60 mg once daily, for major depressive disorder: a randomized double-blind placebo-controlled trial. *J Clin Psychiatry* 2002; **63**:308–315.

15. He H, et al. Efficacy and tolerability of different doses of three new antidepressants for treating major depressive disorder: a PRISMA-compliant meta-analysis. *J Psychiatr Res* 2018; **96**:247–259.

16. Furukawa TA, et al. No benefit from flexible titration above minimum licensed dose in prescribing antidepressants for major depression: systematic review. *Acta Psychiatr Scand* 2020; **141**:401–409.

17. Priest RG, et al. Moclobemide in the treatment of depression. *Rev Contemporary Pharmacother* 1994; **5**:35–43.

18. Schatzberg AF. Clinical efficacy of reboxetine in major depression. *J Clin Psychiatry* 2000; **61 Suppl 10**:31–38.

19. Brogden RN, et al. Trazodone: a review of its pharmacological properties and therapeutic use in depression and anxiety. *Drugs* 1981; **21**:401–429.

20. Feighner JP, et al. Efficacy of once-daily venlafaxine extended release (XR) for symptoms of anxiety in depressed outpatients. *J Affect Disord* 1998; **47**:55–62.

Drug treatment of depression

The drug treatment of depression has been summarised in Figure 3.1.

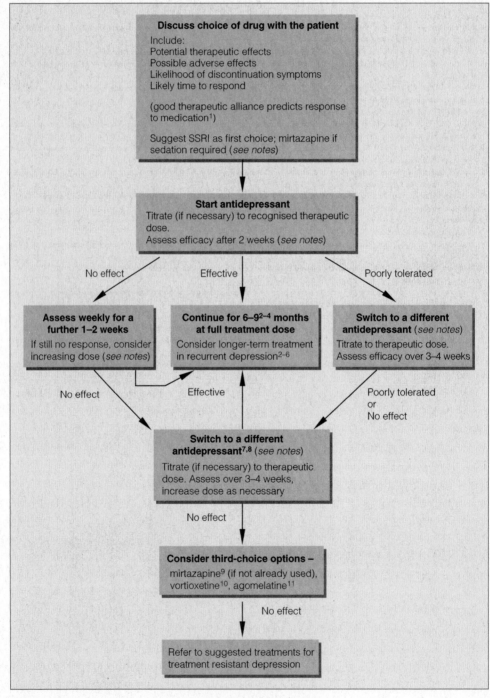

Figure 3.1 Drug treatment of depression

Notes

- Tools such as the Montgomery–Asberg Depression Rating Scale (MADRS)[12] and the Hamilton Depression Rating Scale (HDRS)[13] are used in trials to assess drug effect. The HDRS is now somewhat anachronistic, and few clinicians are familiar with the MADRS (although it is probably the best scale to measure severity and change). The Patient Health Questionnaire-9 (PHQ-9)[14] is simple to use and is recommended for assessing symptom change in depression (although it better measures frequency rather than severity of symptoms).
- Choice of antidepressant is governed largely by patient and clinician preference, but most authorities recommend an SSRI, or mirtazapine where sedation is required. The largest network meta-analysis[15] suggested that drugs with effects on both norepinephrine and serotonin uptake are the most effective (5 of the top 6 ranked drugs are dual-action drugs), whereas agomelatine and SSRIs have the lowest drop-out rates. A 2018 network meta-analysis[16] of newer antidepressants suggested few, if any, clear advantages over older drugs for levomilnacipran, vilazodone and vortioxetine.
- Assessment at two weeks has some utility in determining eventual outcome.[17] Only around 30% of those not reaching accepted symptom score threshold for improvement at two weeks will ultimately respond. Even fewer people go on to respond if there is no improvement at all or deterioration at 2 weeks.
- Switching between drug classes in cases of poor tolerability is supported by some studies[18] and has a strong theoretical basis. Having said that, in practice, many patients who cannot tolerate one SSRI will readily tolerate another.
- In cases of non-response, there is some evidence that switching within a drug class is effective,[8,19–22] but switching between classes is, in practice, the most common option and is supported by some analyses.[23] The APA recommend both options.[2] The 2018 NICE draft guidelines[24] suggested that there is little cogent evidence for switching between antidepressants (an observation in another analysis[25]) and that combining antidepressants or adding an second-generation antipsychotic (SGA) are better-supported options at this stage. The strongest evidence in support of switching after the failure of one treatment is probably for vortioxetine.[10]
- There is minimal evidence to recommend increasing the dose of most SSRIs in depression, at least when severity is measured using total rating scale scores.[26] Examining only the mood item on the HAMD suggests some dose-response relationship for SSRIs.[27] Other evidence suggests that increasing the dose of venlafaxine, escitalopram and tricyclics may be helpful.[3] Generally speaking, gains in efficacy afforded by dose increases are small (SSRIs, venlafaxine) or non-existent (e.g. mirtazapine above 30mg/day) while effects on tolerability are reliably and starkly detrimental.[28]
- Switch treatments early (e.g. after a week or two) if adverse effects are intolerable or if no improvement *at all* is seen by 3–4 weeks. Opinions on when to switch vary somewhat, but it is clear that antidepressants have a fairly prompt onset of action[29–31] and that non-response at 2–6 weeks is a good predictor of overall non-response.[32–34] The absence of any improvement *at all* at 3–4 weeks should normally provoke a change in treatment (British Association for Psychopharmacology [BAP] guidelines suggest 4 weeks[3]). If there is some improvement at this time, continue and assess for a further 2–3 weeks (see the section on 'Antidepressants: general overview', this chapter).

References

1. Leuchter AF, et al. Role of pill-taking, expectation and therapeutic alliance in the placebo response in clinical trials for major depression. *Br J Psychiatry* 2014; 205:443–449.
2. American Psychiatric Association. *Practice guideline for the treatment of patients with major depressive disorder*. Third Edition. Washington, USA: American Psychiatric Association; 2010.
3. Anderson IM, et al. Evidence-based guidelines for treating depressive disorders with antidepressants: a revision of the 2000 British Association for Psychopharmacology guidelines. *J Psychopharmacology* 2008; 22:343–396.
4. Crismon ML, et al. The Texas medication algorithm project: report of the Texas consensus conference panel on medication treatment of major depressive disorder. *J Clin Psychiatry* 1999; 60:142–156.
5. Kocsis JH, et al. Maintenance therapy for chronic depression. A controlled clinical trial of desipramine. *Arch Gen Psychiatry* 1996; 53:769–774.
6. Dekker J, et al. The use of antidepressants after recovery from depression. *Eur J Psychiatry* 2000; 14:207–212.
7. Nelson JC. Treatment of antidepressant nonresponders: augmentation or switch? *J Clin Psychiatry* 1998; 59 Suppl 15:35–41.
8. Joffe RT. Substitution therapy in patients with major depression. *CNS Drugs* 1999; 11:175–180.
9. National Institute for Health and Care Excellence. Depression in adults: recognition and management. Clinical Guidance [CG90]. 2009 (reviewed December 2013); http://www.nice.org.uk/Guidance/cg90.

10. Montgomery SA, et al. A randomised, double-blind study in adults with major depressive disorder with an inadequate response to a single course of selective serotonin reuptake inhibitor or serotonin-noradrenaline reuptake inhibitor treatment switched to vortioxetine or agomelatine. *Human Psychopharmacology* 2014; **29**:470–482.

11. Sparshatt A, et al. A naturalistic evaluation and audit database of agomelatine: clinical outcome at 12 weeks. *Acta Psychiatr Scand* 2013; **128**:203–211.

12. Montgomery SA, et al. A new depression scale designed to be sensitive to change. *Br J Psychiatry* 1979; **134**:382–389.

13. Hamilton M. Development of a rating scale for primary depressive illness. *Br J Soc Clin Psychol* 1967; **6**:278–296.

14. Kroenke K, et al. The PHQ-9: validity of a brief depression severity measure. *J Gen Intern Med* 2001; **16**:606–613.

15. Cipriani A, et al. Comparative efficacy and acceptability of 21 antidepressant drugs for the acute treatment of adults with major depressive disorder: a systematic review and network meta-analysis. *Lancet* 2018; **391**:1357–1366.

16. Wagner G, et al. Efficacy and safety of levomilnacipran, vilazodone and vortioxetine compared with other second-generation antidepressants for major depressive disorder in adults: a systematic review and network meta-analysis. *J Affect Disord* 2018; **228**:1–12.

17. de Vries YA, et al. Predicting antidepressant response by monitoring early improvement of individual symptoms of depression: individual patient data meta-analysis. *Br J Psychiatry* 2019; **214**:4–10.

18. Köhler-Forsberg O, et al. Efficacy of anti-inflammatory treatment on major depressive disorder or depressive symptoms: meta-analysis of clinical trials. *Acta Psychiatr Scand* 2019; **139**:404–419.

19. Thase ME, et al. Citalopram treatment of fluoxetine nonresponders. *J Clin Psychiatry* 2001; **62**:683–687.

20. Rush AJ, et al. Bupropion-SR, sertraline, or venlafaxine-XR after failure of SSRIs for depression. *N Engl J Med* 2006; **354**:1231–1242.

21. Ruhe HG, et al. Switching antidepressants after a first selective serotonin reuptake inhibitor in major depressive disorder: a systematic review. *J Clin Psychiatry* 2006; **67**:1836–1855.

22. Brent D, et al. Switching to another SSRI or to venlafaxine with or without cognitive behavioral therapy for adolescents with SSRI-resistant depression: the TORDIA randomized controlled trial. *JAMA* 2008; **299**:901–913.

23. Papakostas GI, et al. Treatment of SSRI-resistant depression: a meta-analysis comparing within- versus across-class switches. *Biol Psychiatry* 2008; **63**:699–704.

24. National Institute for Health and Care Excellence. Depression in adults: treatment and management – Full guideline (Draft for Consultation). 2017; https://www.nice.org.uk/guidance/GID-CGWAVE0725/documents/draft-guideline.

25. Bschor T, et al. Switching the antidepressant after nonresponse in adults with major depression: a systematic literature search and meta-analysis. *J Clin Psychiatry* 2018; **79**.

26. Adli M, et al. Is dose escalation of antidepressants a rational strategy after a medium-dose treatment has failed? A systematic review. *Eur Arch Psychiatry Clin Neurosci* 2005; **255**:387–400.

27. Hieronymus F, et al. A mega-analysis of fixed-dose trials reveals dose-dependency and a rapid onset of action for the antidepressant effect of three selective serotonin reuptake inhibitors. *Trans Psychiatry* 2016; **6**:e834.

28. Furukawa TA, et al. Optimal dose of selective serotonin reuptake inhibitors, venlafaxine, and mirtazapine in major depression: a systematic review and dose-response meta-analysis. *Lancet Psychiatry* 2019; **6**:601–609.

29. Papakostas GI, et al. A meta-analysis of early sustained response rates between antidepressants and placebo for the treatment of major depressive disorder. *J Clin Psychopharmacol* 2006; **26**:56–60.

30. Taylor MJ, et al. Early onset of selective serotonin reuptake inhibitor antidepressant action: systematic review and meta-analysis. *Arch Gen Psychiatry* 2006; **63**:1217–1223.

31. Posternak MA, et al. Is there a delay in the antidepressant effect? A meta-analysis. *J Clin Psychiatry* 2005; **66**:148–158.

32. Szegedi A, et al. Early improvement in the first 2 weeks as a predictor of treatment outcome in patients with major depressive disorder: a meta-analysis including 6562 patients. *J Clin Psychiatry* 2009; **70**:344–353.

33. Baldwin DS, et al. How long should a trial of escitalopram treatment be in patients with major depressive disorder, generalised anxiety disorder or social anxiety disorder? An exploration of the randomised controlled trial database. *Human Psychopharmacology* 2009; **24**:269–275.

34. Nierenberg AA, et al. Early nonresponse to fluoxetine as a predictor of poor 8-week outcome. *Am J Psychiatry* 1995; **152**:1500–1503.

Management of treatment-resistant depression – first choice

Resistant depression is difficult to treat successfully, and outcomes are often poor,[1-3] especially if evidence-based protocols are not followed.[4] Treatment-resistant depression is not a uniform entity but a complex spectrum of severity which can be graded[5] and in which outcome is closely linked to grading.[6] A significant minority of apparently resistant unipolar depression may in fact be bipolar depression[7,8] which is often unresponsive to standard antidepressants[9,10] (see section on 'Bipolar depression' in Chapter 2). Recently there has been a move to characterise treatment-resistant depression as 'difficult-to-treat' depression on the basis that the former description implies that depression treatments are normally effective and that non-response is therefore somehow abnormal.[11] Others suggest abandoning treatment-resistant depression as a diagnosis (again proposing 'difficult-to-treat' depression) because it propels clinicians to try more and more drugs in increasingly complex regimens rather than managing expectations of recovery to a more realistic level.[12]

Management of treatment-resistant depression has been informed by the STAR*D programme (Sequenced Treatment Alternatives to Relieve Depression). This was a pragmatic effectiveness study which used remission of symptoms as its main outcome. At stage 1,[13] 2,786 subjects received citalopram (mean dose 41.8mg/day) for 14 weeks;

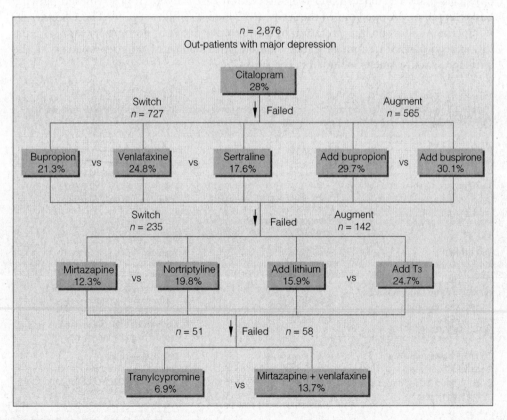

Figure 3.2 Remission rates in STAR*D

CHAPTER 3

remission was seen in 28% (response [50% reduction in symptoms score] in 47%). Subjects who failed to remit were entered into the continued study of sequential treatments.[14–18] Remission rates are given in Figure 3.2. Very few statistically significant differences were noted from this point on. At stage 3,[17] T_3 was found to be significantly better tolerated than lithium. At stage 4,[18] tranylcypromine was less effective and less well tolerated than the mirtazapine/venlafaxine combination. Overall, remission rates, as can be seen, were worryingly low, although it should be noted that the trial consisted of participants with long histories of recurrent depression.

STAR*D demonstrated that the treatment for resistant depression requires a flexible approach and that response to a particular treatment option is not readily predicted by pharmacology or previous treatments. The programme established bupropion and buspirone augmentation as worthwhile options and resurrected from some obscurity the use of T_3 augmentation and of nortriptyline. It also, to some extent, confirmed the safety and (to a lesser extent) efficacy of the combination of mirtazapine and venlafaxine.

It should be noted that there are numerous valid criticisms of the STAR*D programme. These include: the absence of a placebo group; the open nature of treatment and some assessments; the failure to account for patients withdrawing after their first visit; the unexplained use of an *a priori* secondary measure as the main outcome metric; payments made to subjects; and the observation that 93% of 1,518 remitted patients had relapsed or dropped out of the study at 12 months' follow-up.[19,20] These factors do not, perhaps, alter the interpretation of comparative data but do further emphasise the low expectations of treatment of long-standing, treatment-resistant depression with the antidepressant regimens included in the study.

Table 3.3 Treatment-resistant depression – first choice: commonly used treatments generally well supported by published literature (no preference implied by order)

Treatment	Advantages	Disadvantages
Add **aripiprazole**[21–27] (2–20mg/day) to antidepressant	■ Good evidence base ■ Usually well tolerated and safe ■ Low doses (2–10mg/day) may be effective ■ Supported by a recent meta-analysis[28]	■ Akathisia and restlessness common at standard doses (≥10mg/day) ■ Insomnia may be problematic
Add **lithium**[29] Aim for plasma level of 0.4–0.8mmol/L initially, increasing to up to 1.0mmol/L if sub-optimal response	■ Well established ■ Well supported in the literature ■ Recommended by NICE[30] ■ Supported by a recent meta-analysis[28]	■ Sometimes poorly tolerated at higher plasma levels ■ Potentially toxic ■ Usually needs a specialist referral ■ Plasma level monitoring is essential (and TFTs; eGFR) ■ May not be effective in patients resistant to multiple treatments
Combine **olanzapine** and **fluoxetine**[31] (6.25–12.5mg + 25–50mg daily US licensed dose)*	■ Well researched ■ Usually well tolerated ■ Olanzapine + TCA may also be effective[32] ■ Olanzapine alone may be effective[33,34]	■ Risk of weight gain ■ Limited clinical experience outside USA ■ Most data relate to bipolar depression

(Continued)

Table 3.3 (Continued)

Treatment	Advantages	Disadvantages
Add **quetiapine**[35-40] (150mg or 300mg a day) to SSRI/SNRI	▪ Good evidence base ▪ Usually well tolerated ▪ Plausible explanation for antidepressant effect ▪ Possibly more effective than lithium	▪ Dry mouth, sedation, constipation can be problematic ▪ Weight gain risk in the longer term
SSRI + Bupropion[15,41-45] up to 400mg/day	▪ Supported by STAR*D ▪ Well tolerated ▪ May improve sexual adverse effects	▪ Not licensed for depression in the UK
SSRI or **venlafaxine** + **mianserin** (30mg/day) or **mirtazapine**[18,45-48] (30–45mg/day)	▪ Recommended by NICE ▪ Usually well tolerated ▪ Widely used	▪ Theoretical risk of serotonin syndrome (inform patient) ▪ Risk of blood dyscrasia with mianserin ▪ Weight gain and sedation with mirtazapine ▪ Recent large RCT shows no advantage for mirtazapine added to SSRI/SNRIs in prior non-response[49]

* 5mg + 20mg rising to 10mg + 40mg seems reasonable where combination formulations not available.
eGFR, estimated glomerular filtration rate; NICE, National Institute for Health and Care Excellence; SNRI, serotonin–noradrenaline reuptake inhibitor; SSRI, selective serotonin reuptake inhibitor; STAR*D, Sequenced Treatment Alternatives to Relieve Depression; TCA, tricyclic antidepressant; TFT, thyroid function test.

References

1. Dunner DL, et al. Prospective, long-term, multicenter study of the naturalistic outcomes of patients with treatment-resistant depression. *J Clin Psychiatry* 2006; **67**:688–695.
2. Wooderson SC, et al. Prospective evaluation of specialist inpatient treatment for refractory affective disorders. *J Affect Disord* 2011; **131**:92–103.
3. Fekadu A, et al. What happens to patients with treatment-resistant depression? A systematic review of medium to long term outcome studies. *J Affect Disord* 2009; **116**:4–11.
4. Trivedi MH, et al. Clinical results for patients with major depressive disorder in the Texas Medication Algorithm Project. *Arch Gen Psychiatry* 2004; **61**:669–680.
5. Fekadu A, et al. A multidimensional tool to quantify treatment resistance in depression: the Maudsley staging method. *J Clin Psychiatry* 2009; **70**:177–184.
6. Fekadu A, et al. The Maudsley Staging Method for treatment-resistant depression: prediction of longer-term outcome and persistence of symptoms. *J Clin Psychiatry* 2009; **70**:952–957.
7. Angst J, et al. Toward a re-definition of subthreshold bipolarity: epidemiology and proposed criteria for bipolar-II, minor bipolar disorders and hypomania. *J Affect Disord* 2003; **73**:133–146.
8. Smith DJ, et al. Unrecognised bipolar disorder in primary care patients with depression. *British J Psychiatry* 2011; **199**:49–56.
9. Sidor MM, et al. Antidepressants for the acute treatment of bipolar depression: a systematic review and meta-analysis. *J Clin Psychiatry* 2011; **72**:156–167.
10. Taylor DM, et al. Comparative efficacy and acceptability of drug treatments for bipolar depression: a multiple-treatments meta-analysis. *Acta Psychiatr Scand* 2014; **130**:452–469.
11. Cosgrove L, et al. Reconceptualising treatment-resistant depression as difficult-to-treat depression. *Lancet Psychiatry* 2021; **8**:11–13.
12. Rush AJ, et al. Difficult-to-treat depression: a clinical and research roadmap for when remission is elusive. *Aust N Z J Psychiatry* 2019; **53**:109–118.
13. Trivedi MH, et al. Evaluation of outcomes with citalopram for depression using measurement-based care in STAR*D: implications for clinical practice. *Am J Psychiatry* 2006; **163**:28–40.
14. Rush AJ, et al. Bupropion-SR, sertraline, or venlafaxine-XR after failure of SSRIs for depression. *N Engl J Med* 2006; **354**:1231–1242.
15. Trivedi MH, et al. Medication augmentation after the failure of SSRIs for depression. *N Engl J Med* 2006; **354**:1243–1252.
16. Fava M, et al. A comparison of mirtazapine and nortriptyline following two consecutive failed medication treatments for depressed outpatients: a STAR*D report. *Am J Psychiatry* 2006; **163**:1161–1172.
17. Nierenberg AA, et al. A comparison of lithium and T(3) augmentation following two failed medication treatments for depression: a STAR*D report. *Am J Psychiatry* 2006; **163**:1519–1530.

CHAPTER 3

18. McGrath PJ, et al. Tranylcypromine versus venlafaxine plus mirtazapine following three failed antidepressant medication trials for depression: a STAR*D report. *Am J Psychiatry* 2006; **163**:1531–1541.

19. Pigott HE, et al. Efficacy and effectiveness of antidepressants: current status of research. *Psychother Psychosom* 2010; **79**:267–279.

20. Pigott HE. The STAR*D trial: it is time to reexamine the clinical beliefs that guide the treatment of major depression. *Can J Psychiatry* 2015; **60**:9–13.

21. Marcus RN, et al. The efficacy and safety of aripiprazole as adjunctive therapy in major depressive disorder: a second multicenter, randomized, double-blind, placebo-controlled study. *J Clin Psychopharmacol* 2008; **28**:156–165.

22. Hellerstein DJ, et al. Aripiprazole as an adjunctive treatment for refractory unipolar depression. *Prog Neuropsychopharmacol Biol Psychiatry* 2008; **32**:744–750.

23. Simon JS, et al. Aripiprazole augmentation of antidepressants for the treatment of partially responding and nonresponding patients with major depressive disorder. *J Clin Psychiatry* 2005; **66**:1216–1220.

24. Papakostas GI, et al. Aripiprazole augmentation of selective serotonin reuptake inhibitors for treatment-resistant major depressive disorder. *J Clin Psychiatry* 2005; **66**:1326–1330.

25. Berman RM, et al. Aripiprazole augmentation in major depressive disorder: a double-blind, placebo-controlled study in patients with inadequate response to antidepressants. *CNS Spectr* 2009; **14**:197–206.

26. Fava M, et al. A double-blind, placebo-controlled study of aripiprazole adjunctive to antidepressant therapy among depressed outpatients with inadequate response to prior antidepressant therapy (ADAPT-A Study). *PsychotherPsychosom* 2012; **81**:87–97.

27. Jon DI, et al. Augmentation of aripiprazole for depressed patients with an inadequate response to antidepressant treatment: a 6-week prospective, open-label, multicenter study. *Clin Neuropharmacol* 2013; **36**:157–161.

28. Strawbridge R, et al. Augmentation therapies for treatment-resistant depression: systematic review and meta-analysis. *Br J Psychiatry* 2019; **214**:42–51.

29. Undurraga J, et al. Lithium treatment for unipolar major depressive disorder: systematic review. *J Psychopharmacology (Oxford, England)* 2019; **33**:167–176.

30. National Institute for Clinical Excellence. Depression: the treatment and management of depression in adults. Clinical Guidance [CG90]. 2009 (last reviewed Dec 2013); https://www.nice.org.uk/guidance/cg90.

31. Luan S, et al. Efficacy and safety of olanzapine/fluoxetine combination in the treatment of treatment-resistant depression: a meta-analysis of randomized controlled trials. *Neuropsychiatr Dis Treat* 2017; **13**:609–620.

32. Takahashi H, et al. Augmentation with olanzapine in TCA-refractory depression with melancholic features: a consecutive case series. *Human Psychopharmacology* 2008; **23**:217–220.

33. Corya SA, et al. A randomized, double-blind comparison of olanzapine/fluoxetine combination, olanzapine, fluoxetine, and venlafaxine in treatment-resistant depression. *Depress Anxiety* 2006; **23**:364–372.

34. Thase ME, et al. A randomized, double-blind comparison of olanzapine/fluoxetine combination, olanzapine, and fluoxetine in treatment-resistant major depressive disorder. *J Clin Psychiatry* 2007; **68**:224–236.

35. Jensen NH, et al. N-desalkylquetiapine, a potent norepinephrine reuptake inhibitor and partial 5-HT1A agonist, as a putative mediator of quetiapine's antidepressant activity. *Neuropsychopharmacology* 2008; **33**:2303–2312.

36. El-Khalili N, et al. Extended-release quetiapine fumarate (quetiapine XR) as adjunctive therapy in major depressive disorder (MDD) in patients with an inadequate response to ongoing antidepressant treatment: a multicentre, randomized, double-blind, placebo-controlled study. *Int J Neuropsychopharmacol* 2010; **13**:917–932.

37. Bauer M, et al. Extended-release quetiapine as adjunct to an antidepressant in patients with major depressive disorder: results of a randomized, placebo-controlled, double-blind study. *J Clin Psychiatry* 2009; **70**:540–549.

38. Bauer M, et al. A pooled analysis of two randomised, placebo-controlled studies of extended release quetiapine fumarate adjunctive to antidepressant therapy in patients with major depressive disorder. *J Affect Disord* 2010; **127**:19–30.

39. Montgomery S, et al. P01-75 – Quetiapine XR or lithium combination with antidepressants in treatment resistant depression. *Eur Psychiatry* 2010; **25**:296–296.

40. Doree JP, et al. Quetiapine augmentation of treatment-resistant depression: a comparison with lithium. *Curr Med Res Opin* 2007; **23**:333–341.

41. Zisook S, et al. Use of bupropion in combination with serotonin reuptake inhibitors. *Biol Psychiatry* 2006; **59**:203–210.

42. Fatemi SH, et al. Venlafaxine and bupropion combination therapy in a case of treatment-resistant depression. *Ann Pharmacother* 1999; **33**:701–703.

43. Lam RW, et al. Citalopram and bupropion-SR: combining versus switching in patients with treatment-resistant depression. *J Clin Psychiatry* 2004; **65**:337–340.

44. Papakostas GI, et al. The combination of duloxetine and bupropion for treatment-resistant major depressive disorder. *Depress Anxiety* 2006; **23**:178–181.

45. Henssler J, et al. Combining antidepressants in acute treatment of depression: a meta-analysis of 38 studies including 4511 patients. *Can J Psychiatry* 2016; **61**:29–43.

46. Carpenter LL, et al. A double-blind, placebo-controlled study of antidepressant augmentation with mirtazapine. *Biol Psychiatry* 2002; **51**:183–188.

47. Carpenter LL, et al. Mirtazapine augmentation in the treatment of refractory depression. *J Clin Psychiatry* 1999; **60**:45–49.

48. Ferreri M, et al. Benefits from mianserin augmentation of fluoxetine in patients with major depression non-responders to fluoxetine alone. *Acta Psychiatr Scand* 2001; **103**:66–72.

49. Kessler DS, et al. Mirtazapine added to SSRIs or SNRIs for treatment resistant depression in primary care: phase III randomised placebo controlled trial (MIR). *BMJ* 2018; **363**:k4218.

Management of treatment-resistant depression – second choice

Table 3.4 Second choice: less commonly used, variably supported by published evaluations (no preference implied by order)

Treatment	Advantages	Disadvantages
Add **ketamine** (0.5mg/kg IV over 40 minutes)[1] Intranasal **esketamine** (licensed in most countries) dose is 28–84mg[2] See section on ketamine preparations in this chapter	▪ Very rapid response (within hours) – including effects on suicidality[3,4] ▪ High remission rate ▪ Some evidence of maintained response if repeated doses given ▪ Usually well tolerated at this sub-anaesthetic dose	▪ IV needs to be administered in hospital environment ▪ Cognitive effects (confusion, dissociation) and other psychiatric symptoms[5] ▪ Associated with transient increases in BP, tachycardia and arrhythmias. Pre-treatment ECG required with IV form.[6] ▪ Adverse effects may have been underestimated[7] ▪ Repeated treatment may be necessary to maintain effect
Add **lamotrigine** (100mg, 200mg and 400mg a day have been used)[8]	▪ Reasonably well researched ▪ Quite widely used ▪ Probably best tolerated augmentation strategy[9]	▪ Slow titration ▪ Risk of rash ▪ Appropriate dosing unclear
ECT[10–12]	▪ Well established ▪ Effective ▪ Well supported in the literature	▪ Poor reputation in public domain ▪ Necessitates general anaesthetic ▪ Needs specialist referral ▪ Usually reserved for last-line treatment or if rapid response needed ▪ Usually combined with other treatments
Add **tri-iodothyronine** (20–50µg/day) Higher doses have been safely used[13–19]	▪ Usually well tolerated ▪ Reasonable literature support ▪ May be effective in bipolar depression	▪ Clinical and biochemical TFT monitoring required ▪ Usually needs specialist referral ▪ Some negative studies ▪ No advantage over antidepressant alone in non-refractory illness[20]

CHAPTER 3

References

1. Marcantoni WS, et al. A systematic review and meta-analysis of the efficacy of intravenous ketamine infusion for treatment resistant depression: January 2009–January 2019. *J Affect Disord* 2020; 277:831–841.
2. Papakostas GI, et al. Efficacy of esketamine augmentation in major depressive disorder: a meta-analysis. *J Clin Psychiatry* 2020; 81:19r12889.
3. Wilkinson ST, et al. The effect of a single dose of intravenous ketamine on suicidal ideation: a systematic review and individual participant data meta-analysis. *Am J Psychiatry* 2018; 175:150–158.
4. Witt K, et al. Ketamine for suicidal ideation in adults with psychiatric disorders: a systematic review and meta-analysis of treatment trials. *Aust N Z J Psychiatry* 2020; 54:29–45.
5. Beck K, et al. Association of ketamine with psychiatric symptoms and implications for its therapeutic use and for understanding schizophrenia: a systematic review and meta-analysis. *JAMA Network Open* 2020; 3:e204693.
6. Aan Het Rot M, et al. Safety and efficacy of repeated-dose intravenous ketamine for treatment-resistant depression. *Biol Psychiatry* 2010; 67:139–145.
7. Short B, et al. Side-effects associated with ketamine use in depression: a systematic review. *Lancet Psychiatry* 2018; 5:65–78.
8. Goh KK, et al. Lamotrigine augmentation in treatment-resistant unipolar depression: a comprehensive meta-analysis of efficacy and safety. *J Psychopharmacology* 2019; 33:700–713.
9. Papadimitropoulou K, et al. Comparative efficacy and tolerability of pharmacological and somatic interventions in adult patients with treatment-resistant depression: a systematic review and network meta-analysis. *Curr Med Res Opin* 2017; 33:701–711.
10. Folkerts HW, et al. Electroconvulsive therapy vs. paroxetine in treatment-resistant depression – a randomized study. *Acta Psychiatr Scand* 1997; 96:334–342.
11. Gonzalez-Pinto A, et al. Efficacy and safety of venlafaxine-ECT combination in treatment-resistant depression. *J Neuropsychiatry Clin Neurosci* 2002; 14:206–209.
12. Eranti S, et al. A randomized, controlled trial with 6-month follow-up of repetitive transcranial magnetic stimulation and electroconvulsive therapy for severe depression. *Am J Psychiatry* 2007; 164:73–81.
13. Joffe RT, et al. A comparison of triiodothyronine and thyroxine in the potentiation of tricyclic antidepressants. *Psychiatry Res* 1990; 32:241–251.
14. Anderson IM. Drug treatment of depression: reflections on the evidence. *Adv Psychiatric Treatment* 2003; 9:11–20.
15. Nierenberg AA, et al. A comparison of lithium and T(3) augmentation following two failed medication treatments for depression: a STAR*D report. *Am J Psychiatry* 2006; 163:1519–1530.
16. Iosifescu DV, et al. An open study of triiodothyronine augmentation of selective serotonin reuptake inhibitors in treatment-resistant major depressive disorder. *J Clin Psychiatry* 2005; 66:1038–1042.
17. Abraham G, et al. T3 augmentation of SSRI resistant depression. *J Affect Disord* 2006; 91:211–215.
18. Kelly TF, et al. Long term augmentation with T3 in refractory major depression. *J Affect Disord* 2009; 115:230–233.
19. Parmentier T, et al. The use of triiodothyronine (T3) in the treatment of bipolar depression: a review of the literature. *J Affect Disord* 2018; 229:410–414.
20. Garlow SJ, et al. The combination of triiodothyronine (T3) and sertraline is not superior to sertraline monotherapy in the treatment of major depressive disorder. *J Psychiatr Res* 2012; 46:1406–1413.

CHAPTER 3

Treatment-resistant depression – other reported treatments

A very wide range of treatments have been investigated as potential therapy for treatment-resistant depression. Table 3.5 in this section briefly describes strategies that have limited support for their use but may be worth trying in exceptional circumstances. Prescribers should familiarise themselves with the primary literature before using these strategies.

Table 3.5 Other reported treatments (alphabetical order – no preference implied)

Treatment	Comments
Amantadine[1] (up to 300mg/day)	Limited data
Ayahuasca[2,3]	Effective but specialist use only
Buprenorphine[4] (0.8–2mg/day)	Reasonable evidence but obvious contraindications
Carbergoline[5] 2mg/day	Very limited data
D-cycloserine[6] 1000mg/day	One small RCT showing useful effect
Dexamethasone[7,8] 3–4mg/day	Limited data
Dextromethorphan + quinidine[9,10] 45/10mg BD	Promising novel treatment. NDMA antagonist. Quinidine is needed as CYP2D6 inhibitor to prolong action of dextromethorphan[11]
Folate/methyl folate[12–14] (2mg/day folate?)	Possible benefit but poor-quality trials
Hyoscine[15] (Scopolomine) (4mcg/kg IV)	Growing evidence base of prompt and sizeable effect
Ketoconazole[16] 400–800mg/day	Rarely used. Risk of hepatotoxicity
MAOI and TCA[17–19] e.g. trimipramine and phenelzine	Formerly very widely used, but great care needed
Mecamylamine[20,21] up to 10mg/day	One pilot study of 21 patients
Minocycline 200mg/day	Several positive meta-analyses in both animals[22] and humans.[23,24] Recent failed RCT in bipolar depression[25]
Modafinil[26–30] 100–400mg/day	See section on 'Psychostimulants in depression' (this chapter)
Naltrexone[31,32] 100mg/day	No studies in non-opiate misuers
Nemifitide[33] 40–240mg/day SC	One pilot study in 25 patients
Nortriptyline ± lithium[34–37]	Re-emergent treatment option
Oestrogens[38] (various regimens)	Limited data

(Continued)

CHAPTER 3

Table 3.5 (Continued)

Treatment	Comments
Omega–3-triglycerides EPA[39]	Usually added to antidepressant treatment. Effect is possibly dose-sensitive – total dose should be <1g a day and EPA content >60%
Pindolol[30,40–44] 5mg tds or 7.5mg once daily	Well tolerated, can be initiated in primary care. Data mainly relate to acceleration of response. Refractory data somewhat contradictory
Pramipexole[38,39] 0.125–5mg/day	One good RCT showing clear effect
Psilocybin[45] 10/25mg one week apart	Effective but specialist use only
Risperidone[46–51] 0.5–3mg/day to antidepressant	Generally less robust RCT support than for other SGAs
***S*-adenosyl-l-methionine**[52–54] 400mg/day IM; 1600mg/day oral	Limited data in treatment-resistant depression Use weakly supported by a Cochrane review[55]
SSRI + Buspirone[56,57] Up to 60mg/day	Supported by STAR*D Higher doses required poorly tolerated (dizziness common)
SSRI + TCA[58]	Formerly widely used
Stimulants: amfetamine; methylphenidate	Varied outcomes. See section on 'Psychostimulants in depression' (this chapter)
TCA – high dose[59]	Formerly widely used. Cardiac monitoring essential
Testosterone gel[30,60]	Effective in those with low testosterone levels
Tianeptine[61,62] 25–50mg/day	Tiny database. Tianeptine not available in many countries
Tryptophan[63–66] 2–3g TDS	Long history of successful use
Venlafaxine[67–70] >200mg/day	Can be initiated in primary care Recommended by NICE[71] Nausea and vomiting; discontinuation reactions more common. Blood pressure monitoring essential
Venlafaxine – very high dose (up to 600mg/day)[72]	See above entry. Cardiac monitoring essential
Venlafaxine + IV clomipramine[73]	Cardiac monitoring essential
Zinc[74] 25mg Zn +/day	One RCT (*n* = 60) showed good results in refractory depression
Ziprasidone[75–77] Up to 160mg/day	Poorly supported. Probably has no antidepressant effects

Note: Other non-drug treatments are available, including various psychological approaches, repetitive transcranial magnetic stimulation (rTMS), vagus nerve stimulation, deep brain stimulation and psychosurgery. Discussion of these is beyond the scope of the book.

EPA, eicosapentanoic acid; IM, intramuscular; IV, intravenous; MAOI, monoamine oxidase inhibitor; RCT, randomised controlled trial; SC, subcutaneous; SSRI, selective serotonin reuptake inhibitor; TCA, tricyclic antidepressant; tds, three times a day.

References

1. Stryjer R, et al. Amantadine as augmentation therapy in the management of treatment-resistant depression. *Int Clin Psychopharmacol* 2003; 18:93–96.

2. Santos RGD, et al. Long-term effects of ayahuasca in patients with recurrent depression: a 5-year qualitative follow-up. *Arch Clin Psychiatry* 2018; 45:22–24.

3. Palhano-Fontes F, et al. Rapid antidepressant effects of the psychedelic ayahuasca in treatment-resistant depression: a randomized placebo-controlled trial. *Psychol Med* 2019; 49:655–663.

4. Stanciu CN, et al. Use of buprenorphine in treatment of refractory depression-A review of current literature. *Asian J Psychiatr* 2017; 26:94–98.

5. Takahashi H, et al. Addition of a dopamine agonist, cabergoline, to a serotonin-noradrenalin reuptake inhibitor, milnacipran as a therapeutic option in the treatment of refractory depression: two case reports. *Clin Neuropharmacol* 2003; 26:230–232.

6. Heresco-Levy U, et al. A randomized add-on trial of high-dose D-cycloserine for treatment-resistant depression. *Int J Neuropsychopharmacol* 2013; 16:501–506.

7. Dinan TG, et al. Dexamethasone augmentation in treatment-resistant depression. *Acta Psychiatr Scand* 1997; 95:58–61.

8. Bodani M, et al. The use of dexamethasone in elderly patients with antidepressant-resistant depressive illness. *J Psychopharmacology* 1999; 13:196–197.

9. Murrough JW, et al. Dextromethorphan/quinidine pharmacotherapy in patients with treatment resistant depression: a proof of concept clinical trial. *J Affect Disord* 2017; 218:277–283.

10. Kelly TF, et al. The utility of the combination of dextromethorphan and quinidine in the treatment of bipolar II and bipolar NOS. *J Affect Disord* 2014; 167:333–335.

11. Nofziger JL, et al. Evaluation of dextromethorphan with select antidepressant therapy for the treatment of depression in the acute care psychiatric setting. *Ment Health Clin* 2019; 9:76–81.

12. Firth J, et al. The efficacy and safety of nutrient supplements in the treatment of mental disorders: a meta-review of meta-analyses of randomized controlled trials. *World Psychiatry* 2019; 18:308–324.

13. Roberts E, et al. Caveat emptor: folate in unipolar depressive illness, a systematic review and meta-analysis. *J Psychopharmacology* 2018; 32:377–384.

14. Abou-Saleh MT, et al. Folic acid and the treatment of depression. *J Psychosom Res* 2006; 61:285–287.

15. Drevets WC, et al. Antidepressant effects of the muscarinic cholinergic receptor antagonist scopolamine: a review. *Biol Psychiatry* 2013; 73:1156–1163.

16. Wolkowitz OM, et al. Antiglucocorticoid treatment of depression: double-blind ketoconazole. *Biol Psychiatry* 1999; 45:1070–1074.

17. White K, et al. The combined use of MAOIs and tricyclics. *J Clin Psychiatry* 1984; 45:67–69.

18. Kennedy N, et al. Treatment and response in refractory depression: results from a specialist affective disorders service. *J Affect Disord* 2004; 81:49–53.

19. Connolly KR, et al. If at first you don't succeed: a review of the evidence for antidepressant augmentation, combination and switching strategies. *Drugs* 2011; 71:43–64.

20. George TP, et al. Nicotinic antagonist augmentation of selective serotonin reuptake inhibitor-refractory major depressive disorder: a preliminary study. *J Clin Psychopharmacol* 2008; 28:340–344.

21. Bacher I, et al. Mecamylamine – a nicotinic acetylcholine receptor antagonist with potential for the treatment of neuropsychiatric disorders. *Expert Opin Pharmacother* 2009; 10:2709–2721.

22. Reis DJ, et al. The antidepressant impact of minocycline in rodents: a systematic review and meta-analysis. *Sci Rep* 2019; 9:261.

23. Zazula R, et al. Minocycline as adjunctive treatment for major depressive disorder: pooled data from two randomized controlled trials. *Aust N Z J Psychiatry* 2020; 4867420965697.

24. Strawbridge R, et al. Augmentation therapies for treatment-resistant depression: systematic review and meta-analysis. *Br J Psychiatry* 2019; 214:42–51.

25. Husain MI, et al. Minocycline and celecoxib as adjunctive treatments for bipolar depression: a multicentre, factorial design randomised controlled trial. *Lancet Psychiatry* 2020; 7:515–527.

26. DeBattista C, et al. A prospective trial of modafinil as an adjunctive treatment of major depression. *J Clin Psychopharmacol* 2004; 24:87–90.

27. Ninan PT, et al. Adjunctive modafinil at initiation of treatment with a selective serotonin reuptake inhibitor enhances the degree and onset of therapeutic effects in patients with major depressive disorder and fatigue. *J Clin Psychiatry* 2004; 65:414–420.

28. Menza MA, et al. Modafinil augmentation of antidepressant treatment in depression. *J Clin Psychiatry* 2000; 61:378–381.

29. Taneja I, et al. A randomized, double-blind, crossover trial of modafinil on mood. *J Clin Psychopharmacol* 2007; 27:76–78.

30. Kleeblatt J, et al. Efficacy of off-label augmentation in unipolar depression: a systematic review of the evidence. *Eur Neuropsychopharmacol* 2017; 27:423–441.

31. Pettinati HM, Ph.D., et al. A double-blind, placebo-controlled trial combining sertraline and naltrexone for treating co-occurring depression and alcohol dependence. *Am J Psychiatry* 2010; 167:668–675.

32. Browne CA, et al. Novel targets to treat depression: opioid-based therapeutics. *Harv Rev Psychiatry* 2020; 28:40–59.

33. Feighner JP, et al. Clinical effect of nemifitide, a novel pentapeptide antidepressant, in the treatment of severely depressed refractory patients. *Int Clin Psychopharmacol* 2008; 23:29–35.

34. Nierenberg AA, et al. Nortriptyline for treatment-resistant depression. *J Clin Psychiatry* 2003; 64:35–39.

35. Nierenberg AA, et al. Lithium augmentation of nortriptyline for subjects resistant to multiple antidepressants. *J Clin Psychopharmacol* 2003; 23:92–95.

36. Fava M, et al. A comparison of mirtazapine and nortriptyline following two consecutive failed medication treatments for depressed outpatients: a STAR*D report. *Am J Psychiatry* 2006; 163:1161–1172.

37. Shelton RC, et al. Olanzapine/fluoxetine combination for treatment-resistant depression: a controlled study of SSRI and nortriptyline resistance. *J Clin Psychiatry* 2005; 66:1289–1297.

38. Stahl SM. Basic psychopharmacology of antidepressants, part 2: oestrogen as an adjunct to antidepressant treatment. *J Clin Psychiatry* 1998; 59 Suppl 4:15–24.

39. Liao Y, et al. Efficacy of omega-3 PUFAs in depression: a meta-analysis. *Trans Psychiatry* 2019; 9:190.

40. McAskill R, et al. Pindolol augmentation of antidepressant therapy. *Br J Psychiatry* 1998; 173:203–208.

41. Rasanen P, et al. Mitchell B. Balter award–1998. Pindolol and major affective disorders: a three-year follow-up study of 30,485 patients. *J Clin Psychopharmacol* 1999; 19:297–302.

42. Perry EB, et al. Pindolol augmentation in depressed patients resistant to selective serotonin reuptake inhibitors: a double-blind, randomized, controlled trial. *J Clin Psychiatry* 2004; 65:238–243.

43. Sokolski KN, et al. Once-daily high-dose pindolol for SSRI-refractory depression. *Psychiatry Res* 2004; 125:81–86.

44. Whale R, et al. Pindolol augmentation of serotonin reuptake inhibitors for the treatment of depressive disorder: a systematic review. *J Psychopharmacology* 2010; 24:513–520.

45. Carhart-Harris RL, et al. Psilocybin with psychological support for treatment-resistant depression: an open-label feasibility study. *Lancet Psychiatry* 2016; 3:619–627.

46. Yoshimura R, et al. Addition of risperidone to sertraline improves sertraline-resistant refractory depression without influencing plasma concentrations of sertraline and desmethylsertraline. *Human Psychopharmacology* 2008; 23:707–713.

47. Mahmoud RA, et al. Risperidone for treatment-refractory major depressive disorder: a randomized trial. *Ann Intern Med* 2007; 147:593–602.

48. Ostroff RB, et al. Risperidone augmentation of selective serotonin reuptake inhibitors in major depression. *J Clin Psychiatry* 1999; 60:256–259.

49. Rapaport MH, et al. Effects of risperidone augmentation in patients with treatment-resistant depression: results of open-label treatment followed by double-blind continuation. *Neuropsychopharmacology* 2006; 31:2505–2513.

50. Stoll AL, et al. Tranylcypromine plus risperidone for treatment-refractory major depression. *J Clin Psychopharmacol* 2000; 20:495–496.

51. Keitner GI, et al. A randomized, placebo-controlled trial of risperidone augmentation for patients with difficult-to-treat unipolar, non-psychotic major depression. *J Psychiatr Res* 2009; 43:205–214.

52. Pancheri P, et al. A double-blind, randomized parallel-group, efficacy and safety study of intramuscular S-adenosyl-L-methionine 1,4-butanedisulphonate (SAMe) versus imipramine in patients with major depressive disorder. *Int J Neuropsychopharmacol* 2002; 5:287–294.

53. Alpert JE, et al. S-adenosyl-L-methionine (SAMe) as an adjunct for resistant major depressive disorder: an open trial following partial or nonresponse to selective serotonin reuptake inhibitors or venlafaxine. *J Clin Psychopharmacol* 2004; 24:661–664.

54. Sharma A, et al. S-adenosylmethionine (SAMe) for neuropsychiatric disorders: a clinician-oriented review of research. *J Clin Psychiatry* 2017; 78:e656–e667.

55. Galizia I, et al. S-adenosyl methionine (SAMe) for depression in adults. *Cochrane Database Syst Rev* 2016; 10:Cd011286.

56. Trivedi MH, et al. Medication augmentation after the failure of SSRIs for depression. *N Engl J Med* 2006; 354:1243–1252.

57. Appelberg BG, et al. Patients with severe depression may benefit from buspirone augmentation of selective serotonin reuptake inhibitors: results from a placebo-controlled, randomized, double-blind, placebo wash-in study. *J Clin Psychiatry* 2001; 62:448–452.

58. Taylor D. Selective serotonin reuptake inhibitors and tricyclic antidepressants in combination – interactions and therapeutic uses. *Br J Psychiatry* 1995; 167:575–580.

59. Malhi GS, et al. Management of resistant depression. *Int J Psychiatry Clin Pract* 1997; 1:269–276.

60. Pope HG, Jr., et al. Testosterone gel supplementation for men with refractory depression: a randomized, placebo-controlled trial. *Am J Psychiatry* 2003; 160:105–111.

61. Tobe EH, et al. Possible usefulness of tianeptine in treatment-resistant depression. *Int J Psychiatry Clin Pract* 2013; 17:313–316.

62. Woo YS, et al. Tianeptine combination for partial or non-response to selective serotonin re-uptake inhibitor monotherapy. *Psychiatry Clin Neurosci* 2013; 67:219–227.

63. Angst J, et al. The treatment of depression with L-5-hydroxytryptophan versus imipramine. Results of two open and one double-blind study. *Arch Psychiatr Nervenkr* 1977; 224:175–186.

64. Alino JJ, et al. 5-Hydroxytryptophan (5-HTP) and a MAOI (nialamide) in the treatment of depressions. A double-blind controlled study. *Int Pharmacopsychiatry* 1976; 11:8–15.

65. Hale AS, et al. Clomipramine, tryptophan and lithium in combination for resistant endogenous depression: seven case studies. *Br J Psychiatry* 1987; 151:213–217.

66. Young SN. Use of tryptophan in combination with other antidepressant treatments: a review. *J Psychiatry Neurosci* 1991; 16:241–246.

67. Poirier MF, et al. Venlafaxine and paroxetine in treatment-resistant depression. Double-blind, randomised comparison. *Br J Psychiatry* 1999; 175:12–16.

68. Nierenberg AA, et al. Venlafaxine for treatment-resistant unipolar depression. *J Clin Psychopharmacol* 1994; 14:419–423.

69. Smith D, et al. Efficacy and tolerability of venlafaxine compared with selective serotonin reuptake inhibitors and other antidepressants: a meta-analysis. *Br J Psychiatry* 2002; 180:396–404.

70. Rush AJ, et al. Bupropion-SR, sertraline, or venlafaxine-XR after failure of SSRIs for depression. *N Engl J Med* 2006; 354:1231–1242.

71. National Institute for Clinical Excellence. Depression: the treatment and management of depression in adults. Clinical Guidance [CG90]. 2009 (last reviewed Dec 2013); https://www.nice.org.uk/guidance/cg90.

72. Harrison CL, et al. Tolerability of high-dose venlafaxine in depressed patients. *J Psychopharmacology* 2004; **18**:200–204.

73. Fountoulakis KN, et al. Combined oral venlafaxine and intravenous clomipramine-A: successful temporary response in a patient with extremely refractory depression. *Can J Psychiatry* 2004; **49**:73–74.

74. Siwek M, et al. Zinc supplementation augments efficacy of imipramine in treatment resistant patients: a double blind, placebo-controlled study. *J Affect Disord* 2009; **118**:187–195.

75. Papakostas GI, et al. Ziprasidone augmentation of selective serotonin reuptake inhibitors (SSRIs) for SSRI-resistant major depressive disorder. *J Clin Psychiatry* 2004; **65**:217–221.

76. Dunner DL, et al. Efficacy and tolerability of adjunctive ziprasidone in treatment-resistant depression: a randomized, open-label, pilot study. *J Clin Psychiatry* 2007; **68**:1071–1077.

77. Papakostas GI, et al. A 12-week, randomized, double-blind, placebo-controlled, sequential parallel comparison trial of ziprasidone as monotherapy for major depressive disorder. *J Clin Psychiatry* 2012; **73**:1541–1547.

CHAPTER 3

Ketamine

Background

Over the last two decades, ketamine, an uncompetitive N-Methyl-D-Aspartate (NMDA) receptor antagonist and dissociative anaesthetic, has emerged as a novel and effective rapid-acting antidepressant. In 2000, Berman and colleagues reported findings from a landmark RCT, administering a single subanaesthetic dose of intravenous (IV) ketamine (0.5mg/kg over 40 minutes) to individuals with major depressive disorder (MDD).[1] Ketamine produced a significant antidepressant effect within hours after the infusion that increased progressively up to 3 days after administration. This finding has since been replicated in several trials in both unipolar and bipolar depression (including treatment-resistant individuals).[2-6]

Ketamine is a racemic mixture that is composed of equal amounts of the two enantiomers (S)-ketamine and (R)-ketamine (esketamine and arketamine), with esketamine binding more potently to the NMDA receptor. Although ketamine currently remains an off-label treatment for treatment-resistant depression (TRD), an esketamine nasal spray (Spravato™) has been developed and approved for use in TRD (in conjunction with an oral antidepressant) in Europe and the United States.

Mechanism

At present, the precise mechanisms of action for the rapid antidepressant effects of ketamine and esketamine are not clear, but it has been proposed that these effects are mediated via blockade of NMDA receptors on γ-amynobutyric acid (GABA)ergic interneurons that normally act to suppress glutamate release from glutamatergic neurons.[7] This disinhibition results in an acute cortical glutamate surge, activation of post-synaptic α-amino-3-hydroxy-5-methyl-4-isoxazolepropionic acid (AMPA) receptors, with downstream effects on synaptogenesis and neuroplastic pathways.[7]

Route

The optimal method for administering ketamine for TRD is not fully established; however, there are now approved dosing guidelines for intranasal esketamine (Table 3.6). IV ketamine (0.5mg/kg over 40 minutes) is the gold standard for off-label ketamine administration, with the best supporting evidence for efficacy. Other routes of administration have also been proposed including subcutaneous (SC), intramuscular (IM), oral and sublingual (SL), although further research is needed to qualify the relative efficacy and safety of these routes, as well as the optimal dosing regime in each case. Each route has its own advantages and challenges in terms of bioavailability, duration of effect, practicality and patient comfort. While no fixed dosing strategy for ketamine has been established across the different routes and doses tested, in Table 3.6 we provide a summary of dosing recommendations, considering available evidence and clinical experience.

Adverse effects

Ketamine generally leads to significant dissociative symptoms when given at antidepressant doses.[8] These include perceptual distortions and can lead to significant anxiety. As a result, it is necessary that any patients administered ketamine should be observed by a trained clinician during dosing and for an hour after administration. Furthermore, although a rare event, ketamine has been reported to induce laryngospasm and so the observing clinician should be trained in intermediate or advanced life support. When ketamine is given at lower doses by oral or sublingual routes, it is less likely to induce strong dissociative symptoms, and so once a test dose has been given under clinical supervision, it may be possible for administration to take place in a non-clinical (home) setting although patients should be advised not to drive, operate heavy machinery or partake in other high risk activities for at least an hour after administration. In addition, consideration must be given by the prescribing clinician to the risks of diversion and illegal use.

Ketamine can have significant effects on blood pressure and heart rate, and before administration, a physical examination including baseline blood pressure, full blood count, liver function test, thyroid function test plus ECG is recommended. Furthermore, physical monitoring (blood pressure and heart rate) during and after ketamine administration is also indicated.

Table 3.6 Dosing recommendations for different routes of ketamine administration and intranasal esketamine in TRD

Route	Dose	Details	Frequency	Comments
IV[2-6]	▪ 0.5mg/kg, increasing up to 1.0mg/kg if no response ▪ (titrate from 0.25mg/kg in older people)	▪ Infuse over 40 minutes	▪ Induction phase: once or twice a week ▪ Maintenance phase: according to response, weekly and then every 2 weeks, or even monthly (consider supplementing with oral/sublingual doses between IV treatments)	▪ Needs to be administered in clinical setting. ▪ Cognitive effects (confusion, dissociation, etc.) do occasionally occur. ▪ Associated with transient increase in BP, tachycardia and arrhythmias. Pre-treatment ECG required. Monitor BP before and after infusion. ▪ Observe during and for 1 hour after infusion.
SC[9,10]	▪ 0.5mg/kg, increasing up to 1.0mg/kg if no response ▪ (titrate from 0.25mg/kg in older people)	▪ SC bolus injection to appropriate SC site	▪ As per IV above	▪ As per IV above. ▪ May be better tolerated than IV or IM routes.[9]

(Continued)

CHAPTER 3

Table 3.6 (Continued)

Route	Dose	Details	Frequency	Comments
IM[11,12]	• 0.5mg/kg, increasing up to 1.0mg/kg if no response • (titrate from 0.25mg/kg in older people)	• IM bolus injection to appropriate IM site	• As per IV above	• As per IV above.
Oral[13–15]	• 0.5–5.0mg/kg depending on dosing strategy	• Oral capsules	• Regular lower doses: ▪ 0.5–2.0mg/kg every 1–3 days • Intermittent higher doses to supplement IV/SC/IM treatment: ▪ 2.0–5.0mg/kg once or twice a week	• Can be taken at home. • Lower doses show good tolerability; however, antidepressant effects not as rapid as IV/SC/IM. • Higher doses may be used as practical alternative to maintain response to IV/SC/IM treatment. Titrate dose according to response/side effects.
Sublingual[15–17]	• 0.5–3.0mg/kg depending on dosing strategy	• Ketamine solution (held under tongue for 5 minutes and swallowed) • Sublingual ketamine lozenges	• Regular lower doses: ▪ 0.5–1.5mg/kg every 1–3 days ▪ Limited evidence for very low sublingual dosing (10mg every 2–3 days or weekly)[18] • Intermittent higher doses to supplement IV/SC/IM treatment: ▪ 1.5–3.0mg/kg once or twice a week	• Can be taken at home. • Lower doses show good tolerability; however, putative antidepressant effects not as rapid as IV/SC/IM. • Higher doses may be used as practical alternative to maintain response to IV/SC/IM treatment. Titrate dose according to response/side effects.
Intranasal esketamine[19–22]	• 56–84mg • (28mg in older people) • *Treatment in conjunction with oral antidepressant*	• 28mg in two sprays (one spray per nostril) • Repeat after 5 minutes intervals, depending on total dose required.	• Twice weekly, then weekly then every 2 weeks	• Needs to be administered in clinical setting. • Cognitive effects (confusion, dissociation, etc.) do occasionally occur. • Associated with transient increase in BP, tachycardia and arrhythmias. Pretreatment ECG recommended. Monitor BP before and after dose. • Observe for approximately 2 hours after dose.

CI, contraindicated; CV, cardiovascular; CVD, cardiovascular disease; ECG, electrocardiogram; LVF, left ventricular fraction; MAOI, monoamine oxidase inhibitor; MI, myocardial infarction; SPC, summary of product characteristics; SSRI, selective serotonin reuptake inhibitor; TCA, tricyclic antidepressant.

References

1. Berman RM, et al. Antidepressant effects of ketamine in depressed patients. *Biol Psychiatry* 2000; **47**:351–354.
2. Zarate CA, Jr., et al. A randomized trial of an N-methyl-D-aspartate antagonist in treatment-resistant major depression. *Arch Gen Psychiatry* 2006; **63**:856–864.
3. Diazgranados N, et al. A randomized add-on trial of an N-methyl-D-aspartate antagonist in treatment-resistant bipolar depression. *Arch Gen Psychiatry* 2010; **67**:793–802.
4. Murrough JW, et al. Antidepressant efficacy of ketamine in treatment-resistant major depression: a two-site randomized controlled trial. *Am J Psychiatry* 2013; **170**:1134–1142.
5. Singh JB, et al. A double-blind, randomized, placebo-controlled, dose-frequency study of intravenous ketamine in patients with treatment-resistant depression. *Am J Psychiatry* 2016; **173**:816–826.
6. Fava M, et al. Double-blind, placebo-controlled, dose-ranging trial of intravenous ketamine as adjunctive therapy in treatment-resistant depression (TRD). *Mol Psychiatry* 2020; **25**:1592–1603.
7. Lener MS, et al. Glutamate and gamma-aminobutyric acid systems in the pathophysiology of major depression and antidepressant response to ketamine. *Biol Psychiatry* 2017; **81**:886–897.
8. Beck K, et al. Association of ketamine with psychiatric symptoms and implications for its therapeutic use and for understanding schizophrenia: a systematic review and meta-analysis. *JAMA Netw Open* 2020; **3**:e204693.
9. Loo CK, et al. Placebo-controlled pilot trial testing dose titration and intravenous, intramuscular and subcutaneous routes for ketamine in depression. *Acta Psychiatr Scand* 2016; **134**:48–56.
10. George D, et al. Pilot randomized controlled trial of titrated subcutaneous ketamine in older patients with treatment-resistant depression. *Am J Geriatr Psychiatry* 2017; **25**:1199–1209.
11. Glue P, et al. Dose- and exposure-response to ketamine in depression. *Biol Psychiatry* 2011; **70**:e9–e10; author reply e11–e12.
12. Cusin C, et al. Long-term maintenance with intramuscular ketamine for treatment-resistant bipolar II depression. *Am J Psychiatry* 2012; **169**:868–869.
13. Arabzadeh S, et al. Does oral administration of ketamine accelerate response to treatment in major depressive disorder? Results of a double-blind controlled trial. *J Affect Disord* 2018; **235**:236–241.
14. Domany Y, et al. Repeated oral ketamine for out-patient treatment of resistant depression: randomised, double-blind, placebo-controlled, proof-of-concept study. *Br J Psychiatry* 2019; **214**:20–26.
15. Rosenblat JD, et al. Oral ketamine for depression: a systematic review. *J Clin Psychiatry* 2019; **80**:18r12475.
16. Swainson J, et al. Sublingual ketamine: an option for increasing accessibility of ketamine treatments for depression? *J Clin Psychiatry* 2020; **81**:19lr13146.
17. Nguyen L, et al. Off-label use of transmucosal ketamine as a rapid-acting antidepressant: a retrospective chart review. *Neuropsychiatr Dis Treat* 2015; **11**:2667–2673.
18. Lara DR, et al. Antidepressant, mood stabilizing and procognitive effects of very low dose sublingual ketamine in refractory unipolar and bipolar depression. *Int J Neuropsychopharmacol* 2013; **16**:2111–2117.
19. Canuso CM, et al. Efficacy and safety of intranasal esketamine for the rapid reduction of symptoms of depression and suicidality in patients at imminent risk for suicide: results of a double-blind, randomized, placebo-controlled study. *Am J Psychiatry* 2018; **175**:620–630.
20. Daly EJ, et al. Efficacy and safety of intranasal esketamine adjunctive to oral antidepressant therapy in treatment-resistant depression: a randomized clinical trial. *JAMA Psychiatry* 2018; **75**:139–148.
21. Popova V, et al. Efficacy and safety of flexibly dosed esketamine nasal spray combined with a newly initiated oral antidepressant in treatment-resistant depression: a randomized double-blind active-controlled study. *Am J Psychiatry* 2019; **176**:428–438.
22. Daly EJ, et al. Efficacy of esketamine nasal spray plus oral antidepressant treatment for relapse prevention in patients with treatment-resistant depression: a randomized clinical trial. *JAMA Psychiatry* 2019; **76**:893–903.

Psychotic depression

Although psychotic symptoms can occur across the whole spectrum of depression severity,[1] those patients who have psychotic symptoms are generally more severely unwell than those who do not have psychotic symptoms.[2] Despite this, psychotic depression is an under-identified disorder[3] and may have a life-time risk of up to 1%.[4] Combined treatment with an antidepressant and antipsychotic is often recommended first line,[5] but until fairly recently the data underpinning this practice has been weak.[6,7]

When given in adequate doses, TCAs are probably more effective than newer antidepressants in the treatment of psychotic depression.[6,8,9] Prior failure to respond to previous adequate treatment predicts a reduced chance of response to subsequent treatment.[10]

There are few studies of newer antidepressants and atypical antipsychotics, either alone or in combination, specifically for psychotic depression. One large RCT showed response rates of 64% for combined olanzapine and fluoxetine compared to 35% for olanzapine alone and 28% for placebo.[11] Another, the study of pharmacotherapy of psychotic depression (STOP-PD) study, showed a remission rate of 42% with olanzapine plus sertraline compared with 24% with olanzapine alone.[12] There was no antidepressant alone group in either study. Small open studies have found quetiapine,[13] aripiprazole[14] and amisulpride[15] augmentation of an antidepressant to be effective and relatively well tolerated, but again there were no data available for antidepressant treatment alone. One RCT ($n = 122$)[9] found venlafaxine plus quetiapine to be more effective than venlafaxine alone but not more effective than imipramine alone. These findings could be interpreted as supporting the increased efficacy of a TCA over venlafaxine and supporting combined antidepressant-antipsychotic treatment over an antidepressant drug alone.

A review of all combination studies concluded that an antipsychotic + antidepressant was superior to either alone (four of nine studies showed some advantage for combination[16]). A meta-analysis concluded that a combination of an antipsychotic and an antidepressant is more effective than either an antipsychotic alone (NNT 5) or an antidepressant alone (NNT 7).[17] NICE[18] recommends that consideration should be given to augmenting an antidepressant with an antipsychotic in the treatment of an acute episode of psychotic depression. Cochrane is in agreement but with reservations regarding the number and quality of trials.[19] Note that these data relate to acute treatment.

Virtually nothing is known of the optimum duration of treatment with a combination of an antidepressant and antipsychotic. NICE recommends augmentation of an antidepressant with an antipsychotic in non-psychotic depression that does not respond adequately to an antidepressant alone and state that if one agent is to be stopped during the maintenance phase it should usually be the augmenting agent. In psychotic depression, there is evidence from the continuation phase of the STOP-PD study that withdrawal of olanzapine from sertraline co-therapy worsens outcome in the longer term.[20,21] This is perhaps sufficient evidence to suggest continuing co-therapy after resolution of the acute illness, but there is no consensus on this question.[22] An important consideration is the substantial weight gain seen in younger people allocated olanzapine in the STOP-PD study.[23]

In clinical practice, at least until recent years, only a small proportion of patients with psychotic depression received an antipsychotic drug,[24] perhaps reflecting clinicians' uncertainty regarding the risk–benefit ratio of this treatment strategy and the lack of consensus across published guidelines.[25] Under-diagnosis (and hence inadequacy of treatment) of psychotic symptoms in depression is also a significant problem.[3,26] Nonetheless, some antipsychotic drugs such as quetiapine and olanzapine have useful antidepressant effects (as well as being antipsychotic) and so there is an empiric basis (in addition to the trial outcomes above) for their use as additive agents to antidepressant treatment.

Long-term outcome is generally poorer for psychotic than non-psychotic depression.[27,28] Patients with psychotic depression may also have a poorer response to combined pharmacological and psychological treatment than those with non-psychotic depression.[29] People with psychotic depression are much more likely than those with non-psychotic depression to attempt and complete suicide.[30]

Psychotic depression is one of the indications for ECT. Not only is ECT effective, it may also be more protective against relapse in psychotic depression than in non-psychotic depression.[31] One small RCT demonstrated superiority of maintenance ECT plus nortriptyline over nortriptyline alone at 2 years.[32]

Another approach is that based on antiglucocorticoid strategies, since HPA axis hyperactivity is more common in psychotic depression. One small open study found rapid effects of the glucocorticoid receptor antagonist mifepristone,[33] although these findings have been criticised.[34] Response may be related to mifepristone plasma levels (>1800ng/mL).[35] Another analysis suggested a plasma concentration of above 1637ng/mL was robustly associated with response,[36] albeit in a trial stopped early because of lack of efficacy of mifepristone.

There is an anecdotal report of the successful use of methylphenidate in a patient who did not respond to robust doses of an antidepressant and antipsychotic combined.[37] Other case reports describe successful outcome with lamotrigine[38] and a combination of phenelzine, aripiprazole and quetiapine.[39] Minocycline has also shown good effect, albeit in an open study.[40]

Ketamine may also be effective in psychotic depression. One report[41] describes successful use of intravenous ketamine (0.5mg/kg) in two patients unresponsive to standard treatments (one of the two patients had a diagnosis of schizoaffective disorder). Another[42] outlines rapid response to esketamine (0.5mg/kg) given intravenously or subcutaneously) in four patients, two of whom had a primary diagnosis of unipolar depression.

There is no specific indication for other therapies or augmentation strategies in psychotic depression over and above that for resistant depression or psychosis described elsewhere.

Summary

- TCAs are probably drugs of first choice in psychotic depression.
- SSRIs/SNRIs are a second-line alternative when TCAs are poorly tolerated.
- Augmentation of an antidepressant with olanzapine or quetiapine is recommended.
- The optimum dose and duration of antipsychotic augmentation are unknown.

CHAPTER 3

- If one treatment is to be stopped during the maintenance phase, this should usually be the antipsychotic, but there is some evidence that this worsens outcome.
- ECT should always be considered where a rapid response is required or where other treatments have failed.

References

1. Forty L, et al. Is depression severity the sole cause of psychotic symptoms during an episode of unipolar major depression? A study both between and within subjects. *J Affect Disord* 2009; **114**:103–109.
2. Gaudiano BA, et al. Depressive symptom profiles and severity patterns in outpatients with psychotic vs nonpsychotic major depression. *Compr Psychiatry* 2008; **49**:421–429.
3. Heslin M, et al. Psychotic major depression: challenges in clinical practice and research. *Br J Psychiatry* 2018; **212**:131–133.
4. Jääskeläinen E, et al. Epidemiology of psychotic depression – systematic review and meta-analysis. *Psychol Med* 2018; **48**:905–918.
5. Cleare A, et al. Evidence-based guidelines for treating depressive disorders with antidepressants: a revision of the 2008 British Association for Psychopharmacology guidelines. *J Psychopharmacology* 2015; **29**:459–525.
6. Wijkstra J, et al. Pharmacological treatment for unipolar psychotic depression: systematic review and meta-analysis. *Br J Psychiatry* 2006; **188**:410–415.
7. Mulsant BH, et al. A double-blind randomized comparison of nortriptyline plus perphenazine versus nortriptyline plus placebo in the treatment of psychotic depression in late life. *J Clin Psychiatry* 2001; **62**:597–604.
8. Birkenhager TK, et al. Efficacy of imipramine in psychotic versus nonpsychotic depression. *J Clin Psychopharmacol* 2008; **28**:166–170.
9. Wijkstra J, et al. Treatment of unipolar psychotic depression: a randomized, double-blind study comparing imipramine, venlafaxine, and venlafaxine plus quetiapine. *Acta Psychiatr Scand* 2010; **121**:190–200.
10. Blumberger DM, et al. Impact of prior pharmacotherapy on remission of psychotic depression in a randomized controlled trial. *J Psychiatr Res* 2011; **45**:896–901.
11. Rothschild AJ, et al. A double-blind, randomized study of olanzapine and olanzapine/fluoxetine combination for major depression with psychotic features. *J Clin Psychopharmacol* 2004; **24**:365–373.
12. Meyers BS, et al. A double-blind randomized controlled trial of olanzapine plus sertraline vs olanzapine plus placebo for psychotic depression: the study of pharmacotherapy of psychotic depression (STOP-PD). *Arch Gen Psychiatry* 2009; **66**:838–847.
13. Konstantinidis A, et al. Quetiapine in combination with citalopram in patients with unipolar psychotic depression. *Prog Neuropsychopharmacol Biol Psychiatry* 2007; **31**:242–247.
14. Matthews JD, et al. An open study of aripiprazole and escitalopram for psychotic major depressive disorder. *J Clin Psychopharmacol* 2009; **29**:73–76.
15. Politis AM, et al. Combination therapy with amisulpride and antidepressants: clinical observations in case series of elderly patients with psychotic depression. *Prog Neuropsychopharmacol Biol Psychiatry* 2008; **32**:1227–1230.
16. Rothschild AJ. Challenges in the treatment of major depressive disorder with psychotic features. *Schizophr Bull* 2013; **39**:787–796.
17. Farahani A, et al. Are antipsychotics or antidepressants needed for psychotic depression? A systematic review and meta-analysis of trials comparing antidepressant or antipsychotic monotherapy with combination treatment. *J Clin Psychiatry* 2012; **73**:486–496.
18. National Institute for Health and Care Excellence. Depression in adults: recognition and management. Clinical guideline [CG90]. 2009 (Last updated: December 2013); https://www.nice.org.uk/Guidance/cg90.
19. Wijkstra J, et al. Pharmacological treatment for psychotic depression. *Cochrane Database Syst Rev* 2015; Cd004044.
20. Bingham KS, et al. Stabilization treatment of remitted psychotic depression: the STOP-PD study. *Acta Psychiatr Scand* 2018; **138**:267–273.
21. Flint AJ, et al. Effect of continuing olanzapine vs placebo on relapse among patients with psychotic depression in remission: the STOP-PD II randomized clinical trial. *JAMA* 2019; **322**:622–631.
22. Dubovsky SL, et al. Psychotic depression: diagnosis, differential diagnosis, and treatment. *Psychother Psychosom* 2020; 1–18. [Epub ahead print].
23. Flint AJ, et al. Effect of older vs younger age on anthropometric and metabolic variables during treatment of psychotic depression with sertraline plus olanzapine: the STOP-PD II Study. *Am J Geriatr Psychiatry* 2020:S1064-7481(20)30546-7.
24. Andreescu C, et al. Persisting low use of antipsychotics in the treatment of major depressive disorder with psychotic features. *J Clin Psychiatry* 2007; **68**:194–200.
25. Leadholm AK, et al. The treatment of psychotic depression: is there consensus among guidelines and psychiatrists? *J Affect Disord* 2013; **145**:214–220.
26. Rothschild AJ, et al. Missed diagnosis of psychotic depression at 4 academic medical centers. *J Clin Psychiatry* 2008; **69**:1293–1296.
27. Flint AJ, et al. Two-year outcome of psychotic depression in late life. *Am J Psychiatry* 1998; **155**:178–183.
28. Maj M, et al. Phenomenology and prognostic significance of delusions in major depressive disorder: a 10-year prospective follow-up study. *J Clin Psychiatry* 2007; **68**:1411–1417.
29. Gaudiano BA, et al. Differential response to combined treatment in patients with psychotic versus nonpsychotic major depression. *J Nerv Ment Dis* 2005; **193**:625–628.
30. Gournellis R, et al. Psychotic (delusional) depression and suicidal attempts: a systematic review and meta-analysis. *Acta Psychiatr Scand* 2018; **137**:18–29.

CHAPTER 3

31. Birkenhager TK, et al. One-year outcome of psychotic depression after successful electroconvulsive therapy. *J ECT* 2005; **21**:221–226.

32. Navarro V, et al. Continuation/maintenance treatment with nortriptyline versus combined nortriptyline and ECT in late-life psychotic depression: a two-year randomized study. *Am J Geriatr Psychiatry* 2008; **16**:498–505.

33. Belanoff JK, et al. An open label trial of C-1073 (mifepristone) for psychotic major depression. *Biol Psychiatry* 2002; **52**:386–392.

34. Rubin RT. Dr. Rubin replies (Letter). *Am J Psychiatry* 2004; **161**:1722.

35. Blasey CM, et al. A multisite trial of mifepristone for the treatment of psychotic depression: a site-by-treatment interaction. *Contemp Clin Trials* 2009; **30**:284–288.

36. Block T, et al. Mifepristone plasma level and glucocorticoid receptor antagonism associated with response in patients with psychotic depression. *J Clin Psychopharmacol* 2017; **37**:505–511.

37. Huang CC, et al. Adjunctive use of methylphenidate in the treatment of psychotic unipolar depression. *Clin Neuropharmacol* 2008; **31**:245–247.

38. Kajiya T, et al. Effect of lamotrigine in the treatment of bipolar depression with psychotic features: a case report. *Ann General Psychiatry* 2017; **16**:31.

39. Meyer JM, et al. Augmentation of phenelzine with aripiprazole and quetiapine in a treatment-resistant patient with psychotic unipolar depression: case report and literature review. *CNS Spectr* 2017; **22**:391–396.

40. Miyaoka T, et al. Minocycline as adjunctive therapy for patients with unipolar psychotic depression: an open-label study. *Prog Neuropsychopharmacol Biol Psychiatry* 2012; **37**:222–226.

41. Ribeiro CM, et al. The use of ketamine for the treatment of depression in the context of psychotic symptoms: to the editor. *Biol Psychiatry* 2016; **79**:e65–e66.

42. Ajub E, et al. Efficacy of esketamine in the treatment of depression with psychotic features: a case series. *Biol Psychiatry* 2018; **83**:e15–e16.

CHAPTER 3

Switching antidepressants

General guidelines

- When changing from one antidepressant to another, abrupt withdrawal should be avoided unless there has been a serious adverse event. Cross-tapering is preferred, in which the dose of the ineffective or poorly tolerated drug is slowly reduced while the new drug is slowly introduced.

Example		Week1	Week 2	Week 3	Week 4
Withdrawing citalopram	40mg OD	20mg OD	10mg OD	5mg	2.5mg
Introducing mirtazapine	Nil	15mg OD	30mg OD	30mg OD	45mg OD (if required)

OD, omnie die, once a day

- The speed of cross-tapering is best judged by monitoring patient tolerability. Few studies have been done, so caution is required. Extended periods may be necessary to mitigate withdrawal symptoms.
- Note that the co-administration of some antidepressants, even when cross-tapering, is absolutely contraindicated. In other cases, theoretical risks or lack of experience preclude recommending cross-tapering.
- The switching strategy depends not only on the reason for switching – inadequate or non-response, poor tolerability or adverse effects—but also on the pharmacokinetic and pharmacodynamic properties of the antidepressants involved.[1-3]
- In some cases, cross-tapering may not be necessary. An example is when switching from one SSRI to another: their effects are so similar that administration of the second drug is likely to ameliorate withdrawal effects of the first. In fact, the use of fluoxetine has been advocated as an abrupt switch treatment for SSRI discontinuation symptoms.[4] Abrupt cessation may also be acceptable when switching to a drug with a similar, but not identical, mode of action.[5] Thus, in some cases, abruptly stopping one antidepressant and starting another antidepressant at the usual dose may not only be well tolerated, but may also reduce the risk and severity of discontinuation symptoms.
- Potential dangers of simultaneously administering two antidepressants include pharmacodynamic interactions (serotonin syndrome, hypotension, drowsiness; depending on the drugs involved) and pharmacokinetic interactions (e.g. elevation of tricyclic plasma levels by some SSRIs).

- Agomelatine does not seem to be associated with a discontinuation syndrome,[6] but slow withdrawal when switching is nonetheless recommended. Given agomelatine's mode of action (melatonin agonism; $5HT_{2C}$ antagonism), it is not expected to mitigate discontinuation reactions of other antidepressants. There is no theoretical basis to suggest that pharmacodynamic interactions might occur between agomelatine and other co-administered antidepressants, but caution is advised in the absence of useful data. Some pharmacokinetic interactions do occur, and agomelatine should not be administered with fluvoxamine.
- Serotonin syndrome can occur with a single serotonergic drug at a therapeutic dose or more frequently in combination of serotonergic drugs or in overdose. Most severe cases of serotonin syndrome involve an MAOI (including moclobemide) plus an SSRI.[7,8] Caution is advised when switching strategies call for the combining of serotonergic drugs.

Serotonin syndrome – symptoms[11]

Increasing severity

Severity	Symptoms
Mild	Insomnia, anxiety, nausea, diarrhoea, hypertension, tachycardia, hyper-reflexia
Moderate	Agitation, myoclonus, tremor, mydriasis, flushing, diaphoresis, low fever (<38.5°C)
Severe	Severe hyperthermia, confusion, rigidity, respiratory failure, coma, death

The advice given in Table 3.7 should be treated with caution and patients should be very carefully monitored when switching.

CHAPTER 3

Table 3.7 Antidepressants – swapping and stopping*

From \ To	Agomelatine	Bupropion	Clomipramine	Fluoxetine	Fluvoxamine	MAOIs Phenelzine Tranylcypromine Selegiline
Agomelatine[a]		Stop agomelatine then start bupropion	Stop agomelatine then start clomipramine	Stop agomelatine then start fluoxetine	Stop agomelatine then start fluvoxamine	Stop agomelatine then start MAOIs
Bupropion[b]	Cross-taper cautiously		Cross-taper cautiously with low dose clomipramine	Cross-taper cautiously	Cross-taper cautiously	Taper and stop then wait for 2 weeks then start MAOIs
Clomipramine	Cross-taper cautiously	Cross-taper cautiously		Taper and stop then start fluoxetine at 10mg/day	Taper and stop then start low dose fluvoxamine	Taper and stop then wait for 3 weeks then start MAOIs
Fluoxetine[c]	Cross-taper cautiously	Stop fluoxetine. Wait 4–7 days then start bupropion	Stop fluoxetine. Wait 2 weeks then start low dose clomipramine		Stop fluoxetine. Wait 4–7 days then start fluvoxamine	Stop fluoxetine then wait for 5–6 weeks then start MAOIs
Fluvoxamine[d]	Taper and stop then wait for 4 days	Cross-taper cautiously	Taper and stop then start low dose clomipramine	Direct switch possible		Taper and stop then wait for 1 week then start MAOIs
MAOIs Phenelzine Tranylcypromine Selegiline	Cross-taper cautiously	Taper and stop then wait for 2 weeks	Taper and stop then wait for 3 weeks	Taper and stop then wait for 2 weeks	Taper and stop then wait for 2 weeks	Taper and stop then wait for 2 weeks
Moclobemide	Taper and stop then wait 24 hours	Taper and stop then wait 24 hours	Taper and stop then wait 24 hours	Taper and stop then wait 24 hours	Taper and stop then wait 24 hours	Taper and stop, wait 24 hours then start MAOIs
Mirtazapine	Cross-taper cautiously	Cross-taper cautiously	Cross-taper cautiously	Cross-taper cautiously	Cross-taper cautiously	Taper and stop then wait for 2 weeks
Reboxetine[e]	Cross-taper cautiously	Cross-taper cautiously	Cross-taper cautiously	Cross-taper cautiously	Cross-taper cautiously	Taper and stop then wait for 1 week then start MAOIs

CHAPTER 3

Moclobemide	Mirtazapine	Reboxetine	Trazodone	Other SSRIs,[f] Vortioxetine	SNRIs Duloxetine Venlafaxine Desvenlaxine	TCAs (except clomipramine)
Stop agomelatine then start moclobemide	Stop agomelatine then start mirtazapine	Stop agomelatine then start reboxetine	Stop agomelatine then start trazodone	Stop agomelatine then start SSRI	Stop agomelatine then start SNRI	Stop agomelatine then start TCA
Taper and stop then start moclobemide	Cross-taper cautiously	Cross-taper cautiously	Cross-taper cautiously	Cross-taper cautiously	Cross-taper cautiously	Cross-taper cautiously with low dose TCA
Taper and stop then wait for 1 week then start moclobemide	Cross-taper cautiously	Cross-taper cautiously	Cross-taper cautiously	Taper and stop then start low dose	Taper and stop. Start low dose SNRI	Cross-taper cautiously
Stop fluoxetine then wait for 5–6 weeks then start moclobemide	Cross-taper cautiously	Cross-taper cautiously	Cross-taper cautiously	Stop fluoxetine. Wait 4–7 days then start low dose	Stop fluoxetine. Wait 4–7 days then start SNRI	Stop fluoxetine. Wait 4–7 days then start low dose TCA
Taper and stop then wait for 1 week then start moclobemide	Cross-taper cautiously. Start mirtazapine at 15mg	Cross-taper cautiously	Cross-taper cautiously	Direct switch possible	Direct switch possible	Cross-taper cautiously with low dose TCA
Taper and stop then wait for 2 weeks then start moclobemide	Taper and stop then wait for 2 weeks	Taper and stop then wait for 2 weeks	Taper and stop then wait for 2 weeks	Taper and stop then wait for 2 weeks	Taper and stop then wait for 2 weeks	Taper and stop then wait for 2 weeks[j]
	Taper and stop then wait 24 hours	Taper and stop then wait 24 hours	Taper and stop then wait 24 hours	Taper and stop then wait 24 hours	Taper and stop then wait 24 hours	Taper and stop then wait 24 hours
Taper and stop then wait for 1 week then start moclobemide		Cross-taper cautiously	Cross-taper cautiously	Cross-taper cautiously	Cross-taper cautiously	Cross-taper cautiously
Taper and stop then wait for 1 week then start moclobemide	Cross-taper cautiously		Cross-taper cautiously	Cross-taper cautiously	Cross-taper cautiously	Cross-taper cautiously

(Continued)

CHAPTER 3

Table 3.7 (*Continued*)

From \ To	Agomelatine	Bupropion	Clomipramine	Fluoxetine	Fluvoxamine	MAOIs Phenelzine Tranylcypromine Selegiline
Trazodone	Cross-taper cautiously	Cross-taper cautiously	Cross-taper cautiously with low dose clomipramine	Cross-taper cautiously	Cross-taper cautiously	Taper and stop then wait for 1 week
Other SSRIs[f], Vortioxetine[g]	Cross-taper cautiously	Cross-taper cautiously	Taper and stop then start low dose clomipramine	Direct switch possible	Direct switch possible	Taper and stop then wait for 1 week[h]
SNRI Duloxetine[i] Venlafaxine Desvenlaxine	Cross-taper cautiously	Cross-taper cautiously	Taper and stop then start low dose clomipramine	Direct switch possible	Direct switch possible	Taper and stop then wait for 1 week
Tricyclics	Cross-taper cautiously	Halve dose and add bupropion and then slow withdrawal	Direct switch possible	Halve dose and add fluoxetine and then slow withdrawal	Cross-taper cautiously	Taper and stop then wait for 2 weeks[j]

CHAPTER 3

Moclobemide	Mirtazapine	Reboxetine	Trazodone	Other SSRIs,[f] Vortioxetine	SNRIs Duloxetine Venlafaxine Desvenlaxine	TCAs (except clomipramine)
Taper and stop then wait for 1 week then start moclobemide	Cross-taper cautiously	Cross-taper cautiously		Cross-taper cautiously	Cross-taper cautiously	Cross-taper cautiously with low dose TCA
Taper and stop then wait for 1 week then start moclobemide	Cross-taper cautiously	Cross-taper cautiously	Cross-taper cautiously	Direct switch possible	Direct switch possible	Cross-taper cautiously with low dose TCA
Taper and stop then wait for 1 week then start moclobemide	Cross-taper cautiously	Cross-taper cautiously	Cross-taper cautiously	Direct switch possible	Direct switch possible	Cross-taper cautiously with low dose TCA
Taper and stop then wait for 1 week then start moclobemide	Cross-taper cautiously	Cross-taper cautiously	Halve dose and add trazodone and then slow withdrawal	Halve dose and add SSRI then slow withdrawal	Cross-taper cautiously starting with low dose SNRI	Direct switch possible

Notes:

*Advice given in this table is partly derived from manufacturers' information and available published data and partly theoretical. There are several factors that affect individual drug handling and caution is required in every instance Cross taper cautiously – usually over 2–4 weeks as per example

[a]Agomelatine has no effect on monoamine uptake and no affinity for α, β adrenergic, histaminergic, cholinergic, dopaminergic and benzodiazepine receptors. The potential for interactions between agomelatine and other antidepressants is low and it is not expected to mitigate discontinuation reactions of other antidepressants. Some crossover with other antidepressants might be cautiously attempted when switching from agomelatine.

[b]Bupropion is licensed for smoking cessation but unlicensed for the treatment of depression in the UK. It is a CYP2D6 inhibitor and particular caution required when cross-tapering with drugs metabolised by this enzyme.

[c]Beware: interactions with fluoxetine may still occur for 5 weeks after stopping fluoxetine because of its metabolite's long half-life.

[d]Fluvoxamine is a potent inhibitor of CYP1A2, and to a lesser extent of CYP2C and CYP3A4 and has a high potential for interactions hence extra precaution is required.

[e]Switching to reboxetine as antidepressant monotherapy is no longer recommended.

[f]Citalopram, escitalopram, paroxetine and sertraline.

[g]Limited experience with vortioxetine and extra precaution required. Particular care when switching to or from bupropion and other CYP2D6 inhibitors such as fluoxetine and paroxetine.[9]

[h] Wait 3 weeks in the case of vortioxetine.[10]

[i] Abrupt switch from SSRIs and venlafaxine to duloxetine is possible starting at 60mg/day.[5]

[j] Wait 3 weeks in the case of imipramine.

CHAPTER 3

References

1. Cleare A, et al. Evidence-based guidelines for treating depressive disorders with antidepressants: a revision of the 2008 British Association for Psychopharmacology guidelines. *J Psychopharmacology* 2015; 29:459–525.
2. Harvey BH, et al. New insights on the antidepressant discontinuation syndrome. *Human Psychopharmacology* 2014; 29:503–516.
3. Malhi GS, et al. Royal Australian and New Zealand College of Psychiatrists clinical practice guidelines for mood disorders. *Aust N Z J Psychiatry* 2015; 49:1087–1206.
4. Benazzi F. Fluoxetine for the treatment of SSRI discontinuation syndrome. *Int J Neuropsychopharmacol* 2008; 11:725–726.
5. Perahia DG, et al. Switching to duloxetine from selective serotonin reuptake inhibitor antidepressants: a multicenter trial comparing 2 switching techniques. *J Clin Psychiatry* 2008; 69:95–105.
6. Goodwin GM, et al. Agomelatine prevents relapse in patients with major depressive disorder without evidence of a discontinuation syndrome: a 24-week randomized, double-blind, placebo-controlled trial. *J Clin Psychiatry* 2009; 70:1128–1137.
7. Buckley NA, et al. Serotonin syndrome. *BMJ* 2014; 348:g1626.
8. Abadie D, et al. Serotonin syndrome: analysis of cases registered in the French pharmacovigilance database. *J Clin Psychopharmacol* 2015; 35:382–388.
9. Chen G, et al. Pharmacokinetic drug interactions involving vortioxetine (Lu AA21004), a multimodal antidepressant. *Clin Drug Investig* 2013; 33:727–736.
10. Citrome L. Vortioxetine for major depressive disorder: a systematic review of the efficacy and safety profile for this newly approved antidepressant – what is the number needed to treat, number needed to harm and likelihood to be helped or harmed? *Int J Clin Pract* 2014; 68:60–82.

Antidepressant withdrawal symptoms

Background

Many medications are associated with withdrawal symptoms on discontinuation, including antidepressants. The term 'discontinuation symptoms' (or syndrome), distinct from 'withdrawal', was coined to describe symptoms on stopping experienced on stopping antidepressants.[1,2] There is a semantic difference between 'discontinuation' and 'withdrawal' symptoms – the latter implies addiction; the former does not. While antidepressants are not addictive substances (they do not provoke craving, for example), the categorical and semantic differences may be irrelevant to patient experience. Withdrawal symptoms can be explained in the context of 'receptor rebound'[3] – for example, an antidepressant with potent anticholinergic side effects may be associated with diarrhoea on discontinuation.

Signs and symptoms

Antidepressant withdrawal symptoms may be entirely new or similar to some of the original symptoms of the illness for which the medication was originally given. Withdrawal symptoms can be distinguished from a relapse or reoccurrence of the underlying disorder by their rapid onset (days, rather than weeks, or within 3–5 half-lives of the drug[4]), the rapid response to reintroduction of the antidepressant (generally within hours, certainly within days), and the presence of somatic and psychological symptoms distinct from the original illness (e.g. brain zaps, dizziness, nausea).[1] The wide variety of symptoms reported with SSRI and related drugs (e.g. SNRIs and other serotonin reuptake inhibitors) is summarised in Figure 3.3. Symptoms reported with other antidepressants are summarised in Table 3.8.

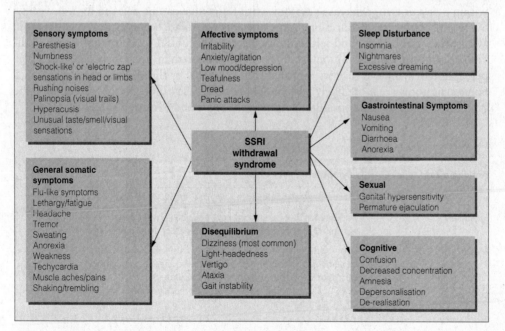

Figure 3.3 Common withdrawal symptoms

Table 3.8 Factors influencing the incidence and severity of antidepressant withdrawal symptoms

Pharmacological factors
  – Pharmacokinetics
  – Drug half life
  – Pharmacodynamics
  – Receptor affinities
Treatment factors
  – Duration of treatment
  – Dose
  – Method of tapering
Patient specific factors
  – Prior experience and
    anticipation effects
	■ Drug half-lives – correlate with the severity and onset of symptoms. Symptoms typically more severe with shorter half-life drugs (e.g. venlafaxine, paroxetine)
	■ Other pharmacokinetic factors: non-linear pharmacokinetics
	■ Receptor affinities: higher affinity for the serotonin transporter may confer higher risk of withdrawal symptoms

Incidence and severity

Antidepressant discontinuation symptoms occur in many patients: incidence rates from 14 studies that examined antidepressant withdrawal ranged from 27% to 86%, with a weighted average of 56%.[5] Though reported incidence rates vary widely between studies of differing drugs and methodologies (9% to 77% for fluoxetine, and from 42% to 100% with paroxetine[5]), symptoms are seen to some extent with all antidepressants, with the possible exception of agomelatine.[4]

Time Course

The onset and severity of symptoms are related to the half-life of the antidepressant. Short half-life antidepressants like paroxetine and venlafaxine produce symptoms within a day or two, whereas symptoms with fluoxetine can be delayed by 2–6 weeks.[1] Symptoms can vary in duration, form and intensity and occur in any combination. Whilst they can be mild and self-limiting, there is substantial variation in between individuals, and for some symptoms can last much longer than previously reported.[6] The perception of symptom severity is probably made worse by the absence of forewarnings. Some symptoms are more likely with individual drugs (see Table 3.9). Symptoms can be quantified using the Discontinuation–Emergent Signs and Symptoms (DESS) scale.[7]

Table 3.9 Symptoms reported with other (non-SSRI) antidepressants

Antidepressant type	Symptoms
Agomelatine	Seems to be associated with a very low, if any, risk of discontinuation symptoms[4]
Bupropion	Uncommon, but case reports have described anxiety, headache, insomnia, irritability, and myalgias;[8,9] single case report of acute dystonia[10]
MAOIs*	Common: agitation, irritability, ataxia, movement disorders, insomnia, somnolence, vivid dreams, cognitive impairment, slowed speech, pressured speech; Occasionally: Hallucinations, paranoid delusions RIMAs: Flu like symptoms reported with moclobemide[11]

(Continued)

Antidepressant type	Symptoms
NaSSAs (e.g. mirtazapine)	Panic, anxiety, restlessness, irritability, hypomania, insomnia, dizziness, paresthesia, nausea, vomiting[10]
Serotonin modulators (vortioxetine, vilazodone)	None reported,[10] though these are relatively new antidepressants with less clinical experience. Shared pharmacological actions with other antidepressants (SSRIs) so possibility of withdrawal symptoms cannot be discounted[10]
TCAs	General somatic and GI distress, sleep disturbances characterised by initial and middle insomnia or excessively vivid and frightening dreams, akathisia or parkinsonism, hypomania or mania, cardiac arrhythmia[10]
Trazodone	Hypomania, anxiety, restless sleep, nightmares, depersonalisation, formication, headache[10]

*Tranylcypromine may have amfetamine-like properties at higher doses[12] and therefore could be associated with a true 'withdrawal syndrome'. Delirium may occur.[13]

CHAPTER 3

Clinical relevance[14,15]

The symptoms of a withdrawal reaction may be mistaken for a relapse of illness or the emergence of a new physical illness[16] leading to unnecessary investigations or reintroduction of the antidepressant. Symptoms may be severe enough to interfere with daily functioning, and those who have experienced discontinuation symptoms may reason (perhaps appropriately) that antidepressants are 'addictive' and not wish to accept treatment. There is also evidence of emergent suicidal thoughts on discontinuation with paroxetine.[17]

Who is most at risk?[10,14–16,18]

Although anyone can experience discontinuation symptoms, the risk is increased in those prescribed short half-life drugs[7] (e.g. paroxetine, venlafaxine), particularly if they do not take them regularly. Two-thirds of patients prescribed antidepressants skip a few doses from time to time,[19] and many patients stop their antidepressant abruptly.[20] The risk is also increased in those who have been taking antidepressants for 8 weeks or longer,[21] those taking antidepressants at higher doses, those who have developed anxiety symptoms at the start of antidepressant therapy (particularly with SSRIs), those receiving other centrally acting medication (e.g. antihypertensives, antihistamines, antipsychotics), children and adolescents,[7] younger patients[22] and those who have experienced withdrawal symptoms before.

Antidepressant withdrawal symptoms are common in neonates born to women taking antidepressants (see section on 'Pregnancy' in Chapter 7).

How to avoid[14–16,18]

Generally, antidepressant therapy should be discontinued gradually.[6] Readers are referred to the section on 'Stopping antidepressants' in this chapter for advice on specific antidepressants. The shorter the half-life of the drug, the more important that this rule is followed. The end of the taper may need to be slower, as symptoms may not

CHAPTER 3

appear until the reduction in the total daily dosage of the antidepressant is (proportionately) substantial. Patients receiving MAOIs may need to be tapered over a longer period. Tranylcypromine may be particularly difficult to stop.[13] At-risk patients (see above) may need a slower taper. Agomelatine can probably be stopped abruptly without provoking withdrawal symptoms but should be slowly withdrawn as a matter of principle – all psychotropic drugs should be slowly withdrawn where possible.

Many people suffer symptoms despite slow withdrawal and even if they have received adequate education regarding withdrawal symptoms.[7,17] This may be because hyperbolic tapering is not employed (see section on 'Stopping antidepressants' in this chapter).

How to treat[14–16,23]

There are few systematic studies in this area. Treatment is pragmatic. If symptoms are mild, reassure the patient that these symptoms are common after discontinuing an antidepressant and will pass in a few days or weeks. If symptoms are severe, reintroduce the original antidepressant (or another with a longer half-life from the same class) and taper gradually while monitoring for symptoms.[6]

Some evidence supports the use of anticholinergic agents in tricyclic withdrawal[24] and fluoxetine for symptoms associated with stopping paroxetine,[25] sertraline,[25] clomipramine[26] or venlafaxine[27] – fluoxetine, having a longer plasma half-life, seems to be associated with a lower incidence of discontinuation symptoms than other similar drugs.[7] The use of alternative classes of medications (e.g. short term of symptomatic use of a benzodiazepine) has been suggested for the treatment of anxiety and insomnia.[28]

Key points that patients should know

- Antidepressants are not addictive according to the medical definition of the word. (Patients most frequently mentioned reason for a negative opinion on antidepressants is addiction,[29] and a survey of 1,946 people across the United Kingdom conducted in 1997 found that 74% thought that antidepressants were addictive.[30]) Note, however, that the semantic and categorical distinctions between addiction and the withdrawal symptoms seen with antidepressants may be unimportant to patients.
- Patients should be informed that they may experience withdrawal symptoms (and the most likely symptoms associated with the drug that they are taking) when they stop their antidepressant.
- Antidepressants should not generally be stopped abruptly: withdrawal symptoms are more likely and relapse more common.[31]
- Discontinuation symptoms can occur after missed or late doses if the antidepressant prescribed has a short half-life. A very few patients experience pre-dose discontinuation symptoms which provoke the taking of the antidepressant at an earlier time each day.

References

1. Horowitz MA, et al. Tapering of SSRI treatment to mitigate withdrawal symptoms. *Lancet Psychiatry* 2019; 6:538–546.
2. Massabki I, et al. Selective serotonin reuptake inhibitor 'discontinuation syndrome' or withdrawal. *Br J Psychiatry* 2020; 6:1–4.
3. Zabegalov KN, et al. Understanding antidepressant discontinuation syndrome (ADS) through preclinical experimental models. *Eur J Pharmacol* 2018; 829:129–140.
4. Henssler J, et al. Antidepressant withdrawal and rebound phenomena. *Dtsch Arztebl Int* 2019; 116:355–361.
5. Davies J, et al. A systematic review into the incidence, severity and duration of antidepressant withdrawal effects: are guidelines evidence-based? *Addict Behav* 2019; 97:111–121.
6. National Institute for Health and Care Excellence. Depression in adults: recognition and management. Clinical guideline [CG90]. 2009 (Last updated: December 2013); https://www.nice.org.uk/Guidance/cg90.
7. Fava GA, et al. Withdrawal symptoms after selective serotonin reuptake inhibitor discontinuation: a systematic review. *Psychother Psychosom* 2015; 84:72–81.
8. Berigan TR. Bupropion-associated withdrawal symptoms revisited: a case report. *Prim Care Companion J Clin Psychiatry* 2002; 4:78.
9. Berigan TR, et al. Bupropion-associated withdrawal symptoms: a case report. *Prim Care Companion J Clin Psychiatry* 1999; 1:50–51.
10. Cosci F, et al. Acute and persistent withdrawal syndromes following discontinuation of psychotropic medications. *Psychother Psychosom* 2020; 89:283–306.
11. Curtin F, et al. Moclobemide discontinuation syndrome predominantly presenting with influenza-like symptoms. *J Psychopharmacology* 2002; 16:271–272.
12. Ricken R, et al. Tranylcypromine in mind (Part II): review of clinical pharmacology and meta-analysis of controlled studies in depression. *Eur Neuropsychopharmacol* 2017; 27:714–731.
13. Gahr M, et al. Withdrawal and discontinuation phenomena associated with tranylcypromine: a systematic review. *Pharmacopsychiatry* 2013; 46:123–129.
14. Lejoyeux M, et al. Antidepressant withdrawal syndrome: recognition, prevention and management. *CNS Drugs* 1996; 5:278–292.
15. Haddad PM, et al. Recognising and managing antidepressant discontinuation symptoms. *Adv Psychiatric Treatment* 2007; 13:447–457.
16. Haddad PM. Antidepressant discontinuation syndromes. *Drug Saf* 2001; 24:183–197.
17. Tint A, et al. The effect of rate of antidepressant tapering on the incidence of discontinuation symptoms: a randomised study. *J Psychopharmacology* 2008; 22:330–332.
18. Ogle NR, et al. Guidance for the discontinuation or switching of antidepressant therapies in adults. *J Pharm Pract* 2013; 26:389–396.
19. Meijer WE, et al. Spontaneous lapses in dosing during chronic treatment with selective serotonin reuptake inhibitors. *Br J Psychiatry* 2001; 179:519–522.
20. van Geffen EC, et al. Discontinuation symptoms in users of selective serotonin reuptake inhibitors in clinical practice: tapering versus abrupt discontinuation. *Eur J Clin Pharmacol* 2005; 61:303–307.
21. Kramer JC, et al. Withdrawal symptoms following discontinuation of imipramine therapy. *Am J Psychiatry* 1961; 118:549–550.
22. Read J. How common and severe are six withdrawal effects from, and addiction to, antidepressants? The experiences of a large international sample of patients. *Addict Behav* 2020; 102:106–157.
23. Wilson E, et al. A review of the management of antidepressant discontinuation symptoms. *Ther Adv Psychopharmacol* 2015; 5:357–368.
24. Dilsaver SC, et al. Antidepressant withdrawal symptoms treated with anticholinergic agents. *Am J Psychiatry* 1983; 140:249–251.
25. Benazzi F. Re: selective serotonin reuptake inhibitor discontinuation syndrome: putative mechanisms and prevention strategies. *Can J Psychiatry* 1999; 44:95–96.
26. Benazzi F. Fluoxetine for clomipramine withdrawal symptoms. *Am J Psychiatry* 1999; 156:661–662.
27. Giakas WJ, et al. Intractable withdrawal from venlafaxine treated with fluoxetine. *Psychiatric Annals* 1997; 27:85–93.
28. Fava GA, et al. Understanding and managing withdrawal syndromes after discontinuation of antidepressant drugs. *J Clin Psychiatry* 2019; 80.
29. Gibson K, et al. Patient-centered perspectives on antidepressant use. *Int J Mental Health* 2014; 43:81–99.
30. Paykel ES, et al. Changes in public attitudes to depression during the Defeat Depression Campaign. *Br J Psychiatry* 1998; 173:519–522.
31. Baldessarini RJ, et al. Illness risk following rapid versus gradual discontinuation of antidepressants. *Am J Psychiatry* 2010; 167:934–941.

Further Reading

Fava GA, et al. Withdrawal Symptoms after Selective Serotonin Reuptake Inhibitor Discontinuation: A Systematic Review. *Psychother Psychosom* 2015; 84:72–81.

Haddad PM, et al. Recognising and managing antidepressant discontinuation symptoms. *Advances in Psychiatric Treatment* 2007; 13:447–457.

Schatzberg AF, et al. Antidepressant discontinuation syndrome: consensus panel recommendations for clinical management and additional research. *J Clin Psychiatry* 2006; 67 Suppl 4:27–30.

Shelton RC. The nature of the discontinuation syndrome associated with antidepressant drugs. *J Clin Psychiatry* 2006; 67 Suppl 4:3–7.

Stopping antidepressants

Approximately half of patients will experience withdrawal symptoms on reducing or stopping their antidepressant.[1] For some of these patients the symptoms will be severe (possibly up to half)[1] and can be long-lasting (for months, or years).[1,2] For others they may be mild and self-limiting. Some have identified a separate category of withdrawal, known as post-acute withdrawal syndrome (PAWS), which can last for years and involve myriad, sometimes debilitating symptoms, but the pathophysiology is poorly understood.[3]

There are a number of characteristics of antidepressant use that influence the likelihood of withdrawal effects. Patients who have been on antidepressants for longer periods and higher doses are more likely to have withdrawal effects.[4,5] Antidepressants with short half-lives and cholinergic or noradrenergic effects tend to be associated with more severe withdrawal – venlafaxine, duloxetine and paroxetine are the most often implicated.[6,7] Patients who stop abruptly or rapidly have more withdrawal effects.[8–10] There are likely to be a range of individual physiological (and psychological) differences, as yet poorly understood, which also determine withdrawal severity.[11]

Theoretical basis for tapering

There is some evidence that tapering slowly can reduce the chance of intolerable withdrawal symptoms, by spreading out symptoms over a longer period.[9,10,12] Randomised studies show that tapering for up to 14 days either demonstrated no[13] or minimal[14] improvement in withdrawal symptom severity over abrupt discontinuation.[15] It has generally been concluded from these studies that longer tapering regimes are required.[16,17] Tapering over months[9,10,12] seems to reduce the risk of withdrawal symptoms, but some patients take years. Clinical experience suggests that most patients take between 3 months and 2 years to withdraw in a tolerable manner from long-term antidepressant treatment.

Although reducing by linear amounts (e.g. 50mg, 37.5mg, 25mg, 12.5mg, 0 for sertraline) seems intuitively reasonable (and practical, through splitting tablets), because of the hyperbolic relationship between dose of antidepressant and effect on its principal target, the serotonin receptor (SERT), (following the law of mass action)[18] this is likely to produce increasingly severe withdrawal symptoms (Figure 3.4a).[11] This is consistent with patient reports that reducing at small doses is the most difficult aspect of the process.

It makes more sense to reduce the drug in such a way that produces an 'even' amount of reduction in effect on target receptors: this entails hyperbolic dose reductions (Figure 3.4b). This is most easily approximated by exponential (proportional) reductions of dose – for example, reducing by between 10% and 20% of the most recent dose every 2–4 weeks (Table 3.10). The final dose before completely stopping will need to be very small (<1mg) to prevent the reduction to zero being a bigger 'drop' than previously tolerated reductions. This is supported by evidence that tapering down to doses much lower than common therapeutic doses (e.g. 0.5mg for sertraline) improves the chance that people will be able to stop antidepressants,[12,19] and remain off them.[20]

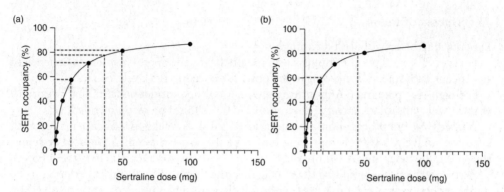

Figure 3.4 (a) Linear reductions of dose cause increasingly large reductions in effect on receptor targets, probably associated with more withdrawal effects. (b) Even reductions of effect at target receptors require hyperbolic dose reductions. The final dose before stopping will need to be very small.

Practical application of tapering

Before tapering

All patients should be informed of the risk of withdrawal symptoms on stopping any antidepressant. Some antidepressants, such as paroxetine and venlafaxine, are more commonly associated with severe withdrawal symptoms.

Patient should be warned not to stop antidepressants abruptly, because this is the method thought to be most likely to give rise to severe and long-lasting withdrawal symptoms and to an increased risk of relapse.

Although stopping antidepressants can cause some unpleasant symptoms, patients should be told that if they are tapered gradually and carefully that withdrawal symptoms can be maintained at tolerable levels. As patients may have had negative experiences of too rapid tapering in the past, reassurance may be required.

It is difficult to predict the exact period required for an individual to taper off antidepressant medication, but most long-standing patients take around 3 months and some up to 2 years. This may help to set expectations.

Patients' past experience of stopping should be explored as this can be informative for predicting what symptoms may arise again on tapering. Careful consideration of past attempts to stop may detect withdrawal symptoms being mis-diagnosed as relapse.

Often patients will require some preparation for antidepressant tapering. This might include arrangements for lightening work or family duties or increased focus on non-pharmacological coping skills (patients have found a wide variety useful including acceptance, breathing exercises, exercise, hobbies, diary keeping and de-catastrophising).[21,22] Mindfulness-based cognitive therapy (MB-CT) has evidence that it is helpful in the process of stopping antidepressants.[23]

Both doctors and patients should be aware that patients can experience negative psychological and physical symptoms during withdrawal that need not indicate that the full dose of the drug is needed (but may indicate that the taper rate needs to be slowed). Familiarity of the patient and the doctor with the wide variety of withdrawal symptoms (Figure 3.4) may help to mitigate unnecessary anxiety when symptoms arise. Patients may require more support during the process, that may be professional or otherwise.[22]

CHAPTER 3

The process of tapering

Patients may be broadly risk-stratified:

For low-risk patients (<6 months use, long half-life antidepressant, no experience of significant withdrawal symptoms in the past), a test reduction could be made (of 25%).

For high-risk patients (>6 months use, short half-life antidepressant, past history of withdrawal symptoms), a test reduction of 5–10% should be recommended.

Withdrawal symptoms should be monitored for 2–4 weeks for all patients, or until symptoms have resolved. Monitoring may take the form of simple measures of symptoms each day (e.g. out of 10) or using standardised measurement such as the DESS.[24]

Further reductions should be titrated against the tolerability of this experience. If the initial reduction was tolerable and withdrawal symptoms absent or have resolved by the end of this monitoring period, continue reducing dose by the same *proportion* (note this is worked out on the last dose used) and the same rate. See example regimens in Table 3.10. If symptoms were intolerable, then the taper should proceed at a slower rate; if severe, this may require re-instatement of the previous dose, a period of stabilisation and then a more cautious reduction schedule.

Troubleshooting

If withdrawal symptoms become intolerable at any point, either hold the current dose for longer to allow them to resolve, or if very unpleasant, increase to the last dose at which the symptoms were tolerable, and remain there until symptoms resolve. After stabilisation, tapering will need to be more gradual, with reduction in smaller amounts and/or longer periods in between reductions. Some patients find that they cannot reduce at more than 5% of the last dose a month.

It is important to remember that if a patient experiences distressing withdrawal symptoms, it does not indicate that they cannot stop antidepressants, but that they will need to taper more slowly, with smaller reductions than they have been undertaking.

Owing to long half-life of fluoxetine, withdrawal symptoms can be delayed by weeks, and so careful attention should be paid to this. As the withdrawal period is spread out over a longer period, larger reductions of fluoxetine may be relatively tolerable.[11] Fluoxetine dose can also be reduced by decreasing the frequency of dosing (e.g. 20mg a day for 6 days a week, then 20mg a day for 5 days a week, and so on).

Unfortunately, current tablet formulations of antidepressants do not permit pharmacologically informed tapering regimens, and so patients will require liquid formulations of their antidepressant (or access to Dutch tapering strips).[19] For those antidepressants that do not come in liquid formulations, liquid will have to be compounded or patients can be switched to medications with liquid formulations. Many patients report cutting up fragments of tablets and weighing them or making their own solutions from crushed tablets, but this approach cannot be recommended.

Final doses before completely stopping the drug may need to be very small to avoid a larger reduction in effect on transmitter systems. For many drugs, the final dose will need to be much less than 1mg. For example, for a patient reducing sertraline at 10% per month, the final dose will need to be 0.1mg to bring about the same reduction in effect on serotonin transporter inhibition as previous reductions.[11]

Box 3.1 A simplified guide to tapering sertraline according to an exponential pattern. The range of reductions provided is equivalent to about 10–20% dose reductions at each step. Some patients may require smaller reductions, and others may tolerate larger reductions at a faster rate

- Reduce dose by 12.5–25mg every 2–4 weeks until reaching 50mg per day
- Reduce by 2–5mg every 2–4 weeks until reaching 15mg per day, then
- Reduce by 1–2mg every 2–4 weeks until reaching 9mg per day, then
- Reduce by 0.4–1mg every 2–4 weeks until reaching 4mg per day, then
- Reduce by 0.2–0.4mg every 2–4 weeks until reaching 2mg per day, then
- Reduce by 0.1–0.25mg every 2–4 weeks until completely stopped.

This process normally takes between 3 months and 2 years but in some people can require longer periods.

Table 3.10 An example reduction schedule for sertraline consisting of 20% reductions (based on the last dose) each period.

Period*	Dose (mg)	Period	Dose (mg)	Period	Dose (mg)
1	200	12	17	23	1.5
2	160	13	14	24	1.2
3	128	14	11	25	0.9
4	102	15	9	26	0.75
5	82	16	7	27	0.6
6	66	17	5.5	28	0.5
7	52	18	4.5	29	0.4
8	42	19	3.6	30	0.3
9	34	20	2.9	31	0.25
10	27	21	2.3	32	0
11	21	22	1.8		

Many patients reduce with even greater number of steps than this – as little as 5–10% of the most recent dose every month.

*2–4 weeks may be tolerable; others might require longer. The reduction from 0.25mg to 0mg will be equivalent to the size of the previous reductions (20% reductions are approximately equal to 3 percentage point reductions of serotonin transporter inhibition)

CHAPTER 3

References

1. Davies J, et al. A systematic review into the incidence, severity and duration of antidepressant withdrawal effects: are guidelines evidence-based? *Addict Behav* 2019; 97:111–121.
2. Stockmann T, et al. SSRI and SNRI withdrawal symptoms reported on an internet forum. *Int J Risk Saf Med* 2018; 29:175–180.
3. Cosci F, et al. Acute and persistent withdrawal syndromes following discontinuation of psychotropic medications. *Psychother Psychosom* 2020; 89:283–306.
4. Weller I, et al. Report of the CSM expert working group on the safety of selective serotonin reuptake inhibitors antidepressants. 2005; https://www.neuroscience.ox.ac.uk/publications/474047.
5. Read J, et al. Adverse effects of antidepressants reported by a large international cohort: emotional blunting, suicidality, and withdrawal effects. *Current Drug Safety* 2018; 13:176–186.
6. Taylor D, et al. Antidepressant withdrawal symptoms-telephone calls to a national medication helpline. *J Affect Disord* 2006; 95:129–133.
7. Henssler J, et al. Antidepressant withdrawal and rebound phenomena. *Dtsch Arztebl Int* 2019; 116:355–361.
8. Himei A, et al. Discontinuation syndrome associated with paroxetine in depressed patients: a retrospective analysis of factors involved in the occurrence of the syndrome. *CNS Drugs* 2006; 20:665–672.
9. Murata Y, et al. Effects of the serotonin 1A, 2A, 2C, 3A, and 3B and serotonin transporter gene polymorphisms on the occurrence of paroxetine discontinuation syndrome. *J Clin Psychopharmacol* 2010; 30:11–17.
10. van Geffen EC, et al. Discontinuation symptoms in users of selective serotonin reuptake inhibitors in clinical practice: tapering versus abrupt discontinuation. *Eur J Clin Pharmacol* 2005; 61:303–307.
11. Horowitz MA, et al. Tapering of SSRI treatment to mitigate withdrawal symptoms. *Lancet Psychiatry* 2019; 6:538–546.
12. Groot PC, et al. Antidepressant tapering strips to help people come off medication more safely. *Psychosis* 2018; 10:142–145.
13. Tint A, et al. The effect of rate of antidepressant tapering on the incidence of discontinuation symptoms: a randomised study. *J Psychopharmacology* 2008; 22:330–332.
14. Baldwin DS, et al. A double-blind, randomized, parallel-group, flexible-dose study to evaluate the tolerability, efficacy and effects of treatment discontinuation with escitalopram and paroxetine in patients with major depressive disorder. *Int Clin Psychopharmacol* 2006; 21:159–169.
15. Montgomery SA, et al. Absence of discontinuation symptoms with agomelatine and occurrence of discontinuation symptoms with paroxetine: a randomized, double-blind, placebo-controlled discontinuation study. *Int Clin Psychopharmacol* 2004; 19:271–280.
16. Haddad PM, et al. Recognising and managing antidepressant discontinuation symptoms. *Adv Psychiatric Treatment* 2007; 13:447–457.
17. Phelps J. Tapering antidepressants: is 3 months slow enough? *Med Hypotheses* 2011; 77:1006–1008.
18. Holford N. Pharmacodynamic principles and the time course of delayed and cumulative drug effects. *Trans Clin Pharmacology* 2018; 26:56–59.
19. Groot PC, et al. How user knowledge of psychotropic drug withdrawal resulted in the development of person-specific tapering medication. *Ther Adv Psychopharmacol* 2020; 10:2045125320932452.
20. Groot PC, et al. Outcome of antidepressant drug discontinuation with taperingstrips after 1–5 years. *Ther Adv Psychopharmacol* 2020; 10:2045125320954609.
21. Inner Compass Initiative Inc. The withdrawal project. 2019; https://withdrawal.theinnercompass.org.
22. Guy A, et al. *Guidance for psychological therapists: enabling conversations with clients taking or withdrawing from prescribed psychiatric drugs.* London: APPG for Prescribed Drug Dependence; 2019.
23. Maund E, et al. Managing antidepressant discontinuation: a systematic review. *Ann Fam Med* 2019; 17:52–60.
24. Rosenbaum JF, et al. Selective serotonin reuptake inhibitor discontinuation syndrome: a randomized clinical trial. *Biol Psychiatry* 1998; 44:77–87.

Electroconvulsive therapy (ECT) and psychotropic drugs

Psychotropics are often continued during ECT, and some agents (particularly antidepressants[1,2]) enhance its efficacy.

Table 3.11 summarises the effect of various psychotropics on seizure duration during ECT. Note that there are few well-controlled studies in this area, and so recommendations should be viewed with this in mind.

Be aware also that choice of anaesthetic agent profoundly affects seizure duration[3-8] as well as the severity of post-ictal confusion and ECT efficacy.[9,10] The use of ketamine as an anaesthetic does not ultimately improve outcome with ECT,[11,12] but it may provide short-term benefits in improving depressive symptoms at the early stages of ECT.[13] Aside from concurrent medication, there are many factors that influence seizure threshold and duration.[14]

Table 3.11 Effect of psychotropic drugs on seizure duration in ECT

Drug	Effect on ECT seizure duration	Comments[3,15–18]
Benzodiazepines[19]	Reduced Mixed evidence and clinical implications unclear	All may raise seizure threshold and so should be avoided where possible. Many are long-acting and may need to be discontinued some days before ECT. Benzodiazepines may also complicate anaesthesia and may reduce efficacy of ECT. If sedation is required, consider hydroxyzine. If benzodiazepine use is very long term and essential, continue and use higher stimulus, bilaterally.
SSRIs[2,20–23]	Minimal effect; small increase possible	Generally considered safe to use during ECT. Beware complex pharmacokinetic interactions with anaesthetic agents. Isolated case reports of serotonin syndrome with fluoxetine and paroxetine with ECT.[24,25]
Venlafaxine[26]	Minimal effect at standard doses	Limited data suggest no effect on seizure duration but possibility of increased risk of asystole with doses above 300mg/day.[27] Clearly epileptogenic in higher doses. ECG advised.
Mirtazapine[2,28]	Minimal effect – small increase	Apparently safe in ECT and, like other antidepressants, may enhance ECT efficacy. May reduce post ECT nausea and headache.
Duloxetine[29,30]	Not known	One case report suggests duloxetine does not complicate ECT. Another links its use to ventricular tachycardia.
TCAs[2,21,31]	Possibly increased	Few data relevant to ECT but many TCAs lower seizure threshold. TCAs are associated with arrhythmia following ECT and should be avoided in elderly patients and those with cardiac disease. In others, it is preferable to continue TCA treatment during ECT. Close monitoring is essential. Beware hypotension and risk of prolonged seizures.
MAOIs[32]	Minimal effect	Data relating to ECT very limited but long history of ECT use during MAOI therapy. MAOIs probably do not affect seizure duration but interactions with sympathomimetics occasionally used in anaesthesia are possible and may lead to hypertensive crisis. Transdermal selegiline seems safe.[33] MAOIs may be continued during ECT, but the anaesthetist must be informed. Beware hypotension.

(Continued)

CHAPTER 3

Table 3.11 *(Continued)*

Drug	Effect on ECT seizure duration	Comments[3,15–18]
Lithium[34–37,]	Possibly increased	Conflicting data on lithium and ECT. The combination may be more likely to lead to delirium and confusion, and some authorities suggest discontinuing lithium 48 hours before ECT. In the UK, ECT is often used during lithium therapy but starting with a low stimulus and with very close monitoring. The combination is generally well tolerated.[38] Note that lithium potentiates the effects of non-depolarising neuromuscular blockers such as suxamethonium. Concomitant use of thiopentone or propofol with lithium treatment lowers seizure threshold.[39]
Antipsychotics[40–44]	Variable – increased with phenothiazines and clozapine Others – no obvious effect reported	Few published data but widely used. Phenothiazines and clozapine are perhaps most likely to prolong seizures, and some suggest withdrawal before ECT. However, safe concurrent use has been reported (particularly with clozapine[45,46] which is now usually continued). ECT is effective in clozapine non-response.[47] ECT and antipsychotics appear generally to be a safe combination. Few data on aripiprazole, quetiapine and ziprasidone, but they too appear to be safe. One case series[48] suggests antipsychotics increase post ictal cognitive dysfunction.
Antiseizure medications[49–52]	Reduced	If used as a mood-stabiliser, continue but be prepared to use higher energy stimulus (not always required). If used for epilepsy, their effect is to normalise seizure threshold. Interactions are possible. Valproate may prolong the effect of thiopental; carbamazepine may inhibit neuromuscular blockade. A small RCT found no significant difference between carbamazepine and valproate (full dose vs half dose) in seizure duration, seizure threshold and cognition outcomes.[53] Lamotrigine is reported to cause no problems.
Barbiturates	Reduced	All barbiturates reduce seizure duration in ECT but are widely used as sedative anaesthetic agents. Thiopental and methohexital may be associated with cardiac arrhythmia.

For drugs known to lower seizure threshold, treatment is best begun with a low-energy stimulus (50mC). Staff should be alerted to the possibility of prolonged seizures and IV diazepam should be available. With drugs known to elevate seizure threshold, higher stimuli may, of course, be required. Methods are available to lower seizure threshold or prolong seizures,[54] but discussion of these is beyond the scope of this book.

ECT frequently causes confusion and disorientation; more rarely, it causes delirium. Concurrent lithium may increase the risk of delirium.[34] There have also been two case reports of serotonin syndrome; one occurred after ECT in a patient on combination of trazodone, bupropion and quetiapine[55] and the other in a patient receiving lithium duringECT therapy.[56] Close observation is essential. Very limited data support the use of thiamine (200mg daily) in reducing post-ECT confusion.[57] Nortriptyline seems to enhance ECT efficacy and reduce cognitive adverse effects.[1] Cognitive enhancers (donepezil, memantine, rivastigmine) might improve cognitive function and reduce ECT-induced cognitive side effects (and appear to be safe).[58,59] Ibuprofen may be used to prevent headache,[60] and intranasal sumatriptan[61] can be used to treat it.

References

1. Sackeim HA, et al. Effect of concomitant pharmacotherapy on electroconvulsive therapy outcomes: short-term efficacy and adverse effects. *Arch Gen Psychiatry* 2009; **66**:729–737.

2. Baghai TC, et al. The influence of concomitant antidepressant medication on safety, tolerability and clinical effectiveness of electroconvulsive therapy. *World J Biol Psychiatry* 2006; **7**:82–90.

3. Avramov MN, et al. The comparative effects of methohexital, propofol, and etomidate for electroconvulsive therapy. *Anesth Analg* 1995; **81**:596–602.

4. Stadtland C, et al. A switch from propofol to etomidate during an ECT course increases EEG and motor seizure duration. *J ECT* 2002; **18**:22–25.

5. Gazdag G, et al. Etomidate versus propofol for electroconvulsive therapy in patients with schizophrenia. *J ECT* 2004; **20**:225–229.

6. Conca A, et al. Etomidate vs. thiopentone in electroconvulsive therapy. An interdisciplinary challenge for anesthesiology and psychiatry. *Pharmacopsychiatry* 2003; **36**:94–97.

7. Rasmussen KG, et al. Seizure length with sevoflurane and thiopental for induction of general anesthesia in electroconvulsive therapy: a randomized double-blind trial. *J ECT* 2006; **22**:240–242.

8. Bundy BD, et al. Influence of anesthetic drugs and concurrent psychiatric medication on seizure adequacy during electroconvulsive therapy. *J Clin Psychiatry* 2010; **71**:775–777.

9. Stripp TK, et al. Anaesthesia for electroconvulsive therapy – new tricks for old drugs: a systematic review. *Acta Neuropsychiatr* 2018; **30**:61–69.

10. Eser D, et al. The influence of anaesthetic medication on safety, tolerability and clinical effectiveness of electroconvulsive therapy. *World J Biol Psychiatry* 2010; **11**:447–456.

11. McGirr A, et al. Adjunctive ketamine in electroconvulsive therapy: updated systematic review and meta-analysis. *Br J Psychiatry* 2017; **210**:403–407.

12. Fernie G, et al. Ketamine as the anaesthetic for electroconvulsive therapy: the KANECT randomised controlled trial. *Br J Psychiatry* 2017; **210**:422–428.

13. Zheng W, et al. Adjunctive ketamine and electroconvulsive therapy for major depressive disorder: a meta-analysis of randomized controlled trials. *J Affect Disord* 2019; **250**:123–131.

14. van Waarde JA, et al. Clinical predictors of seizure threshold in electroconvulsive therapy: a prospective study. *Eur Arch Psychiatry Clin Neurosci* 2013; **263**:167–175.

15. Royal College of Psychiatrists. The ECT Handbook (4th Edition) – rCPsych Publications: rCPsych Publications 2019.

16. Kellner CH, et al. ECT–drug interactions: a review. *Psychopharmacol Bull* 1991; **27**:595–609.

17. Naguib M, et al. Interactions between psychotropics, anaesthetics and electroconvulsive therapy: implications for drug choice and patient management. *CNS Drugs* 2002; **16**:229–247.

18. Maidment I. The interaction between psychiatric medicines and ECT. *Hosp Pharm* 1997; **4**:102–105.

19. Tang VM, et al. Should benzodiazepines and anticonvulsants be used during electroconvulsive therapy?: a case study and literature review. *J ECT* 2017; **33**:237–242.

20. Masdrakis VG, et al. The safety of the electroconvulsive therapy-escitalopram combination. *J ECT* 2008; **24**:289–291.

21. Dursun SM, et al. Effects of antidepressant treatments on first-ECT seizure duration in depression. *Prog Neuropsychopharmacol Biol Psychiatry* 2001; **25**:437–443.

22. Jarvis MR, et al. Novel antidepressants and maintenance electroconvulsive therapy: a review. *Ann Clin Psychiatry* 1992; **4**:275–284.

23. Papakostas YG, et al. Administration of citalopram before ECT: seizure duration and hormone responses. *J ECT* 2000; **16**:356–360.

24. Okamoto N, et al. Transient serotonin syndrome by concurrent use of electroconvulsive therapy and selective serotonin reuptake inhibitor: a case report and review of the literature. *Case Reports in Psychiatry* 2012; **2012**:215214.

25. Klysner R, et al. Transient serotonin toxicity evoked by combination of electroconvulsive therapy and fluoxetine. *Case Rep Psychiatry* 2014; **2014**:162502.

26. Gonzalez-Pinto A, et al. Efficacy and safety of venlafaxine-ECT combination in treatment-resistant depression. *J Neuropsychiatry Clin Neurosci* 2002; **14**:206–209.

27. Kranaster L, et al. Venlafaxine-associated post-ictal asystole during electroconvulsive therapy. *Pharmacopsychiatry* 2012; **45**:122–124.

28. Li TC, et al. Mirtazapine relieves post-electroconvulsive therapy headaches and nausea: a case series and review of the literature. *J ECT* 2011; **27**:165–167.

29. Hanretta AT, et al. Combined use of ECT with duloxetine and olanzapine: a case report. *J ECT* 2006; **22**:139–141.

30. Heinz B, et al. Postictal ventricular tachycardia after electroconvulsive therapy treatment associated with a lithium-duloxetine combination. *J ECT* 2013; **29**:e33–e35.

31. Birkenhager TK, et al. Possible synergy between electroconvulsive therapy and imipramine: a case report. *J Psychiatr Pract* 2016; **22**:478–480.

32. Dolenc TJ, et al. Electroconvulsive therapy in patients taking monoamine oxidase inhibitors. *J ECT* 2004; **20**:258–261.

33. Horn PJ, et al. Transdermal selegiline in patients receiving electroconvulsive therapy. *Psychosomatics* 2010; **51**:176–178.

34. Patel RS, et al. Combination of lithium and electroconvulsive therapy (ECT) is associated with higher odds of delirium and cognitive problems in a large national sample across the United States. *Brain Stimul* 2020; **13**:15–19.

35. Jha AK, et al. Negative interaction between lithium and electroconvulsive therapy–a case-control study. *Br J Psychiatry* 1996; **168**:241–243.

36. Rucker J, et al. A case of prolonged seizure after ECT in a patient treated with clomipramine, lithium, L-tryptophan, quetiapine, and thyroxine for major depression. *J ECT* 2008; 24:272–274.

37. Dolenc TJ, et al. The safety of electroconvulsive therapy and lithium in combination: a case series and review of the literature. *J ECT* 2005; 21:165–170.

38. Thirthalli J, et al. A prospective comparative study of interaction between lithium and modified electroconvulsive therapy. *World J Biol Psychiatry* 2011; 12:149–155.

39. Galvez V, et al. Predictors of seizure threshold in right unilateral ultrabrief electroconvulsive therapy: role of concomitant medications and anaesthesia used. *Brain Stimul* 2015; 8:486–492.

40. Havaki-Kontaxaki BJ, et al. Concurrent administration of clozapine and electroconvulsive therapy in clozapine-resistant schizophrenia. *Clin Neuropharmacol* 2006; 29:52–56.

41. Nothdurfter C, et al. The influence of concomitant neuroleptic medication on safety, tolerability and clinical effectiveness of electroconvulsive therapy. *World J Biol Psychiatry* 2006; 7:162–170.

42. Gazdag G, et al. The impact of neuroleptic medication on seizure threshold and duration in electroconvulsive therapy. *Ideggyogy Sz* 2004; 57:385–390.

43. Masdrakis VG, et al. The safety of the electroconvulsive therapy-aripiprazole combination: four case reports. *J ECT* 2008; 24:236–238.

44. Oulis P, et al. Corrected QT interval changes during electroconvulsive therapy-antidepressants-atypical antipsychotics coadministration: safety issues. *J ECT* 2011; 27:e4–e6.

45. Grover S, et al. Combined use of clozapine and ECT: a review. *Acta Neuropsychiatr* 2015; 27:131–142.

46. Flamarique I, et al. Electroconvulsive therapy and clozapine in adolescents with schizophrenia spectrum disorders: is it a safe and effective combination? *J Clin Psychopharmacol* 2012; 32:756–766.

47. Arumugham SS, et al. Efficacy and safety of combining clozapine with electrical or magnetic brain stimulation in treatment-refractory schizophrenia. *Expert Rev Clin Pharmacol* 2016; 9:1245–1252.

48. van Waarde JA, et al. Patient, treatment, and anatomical predictors of outcome in electroconvulsive therapy: a prospective study. *J ECT* 2013; 29:113–121.

49. Penland HR, et al. Combined use of lamotrigine and electroconvulsive therapy in bipolar depression: a case series. *J ECT* 2006; 22:142–147.

50. Zarate CA, Jr., et al. Combined valproate or carbamazepine and electroconvulsive therapy. *Ann Clin Psychiatry* 1997; 9:19–25.

51. Sienaert P, et al. Concurrent use of lamotrigine and electroconvulsive therapy. *J ECT* 2011; 27:148–152.

52. Jahangard L, et al. Comparing efficacy of ECT with and without concurrent sodium valproate therapy in manic patients. *J ECT* 2012; 28:118–123.

53. Rakesh G, et al. Concomitant anticonvulsants with bitemporal electroconvulsive therapy: a randomized controlled trial with clinical and neurobiological application. *J ECT* 2017; 33:16–21.

54. Datto C, et al. Augmentation of seizure induction in electroconvulsive therapy: a clinical reappraisal. *J ECT* 2002; 18:118–125.

55. Cheng YC, et al. Serotonin syndrome after electroconvulsive therapy in a patient on trazodone, bupropion, and quetiapine: a case report. *Clin Neuropharmacol* 2015; 38:112–113.

56. Deuschle M, et al. Electroconvulsive therapy induces transient sensitivity for a serotonin syndrome: a case report. *Pharmacopsychiatry* 2017; 50:41–42.

57. Linton CR, et al. Using thiamine to reduce post-ECT confusion. *Int J Geriatr Psychiatry* 2002; 17:189–192.

58. Prakash J, et al. Therapeutic and prophylactic utility of the memory-enhancing drug donepezil hydrochloride on cognition of patients undergoing electroconvulsive therapy: a randomized controlled trial. *J ECT* 2006; 22:163–168.

59. Niu Y, et al. Prophylactic cognitive enhancers for improvement of cognitive function in patients undergoing electroconvulsive therapy: a systematic review and meta-analysis. *Medicine (Baltimore)* 2020; 99:e19527.

60. Leung M, et al. Pretreatment with ibuprofen to prevent electroconvulsive therapy-induced headache. *J Clin Psychiatry* 2003; 64:551–553.

61. Markowitz JS, et al. Intranasal sumatriptan in post-ECT headache: results of an open-label trial. *J ECT* 2001; 17:280–283.

Psychostimulants in depression

Psychostimulants reduce fatigue, promote wakefulness and are mood-elevating (as distinct from antidepressant). Amfetamines have been used as treatments for depression since the 1930s,[1] and more recently modafinil has been evaluated as an adjunct to standard antidepressants.[2] Amfetamines are now rarely used in depression because of their propensity for the development of tolerance and dependence. Prolonged use of high doses is associated with paranoid psychosis.[3] Methylphenidate is now more widely used but may have similar shortcomings. Modafinil seems not to induce tolerance, dependence or psychosis but lacks the marked euphoric effects of amfetamines. Armodafinil, the longer acting isomer of modafinil, is available in some countries.

Psychostimulants differ importantly from standard antidepressants in that their mood-elevating effects are usually seen within a few hours, but their antidepressant action may be short-lived. Amfetamines and methylphenidate may thus be useful where a prompt effect is required and where dependence would not be problematic (e.g. in depression associated with terminal illness), although ketamine might also be considered (if available). Their use might also be justified in severe, prolonged depression unresponsive to standard treatments (e.g. in those considered for psychosurgery). Modafinil might justifiably be used as an adjunct to antidepressants in a wider range of patients and as a specific treatment for hypersomnia and fatigue.[4]

Table 3.12 outlines support (or the absence of it) for the use of psychostimulants in various clinical situations. Generally speaking, data relating to stimulants in depression are rather poor and inconclusive.[5–7] Careful consideration should be given to any use of any psychostimulant in depression since their short- and long-term safety have not been clearly established. Inclusion of individual drugs in Table 3.11 should not in itself be considered a recommendation for their use.

Table 3.12 Stimulants in depression

Clinical use	Regimens evaluated	Comments	Recommendations
Monotherapy in uncomplicated depression	Modafinil 100–200mg a day[8,9]	Case reports only – efficacy unproven	Standard antidepressants preferred. Avoid psychostimulants as monotherapy in uncomplicated depression.[10] Meta-analysis found adjunctive therapy but not monotherapy to be associated with clinically significant improvements.[7]
	Methylphenidate 20–40mg a day[11,12]	Minimal efficacy	
	Dexamphetamine 20mg a day[11]	Minimal efficacy	
Adjunctive therapy to accelerate or improve response	SSRI + methylphenidate 10–20mg a day[13,14]	No clear effect on time to response	Psychostimulants in general not recommended, but modafinil may be useful.
	SSRI + modafinil 400mg/day[15]	Improved response over SSRI alone	
	Tricyclic + methylphenidate 5–15mg a day[16]	Single open-label trial suggests faster response	
	SSRI or SNRI + lisdexamfetamine 20–70mg/day[17]	No superiority over placebo	

(Continued)

CHAPTER 3

CHAPTER 3

Table 3.12 (Continued)

Clinical use	Regimens evaluated	Comments	Recommendations
Adjunctive treatment of depression with fatigue and hypersomnia	SSRI + modafinil 200mg/day[18,19]	Beneficial effect only on hypersomnia. Modafinil may induce suicidal ideation	Possible effect on fatigue, but weak evidence base. An option where fatigue is prominent and otherwise unresponsive.
	SSRI + methylphenidate 10–40mg/day[20]	Clear effect on fatigue in hospice patients	
Adjunctive therapy in treatment resistant depression	SSRI + modafinil 100–400mg a day[7,21–26]	Effect mainly on fatigue and daytime sleepiness. Meta-analysis of 10 trials suggested clinically significant improvement in depressive symptoms[7]	Data limited. Modafinil may be useful for fatigue[27] and cognition.[28]
	MAOI + dexamfetamine 7.5–40mg a day[29] or lisdexamfetamine 50mg/day[30]	Support from single case series and one case report	Stimulants an option in refractory illness but other options better supported. One naturalistic study suggests methylphenidate may reduce self-harm or suicide attempts.[31]
	Methylphenidate or dexamfetamine ± antidepressant[32]	Large case series (n = 50) suggests benefit in the majority	
	Lisdexamfetamine 20–70mg/day + antidepressant[7,17,33]	Two meta-analyses found a small, non-significant effect on depressive symptoms compared to placebo	
Adjunctive treatment in bipolar depression[34,35]	Mood stabiliser and/or antidepressants + modafinil 100–200mg/day[36]	Significantly superior to placebo	Possible treatment option where other standard treatments fail. Meta-analysis of trials referenced here found stimulants well tolerated and an overall benefit versus placebo.[37] No evidence of treatment-emergent mania.[34,37,38]
	Mood stabiliser + armodafinil 150–200mg/day[38]	Superior to placebo on some measures	
	Mood stabiliser + methylphenidate 10–40mgday[39]	Mixed results, mainly positive	
	Mood stabiliser and/or antipsychotic + lisdexamfetamine 20–70mg/day[40]	Greater rates of improvement compared to placebo on patient-rated measures	

Table 3.12 (*Continued*)

Clinical use	Regimens evaluated	Comments	Recommendations
Monotherapy or add-on treatment in late-stage terminal cancer	Methylphenidate 5–30mg a day[41–45]	Case series and open prospective studies	Useful treatment options in those expected to live only for a few weeks.
	Dexamfetamine 2.5–20mg a day[46,47]	Beneficial effects seen on mood, fatigue and pain	
	Methylphenidate 20mg/day + mirtazapine 30mg/day[48]	RCT shows benefit for combination from third day of treatment	
	Methylphenidate 20mg/day + SSRI[49]	RCT failed to show benefit for combination	
	Modafinil 200mg/day[50]	Benefit to depression scores only in those also experiencing severe cancer-related fatigue	
Monotherapy or add-on treatment for depression in the elderly	Methylphenidate 1.25–20mg a day[51–53]	Use supported by three placebo-controlled studies. Rapid effect observed on mood and activity	Recommended only where patients fail to tolerate standard antidepressants or where contra-indications apply.
	Methylphenidate 5–40mg + citalopram 20–60mg/day[54]	One placebo-controlled study. Faster rate of response with combination compared to monotherapy with either drug	Monitor for increased heart rate – significant increase seen in one trial.[54]
Monotherapy in post-stroke depression	Methylphenidate 5–40mg a day[55–58]	Variable support but including two placebo-controlled trials.[55,58] Effect on mood evident after a few days	Standard antidepressants preferred. Further investigation required: stimulants may improve cognition and motor function.
	Modafinil 100mg/day[59]	Single case report	
Monotherapy in depression secondary to medical illness	Methylphenidate 5–20mg/day[60]	Limited data	Psychostimulants not appropriate therapy. Standard antidepressant preferred.
	Dexamfetamine 2.5–30mg/day[61,62]		
Monotherapy in depression and fatigue associated with HIV	Dexamfetamine 2.5–40mg/day[63,64]	Supported by one good, controlled study[64] Beneficial effect on mood and fatigue	Possible treatment option where fatigue is not responsive to standard antidepressants.
Monotherapy in depression in traumatic brain injury	Methylphenidate 5–20mg/day[65,66]	Improves depressive symptoms, daytime sleepiness and cognitive function	Appears to outperform antidepressants for this indication, but data are limited to two studies.

References

1. Satel SL, et al. Stimulants in the treatment of depression: a critical overview. *J Clin Psychiatry* 1989; **50**:241–249.
2. Menza MA, et al. Modafinil augmentation of antidepressant treatment in depression. *J Clin Psychiatry* 2000; **61**:378–381.
3. Warneke L. Psychostimulants in psychiatry. *Canadian J Psychiatry* 1990; **35**:3–10.
4. Goss AJ, et al. Modafinil augmentation therapy in unipolar and bipolar depression: a systematic review and meta-analysis of randomized controlled trials. *J Clin Psychiatry* 2013; **74**:1101–1107.
5. Candy M, et al. Psychostimulants for depression. *Cochrane Database Syst Rev* 2008; CD006722.
6. Hardy SE. Methylphenidate for the treatment of depressive symptoms, including fatigue and apathy, in medically ill older adults and terminally ill adults. *Am J Geriatr Pharmacother* 2009; **7**:34–59.
7. McIntyre RS, et al. The efficacy of psychostimulants in major depressive episodes: a systematic review and meta-analysis. *J Clin Psychopharmacol* 2017; **37**:412–418.
8. Lundt L. Modafinil treatment in patients with seasonal affective disorder/winter depression: an open-label pilot study. *J Affect Disord* 2004; **81**:173–178.
9. Kaufman KR, et al. Modafinil monotherapy in depression. *Eur Psychiatry* 2002; **17**:167–169.
10. Hegerl U, et al. Why do stimulants not work in typical depression? *Aust N Z J Psychiatry* 2017; **51**:20–22.
11. Little KY. d-Amphetamine versus methylphenidate effects in depressed inpatients. *J Clin Psychiatry* 1993; **54**:349–355.
12. Robin AA, et al. A controlled trial of methylphenidate (ritalin) in the treatment of depressive states. *J Neurol Neurosurg Psychiatry* 1958; **21**:55–57.
13. Lavretsky H, et al. Combined treatment with methylphenidate and citalopram for accelerated response in the elderly: an open trial. *J Clin Psychiatry* 2003; **64**:1410–1414.
14. Postolache TT, et al. Early augmentation of sertraline with methylphenidate. *J Clin Psychiatry* 1999; **60**:123–124.
15. Abolfazli R, et al. Double-blind randomized parallel-group clinical trial of efficacy of the combination fluoxetine plus modafinil versus fluoxetine plus placebo in the treatment of major depression. *Depress Anxiety* 2011; **28**:297–302.
16. Gwirtsman HE, et al. The antidepressant response to tricyclics in major depressives is accelerated with adjunctive use of methylphenidate. *Psychopharmacol Bull* 1994; **30**:157–164.
17. Giacobbe P, et al. Efficacy and tolerability of lisdexamfetamine as an antidepressant augmentation strategy: a meta-analysis of randomized controlled trials. *J Affect Disord* 2018; **226**:294–300.
18. Dunlop BW, et al. Coadministration of modafinil and a selective serotonin reuptake inhibitor from the initiation of treatment of major depressive disorder with fatigue and sleepiness: a double-blind, placebo-controlled study. *J Clin Psychopharmacol* 2007; **27**:614–619.
19. Fava M, et al. Modafinil augmentation of selective serotonin reuptake inhibitor therapy in MDD partial responders with persistent fatigue and sleepiness. *Ann Clin Psychiatry* 2007; **19**:153–159.
20. Kerr CW, et al. Effects of methylphenidate on fatigue and depression: a randomized, double-blind, placebo-controlled trial. *J Pain Symptom Manage* 2012; **43**:68–77.
21. DeBattista C, et al. Adjunct modafinil for the short-term treatment of fatigue and sleepiness in patients with major depressive disorder: a preliminary double-blind, placebo-controlled study. *J Clin Psychiatry* 2003; **64**:1057–1064.
22. Fava M, et al. A multicenter, placebo-controlled study of modafinil augmentation in partial responders to selective serotonin reuptake inhibitors with persistent fatigue and sleepiness. *J Clin Psychiatry* 2005; **66**:85–93.
23. Rasmussen NA, et al. Modafinil augmentation in depressed patients with partial response to antidepressants: a pilot study on self-reported symptoms covered by the major depression inventory (MDI) and the symptom checklist (SCL-92). *Nordic J Psychiatry* 2005; **59**:173–178.
24. DeBattista C, et al. A prospective trial of modafinil as an adjunctive treatment of major depression. *J Clin Psychopharmacol* 2004; **24**:87–90.
25. Markovitz PJ, et al. An open-label trial of modafinil augmentation in patients with partial response to antidepressant therapy. *J Clin Psychopharmacol* 2003; **23**:207–209.
26. Ravindran AV, et al. Osmotic-release oral system methylphenidate augmentation of antidepressant monotherapy in major depressive disorder: results of a double-blind, randomized, placebo-controlled trial. *J Clin Psychiatry* 2008; **69**:87–94.
27. Ghanean H, et al. Fatigue in patients with major depressive disorder: prevalence, burden and pharmacological approaches to management. *CNS Drugs* 2018; **32**:65–74.
28. Vaccarino SR, et al. The potential procognitive effects of modafinil in major depressive disorder: a systematic review. *J Clin Psychiatry* 2019; **80**:19r12767.
29. Fawcett J, et al. CNS stimulant potentiation of monoamine oxidase inhibitors in treatment refractory depression. *J Clin Psychopharmacol* 1991; **11**:127–132.
30. Israel JA. Combining stimulants and monoamine oxidase inhibitors: a reexamination of the literature and a report of a new treatment combination. *Prim Care Companion CNS Disord* 2015; **17**:10.4088/PCC.15br01836.
31. Rohde C, et al. The use of stimulants in depression: results from a self-controlled register study. *Aust N Z J Psychiatry* 2020; **54**:808–817.
32. Parker G, et al. Do the old psychostimulant drugs have a role in managing treatment-resistant depression? *Acta Psychiatr Scand* 2010; **121**:308–314.
33. Richards C, et al. A randomized, double-blind, placebo-controlled, dose-ranging study of lisdexamfetamine dimesylate augmentation for major depressive disorder in adults with inadequate response to antidepressant therapy. *J Psychopharmacology* 2017; **31**:1190–1203.
34. Szmulewicz AG, et al. Dopaminergic agents in the treatment of bipolar depression: a systematic review and meta-analysis. *Acta Psychiatr Scand* 2017; **135**:527–538.

35. Perugi G, et al. Use of stimulants in bipolar disorder. *Curr Psychiatry Rep* 2017; **19**:7.

36. Frye MA, et al. A placebo-controlled evaluation of adjunctive modafinil in the treatment of bipolar depression. *Am J Psychiatry* 2007; **164**:1242–1249.

37. Tsapakis EM, et al. Adjunctive treatment with psychostimulants and stimulant-like drugs for resistant bipolar depression: a systematic review and meta-analysis. *CNS Spectr* 2020: 1–12. [Epub ahead of print].

38. Nunez NA, et al. Efficacy and tolerability of adjunctive modafinil/armodafinil in bipolar depression: a meta-analysis of randomized controlled trials. *Bipolar Disord* 2020; **22**:109–120.

39. Dell'Osso B, et al. Assessing the roles of stimulants/stimulant-like drugs and dopamine-agonists in the treatment of bipolar depression. *Curr Psychiatry Rep* 2013; **15**:378.

40. McElroy SL, et al. Adjunctive lisdexamfetamine in bipolar depression: a preliminary randomized, placebo-controlled trial. *Int Clin Psychopharmacol* 2015; **30**:6–13.

41. Fernandez F, et al. Methylphenidate for depressive disorders in cancer patients. *Psychosomatics* 1987; **28**:455–461.

42. Macleod AD. Methylphenidate in terminal depression. *J Pain Symptom Manage* 1998; **16**:193–198.

43. Homsi J, et al. Methylphenidate for depression in hospice practice. *Am J Hosp Palliat Care* 2000; **17**:393–398.

44. Sarhill N, et al. Methylphenidate for fatigue in advanced cancer: a prospective open-label pilot study. *Am J Hosp Palliat Care* 2001; **18**:187–192.

45. Homsi J, et al. A phase II study of methylphenidate for depression in advanced cancer. *Am J Hosp Palliat Care* 2001; **18**:403–407.

46. Burns MM, et al. Dextroamphetamine treatment for depression in terminally ill patients. *Psychosomatics* 1994; **35**:80–83.

47. Olin J, et al. Psychostimulants for depression in hospitalized cancer patients. *Psychosomatics* 1996; **37**:57–62.

48. Ng CG, et al. Rapid response to methylphenidate as an add-on therapy to mirtazapine in the treatment of major depressive disorder in terminally ill cancer patients: a four-week, randomized, double-blinded, placebo-controlled study. *Eur Neuropsychopharmacol* 2014; **24**:491–498.

49. Sullivan DR, et al. Randomized, double-blind, placebo-controlled study of methylphenidate for the treatment of depression in SSRI-treated cancer patients receiving palliative care. *Psychooncology* 2017; **26**:1763–1769.

50. Conley CC, et al. Modafinil moderates the relationship between cancer-related fatigue and depression in 541 patients receiving chemotherapy. *J Clin Psychopharmacol* 2016; **36**:82–85.

51. Padala PR, et al. Methylphenidate for apathy in community-dwelling older veterans with mild Alzheimer's disease: a double-blind, randomized, placebo-controlled trial. *Am J Psychiatry* 2018; **175**:159–168.

52. Kaplitz SE. Withdrawn, apathetic geriatric patients responsive to methylphenidate. *J Am Geriatr Soc* 1975; **23**:271–276.

53. Wallace AE, et al. Double-blind, placebo-controlled trial of methylphenidate in older, depressed, medically ill patients. *Am J Psychiatry* 1995; **152**:929–931.

54. Lavretsky H, et al. Citalopram, methylphenidate, or their combination in geriatric depression: a randomized, double-blind, placebo-controlled trial. *Am J Psychiatry* 2015; **172**:561–569.

55. Grade C, et al. Methylphenidate in early poststroke recovery: a double-blind, placebo-controlled study. *Arch Phys Med Rehabil* 1998; **79**:1047–1050.

56. Lazarus LW, et al. Efficacy and side effects of methylphenidate for poststroke depression. *J Clin Psychiatry* 1992; **53**:447–449.

57. Lingam VR, et al. Methylphenidate in treating poststroke depression. *J Clin Psychiatry* 1988; **49**:151–153.

58. Delbari A, et al. Effect of methylphenidate and/or levodopa combined with physiotherapy on mood and cognition after stroke: a randomized, double-blind, placebo-controlled trial. *Eur Neurol* 2011; **66**:7–13.

59. Sugden SG, et al. Modafinil monotherapy in poststroke depression. *Psychosomatics* 2004; **45**:80–81.

60. Rosenberg PB, et al. Methylphenidate in depressed medically ill patients. *J Clin Psychiatry* 1991; **52**:263–267.

61. Woods SW, et al. Psychostimulant treatment of depressive disorders secondary to medical illness. *J Clin Psychiatry* 1986; **47**:12–15.

62. Kaufmann MW, et al. The use of d-amphetamine in medically ill depressed patients. *J Clin Psychiatry* 1982; **43**:463–464.

63. Wagner GJ, et al. Dexamphetamine as a treatment for depression and low energy in AIDS patients: a pilot study. *J Psychosom Res* 1997; **42**:407–411.

64. Wagner GJ, et al. Effects of dextroamphetamine on depression and fatigue in men with HIV: a double-blind, placebo-controlled trial. *J Clin Psychiatry* 2000; **61**:436–440.

65. Zhang WT, et al. Efficacy of methylphenidate for the treatment of mental sequelae after traumatic brain injury. *Medicine (Baltimore)* 2017; **96**:e6960.

66. Lee H, et al. Comparing effects of methylphenidate, sertraline and placebo on neuropsychiatric sequelae in patients with traumatic brain injury. *Human Psychopharmacology* 2005; **20**:97–104.

Post-stroke depression

Depression itself is a well-established risk factor for stroke.[1-4] In addition, depression is seen in at least 30–40% of survivors of stroke[5,6] and post-stroke depression is known to slow functional rehabilitation.[7] Antidepressants may reduce depressive symptoms[8] and thereby facilitate faster rehabilitation.[9] They may also improve global cognitive functioning,[10,11] enhance motor recovery[12,13] and even reduce mortality.[14] Despite these benefits post-stroke depression often goes untreated.[15]

Prophylaxis

The high incidence of depression after stroke makes prophylaxis worthy of consideration. Pooled data suggest a robust prophylactic effect for antidepressants.[16,17] Nortriptyline, fluoxetine, escitalopram, duloxetine and sertraline appear to prevent post-stroke depression.[18-22] Mirtazapine may both protect against depressive episodes and treat them.[23] A well-designed, multicentre, placebo-controlled RCT found escitalopram to reduce the incidence of mild depressive symptoms but not moderate or severe symptoms.[24]

A large cohort study that examined adverse outcomes in elderly patients treated with antidepressants reported that mirtazapine (and venlafaxine) may be associated with an increased risk of a new stroke compared with SSRIs or TCAs.[25]

Mianserin seems ineffective in the treatment of post-stroke depression.[26] Amitriptyline[27] and duloxetine[28] are effective in treating central post-stroke pain.

Routine use of antidepressants for the prevention of post-stroke depression is not recommended – Cochrane suggests that there may be a benefit, but note that the evidence is poor.[29] Three recent large multicentre RCTs (not included in the Cochrane review) showed the risks of prescribing fluoxetine (bone fractures, falls, seizures) to outweigh benefits in the reduction in incident depression.[30-32]

Treatment

Treatment is complicated by medical co-morbidity and by the potential for interaction with other co-prescribed drugs (especially warfarin – see Box 3.2). Contraindication to antidepressant treatment is more likely with tricyclics than with SSRIs.[33] Fluoxetine,[12,30,34,35] citalopram[10,36-38] and nortriptyline[39,40] are probably the most studied[41] and seem to be effective and safe.[42] SSRIs and nortriptyline are widely recommended for post-stroke depression. Reboxetine (which, like nortriptyline, does not affect platelet activity) may also be effective and well tolerated,[43] although its effects overall are doubtful.[44] Vortioxetine may be of particular interest owing to its additional benefits on cognition (independent of effects on depressive symptoms). It also does not appear to adversely affect cardiovascular parameters or interact with warfarin or aspirin, but there are currently no data to support its use specifically in post-stroke depression.

Despite fears, SSRIs seem not to increase risk of stroke[45] (post-stroke), although some doubt remains.[46-49] (Stroke can be embolic or haemorrhagic – SSRIs may protect against the former[50,51] and provoke the latter[52,53] although the evidence base for this is rather weak[54] – see section on 'SSRIs and Bleeding' in this chapter). Other side effects may also be problematic – specifically falls, bone fractures and epileptic seizures.[30–32]

Antidepressants are clearly effective in post-stroke depression,[42,55] and treatment should not usually be withheld (even though Cochrane is rather lukewarm about the benefits of antidepressants[29]). Inadequate treatment of depression increases the risk of stroke.[14,56] Two multiple-treatments meta-analyses suggested that paroxetine might be the drug of choice when considering both efficacy and tolerability post-stroke, although small sample sizes and a lack of high-quality studies in this area limit the strength of this recommendation[57,58] (each analysis included only one paroxetine trial, whereas a meta-analysis of four trials of paroxetine found no benefit[59]). A recent large multiple treatments meta-analysis of 51 trials ranked mirtazapine first for response rate, followed by venlafaxine and escitalopram, although the studies were limited to Chinese patients and so may lack generalisability.[60]

Box 3.2 Post-stroke depression – recommended drugs

SSRIs*

Nortriptyline

---

* Caution is clearly required if the index stroke was known to be haemorrhagic because SSRIs increase the risk of *de novo* haemorrhagic stroke (although absolute risk is low), especially when combined with warfarin or other anti-platelet drugs.[61,62] If patient is taking warfarin, suggest citalopram or escitalopram (probably lowest interaction potential[63]) and use the lowest effective dose.[49] Little is known of the pharmacokinetic interaction potential with direct-acting oral anticoagulants (DOACs). Citalopram or escitalopram may again be preferred as neither drug affects enzymes associated with DOAC metabolism.[64]

Where SSRIs are given in any anticoagulated or aspirin-treated patient, consideration should be given to the prescription of a proton-pump inhibitor for gastric protection. Nortriptyline, which does not appear to increase risk of bleeding, is an alternative.

References

1. Wium-Andersen MK, et al. An attempt to explain the bidirectional association between ischaemic heart disease, stroke and depression: a cohort and meta-analytic approach. *Br J Psychiatry* 2020; **217**:434–441.
2. Pan A, et al. Depression and risk of stroke morbidity and mortality: a meta-analysis and systematic review. *JAMA* 2011; **306**:1241–1249.
3. Pequignot R, et al. Depressive symptoms, antidepressants and disability and future coronary heart disease and stroke events in older adults: the Three City Study. *Eur J Epidemiol* 2013; **28**:249–256.
4. Li CT, et al. Major depressive disorder and stroke risks: a 9-year follow-up population-based, matched cohort study. *PLoS One* 2012; **7**:e46818.
5. Gainotti G, et al. Relation between depression after stroke, antidepressant therapy, and functional recovery. *J Neurol Neurosurg Psychiatry* 2001; **71**:258–261.
6. Hayee MA, et al. Depression after stroke-analysis of 297 stroke patients. *Bangladesh Med Res Counc Bull* 2001; **27**:96–102.
7. Paolucci S, et al. Post-stroke depression, antidepressant treatment and rehabilitation results. A case-control study. *Cerebrovasc Dis* 2001; **12**:264–271.
8. Xu XM, et al. Efficacy and feasibility of antidepressant treatment in patients with post-stroke depression. *Medicine (Baltimore)* 2016; **95**:e5349.

9. Gainotti G, et al. Determinants and consequences of post-stroke depression. *Curr Opin Neurol* 2002; **15**:85–89.

10. Jorge RE, et al. Escitalopram and enhancement of cognitive recovery following stroke. *Arch Gen Psychiatry* 2010; **67**:187–196.

11. Gu SC, et al. Early selective serotonin reuptake inhibitors for recovery after stroke: a meta-analysis and trial sequential analysis. *J Stroke Cerebrovasc Dis* 2018; **27**:1178–1189.

12. Chollet F, et al. Fluoxetine for motor recovery after acute ischaemic stroke (FLAME): a randomised placebo-controlled trial. *Lancet Neurol* 2011; **10**:123–130.

13. Thilarajah S, et al. Factors associated with post-stroke physical activity: a systematic review and meta-analysis. *Arch Phys Med Rehabil* 2018; **99**:1876–1889.

14. Krivoy A, et al. Low adherence to antidepressants is associated with increased mortality following stroke: a large nationally representative cohort study. *Eur Neuropsychopharmacol* 2017; **27**:970–976.

15. El Husseini N, et al. Depression and antidepressant use after stroke and transient ischemic attack. *Stroke* 2012; **43**:1609–1616.

16. Farooq S, et al. Pharmacological interventions for prevention of depression in high risk conditions: systematic review and meta-analysis. *J Affect Disord* 2020; **269**:58–69.

17. Chen Y, et al. Antidepressant prophylaxis for poststroke depression: a meta-analysis. *Int Clin Psychopharmacol* 2007; **22**:159–166.

18. Feng R, et al. Effect of sertraline in the treatment and prevention of poststroke depression: a meta-analysis. *Medicine (Baltimore)* 2018; **97**:e13453.

19. Narushima K, et al. Preventing poststroke depression: a 12-week double-blind randomized treatment trial and 21-month follow-up. *J Nerv Ment Dis* 2002; **190**:296–303.

20. Robinson RG, et al. Escitalopram and problem-solving therapy for prevention of poststroke depression: a randomized controlled trial. *JAMA* 2008; **299**:2391–2400.

21. Almeida OP, et al. Preventing depression after stroke: results from a randomized placebo-controlled trial. *J Clin Psychiatry* 2006; **67**:1104–1109.

22. Zhang LS, et al. Prophylactic effects of duloxetine on post-stroke depression symptoms: an open single-blind trial. *Eur Neurol* 2013; **69**:336–343.

23. Niedermaier N, et al. Prevention and treatment of poststroke depression with mirtazapine in patients with acute stroke. *J Clin Psychiatry* 2004; **65**:1619–1623.

24. Kim JS, et al. Efficacy of early administration of escitalopram on depressive and emotional symptoms and neurological dysfunction after stroke: a multicentre, double-blind, randomised, placebo-controlled study. *Lancet Psychiatry* 2017; **4**:33–41.

25. Coupland C, et al. Antidepressant use and risk of adverse outcomes in older people: population based cohort study. *BMJ* 2011; **343**:d4551.

26. Palomaki H, et al. Prevention of poststroke depression: 1 year randomised placebo controlled double blind trial of mianserin with 6 month follow up after therapy. *J Neurol Neurosurg Psychiatry* 1999; **66**:490–494.

27. Lampl C, et al. Amitriptyline in the prophylaxis of central poststroke pain. Preliminary results of 39 patients in a placebo-controlled, long-term study. *Stroke* 2002; **33**:3030–3032.

28. Kim NY, et al. Effect of duloxetine for the treatment of chronic central poststroke pain. *Clin Neuropharmacol* 2019; **42**:73–76.

29. Allida S, et al. Pharmacological, psychological and non-invasive brain stimulation interventions for preventing depression after stroke. *Cochrane Database Syst Rev* 2020; **5**:Cd003689.

30. EFFECTS Trial Collaboration. Safety and efficacy of fluoxetine on functional recovery after acute stroke (EFFECTS): a randomised, double-blind, placebo-controlled trial. *Lancet Neurol* 2020; **19**:661–669.

31. FOCUS Trial Collaboration. Effects of fluoxetine on functional outcomes after acute stroke (FOCUS): a pragmatic, double-blind, randomised, controlled trial. *Lancet* 2019; **393**:265–274.

32. AFFINITY Trial Collaboration. Safety and efficacy of fluoxetine on functional outcome after acute stroke (AFFINITY): a randomised, double-blind, placebo-controlled trial. *Lancet Neurol* 2020; **19**:651–660.

33. Cole MG, et al. Feasibility and effectiveness of treatments for post-stroke depression in elderly inpatients: systematic review. *J Geriatr Psychiatry Neurol* 2001; **14**:37–41.

34. Wiart L, et al. Fluoxetine in early poststroke depression: a double-blind placebo-controlled study. *Stroke* 2000; **31**:1829–1832.

35. Choi-Kwon S, et al. Fluoxetine improves the quality of life in patients with poststroke emotional disturbances. *Cerebrovasc Dis* 2008; **26**:266–271.

36. Andersen G, et al. Effective treatment of poststroke depression with the selective serotonin reuptake inhibitor citalopram. *Stroke* 1994; **25**:1099–1104.

37. Tan S, et al. Efficacy and safety of citalopram in treating post-stroke depression: a meta-analysis. *Eur Neurol* 2015; **74**:188–201.

38. Cui M, et al. Efficacy and safety of citalopram for the treatment of poststroke depression: a meta-analysis. *J Stroke Cerebrovasc Dis* 2018; **27**:2905–2918.

39. Robinson RG, et al. Nortriptyline versus fluoxetine in the treatment of depression and in short-term recovery after stroke: a placebo-controlled, double-blind study. *Am J Psychiatry* 2000; **157**:351–359.

40. Zhang WH, et al. Nortriptyline protects mitochondria and reduces cerebral ischemia/hypoxia injury. *Stroke* 2008; **39**:455–462.

41. Starkstein SE, et al. Antidepressant therapy in post-stroke depression. *Expert Opin Pharmacother* 2008; **9**:1291–1298.

42. Mead GE, et al. Selective serotonin reuptake inhibitors for stroke recovery. *JAMA* 2013; **310**:1066–1067.

43. Rampello L, et al. An evaluation of efficacy and safety of reboxetine in elderly patients affected by 'retarded' post-stroke depression. A random, placebo-controlled study. *Arch Gerontol Geriatr* 2005; **40**:275–285.

44. Eyding D, et al. Reboxetine for acute treatment of major depression: systematic review and meta-analysis of published and unpublished placebo and selective serotonin reuptake inhibitor controlled trials. *BMJ* 2010; **341**:c4737.

45. Douglas I, et al. The use of antidepressants and the risk of haemorrhagic stroke: a nested case control study. *Br J Clin Pharmacol* 2011; **71**:116–120.

46. Trajkova S, et al. Use of antidepressants and risk of incident stroke: a systematic review and meta-analysis. *Neuroepidemiology* 2019; **53**:142–151.

47. Hoirisch-Clapauch S, et al. Antidepressants: bleeding or thrombosis? *Thromb Res* 2019; **181 Suppl 1**:S23–S28.

48. Hackam DG, et al. Selective serotonin reuptake inhibitors and brain hemorrhage: a meta-analysis. *Neurology* 2012; **79**:1862–1865.

49. Kim JH, et al. Major adverse cardiovascular events in antidepressant users within patients with ischemic heart diseases: a nationwide cohort study. *J Clin Psychopharmacol* 2020; **40**:475–481.

50. He Y, et al. Effect of fluoxetine on three-year recurrence in acute ischemic stroke: a randomized controlled clinical study. *Clin Neurol Neurosurg* 2018; **168**:1–6.

51. Douros A, et al. Degree of serotonin reuptake inhibition of antidepressants and ischemic risk: a cohort study. *Neurology* 2019; **93**:e1010–e1020.

52. Trifiro G, et al. Risk of ischemic stroke associated with antidepressant drug use in elderly persons. *J Clin Psychopharmacol* 2010; **30**:252–258.

53. Wu CS, et al. Association of cerebrovascular events with antidepressant use: a case-crossover study. *Am J Psychiatry* 2011; **168**:511–521.

54. Mortensen JK, et al. Safety of selective serotonin reuptake inhibitor treatment in recovering stroke patients. *Exp Opin Drug Saf* 2015; **14**:911–919.

55. Chen Y, et al. Treatment effects of antidepressants in patients with post-stroke depression: a meta-analysis. *Ann Pharmacother* 2006; **40**:2115–2122.

56. Bangalore S, et al. Cardiovascular hazards of insufficient treatment of depression among patients with known cardiovascular disease: a propensity score adjusted analysis. *Eur Heart J Qual Care Clin Outcomes* 2018; **4**:258–266.

57. Sun Y, et al. Comparative efficacy and acceptability of antidepressant treatment in poststroke depression: a multiple-treatments meta-analysis. *BMJ Open* 2017; **7**:e016499.

58. Deng L, et al. Interventions for management of post-stroke depression: a Bayesian network meta-analysis of 23 randomized controlled trials. *Sci Rep* 2017; **7**:16466.

59. Li L, et al. Effectiveness of paroxetine for poststroke depression: a meta-analysis. *J Stroke Cerebrovasc Dis* 2020; **29**:104664.

60. Li X, et al. Comparative efficacy of nine antidepressants in treating Chinese patients with post-stroke depression: a network meta-analysis. *J Affect Disord* 2020; **266**:540–548.

61. Jeong HE, et al. Risk of major adverse cardiovascular events associated with concomitant use of antidepressants and non-steroidal anti-inflammatory drugs: a retrospective cohort study. *CNS Drugs* 2020; **34**:1063–1074.

62. Quinn GR, et al. Effect of selective serotonin reuptake inhibitors on bleeding risk in patients with atrial fibrillation taking warfarin. *Am J Cardiol* 2014; **114**:583–586.

63. Sayal KS, et al. Psychotropic interactions with warfarin. *Acta Psychiatr Scand* 2000; **102**:250–255.

64. Fitzgerald JL, et al. Drug interactions of direct-acting oral anticoagulants. *Drug Saf* 2016; **39**:841–845.

Further reading

Castilla-Guerra. Pharmacological management of post-stroke depression. *Expert Rev Neurother* 2020; **20**:157–166.

CHAPTER 3

Antidepressants – alternative routes of administration

In rare cases, patients may be unable or unwilling to take antidepressants orally, or gastrointestinal absorption of medication may be compromised, and alternative treatments including psychological interventions and electroconvulsive therapy (ECT) are either impractical or contra-indicated.

One such scenario is depression in the medically ill,[1] particularly those who have undergone surgical resection procedures affecting the gastrointestinal tract. Such patients often have feeding tubes inserted. Where the intra-gastric (IG) route is used, antidepressants can usually be crushed and administered. If an intra-jejunal (IJ) tube is used then more care is required because of changes in the rate or extent of absorption. Where available, plasma level monitoring may be helpful in differentiating between non-response and lack of absorption.

Very few non-oral formulations are available as commercial products. Most formulations do not have UK licences and may be very difficult to obtain, being available only through pharmaceutical importers or from Specials manufacturers. In addition, the use of these preparations beyond their licence or in an absence of a licence usually means that accountability for adverse effects lies with the prescriber. As a consequence, non-oral administration of antidepressants should be undertaken only when absolutely necessary. It is worth considering that some psychotropics that are not conventionally labelled 'antidepressants' may possess pharmacological antidepressant activity and be more readily available in non-oral formulations. Many of the atypical antipsychotics are available as intramuscular injections, although data supporting use in depression are limited to oral adjunct of standard antidepressants.

Alternative antidepressant delivery methods

Sublingual

There are a small number of case reports supporting the effectiveness of **fluoxetine** liquid used sublingually in depressed, medically compromised patients.[2] In these reports, doses of up to 60mg a day produced plasma fluoxetine and norfluoxetine levels towards the lower end of the proposed therapeutic range.[2] Ketamine injection has also been used sublingually, with apparent good efficacy.[3] It may be better tolerated than other routes of administration (IV or SC).[3]

Buccal

Selegiline is available as oral lyophilisates for absorption in the buccal cavity (licensed for the treatment of Parkinson's disease) but is selective for MAO-B inhibition at the 1.25mg doses available – lack of action at MAO-A in the central nervous system at these doses is thought to preclude antidepressant activity.[4] A very small study of orally disintegrating 10mg/day selegiline, however, showed significant inhibition of brain MAO-A, but clinical antidepressant activity has not been investigated.[5]

Various studies have investigated development of a buccal-adhesive delivery system for doxepin,[6,7] but no commercial product is yet available. One case report describes buccal administration of amitriptyline tablets[8] achieving therapeutic plasma levels. Another case used orodispersible mirtazapine, assuming buccal absorption,[9] although no plasma levels were reported, and no information is available to suggest that orodispersible mirtazapine is actually absorbed through the buccal mucosa (as opposed to dispersing in saliva that is then swallowed).

Intravenous and intramuscular injections

Intravenous formulations avoid the first-pass effect, leading to somewhat higher drug plasma levels[10,11] and perhaps greater response[11,12] but not necessarily faster onset of action.[12–14] The placebo effect associated with IV administration is known to be large.[15] Note that calculating the correct parenteral dose of antidepressants is difficult given the variable first-pass effect to which oral drugs are usually subject. Parenteral doses can be expected to be much lower than oral doses and give the same effect.

Intravenous **citalopram** followed by maintenance oral citalopram may be a clinically useful treatment strategy for severely depressed, hospitalised patients.[13] Better efficacy and faster response (compared with oral doses) have also been demonstrated when using IV citalopram in treating symptoms of obsessive compulsive disorder.[16] The IV preparation appears to be well-tolerated, with the most common adverse events being nausea, headache, tremor and somnolence – similar to oral administration.[17,18] A case report of a 65-year-old man describes acute hyperkinetic delirium associated with IV citalopram.[19] Intravenous **escitalopram** also exists although studies reported to date are pharmacokinetic analyses.[20] Note that oral citalopram is associated with a higher risk of QTc prolongation than other SSRIs. If used IV in a medically compromised patient, ECG monitoring is recommended.

Mirtazapine is also available as an intravenous preparation. It has been administered by slow infusion at a dose of 15mg a day for 14 days in two studies and was well tolerated in depressed patients.[21,22] There are reports of IV mirtazapine 6–30mg/day being used to treat hyperemesis gravidarum.[23,24]

Amitriptyline was available as both an IV and IM injection (IM injection has been given IV), and both routes have been used in the treatment of post-operative pain and depression.[25] The concentration of the IM preparation (10mg/mL) may mean that a high volume injection is needed to achieve antidepressant doses, and this clearly militates against its use intramuscularly.[26] It is no longer available in most parts of the world. **Clomipramine** is probably the most widely studied IV antidepressant. Pulse loading doses of intravenous clomipramine have been shown to produce a larger more rapid decrease in obsessive compulsive disorder symptoms compared with oral doses.[10,27] The potential for serious cardiac side effects when using any tricyclic antidepressant intravenously necessitates monitoring of pulse, blood pressure and ECG.

Allopregnanolone (marketed as brexanolone) is an endogenous progesterone metabolite licensed in the USA for intravenous treatment of postpartum depression. Given the unique mechanism of action, it is not suitable for treatment of other types of depression.

Intravenous **vortioxetine** has been used to accelerate response to the oral formulation,[28] but this is not a commercially available preparation.

CHAPTER 3

One attraction of IV administration of antidepressants may be a more rapid onset of action, but this is not consistently demonstrated in controlled studies.[29]

Extensive studies of IV **ketamine**, a glutamate N-methyl-d-aspartate (NMDA) receptor antagonist have demonstrated rapid, albeit short-lived antidepressant effects.[30] Concerns over long-term duration of response may be less relevant for acutely medically unwell patients. Ketamine has also been delivered via intranasal,[31] IM and SC routes,[32,33] sublingually[3,34] and via transmucosal routes.[35] IV **scopolamine (hyoscine)** as an antidepressant has also been investigated and has produced rapid antidepressant effects within 72 hours in both unipolar and bipolar depression.[36–38]

Transdermal

Amitriptyline gel is used in pain clinics as an adjuvant in the treatment of a variety of chronic pain conditions.[39,40] It is usually prepared as a 50mmol/L or 100mmol/L gel with or without lidocaine, and although it has proven analgesic activity there are no published data on the plasma levels attained via this route. **Nortriptyline** hydrochloride has been formulated as a transdermal patch for smoking cessation.[41] Nanoemulsion formulations of **imipramine** and of **doxepin** have also been formulated for transdermal delivery for use as analgesics.[42] At the time of writing there are no published studies on nortriptyline patches or imipramine or doxepin nanoemulsions in depression. It is unlikely that any of these formulations achieve plasma concentrations high enough to elicit antidepressant effects.

Oral selegiline at doses greater than 20mg/day may be antidepressant, but enzyme selectivity is lost at these doses, necessitating a tyramine-restricted diet.[43,44] **Selegiline** can be administered transdermally. It is efficacious and tolerable and delivers 25–30% of the selegiline content over 24 hours and steady-state plasma concentrations are achieved within 5 days of daily dosing.[45] This route bypasses first-pass metabolism, thereby providing a higher, more sustained, plasma concentration of selegiline while being relatively sparing of the gastrointestinal MAO-A system.[46,47] There seems to be no need for tyramine restriction when the lower dose patch (6mg/24 hours) is used, and there have been no reports of hypertensive reactions even with the higher dose patch. Patients using the higher strength patches (9mg or 12mg/24 hours) should avoid very high tyramine content food substances,[48] but generally transdermal selegiline is well tolerated.

Rectal

The rectal mucosa lacks the extensive villi and microvilli of other parts of the gastrointestinal tract limiting its surface area. Therefore, rectal agents need to be in a formulation that maximises the extent of contact the active ingredient will have with the mucosa. There are no readily available antidepressant suppositories, but extemporaneous preparation is possible. For example, **amitriptyline** (in cocoa butter) suppositories have been manufactured by a hospital pharmacy and administered in a dose of 50mg twice daily with some subjective success.[49,50] **Doxepin** capsules have been administered via the rectal route directly in the treatment of cancer-related pain (without a special formulation) and produced plasma concentrations within the supposed therapeutic range.[51] Similarly, it has been reported that extemporaneously manufactured **imipramine** and **clomipramine** suppositories produced plasma levels comparable with the oral route of administration.[52] **Trazodone** has also been successfully administered in a suppository formulation post-operatively for a patient who was stable on the oral formulation prior to surgery.[50,51] **Sertraline** tablets administered rectally have also been used with success in a critically ill patient with bowel compromise.[53]

Intranasal

Esketamine is available as a nasal spray (Spravato) and was licensed in the United Kingdom in 2019 and in the United States of America in 2020 for treatment-resistant major depressive disorder. It requires specific administration practices (tilting of the head), which may not be possible to adhere to in medically unwell patients. At the time of writing, the UK National Institute of Health and Care Excellence had not recommended intranasal esketamine for use in treatment-resistant depression due to concerns over clinical and cost-effectiveness (in long-term use). This may make it difficult to obtain in UK hospitals where ketamine (in other formulations) is cheap and readily available (see Table 3.13).

Table 3.13 Alternative formulations and routes of administration of antidepressants

Drug name and route	Dosing information	Manufacturer	Notes
Sublingual fluoxetine	Doses up to 60mg a day	Use liquid fluoxetine preparation	Plasma levels may be slightly lower compared with oral dosing
Buccal selegiline (oral lyophilisate)	10mg (8 × 1.25mg lyophilisates) daily	Cephalon UK Limited	Orally disintegrating freeze-dried formulation (Zelapar®) is licensed for treatment of Parkinson's disease. Trial data showed that 10mg of the lyophilizate formulation was required for MAO-A inhibition[5] – this may be practically difficult to administer
Buccal amitriptyline	Initiated at 25mg nocte and titrated up to 125mg daily	Generic amitriptyline	Tablets were crushed and allowed to dissolve in patient's mouth to promote buccal absorption. Authors report a decrease in the patient's depression[8]
Intravenous amitriptyline	25–100mg given in 250mL NaCl 0.9% by slow infusion over 120 minutes	Contact local importer	Adverse effects tend to be dose-related and are largely similar to the oral formulation. At higher doses drowsiness and dizziness occur. Bradycardia may occur with doses around 100mg. ECG monitoring is recommended

(Continued)

Table 3.13 (Continued)

Drug name and route	Dosing information	Manufacturer	Notes
Intravenous clomipramine	25mg/2mL injection Starting dose is 25mg diluted in 500mL NaCl 0.9% by slow infusion over 90 minutes. Increased to 250–300mg in increments of 25mg/day over 10–14 days[54,55]	Novartis Defiante	The most common reported side effects are similar to the oral formulation, which included nausea, sweating, restlessness, flushing, drowsiness, fatigue, abdominal distress and nervousness. ECG monitoring recommended
	Another report used starting dose of 50mg IV per day and titrated up to a maximum dose of 225mg/day over 5–7 days[56]		Reduction of symptoms was detected after one week of the first IV dose
Intravenous citalopram	40mg/mL injection Doses from 20 to 40mg in 250mL NaCL 0.9% or Glucose 5% Doses up to 80mg have been used for OCD Rate of infusion is 20mg per hour	Lundbeck – available in some countries. Not licensed in the UK, can be imported from Germany but may take 3–4 weeks to obtain	The most commonly reported side effects are nausea, headache, tremor and somnolence similar to adverse effects of the oral preparation. A case of acute hyperkinetic delirium has also been reported. Used for depression and obsessive compulsive disorder. ECG monitoring recommended
Intravenous escitalopram	10mg slow infusion over 60 minutes	Lundbeck – not marketed anywhere in the world	Studies to date have only looked at pharmacokinetic profile. ECG monitoring recommended
Intravenous mirtazapine	6mg/2mL infusion solution 15mg/5mL infusion solution Dose 15mg in Glucose 5% over 60 minutes	Contact local importer	The most common reported side effects are nausea, sedation and dizziness similar to side effects of the oral preparation
Intravenous trazodone[57]	25–100mg in 250mL of saline daily for 1 week, lasting approximately 1.5 hours. IV doses were decided according to the severity of depressive symptoms	Available only in Italy	Trazodone showed a significant improvement of symptoms only after one week of IV treatment and was better tolerated than clomipramine
Intramuscular flupentixol decanoate depot[58]	5–10mg/2 weeks	Lundbeck Mylan	IM flupentixol had a mood-elevating effect and is well tolerated at these doses. Extrapyramidal effects are rarely seen. Side-effects reported include dry mouth, dizziness and drowsiness

Table 3.13 (*Continued*)

Drug name and route	Dosing information	Manufacturer	Notes
Transdermal selegiline	6mg/24 hours, 9mg/24 hours, 12mg/24 hours Starting dose is 6mg/24 hours. Titration to higher doses in 3mg/24 hours increments at ≥2-week intervals, up to a maximum dose of 12mg/24 hours[59]	Bristol Myers Squib, available via Alliance Wholesaler	The 6mg/24 hours dose does not require a tyramine restricted diet At higher doses, although no hypertensive crisis reactions have been reported, the manufacturer recommends avoiding high tyramine content food substances Application site reactions and insomnia are the most common reported side effects
Rectal amitriptyline	Doses up to 50mg bd	Suppositories have been manufactured by pharmacies	Case reports only
Rectal clomipramine	No detailed information available		
Rectal imipramine	No detailed information available		
Rectal doxepin	No detailed information available	Capsules have been used rectally	
Rectal sertraline	Starting dose: a 25mg tablet was placed inside the rectal chamber daily. This was titrated up at 3-day intervals to a maximal dose of 100mg on day 10	Tablets have been used rectally	Levels at the 100mg steady-state dose revealed detectable serum levels of sertraline, but not the metabolite. The levels fell within the reported range of levels for orally administered sertraline. No adverse effects were recorded
Rectal trazodone	No detailed information available	Suppositories have been manufactured by pharmacies	Trazodone in the rectal formulation has been used for post-operative or cancer pain control rather than antidepressant activity
Ketamine	IV: 0.5mg/kg over 40 minutes SC: first dose 0.25mg/kg bolus (range 12.5–25mg), standard treatment dose 0.5mg/kg bolus (range 25–50mg) SL: 1.5mg/kg	IV preparation is widely available	SC ketamine is less likely to cause side effects (dissociative symptoms or blood pressure changes) compared to IV. SL apparently also well tolerated. Experience is increasing with ketamine, but expert advice before commencing is recommended

Note: Availability of all preparations listed varies over time and from country to country.

bd, bis die (twice a day).

CHAPTER 3

References

1. Cipriani A, et al. Metareview on short-term effectiveness and safety of antidepressants for depression: an evidence-based approach to inform clinical practice. *Can J Psychiatry* 2007; 52:553–562.

2. Pakyurek M, et al. Sublingually administered fluoxetine for major depression in medically compromised patients. *Am J Psychiatry* 1999; 156:1833–1834.

3. Swainson J, et al. Sublingual ketamine: an option for increasing accessibility of ketamine treatments for depression? *J Clin Psychiatry* 2020; 81:19lr13146.

4. Morgan PT. Treatment-resistant depression: response to low-dose transdermal but not oral selegiline. *J Clin Psychopharmacol* 2007; 27:313–314.

5. Fowler JS, et al. Evidence that formulations of the selective MAO-B inhibitor, selegiline, which bypass first-pass metabolism, also inhibit MAO-A in the human brain. *Neuropsychopharmacology* 2015; 40:650–657.

6. Laffleur F, et al. Modified biomolecule as potential vehicle for buccal delivery of doxepin. *Ther Deliv* 2016; 7:683–689.

7. Sanz R, et al. Development of a buccal doxepin platform for pain in oral mucositis derived from head and neck cancer treatment. *Eur J Pharm Biopharm* 2017; 117:203–211.

8. Robbins B, et al. Amitriptyline absorption in a patient with short bowel syndrome. *Am J Gastroenterol* 1999; 94:2302–2304.

9. Das A, et al. Options when anti-depressants cannot be used in conventional ways. Clinical case and review of literature. *Personal Med Psychiatry* 2019; 15–16:22–27.

10. Deisenhammer EA, et al. Intravenous versus oral administration of amitriptyline in patients with major depression. *J Clin Psychopharmacol* 2000; 20:417–422.

11. Koran LM, et al. Rapid benefit of intravenous pulse loading of clomipramine in obsessive-compulsive disorder. *Am J Psychiatry* 1997; 154:396–401.

12. Svestka J, et al. [Citalopram (Seropram) in tablet and infusion forms in the treatment of major depression]. *Cesk Psychiatr* 1993; 89:331–339.

13. Baumann P, et al. A double-blind double-dummy study of citalopram comparing infusion versus oral administration. *J Affect Disord* 1998; 49:203–210.

14. Pollock BG, et al. Acute antidepressant effect following pulse loading with intravenous and oral clomipramine. *Arch Gen Psychiatry* 1989; 46:29–35.

15. Sallee FR, et al. Pulse intravenous clomipramine for depressed adolescents: double-blind, controlled trial. *Am J Psychiatry* 1997; 154:668–673.

16. Bhikram TP, et al. The effect of intravenous citalopram on the neural substrates of obsessive-compulsive disorder. *J Neuropsychiatry Clin Neurosci* 2016; 28:243–247.

17. Guelfi JD, et al. Efficacy of intravenous citalopram compared with oral citalopram for severe depression. Safety and efficacy data from a double-blind, double-dummy trial. *J Affect Disord* 2000; 58:201–209.

18. Kasper S, et al. Intravenous antidepressant treatment: focus on citalopram. *Eur Arch Psychiatry Clin Neurosci* 2002; 252:105–109.

19. Delic M, et al. Delirium during i. v. citalopram treatment: a case report. *Pharmacopsychiatry* 2013; 46:37–38.

20. Sogaard B, et al. The pharmacokinetics of escitalopram after oral and intravenous administration of single and multiple doses to healthy subjects. *J Clin Pharmacol* 2005; 45:1400–1406.

21. Konstantinidis A, et al. Intravenous mirtazapine in the treatment of depressed inpatients. *Eur Neuropsychopharmacol* 2002; 12:57–60.

22. Muhlbacher M, et al. Intravenous mirtazapine is safe and effective in the treatment of depressed inpatients. *Neuropsychobiology* 2006; 53:83–87.

23. Guclu S, et al. Mirtazapine use in resistant hyperemesis gravidarum: report of three cases and review of the literature. *ArchGynecolObstet* 2005; 272:298–300.

24. Schwarzer V, et al. Treatment resistant hyperemesis gravidarum in a patient with type 1 diabetes mellitus: neonatal withdrawal symptoms after successful antiemetic therapy with mirtazapine. *Arch Gynecol Obstet* 2008; 277:67–69.

25. Collins JJ, et al. Intravenous amitriptyline in pediatrics. *J Pain SymptomManage* 1995; 10:471–475.

26. RX List. Elavil. 2021; http://www.rxlist.com.

27. Koran LM, et al. Pulse loading versus gradual dosing of intravenous clomipramine in obsessive-compulsive disorder. *Eur Neuropsychopharmacol* 1998; 8:121–126.

28. Vieta E, et al. Intravenous vortioxetine to accelerate onset of effect in major depressive disorder: a 2-week, randomized, double-blind, placebo-controlled study. *Int Clin Psychopharmacol* 2019; 34:153–160.

29. Moukaddam NJ, et al. Intravenous antidepressants: a review. *Depress Anxiety* 2004; 19:1–9.

30. Murrough JW, et al. Antidepressant efficacy of ketamine in treatment-resistant major depression: a two-site randomized controlled trial. *Am J Psychiatry* 2013; 170:1134–1142.

31. Lapidus KA, et al. A randomized controlled trial of intranasal ketamine in major depressive disorder. *Biol Psychiatry* 2014; 76:970–976.

32. Loo CK, et al. Placebo-controlled pilot trial testing dose titration and intravenous, intramuscular and subcutaneous routes for ketamine in depression. *Acta Psychiatr Scand* 2016; 134:48–56.

33. George D, et al. Pilot randomized controlled trial of titrated subcutaneous ketamine in older patients with treatment-resistant depression. *Am J Geriatr Psychiatry* 2017; 25:1199–1209.

34. Lara DR, et al. Antidepressant, mood stabilizing and procognitive effects of very low dose sublingual ketamine in refractory unipolar and bipolar depression. *Int J Neuropsychopharmacol* 2013; 16:2111–2117.

35. Nguyen L, et al. Off-label use of transmucosal ketamine as a rapid-acting antidepressant: a retrospective chart review. *Neuropsychiatr Dis Treat* 2015; 11:2667–2673.

36. Jaffe RJ, et al. Scopolamine as an antidepressant: a systematic review. *Clin Neuropharmacol* 2013; 36:24–26.

37. Furey ML, et al. Pulsed intravenous administration of scopolamine produces rapid antidepressant effects and modest side effects. *J Clin Psychiatry* 2013; 74:850–851.

38. Drevets WC, et al. Replication of scopolamine's antidepressant efficacy in major depressive disorder: a randomized, placebo-controlled clinical trial. *Biol Psychiatry* 2010; 67:432–438.

39. Gerner P, et al. Topical amitriptyline in healthy volunteers. *Reg Anesth Pain Med* 2003; 28:289–293.

40. Ho KY, et al. Topical amitriptyline versus lidocaine in the treatment of neuropathic pain. *Clin J Pain* 2008; 24:51–55.

41. Melero A, et al. Nortriptyline for smoking cessation: release and human skin diffusion from patches. *Int J Pharm* 2009; 378:101–107.

42. Sandig AG, et al. Transdermal delivery of imipramine and doxepin from newly oil-in-water nanoemulsions for an analgesic and anti-allodynic activity: development, characterization and in vivo evaluation. *Colloids SurfB Biointerfaces* 2013; 103:558–565.

43. Sunderland T, et al. High-dose selegiline in treatment-resistant older depressive patients. *Arch Gen Psychiatry* 1994; 51:607–615.

44. Mann JJ, et al. A controlled study of the antidepressant efficacy and side effects of (-)-deprenyl. A selective monoamine oxidase inhibitor. *Arch Gen Psychiatry* 1989; 46:45–50.

45. Viatris. EMSAM®* (selegiline transdermal system). 2021; https://www.viatris.com/en-us/lm/countryhome/us-products/productcatalog/productdetails?id=bcd487dc-1180-48d3-a0ca-4ac8927c6980.

46. Wecker L, et al. Transdermal selegiline: targeted effects on monoamine oxidases in the brain. *Biol Psychiatry* 2003; 54:1099–1104.

47. Azzaro AJ, et al. Pharmacokinetics and absolute bioavailability of selegiline following treatment of healthy subjects with the selegiline transdermal system (6 mg/24 h): a comparison with oral selegiline capsules. *J Clin Pharmacol* 2007; 47:1256–1267.

48. Amsterdam JD, et al. Selegiline transdermal system in the prevention of relapse of major depressive disorder: a 52-week, double-blind, placebo-substitution, parallel-group clinical trial. *J Clin Psychopharmacol* 2006; 26:579–586.

49. Adams S. Amitriptyline suppositories. *N Engl J Med* 1982; 306:996.

50. Mirassou MM. Rectal antidepressant medication in the treatment of depression. *J Clin Psychiatry* 1998; 59:29.

51. Storey P, et al. Rectal doxepin and carbamazepine therapy in patients with cancer. *N Engl J Med* 1992; 327:1318–1319.

52. Chaumeil JC, et al. Formulation of suppositories containing imipramine and clomipramine chlorhydrates. *Drug Dev Ind Pharm* 1988; 15–17:2225–2239.

53. Leung JG, et al. Rectal bioavailability of sertraline tablets in a critically ill patient with bowel compromise. *J Clin Psychopharmacol* 2017; 37:372–373.

54. Lopes R, et al. The utility of intravenous clomipramine in a case of Cotard's syndrome. *Rev Bras Psiquiatr* 2013; 35:212–213.

55. Fallon BA, et al. Intravenous clomipramine for obsessive-compulsive disorder refractory to oral clomipramine: a placebo-controlled study. *Arch Gen Psychiatry* 1998; 55:918–924.

56. Karameh WK, et al. Intravenous clomipramine for treatment-resistant obsessive-compulsive disorder. *Int J Neuropsychopharmacol* 2015; 19:pyv084.

57. Buoli M, et al. Is trazodone more effective than clomipramine in major depressed outpatients? A single-blind study with intravenous and oral administration. *CNS Spectr* 2019; 24:258–264.

58. Maragakis BP. A double-blind comparison of oral amitriptyline and low-dose intramuscular flupenthixol decanoate in depressive illness. *Curr Med Res Opin* 1990; 12:51–57.

59. Nandagopal JJ, et al. Selegiline transdermal system: a novel treatment option for major depressive disorder. *Exp Opin Pharmacother* 2009; 10:1665–1673.

CHAPTER 3

Antidepressant prophylaxis

First episode

A single episode of depression should be treated for at least 6–9 months after full remission.[1] If antidepressant therapy is stopped immediately on recovery, 50% of patients experience a return of depressive symptoms within 3–6 months.[1] A landmark study of fluoxetine maintenance[2] demonstrated that stopping successful treatment at 12 weeks gave the worst relapse outcome, followed by withdrawal at 26 weeks and then withdrawal at 50 weeks (at which point placebo and active treatment did not differ in respect to relapse risk). Another trial suggested that withdrawal should only be attempted when patients had been 'free of significant symptoms for 16–20 weeks'[3] Even non-continuous use of antidepressants during the first 6 months of treatment predicts higher rates of relapse.[4]

Recurrent depression

Major depressive disorder is unremitting in 15% of cases and recurrent in 35%. About half of those with a first-onset episode recover and have no further episodes.[5] Many factors are known to increase the risk of recurrence, including a family history of depression, recurrent dysthymia, concurrent non-affective psychiatric illness, female gender, long episode duration, degree of treatment resistance,[6] chronic medical illness and social factors (e.g. lack of confiding relationships and psychosocial stressors). Some prescription drugs may precipitate depression.[6,7]

Figure 3.5 outlines the risk of recurrence for multiple-episode patients: those recruited to the study had already experienced at least three episodes of depression, with 3 years or less between episodes.[8,9] People with depression are at increased risk of cardiovascular disease.[10] Suicide mortality is significantly increased over population norms.

A meta-analysis of antidepressant continuation studies[11] concluded that continuing treatment with antidepressants reduces the odds of depressive relapse by around

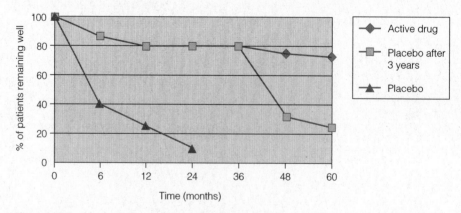

Figure 3.5 The risk of recurrence of depression in multi-episode patients. Patients had experienced at least three episodes of depression with 3 years or less between episodes

two-thirds, which is approximately equal to halving the absolute risk. A later meta-analysis of 54 studies produced almost exactly the same results: odds of relapse were reduced by 65%.[12] The risk of relapse is greatest in the first few months after discontinuation; this holds true irrespective of the duration of prior treatment.[13] Benefits persist at 36 months and beyond and seem to be similar across heterogeneous patient groups (first episode, multiple episode and chronic), although none of the studies included first-episode patients only. Specific studies in first-episode patients are required to confirm that treatment beyond 6–9 months confers additional benefit in this patient group. Most data are for non-elderly adults.

An RCT of maintenance treatment in elderly patients, many of whom were first episode, found continuation treatment with antidepressants beneficial over 2 years with a similar effect size to that seen in adults.[14] One small RCT ($n = 22$) demonstrated benefit from prophylactic antidepressants in adolescents.[15]

Many patients who might benefit from maintenance treatment with antidepressants do not receive them.[16] Assuring optimal management of long-term depression vastly reduces mortality associated with the condition.[17]

A minority view is that the prophylactic effects of antidepressants have been overestimated because of confounding in maintenance trials – effective drug treatment may be abruptly withdrawn, and it is the manner of this withdrawal (not necessarily the withdrawal itself) which increases the risk of relapse.[18,19] Thus, at least part of the advantage seen for continuation treatment is derived from suboptimal treatment in patients switched to placebo. More recent studies employ longer periods (a month or more) of withdrawal from active treatment,[20] but even this may not be long enough to allow complete abolition of the negative effects of withdrawal.[21] There is also a minority school of thought which posits that antidepressant may ultimately worsen the conditions they treat.[22] Some support for this theory comes from the observation that response to antidepressant reduces in line with the number of antidepressants previously prescribed.[23]

Other potential disadvantages of long-term antidepressants include an increased risk of GI and cerebral haemorrhage (see section on 'SSRIs and bleeding' in this chapter) and an additional risk of interaction with co-prescribed drugs likely to increase risk of bleeding or hyponatraemia.

These observations, alongside awareness that maintenance trials have been conducted largely in those in remission, strongly suggest that antidepressant treatment should be continued only where there is clear evidence of substantial efficacy. This may seem like an obvious point but clinical experience suggests that long-term, ineffective or partially effective antidepressant treatment is commonplace. The aim treatment should be the achieving and maintenance of remission. Residual symptoms portend poor outcome and higher risk of relapse.[24]

NICE recommend that:[25]

- Patients who have had two or more episodes of depression in the recent past, and who have experienced significant functional impairment during these episodes, should be advised to continue antidepressants for at least two years.
- Patients on maintenance treatment should be re-evaluated, taking into account age, co-morbid conditions and other risk factors in the decision to continue maintenance treatment beyond two years.

Dose for prophylaxis

Adults should receive the same dose as used for acute treatment.[26] There is some evidence to support the use of lower doses in elderly patients: dosulepin 75mg/day offers effective prophylaxis[27] but is now rarely used and is reserved for specialist use. There is no evidence to support the use of lower than standard doses of SSRIs.[28]

Relapse rates after ECT are similar to those after stopping antidepressants.[29] Antidepressant prophylaxis will be required, ideally with a different drug from the one that failed to get the patient well in the first instance, although good data in this area are lacking.

Lithium also have some efficacy in the prophylaxis of unipolar depression; efficacy relative to antidepressants is unknown.[30] However, lithium treatment has been shown to be associated with the best outcomes of any treatment for unipolar depression.[31] NICE recommend that lithium should not be used as the sole prophylactic drug in unipolar depression.[25] There is some support for the use of a combination of lithium and nortriptyline.[32]

Maintenance treatment with lithium protects against suicide.[26]

Key points that patients should know

- A single episode of depression should be treated for 6–9 months after remission.
- The risk of recurrence of depressive illness is high and increases with each episode.
- Those who have had multiple episodes may require treatment for many years.
- The chances of staying well are greatly increased by taking antidepressants.
- Antidepressants are:
  - effective
  - not addictive (although withdrawal symptoms can be expected)
  - not known to lose their efficacy over time
  - not known to cause new long-term side-effects.
- Medication needs to be continued at the treatment dose. If side effects are intolerable, it may be possible to find a more suitable alternative.
- If patients decide to stop their medication, this must not be done abruptly, as this may lead to unpleasant discontinuation effects (see 'Antidepressant withdrawal symptoms' in this chapter) and confers a higher risk of relapse.[33] The medication needs to be reduced slowly under specialist supervision.[21]

References

1. Cleare A, et al. Evidence-based guidelines for treating depressive disorders with antidepressants: a revision of the 2008 British Association for Psychopharmacology guidelines. *J Psychopharmacology* 2015; **29**:459–525.

2. Reimherr FW, et al. Optimal length of continuation therapy in depression: a prospective assessment during long-term fluoxetine treatment. *Am J Psychiatry* 1998; **155**:1247–1253.

3. Prien RF, et al. Continuation drug therapy for major depressive episodes: how long should it be maintained? *Am J Psychiatry* 1986; **143**:18–23.

4. Kim KH, et al. The effects of continuous antidepressant treatment during the first 6months on relapse or recurrence of depression. *J Affect Disord* 2011; **132**:121–129.

5. Eaton WW, et al. Population-based study of first onset and chronicity in major depressive disorder. *Arch Gen Psychiatry* 2008; **65**:513–520.

6. National Institute for Health and Clinical Excellence. Depression in adults with a chronic physical health problem: recognition and management. Clinical Guidance [CG91]. 2009; http://www.nice.org.uk/CG91.

7. Patten SB, et al. Drug-induced depression. *Psychother Psychosom* 1997; **66**:63–73.

8. Frank E, et al. Three-year outcomes for maintenance therapies in recurrent depression. *Arch Gen Psychiatry* 1990; **47**:1093–1099.

9. Kupfer DJ, et al. Five-year outcome for maintenance therapies in recurrent depression. *Arch Gen Psychiatry* 1992; **49**:769–773.

10. Taylor D. Antidepressant drugs and cardiovascular pathology: a clinical overview of effectiveness and safety. *Acta Psychiatr Scand* 2008; **118**:434–442.

11. Geddes JR, et al. Relapse prevention with antidepressant drug treatment in depressive disorders: a systematic review. *Lancet* 2003; **361**:653–661.

12. Glue P, et al. Meta-analysis of relapse prevention antidepressant trials in depressive disorders. *Aust N Z J Psychiatry* 2010; **44**:697–705.

13. Keller MB, et al. The prevention of recurrent episodes of depression with venlafaxine for two years (PREVENT) study: outcomes from the 2-year and combined maintenance phases. *J Clin Psychiatry* 2007; **68**:1246–1256.

14. Reynolds CF, III, et al. Maintenance treatment of major depression in old age. *N Engl J Med* 2006; **354**:1130–1138.

15. Cheung A, et al. Maintenance study for adolescent depression. *J Child Adolesc Psychopharmacol* 2008; **18**:389–394.

16. Holma IA, et al. Maintenance pharmacotherapy for recurrent major depressive disorder: 5-year follow-up study. *Br J Psychiatry* 2008; **193**:163–164.

17. Gallo JJ, et al. Long term effect of depression care management on mortality in older adults: follow-up of cluster randomized clinical trial in primary care. *BMJ* 2013; **346**:f2570.

18. Cohen D, et al. Withdrawal effects confounding in clinical trials: another sign of a needed paradigm shift in psychopharmacology research. *Ther Adv Psychopharmacol* 2020; **10**:2045125320964097.

19. Hengartner MP. Editorial: antidepressant prescriptions in children and adolescents. *Front Psychiatry* 2020; **11**:600283.

20. DeRubeis RJ, et al. Prevention of recurrence after recovery from a major depressive episode with antidepressant medication alone or in combination with cognitive behavioral therapy: phase 2 of a 2-phase randomized clinical trial. *JAMA Psychiatry* 2020; **77**:237–245.

21. Horowitz MA, et al. Tapering of SSRI treatment to mitigate withdrawal symptoms. *Lancet Psychiatry* 2019; **6**:538–546.

22. Fava GA. May antidepressant drugs worsen the conditions they are supposed to treat? The clinical foundations of the oppositional model of tolerance. *Ther Adv Psychopharmacol* 2020; **10**:2045125320970325.

23. Amsterdam JD, et al. Prior antidepressant treatment trials may predict a greater risk of depressive relapse during antidepressant maintenance therapy. *J Clin Psychopharmacol* 2019; **39**:344–350.

24. Kennedy N, et al. Residual symptoms at remission from depression: impact on long-term outcome. *J Affect Disord* 2004; **80**:135–144.

25. National Institute for Clinical Excellence. Depression: the treatment and management of depression in adults. Clinical Guidance [CG90]; 2009 (last reviewed December 2013); https://www.nice.org.uk/guidance/cg90.

26. Anderson IM, et al. Evidence-based guidelines for treating depressive disorders with antidepressants: a revision of the 2000 British Association for Psychopharmacology guidelines. *J Psychopharmacology* 2008; **22**:343–396.

27. Old Age Depression Interest Group. How long should the elderly take antidepressants? A double-blind placebo-controlled study of continuation/prophylaxis therapy with dothiepin. *Br J Psychiatry* 1993; **162**:175–182.

28. Franchini L, et al. Dose-response efficacy of paroxetine in preventing depressive recurrences: a randomized, double-blind study. *J Clin Psychiatry* 1998; **59**:229–232.

29. Nobler MS, et al. *Refractory depression and electroconvulsive therapy*. Chichester: John Wiley & Sons Ltd; 1994.

30. Cipriani A, et al. Lithium versus antidepressants in the long-term treatment of unipolar affective disorder. *Cochrane Database Syst Rev* 2006; CD003492.

31. Young AH. Lithium for long-term treatment of unipolar depression. *Lancet Psychiatry* 2017; **4**:511–512.

32. Sackeim HA, et al. Continuation pharmacotherapy in the prevention of relapse following electroconvulsive therapy: a randomized controlled trial. *JAMA* 2001; **285**:1299–1307.

33. Baldessarini RJ, et al. Illness risk following rapid versus gradual discontinuation of antidepressants. *Am J Psychiatry* 2010; **167**:934–941.

CHAPTER 3

Drug interactions with antidepressants

Drugs can interact with each other in two different ways:

- **Pharmacokinetic interactions** where one drug interferes with the absorption, distribution, metabolism or elimination of another drug. This may result in a subtherapeutic effect or toxicity. The largest group of pharmacokinetic interactions involves drugs that inhibit or induce hepatic CYP450 enzymes (see Tables 3.14 and 3.15). Other enzyme systems include FMO[1] and UGT.[2] While both of these latter enzyme systems are involved in the metabolism of psychotropic drugs, the potential for drugs to inhibit or induce these enzyme systems has been less well studied.

The clinical consequences of pharmacokinetic interactions in an individual patient can be difficult to predict. Some are highly clinically significant; for example, when paroxetine (a potent *CYP2D6* inhibitor) is taken with tamoxifen, up to 1 extra woman in 20 will die within 5 years of stopping tamoxifen.[3] The following factors affect outcome of interactions: the degree of enzyme inhibition or induction, the pharmacokinetic properties of the affected drug and other co-administered drugs, the relationship between plasma level and pharmacodynamic effect for the affected drug, and patient-specific factors such as variability in the role of primary and secondary metabolic pathways and the presence of co-morbid physical illness.[4]

Table 3.14 Summary of antidepressant effects on CYP enzymes[5–7]

Antidepressant		Substrate for	Inhibits
SSRIs			
	Citalopram	*CYP2C19*, CYP2D6, CYP3A4	CYP2D6 (weak)
	Escitalopram	*CYP2C19*, CYP2D6, CYP3A4	CYP2D6 (weak)
	Fluoxetine	*CYP2D6*, CYP3A4	*CYP2D6 (moderate to potent)*, CYP2C9 (moderate), CYP3A4 (weak)
	Fluvoxamine	*CYP2D6*; others possibly involved	*CYP1A2* (potent), *CYP2C19* (potent), CYP3A4 (weak), CYP2C9 (weak)
	Paroxetine	*CYP2D6*	*CYP2D6* (potent)
	Sertraline	*CYP3A4*, CYP2D6 (minor) and possibly other pathways	*CYP2D6* (weak)
SNRIs			
	Desvenlafaxine	*CYP3A4*	CYP2D6 (weak)
	Duloxetine	*CYP1A2, CYP2D6*	CYP2D6 (moderate)
	Levomilnacipran	*CYP3A4*, CYP2C8, CYP2C19, CYP2D6	
	Venlafaxine	*CYP2D6*, CYP3A4	CYP2D6 (weak)

(Continued)

Table 3.14 (Continued)

Antidepressant		Substrate for	Inhibits
TCAs			
	Amitriptyline	**CYP1A2, CYP2D6,** CYP3A4, CYP2C19	
	Clomipramine		
	Desipramine	**CYP2D6**	
	Dosulepin	CYP2D6 and possibly other pathways	
	Doxepin	CYP2D6, CYP1A2 (minor), CYP3A4 (minor)	
	Imipramine	**CYP1A2, CYP2D6,** CYP3A4, CYP2C19	
	Nortriptyline	**CYP2D6**	
	Trimipramine	**CYP2D6**	
Others			
	Agomelatine	**CYP1A2**	
	Bupropion	**CYP2B6**	**CYP2D6 (potent)**
	Esketamine	**CYP3A4, CYP2B6**	
	Mianserin	CYP2D6	
	Mirtazapine	CYP1A2, CYP2D6, CYP3A4	CYP2D6 (weak)
	Reboxetine	**CYP3A4**	
	Trazodone	**CYP3A4**	
	Vortioxetine	**CYP2D6,** CYP2A6, CYP2B6, CYP2C8, CYP2C9, CYP2C19, CYP3A4	
	Vilazodone	**CYP3A4**	CYP2C8

CYP enzymes highlighted in **bold** indicate:
- predominant metabolic enzyme pathway or
- predominant enzyme activity.

- **Pharmacodynamic interactions** where the effects of one drug are altered by another drug via physiological mechanisms such as direct competition at receptor sites (e.g. dopamine agonists with dopamine blockers may negate any therapeutic effect), augmentation of the same neurotransmitter pathway (e.g. fluoxetine with tramadol or a triptan can lead to serotonin syndrome) or an effect on the physiological functioning of an organ/organ system in different ways (e.g. SSRIs impair clotting and NSAIDs irritate the gastric mucosa so when these drugs are used together, the risk of GI bleeds is increased). Up-to-date interaction tables are readily available online and most known interactions are described in an individual product's literature.

Pharmacodynamic interactions

Tricyclic antidepressants[7–10]

- are H_1 blockers (sedative). This effect can be exacerbated by other sedative drugs or alcohol. Beware respiratory depression

- are anticholinergic (dry mouth, blurred vision, constipation). This effect can be exacerbated by other anticholinergic drugs such as antihistamines or antipsychotics. Beware cognitive impairment and gastrointestinal obstruction
- are adrenergic α_1 blockers (postural hypotension). This effect can be exacerbated by other drugs that block α_1-receptors and by antihypertensive drugs in general. Beware falls. Adrenaline in combination with α_1-blockers can lead to hypertension
- are arrhythmogenic. Caution is required with other drugs that can alter cardiac conduction directly or indirectly. See section on 'Antidepressant-induced arrhythmia' in this chapter
- lower the seizure threshold. Caution is required with other proconvulsive drugs (e.g. antipsychotics) and particularly if the patient is being treated for epilepsy. See section on 'Epilepsy' (Chapter 10)
- possess varying degrees of serotonin reuptake inhibition (e.g. imipramine and clomipramine in particular). There is the potential for these drugs to interact with other serotonergic drugs (e.g. tramadol, SSRIs, MAOIs, triptans) to cause serotonin syndrome

SSRIs/SNRIs[7–9,11,12]

- increase serotonergic neurotransmission. The main concern when co-prescribed with other serotonergic drugs is serotonin syndrome
- inhibit platelet aggregation and increase the risk of bleeding, particularly of the upper GI tract. This effect is exacerbated by aspirin and NSAIDs (see section on 'SSRIs and bleeding' in this chapter)
- may be more likely than other antidepressants to cause hyponatraemia (see section on 'Antidepressant-induced hyponatraemia' in this chapter). This may exacerbate electrolyte disturbances caused by other drugs such as diuretics.
- may cause osteopenia. This adds to the negative effects prolactin elevating drugs have on bone mineral density and increases the risks of clinical harm should the patient have a fall.

MAOIs[13,14]

- prevent the destruction of monoamine neurotransmitters (e.g. serotonin). Co-prescription with serotonergic drugs (in particular, sertonin reuptake inhibitors or releasing agents) risks potentially fatal serotonin syndrome. Examples include SSRI and related antidepressants but also certain over-the-counter medicines (e.g. chlorphenamine, dextromethorphan), opioids (e.g. tramadol, pethidine) and drugs of misuse (e.g. MDMA)
- prevent the destruction of other monoamine neurotransmitters (e.g. catecholamines). Co-prescription with sympathomimetic drugs that raise blood pressure (e.g. psychostimulants) can cause hypertensive crises. MAOIs also prevent the breakdown of dietary tyramine (high levels present in aged and fermented foods), which acts as a catecholamine releasing agent leading to similar hypertensive reactions

Table 3.15 Pharmacokinetic interactions – a brief summary of important interactions[3,15]

CYP1A2	CYP2B6	CYP2C9	CYP2C19	CYP2D6	CYP3A4/5/7
Genetic polymorphism Ultra-rapid metabolisers possible	2–10% of total hepatic CYP content[16]	5–10% of Caucasians poor metabolisers	~20% of Asians and 3–5% Caucasians are poor metabolisers	3–5% of Caucasians poor metabolisers	60% p450 content
Induced by:	*Induced by:*	*Induced by:*	*Induced by:*	*Induced by:*	*Induced by:*
Carbamazepine Charcoal cooking Tobacco smoke Omeprazole Phenobarbital Phenytoin	Carbamazepine Efavirenz Lopinavir Rifampicin Ritonavir	Phenytoin Rifampicin	Apalutamide Rifampicin Enzalutamide Artemisinin Efavirenz	Carbamazepine Phenytoin	Carbamazepine Phenytoin Prednisolone Rifampicin
Inhibited by:	*Inhibited by:*	*Inhibited by:*	*Inhibited by:*	*Inhibited by:*	*Inhibited by:*
Cimetidine Ciprofloxacin Erythromycin Fluvoxamine	Clopidogrel Ticlopidine Voriconazole	Cimetidine Fluoxetine Fluvoxamine Moclobemide Sertraline	Fluconazole Fluoxetine Fluvoxamine Esomeprazole Moclobemide Omeprazole Voriconazole Armodafinil Etravirine Isoniazid Modafinil Cimetidine	Chlorpromazine Bupropion Duloxetine Fluoxetine Fluphenazine Haloperidol Paroxetine Sertraline Tricyclics	Erythromycin Fluoxetine Fluvoxamine Grapefruit Juice Ketoconazole Norfluoxetine Paroxetine Sertraline Tricyclics
Metabolises:	*Metabolises:*	*Metabolises:*	*Metabolises:*	*Metabolises:*	*Metabolises:*
Agomelatine Benzodiazepines Caffeine Clozapine Duloxetine Haloperidol Mirtazapine Olanzapine Ramelteon Theophylline Tizanidine Tricyclics Warfarin	Bupropion Methadone Tramadol	Agomelatine Bupropion Citalopram Diazepam Omeprazole Phenytoin Tricyclics Warfarin	Citalopram Diazepam Moclobemide	Clozapine Codeine Donepezil Duloxetine Haloperidol Phenothiazines Risperidone Tamoxifen Tricyclics Tramadol Trazodone Venlafaxine Vortioxetine	Calcium Blockers Carbamazepine Clozapine Donepezil Erythromycin Galantamine Methadone Levomilnacipran Mirtazapine Reboxetine Risperidone Statins Tricyclics Valproate Venlafaxine Vilazodone Vortioxetine Z-hypnotics

CHAPTER 3

Overall

Avoid/minimise problems by:

- where antidepressant polypharmacy is used, select drugs that are safer to use together and monitor carefully for side effects when the second antidepressant is initiated
- avoiding the co-prescription of other drugs with a similar pharmacology but not marketed as antidepressants (e.g. atomoxetine, bupropion)

References

1. Cashman JR. Human flavin-containing monooxygenase: substrate specificity and role in drug metabolism. *Curr Drug Metabol* 2000; 1:181–191.
2. Anderson GD. A mechanistic approach to antiepileptic drug interactions. *Ann Pharmacother* 1998; 32:554–563.
3. Kelly CM, et al. Selective serotonin reuptake inhibitors and breast cancer mortality in women receiving tamoxifen: a population based cohort study. *BMJ* 2010; 340:c693.
4. Devane CL. Antidepressant-drug interactions are potentially but rarely clinically significant. *Neuropsychopharmacology* 2006; 31:1594–1604.
5. Andrade C. Ketamine for depression, 5: potential pharmacokinetic and pharmacodynamic drug interactions. *J Clin Psychiatry* 2017; 78:e858–e861.
6. Preskorn SH. Drug-drug interactions (DDIs) in psychiatric practice, part 9: interactions mediated by drug-metabolizing cytochrome P450 enzymes. *J Psychiatr Pract* 2020; 26:126–134.
7. Medicines Complete. Stockley's drug interactions. 2020; https://www.medicinescomplete.com.
8. Preskorn SH. Drug-drug interactions (DDIs) in psychiatric practice, part 8: relative receptor binding affinity as a way of understanding the differential pharmacology of currently available antidepressants. *J Psychiatr Pract* 2020; 26:46–51.
9. BNF Online. British national formulary. 2020; https://www.medicinescomplete.com/mc/bnf/current.
10. Gillman PK. Tricyclic antidepressant pharmacology and therapeutic drug interactions updated. *Br J Pharmacol* 2007; 151:737–748.
11. Preskorn SH. Drug-drug interactions (DDIs) in psychiatric practice, part 6: pharmacodynamic considerations. *J Psychiatr Pract* 2019; 25:290–297.
12. Williams LJ, et al. Selective serotonin reuptake inhibitor use and bone mineral density in women with a history of depression. *Int Clin Psychopharmacol* 2008; 23:84–87.
13. Gillman PK. Advances pertaining to the pharmacology and interactions of irreversible nonselective monoamine oxidase inhibitors. *J Clin Psychopharmacol* 2011; 31:66–74.
14. Grady MM, et al. Practical guide for prescribing MAOIs: debunking myths and removing barriers. *CNS Spectr* 2012; 17:2–10.
15. Mitchell PB. Drug interactions of clinical significance with selective serotonin reuptake inhibitors. *Drug Saf* 1997; 17:390–406.
16. Hedrich WD, et al. Insights into CYP2B6-mediated drug-drug interactions. *Acta Pharm Sin B* 2016; 6:413–425.

CHAPTER 3

Cardiac effects of antidepressants – summary

The cardiac effects of antidepressants are summarised in Table 3.16.

Table 3.16 Cardiac effect of antidepressants

Drug	Heart rate	Blood pressure	QTc	Arrhythmia	Conduction disturbance	Licensed restrictions post-MI	Comments
Agomelatine[1,2]	No changes reported	No changes reported	Single case of QTc prolongation	No arrhythmia reported	Unclear	No specific contra-indication	Cautiously recommended
Bupropion*[3-6]	Slight increase	Slight increases in blood pressure but can sometimes be significant. Rarely postural hypotension	QTc shortening, but prolongation has been reported in cases of overdose	No effect. Rare reports in overdose	None	Well tolerated for smoking cessation in post MI patients	Be aware of interaction potential. Monitor blood pressure
Citalopram[7-11] (assume same for escitalopram)	Small decrease in heart rate	Slight drop in systolic blood pressure	Dose-related increase in QTc	Torsade de Pointes reported, mainly in overdose	None	Caution in patients with recent MI or uncompensated heart failure. But some evidence of safety in CVD	Minor metabolite which increases QTc interval. No clear evidence of increased risk of arrhythmia at any licensed dose
Duloxetine[12-17]	Slight increase	Important effect (see SPC) Caution in hypertension	Isolated reports of QT prolongation	Isolated reports of toxicity	Isolated reports of toxicity	Caution in patients with 'whose conditions could be compromised by an increased heart rate or by an increase in blood pressure'	Not recommended ion cardiac disease
Fluoxetine[18-21]	Small decrease in mean heart rate	Minimal effect on blood pressure	No effect on QTc interval	None	None	Caution in patients with acute MI or uncompensated heart failure	Evidence of safety post MI
Fluvoxamine[22,23]	Minimal effect on heart rate	Small drop in systolic blood pressure	No significant effect on QTc	None	None	Caution	Limited changes in ECG have been observed

(Continued)

Table 3.16 (Continued)

Drug	Heart rate	Blood pressure	QTc	Arrhythmia	Conduction disturbance	Licensed restrictions post-MI	Comments
Levomilnacipran[24,25]	Slight increase	Small increase	No effect on QTc interval	Pre-existing tachyarrhythmias should be treated before initiating treatment	None	Caution in cardiac patients	Monitor heart rate and blood pressure
Lofepramine[26,27]	Modest increase in heart rate	Less decrease in postural blood pressure compared with other TCAs	Can possibly prolong QTc interval at higher doses	May occur at higher doses, but rare	Unclear	CI in patients with recent MI	Less cardiotoxic than other TCAs. Reasons unclear
MAOIs[26,28]	Decrease in heart rate	Postural hypotension Risk of hypertensive crisis	Unclear but may shorten QTc interval	May cause arrhythmia and decrease LVF	No clear effect on cardiac conduction	Use with caution in patients with cardiovascular disease	Not recommended in CV disease
Milnacipran[29,30]	Slight increase in heart rate (c.10 bpm)	Small increases in systolic and diastolic BP	No effect on QTc	None	None	Caution	Avoid in hypertension and heart failure
Mirtazapine[31,32]	Minimal change in heart rate	Minimal effect on blood pressure	No effect on QTc	None	None	Caution in patients with recent MI	Evidence of safety post MI. Good alternative to SSRIs
Moclobemide[33–35]	Marginal decrease in heart rate	Minimal effect on blood pressure. Isolated cases of hypertensive episodes	No effect on QTc interval in normal doses. Prolongation in overdose	None	None	General caution in patients with a history of cardiac disorders	Possibly arrhythmogenic in overdose
Paroxetine[36,37]	Small decrease in mean heart rate	Minimal effect on blood pressure	No effect on QTc interval	None	None	General caution in cardiac patients	Probably safe post MI
Reboxetine[38–40]	Significant increase in heart rate	Marginal increase in both systolic and diastolic blood pressure. Postural decrease at higher doses	No effect on QTc	Rhythm abnormalities may occur	Atrial and ventricular ectopic beats, especially in the elderly	Caution in patients with cardiac disease	Probably best avoided in coronary disease

(Continued)

Table 3.16 (Continued)

Drug	Heart rate	Blood pressure	QTc	Arrhythmia	Conduction disturbance	Licensed restrictions post-MI	Comments
Sertraline[41–45]	Minimal effect on heart rate	Minimal effect on blood pressure	No effect on QTc interval at standard doses. Small increase (<10ms) at 400mg/day.[46]	None	None	Drug of choice post MI but formal labelling acknowledges effect on QT cautions against use in patients with additional risk factors for QTc prolongation	Safe post MI and in heart failure
Trazodone[26,47,48]	Decrease in heart rate more common, although increase can also occur	Can cause significant postural hypotension	Can prolong QTc interval	Several case reports of prolonged QT and arrhythmia	Unclear	Contraindicated in patients with acute MI	May be arrhythmogenic in patients with pre-existing cardiac disease
Tricyclics[26,49–51]	Increase in heart rate	Postural hypotension	Prolongation of QTc interval and QRS interval	Ventricular arrhythmia common in overdose. Torsade de Pointes reported	Slows cardiac conduction – blocks cardiac Na/K channels	Contraindicated in patients with recent MI	TCAs affect cardiac contractility. Some TCAs linked to ischaemic heart disease and sudden cardiac death. Avoid in coronary artery disease
Venlafaxine[15,52–56] (assume same for desvenlafaxine)	Marginally increased	Some increase in postural blood pressure. At higher doses increase in blood pressure	Possible prolongation in overdose, but very rare	Rare reports of cardiac arrhythmia in overdose	Rare reports of conduction abnormalities	Has not been evaluated in post-MI patients. Caution advised	Evidence for arrhythmogenic potential is slim, but avoid in coronary disease
Vilazodone[57–59]	Increased in overdose	Increased in overdose	No effect, even in overdose	No reports, even in overdose	No effect	No specific contra-indication	Probably no effect on CV function in clinical doses
Vortioxetine[60–62]	No effect	No effect	No effect	No effect	No effect	No specific contra-indication	Trial data suggest no effect on QTc or on coagulation parameters

SSRIs are generally recommended in cardiac disease but beware anti-platelet activity and cytochrome-medicated interactions with co-administered cardiac drugs. Mirtazapine has been suggested as a suitable alternative,[32] but analysis suggests that it too is associated with bleeding disorders.[63]

SSRIs may protect against myocardial infarction,[64,65] and untreated depression worsens prognosis in cardiovascular disease.[66] Post MI, SSRIs and mirtazapine have either a neutral or beneficial effect on mortality.[67] Treatment of depression with SSRIs should not therefore be withheld post-MI. Protective effects of treatment of depression post-MI appear to relate to antidepressant administration possibly because of an anti-coagulant effect or because of indirect reduction in arrhythmia frequency.[45,68] CBT may be ineffective in this respect.[69] Note that the anti-platelet effect of SSRIs may have adverse consequences too (see section on 'SSRIs and bleeding' – this chapter).

References

1. Dolder CR, et al. Agomelatine treatment of major depressive disorder. *Ann Pharmacotherapy* 2008; **42**:1822–1831.
2. Kozian R, et al. [QTc prolongation during treatment with agomelatine]. *Psychiatr Prax* 2010; **37**:405–407.
3. Roose SP, et al. Pharmacologic treatment of depression in patients with heart disease. *Psychosom Med* 2005; **67 Suppl 1**:S54–S57.
4. Dwoskin LP, et al. Review of the pharmacology and clinical profile of bupropion, an antidepressant and tobacco use cessation agent. *CNSDrug Rev* 2006; **12**:178–207.
5. Castro VM, et al. QT interval and antidepressant use: a cross sectional study of electronic health records. *BMJ* 2013; **346**:f288.
6. Eisenberg MJ, et al. Bupropion for smoking cessation in patients hospitalized with acute myocardial infarction: a randomized, placebo-controlled trial. *J Am Coll Cardiol* 2013; **61**:524–532.
7. Rasmussen SL, et al. Cardiac safety of citalopram: prospective trials and retrospective analyses. *J Clin Psychopharmacol* 1999; **19**:407–415.
8. Catalano G, et al. QTc interval prolongation associated with citalopram overdose: a case report and literature review. *Clin Neuropharmacol* 2001; **24**:158–162.
9. Lesperance F, et al. Effects of citalopram and interpersonal psychotherapy on depression in patients with coronary artery disease: the Canadian Cardiac Randomized Evaluation of Antidepressant and Psychotherapy Efficacy (CREATE) trial. *JAMA* 2007; **297**:367–379.
10. Astrom-Lilja C, et al. Drug-induced torsades de pointes: a review of the Swedish pharmacovigilance database. *Pharmacoepidemiol Drug Saf* 2008; **17**:587–592.
11. Zivin K, et al. Evaluation of the FDA warning against prescribing citalopram at doses exceeding 40 mg. *Am J Psychiatry* 2013; **170**:642–650.
12. Sharma A, et al. Pharmacokinetics and safety of duloxetine, a dual-serotonin and norepinephrine reuptake inhibitor. *J Clin Pharmacol* 2000; **40**:161–167.
13. Schatzberg AF. Efficacy and tolerability of duloxetine, a novel dual reuptake inhibitor, in the treatment of major depressive disorder. *J Clin Psychiatry* 2003; **64 Suppl 13**:30–37.
14. Detke MJ, et al. Duloxetine, 60 mg once daily, for major depressive disorder: a randomized double-blind placebo-controlled trial. *J Clin Psychiatry* 2002; **63**:308–315.
15. Colucci VJ, et al. Heart failure worsening and exacerbation after venlafaxine and duloxetine therapy. *Ann Pharmacother* 2008; **42**:882–887.
16. Stuhec M. Duloxetine-induced life-threatening long QT syndrome. *Wien Klin Wochenschr* 2013; **125**:165–166.
17. Orozco BS, et al. Duloxetine: an uncommon cause of fatal ventricular arrhythmia. *Clin Toxicol* 2014; **51**:672–672.
18. Fisch C. Effect of fluoxetine on the electrocardiogram. *J Clin Psychiatry* 1985; **46**:42–44.
19. Ellison JM, et al. Fluoxetine-induced bradycardia and syncope in two patients. *J Clin Psychiatry* 1990; **51**:385–386.
20. Roose SP, et al. Cardiovascular effects of fluoxetine in depressed patients with heart disease. *Am J Psychiatry* 1998; **155**:660–665.
21. Strik JJ, et al. Efficacy and safety of fluoxetine in the treatment of patients with major depression after first myocardial infarction: findings from a double-blind, placebo-controlled trial. *Psychosom Med* 2000; **62**:783–789.
22. Strik JJ, et al. Cardiac side-effects of two selective serotonin reuptake inhibitors in middle-aged and elderly depressed patients. *Int Clin Psychopharmacol* 1998; **13**:263–267.
23. Stirnimann G, et al. Brugada syndrome ECG provoked by the selective serotonin reuptake inhibitor fluvoxamine. *Europace* 2010; **12**:282–283.
24. Mago R, et al. Safety and tolerability of levomilnacipran ER in major depressive disorder: results from an open-label, 48-week extension study. *Clin Drug Investig* 2013; **33**:761–771.

25. U.S. Food & Drug Administration. Highlights of Prescribing Information. Fetzima (levomilnacipran) extended-release capsules for oral use. 2019; https://www.accessdata.fda.gov/drugsatfda_docs/label/2019/204168s006lbl.pdf.

26. Warrington SJ, et al. The cardiovascular effects of antidepressants. *Psychol Med Monogr Suppl* 1989; **16**:i-40.

27. Stern H, et al. Cardiovascular effects of single doses of the antidepressants amitriptyline and lofepramine in healthy subjects. *Pharmacopsychiatry* 1985; **18**:272–277.

28. WS W, et al. Acute myocarditis after massive phenelzine overdose. *Eur J Clin Pharmacol* 2007; **63**:1007–1009.

29. Periclou A, et al. Effects of milnacipran on cardiac repolarization in healthy participants. *J Clin Pharmacol* 2010; **50**:422–433.

30. U.S Food & Drug Administration. Highlights of Prescribing Information. Savella (milnacipran HCl) Tablets. 2009; https://www.accessdata.fda.gov/drugsatfda_docs/label/2011/022256s011lbl.pdf.

31. Montgomery SA. Safety of mirtazapine: a review. *Int Clin Psychopharmacol* 1995; **10 Suppl 4**:37–45.

32. Honig A, et al. Treatment of post-myocardial infarction depressive disorder: a randomized, placebo-controlled trial with mirtazapine. *Psychosom Med* 2007; **69**:606–613.

33. Moll E, et al. Safety and efficacy during long-term treatment with moclobemide. *Clin Neuropharmacol* 1994; **17 Suppl 1**:S74–S87.

34. Hilton S, et al. Moclobemide safety: monitoring a newly developed product in the 1990s. *J Clin Psychopharmacol* 1995; **15**:76S–83S.

35. Downes MA, et al. QTc abnormalities in deliberate self-poisoning with moclobemide. *Intern Med J* 2005; **35**:388–391.

36. Kuhs H, et al. Cardiovascular effects of paroxetine. *Psychopharmacology (Berl)* 1990; **102**:379–382.

37. Roose SP, et al. Comparison of paroxetine and nortriptyline in depressed patients with ischemic heart disease. *JAMA* 1998; **279**:287–291.

38. Mucci M. Reboxetine: a review of antidepressant tolerability. *J Psychopharmacology* 1997; **11**:S33–S37.

39. KJ H, et al. Reboxetine: a review of its use in depression. *CNS Drugs* 1999; **12**:65–83.

40. Fleishaker JC, et al. Lack of effect of reboxetine on cardiac repolarization. *Clin Pharmacol Ther* 2001; **70**:261–269.

41. Shapiro PA, et al. An open-label preliminary trial of sertraline for treatment of major depression after acute myocardial infarction (the SADHAT Trial). Sertraline Anti-Depressant Heart Attack Trial. *Am Heart J* 1999; **137**:1100–1106.

42. Glassman AH, et al. Sertraline treatment of major depression in patients with acute MI or unstable angina. *JAMA* 2002; **288**:701–709.

43. Winkler D, et al. Trazodone-induced cardiac arrhythmias: a report of two cases. *Human Psychopharmacology* 2006; **21**:61–62.

44. Jiang W, et al. Safety and efficacy of sertraline for depression in patients with CHF (SADHART-CHF): a randomized, double-blind, placebo-controlled trial of sertraline for major depression with congestive heart failure. *Am Heart J* 2008; **156**:437–444.

45. Leftheriotis D, et al. The role of the selective serotonin re-uptake inhibitor sertraline in nondepressive patients with chronic ischemic heart failure: a preliminary study. *Pacing Clin Electrophysiol* 2010; **33**:1217–1223.

46. Abbas R, et al. A thorough QT study to evaluate the effects of a supratherapeutic dose of sertraline on cardiac repolarization in healthy subjects. *Clin Pharmacol Drug Develop* 2020; **9**:307–320.

47. JA S, et al. QT Prolongation and delayed atrioventricular conduction caused by acute ingestion of trazodone. *Clin Toxicol (Phila)* 2008; **46**:71–73.

48. Dattilo PB, et al. Prolonged QT associated with an overdose of trazodone. *J Clin Psychiatry* 2007; **68**:1309–1310.

49. Hippisley-Cox J, et al. Antidepressants as risk factor for ischaemic heart disease: case-control study in primary care. *BMJ* 2001; **323**:666–669.

50. Whyte IM, et al. Relative toxicity of venlafaxine and selective serotonin reuptake inhibitors in overdose compared to tricyclic antidepressants. *QJM* 2003; **96**:369–374.

51. van Noord C, et al. Psychotropic drugs associated with corrected QT interval prolongation. *J Clin Psychopharmacol* 2009; **29**:9–15.

52. Khawaja IS, et al. Cardiovascular effects of selective serotonin reuptake inhibitors and other novel antidepressants. *Heart Dis* 2003; **5**:153–160.

53. Pfizer Limited. Summary of product characteristics. Efexor XL 75 mg hard prolonged release capsules. https://www.medicines.org.uk/2013.

54. Letsas K, et al. QT interval prolongation associated with venlafaxine administration. *Int J Cardiol* 2006; **109**:116–117.

55. Taylor D, et al. Volte-face on venlafaxine–reasons and reflections. *Journal of Psychopharmacology* 2006; **20**:597–601.

56. Cooper JM, et al. Desvenlafaxine overdose and the occurrence of serotonin toxicity, seizures and cardiovascular effects. *Clin Toxicol (Phila)* 2017; **55**:18–24.

57. Edwards J, et al. Vilazodone lacks proarrhythmogenic potential in healthy participants: a thorough ECG study. *Int J Clin Pharmacol Ther* 2013; **51**:456–465.

58. Heise CW, et al. A review of vilazodone exposures with focus on serotonin syndrome effects. *Clin Toxicol (Phila)* 2017; **55**:1004–1007.

59. Gaw CE, et al. Evaluation of dose and outcomes for pediatric vilazodone ingestions. *Clin Toxicol (Phila)* 2018; **56**:113–119.

60. Citrome L. Vortioxetine for major depressive disorder: a systematic review of the efficacy and safety profile for this newly approved antidepressant – what is the number needed to treat, number needed to harm and likelihood to be helped or harmed? *Int J Clin Pract* 2014; **68**:60–82.

61. Takeda Pharmaceuticals America Inc. Highlights of prescribing information. BRINTELLIX (vortioxetine) tablets. 2014; http://www.us.brintellix.com.

62. Baldwin DS, et al. The safety and tolerability of vortioxetine: analysis of data from randomized placebo-controlled trials and open-label extension studies. *J Psychopharmacology* 2016; **30**:242–252.

63. Na K-S, et al. Can we recommend mirtazapine and bupropion for patients at risk for bleeding?: a systematic review and meta-analysis. *J Affect Disord* 2018; **225**:221–226.

64. Alqdwah-Fattouh R, et al. Differential effects of antidepressant subgroups on risk of acute myocardial infarction: a nested case-control study. *Br J Clin Pharmacol* 2020; **86**:2040–2050.

65. Sauer WH, et al. Selective serotonin reuptake inhibitors and myocardial infarction. *Circulation* 2001; **104**:1894–1898.

66. Davies SJ, et al. Treatment of anxiety and depressive disorders in patients with cardiovascular disease. *BMJ* 2004; **328**:939–943.

67. Taylor D, et al. Pharmacological interventions for people with depression and chronic physical health problems: systematic review and meta-analyses of safety and efficacy. *British J Psychiatry* 2011; **198**:179–188.

68. Chen S, et al. Serotonin and catecholaminergic polymorphic ventricular tachycardia: a possible therapeutic role for SSRIs? *Cardiovasc J Afr* 2010; **21**:225–228.

69. Berkman LF, et al. Effects of treating depression and low perceived social support on clinical events after myocardial infarction: the Enhancing Recovery in Coronary Heart Disease Patients (ENRICHD) Randomized Trial. *JAMA* 2003; **289**:3106–3116.

Antidepressant-induced arrhythmia

Depression confers an increased risk of cardiovascular disease[1] and sudden cardiac death[2] perhaps because of platelet activation,[3] decreased heart rate variability,[4] reduced physical activity,[5] an association with an increased risk of diabetes and/or other factors.

Tricyclic antidepressants (TCAs) have established arrhythmogenic activity which arises as a result of potent blockade of cardiac sodium channels and variable activity at potassium channels.[6] ECG changes produced include PR, QRS and QT prolongation and the Brugada syndrome.[7] Normal clinical use of nortriptyline has been associated in one study with an increased risk of cardiac arrest,[8] although a large cohort study did not confirm this finding.[9] **Lofepramine**, for reasons unknown, seems to lack the over-dose arrhythmogenicity of other TCAs, despite its major metabolite, desipramine, being a potent potassium channel blocker.[10] Oddly, in one study,[11] clinical use of lofepramine was associated with an increased risk of myocardial infarction, whereas other antide-pressants were not. In patients taking tricyclics, ECG monitoring is a more meaningful and useful measure of toxicity than plasma level monitoring.

There is limited evidence that **venlafaxine** is a sodium channel antagonist[12] and a weak antagonist at hERG potassium channels. Arrhythmia is a rare occurrence even after massive overdose,[13-16] and ECG changes no more common than with SSRIs.[17] No ECG changes are seen in therapeutic dosing,[18] and sudden cardiac death in clinical use is no more common than with fluoxetine or citalopram.[9,19] **Desvenlafaxine** does not appear to prolong QT even in overdose.[20]

Moclobemide,[21] **citalopram**,[22,23] **escitalopram**,[24] **bupropion** (amfebutamone),[25] **trazo-done**[26,27] and **sertraline**,[28] amongst others,[1] have been reported to prolong the QTc inter-val in overdose, but the clinical consequences of this are uncertain. Sertraline prolongs QT by 5–10ms at 400mg a day,[29] but QT changes are not usually seen with most SSRIs at normal clinical doses.[30,31] Nonetheless, an association between SSRIs (as a group) and QT changes in normal dosing can be shown,[32] but this seems largely to be driven by the effects of citalopram and escitalopram.[33] The effect is dose-related[33] but mod-est.[32] Neither a large database study[9] nor a large cohort study[34] found any association between citalopram treatment and arrhythmia or cardiac mortality in routine clinical practice; in fact, higher doses of citalopram (>40mg) were associated with fewer adverse outcomes than were lower doses.[34] A large study found no excess risk of cardiac arrest and sudden death for citalopram or escitalopram,[35] but a more recent Taiwanese study showed a small increase in mortality with these drugs.[36]

Vortioxetine seems to have no effect on QT,[37-39] similarly, **agomelatine** has no effect, even at supratherapeutic doses.[40] **Vilazodone** has no effect on cardiac conduction.[41] **Levomilnacipran**[42] and **milnacipran**[43] probably have no effect on QT, at least at thera-peutic doses.

Use in at-risk patients

There is clear evidence for the safety of sertraline[44] and mirtazapine[45] (and to a lesser extent, citalopram,[45] fluoxetine[46] and bupropion[47]) in subjects at risk of arrhythmia due to recent myocardial infarction. One trial found that SSRIs and trazodone decrease the risk of MI,[48] another suggested no effect in either direction for any antidepressant.[49]

One study supports the safety of citalopram in patients with coronary artery disease[50] (although citalopram is linked to a risk of torsades de pointes[51]). Escitalopram did not affect mortality in a trial in patients with heart failure,[52] and a later systematic review found no adverse effect on mortality for any SSRIs in heart failure.[53] Sertraline may help improve cardiovascular risk factors,[54] but in older people, there is an indication that all modern antidepressants confer an increased risk of arrhythmia.[55]

Relative cardiotoxicity

Relative cardiotoxicity of antidepressants is difficult to establish with any precision. Surveillance monitoring data suggest that all marketed antidepressants have been linked to arrhythmia (ranging from clinically insignificant to life threatening) and sudden cardiac death. For a substantial proportion of drugs these figures are more likely to reflect coincidence rather than causation.

The Fatal Toxicity Index (FTI) may provide some means for comparison. This is a measure of the number of overdose deaths per million (FP10) prescriptions issued. FTI figures suggest high toxicity for tricyclic drugs (especially dosulepin but not lofepramine), medium toxicity for venlafaxine and moclobemide, and low toxicity for SSRIs, mirtazapine and reboxetine.[56-60] However, FTI does not necessarily reflect only cardiotoxicity (antidepressants variously cause serotonin syndrome, seizures and coma) and is, in any case, open to other influences. This is best evidenced in the change in FTI over time. A good example here is nortriptyline, the FTI of which has been estimated at 0.6[16] and 39.2[12] and several values in between.[56,57,59] This change probably reflects changes in the type of patient prescribed nortriptyline, but 'double-counting' (nortriptyline is a metabolite of amitriptyline) at post-mortem also plays a part. There is good evidence that venlafaxine is relatively more often prescribed to patients with more severe depression and who are relatively more likely to attempt suicide.[61-63] This is likely to inflate venlafaxine's FTI and erroneously suggest greater inherent toxicity. Drugs with consistently low FTIs can probably be assumed to have very low risk of arrhythmias.

Citalopram and escitalopram have very low overdose toxicity despite QT prolongation occurring in about one-third of reported overdoses.[64] Standard doses of citalopram may be linked to an increased risk of cardiac arrest,[8] but as mentioned earlier, other data suggest no increased risk of arrhythmia or death with standard and higher licensed doses of citalopram and escitalopram.[34] Citalopram and escitalopram are probably the most cardiotoxic of the SSRIs, but their toxicity is modest at worst, and possibly insignificant.

Summary

- Tricyclics (but not lofepramine) have an established link to ion channel blockade and cardiac arrhythmia.
- Non-tricyclics generally have a very low risk of inducing arrhythmia.
- Sertraline is recommended post MI, but other SSRIs and mirtazapine are also likely to be safe.
- Bupropion, citalopram, escitalopram, moclobemide, lofepramine and venlafaxine should be used with caution or avoided in those at risk of serious arrhythmia (those with heart failure, left ventricular hypertrophy; previous arrhythmia or MI). An ECG should be performed at baseline and 1 week after every increase in dose if any of these drugs are used in at-risk patients.

▪ TCAs (with the exception of lofepramine) are best avoided completely in patients at risk of serious arrhythmia. If the use of a TCA cannot be avoided, an ECG should be performed at baseline, one week after each increase in dose and periodically throughout treatment. Frequency will be determined by the stability of the cardiac disorder and the TCA (and dose) being used; advice from cardiology should be sought.

▪ The arrhythmogenic potential of TCAs and other antidepressants is dose-related. Consideration should be given to ECG monitoring of all patients prescribed doses towards the top of the licensed range and those who are prescribed other drugs that through pharmacokinetic (e.g. fluoxetine) or pharmacodynamic (e.g. diuretics) mechanisms may add to the risk posed by the TCA.

References

1. Taylor D. Antidepressant drugs and cardiovascular pathology: a clinical overview of effectiveness and safety. *Acta Psychiatr Scand* 2008; 118:434–442.
2. Whang W, et al. Depression and risk of sudden cardiac death and coronary heart disease in women: results from the Nurses' Health Study. *J Am Coll Cardiol* 2009; 53:950–958.
3. Ziegelstein RC, et al. Platelet function in patients with major depression. *Intern Med J* 2009; 39:38–43.
4. Glassman AH, et al. Heart rate variability in acute coronary syndrome patients with major depression: influence of sertraline and mood improvement. *Arch Gen Psychiatry* 2007; 64:1025–1031.
5. Whooley MA, et al. Depressive symptoms, health behaviors, and risk of cardiovascular events in patients with coronary heart disease. *JAMA* 2008; 300:2379–2388.
6. Thanacoody HK, et al. Tricyclic antidepressant poisoning: cardiovascular toxicity. *Toxicol Rev* 2005; 24:205–214.
7. Sicouri S, et al. Sudden cardiac death secondary to antidepressant and antipsychotic drugs. *Exp Opin Drug Saf* 2008; 7:181–194.
8. Weeke P, et al. Antidepressant use and risk of out-of-hospital cardiac arrest: a nationwide case-time-control study. *Clin Pharmacol Ther* 2012; 92:72–79.
9. Leonard CE, et al. Antidepressants and the risk of sudden cardiac death and ventricular arrhythmia. *Pharmacoepidemiol Drug Saf* 2011; 20:903–913.
10. Hong HK, et al. Block of the human ether-a-go-go-related gene (hERG) K+ channel by the antidepressant desipramine. *Biochem Biophys Res Commun* 2010; 394:536–541.
11. Coupland C, et al. Antidepressant use and risk of cardiovascular outcomes in people aged 20 to 64: cohort study using primary care database. *BMJ* 2016; 352:i1350.
12. Khalifa M, et al. Mechanism of sodium channel block by venlafaxine in guinea pig ventricular myocytes. *J Pharmacol Exp Ther* 1999; 291:280–284.
13. Colbridge MG, et al. Venlafaxine in overdose – experience of the National Poisons Information Service (London centre). *J Toxicol Clin Toxicol* 1999; 37:383.
14. Blythe D, et al. Cardiovascular and neurological toxicity of venlafaxine. *Hum Exp Toxicol* 1999; 18:309–313.
15. Combes A, et al. Conduction disturbances associated with venlafaxine. *Ann Intern Med* 2001; 134:166–167.
16. Isbister GK. Electrocardiogram changes and arrhythmias in venlafaxine overdose. *Br J Clin Pharmacol* 2009; 67:572–576.
17. Whyte IM, et al. Relative toxicity of venlafaxine and selective serotonin reuptake inhibitors in overdose compared to tricyclic antidepressants. *QJM* 2003; 96:369–374.
18. Feighner JP. Cardiovascular safety in depressed patients: focus on venlafaxine. *J Clin Psychiatry* 1995; 56:574–579.
19. Martinez C, et al. Use of venlafaxine compared with other antidepressants and the risk of sudden cardiac death or near death: a nested case-control study. *BMJ* 2010; 340:c249.
20. Cooper JM, et al. Desvenlafaxine overdose and the occurrence of serotonin toxicity, seizures and cardiovascular effects. *Clin Toxicol (Phila)* 2017; 55:18–24.
21. Downes MA, et al. QTc abnormalities in deliberate self-poisoning with moclobemide. *Intern Med J* 2005; 35:388–391.
22. Kelly CA, et al. Comparative toxicity of citalopram and the newer antidepressants after overdose. *J Toxicol Clin Toxicol* 2004; 42:67–71.
23. Grundemar L, et al. Symptoms and signs of severe citalopram overdose. *Lancet* 1997; 349:1602.
24. Mohammed R, et al. Prolonged QTc interval due to escitalopram overdose. *J MissState Med Assoc* 2010; 51:350–353.
25. Isbister GK, et al. Bupropion overdose: qTc prolongation and its clinical significance. *Ann Pharmacother* 2003; 37:999–1002.
26. Service JA, et al. QT Prolongation and delayed atrioventricular conduction caused by acute ingestion of trazodone. *Clin Toxicol (Phila)* 2008; 46:71–73.
27. Dattilo PB, et al. Prolonged QT associated with an overdose of trazodone. *J Clin Psychiatry* 2007; 68:1309–1310.
28. de Boer RA, et al. QT interval prolongation after sertraline overdose: a case report. *BMC Emerg Med* 2005; 5:5.
29. Abbas R, et al. A thorough QT study to evaluate the effects of a supratherapeutic dose of sertraline on cardiac repolarization in healthy subjects. *Clin Pharmacol Drug Develop* 2020; 9:307–320.
30. Maljuric NM, et al. Use of selective serotonin re-uptake inhibitors and the heart rate corrected QT interval in a real-life setting: the population-based Rotterdam Study. *Br J Clin Pharmacol* 2015; 80:698–705.

CHAPTER 3

31. van Haelst IM, et al. QT interval prolongation in users of selective serotonin reuptake inhibitors in an elderly surgical population: a cross-sectional study. *J Clin Psychiatry* 2014; 75:15–21.

32. Beach SR, et al. Meta-analysis of selective serotonin reuptake inhibitor-associated QTc prolongation. *J Clin Psychiatry* 2014; 75:e441–e449.

33. Castro VM, et al. QT interval and antidepressant use: a cross sectional study of electronic health records. *BMJ* 2013; 346:f288.

34. Zivin K, et al. Evaluation of the FDA warning against prescribing citalopram at doses exceeding 40 mg. *Am J Psychiatry* 2013; 170:642–650.

35. Ray WA, et al. High-dose citalopram and escitalopram and the risk of out-of-hospital death. *J Clin Psychiatry* 2017; 78:190–195.

36. Lin YT, et al. Selective serotonin reuptake inhibitor use and risk of arrhythmia: a nationwide, population-based cohort study. *Clin Ther* 2019; 41:1128–1138.e1128.

37. Dubovsky SL. Pharmacokinetic evaluation of vortioxetine for the treatment of major depressive disorder. *Exp Opin Drug Metab Toxicol* 2014; 10:759–766.

38. Alam MY, et al. Safety, tolerability, and efficacy of vortioxetine (Lu AA21004) in major depressive disorder: results of an open-label, flexible-dose, 52-week extension study. *Int Clin Psychopharmacol* 2014; 29:36–44.

39. Wang Y, et al. Effect of vortioxetine on cardiac repolarization in healthy adult male subjects: results of a thorough QT/QTc study. *Clin Pharmacol Drug Develop* 2013; 2:298–309.

40. Donazzolo Y, et al. Evaluation of the effects of therapeutic and supra-therapeutic doses of agomelatine on the QT/QTc interval – A phase I, randomised, double-blind, placebo-controlled and positive-controlled, cross-over thorough QT/QTc study conducted in healthy volunteers. *J Cardiovasc Pharmacol* 2014; 64:440–451.

41. Edwards J, et al. Vilazodone lacks proarrhythmogenic potential in healthy participants: a thorough ECG study. *Int J Clin Pharmacol Ther* 2013; 51:456–465.

42. Mago R, et al. Safety and tolerability of levomilnacipran ER in major depressive disorder: results from an open-label, 48-week extension study. *Clin Drug Investig* 2013; 33:761–771.

43. Periclou A, et al. Effects of milnacipran on cardiac repolarization in healthy participants. *J Clin Pharmacol* 2010; 50:422–433.

44. Glassman AH, et al. Sertraline treatment of major depression in patients with acute MI or unstable angina. *JAMA* 2002; 288:701–709.

45. van Melle JP, et al. Effects of antidepressant treatment following myocardial infarction. *Br J Psychiatry* 2007; 190:460–466.

46. Strik JJ, et al. Efficacy and safety of fluoxetine in the treatment of patients with major depression after first myocardial infarction: findings from a double-blind, placebo-controlled trial. *Psychosom Med* 2000; 62:783–789.

47. Rigotti NA, et al. Bupropion for smokers hospitalized with acute cardiovascular disease. *Am J Med* 2006; 119:1080–1087.

48. Alqdwah-Fattouh R, et al. Differential effects of antidepressant subgroups on risk of acute myocardial infarction: a nested case-control study. *Br J Clin Pharmacol* 2020; 86:2040–2050.

49. Wu CS, et al. Use of antidepressants and risk of hospitalization for acute myocardial infarction: a nationwide case-crossover study. *J Psychiatr Res* 2017; 94:7–14.

50. Lesperance F, et al. Effects of citalopram and interpersonal psychotherapy on depression in patients with coronary artery disease: the Canadian Cardiac Randomized Evaluation of Antidepressant and Psychotherapy Efficacy (CREATE) trial. *JAMA* 2007; 297:367–379.

51. Astrom-Lilja C, et al. Drug-induced torsades de pointes: a review of the Swedish pharmacovigilance database. *Pharmacoepidemiol Drug Saf* 2008; 17:587–592.

52. Angermann CE, et al. Effect of escitalopram on all-cause mortality and hospitalization in patients with heart failure and depression: the MOOD-HF randomized clinical trial. *JAMA* 2016; 315:2683–2693.

53. Hedrick R, et al. The impact of antidepressants on depressive symptom severity, quality of life, morbidity, and mortality in heart failure: a systematic review. *Drugs Context* 2020; 9.

54. Sherwood A, et al. Effects of exercise and sertraline on measures of coronary heart disease risk in patients with major depression: results from the SMILE-II randomized clinical trial. *Psychosom Med* 2016; 78:602–609.

55. Biffi A, et al. Antidepressants and the risk of arrhythmia in elderly affected by a previous cardiovascular disease: a real-life investigation from Italy. *Eur J Clin Pharmacol* 2018; 74:119–129.

56. Crome P. The toxicity of drugs used for suicide. *Acta Psychiatr Scand Suppl* 1993; 371:33–37.

57. Cheeta S, et al. Antidepressant-related deaths and antidepressant prescriptions in England and Wales, 1998–2000. *Br J Psychiatry* 2004; 184:41–47.

58. Buckley NA, et al. Fatal toxicity of serotoninergic and other antidepressant drugs: analysis of United Kingdom mortality data. *BMJ* 2002; 325:1332–1333.

59. Buckley NA, et al. Greater toxicity in overdose of dothiepin than of other tricyclic antidepressants. *Lancet* 1994; 343:159–162.

60. Morgan O, et al. Fatal toxicity of antidepressants in England and Wales, 1993–2002. *Health Stat Q* 2004; 18–24.

61. Egberts ACG, et al. Channeling of three newly introduced antidepressants to patients not responding satisfactorily to previous treatment. *J Clin Psychopharmacol* 1997; 17:149–155.

62. Mines D, et al. Prevalence of risk factors for suicide in patients prescribed venlafaxine, fluoxetine, and citalopram. *Pharmacoepidemiol Drug Saf* 2005; 14:367–372.

63. Chan AN, et al. A comparison of venlafaxine and SSRIs in deliberate self-poisoning. *J Med Toxicol* 2010; 6:116–121.

64. Hasnain M, et al. Escitalopram and QTc prolongation. *J Psychiatry Neurosci* 2013; 38:E11.

Antidepressant-induced hyponatraemia

Most antidepressants have been associated with hyponatraemia. The onset is usually within 30 days of starting treatment (median 11 days).[1-3] The effect appears not to be dose-related[1,4] although some case reports suggest otherwise.[5,6] The most likely mechanism of this adverse effect is the syndrome of inappropriate secretion of antidiuretic hormone (SIADH). Risk of hospitalisation with hyponatraemia is elevated from 1 in 1600 in the general population to 1 in 300 for those on an antidepressant.[7] Hyponatraemia is a potentially serious adverse effect of antidepressants that demands careful monitoring,[8] particularly in those patients at greatest risk. Hyponatraemia of all severities is associated with increased mortality.[9]

Antidepressants

No antidepressant has been definitively shown *not* to be linked with hyponatraemia, and almost all have a reported association.[10] It has been suggested that serotonergic drugs are relatively more likely than noradrenergic drugs to cause hyponatraemia,[11,12] although this is disputed.[13] One review of the literature suggests SSRIs are more likely to cause hyponatraemia than TCAs or mirtazapine,[14] and that older women who are co-prescribed other medication known to reduce plasma sodium are at the greatest risk.[15]

None of the more recently introduced serotonergic drugs is free of an association with hyponatraemia – cases have been described with mirtazapine[16-19] (although the reported incidence overall is very low[15]), escitalopram[5,20-22] and duloxetine.[4,23-28] Vortioxetine has also been linked to hyponatraemia,[29,30] as has desvenlafaxine[31] and vilazodone.[6] Noradrenergic antidepressants are also clearly linked to hyponatraemia,[32-38] albeit at a lower frequency than with SSRIs. There are notably few reports for MAOIs.[39,40]

One French pharmacovigilance database study found an association of hyponatraemia with agomelatine, contrasting with most other studies.[41] Another database study using FDA data found the strongest association between hyponatraemia and antidepressants to be for mirtazapine, also in contrast to most other reports,[42] and a further French database study found the greatest risk to be with duloxetine.[43] However, extrapolating from incident report databases to estimate relative or absolute risk of hyponatremia is fraught with difficulty. Problems include disproportionate reporting for antidepressants for which the side effect is felt to be rare, the inability to adjust for confounding by indication (drugs perceived to be of low risk are more likely to be prescribed to patients at already at high risk of hyponatraemia), and the impact of concomitant prescriptions.

CYP2D6 poor metabolisers may be at increased risk[44] of antidepressant-induced hyponatraemia, although evidence is somewhat inconsistent (Table 3.17).[45]

Table 3.17 Summary of risk of hyponatraemia with antidepressants[7,14,46–48]

Drug/drug group	Risk of ↓Na	Level of supporting evidence
SSRIs	High	Strong
SNRIs	High	Strong
Tricyclics	Moderate	Strong
MAOIs	Low	Weak
NaSSas (mirtazapine, mianserin)	Low	Strong
Bupropion	Low	Moderate
Agomelatine	Low	Weak

Monitoring[1,14,15,49–53]

All patients taking antidepressants should be informed of and observed for signs of hyponatraemia (dizziness, nausea, lethargy, confusion, cramps, seizures). The risk is highest in the first 2–4 weeks of starting antidepressants and diminishes over time until by 3–6 months the risk is the same as for patients who do not take antidepressants.[47,48] Serum sodium should be determined (at baseline and 2 and 4 weeks, and then 3-monthly[54]) for those at high risk of drug-induced hyponatraemia. High-risk factors are as follows:

- Older age
- Female sex
- Major surgery
- History of hyponatraemia or a low baseline sodium concentration
- Co-therapy with other drugs known to be associated with hyponatraemia (*e.g. diuretics, NSAIDs, antipsychotics, carbamazepine, cancer chemotherapy, calcium antagonists, ACE inhibitors and laxatives*)
- Reduced renal function (GFR < 50mL/min)
- Medical co-morbidity (e.g. hypothyroidism, diabetes, COPD, hypertension, head injury, CCF, CVA, various cancers)
- Low body weight

Age is perhaps the most important risk factor, so for older people (especially women) monitoring is essential.[15,47,55,56]

Treatment[56]

It may be possible to manage mild hyponatraemia with fluid restriction.[50] Some suggest increasing sodium intake,[4] although this is likely to be impractical. If symptoms persist, the antidepressant should be discontinued.

- The normal range for serum sodium is 136–145mmol/L.
- If serum sodium is >125mmol/L – monitor sodium daily until normal. Symptoms include headache, nausea, vomiting, muscle cramps, restlessness, lethargy, confusion and disorientation. Consider withdrawing the offending antidepressant.

- If serum sodium is <125mmol/L, refer urgently to specialist medical care. There is an increased risk of life-threatening symptoms such as seizures, coma and respiratory arrest. The antidepressant should be discontinued immediately. (Note risk of discontinuation symptoms which may complicate the clinical picture.) Over rapid correction of hyponatraemia may be harmful.[19]

Restarting treatment

- For those who develop hyponatraemia with an SSRI, there are many case reports of recurrent hyponatraemia on rechallenge with the same, or a different SSRI, and relatively fewer reports of recurrence occurring with an antidepressant from another class.[15,17] There are also a handful of case reports of successful rechallenge.[1]
- Consider withdrawing other drugs associated with hyponatraemia (risk increases exponentially when antidepressants are combined with diuretics[3]).
- Prescribe a drug from a different class. Consider noradrenergic drugs such as nortriptyline and lofepramine, mirtazapine or an MAOI such as moclobemide. Agomelatine or bupropion[57] might also be considered. Begin with a low dose, increasing slowly, and monitor closely. If hyponatraemia recurs and continued antidepressant use is essential, consider water restriction and/or careful use of demeclocycline (see BNF).
- Consider ECT.

Other prescribed drugs

Carbamazepine has a well-known association with SIADH.[58] Note also that antipsychotic use has been linked to hyponatraemia[59-61] (See in section Hyponatraemia in chapter 1). Other commonly prescribed drugs such as thiazide diuretics, opiates, NSAIDs, tramadol, cytotoxics, omeprazole and trimethoprim can also cause hyponatraemia.[2,51,58]

CHAPTER 3

References

1. Egger C, et al. A review on hyponatremia associated with SSRIs, reboxetine and venlafaxine. *Int J Psychiatry Clin Pract* 2006; **10**:17–26.
2. Liamis G, et al. A review of drug-induced hyponatremia. *Am J Kidney Dis* 2008; **52**:144–153.
3. Letmaier M, et al. Hyponatraemia during psychopharmacological treatment: results of a drug surveillance programme. *Int J Neuropsychopharmacol* 2012; **15**:739–748.
4. Kruger S, et al. Duloxetine and hyponatremia: a report of 5 cases. *J Clin Psychopharmacol* 2007; **27**:101–104.
5. Naschitz JE. Escitalopram dose-dependent hyponatremia. *J Clin Pharmacol* 2018; **58**:834–835.
6. Das S, et al. Dose dependent hyponatremia caused by Vilazodone: a case report. *Asian J Psychiatr* 2019; **43**:213.
7. Gandhi S, et al. Second-generation antidepressants and hyponatremia risk: a population-based cohort study of older adults. *Am J Kidney Dis* 2017; **69**:87–96.
8. Mohan S, et al. Prevalence of hyponatremia and association with mortality: results from NHANES. *Am J Med* 2013; **126**:1127–1137.e1121.
9. Selmer C, et al. Hyponatremia, all-cause mortality, and risk of cancer diagnoses in the primary care setting: a large population study. *Eur J Intern Med* 2016; **36**:36–43.
10. Thomas A, et al. Hyponatraemia and the syndrome of inappropriate antidiuretic hormone secretion associated with drug therapy in psychiatric patients. *CNS Drugs* 1995; **5**:357–369.
11. Movig KL, et al. Serotonergic antidepressants associated with an increased risk for hyponatraemia in the elderly. *Eur J Clin Pharmacol* 2002; **58**:143–148.
12. Movig KL, et al. Association between antidepressant drug use and hyponatraemia: a case-control study. *Br J Clin Pharmacol* 2002; **53**:363–369.
13. Kirby D, et al. Hyponatraemia and selective serotonin re-uptake inhibitors in elderly patients. *Int J Geriatr Psychiatry* 2001; **16**:484–493.
14. De Picker L, et al. Antidepressants and the risk of hyponatremia: a class-by-class review of literature. *Psychosomatics* 2014; **55**:536–547.
15. Dirks AC, et al. Recurrent hyponatremia after substitution of citalopram with duloxetine. *J Clin Psychopharmacol* 2007; **27**:313.
16. Lim SY, et al. Hyponatraemia: the importance of obtaining a detailed history and corroborating point-of-care analysis with laboratory testing. *BMJ Case Rep* 2019; **12**:e229221.
17. Bavbek N, et al. Recurrent hyponatremia associated with citalopram and mirtazapine. *Am J Kidney Dis* 2006; **48**:e61–e62.
18. Ladino M, et al. Mirtazapine-induced hyponatremia in an elderly hospice patient. *J Palliat Med* 2006; **9**:258–260.
19. Cheah CY, et al. Mirtazapine associated with profound hyponatremia: two case reports. *Am J Geriatr Pharmacother* 2008; **6**:91–95.
20. Grover S, et al. Escitalopram-associated hyponatremia. *Psychiatry Clin Neurosci* 2007; **61**:132–133.
21. Covyeou JA, et al. Hyponatremia associated with escitalopram. *N Engl J Med* 2007; **356**:94–95.
22. Vidyasagar S, et al. Escitalopram induced SIADH in an elderly female: a case study. *Psychopharmacol Bull* 2017; **47**:64–67.
23. Şahan E, et al. Duloxetine induced hyponatremia. *Turk Psikiyatri Dergisi* 2019; **30**:287–289.
24. Sun CF, et al. Duloxetine-induced hyponatremia in an elderly male patient with treatment-refractory major depressive disorder. *Case Rep Psychiatry* 2019; **2019**:4109150.
25. Hu D, et al. Hyponatremia induced by duloxetine: a case report. *Consult Pharm* 2018; **33**:446–449.
26. Yoshida K, et al. Acute hyponatremia resulting from duloxetine-induced syndrome of inappropriate antidiuretic hormone secretion. *Intern Med* 2019; **58**:1939–1942.
27. Wang D, et al. Rapid-onset hyponatremia and delirium following duloxetine treatment for postherpetic neuralgia: case report and literature review. *Medicine (Baltimore)* 2018; **97**:e13178.
28. Takayama A, et al. Duloxetine and angiotensin II receptor blocker combination potentially induce severe hyponatremia in an elderly woman. *Intern Med* 2019; **58**:1791–1794.
29. Pelayo-Terán JM, et al. Safety in the use of antidepressants: vortioxetine-induce hyponatremia in a case report. *Revista de psiquiatria y salud mental* 2017; **10**:219–220.
30. Lundbeck Limited. Summary of product characteristics. Brintellix (vortioxetine) tablets 5, 10 and 20mg. 2020; https://www.medicines.org.uk/emc/medicine/30904.
31. Lee G, et al. Syndrome of inappropriate secretion of antidiuretic hormone due to desvenlafaxine. *Gen Hosp Psychiatry* 2013; **35**:574.e571–573.
32. O'Sullivan D, et al. Hyponatraemia and lofepramine. *Br J Psychiatry* 1987; **150**:720–721.
33. Wylie KR, et al. Lofepramine-induced hyponatraemia. *Br J Psychiatry* 1989; **154**:419–420.
34. Ranieri P, et al. Reboxetine and hyponatremia. *N Engl J Med* 2000; **342**:215–216.
35. Miller MG. Tricyclics as a possible cause of hyponatremia in psychiatric patients. *Am J Psychiatry* 1989; **146**:807.
36. Colgate R. Hyponatraemia and inappropriate secretion of antidiuretic hormone associated with the use of imipramine. *Br J Psychiatry* 1993; **163**:819–822.
37. Koelkebeck K, et al. A case of non-SIADH-induced hyponatremia in depression after treatment with reboxetine. *World J Biol Psychiatry* 2009; **10**:609–611.
38. Kate N, et al. Bupropion-induced hyponatremia. *Gen Hosp Psychiatry* 2013; **35**:681.e611–682.
39. Mercier S, et al. Severe hyponatremia induced by moclobemide (in French). *Therapie* 1997; **52**:82–83.
40. Peterson JC, et al. Inappropriate antidiuretic hormone secondary to a monamine oxidase inhibitor. *JAMA* 1978; **239**:1422–1423.
41. Rochoy M, et al. [Antidepressive agents and hyponatremia: a literature review and a case/non-case study in the French Pharmacovigilance database]. *Therapie* 2018; **73**:389–398.

42. Mazhar F, et al. Association of hyponatraemia and antidepressant drugs: a pharmacovigilance-pharmacodynamic assessment through an analysis of the US food and drug administration adverse event reporting system (FAERS) database. *CNS Drugs* 2019; 33:581–592.
43. Revol R, et al. [Hyponatremia associated with SSRI/NRSI: descriptive and comparative epidemiological study of the incidence rates of the notified cases from the data of the French National Pharmacovigilance Database and the French National Health Insurance]. *Encephale* 2018; 44:291–296.
44. Kwadijk-de GS, et al. Variation in the CYP2D6 gene is associated with a lower serum sodium concentration in patients on antidepressants. *Br J Clin Pharmacol* 2009; 68:221–225.
45. Stedman CA, et al. Cytochrome P450 2D6 genotype does not predict SSRI (fluoxetine or paroxetine) induced hyponatraemia. *Human Psychopharmacology* 2002; 17:187–190.
46. Leth-Moller KB, et al. Antidepressants and the risk of hyponatremia: a Danish register-based population study. *BMJ Open* 2016; 6:e011200.
47. Lien YH. Antidepressants and hyponatremia. *Am J Med* 2018; 131:7–8.
48. Farmand S, et al. Differences in associations of antidepressants and hospitalization due to hyponatremia. *Am J Med* 2018; 131:56–63.
49. Jacob S, et al. Hyponatremia associated with selective serotonin-reuptake inhibitors in older adults. *Ann Pharmacother* 2006; 40:1618–1622.
50. Roxanas M, et al. Venlafaxine hyponatraemia: incidence, mechanism and management. *Aust N Z J Psychiatry* 2007; 41:411–418.
51. Reddy P, et al. Diagnosis and management of hyponatremia in hospitalised patients. *Int J Clin Pract* 2009; 63:1494–1508.
52. Siegler EL, et al. Risk factors for the development of hyponatremia in psychiatric inpatients. *Arch Intern Med* 1995; 155:953–957.
53. Mannesse CK, et al. Characteristics, prevalence, risk factors, and underlying mechanism of hyponatremia in elderly patients treated with antidepressants: a cross-sectional study. *Maturitas* 2013; 76:357–363.
54. Arinzon ZH, et al. Delayed recurrent SIADH associated with SSRIs. *Ann Pharmacother* 2002; 36:1175–1177.
55. Fabian TJ, et al. Paroxetine-induced hyponatremia in the elderly due to the syndrome of inappropriate secretion of antidiuretic hormone (SIADH). *J Geriatr Psychiatry Neurol* 2003; 16:160–164.
56. Sharma H, et al. Antidepressant-induced hyponatraemia in the aged. Avoidance and management strategies. *Drugs Aging* 1996; 8:430–435.
57. Varela Piñón M, et al. Selective serotonin reuptake inhibitor-induced hyponatremia: clinical implications and therapeutic alternatives. *Clin Neuropharmacol* 2017; 40:177–179.
58. Shepshelovich D, et al. Medication-induced SIADH: distribution and characterization according to medication class. *Br J Clin Pharmacol* 2017; 83:1801–1807.
59. Ohsawa H, et al. An epidemiological study on hyponatremia in psychiatric patients in mental hospitals in Nara Prefecture. *Jpn J Psychiatry Neurol* 1992; 46:883–889.
60. Leadbetter RA, et al. Differential effects of neuroleptic and clozapine on polydipsia and intermittent hyponatremia. *J Clin Psychiatry* 1994; 55 Suppl B:110–113.
61. Collins A, et al. SIADH induced by two atypical antipsychotics. *Int J Geriatr Psychiatry* 2000; 15:282–283.

CHAPTER 3

Antidepressants and hyperprolactinaemia

Prolactin release is controlled by endogenous dopamine but is also indirectly modulated by serotonin via stimulation of $5HT_{1C}$ and $5HT_2$ receptors.[1,2] Long-standing increased plasma prolactin (with or without symptoms) is very occasionally seen with antidepressant use.[3] Where antidepressant-induced hyperprolactinaemia does occur, rises in prolactin are usually small and short-lived[4] and so symptoms are very rare. There is no association between SSRI use and breast cancer.[5]

Routine monitoring of prolactin is not recommended, but where symptoms suggest the possibility of hyperprolactinaemia, then measurement of plasma prolactin is essential. Where symptomatic hyperprolactinaemia is confirmed, a switch to mirtazapine is recommended (see below), although there is also evidence that switching to an alternative SSRI can resolve symptoms.[6,7]

Some details of associations between antidepressants and increased prolactin are given in Table 3.18.

Table 3.18 Reported associations between antidepressants and increased prolactin

Drug/group	Prospective studies	Case reports/series
Agomelatine	No mention of prolactin changes in clinical trials[8] Melatonin itself may inhibit prolactin production[9]	None
Bupropion	Single doses of up to 100mg seem not to affect prolactin[10] May decrease prolactin[11]	None
MAOIs	Small mean changes observed with phenelzine[11] and tranylcypromine[12]	Very occasional reports of increased prolactin[11]
Mirtazapine	Strong evidence that mirtazapine has no effect on prolactin[13–15]	Occasional reports of galactorrhoea[16] and gynaecomastia[17]
SNRIs	Clear association observed between venlafaxine and duloxetine and prolactin elevation[18–20]	Galactorrhoea reported with venlafaxine[21,22] and duloxetine.[23,24] Duloxetine-linked hyperprolactinaemia has been treated with aripiprazole[18]
SSRIs	Prospective studies generally show no change in prolactin.[25–27] Some evidence from prescription event monitoring that SSRIs are associated with higher risk of non-puerperal lactation.[28] In a French study, 1.6% of adverse event reports for SSRIs were of hyperprolactinaemia[3]	Galactorrhoea reported with fluoxetine[6,29] and paroxetine[30,31] Euprolactinaemic galactorrhoea and amenorrhoea[32] reported with escitalopram[33] and fluvoxamine[34] Hyperprolactinaemia reported with sertraline[7,35]

(Continued)

Table 3.18 (*Continued*)

Drug/group	Prospective studies	Case reports/series
Tricyclics	Small mean changes seen in some studies[11,36,37] but no changes in others[11,38]	Symptomatic hyperprolactinaemia reported with imipramine,[33] dosulepin[39] and clomipramine[40,41] Galactorrhoea reported with nortriptyline[42] and when trazodone was added to citalopram[43] Raised prolactin may be linked to response to amitriptyline[36]
Vortioxetine	No mention of prolactin changes in clinical trials[44,45]	None One review suggests 'probable relation between vortioxetine and galactorrhea'[46]

References

1. Emiliano AB, et al. From galactorrhea to osteopenia: rethinking serotonin-prolactin interactions. *Neuropsychopharmacology* 2004; **29**:833–846.
2. Rittenhouse PA, et al. Neurons in the hypothalamic paraventricular nucleus mediate the serotonergic stimulation of prolactin secretion via 5-HT1c/2 receptors. *Endocrinology* 1993; **133**:661–667.
3. Trenque T, et al. Serotonin reuptake inhibitors and hyperprolactinaemia: a case/non-case study in the French pharmacovigilance database. *Drug Saf* 2011; **34**:1161–1166.
4. Voicu V, et al. Drug-induced hypo- and hyperprolactinemia: mechanisms, clinical and therapeutic consequences. *Exp Opin Drug Metab Toxicol* 2013; **9**:955–968.
5. Ashbury JE, et al. Selective serotonin reuptake inhibitor (SSRI) antidepressants, prolactin and breast cancer. *Front Oncol* 2012; **2**:177.
6. Mondal S, et al. A new logical insight and putative mechanism behind fluoxetine-induced amenorrhea, hyperprolactinemia and galactorrhea in a case series. *Ther Adv Psychopharmacol* 2013; **3**:322–334.
7. Strzelecki D, et al. Hyperprolactinemia and bleeding following use of sertraline but not use of citalopram and paroxetine: a case report. *Arch Psychiatry Psychotherapy* 2012; **1**:45–48.
8. Taylor D, et al. Antidepressant efficacy of agomelatine: meta-analysis of published and unpublished studies. *BMJ* 2014; **348**:g1888.
9. Chu YS, et al. Stimulatory and entraining effect of melatonin on tuberoinfundibular dopaminergic neuron activity and inhibition on prolactin secretion. *J Pineal Res* 2000; **28**:219–226.
10. Whiteman PD, et al. Bupropion fails to affect plasma prolactin and growth hormone in normal subjects. *Br J Clin Pharmacol* 1982; **13**:745.
11. Meltzer HY, et al. Effect of antidepressants on neuroendocrine axis in humans. *Adv Biochem Psychopharmacol* 1982; **32**:303–316.
12. Price LH, et al. Effects of tranylcypromine treatment on neuroendocrine, behavioral, and autonomic responses to tryptophan in depressed patients. *Life Sci* 1985; **37**:809–818.
13. Laakmann G, et al. Effects of mirtazapine on growth hormone, prolactin, and cortisol secretion in healthy male subjects. *Psychoneuroendocrinology* 1999; **24**:769–784.
14. Laakmann G, et al. Mirtazapine: an inhibitor of cortisol secretion that does not influence growth hormone and prolactin secretion. *J Clin Psychopharmacol* 2000; **20**:101–103.
15. Schule C, et al. The influence of mirtazapine on anterior pituitary hormone secretion in healthy male subjects. *Psychopharmacology (Berl)* 2002; **163**:95–101.
16. Schroeder K, et al. Mirtazapine-induced galactorrhea: a case report. *J Neuropsychiatry Clin Neurosci* 2013; **25**:E13–E14.
17. Lynch A, et al. [Gynecomastia-galactorrhea during treatment with mirtazapine]. *Presse Med* 2004; **33**:458.
18. Luo T, et al. Aripiprazole for the treatment of duloxetine-induced hyperprolactinemia: a case report. *J Affect Disord* 2019; **250**:330–332.
19. Daffner-Bugia C, et al. The neuroendocrine effects of venlafaxine in healthy subjects. *Human Psychopharmacology* 1996; **11**:1–9.
20. McGrane IR, et al. Probable galactorrhea associated with sequential trials of escitalopram and duloxetine in an adolescent female. *J Child Adolesc Psychopharmacol* 2019; **29**:788–789.
21. Sternbach H. Venlafaxine-induced galactorrhea. *J Clin Psychopharmacol* 2003; **23**:109–110.
22. Demir EY, et al. Hyperprolactinemia connected with venlafaxine: a case report. *Anatolian J Psychiatry* 2014; **15**:S10–S14.
23. Ashton AK, et al. Hyperprolactinemia and galactorrhea induced by serotonin and norepinephrine reuptake inhibiting antidepressants. *Am J Psychiatry* 2007; **164**:1121–1122.
24. Korkmaz S, et al. Galactorrhea during duloxetine treatment: a case report. *Turk Psikiyatri Dergisi* 2011; **22**:200–201.
25. Sagud M, et al. Effects of sertraline treatment on plasma cortisol, prolactin and thyroid hormones in female depressed patients. *Neuropsychobiology* 2002; **45**:139–143.

CHAPTER 3

26. Schlosser R, et al. Effects of subchronic paroxetine administration on night-time endocrinological profiles in healthy male volunteers. *Psychoneuroendocrinology* 2000; **25**:377–388.

27. Nadeem HS, et al. Comparison of the effects of citalopram and escitalopram on 5-Ht-mediated neuroendocrine responses. *Neuropsychopharmacology* 2004; **29**:1699–1703.

28. Egberts AC, et al. Non-puerperal lactation associated with antidepressant drug use. *Br J Clin Pharmacol* 1997; **44**:277–281.

29. Peterson MC. Reversible galactorrhea and prolactin elevation related to fluoxetine use. *Mayo Clin Proc* 2001; **76**:215–216.

30. Morrison J, et al. Galactorrhea induced by paroxetine. *Can J Psychiatry* 2001; **46**:88–89.

31. Evrensel A, et al. A case of galactorrhea during paroxetine treatment. *Int J Psychiatry Med* 2016; **51**:302–305.

32. Selvaraj V, et al. Escitalopram-induced amenorrhea and false positive urine pregnancy test. *Korean J Fam Med* 2017; **38**:40–42.

33. Mahasuar R, et al. Euprolactinemic galactorrhea associated with use of imipramine and escitalopram in a postmenopausal woman. *Gen Hosp Psychiatry* 2010; **32**:341–343.

34. Vispute C, et al. Fluvoxamine-induced reversible euprolactinemic galactorrhea in a case of obsessive-compulsive disorder. *Ann Indian Psychiatry* 2017; **1**:127–128.

35. Ekinci N, et al. Sertraline-related amenorrhea in an adolescent. *Clin Neuropharmacol* 2019; **42**:99–100.

36. Fava GA, et al. Prolactin, cortisol, and antidepressant treatment. *Am J Psychiatry* 1988; **145**:358–360.

37. Orlander H, et al. Imipramine induced elevation of prolactin levels in patients with HIV/AIDS improved their immune status. *West Indian Med J* 2009; **58**:207–213.

38. Meltzer HY, et al. Lack of effect of tricyclic antidepressants on serum prolactin levels. *Psychopharmacology (Berl)* 1977; **51**:185–187.

39. Gadd EM, et al. Antidepressants and galactorrhoea. *Int Clin Psychopharmacol* 1987; **2**:361–363.

40. Anand VS. Clomipramine–induced galactorrhoea and amenorrhoea. *Br J Psychiatry* 1985; **147**:87–88.

41. Fowlie S, et al. Hyperprolactinaemia and nonpuerperal lactation associated with clomipramine. *Scott Med J* 1987; **32**:52.

42. Kukreti P, et al. Rising trend of use of antidepressants induced non- puerperal lactation: a case report. *JCDR* 2016; **10**:Vd01–vd02.

43. Arslan FC, et al. Trazodone induced galactorrhea: a case report. *Gen Hosp Psychiatry* 2015; **37**:373.e371–372.

44. Mahableshwarkar AR, et al. A randomized, double-blind, fixed-dose study comparing the efficacy and tolerability of vortioxetine 2.5 and 10 mg in acute treatment of adults with generalized anxiety disorder. *Human Psychopharmacology* 2014; **29**:64–72.

45. Baldwin DS, et al. Vortioxetine (Lu AA21004) in the long-term open-label treatment of major depressive disorder. *Curr Med Res Opin* 2012; **28**:1717–1724.

46. Verma A, et al. Risks associated with vortioxetine in the established therapeutic indication. *Curr Neuropharmacol* 2020. [Epub ahead of print].

Antidepressants and diabetes mellitus

Depression and diabetes

There is an established link between diabetes and depression.[1] Prevalence rates of co-morbid depressive symptoms in diabetic patients have been reported to range from 9 to 60%, depending on the study design and screening method used.[2] Moreover, having diabetes doubles the odds of co-morbid depression,[2] and a diagnosis of diabetes is linked to an increased likelihood of antidepressant prescription.[3,4] Patients with depression and diabetes have a high number of cardiovascular risk factors and increased and 50% increased risk of mortality.[5,6] The presence of depression has a negative impact on metabolic control and likewise poor metabolic control may worsen depression.[7] Considering all of this, the treatment of co-morbid depression in patients with diabetes is of vital importance, and drug choice should take into account likely effects on metabolic control (see Table 3.19). Cochrane[8] suggests that antidepressants are effective and moderately improve glycaemic control. Be aware, however, that the prescribing of antidepressants may be associated with reduced adherence to antidiabetic medication.[9]

Table 3.19 Effect of antidepressants on glucose homeostasis and weight

Antidepressant class	Effect on glucose homeostasis and weight
SSRIs[10–23]	■ Studies indicate that SSRIs have a favourable effect on diabetic parameters in patients with type II diabetes. Insulin requirements may be decreased ■ Fluoxetine has been associated with improvement in HbA1c levels, reduced insulin requirements, weight loss and enhanced insulin sensitivity. Its effect on insulin sensitivity is independent of its effect on weight loss. Sertraline may also reduce HbA1c ■ Escitalopram also seems to improve glycaemic control ■ Some evidence that long-term SSRIs may increase the risk of diabetes in general[24] and gestational diabetes, in particular,[25] but there is also evidence of no effect either way[26]
TCAs[16,17,27–29]	■ TCAs are associated with increased appetite, weight gain and hyperglycaemia ■ Nortriptyline improved depression but worsened glycaemic control in diabetic patients in one study. Overall improvement in depression had a beneficial effect on HbA1c. Clomipramine reported to precipitate diabetes ■ Long-term use of TCAs seems to increase risk of diabetes
MAOIs[30,31]	■ Irreversible MAOIs have a tendency to cause extreme hypoglycaemic episodes and weight gain ■ No known effects with moclobemide
SNRIs[28,32,33]	■ SNRIs do not appear to disrupt glycaemic control and have minimal impact on weight ■ Studies of duloxetine in the treatment of diabetic neuropathy show that it has little influence on glycaemic control. No data on depression and diabetes ■ Limited data on venlafaxine ■ One report of hyperglycaemia with desvenlafaxine[34]
Mirtazapine[35,36]	■ Mirtazapine does not appear to impair glucose tolerance in non-diabetic depressed patients ■ Improvement in HbA1c was seen with short-term use but HbA1c worsened during a 1-year follow-up ■ Mirtazapine was associated with an increase in body mass index (BMI) in diabetic patients both in the short and long term
Agomelatine[22,23,37,38]	■ A few studies suggest agomelatine is effective with some improvement or no worsening of glycaemic parameters ■ Agomelatine also demonstrated a minimum effect on body weight
Reboxetine, trazodone and vortioxetine	■ No data in patients with diabetes ■ One study revealed 20% increased risk of type 2 diabetes in people prescribed trazodone[24]

CHAPTER 3

Recommendations

- All patients with a diagnosis of depression should be screened for diabetes.

In those who are diabetic:

- Use SSRIs first line; data support sertraline, escitalopram and fluoxetine.
- SNRIs are also likely to be safe, but there are fewer supporting data.
- Agomelatine seems promising with limited data available.
- Avoid TCAs and MAOIs if possible due to their effects on weight and glucose homeostasis.
- Monitor blood glucose and HbA1c carefully when antidepressant treatment is initiated, when the dose is changed and after discontinuation.

References

1. Katon WJ. The comorbidity of diabetes mellitus and depression. *Am J Med* 2008; **121 Suppl** 2:S8–S15.
2. Anderson RJ, et al. The prevalence of comorbid depression in adults with diabetes: a meta-analysis. *Diabetes Care* 2001; **24**:1069–1078.
3. Musselman DL, et al. Relationship of depression to diabetes types 1 and 2: epidemiology, biology, and treatment. *Biol Psychiatry* 2003; **54**:317–329.
4. Knol MJ, et al. Antidepressant use before and after initiation of diabetes mellitus treatment. *Diabetologia* 2009; **52**:425–432.
5. Katon WJ, et al. Cardiac risk factors in patients with diabetes mellitus and major depression. *J Gen Intern Med* 2004; **19**:1192–1199.
6. van Dooren FE, et al. Depression and risk of mortality in people with diabetes mellitus: a systematic review and meta-analysis. *PLoS One* 2013; **8**:e57058.
7. Lustman PJ, et al. Depression in diabetic patients: the relationship between mood and glycemic control. *J Diabetes Complications* 2005; **19**:113–122.
8. Baumeister H, et al. Psychological and pharmacological interventions for depression in patients with diabetes mellitus and depression. *Cochrane Database Syst Rev* 2012; **12**:Cd008381.
9. Lunghi C, et al. The association between depression and medication nonpersistence in new users of antidiabetic drugs. *Value Health* 2017; **20**:728–735.
10. Maheux P, et al. Fluoxetine improves insulin sensitivity in obese patients with non-insulin-dependent diabetes mellitus independently of weight loss. *Int J Obes Relat Metab Disord* 1997; **21**:97–102.
11. Gulseren L, et al. Comparison of fluoxetine and paroxetine in type II diabetes mellitus patients. *Arch Med Res* 2005; **36**:159–165.
12. Lustman PJ, et al. Sertraline for prevention of depression recurrence in diabetes mellitus: a randomized, double-blind, placebo-controlled trial. *Arch Gen Psychiatry* 2006; **63**:521–529.
13. Gray DS, et al. A randomized double-blind clinical trial of fluoxetine in obese diabetics. *Int J Obes Relat Metab Disord* 1992; **16 Suppl** 4:S67–S72.
14. Knol MJ, et al. Influence of antidepressants on glycaemic control in patients with diabetes mellitus. *Pharmacoepidemiol Drug Saf* 2008; **17**:577–586.
15. Briscoe VJ, et al. Effects of a selective serotonin reuptake inhibitor, fluoxetine, on counterregulatory responses to hypoglycemia in healthy individuals. *Diabetes* 2008; **57**:2453–2460.
16. Andersohn F, et al. Long-term use of antidepressants for depressive disorders and the risk of diabetes mellitus. *Am J Psychiatry* 2009; **166**:591–598.
17. Kivimaki M, et al. Antidepressant medication use, weight gain, and risk of type 2 diabetes: a population-based study. *Diabetes Care* 2010; **33**:2611–2616.
18. Rubin RR, et al. Antidepressant medicine use and risk of developing diabetes during the diabetes prevention program and diabetes prevention program outcomes study. *Diabetes Care* 2010; **33**:2549–2551.
19. Echeverry D, et al. Effect of pharmacological treatment of depression on A1C and quality of life in low-income Hispanics and African Americans with diabetes: a randomized, double-blind, placebo-controlled trial. *Diabetes Care* 2009; **32**:2156–2160.
20. Dhavale HS, et al. Depression and diabetes: impact of antidepressant medications on glycaemic control. *J Assoc Physicians India* 2013; **61**:896–899.
21. Mojtabai R. Antidepressant use and glycemic control. *Psychopharmacology (Berl)* 2013; **227**:467–477.
22. Salman MT, et al. Comparative effect of agomelatine versus escitalopram on glycemic control and symptoms of depression in patients with type 2 diabetes mellitus and depression. 2015; **6**:4304-09.
23. Kang R, et al. Comparison of paroxetine and agomelatine in depressed type 2 diabetes mellitus patients: a double-blind, randomized, clinical trial. *Neuropsychiatr Dis Treat* 2015; **11**:1307–1311.
24. Nguyen TTH, et al. Role of serotonin transporter in antidepressant-induced diabetes mellitus: a pharmacoepidemiological-pharmacodynamic study in VigiBase(®). *Drug Saf* 2018; **41**:1087–1096.

25. Dandjinou M, et al. Antidepressant use during pregnancy and the risk of gestational diabetes mellitus: a nested case-control study. *BMJ Open* 2019; 9:e025908.

26. Kuo HY, et al. Antidepressants and risk of type 2 diabetes mellitus: a population-based nested case-control study. *J Clin Psychopharmacol* 2020; 40:359–365.

27. Lustman PJ, et al. Effects of nortriptyline on depression and glycemic control in diabetes: results of a double-blind, placebo-controlled trial. *Psychosom Med* 1997; 59:241–250.

28. McIntyre RS, et al. The effect of antidepressants on glucose homeostasis and insulin sensitivity: synthesis and mechanisms. *Expert Opinion on Drug Safety* 2006; 5:157–168.

29. Mumoli N, et al. Clomipramine-induced diabetes. *Ann Intern Med* 2008; 149:595–596.

30. Goodnick PJ. Use of antidepressants in treatment of comorbid diabetes mellitus and depression as well as in diabetic neuropathy. *Ann Clin Psychiatry* 2001; 13:31–41.

31. McIntyre RS, et al. Mood and psychotic disorders and type 2 diabetes: a metabolic triad. *Canadian Journal of Diabetes* 2005; 29:122–132.

32. Raskin J, et al. Duloxetine versus routine care in the long-term management of diabetic peripheral neuropathic pain. *J Palliat Med* 2006; 9:29–40.

33. Crucitti A, et al. Duloxetine treatment and glycemic controls in patients with diagnoses other than diabetic peripheral neuropathic pain: a meta-analysis. *Curr Med Res Opin* 2010; 26:2579–2588.

34. Mekonnen AD, et al. Desvenlafaxine-associated hyperglycemia: a case report and literature review. *Ment Health Clin* 2020; 10:85–89.

35. Song HR, et al. Does mirtazapine interfere with naturalistic diabetes treatment? *J Clin Psychopharmacol* 2014; 34:588–594.

36. Song HR, et al. Effects of mirtazapine on patients undergoing naturalistic diabetes treatment: a follow-up study extended from 6 to 12 months. *J Clin Psychopharmacol* 2015; 35:730–731.

37. Karaiskos D, et al. Agomelatine and sertraline for the treatment of depression in type 2 diabetes mellitus. *Int J Clin Pract* 2013; 67:257–260.

38. Vasile D, et al. P.2.c.002 Agomelatine versus selective serotoninergic reuptake inhibitors in major depressive disorder and comorbid diabetes mellitus. *Eur Neuropsychopharmacol* 2011; 21:S383–S384.

CHAPTER 3

Antidepressants and sexual dysfunction

Sexual dysfunction is common in the general population, although reliable, precise data are lacking.[1] Reported prevalence rates vary depending on how sexual dysfunction is defined, assessed and also the method of data collection.[1] Physical illness, psychiatric illness, substance misuse and prescribed drug treatment can all cause sexual dysfunction.[2] People with depression are more likely to be obese,[3] have diabetes[4] and have cardiovascular disease[5] than the general population, making them more likely to suffer sexual dysfunction outside any influence of depression itself.

Before prescribing, baseline sexual functioning should be determined because treatment-emergent sexual dysfunction adversely affects the quality of life and may contribute to reduced compliance.[6] Questionnaires or rating scales may be useful (for example, the Arizona Sexual Experience Scale[7]). If scales are not used then direct questioning should be employed as it is much more effective than relying on spontaneous patient reporting.[8] Complaints of sexual dysfunction may also indicate progression or inadequate treatment of underlying medical or psychiatric conditions. It may also be the result of drug treatment and intervention may greatly improve quality of life.[6]

Effects of depression

Both depression and the drugs used to treat it can cause disorders of desire, arousal and orgasm. The precise nature of the sexual dysfunction may indicate whether depression or treatment is the more likely cause. For example, 40–50% of people with depression report diminished libido and problems regarding sexual arousal in the month before diagnosis, but only 15–20% experience orgasm problems before taking an antidepressant.[9] The prevalence for loss of libido appears to correlate with depression severity.[10]

Although many patients experience treatment-emergent sexual dysfunction whilst taking antidepressants, in others the reduction in depressive symptoms can be accompanied by improvements in sexual desire and satisfaction.[6] Improvements appear more commonly among those who respond to antidepressant treatment.[6] For example, a post-hoc analysis of data from the STAR*D study revealed that sexual dysfunction was problematic in 21% of patients whose depression remitted with citalopram treatment compared with 61% of those whose depression did not remit.[11]

Effects of antidepressant drugs

Antidepressants can cause sedation, hormonal changes, disturbance of cholinergic/adrenergic balance, peripheral alpha-adrenergic agonism, inhibition of nitric oxide and increased serotonin neurotransmission, all of which can result in sexual dysfunction. Sexual dysfunction has been reported as a side effect of all antidepressants, although rates vary (see Table 3.20). Individual susceptibility also varies and may be at least partially genetically determined.[12]

Sexual dysfunction with antidepressants is likely to be dose-dependent,[12] and is generally considered to be fully reversible.[12] However, there have been reports of long-lasting sexual dysfunction where the symptoms have continued despite discontinuation of SSRIs/SNRI.[13] The term 'post-SSRI sexual dysfunction' (PSSD) has been used to describe these symptoms. The prevalence and pathophysiology of PSSD remain uncertain.[14]

Not all of the sexual side effects of antidepressants are undesirable: serotonergic antidepressants including clomipramine are effective in the treatment of premature ejaculation[6] and may also be beneficial in paraphilias. The short-acting SSRI dapoxetine is an effective treatment for premature ejaculation and is licensed for this indication in many countries.[6,15] A systematic review of RCTs with trazodone showed benefit for reducing 'psychogenic erectile dysfunction'.[6]

Sexual side effects can be minimised by careful selection of the antidepressant drug. Note that the assessment of sexual side-effects in clinical trials is generally inadequate, often relying on spontaneous reports rather than using validated questionnaires and lacking positive controls.[16] Where possible, information has been obtained from studies where sexual side effects are purposefully and directly investigated. Management strategies for people who do develop sexual dysfunction on antidepressants are summarised in Table 3.21. No single approach can be considered 'ideal',[6] so individual assessment case-by-case is recommended.

Table 3.20 Relative frequency sexual dysfunction (SD) with antidepressants[10,12,17–19].

	Impact on sexual response			
Antidepressant	Sexual desire*	Sexual arousal†	Orgasm‡	Comments[12]
Agomelatine	–	–	–	Rates of SD may be similar to placebo.[6]
Bupropion	–	+/–	–	Low rates of SD compared to some other antidepressants.[20] Overall, considerable evidence that SD occurs at or below the rate of placebo.
Duloxetine	++	+	++	Rate of SD similar to some SSRIs and venlafaxine in one meta-analysis.[20]
Levomilnacipran	?	++	++	Limited comparative studies with other antidepressants[21] so relative frequency of SD is uncertain. Erectile dysfunction and disorders of ejaculation shown in RCTs against placebo.
MAOIs	++	++	++	Limited evidence though reported incidence of SD ranges from 20% to 42%. Rates of SD with transdermal selegiline are comparable to placebo.
Mirtazapine	+	–	–	Causes less SD than SSRIs.[22]
Moclobemide	–	–	–	Consistently shown to have a low risk of SD.
Reboxetine	–	+	–	Probably causes less SD than SSRIs/SNRIs though efficacy has been questioned.[23]
SSRIs	++	++	++	Overall evidence suggests relatively high rates of SD across all the SSRIs (although reported incidence varies widely).[12] Rates of anorgasmia may be lower with fluvoxamine.[24]
Trazodone	–	+	+	Priapism reported in case studies; however, overall reports of SD seem to be low. Earlier case reports document increased sexual desire.

(Continued)

Table 3.20 (Continued)

Antidepressant	Sexual desire*	Sexual arousal†	Orgasm‡	Comments[12]
Tricyclics	++	++	++	SD more common with clomipramine (particularly anorgasmia), amitriptyline and imipramine. Less common with secondary amine TCAs (desipramine, nortriptyline).
Venlafaxine	++	++	++	High rates of SD. Isolated case reports of increased libido, orgasm and spontaneous erections.
Vilazodone	+	+	+	Rates of SD possibly lower than citalopram and similar to placebo in RCTs. However, a clear advantage over other antidepressants remains uncertain.[21]
Vortioxetine	–	+	+	Incidence of SD reportedly similar to placebo at doses 10mg/day or less;[23,25] however, a clear advantage over other antidepressants remains uncertain.[21,26]

Key: ++, common; +, may occur; –, absent or rare; ?, unknown/insufficient information*
Or sex drive.
† Ease of arousal and ability to achieve lubrication or erections.
‡ Ease of reaching orgasm and orgasm satisfaction.

Table 3.21 Management of sexual adverse effects

Strategy	Details
1. Rule out other possible causes[27]	▪ Depressive symptoms are associated with impaired sexual functioning. Compare sexual functioning on antidepressants with sexual functioning before antidepressants, not before the onset of depressive illness. ▪ Consider other possible contributing causes (e.g. alcohol/substance misuse, diabetes, atherosclerosis, cardiac disease, and central and peripheral nervous system conditions). Other medications could be implicated, including both non-psychotropics (e.g. diuretics, beta-blockers) and other psychotropics (summarised elsewhere in the *Guidelines*).
2. Switch to a lower risk antidepressant[23]	▪ Lower risk antidepressants include agomelatine, bupropion, mirtazapine, vilazodone, vortioxetine and moclobemide.[12] Of these, agomelatine, bupropion and vortioxetine have the best evidence supporting a more favourable sexual side effect profile.[12]
Non-pharmacological treatment strategies	▪ **Waiting for spontaneous remission:** widely used though least effective method.[24] May occur in a small number of people (5–10%) but can take up to 4–6 months.[12] Impractical for many patients, though it might be considered in milder cases.[13] ▪ **Dose reduction:** can be considered in patients who have achieved full remission on an antidepressant.[6] ▪ **Drug holidays:** intermittently missing one or two doses prior to planned sexual activity may possibly help but risks discontinuation symptoms.[12] Not an effective strategy with fluoxetine due to its long half-life.[12] Lowering doses to a half for two consecutive days prior to sexual activity could be another possible strategy.[24]

(Continued)

CHAPTER 3

Table 3.21 (*Continued*)

Strategy	Details
Pharmacological treatments	▪ **Phosphodiesterase inhibitors:** both sildenafil and tadalafil have been shown to improve sexual functioning in men with antidepressant-related erectile dysfunction.[23,28] Limited evidence in women though one RCT found benefits.[23] ▪ **Bupropion:** may be useful in women at higher doses (300mg/day).[28] Lower doses appear to be ineffective.[23] A positive RCT in men[29] was later retracted. ▪ **Mirtazapine:** Evidence is mixed. Open studies suggest some benefit for antidepressant-induced SD, but negative results were reported in one RCT.[27] ▪ **Transdermal testosterone:** RCTs provide evidence of possible efficacy in women with SSRI/SNRI-emergent loss of libido[30] and in men who continue to take serotonergic antidepressants with low or low-normal testosterone levels.[31] ▪ **Others:**[12] many other agents have been studied; however, some of these have little or no evidence of their effectiveness. **Buspirone** was effective in one study for citalopram- or paroxetine-induced sexual dysfunction, but ineffective in another study with fluoxetine. **Cyproheptadine** has been used successfully in case reports of SSRI-induced sexual dysfunction in men, and for anorgasmia in women. **Loratadine** was effective in a small open study for men with SSRI-induced erectile dysfunction. **Amantadine** was effective in earlier studies for SSRI-induced sexual dysfunction, but recent results have been negative. **Yohimbine** may be more effective for medication-induced SD and improvements were reported by patients in two small studies (although results were nonsignificant). **Bethanechol** appears to help with TCA-induced sexual dysfunction when taken before sexual activity. **Granisetron** has been evaluated but the existing data are not definitive. **Flibanserin** and **bremelanotide** are approved by FDA for treatment of HSDD in premenopausal women[32] but there are no data to support use for antidepressant-induced SD. ▪ **Augmenting agents in treatment-resistant depression:** some drugs used as an adjunct for treatment-resistant depression have been associated with improvement in sexual functioning in secondary analyses. **Aripiprazole** improved sexual functioning and desire, though only in women.[24] **Brexpiprazole** was associated with modest improvements in one analysis.[33] **Pimavanserin,** used as an add on treatment to SSRIs/SNRIs, improved sexual functioning in another analysis.[34]

References

1. McCabe MP, et al. Incidence and prevalence of sexual dysfunction in women and men: a consensus statement from the fourth international consultation on sexual medicine 2015. *J Sex Med* 2016; 13:144–152.
2. Chokka PR, et al. Assessment and management of sexual dysfunction in the context of depression. *Ther Adv Psychopharmacol* 2018; 8:13–23.
3. Pereira-Miranda E, et al. Overweight and obesity associated with higher depression prevalence in adults: a systematic review and meta-analysis. *J Am Coll Nutr* 2017; 36:223–233.
4. Semenkovich K, et al. Depression in type 2 diabetes mellitus: prevalence, impact, and treatment. *Drugs* 2015; 75:577–587.
5. Cohen BE, et al. State of the art review: depression, stress, anxiety, and cardiovascular disease. *Am J Hypertens* 2015; 28:1295–1302.
6. Montejo AL, et al. The impact of severe mental disorders and psychotropic medications on sexual health and its implications for clinical management. *World Psychiatry* 2018; 17:3–11.
7. McGahuey CA, et al. The Arizona Sexual Experience Scale (ASEX): reliability and validity. *J Sex Marital Ther* 2000; 26:25–40.
8. Papakostas GI. Identifying patients who need a change in depression treatment and implementing that change. *J Clin Psychiatry* 2016; 77:e1009.
9. Kennedy SH, et al. Sexual dysfunction before antidepressant therapy in major depression. *J Affect Disord* 1999; 56:201–208.
10. Clayton AH, et al. Antidepressants and sexual dysfunction: mechanisms and clinical implications. *Postgrad Med* 2014; 126:91–99.
11. Ishak WW, et al. Sexual satisfaction and quality of life in major depressive disorder before and after treatment with citalopram in the STAR*D study. *J Clin Psychiatry* 2013; 74:256–261.
12. Clayton AH, et al. Sexual dysfunction due to psychotropic medications. *Psychiatr Clin North Am* 2016; 39:427–463.
13. Rothmore J. Antidepressant-induced sexual dysfunction. *Med J Aust* 2020; 212:329–334.
14. Bala A, et al. Post-SSRI sexual dysfunction: a literature review. *Sex Med Rev* 2018; 6:29–34.
15. McMahon CG. Dapoxetine: a new option in the medical management of premature ejaculation. *Ther Adv Urol* 2012; 4:233–251.

16. Khin NA, et al. Regulatory and scientific issues in studies to evaluate sexual dysfunction in antidepressant drug trials. *J Clin Psychiatry* 2015; 76:1060–1063.

17. Serretti A, et al. Treatment-emergent sexual dysfunction related to antidepressants: a meta-analysis. *J Clin Psychopharmacol* 2009; 29:259–266.

18. Chiesa A, et al. Antidepressants and sexual dysfunction: epidemiology, mechanisms and management. *J Psychopathology* 2010; 16:104–113.

19. Lew-Starowicz M, et al. *Impact of psychotropic medications on sexual functioning.* Cham: Springer; 2021:353–371.

20. Reichenpfader U, et al. Sexual dysfunction associated with second-generation antidepressants in patients with major depressive disorder: results from a systematic review with network meta-analysis. *Drug Saf* 2014; 37:19–31.

21. Wagner G, et al. Efficacy and safety of levomilnacipran, vilazodone and vortioxetine compared with other second-generation antidepressants for major depressive disorder in adults: a systematic review and network meta-analysis. *J Affect Disord* 2018; 228:1–12.

22. Watanabe N, et al. Mirtazapine versus other antidepressive agents for depression. *Cochrane Database Syst Rev* 2011; CD006528.

23. Cleare A, et al. Evidence-based guidelines for treating depressive disorders with antidepressants: a revision of the 2008 British Association for Psychopharmacology guidelines. *J Psychopharmacology* 2015; 29:459–525.

24. Montejo AL, et al. Management strategies for antidepressant-related sexual dysfunction: a clinical approach. *J Clin Med* 2019; 8:1640.

25. Jacobsen PL, et al. Treatment-emergent sexual dysfunction in randomized trials of vortioxetine for major depressive disorder or generalized anxiety disorder: a pooled analysis. *CNS Spectr* 2016; 21:367–378.

26. Koesters M, et al. Vortioxetine for depression in adults. *Cochrane Database Syst Rev* 2017; 7:Cd011520.

27. Francois D, et al. Antidepressant-induced sexual side effects: incidence, assessment, clinical implications, and management. *Psychiatric Ann* 2017; 47:154–160.

28. Taylor MJ, et al. Strategies for managing sexual dysfunction induced by antidepressant medication. *CochraneDatabaseSystRev* 2013; 5:CD003382.

29. Safarinejad MR. The effects of the adjunctive bupropion on male sexual dysfunction induced by a selective serotonin reuptake inhibitor: a double-blind placebo-controlled and randomized study. *BJU Int* 2010; 106:840–847.

30. Montejo AL, et al. Sexual side-effects of antidepressant and antipsychotic drugs. *Curr Opin Psychiatry* 2015; 28:418–423.

31. Amiaz R, et al. Testosterone gel replacement improves sexual function in depressed men taking serotonergic antidepressants: a randomized, placebo-controlled clinical trial. *J Sex Marital Ther* 2011; 37:243–254.

32. Bitzer J, et al. *Female sexual dysfunctions.* Cham: Springer; 2021:109–134.

33. Clayton AH, et al. Effect of brexpiprazole on prolactin and sexual functioning: an analysis of short- and long-term study data in major depressive disorder. *J Clin Psychopharmacol* 2020; 40:560–567.

34. Freeman MP, et al. Improvement of sexual functioning during treatment of MDD with adjunctive pimavanserin: a secondary analysis. *Depress Anxiety* 2020; 37:485–495.

Further reading

Montejo, A.L., et al. Management strategies for antidepressant-related sexual dysfunction: a clinical approach. *Journal of clinical medicine* 2019; 8:1640.

SSRIs and bleeding

Serotonin is released from platelets in response to vascular injury, promoting vasoconstriction and morphological changes in platelets that lead to aggregation.[1] SSRIs inhibit the serotonin transporter which is responsible for the uptake of serotonin into platelets. This depletion of platelet serotonin leads to a reduced ability to form clots and a subsequent increase in the risk of bleeding. Broadly speaking, the relative risk of any bleeding event compared with no use of SSRI/SNRI is around 1.4, with the absolute risk being between around 0.5% and 6%[2] (depending on numerous factors, but especially the duration of treatment).

SSRIs may also increase gastric acid secretion and therefore may be indirectly irritant to the gastric mucosa,[3] increasing the risk of peptic ulcer.[4] The risk of abnormal bleeding of any kind with SSRIs is highest during the first 30 days of treatment.[5,6] Effect on bleeding is probably, but not definitely, related to the affinity of individual SSRIs for the serotonin transporter (Table 3.22).[7,8]

Table 3.22 Antidepressants and degree of serotonin reuptake inhibition[6,9]

Degree of serotonin reuptake inhibition	Antidepressant (SSRI)
Strong inhibition	Sertraline, paroxetine, fluoxetine, duloxetine, clomipramine
Intermediate inhibition	Citalopram, escitalopram, fluvoxamine, vilazodone, vortioxetine, venlafaxine Amitriptyline, imipramine
Weak or no inhibition	Agomelatine, dosulepin, doxepin, lofepramine, mirtazapine, moclobemide, nortriptyline, reboxetine, mianserin

Risk factors for bleeding with SSRIs

- Age, particularly those over 65
- Alcohol misuse
- Coronary artery disease
- Drug misuse
- Hypertension
- History of GI bleed
- History of stroke
- History of major bleeding
- Liver disease
- Labile INR
- Medication predisposing to bleeding
- Peptic ulcer
- Renal disease
- Smoking

Caution should be exercised when prescribing serotonergic antidepressants for people with medical conditions such as gout, asthma, COPD, lupus, psoriasis, interferon-induced depression in hepatitis-C patients[10] and arthritis, when patients might also be taking corticosteroids, aspirin or NSAIDS.

Gastrointestinal bleeding

The use of serotonergic antidepressants is an independent risk factor for bleeding events. A population-based study revealed that SSRIs increase the rate of upper gastro-intestinal bleeding (UGIB), with hazard ratio (HR) of 1.97 and lower gastrointestinal bleeding (LGIB) (HR 2.96) after adjusting for all relevant risk factors.[11] In absolute terms, it is likely that SSRIs are responsible for an additional three episodes of bleeding in every 1,000 patient years of treatment,[7,12,13] but this figure masks large variations in risk. For example, 1 in 85 patients with a history of GI bleed will have a further bleed attributable to treatment with an SSRI.[14]

One database study suggests that gastro-protective drugs (PPIs) decrease the risk of GI bleeds associated with SSRIs (either alone or in combination with NSAIDs) although not quite to control levels.[15] A 2020 study found SSRIs increased risk of GI bleeding in people taking direct-acting anticoagulants for atrial fibrillation and that this risk was increased further in those not prescribed PPIs.[16] (Another found no increased risk of bleeding for SSRIs prescribed alongside any anticoagulants.[17])

Other database studies have found that patients who take SSRIs are at significantly increased risk of being admitted to hospital with an upper gastrointestinal (GI) bleed compared with age-and-sex matched controls.[7,15,18,19] This association holds when age, gender, and the effects of other drugs such as aspirin and non-steroidal anti-inflamma-tory drugs (NSAIDs) are controlled for.[2] In addition to this, a meta-analysis of 22 stud-ies concluded that current users of SSRIs are 55% more at risk of UGIB compared with those who do not take SSRIs. This risk was significantly and further increased by con-current use of antiplatelet drugs or NSAIDs.[5]

Co-prescription of low-dose aspirin at least doubles the risk of GI bleeding associ-ated with SSRIs alone and co-prescription of NSAIDs approximately quadruples risk.[20] Combined use of SSRIs and NSAIDs greatly increases the use of anti-acid drugs.[21] The elderly and those with a history of GI bleeding are at greatest risk.[14,15,19]

Some early studies found that in patients who take warfarin, SSRIs increase the risk of a non-GI bleed two to three-fold (similar to the effect size of NSAIDs) but did not seem to increase the risk of a GI bleed.[22,23] A later study[11] showed an increased risk of upper and lower GI bleeding in concomitant users of warfarin and serotonergic antidepressant (see Table 3.23). This effect does not seem to be associated with any change in INR, making it difficult to identify those at highest risk.[23] In keeping with these findings, SSRI use in anti-coagulated patients being treated for acute coronary syndromes may decrease the risk of minor cardiac events at the expense of an increased risk of a bleed.[24] Thus, the increased risk of upper GI bleeds associated with SSRIs may be balanced by a decreased risk of embolic events. One database study failed to find a reduction in the risk of a first myocardial infarc-tion in SSRI treated-patients[25] while another[26] found a reduction in the risk of being admit-ted to hospital with a first MI in smokers on SSRIs. The effect size in the second study was large: approximately 1 in 10 hospitalisations was avoided in SSRI-treated patients.[26] This is similar to the effect size of other antiplatelet therapies such as aspirin.[27]

Table 3.23 Approximate absolute risk of GI bleeding with concomitant use of SSRIs[28]

Drug	Absolute risk of UGIB*	Absolute risk of LGIB**
Aspirin + SSRI	6%	3%
Warfarin + SSRI	4%	3%
NSAID + SSRI	3%	1%
SSRI alone	2%	1%

*Upper gastrointestinal bleeding
**Lower gastrointestinal bleeding
Percentage figures rounded to nearest integer

Many studies do not state changes in absolute risk of intestinal bleeding, and some of those that do fail to provide denominator details (i.e. duration of treatment). Ideally, risk should be defined as the number of additional cases per 1,000 patient years. Table 3.23 shows approximate absolute risks (without a denominator) derived from a single study[11] and personal communication.[28]

Risk decreases to the same level as controls in past users of SSRIs indicating that bleeding is likely to be associated with treatment itself rather than some inherent characteristic of the patients being treated.[7] It also means that the effect of SSRIs disappears after their withdrawal.

The excess risk of bleeding is not confined to upper GI bleeds (see Table 3.23). The risk of lower GI bleeds may also be increased[29] and an increased risk of uterine bleeding (see later) has also been reported.[12]

Intracranial/intracerebral Haemorrhage (ICH)

There is a clear association between the use of SSRIs and ICH, and risk is further increased by concomitant use of NSAIDs and anticoagulants.

Elevated risk of ICH has been observed across all classes of antidepressants with serotonergic activity. In a cohort study of 1,363,990 users of antidepressants,[6] the overall rate of ICH was 3.8 per 10,000 patient years. Current use of SSRI increased the risk of ICH (RR 1.17) compared with TCA with an absolute adjusted rate difference of 6.7 per 100,000 persons per year. Amongst the SSRI group the risk of ICH was 25% greater in those who used strong inhibitors of serotonin reuptake system in comparison to users of weak inhibitors (see Table 3.24). This correlates to an absolute adjusted rate difference of 9.5 events per 100,000 persons per year. Overall risk was highest during the first 30 days of use. A 2018 meta-analysis of 12 studies confirmed an increased risk of ICH for SSRIs (Odds Ratios from 0.8 to 2.42), with an indication that stronger reuptake inhibitors had a greater effect.[30] Since then, one study reported no increased risk of ICH with SSRIs either alone or alongside anticoagulants,[31] whereas another[32] found that SSRIs increased risk of recurrence of ICH by 31%.

One database study[33] also identified an increased risk of ICH in those who have been taking SSRIs alone or in combination with NSAIDs. This and other studies providing data on absolute risk are summarised in Table 3.24.

Table 3.24 gives estimates of absolute risk of ICH derived from 3 studies.

CHAPTER 3

Table 3.24 Absolute risk of intracranial haemorrhage with SSRI with or without anticoagulant or NSAIDs

Study	Risk with SSRI alone	Risk with SSRI + NSAID	Risk with antidepressant + anticoagulant
Shin et al 2015[33]	1 in 632*(0.16%)	1 in 175*(0.57%)	–
Renoux et al 2017[6]	1 in 450** (0.22%)	–	1 in 260** (0.38%)
Smoller et al 2009[34]	1 in 240*** (0.42%)	–	–

*within 30 days of taking antidepressant
**Incident users (no time limit)
***Annual risk (older patients)

Gynaecologic and obstetrical haemorrhage

A multicentre cross-sectional study[35] found an association between the use of antidepressants and menstruation disorders (unusual or excess bleeding, irregular menstruation, menorrhagia, etc.). This study found that the prevalence of menstrual disorder in the study group who were taking SSRIs, venlafaxine or mirtazapine combined with SSRIs or mirtazapine was significantly higher (24.6%) than the control group (12.2%) who did not take any antidepressants.

Abnormal vaginal bleeding

Cases of abnormal vaginal bleeding associated with SSRIs have been reported in a young woman,[36] a postmenopausal woman[37] and in a preadolescent girl aged 11.[38]

Post-partum haemorrhage (PPH)

Whilst one study[39] could not find an increased risk of post-partum haemorrhage with the use of SSRI or non-SSRI antidepressants, a large cohort study[40] found an association between PPH and all classes of antidepressants with a number needed to harm of 80 for current users of SSRIs and 97 for those on other antidepressants. One hospital-based cohort study[41]found an absolute risk of PPH of 18% and an absolute risk of postpartum anaemia of 12.8% after a non-surgical vaginal delivery in women who were current users of SSRIs. The absolute risk of both PPH and postpartum anaemia for those without any exposure to antidepressants was 8.7%. The blood loss during delivery was also higher for those who had SSRI exposure (484mL) compared with those who did not take antidepressants (398mL). The length of hospital stay was also significantly increased for those who had been taking an SSRI. The most recent population study[42] identified that the use of serotonergic medications was associated with 1.5 times increased risk of PPH compared with those who did not take any psychoactive medications. This study highlighted that women who have been taking other psychoactive medications such as antipsychotics and mood stabilisers were three times more at risk of PPH compared to mothers who did not take any medications, suggesting that the occurrence of PPH might not be entirely due to serotonergic activity and that further research is needed to investigate other mechanisms.

In 2021, the UK MHRA issued a warning regarding the use of SSRIs and postpartum blood loss.[43]

Surgical and post-operative bleeding (see Table 3.25)

Use of SSRIs in the pre-operative period has been associated with a 20% increase in inpatient mortality (absolute risk 1 in 1,000), although patient factors rather than drug factors could not be excluded as the cause.[44] One study[45] found that patients prescribed SSRIs who underwent orthopaedic surgery had an almost four-fold risk of requiring a blood transfusion. This equated to one additional patient requiring transfusion for every ten SSRI patients undergoing surgery and was double the risk of patients who were taking NSAIDs alone. It should be noted in this context that treatment with SSRIs has been associated with a 2.4-fold increase in the risk of hip fracture[46] and a two-fold increase of fracture in old age.[47] (Mirtazapine[48] and TCAs[46] also increase risk of hip fracture.) One recent study recognised the preoperative treatment with SSRIs, other antidepressants or antipsychotics as independent risk factors for blood transfusion in elective fast-track hip and knee arthroplasty.[49]

The combination of advanced age, SSRI treatment, orthopaedic surgery and NSAIDs clearly presents a very high risk. However, there does not seem to be an increased risk of bleeding in patients who undergo coronary artery bypass surgery.[50]

Table 3.25 Risk of perioperative blood loss and blood transfusion in SSRI users compared with non-SSRI users[51]

Surgical Procedure	Need for reoperation due to bleeding event in users of SADs* vs non-users	Need for blood product or red blood cell transfusion in users of SADs vs non-users	Increased risk of mortality in users of SADs vs non-users
Coronary artery bypass Graft (CABG)	OR 1.07 (0.66–1.74)	OR 1.06 (0.90–1.24)	OR 1.53 (1.15–2.04)
Breast-cancer directed Surgery	OR 2.7 (1.6–4.56)	–	–
Orthopaedic surgery	–	OR1.61 (0.97–2.68)	OR 0.83 (0.69–1.00)
Major surgery	–	OR 1.19 (1.15–1.23)	OR 1.19 (1.03–1.37)

*Serotonergic antidepressants
OR, odds ratio

During a 10-year review of women who underwent cosmetic breast surgery procedures, the use of SSRIs increased the risk of post-operative bleeding by a factor of 4.14 compared with those who did not take SSRIs. The authors emphasised the importance of balancing the risks and benefits of stopping antidepressants prior to elective surgeries, particularly in psychologically vulnerable patients.[52]

CHAPTER 3

A review of 13 studies found an increased odds ratio (1.21–4.14) of perioperative bleeding with SSRIs.[53] One study noted an increased risk of bleeding in women undergoing breast surgery,[54] and the authors suggest withholding SSRIs for 2 weeks prior to such planned surgery. Others conclude that there is insufficient evidence to support routine discontinuation of SSRIs prior to surgery and call for RCTs to be conducted in this area of care.[55] Venlafaxine may have similar effects,[53] but duloxetine may not affect bleeding risk.[56]

Alternatives to SSRIs/SNRIs

Non-SSRI antidepressants such as mirtazapine and bupropion have been suggested as safer alternatives to SSRIs and SNRIs.[57] Preliminary studies suggest mirtazapine, bupropion and nortriptyline have minimal effects on measurable clotting mechanisms.[58] However, there is little evidence that these drugs are safer, and one meta-analysis found an increased risk of UGI bleeding with mirtazapine (vs. no treatment) and no difference in bleeding risk between mirtazapine or bupropion and SSRIs.[59]

Overall

Serotonergic antidepressants increase the risk of various types of bleeding. Evidence is strongest for SSRIs, and it is likely that risk of bleeding is related to affinity for the serotonin transporter. SSRIs increase the risk of GI bleeding, haemorrhagic stroke, perioperative bleeding, postpartum haemorrhage and uterine bleeding. Their effect is exacerbated by co-prescription with aspirin, anticoagulants and NSAIDs. In most cases, the use of SSRIs increases the risk of an event by a clinically meaningful extent, but especially when co-prescribed with other drugs which affect clotting.

Summary

- SSRIs increase the risk of GI, uterine, cerebral and perioperative bleeding.
- Risk is increased still further in those also receiving aspirin, NSAIDs or oral anticoagulants.
- Try to avoid SSRIs/SNRIs in patients receiving NSAIDs, aspirin or oral anticoagulants or in those with a history of cerebral or GI bleeds.
- Safer alternatives have not been definitively identified, but noradrenergic antidepressants (nortriptyline, bupropion) may be preferred.
- If SSRI/SNRI use cannot be avoided, monitor closely and prescribe gastro-protective proton pump inhibitors.
- Limited evidence suggests risks may be lower with less potent serotonin re-uptake inhibitors.

References

1. Skop BP, et al. Potential vascular and bleeding complications of treatment with selective serotonin reuptake inhibitors. *Psychosomatics* 1996; 37:12–16.

2. Laporte S, et al. Bleeding risk under selective serotonin reuptake inhibitor (SSRI) antidepressants: a meta-analysis of observational studies. *Pharmacol Res* 2017; 118:19–32.

3. Andrade C, et al. Serotonin reuptake inhibitor antidepressants and abnormal bleeding: a review for clinicians and a reconsideration of mechanisms. *J Clin Psychiatry* 2010; 71:1565–1575.

4. Dall M, et al. There is an association between selective serotonin reuptake inhibitor use and uncomplicated peptic ulcers: a population-based case-control study. *Aliment Pharmacol Ther* 2010; 32:1383–1391.

5. Jiang HY, et al. Use of selective serotonin reuptake inhibitors and risk of upper gastrointestinal bleeding: a systematic review and meta-analysis. *Clin Gastroenterol Hepatol* 2015; 13:42–50.

6. Renoux C, et al. Association of selective serotonin reuptake inhibitors with the risk for spontaneous intracranial hemorrhage. *JAMA Neurology* 2017; 74:173–180.

7. Dalton SO, et al. Use of selective serotonin reuptake inhibitors and risk of upper gastrointestinal tract bleeding: a population-based cohort study. *Arch Intern Med* 2003; 163:59–64.

8. Verdel BM, et al. Use of serotonergic drugs and the risk of bleeding. *Clin Pharmacol Ther* 2011; 89:89–96.

9. Tatsumi M, et al. Pharmacological profile of antidepressants and related compounds at human monoamine transporters. *Eur J Pharmacol* 1997; 340:249–258.

10. Weinrieb RM, et al. A critical review of selective serotonin reuptake inhibitor-associated bleeding: balancing the risk of treating hepatitis C-infected patients. *J Clin Psychiatry* 2003; 64:1502–1510.

11. Cheng YL, et al. Use of SSRI, but not SNRI, increased upper and lower gastrointestinal bleeding: a nationwide population-based cohort study in Taiwan. *Medicine (Baltimore)* 2015; 94:e2022.

12. Meijer WE, et al. Association of risk of abnormal bleeding with degree of serotonin reuptake inhibition by antidepressants. *Arch Intern Med* 2004; 164:2367–2370.

13. Yuet WC, et al. Selective serotonin reuptake inhibitor use and risk of gastrointestinal and intracranial bleeding. *J Am Osteopath Assoc* 2019; 119:102–111.

14. van Walraven C, et al. Inhibition of serotonin reuptake by antidepressants and upper gastrointestinal bleeding in elderly patients: retrospective cohort study. *BMJ* 2001; 323:655–658.

15. de Abajo FJ, et al. Risk of upper gastrointestinal tract bleeding associated with selective serotonin reuptake inhibitors and venlafaxine therapy: interaction with nonsteroidal anti-inflammatory drugs and effect of acid-suppressing agents. *Arch Gen Psychiatry* 2008; 65:795–803.

16. Lee MT, et al. Concomitant use of NSAIDs or SSRIs with NOACs requires monitoring for bleeding. *Yonsei Med J* 2020; 61:741–749.

17. Quinn GR, et al. Selective serotonin reuptake inhibitors and bleeding risk in anticoagulated patients with atrial fibrillation: an analysis from the ROCKET AF trial. *J Am Heart Assoc* 2018; 7:e008755.

18. de Abajo FJ, et al. Association between selective serotonin reuptake inhibitors and upper gastrointestinal bleeding: population based case-control study. *BMJ* 1999; 319:1106–1109.

19. Lewis JD, et al. Moderate and high affinity serotonin reuptake inhibitors increase the risk of upper gastrointestinal toxicity. *Pharmacoepidemiol Drug Saf* 2008; 17:328–335.

20. Paton C, et al. SSRIs and gastrointestinal bleeding. *BMJ* 2005; 331:529–530.

21. de Jong JC, et al. Combined use of SSRIs and NSAIDs increases the risk of gastrointestinal adverse effects. *Br J Clin Pharmacol* 2003; 55:591–595.

22. Schalekamp T, et al. Increased bleeding risk with concurrent use of selective serotonin reuptake inhibitors and coumarins. *Arch Intern Med* 2008; 168:180–185.

23. Wallerstedt SM, et al. Risk of clinically relevant bleeding in warfarin-treated patients–influence of SSRI treatment. *Pharmacoepidemiol Drug Saf* 2009; 18:412–416.

24. Ziegelstein RC, et al. Selective serotonin reuptake inhibitor use by patients with acute coronary syndromes. *Am J Med* 2007; 120:525–530.

25. Meier CR, et al. Use of selective serotonin reuptake inhibitors and risk of developing first-time acute myocardial infarction. *Br J Clin Pharmacol* 2001; 52:179–184.

26. Sauer WH, et al. Selective serotonin reuptake inhibitors and myocardial infarction. *Circulation* 2001; 104:1894–1898.

27. Antiplatelet Trialists' Collaboration. Collaborative overview of randomised trials of antiplatelet therapy–I: prevention of death, myocardial infarction, and stroke by prolonged antiplatelet therapy in various categories of patients. *BMJ* 1994; 308:81–106.

28. Cheng YL Personal communication, 2017.

29. Wessinger S, et al. Increased use of selective serotonin reuptake inhibitors in patients admitted with gastrointestinal haemorrhage: a multicentre retrospective analysis. *Aliment Pharmacol Ther* 2006; 23:937–944.

30. Douros A, et al. Risk of intracranial hemorrhage associated with the use of antidepressants inhibiting serotonin reuptake: a systematic review. *CNS Drugs* 2018; 32:321–334.

31. Liu L, et al. Selective serotonin reuptake inhibitors and intracerebral hemorrhage risk and outcome. *Stroke* 2020; 51:1135–1141.

32. Kubiszewski P, et al. Association of selective serotonin reuptake inhibitor use after intracerebral hemorrhage with hemorrhage recurrence and depression severity. *JAMA Neurology* 2020; 78:1–8.

33. Shin JY, et al. Risk of intracranial haemorrhage in antidepressant users with concurrent use of non-steroidal anti-inflammatory drugs: nationwide propensity score matched study. *BMJ (Clinical Research Ed)* 2015; 351:h3517.

34. Smoller JW, et al. Antidepressant use and risk of incident cardiovascular morbidity and mortality among postmenopausal women in the Women's Health Initiative study. *Arch Intern Med* 2009; **169**:2128–2139.

35. Uguz F, et al. Antidepressants and menstruation disorders in women: a cross-sectional study in three centers. *Gen Hosp Psychiatry* 2012; **34**:529–533.

36. Andersohn F, et al. Citalopram-induced bleeding due to severe thrombocytopenia. *Psychosomatics* 2009; **50**:297–298.

37. Durmaz O, et al. Vaginal bleeding associated with antidepressants. *Int J Gynaecol Obstet* 2015; **130**:284.

38. Turkoglu S, et al. Vaginal bleeding and hemorrhagic prepatellar bursitis in a preadolescent girl, possibly related to fluoxetine. *J Child Adolesc Psychopharmacol* 2015; **25**:186–187.

39. Salkeld E, et al. The risk of postpartum hemorrhage with selective serotonin reuptake inhibitors and other antidepressants. *J Clin Psychopharmacol* 2008; **28**:230–234.

40. Palmsten K, et al. Use of antidepressants near delivery and risk of postpartum hemorrhage: cohort study of low income women in the United States. *BMJ* 2013; **347**:f4877.

41. Lindqvist PG, et al. Selective serotonin reuptake inhibitor use during pregnancy increases the risk of postpartum hemorrhage and anemia: a hospital-based cohort study. *J Thromb Haemost* 2014; **12**:1986–1992.

42. Heller HM, et al. Increased postpartum haemorrhage, the possible relation with serotonergic and other psychopharmacological drugs: a matched cohort study. *BMC Pregnancy Childbirth* 2017; **17**:166.

43. Gov.UK. Drug Safety Update. SSRI/SNRI antidepressant medicines: small increased risk of postpartum haemorrhage when used in the month before delivery. 2021; https://www.gov.uk/drug-safety-update/ssri-slash-snri-antidepressant-medicines-small-increased-risk-of-postpartum-haemorrhage-when-used-in-the-month-before-delivery?utm_source=e-shot&utm_medium=email&utm_campaign=DSU_January2021split1.

44. Auerbach AD, et al. Perioperative use of selective serotonin reuptake inhibitors and risks for adverse outcomes of surgery. *JAMA Int Med* 2013; **173**:1075–1081.

45. Movig KL, et al. Relationship of serotonergic antidepressants and need for blood transfusion in orthopedic surgical patients. *Arch Intern Med* 2003; **163**:2354–2358.

46. Liu B, et al. Use of selective serotonin-reuptake inhibitors of tricyclic antidepressants and risk of hip fractures in elderly people. *Lancet* 1998; **351**:1303–1307.

47. Richards JB, et al. Effect of selective serotonin reuptake inhibitors on the risk of fracture. *Arch Intern Med* 2007; **167**:188–194.

48. Leach MJ, et al. The risk of hip fracture due to mirtazapine exposure when switching antidepressants or using other antidepressants as add-on therapy. *Drugs – Real World Outcomes* 2017; **4**:247–255.

49. Gylvin SH, et al. Psychopharmacologic treatment and blood transfusion in fast-track total hip and knee arthroplasty. *Transfusion (Paris)* 2017; **57**:971–976.

50. Andreasen JJ, et al. Effect of selective serotonin reuptake inhibitors on requirement for allogeneic red blood cell transfusion following coronary artery bypass surgery. *Am J Cardiovasc Drugs* 2006; **6**:243–250.

51. Singh I, et al. Influence of pre-operative use of serotonergic antidepressants (SADs) on the risk of bleeding in patients undergoing different surgical interventions: a meta-analysis. *Pharmacoepidemiol Drug Saf* 2015; **24**:237–245.

52. Basile FV, et al. Use of selective serotonin reuptake inhibitors antidepressants and bleeding risk in breast cosmetic surgery. *Aesthetic Plast Surg* 2013; **37**:561–566.

53. Mahdanian AA, et al. Serotonergic antidepressants and perioperative bleeding risk: a systematic review. *Exp Opin Drug Saf* 2014; **13**:695–704.

54. Jeong BO, et al. Use of serotonergic antidepressants and bleeding risk in patients undergoing surgery. *Psychosomatics* 2014; **55**:213–220.

55. Mrkobrada M, et al. Selective serotonin reuptake inhibitors and surgery: to hold or not to hold, that is the question: comment on 'Perioperative use of selective serotonin reuptake inhibitors and risks for adverse outcomes of surgery'. *JAMA Int Med* 2013; **173**:1082–1083.

56. Perahia DG, et al. The risk of bleeding with duloxetine treatment in patients who use nonsteroidal anti-inflammatory drugs (NSAIDs): analysis of placebo-controlled trials and post-marketing adverse event reports. *Drug Healthcare Patient Saf* 2013; **5**:211–219.

57. Bixby AL, et al. Clinical management of bleeding risk with antidepressants. *Ann Pharmacother* 2019; **53**:186–194.

58. Halperin D, et al. Influence of antidepressants on hemostasis. *Dialogues Clin Neurosci* 2007; **9**:47–59.

59. Na K-S, et al. Can we recommend mirtazapine and bupropion for patients at risk for bleeding?: a systematic review and meta-analysis. *J Affect Disord* 2018; **225**:221–226.

St. John's Wort

St. John's Wort (SJW) is the popular name for the plant *Hypericum perforatum*. It contains a combination of at least 10 different components, including hypericin, hyperforin and flavonoids.[1] Preparations of SJW are often unstandardised and this has complicated the interpretation of clinical trials. The active ingredient(s) and mechanism(s) of action of SJW are unclear.[1] Constituents of SJW may inhibit MAO, inhibit the re-uptake of noradrenaline and serotonin, up-regulate serotonin receptors and decrease serotonin receptor expression.[1]

Some preparations of SJW have been granted a traditional herbal registration certificate;[2] note that this is based on traditional use rather than proven efficacy and tolerability. SJW is licensed in Germany for the treatment of depression.[2]

Evidence for SJW in the treatment of depression

A number of trials have examined the efficacy of SJW in the treatment of depression. They have been extensively reviewed,[3-6] and most authors conclude that SJW is likely to be effective in the treatment of mild-to-moderate depression.[3,5-7] For example, Cochrane concludes that SJW is more effective than placebo in the treatment of mild-moderate depression, and is as effective as, and better tolerated than, standard antidepressants.[4] The supporting evidence is not without several limitations. Studies in German-speaking countries showed more favourable results than studies elsewhere.[4] Concerns have also been raised about the inadequate dosing of SSRIs in comparative studies.[8,9] In two reanalyses of data from a large negative RCT of SJW, both participant and clinician beliefs about treatment assignment were more strongly associated with clinical outcomes than the actual treatment received: those who guessed randomisation to active treatment fared better than those who guessed randomisation to placebo.[10,11] Efficacy in severe depression remains uncertain.[4-6] There is little evidence for SJW in postmenopausal depression[12] and in certain pain syndromes.[13]

It should be noted that:

- The active component of SJW for treating depression has not yet been determined. Trials used different preparations of SJW, most of which were standardised according to their total content of hypericins. However, evidence suggests that hypericins alone do not treat depression.[5]
- Many SJW preparations bought over the internet are sold as unregulated food supplements and are often of poor quality or adulterated.[2] One recent analysis of 47 different SJW preparations found that 36% were adulterated with other *Hypericum* species, and 19% adulterated with food dyes.[2]
- Published studies are generally acute treatment studies. There are only preliminary data to support the effectiveness of SJW in the medium term; longer-term and relapse prevention data are lacking.[14]

On balance, SJW should not be prescribed: we lack understanding of what the active ingredient is or what constitutes a therapeutic dose, and most preparations of SJW are unlicensed.

CHAPTER 3

Adverse effects

SJW appears to be well tolerated.[5,6] In a systematic review of existing studies, adverse effects were significantly less than with older antidepressants, slightly less than SSRIs and similar to placebo.[6] The most common, if infrequent, side-effects are nausea, rash, fatigue, restlessness, and photosensitivity.[15] Although severe phototoxic reactions seem to be rare, patients should be informed that SJW can increase light sensitivity.[15] SJW may also share the propensity of SSRIs to increase the risk of bleeding; a case report describes prolonged epistaxis after nasal insertion of SJW.[16] Case reports have described mania, hypomania and mixed states associated with SJW.[17] Onset of manic symptoms range from ranged from 3 days to 2 months.[17] Caution is advised with high doses and those with a known history of bipolar affective disorder.[18]

Drug interactions

SJW is a potent inducer of intestinal and hepatic CYP3A4, CYP2C9, CYP2C19, CYP2E1 and intestinal p-glycoprotein.[15,19] Hyperforin is responsible for this effect.[20] The hyperforin content of SJW preparations varies 50-fold, which will result in a different propensity for drug interactions between brands. Preparations providing a daily dose of <1mg hyperforin are less likely to induce CYP enzymes.[20,21] CYP3A4 activity is induced over 1–2 weeks and returns to normal approximately 7 days after SJW is discontinued.[22]

Studies have shown that SJW significantly reduces plasma concentrations of warfarin,[23] hormonal contraceptives,[24] digoxin and indinavir[15] (a drug used in the treatment of HIV). According to case reports, SJW has lowered the plasma concentrations of clozapine, theophylline, ciclosporin, gliclazide and statins.[15,19,25,26] There is a theoretical risk that SJW may interact with some antiseizure medications.[19] It has also been reported that SJW can increase the effects of clopidogrel (a pro-drug).[19] Serotonin syndrome has been reported when SJW was taken together with sertraline, paroxetine, nefazodone and the triptans.[27,28] SJW should not be taken with any drugs that have a predominantly serotonergic action.

Box 3.3 Key points that patients should know

- Evidence suggests that SJW may be effective in the treatment of mild to moderate depression, but we do not know enough about how much should be taken or what the side-effects are. There is less evidence of benefit in severe depression.
- SJW is not a licensed medicine.
- SJW can interact with other medicines, resulting in serious side-effects. Some important drugs may be metabolised more rapidly and therefore become ineffective with serious consequences (e.g. increased viral load in HIV, failure of oral contraceptives leading to unwanted pregnancy, reduced anticoagulant effect with warfarin leading to thrombosis).
- The symptoms of depression can sometimes be caused by other physical or mental illnesses. It is important that these possible causes are investigated.
- It is always best to consult the doctor if any herbal or natural remedy is being taken or the patient is thinking of taking one.

Many people regard herbal remedies as 'natural' and therefore harmless.[29] Many are not aware of the potential of such remedies for causing side effects or interacting with other drugs. A large study from Germany, ($n = 588$) where SJW is a licensed antidepressant, found that for every prescription written for SJW, one person purchased SJW without seeking the advice of a doctor.[30] Many of these people had severe or persistent depression, but few told their doctor that they took SJW. A small US study ($n = 22$) found that people tend to take SJW because it is easy to obtain alternative medicines and also because they perceive herbal medicines as being purer and safer than prescription medicines. Few would discuss this medication with their conventional health-care provider.[31] Clinicians need to be proactive in asking patients if they use such treatments and try to dispel the myth that natural is the same as safe (see Box 3.3).

References

1. Velingkar VS, et al. A current update on phytochemistry, pharmacology and herb–drug interactions of Hypericum perforatum. *Phytochemistry Rev* 2017; **16**:725–744.
2. Booker A, et al. St John's wort (Hypericum perforatum) products – an assessment of their authenticity and quality. *Phytomedicine* 2018; **40**:158–164.
3. National Institute for Clinical Excellence. Depression: the treatment and management of depression in adults. Clinical Guidance [CG90] 2009 (last reviewed December 2013); https://www.nice.org.uk/guidance/cg90.
4. Linde K, et al. St John's Wort for major depression. *Cochrane Database Syst Rev* 2008; CD000448.
5. Ng QX, et al. Clinical use of Hypericum perforatum (St John's wort) in depression: a meta-analysis. *J Affect Disord* 2017; **210**:211–221.
6. Apaydin EA, et al. A systematic review of St. John's wort for major depressive disorder. *Syst Rev* 2016; **5**:148.
7. Volz HP. Hypericum and Depression, in P Riederer, G Laux, T Nagatsu, W Le, C Riederer eds., *NeuroPsychopharmacotherapy*. Cham: Springer; 2020:1–8.
8. Asher GN, et al. Comparative benefits and harms of complementary and alternative medicine therapies for initial treatment of major depressive disorder: systematic review and meta-analysis. *J Altern Complement Med* 2017; **23**:907–919.
9. Gartlehner G, et al. Pharmacological and non-pharmacological treatments for major depressive disorder: review of systematic reviews. *BMJ Open* 2017; **7**:e014912.
10. Chen JA, et al. Association between patient beliefs regarding assigned treatment and clinical response: reanalysis of data from the Hypericum Depression Trial Study Group. *J Clin Psychiatry* 2011; **72**:1669–1676.
11. Chen JA, et al. Association between physician beliefs regarding assigned treatment and clinical response: re-analysis of data from the Hypericum Depression Trial Study Group. *Asian J Psychiatr* 2015; **13**:23–29.
12. Eatemadnia A, et al. The effect of Hypericum perforatum on postmenopausal symptoms and depression: a randomized controlled trial. *Complement Ther Med* 2019; **45**:109–113.
13. Galeotti N. Hypericum perforatum (St John's wort) beyond depression: a therapeutic perspective for pain conditions. *J Ethnopharmacol* 2017; **200**:136–146.
14. Cleare A, et al. Evidence-based guidelines for treating depressive disorders with antidepressants: a revision of the 2008 British Association for Psychopharmacology guidelines. *J Psychopharmacology* 2015; **29**:459–525.
15. Russo E, et al. Hypericum perforatum: pharmacokinetic, mechanism of action, tolerability, and clinical drug-drug interactions. *Phytother Res* 2014; **28**:643–655.
16. Crampsey DP, et al. Nasal insertion of St John's wort: an unusual cause of epistaxis. *J Laryngol Otol* 2007; **121**:279–280.
17. Bostock E, et al. Mania associated with herbal medicines, other than cannabis: a systematic review and quality assessment of case reports. *Front Psychiatry* 2018; **9**:280.
18. Sarris J. Herbal medicines in the treatment of psychiatric disorders: 10-year updated review. *Phytother Res* 2018; **32**:1147–1162.
19. Soleymani S, et al. Clinical risks of St John's Wort (Hypericum perforatum) co-administration. *Exp Opin Drug Metab Toxicol* 2017; **13**:1047–1062.
20. Chrubasik-Hausmann S, et al. Understanding drug interactions with St John's wort (Hypericum perforatum L.): impact of hyperforin content. *J Pharm Pharmacol* 2018; **71**:129–138.
21. Nicolussi S, et al. Clinical relevance of St. John's wort drug interactions revisited. *Br J Pharmacol* 2020; **177**:1212–1226.
22. Imai H, et al. The recovery time-course of CYP3A after induction by St John's wort administration. *Br J Clin Pharmacol* 2008; **65**:701–707.
23. Choi S, et al. A systematic review of the pharmacokinetic and pharmacodynamic interactions of herbal medicine with warfarin. *PLoS One* 2017; **12**:e0182794.
24. Berry-Bibee EN, et al. Co-administration of St. John's wort and hormonal contraceptives: a systematic review. *Contraception* 2016; **94**:668–677.

25. Xu H, et al. Effects of St John's wort and CYP2C9 genotype on the pharmacokinetics and pharmacodynamics of gliclazide. *Br J Pharmacol* 2008; **153**:1579–1586.

26. Andren L, et al. Interaction between a commercially available St. John's wort product (Movina) and atorvastatin in patients with hypercholesterolemia. *Eur J Clin Pharmacol* 2007; **63**:913–916.

27. Anon. Reminder: St John's Wort (*Hypericum perforatum*) interactions. *Curr Problems Pharmacovigilance* 2000; **26**:6–7.

28. Lantz MS, et al. St. John's wort and antidepressant drug interactions in the elderly. *J Geriatr Psychiatry Neurol* 1999; **12**:7–10.

29. Barnes J, et al. Different standards for reporting ADRs to herbal remedies and conventional OTC medicines: face-to-face interviews with 515 users of herbal remedies. *Br J Clin Pharmacol* 1998; **45**:496–500.

30. Linden M, et al. Self medication with St. John's wort in depressive disorders: an observational study in community pharmacies. *J Affect Disord* 2008; **107**:205–210.

31. Wagner PJ, et al. Taking the edge off: why patients choose St. John's Wort. *J Fam Pract* 1999; **48**:615–619.

Antidepressants: relative adverse effects – a rough guide

Table 3.26 gives a very approximate, unreferenced view of the absolute and relative risk of a small range of adverse effects associated with standard antidepressants.

Table 3.26 Common adverse effects of antidepressants

Drug	Sedation	Postural hypotension§	Cardiac conduction disturbance§	Anticholinergic effects	Nausea/ Vomiting	Sexual dysfunction§
Tricyclics						
Amitriptyline	+++	+++	+++	+++	+	+++
Clomipramine	++	+++	+++	++	++	+++
Dosulepin	+++	+++	+++	++	+	+
Doxepin	+++	++	+++	+++	+	+
Imipramine	++	+++	+++	+++	+	+
Lofepramine	+	+	+	++	+	+
Nortriptyline	+	++	++	+	+	+
Trimipramine	+++	+++	++	++	+	+
Other antidepressants						
Agomelatine	+	–	–	–	–	–
Duloxetine (SNRI)	–	–*	–	–	++	++
Levomilnacipran (SNRI)	–	–*	–	–	++	++
Mianserin	++	–	–	–	–	–
Mirtazapine	+++	+	–	+	+	–
Reboxetine	+	–*	–	+	+	+
Trazodone	+++	+	+	+	+	+
Venlafaxine (SNRI)	–	–*	+	–	+++	+++
Selective serotonin reuptake inhibitors (SSRIs)						
Citalopram	–	–	+	–	++	+++
Escitalopram	–	–	+	–	++	+++
Fluoxetine	–	–	–	–	++	+++
Fluvoxamine	+	–	–	–	+++	+++
Paroxetine	+	–	–	+	++	+++

(Continued)

Table 3.26 (*Continued*)

Drug	Sedation	Postural hypotension[§]	Cardiac conduction disturbance[§]	Anticholinergic effects	Nausea/ Vomiting	Sexual dysfunction[§]
Sertraline	–	–	–	–	++	+++
Vilazodone	–	–	–	–	++	++
Vortioxetine	–	+	–	–	++	+
Monoamine oxidase inhibitors (MAOIs)						
Isocarboxazid	+	++	+	++	+	+
Phenelzine	+	+	+	+	+	+
Tranylcypromine	–	+	+	+	+	+
Reversible inhibitor of monoamine oxidase A (RIMA)						
Moclobemide	–	–	–	–	+	+

KEY:
+++ High incidence/severity
++ Moderate
+ Low– Very low/none
* Hypertension reported.
[§]In some cases, further details can be found in specific sections in this chapter.

Anxiety spectrum disorders

Anxiety disorders can occur in isolation, be co-morbid with other psychiatric disorders (particularly depression), be a consequence of physical illness such as thyrotoxicosis or be drug-induced (e.g. by caffeine). Co-morbidity with other psychiatric disorders is very common.

These disorders tend to be chronic and treatment is often only partially successful. People with anxiety disorders may be especially prone to adverse effects.[1] High initial doses of SSRIs in particular may be poorly tolerated, for example.

Benzodiazepines

Benzodiazepines provide rapid symptomatic relief from acute anxiety states.[2] All guidelines and consensus statements recommend that this group of drugs should be used only to treat anxiety that is severe, disabling, or subjecting the individual to extreme distress. Because of their potential to cause physical dependence and withdrawal symptoms, these drugs should be used at the lowest effective dose for the shortest period of time (maximum 4 weeks), while longer-term treatment strategies are put in place and with caution in patients with substance misuse. For the majority of patients these recommendations are sensible and should be followed. A very small number of patients with severely disabling anxiety may benefit from long-term treatment with a benzodiazepine, and these patients should not be denied treatment. Benzodiazepines are, however, known to be over-prescribed in the long-term for both treatment of anxiety[3] and depression,[4] perhaps especially in the United States where attitudes to benzodiazepines differ markedly from other developed countries.[5]

NICE recommends that benzodiazepines should not be used to treat panic disorder.[6] In other countries, alprazolam is widely used for this indication. Benzodiazepines should be used with extreme care in post-traumatic stress disorder (PTSD).[7]

SSRIs/SNRIs

When used to treat **Generalised Anxiety Disorder (GAD)**, SSRIs should initially be prescribed at half the normal starting dose and titrated to the normal antidepressant dosage range as tolerated (initial worsening of anxiety may be seen when treatment is started[8]). The same advice applies to the use of venlafaxine and duloxetine. Modest benefit is usually seen within 6 weeks and continues to increase over time.[9] The optimal duration of treatment has not been determined but should be at least one year.[10,11] Effective treatment of GAD may prevent the development of major depression.[10]

An early network meta-analysis suggests fluoxetine is the most effective SSRI in GAD and sertraline the best tolerated.[12] More recent analyses suggest that bupropion[13] or agomelatine[14] is the most effective drug in GAD. Neither analysis found clear effects over placebo for lorazepam or vortioxetine.

When used to treat **panic disorder**, the same starting dose and dosage titration as in GAD should be used. Doses of clomipramine,[15] citalopram[16] and sertraline[17] towards the bottom of the antidepressant range give the best balance between efficacy and side-effects, whereas higher doses of paroxetine (40mg and above) may be required.[18] Higher doses of all drugs may be effective when standard doses have failed – efficacy of SSRIs (but not SNRIs) increases across the licensed dose range in anxiety disorders.[19] Onset of action may be as long as 6 weeks. Women may respond better to SSRIs than men.[20] There is some evidence that augmentation with clonazepam leads to a more rapid response (but not a greater magnitude of response overall).[18] The optimal duration of treatment is unknown but should be at least 8 months.[21] A large naturalistic study showed convincing evidence of benefit for at least 3 years.[22] Less than half are likely to remain well after medication is withdrawn.[23]

Lower starting doses are also required in **post-traumatic stress disorder** (PTSD), although high doses (e.g. fluoxetine 60mg) are usually required for full effect. Response is usually seen within 8 weeks, but can take up to 12 weeks.[23] Treatment should be continued for at least 6 months and probably longer.[11,24,25]

Although the doses of SSRIs licensed for the treatment of **obsessive compulsive disorder** (OCD) are higher than those licensed for the treatment of depression (e.g. fluoxetine 60mg, paroxetine 40–60mg), lower (standard antidepressant) doses may be effective, particularly for maintenance treatment.[26] Initial response is usually slower to emerge than in depression (can take 10–12 weeks). Dose should be increased to gain maximal benefit. Treatment should continue for at least 1 year.[11] The relapse rate in those who continue treatment for 2 years is half that of those who stop treatment after initial response (25–40% vs 80%).[27] In most people with OCD, the condition is persistent and symptom severity fluctuates over time.[28] Second-line treatment is usually the addition of either risperidone or aripiprazole.

Body dysmorphic disorder (BDD) should be treated initially with CBT. If symptoms are moderate to severe, adding an SSRI may improve outcome.[29] Buspirone may usefully augment the SSRI,[29] although no RCT has been conducted.

Standard antidepressant starting doses are well tolerated in **social phobia**,[30,31] and dosage titration may benefit some patients but is not always required. Some benefit is usually seen within 8 weeks, and treatment should be continued for at least a year and probably longer.[31] NICE recommends CBT as first-line treatment for Social Anxiety.[32]

All patients treated with SSRIs should be monitored for the development of akathisia, increased anxiety and the emergence of suicidal ideation; the risk is thought to be greatest in those <30 years, those with co-morbid depression and those already known to be at higher risk of suicide.[29,33]

SSRIs should not be stopped abruptly, as patients with anxiety spectrum disorders are particularly sensitive to discontinuation symptoms (see section on Antidepressant withdrawal symptoms). The dose should be reduced as slowly as tolerated over several months.

Pregabalin

Pregabalin is licensed for the treatment of GAD. Several large RCTs have demonstrated its efficacy and tolerability and comparable speed of onset of action to a benzodiazepine.[34] The dose of pregabalin in GAD is initially 150mg, increased gradually to maximum of 600mg in 2 to 3 divided doses. It is widely misused (often alongside opioids[35]), and there is a significant risk of diversion.[36] Pregabalin should not be stopped abruptly as it may precipitate a severe withdrawal syndrome that includes seizures.[37]

Psychological approaches

There is good evidence to support the efficacy of psychological interventions in anxiety spectrum disorders.[11,38] Examples include exposure therapy in OCD and social phobia. Initial drug therapy may be required to help the patient become more receptive to psychological input, although evidence to support this assumption is slim. Some studies suggest that optimal outcome is achieved by combining psychological and drug thera-pies,[6,39] but negative studies also exist.[40,41]

A discussion of the evidence base for psychological interventions is outside the scope of these guidelines. It is recognised that for many patients psychological therapies are the appropriate first-line treatment, and indeed this is supported by NICE.[6]

Summary of NICE guidelines for the treatment of generalised anxiety disorder,[6] panic disorder[6] and OCD[29]

- A 'stepped care' approach is recommended to help in choosing the most effective intervention.
- A comprehensive assessment is recommended that considers the degree of distress and functional impairment; the effect of any co-morbid mental illness, substance mis-use or medical condition; and past response to treatment.
- Treat the primary disorder first.
- Psychological therapy is more effective than pharmacological therapy and should be used as first line where possible. Details of the types of therapy recommended and their duration can be found in the NICE guidelines.
- Pharmacological therapy is also effective. Most evidence supports the use of the SSRIs (sertraline as first line).
- Provide information on the likely benefits and disadvantages of each mode of treatment.
- Consider combination therapy for complex anxiety disorders that are refractory to treatment.

Panic disorder

- Benzodiazepines should not be used.
- An SSRI should be used as first line. If SSRIs are contraindicated or there is no response, imipramine or clomipramine can be used.
- Self-help (based on CBT principles) should be encouraged, as should formal CBT.

Generalised anxiety disorder

- Benzodiazepines should not be used except for crises.
- An SSRI should be used as first-line treatment.
- SNRIs and pregabalin are second and third choices, respectively.
- High-intensity psychological intervention and self-help (based on CBT principles) should be encouraged.
- Antipsychotics should not be offered (presumably this includes quetiapine).

OCD (where there is moderate or severe functional impairment)

- Use an SSRI or intensive CBT.
- Combine the SSRI and CBT if response to single strategy is suboptimal.
- Use clomipramine if SSRIs fail.
- If response is still suboptimal, add an antipsychotic or combine clomipramine and citalopram (see Boxes 3.4–3.8).

CHAPTER 3

CHAPTER 3

Box 3.4 Generalised anxiety disorder

Crisis management

Drug	Comment
Benzodiazepines	Normally for short-term use only: max. 2–4 weeks although some are of the opinion that risks are overstated[42]

First-line drug treatment (In order of preference)[29]

SSRIs (Up to maximum licensed dose)	May initially exacerbate symptoms. A lower starting dose is recommended. Fluoxetine and sertraline are preferred options[12]
SNRIs[14] (Up to maximum licensed dose)	May initially exacerbate symptoms. A lower starting dose is recommended
Pregabalin 150–600mg/day in divided doses	Response may be seen in the first week of treatment.[43] Increasingly misused. Significant withdrawal syndrome

Second-line drug treatment (Less well tolerated or weaker evidence base, no order of preference)

Agomelatine[44] 10–50mg/day	Agomelatine has been shown to prevent relapse over a 6-month period[45]
Betablockers Propranolol 40–120mg/day in divided doses	Initiate at 40mg and titrate dose up to effect if needed. Useful for somatic symptoms, particularly tachycardia[46]
Buspirone 15–60mg/day in divided doses	Has a delayed onset of action, takes up to 6 weeks to show equal efficacy with benzodiazepines[47].
Hydroxyzine 50–100mg/day in divided doses	It is unclear whether hydroxyzine is effective due to an anxiolytic effect or a sedative effect[48]
Quetiapine (MR, 50–300mg)	Recommended as monotherapy. Probably not effective as adjunctive therapy to SSRI/SNRI in treatment resistance[49]
Tricyclic antidepressants Clomipramine 50–250mg/day[50–52] Imipramine 75–200mg/day in divided doses[53]	Initiate clomipramine at 10mg/day and increase the dose gradually Initiate imipramine 25mg every 4 days and when at 100mg can increase in 50mg increments[10]
MAOI Phenelzine 45–90mg/day in divided doses[54]	For mixed anxiety and depressive states. Patients need to avoid food high in tyramine
Mirtazapine 15–30mg nocte[55,56]	

Experimental

Chamomile 220–1500mg/day	Two RCTs, one positive, one negative using standardised doses of chamomile and placebo[57]
Gingko biloba 240mg–480mg/day	One positive RCT using standardised doses of gingko biloba and placebo[58]
Lavender oil preparation 80–160mg/day	One positive RCT using standardised doses of lavender oil compared to placebo and paroxetine[59]
Riluzole 50–100mg/day doses[60]	Liver function monitoring required

nocte, at night

Box 3.5 Panic disorder

Crisis management

Drug	Comment
Benzodiazepines	Rapid effect although panic symptoms return quickly if the drug is withdrawn.[61] NICE do not recommend.[6] Cochrane lukewarm[62]

First-line drug treatment
(In order of preference)[6,63]

SSRIs (Up to maximum licensed dose)	Therapeutic effect can be delayed (this applies to all antidepressants[64]) and patients can experience an initial exacerbation of panic symptoms.[6] Use supported by Cochrane[65]
Venlafaxine MR 75–225mg[63]	Initiate at 37.5mg for 7 days

Second-line treatment (Less well tolerated or weak evidence base, no order of preference)

Mirtazapine 15–60mg/day[66]	A meta-analysis suggests that mirtazapine does not help with panic symptoms but with the anxiety associated with this disorder.[63] Rather limited data overall[67]
Moclobemide 300–600mg/day[68]	One fixed-dose study of 450mg/day and one flexible-dose study suggest efficacy[68,69]
MAOIs Phenelzine 10–60mg/day[64]	No long-term studies, reserve for treatment-resistant cases due to poor tolerability[64]
Tricyclic antidepressants Clomipramine 25–250mg/day[64] Imipramine 25–300mg/day[64] Lofepramine 70–140mg/day in divided doses[70]	Start with a low dose and increase dose according to response and tolerability

Experimental

D-cycloserine 50mg/day	A RCT suggests acceleration of treatment response to CBT, but this advantage is lost at follow-up[71]
Gabapentin 600–3600mg/day	One RCT showed no difference between gabapentin and placebo. However, significant improvement was demonstrated in the more severely ill[72]
Inositol 12g/day[73]	One positive PCT in 21 patients. Equivalent to fluvoxamine in one study.[74] Well tolerated
Levetiracetam 250mg twice daily[67]	Usually well tolerated
Pindolol 7.5mg/day	Efficacy suggested in a small 21-patient DB-PCT where pindolol 2.5mg tds was used to augment fluoxetine in treatment-resistant panic disorder[75]
Valproate 500–2250mg/day	Two very small positive open studies[76,77]
Hydrocortisone	Only acute treatment shown to prevent development of PTSD[78]

DB-PCT, double blind randomised controlled trial, CBT, cognitive behavioural therapy

CHAPTER 3

Box 3.6 Post-traumatic stress disorder (PTSD)

First-line drug treatment
(In order of preference)
(NB psychological approaches should be used before drug treatments[79,80])

SSRIs (Up to maximum licensed doses)	Paroxetine, sertraline or fluoxetine are the preferred SSRIs[81,82] Recommended by NICE[79]
Venlafaxine modified release 37.5mg–300mg[83]	Recommended by NICE[79]

Second-line treatment (Less well tolerated or weak evidence base, no order of preference)

Antipsychotics Olanzapine 5–20mg	Antipsychotics may be effective for the intrusion symptoms (flashbacks and nightmares) but not the avoidance and hyperarousal symptoms of PTSD. Studies done as monotherapy or as adjunctive treatment[84]
Risperidone 0.5–6mg	Risperidone specifically mentioned by NICE[79]
Quetiapine 50–800mg[85]	
Mirtazapine 15–45mg/day[86]	Recommended by NICE[79] Second most effective drug in a network meta-analysis[87]
MAOI Phenelzine 15–75mg/day[88]	Recommended by NICE[79] Most effective drug in a network meta-analysis[87]
Prazosin 2–15mg nocte[89]	For nightmares and sleep disturbances. Initiate at 1mg nocte and titrate dose gradually to reduce the risk of hypotension Supported by a systematic review[90]
Tricyclic antidepressants Amitriptyline 50–300mg/day[91] Imipramine 50–300mg/day	Amitriptyline is recommended by NICE[79] For all TCAs start at a low dose and increase dose according to tolerability Best supporting evidence is for desipramine but this drug is not widely available[87]
IV Ketamine[92,93]	Rapid reduction in symptom severity suggested. Good RCT showing acute and chronic efficacy[94]

Experimental

Duloxetine 60–120mg	Two small open studies suggest efficacy. Start at 30mg for one week[95,96]
Lamotrigine up to 500mg/day	Small double-blind study in 15 patients[97]
Phenytoin plasma concentration 10–20ng/ml[98]	Open-label study in 12 patients
Valproate up to 2.5g[99]	Probably not effective[87]

nocte, at night

Box 3.7 Obsessive compulsive disorder

First-line drug treatment (In order of preference)

Drug	Comments
Any SSRI[39] (Up to maximum licensed dose	If the first SSRI is not tolerated or has a poor response an alternative SSRI may be tried[29]
Clomipramine (Up to 250mg)	Owing to poorer tolerability, recommended trying at least one SSRI first[29]

Second-line drug treatment (Unlicensed or weaker evidence base)

Add antipsychotic to SSRI (Low to moderate doses of antipsychotics used in studies)[100,101]	Most evidence supports the use of aripiprazole or risperidone.[100] Some evidence for haloperidol[101]
Citalopram 40mg with clomipramine 150mg	Based on small randomised open label study[102] Recommended by NICE[29] ECG monitoring required
Acetylcysteine[103] up to 2400mg/day added to SRRI or clomipramine	Gastrointestinal adverse effects may be problematic. Two of five controlled studies negative. Pooled effect shows benefit[104]
Lamotrigine 100mg + added to SSRI[105]	Lamotrigine dose must be titrated gradually as indicated in the SPC May worsen OCD in some[106]
Topiramate up to 400mg added to SSRI[107,108]	Topiramate is not well tolerated, suggested benefits for compulsion but not obsessions.[107] Two trials found topiramate ineffective[109,110]

Experimental

High dose SSRI: Escitalopram 25–50mg[111] Sertraline 250–400mg[112]	Dose titrated gradually according to tolerability. ECG monitoring recommended
Memantine	Good evidence for 20mg/day added to SSRIs[113]
NSAIDS Eg celecoxib 400mg/day	Some supporting evidence[110]
Amantadine 200mg/day	One positive RCT[114]
SNRIs Venlafaxine up to 375mg[115] Duloxetine 60mg[116]	
Mirtazapine 30–60mg[117]	Small trial in 30 patients
5HT3 antagonists Granisetron 1mg with fluvoxamine 200mg[118] Ondansetron 4mg with fluoxetine 20mg[119]	Some evidence for each drug but ondansetron may be the more effective[120]

(Continued)

CHAPTER 3

Box 3.7 (Continued)

Pregabalin 75–225mg/day added to sertraline	One small positive RCT[121]
Riluzole 50mg bd added to existing drug treatment[122]	Variable results in early trials[110]
Anti-androgen – Triptorelin 3.75mg IM every 4 weeks added to existing drug treatment[123]	Open label study done in six men
i.v. treatment Clomipramine IV[124] Ketamine IV[125,126]	Quicker onset of action suggested compared to oral treatments. One clomipramine study suggests clomipramine IV efficacy after failure with oral clomipramine Ketamine – developing evidence base[110]
Once weekly morphine 15–45mg added to existing drug treatment[127]	Small study involving 23 treatment-resistant patients. Positive effects were transient.

bd, bis die (twice a day); CBT (cognitive behavioural therapy)

Box 3.8 Social phobia (social anxiety disorder)

First-line drug treatment[128] (In order of preference)

SSRIs (Up to maximum licensed dose)	If no response to the first SSRI, try an alternative SSRI Supporting meta-analyses for fluvoxamine[129] and citalopram[130] Emerging data for vilazodone[131]
Venlafaxine modified release 75–225mg/day	

Second-line drug treatment (Less well tolerated or weaker evidence base, no order of preference)

Olanzapine 5–20mg[132]	Few studies with antipsychotics. Most evidence with olanzapine
Atenolol 25–100mg/day	Reduces autonomic symptoms in performance situations[132]
Benzodiazepines Clonazepam 0.3–6mg/day[132] Sertraline plus clonazepam up to 3mg/day[133]	Benzodiazepines are helpful on PRN basis. Most evidence for treatment with clonazepam and bromazepam Switching an SSRI to venlafaxine no more effective than adding clonazepam to SSRI[133]
Gabapentin 900–3600mg/day[132]	
Levetiracetam 300–3000mg/day in divided doses[134]	

(Continued)

Box 3.8 *(Continued)*	
Moclobemide 600mg/day in divided doses	Initiate at 300mg/day in divided doses. Moclobemide has a UK licence for Social Phobia. Recommended by NICE[128]
Phenelzine 15–90mg/day[135]	Avoidance of tyramine-rich food important Recommended by NICE[128]
Pregabalin 150–600mg/day[132]	600mg/day superior to placebo[132]
Experimental	
Ketamine 0.5mg.kg IV	One good RCT[136]
Topiramate 25–400mg/day[137]	Small open label study of 23 patients suggests efficacy but poorly tolerated
Valproate 500–2500mg/day[138]	Small open label study of 17 patients suggests efficacy

PRN, pro re nata (as required)

References

1. Nash JR and Nutt DJ. Pharmacotherapy of anxiety. *Handb Exp Pharmacol* 2005; 469–501.
2. Martin JL, et al. Benzodiazepines in generalized anxiety disorder: heterogeneity of outcomes based on a systematic review and meta-analysis of clinical trials. *J Psychopharmacology* 2007; **21**:774–782.
3. Benitez CI, et al. Use of benzodiazepines and selective serotonin reuptake inhibitors in middle-aged and older adults with anxiety disorders: a longitudinal and prospective study. *Am J Geriatr Psychiatry* 2008; **16**:5–13.
4. Demyttenaere K, et al. Clinical factors influencing the prescription of antidepressants and benzodiazepines: results from the European study of the epidemiology of mental disorders (ESEMeD). *J Affect Disord* 2008; **110**:84–93.
5. Hirschtritt ME, et al. Balancing the risks and benefits of benzodiazepines. *JAMA* 2021; **325**:347–348.
6. National Institute for Health and Clinical Excellence. Generalised anxiety disorder and panic disorder in adults: management. Clinical Guideline [CG113]. 2011 (last updated July 2019); http://guidance.nice.org.uk/CG113.
7. Davidson JR. Use of benzodiazepines in social anxiety disorder, generalized anxiety disorder, and posttraumatic stress disorder. *J Clin Psychiatry* 2004; **65 Suppl** 5:29–33.
8. Scott A, et al. Antidepressant drugs in the treatment of anxiety disorders. *Adv Psychiatric Treatment* 2001; **7**:275–282.
9. Ballenger JC. Remission rates in patients with anxiety disorders treated with paroxetine. *J Clin Psychiatry* 2004; **65**:1696–1707.
10. Davidson JR, et al. A psychopharmacological treatment algorithm for generalised anxiety disorder (GAD). *J Psychopharmacology* 2010; **24**:3–26.
11. Baldwin DS, et al. Evidence-based pharmacological treatment of anxiety disorders, post-traumatic stress disorder and obsessive-compulsive disorder: a revision of the 2005 guidelines from the British Association for Psychopharmacology. *J Psychopharmacol* 2014; **28**:403–439.
12. Baldwin D, et al. Efficacy of drug treatments for generalised anxiety disorder: systematic review and meta-analysis. *BMJ* 2011; **342**:d1199.
13. Slee A, et al. Pharmacological treatments for generalised anxiety disorder: a systematic review and network meta-analysis. *Lancet* 2019; **393**:768–777.
14. Kong W, et al. Comparative remission rates and tolerability of drugs for generalised anxiety disorder: a systematic review and network meta-analysis of double-blind randomized controlled trials. *Front Pharmacol* 2020; **11**:580858.
15. Caillard V, et al. Comparative effects of low and high doses of clomipramine and placebo in panic disorder: a double-blind controlled study. French University Antidepressant Group. *Acta Psychiatr Scand* 1999; **99**:51–58.
16. Wade AG, et al. The effect of citalopram in panic disorder. *Br J Psychiatry* 1997; **170**:x549–x553.
17. Londborg PD, et al. Sertraline in the treatment of panic disorder. A multi-site, double-blind, placebo-controlled, fixed-dose investigation. *Br J Psychiatry* 1998; **173**:54–60.
18. Pollack MH, et al. Combined paroxetine and clonazepam treatment strategies compared to paroxetine monotherapy for panic disorder. *J Psychopharmacology* 2003; **17**:276–282.
19. Jakubovski E, et al. Systematic review and meta-analysis: dose-response curve of SSRIs and SNRIs in anxiety disorders. *Depress Anxiety* 2019; **36**:198–212.
20. Clayton AH, et al. Sex differences in clinical presentation and response in panic disorder: pooled data from sertraline treatment studies. *Arch Women's Mental Health* 2006; **9**:151–157.
21. Rickels K, et al. Panic disorder: long-term pharmacotherapy and discontinuation. *J Clin Psychopharmacol* 1998; **18**:12S-18S.

22. Choy Y, et al. Three-year medication prophylaxis in panic disorder: to continue or discontinue? A naturalistic study. *Compr Psychiatry* 2007; **48**:419–425.

23. Michelson D, et al. Continuing treatment of panic disorder after acute response: randomised, placebo-controlled trial with fluoxetine. The Fluoxetine Panic Disorder Study Group. *Br J Psychiatry* 1999; **174**:213–218.

24. Davidson J, et al. Efficacy of sertraline in preventing relapse of posttraumatic stress disorder: results of a 28-week double-blind, placebo-controlled study. *Am J Psychiatry* 2001; **158**:1974–1981.

25. Stein DJ, et al. Pharmacotherapy for post traumatic stress disorder (PTSD). *Cochrane Database Syst Rev* 2006; CD002795.

26. Martenyi F, et al. Fluoxetine v. placebo in prevention of relapse in post-traumatic stress disorder. *Br J Psychiatry* 2002; **181**:315–320.

27. The Expert Consensus Panel for obsessive-compulsive disorder. Treatment of obsessive-compulsive disorder. *J Clin Psychiatry* 1997; **58 Suppl 4**:2–72.

28. Catapano F, et al. Obsessive-compulsive disorder: a 3-year prospective follow-up study of patients treated with serotonin reuptake inhibitors OCD follow-up study. *J Psychiatr Res* 2006; **40**:502–510.

29. National Institute for Clinical Excellence. Surveillance decision. Evidence: obsessive-compulsive disorder and body dysmorphic disorder: treatment. Clinical Guidance [CG31]. 2005 (last updated February 2019); https://www.nice.org.uk/guidance/cg31/resources/2019-surveil lance-of-obsessivecompulsive-disorder-and-body-dysmorphic-disorder-treatment-nice-guideline-cg31-6713804845/chapter/ Surveillance-decision?tab=evidence.

30. Blomhoff S, et al. Randomised controlled general practice trial of sertraline, exposure therapy and combined treatment in generalised social phobia. *Br J Psychiatry* 2001; **179**:23–30.

31. Hood SD and Nutt DJ. 'Psychopharmacological treatments: an overview,' in WR Crozier and LE Alden, eds., *International handbook of social anxiety concepts, research and interventions relating to the self and shyness*. Oxford: John Wiley and Sons Ltd; 2001.

32. Mayo-Wilson E, et al. Psychological and pharmacological interventions for social anxiety disorder in adults: a systematic review and network meta-analysis. *Lancet Psychiatry* 2014; **1**:368–376.

33. National Institute for Clinical Excellence. Depression: the treatment and management of depression in adults. Clinical Guidance [CG90]. 2009 (last reviewed December 2013); https://www.nice.org.uk/guidance/cg90.

34. Pollack MH. Refractory generalized anxiety disorder. *J Clin Psychiatry* 2009; **70 Suppl 2**:32–38.

35. Lancia M, et al. Pregabalin abuse in combination with other drugs: monitoring among methadone patients. *Front Psychiatry* 2019; **10**:1022.

36. Hägg S, et al. Current evidence on abuse and misuse of gabapentinoids. *Drug Saf* 2020; **43**:1235–1254.

37. Naveed S, et al. Pregabalin-associated discontinuation symptoms: a case report. *Cureus* 2018; **10**:e3425.

38. Roberts NP, et al. Early psychological interventions to treat acute traumatic stress symptoms. *Cochrane Database Syst Rev* 2010; CD007944.

39. Skapinakis P, et al. Pharmacological and psychotherapeutic interventions for management of obsessive-compulsive disorder in adults: a systematic review and network meta-analysis. *Lancet Psychiatry* 2016; **3**:730–739.

40. van Apeldoorn FJ, et al. Is a combined therapy more effective than either CBT or SSRI alone? Results of a multicenter trial on panic disorder with or without agoraphobia. *Acta Psychiatr Scand* 2008; **117**:260–270.

41. Marcus SM, et al. A comparison of medication side effect reports by panic disorder patients with and without concomitant cognitive behavior therapy. *Am J Psychiatry* 2007; **164**:273–275.

42. Offidani E, et al. Efficacy and tolerability of benzodiazepines versus antidepressants in anxiety disorders: a systematic review and meta-analysis. *Psychother Psychosom* 2013; **82**:355–362.

43. Generoso MB, et al. Pregabalin for generalized anxiety disorder: an updated systematic review and meta-analysis. *Int Clin Psychopharmacol* 2017; **32**:49–55.

44. Wang SM, et al. Agomelatine for the treatment of generalized anxiety disorder: a meta-analysis. *Clin Psychopharmacol Neurosci* 2020; **18**:423–433.

45. Stein DJ, et al. Agomelatine prevents relapse in generalized anxiety disorder: a 6-month randomized, double-blind, placebo-controlled discontinuation study. *J Clin Psychiatry* 2012; **73**:1002–1008.

46. Hayes PE, et al. Beta-blockers in anxiety disorders. *J Affect Disord* 1987; **13**:119–130.

47. Chessick CA, et al. Azapirones for generalized anxiety disorder. *Cochrane Database Syst Rev* 2006; **3**:CD006115.

48. Guaiana G, et al. Hydroxyzine for generalized anxiety disorder. *Cochrane Database Syst Rev* 2010; Cd006815.

49. Khan A, et al. Extended-release quetiapine fumarate (quetiapine XR) as adjunctive therapy in patients with generalized anxiety disorder and a history of inadequate treatment response: a randomized, double-blind study. *Ann Clin Psychiatry* 2014; **26**:3–18.

50. Wingerson D, et al. Clomipramine treatment for generalized anxiety disorder. *J Clin Psychopharmacol* 1992; **12**:214–215.

51. den Boer JA, et al. Effect of serotonin uptake inhibitors in anxiety disorders; a double-blind comparison of clomipramine and fluvoxamine. *Int Clin Psychopharmacol* 1987; **2**:21–32.

52. Kahn RS, et al. Effect of a serotonin precursor and uptake inhibitor in anxiety disorders; a double-blind comparison of 5-hydroxytryptophan, clomipramine and placebo. *Int Clin Psychopharmacol* 1987; **2**:33–45.

53. Rickels K, et al. Antidepressants for the treatment of generalized anxiety disorder. A Placebo-controlled Comparison of Imipramine, Trazodone, and Diazepam. *Arch Gen Psychiatry* 1993; **50**:884–895.

54. Robinson DS, et al. The monoamine oxidase inhibitor, phenelzine, in the treatment of depressive –anxiety states. A Controlled Clinical Trial. *Arch Gen Psychiatry* 1973; **29**:407–413.

55. Gambi F, et al. Mirtazapine treatment of generalized anxiety disorder: a fixed dose, open label study. *J Psychopharmacology* 2005; **19**:483–487.

56. Sitsen JMA, et al. Mirtazapine, a Novel Antidepressant, in the Treatment of Anxiety Symptoms. *Drug Invest* 1994; **8**:339–344.

57. Amsterdam JD, et al. A randomized, double-blind, placebo-controlled trial of oral Matricaria recutita (chamomile) extract therapy for generalized anxiety disorder. *J Clin Psychopharmacol* 2009; 29:378–382.

58. Woelk H, et al. Ginkgo biloba special extract EGb 761 in generalized anxiety disorder and adjustment disorder with anxious mood: a randomized, double-blind, placebo-controlled trial. *J Psychiatr Res* 2007; 41:472–480.

59. Kasper S, et al. Lavender oil preparation Silexan is effective in generalized anxiety disorder–a randomized, double-blind comparison to placebo and paroxetine. *Int J Neuropsychopharmacol* 2014; 17:859–869.

60. Mathew SJ, et al. Open-label trial of riluzole in generalized anxiety disorder. *Am J Psychiatry* 2005; 162:2379–2381.

61. Otto MW, et al. Discontinuation of benzodiazepine treatment: efficacy of cognitive-behavioral therapy for patients with panic disorder. *Am J Psychiatry* 1993; 150:1485–1490.

62. Breilmann J, et al. Benzodiazepines versus placebo for panic disorder in adults. *Cochrane Database Syst Rev* 2019; 3:Cd010677.

63. Andrisano C, et al. Newer antidepressants and panic disorder: a meta-analysis. *Int Clin Psychopharmacol* 2013; 28:33–45.

64. Batelaan NM, et al. Evidence-based pharmacotherapy of panic disorder: an update. *Int J Neuropsychopharmacol* 2012; 15:403–415.

65. Bighelli I, et al. Antidepressants versus placebo for panic disorder in adults. *Cochrane Database Syst Rev* 2018; 4:Cd010676.

66. Boshuisen ML, et al. The effect of mirtazapine in panic disorder: an open label pilot study with a single-blind placebo run-in period. *Int Clin Psychopharmacol* 2001; 16:363–368.

67. Zulfarina MS, et al. Pharmacological therapy in panic disorder: current guidelines and novel drugs discovery for treatment-resistant patient. *Clin Psychopharmacol Neurosci* 2019; 17:145–154.

68. Tiller JW, et al. Moclobemide for anxiety disorders: a focus on moclobemide for panic disorder. *Int Clin Psychopharmacol* 1997; **12 Suppl** 6:S27–S30.

69. Kruger MB, et al. The efficacy and safety of moclobemide compared to clomipramine in the treatment of panic disorder. *Eur Arch Psychiatry Clin Neurosci* 1999; **249 Suppl 1**:S19–S24.

70. Fahy TJ, et al. The galway study of panic disorder. I: clomipramine and lofepramine in DSM III-R panic disorder: a placebo controlled trial. *J Affect Disord* 1992; 25:63–75.

71. Otto MW, et al. Randomized trial of D-cycloserine enhancement of cognitive-behavioral therapy for panic disorder. *Depress Anxiety* 2016; 33:737–745.

72. Pande AC, et al. Placebo-controlled study of gabapentin treatment of panic disorder. *J Clin Psychopharmacol* 2000; 20:467–471.

73. Benjamin J, et al. Double-blind, placebo-controlled, crossover trial of inositol treatment for panic disorder. *Am J Psychiatry* 1995; 152:1084–1086.

74. Palatnik A, et al. Double-blind, controlled, crossover trial of inositol versus fluvoxamine for the treatment of panic disorder. *J Clin Psychopharmacol* 2001; 21:335–339.

75. Hirschmann S, et al. Pindolol augmentation in patients with treatment-resistant panic disorder: a double-blind, placebo-controlled trial. *J Clin Psychopharmacol* 2000; 20:556–559.

76. Woodman CL, et al. Panic disorder: treatment with valproate. *J Clin Psychiatry* 1994; 55:134–136.

77. Primeau F, et al. Valproic acid and panic disorder. *Can J Psychiatry* 1990; 35:248–250.

78. Astill Wright L, et al. Pharmacological prevention and early treatment of post-traumatic stress disorder and acute stress disorder: a systematic review and meta-analysis. *Trans Psychiatry* 2019; 9:334.

79. National Institute for Clinical Excellence. Post-traumatic stress disorder. NICE Guideline [NG116]. 2018; https://www.nice.org.uk/guidance/NG116.

80. Moore BA, et al. Management of post-traumatic stress disorder in veterans and military service members: a review of pharmacologic and psychotherapeutic interventions since 2016. *Curr Psychiatry Rep* 2021; 23:9.

81. Hoskins M, et al. Pharmacotherapy for post-traumatic stress disorder: systematic review and meta-analysis. *Br J Psychiatry* 2015; 206:93–100.

82. Lee DJ, et al. Psychotherapy versus pharmacotherapy for posttraumatic stress disorder: systematic review and meta-analyses to determine first-line treatments. *Depress Anxiety* 2016; 33:792–806.

83. Davidson J, et al. Treatment of posttraumatic stress disorder with venlafaxine extended release: a 6-month randomized controlled trial. *Arch Gen Psychiatry* 2006; 63:1158–1165.

84. Han C, et al. The potential role of atypical antipsychotics for the treatment of posttraumatic stress disorder. *J Psychiatr Res* 2014; 56:72–81.

85. Villarreal G, et al. Efficacy of quetiapine monotherapy in posttraumatic stress disorder: a randomized, placebo-controlled trial. *Am J Psychiatry* 2016; 173:1205–1212.

86. Davidson JR, et al. Mirtazapine vs. placebo in posttraumatic stress disorder: a pilot trial. *Biol Psychiatry* 2003; 53:188–191.

87. Cipriani A, et al. Comparative efficacy and acceptability of pharmacological treatments for post-traumatic stress disorder in adults: a network meta-analysis. *Psychol Med* 2018; 48:1975–1984.

88. Kosten TR, et al. Pharmacotherapy for posttraumatic stress disorder using phenelzine or imipramine. *J Nerv Ment Dis* 1991; 179:366–370.

89. George KC, et al. Meta-analysis of the efficacy and safety of prazosin versus placebo for the treatment of nightmares and sleep disturbances in adults with posttraumatic stress disorder. *J Trauma & Dissoc* 2016; 17:494–510.

90. Coventry PA, et al. Psychological and pharmacological interventions for posttraumatic stress disorder and comorbid mental health problems following complex traumatic events: systematic review and component network meta-analysis. *PLoS Med* 2020; 17:e1003262.

91. Davidson J, et al. Treatment of posttraumatic stress disorder with amitriptyline and placebo. *Arch Gen Psychiatry* 1990; 47:259–266.

92. Albott CS, et al. Efficacy, safety, and durability of repeated ketamine infusions for comorbid posttraumatic stress disorder and treatment-resistant depression. *J Clin Psychiatry* 2018; 79:17m11634.

CHAPTER 3

93. Feder A, et al. Efficacy of intravenous ketamine for treatment of chronic posttraumatic stress disorder: a randomized clinical trial. *JAMA Psychiatry* 2014; **71**:681–688.

94. Feder A, et al. A randomized controlled trial of repeated ketamine administration for chronic posttraumatic stress disorder. *Am J Psychiatry* 2021; **178**:193–202.

95. Walderhaug E, et al. Effects of duloxetine in treatment-refractory men with posttraumatic stress disorder. *Pharmacopsychiatry* 2010; **43**:45–49.

96. Villarreal G, et al. Duloxetine in military posttraumatic stress disorder. *Psychopharmacol Bull* 2010; **43**:26–34.

97. Hertzberg MA, et al. A preliminary study of lamotrigine for the treatment of posttraumatic stress disorder. *Biol Psychiatry* 1999; **45**:1226–1229.

98. Bremner DJ, et al. Treatment of posttraumatic stress disorder with phenytoin: an open-label pilot study. *J Clin Psychiatry* 2004; **65**:1559–1564.

99. Adamou M, et al. Valproate in the treatment of PTSD: systematic review and meta analysis. *Curr Med Res Opin* 2007; **23**:1285–1291.

100. Veale D, et al. Atypical antipsychotic augmentation in SSRI treatment refractory obsessive-compulsive disorder: a systematic review and meta-analysis. *BMC Psychiatry* 2014; **14**:317.

101. Dold M, et al. Antipsychotic augmentation of serotonin reuptake inhibitors in treatment-resistant obsessive-compulsive disorder: an update meta-analysis of double-blind, randomized, placebo-controlled trials. *Int J Neuropsychopharmacol* 2015; **18**.

102. Pallanti S, et al. Citalopram for treatment-resistant obsessive-compulsive disorder. *Eur Psychiatry* 1999; **14**:101–106.

103. Costa DLC, et al. Randomized, double-blind, placebo-controlled trial of n-acetylcysteine augmentation for treatment-resistant obsessive-compulsive disorder. *J Clin Psychiatry* 2017; **78**:e766–e773.

104. Couto JP, et al. Oral N-acetylcysteine in the treatment of obsessive-compulsive disorder: a systematic review of the clinical evidence. *Prog Neuropsychopharmacol Biol Psychiatry* 2018; **86**:245–254.

105. Bruno A, et al. Lamotrigine augmentation of serotonin reuptake inhibitors in treatment-resistant obsessive-compulsive disorder: a double-blind, placebo-controlled study. *J Psychopharmacology* 2012; **26**:1456–1462.

106. Sharma V, et al. Lamotrigine-induced obsessive-compulsive disorder in patients with bipolar disorder. *CNS Spectr* 2019; **24**:390–394.

107. Berlin HA, et al. Double-blind, placebo-controlled trial of topiramate augmentation in treatment-resistant obsessive-compulsive disorder. *J Clin Psychiatry* 2011; **72**:716–721.

108. Mowla A, et al. Topiramate augmentation in resistant OCD: a double-blind placebo-controlled clinical trial. *CNS Spectr* 2010; **15**:613–617.

109. Afshar H, et al. Topiramate augmentation in refractory obsessive-compulsive disorder: a randomized, double-blind, placebo-controlled trial. *J Res Med Sci* 2014; **19**:976–981.

110. Grassi G, et al. Investigational and experimental drugs to treat obsessive-compulsive disorder. *J Exp Pharmacol* 2020; **12**:695–706.

111. Rabinowitz I, et al. High-dose escitalopram for the treatment of obsessive-compulsive disorder. *Int Clin Psychopharmacol* 2008; **23**:49–53.

112. Ninan PT, et al. High-dose sertraline strategy for nonresponders to acute treatment for obsessive-compulsive disorder: a multicenter double-blind trial. *J Clin Psychiatry* 2006; **67**:15–22.

113. Modarresi A, et al. A systematic review and meta-analysis: memantine augmentation in moderate to severe obsessive-compulsive disorder. *Psychiatry Res* 2019; **282**:112602.

114. Naderi S, et al. Amantadine as adjuvant therapy in the treatment of moderate to severe obsessive-compulsive disorder: a double-blind randomized trial with placebo control. *Psychiatry Clin Neurosci* 2019; **73**:169–174.

115. Dell'Osso B, et al. Serotonin-norepinephrine reuptake inhibitors in the treatment of obsessive-compulsive disorder: a critical review. *J Clin Psychiatry* 2006; **67**:600–610.

116. Mowla A, et al. Duloxetine augmentation in resistant obsessive-compulsive disorder: a double-blind controlled clinical trial. *J Clin Psychopharmacol* 2016; **36**:720–723.

117. Koran LM, et al. Mirtazapine for obsessive-compulsive disorder: an open trial followed by double-blind discontinuation. *J Clin Psychiatry* 2005; **66**:515–520.

118. Askari N, et al. Granisetron adjunct to fluvoxamine for moderate to severe obsessive-compulsive disorder: a randomized, double-blind, placebo-controlled trial. *CNS Drugs* 2012; **26**:883–892.

119. Soltani F, et al. A double-blind, placebo-controlled pilot study of ondansetron for patients with obsessive-compulsive disorder. *Human Psychopharmacology* 2010; **25**:509–513.

120. Sharafkhah M, et al. Comparing the efficacy of ondansetron and granisetron augmentation in treatment-resistant obsessive-compulsive disorder: a randomized double-blind placebo-controlled study. *Int Clin Psychopharmacol* 2019; **34**:222–233. ·

121. Mowla A, et al. Pregabalin augmentation for resistant obsessive-compulsive disorder: a double-blind placebo-controlled clinical trial. *CNS Spectr* 2020; **25**:552–556.

122. Coric V, et al. Riluzole augmentation in treatment-resistant obsessive-compulsive disorder: an open-label trial. *Biol Psychiatry* 2005; **58**:424–428.

123. Eriksson T. Anti-androgenic treatment of obsessive-compulsive disorder: an open-label clinical trial of the long-acting gonadotropin-releasing hormone analogue triptorelin. *Int Clin Psychopharmacol* 2007; **22**:57–61.

124. Fallon BA, et al. Intravenous clomipramine for obsessive-compulsive disorder refractory to oral clomipramine: a placebo-controlled study. *Arch Gen Psychiatry* 1998; **55**:918–924.

125. Rodriguez CI, et al. Randomized controlled crossover trial of ketamine in obsessive-compulsive disorder: proof-of-concept. *Neuropsychopharmacology* 2013; **38**:2475–2483.

126. Bloch MH, et al. Effects of ketamine in treatment-refractory obsessive-compulsive disorder. *Biol Psychiatry* 2012; 72:964–970.

127. Koran LM, et al. Double-blind treatment with oral morphine in treatment-resistant obsessive-compulsive disorder. *J Clin Psychiatry* 2005; 66:353–359.

128. National Institute for Health and Clinical Excellence. Social anxiety disorder: recognition, assessment and treatment. Clinical Guidance [CG159]. 2013 (Last updated March 2020); https://www.nice.org.uk/guidance/cg159

129. Liu X, et al. Efficacy and tolerability of fluvoxamine in adults with social anxiety disorder: a meta-analysis. *Medicine (Baltimore)* 2018; 97:e11547.

130. Baldwin DS, et al. Efficacy of escitalopram in the treatment of social anxiety disorder: a meta-analysis versus placebo. *Eur Neuropsychopharmacol* 2016; 26:1062–1069.

131. Careri JM, et al. A 12-week double-blind, placebo-controlled, flexible-dose trial of vilazodone in generalized social anxiety disorder. *Primary Care Companion CNS Disord* 2015; 17:10.4088/PCC.15m01831.

132. Blanco C, et al. The evidence-based pharmacotherapy of social anxiety disorder. *Int J Neuropsychopharmacol* 2013; 16:235–249.

133. Pollack MH, et al. A double-blind randomized controlled trial of augmentation and switch strategies for refractory social anxiety disorder. *Am J Psychiatry* 2014; 171:44–53.

134. Simon NM, et al. An open-label study of levetiracetam for the treatment of social anxiety disorder. *J Clin Psychiatry* 2004; 65:1219–1222.

135. Blanco C, et al. A placebo-controlled trial of phenelzine, cognitive behavioral group therapy, and their combination for social anxiety disorder. *Arch Gen Psychiatry* 2010; 67:286–295.

136. Taylor JH, et al. Ketamine for social anxiety disorder: a randomized, placebo-controlled crossover trial. *Neuropsychopharmacology* 2018; 43:325–333.

137. Van Ameringen M, et al. An open trial of topiramate in the treatment of generalized social phobia. *J Clin Psychiatry* 2004; 65:1674–1678.

138. Kinrys G, et al. Valproic acid for the treatment of social anxiety disorder. *Int Clin Psychopharmacol* 2003; 18:169–172.

CHAPTER 3

Benzodiazepines in the treatment of psychiatric disorders

Benzodiazepines have a valid place in the treatment of some forms of epilepsy and severe muscle spasm, and as premedication agents in some surgical procedures. However, the vast majority of prescriptions are written for their hypnotic and anxiolytic effects. They are also used for rapid tranquillisation and, usually as adjuncts, in the treatment of depression and schizophrenia. Benzodiazepines are commonly both prescribed and misused. A European study found that almost 10% of adults had taken a benzodiazepine over the previous year[1] and a 2019 US study reported past-year usage of 12.6% amongst adults.[2] Generally speaking, the use of benzodiazepines in psychiatric disorders has gradually become less supportable over the past few decades.[3]

Benzodiazepines are sometimes divided into two groups depending on their half-life: hypnotics (short half-life) or anxiolytics (long half-life), although there are many exceptions (for example, nitrazepam and alprazolam, respectively).

Anxiolytic effect

Benzodiazepines reduce pathological anxiety, agitation and tension. Although useful in the short-term management of generalised anxiety disorder[4] either alone or to augment SSRIs, benzodiazepines are clearly addictive; many patients continue to take these drugs for years[5] with unknown benefits and many likely harms. If a benzodiazepine is prescribed, this should not routinely be for longer than one month.

NICE recommend that benzodiazepines should not be used in patients with generalised anxiety disorder except as a short-term measure during crisis.[6] Evidence is mixed in other anxiety disorders, and potential benefits should be viewed in the context of the known risks associated with benzodiazepine use. A small number of trials report the efficacy of benzodiazepines in social anxiety disorder.[7] Benzodiazepines may be useful in panic disorders,[8] but further studies are needed to draw reliable conclusions about their efficacy and safety with long-term use.[8,9] Benzodiazepines are ineffective or and may be harmful in the treatment of PTSD[10] or phobias.[11]

Repeat prescriptions should be avoided in those with major personality problems whose difficulties are unlikely to resolve, especially in response to drug therapy. Benzodiazepines should also be avoided, if possible, in those with a history of substance misuse.

Hypnotic effect

Benzodiazepines inhibit REM sleep and REM rebound is seen when they are discontinued.[11] There is a debate over the clinical significance of this property.[12]

Benzodiazepines are effective hypnotics, at least in the short term.[13] RCTs support the effectiveness of Z hypnotics over a period of at least 6 months;[13,14] it is unclear if this holds true for benzodiazepine hypnotics. Intermittent use probably extends the period over which benzodiazepines are effective as hypnotics.

Physical causes (pain, dyspnoea, etc.) or substance misuse (most commonly high caffeine consumption) should always be excluded before a hypnotic drug is prescribed. Where possible, behavioural therapies (e.g. CBT for insomnia) should be offered before prescribing hypnotics.[14,15] A high proportion of hospitalised patients are prescribed hypnotics.[16] These should not be routinely continued at discharge.

Use in depression

Benzodiazepines are not a treatment for major depressive illness. The only meta-analysis conducted found no advantage for benzodiazepines over placebo in depression.[17] However, there is some evidence that benzodiazepines may be helpful in preventing relapse of psychotic depression.[18]

In the United Kingdom, the National Service Framework for Mental Health[19] at one time emphasised this point by including a requirement that GPs audit the ratio of benzodiazepines to antidepressants prescribed in their practice. NICE suggests that a benzodiazepine may be helpful for up to 2 weeks early in treatment, particularly in combination with an SSRI (to help with sleep and the management of SSRI-induced agitation).[6] Use beyond this timeframe is discouraged. Limiting initial supply quantities to short periods (1–7 days) may reduce the risk of patients becoming long-term users of benzodiazepines.[20]

Use in psychosis

Benzodiazepines are commonly used for rapid tranquilisation, either alone, or in combination with an antipsychotic.[21] However, a Cochrane review concluded that there is no convincing evidence that combining an antipsychotic and a benzodiazepine offers any advantage over the use of antipsychotics or benzodiazepines alone.[22]

A further Cochrane review in schizophrenia concluded that there are no proven benefits, outside short-term sedation.[23] In contrast, another systematic review using different outcome measures found superiority over placebo for global, psychiatric and behavioural outcomes, but inferiority to antipsychotics on longer-term global outcomes.[24] A significant minority of patients with established psychotic illness fail to respond adequately to antipsychotics alone, and this can result in benzodiazepines being prescribed on a chronic basis.[25] There is, however, no evidence to support benzodiazepine augmentation of antipsychotics in schizophrenia, and use should be reserved for the short-term sedation of acutely agitated patients.[26] Evidence supporting the use of benzodiazepines in tardive dyskinesia is weak,[27] but these drugs remain a treatment option in this condition.

Side effects

Headaches, confusion, ataxia, dysarthria, blurred vision, gastrointestinal disturbances, jaundice and paradoxical excitement are all possible side-effects. Benzodiazepines impair cognition, and long-term use has been associated with a range of cognitive deficits (e.g. memory, attention and processing speed), which may even persist after withdrawal.[28] The use of benzodiazepines has been associated with at least a 50% increase in the risk of hip fracture in the elderly.[29] This is probably because benzodiazepines increase the risk of falls.[30] Patients newly prescribed benzodiazepine have the highest risk.[29] High doses are particularly problematic.[30] This would seem to be a class effect (short-half-life drugs still increase the risk[30]). Benzodiazepines often cause anterograde amnesia and can adversely affect driving performance.[31,32] Benzodiazepines can also cause disinhibition (see the section on disinhibition in this chapter). Benzodiazepines have been linked to aggressive behaviour, though the association is modest, and possibly related to dose and personality factors.[33]

Epidemiologic research has linked benzodiazepine prescribing to serious medical conditions including dementia, infections and cancer.[34–36] However, a causal relationship has not been established, and evidence is conflicting.[35] Also, although benzodiazepine use has been associated with dementia,[37] the absence of a dose-response association argues against a causal link.[38] All studies in this area are confounded by the failure to include illicit use of benzodiazepines.

Respiratory depression is rare with oral therapy but is possible when parenteral routes are used. Buccal and intranasal administration may also cause respiratory depression.[39,40] The use of the specific benzodiazepine antagonist flumazenil is effective in reversing respiratory depression but is not without risk (e.g. convulsions, particularly in mixed overdoses with TCAs), so selective use is recommended.[41] Flumazenil has a much shorter half-life than many benzodiazepines, making close observation of the patient essential for several hours after administration.

IV injections can be painful and lead to thrombophlebitis, because of the low water solubility of benzodiazepines, and therefore it is necessary to use solvents in the preparation of injectable forms. Diazepam is available in emulsion form (Diazemuls in the UK) to overcome these problems.

Drug interactions

Benzodiazepines do not induce microsomal enzymes and so do not frequently precipitate pharmacokinetic interactions with any other drugs. Most benzodiazepines are metabolised by CYP3A4, which is inhibited by erythromycin, several SSRIs and ketoconazole. It is theoretically possible that co-administration of these drugs will result in higher serum levels of benzodiazepines. Pharmacodynamic interactions (usually increased sedation) can occur. Benzodiazepines are associated with an important interaction with methadone and should be used with caution in patients prescribed clozapine (increased risk of cardiopulmonary depression) and not at all with intramuscular olanzapine.

References

1. Demyttenaere K, et al. Clinical factors influencing the prescription of antidepressants and benzodiazepines: results from the European study of the epidemiology of mental disorders (ESEMeD). *J Affect Disord* 2008; 110:84–93.
2. Maust DT, et al. Benzodiazepine use and misuse among adults in the United States. *Psychiatr Serv* 2019; 70:97–106.
3. Hirschtritt ME, et al. Balancing the risks and benefits of benzodiazepines. *JAMA* 2021; 325:347–348.
4. Baldwin DS, et al. Evidence-based pharmacological treatment of anxiety disorders, post-traumatic stress disorder and obsessive-compulsive disorder: a revision of the 2005 guidelines from the British Association for Psychopharmacology. *J Psychopharmacol* 2014; 28:403–439.
5. Kurko TA, et al. Long-term use of benzodiazepines: definitions, prevalence and usage patterns – a systematic review of register-based studies. *Eur Psychiatry* 2015; 30:1037–1047.
6. National Institute for Health and Clinical Excellence. Generalised anxiety disorder and panic disorder in adults: management. Clinical Guideline [CG113] 2011 (last updated July 2019); https://www.nice.org.uk/guidance/cg113.
7. Williams T, et al. Pharmacotherapy for social anxiety disorder (SAnD). *Cochrane Database Syst Rev* 2017; 10:Cd001206.
8. Perna G, et al. Long-term pharmacological treatments of anxiety disorders: an updated systematic review. *Curr Psychiatry Rep* 2016; 18:23.

9. Bighelli I, et al. Antidepressants and benzodiazepines for panic disorder in adults. *Cochrane Database Syst Rev* 2016; **9**:Cd011567.

10. Guina J, et al. Benzodiazepines for PTSD: a systematic review and meta-analysis. *J Psychiatr Pract* 2015; **21**:281–303.

11. Guina J, et al. Benzodiazepines I: upping the care on downers: the evidence of risks, benefits and alternatives. *J Clin Med* 2018; **7**.

12. Roehrs T, et al. Drug-related sleep stage changes: functional significance and clinical relevance. *Sleep Med Clin* 2010; **5**:559–570.

13. Winkler A, et al. Drug treatment of primary insomnia: a meta-analysis of polysomnographic randomized controlled trials. *CNS Drugs* 2014; **28**:799–816.

14. Riemann D, et al. European guideline for the diagnosis and treatment of insomnia. *J Sleep Res* 2017; **26**:675–700.

15. Qaseem A, et al. Management of chronic insomnia disorder in adults: a clinical practice guideline from the American College of Physicians. *Ann Intern Med* 2016; **165**:125–133.

16. Mahomed R, et al. Prescribing hypnotics in a mental health trust: what consultants say and what they do. *Pharm J* 2002; **268**:657–659.

17. Benasi G, et al. Benzodiazepines as a monotherapy in depressive disorders: a systematic review. *Psychother Psychosom* 2018; **87**:65–74.

18. Shiwaku H, et al. Benzodiazepines reduce relapse and recurrence rates in patients with psychotic depression. *J Clin Med* 2020; **9**:1938.

19. Gov.UK. Guidance: national service framework for mental health: modern standards and service models. 1999. https://www.gov.uk/government/publications/quality-standards-for-mental-health-services.

20. Bushnell GA, et al. Simultaneous antidepressant and benzodiazepine new use and subsequent long-term benzodiazepine use in adults with depression, United States, 2001–2014. *JAMA Psychiatry* 2017; **74**:747–755.

21. Baldwin DS, et al. Benzodiazepines: risks and benefits. A reconsideration. *J Psychopharmacology* 2013; **27**:967–971.

22. Zaman H, et al. Benzodiazepines for psychosis-induced aggression or agitation. *Cochrane Database Syst Rev* 2017; **12**:Cd003079.

23. Dold M, et al. Benzodiazepines for schizophrenia. *Cochrane Database Syst Rev* 2012; **11**:Cd006391.

24. Sim F, et al. Re-examining the role of benzodiazepines in the treatment of schizophrenia: a systematic review. *J Psychopharmacology* 2015; **29**:212–223.

25. Paton C, et al. Benzodiazepines in schizophrenia. Is there a trend towards long-term prescribing? *Psychiatric Bull* 2000; **24**:113–115.

26. Dold M, et al. Benzodiazepine augmentation of antipsychotic drugs in schizophrenia: a meta-analysis and Cochrane review of randomized controlled trials. *Eur Neuropsychopharmacol* 2013; **23**:1023–1033.

27. Bergman H, et al. Benzodiazepines for antipsychotic-induced tardive dyskinesia. *Cochrane Database Syst Rev* 2018; **1**:Cd000205.

28. Crowe SF, et al. The residual medium and long-term cognitive effects of benzodiazepine use: an updated meta-analysis. *Arch Clin Neuropsychol* 2018; **33**:901–911.

29. Donnelly K, et al. Benzodiazepines, Z-drugs and the risk of hip fracture: a systematic review and meta-analysis. *PLoS One* 2017; **12**:e0174730.

30. Diaz-Gutierrez MJ, et al. Relationship between the use of benzodiazepines and falls in older adults: a systematic review. *Maturitas* 2017; **101**:17–22.

31. Barbone F, et al. Association of road-traffic accidents with benzodiazepine use. *Lancet* 1998; **352**:1331–1336.

32. Rudisill TM, et al. Medication use and the risk of motor vehicle collisions among licensed drivers: a systematic review. *Accid Anal Prev* 2016; **96**:255–270.

33. Albrecht B, et al. Benzodiazepine use and aggressive behaviour: a systematic review. *Aust N Z J Psychiatry* 2014; **48**:1096–1114.

34. Kim DH, et al. Use of hypnotics and risk of cancer: a meta-analysis of observational studies. *Korean J Fam Med* 2018; **39**:211–218.

35. Brandt J, et al. Benzodiazepines and Z-drugs: an updated review of major adverse outcomes reported on in epidemiologic research. *Drugs in R&D* 2017; **17**:493–507.

36. Peng TR, et al. Hypnotics and risk of cancer: a meta-analysis of observational studies. *Medicina (Kaunas)* 2020; **56**.

37. Lee J, et al. Use of sedative-hypnotics and the risk of Alzheimer's dementia: a retrospective cohort study. *PLoS One* 2018; **13**:e0204413.

38. Gray SL, et al. Benzodiazepine use and risk of incident dementia or cognitive decline: prospective population based study. *BMJ* 2016; **352**:i90.

39. Mula M. The safety and tolerability of intranasal midazolam in epilepsy. *Expert Rev Neurother* 2014; **14**:735–740.

40. Midazolam oral transmucosal route. An alternative to rectal diazepam for some children. *Prescrire Int* 2013; **22**:173–177.

41. Penninga EI, et al. Adverse events associated with flumazenil treatment for the management of suspected benzodiazepine Intoxication–A systematic review with meta-analyses of randomised trials. *Basic Clin Pharmacol Toxicol* 2016; **118**:37–44.

Benzodiazepines, z-drugs and gabapentinoids: dependence, detoxification and discontinuation

In most developed countries, the use of benzodiazepines or z-drugs is restricted to a maximum 2–4 weeks.[1-3] However, long-term use remains common in the United Kingdom, with 300,000 adults taking either a benzodiazepine or z-drug for more than 12 months.[4] Most guidelines, including NICE, recommend that people on long-term benzodiazepines or z-drugs should be advised to stop because tolerance to these drugs (which can develop after 2–4 weeks) means that they are not effectives for insomnia or anxiety over the long term, and because dependence is likely to develop, meaning that treatment is continued only to prevent withdrawal symptoms (Table 3.27).[5]

Gabapentinoids (GABA analogues), with near identical mode of action to benzodiazepines, also can cause addiction, physical dependence and withdrawal over the same time period.[6-8] In total, 1.5 million people in England are prescribed gabapentinoids,[9] and the number of prescriptions for these medications has risen seven-fold in the last 10 years.[10]

Table 3.27 Adverse effects of benzodiazepines

Cognitive*[11-13]	Reactions which can be mistaken for a psychiatric disorder[14]
■ Deficits in memory ■ Deficits in attention ■ Increased reaction time ■ Motor incoordination ■ Drowsiness ■ Nightmares/intrusive thoughts ■ Impaired judgement ■ Perceptual illusions/hallucinations	■ Agitation ■ Emotional lability ■ Restlessness ■ Inter-dose withdrawal
■ **Physical**[15] ■ Motor incoordination/ataxia ■ Dizziness ■ Slurred speech ■ Sensory alterations (tinnitus/strange tastes/paraesthesia/numbness/burning) ■ Rash ■ Autonomic dysfunction (tachycardia/bradycardia/diaphoresis/hypotension/hypertension)	■ **Emotional**[15] ■ Depression/dysphoria ■ Numbness/emotional anaesthesia ■ Anxiety/phobias/panic ■ Anger/irritability/mood lability ■ Excitement/euphoria
■ **Increased morbidity**[12,13] ■ Increased risk of motor vehicle accidents ■ Higher risk of falls (elderly) ■ Delirium (elderly) ■ ?Dementia ■ ?Cancer ■ ?Infections	■ **Behavioural**[15] ■ Insomnia ■ Avoidance/agoraphobia ■ Appetite/weight (anorexia, weight gain) ■ Impulsivity/disinhibition ■ Suicidality ■ Aggression

*Some of these impairments can persist after discontinuation

The majority of people who are dependent on these classes of drugs have not obtained them illegally, but are taking them as prescribed by their physician (so-called 'iatrogenic dependence').

Long-term use of benzodiazepines is associated with a number of problems (Table 3.27), which patients may be unaware of and only appreciate after stopping.[16] Long-term z-drug use is associated with similar risks.[17] Gabapentinoids have been linked to increased risk of suicide, unintentional overdose, road traffic accidents, and head and body injuries,[18] suggesting limitation of their long-term use may also be prudent.

Withdrawal symptoms

Stopping these medications is often difficult (Table 3.28). One study found that 90% of patients experience withdrawal symptoms on stopping, with 32% of people on long half-life benzodiazepines and 42% of people on short half-life benzodiazepines unable to cease their medication because of withdrawal symptoms.[19] Short-acting drugs such as lorazepam are associated with more severe problems on withdrawal than longer-acting drugs such as diazepam.[20,21] As the drugs are ineffective for anxiety and insomnia in the long-term, symptoms which arise on stopping are likely to be withdrawal symptoms as opposed to relapse (though symptoms can be similar).[22] Mental state often improves after withdrawal symptoms abate.[23]

To avoid or reduce the severity of these problems, good practice dictates that benzodiazepines (and z-drugs) should not be prescribed as hypnotics or anxiolytics for longer than 4 weeks. Intermittent use (i.e. not every day) at the lowest possible dose is also prudent. This may also apply to gabapentinoids.

CHAPTER 3

Table 3.28 Withdrawal effects from benzodiazepines[24,25]

Physical	Psychological
■ Stiffness	■ Anxiety/insomnia
■ Fatigue and weakness	■ Terror/panic attacks
■ GI disturbance	■ Nightmares
■ Paraesthesia	■ Depersonalisation/derealisation
■ Flu-like symptoms	■ Delusions and hallucinations
■ Visual disturbances	■ Depression
■ Sensory hypersensitivity	■ Psychosis*
■ Convulsions*	■ Mood instability
■ Cognitive impairment	■ Paranoia
■ Impaired memory	■ Obsessive-compulsive symptoms
■ Tremor	■ Suicidal ideation
■ Dizziness	■ Mania
■ Muscle spasms/cramps	
■ Chest pain	
■ Hypertension	
■ Tachycardia	
■ Photophobia	
■ Confusion, delirium*	

*Usually only from very rapid withdrawal.

There has been limited formal study into the duration of withdrawal symptoms, with some reports of weeks-long duration, but they can last longer than a year, especially in the case of long-term use.[20,23] For a minority, withdrawal symptoms can be protracted and last years, sometimes called the 'post-acute withdrawal syndrome'.[26]

Stopping benzodiazepines

If the patient is in agreement, benzodiazepines should be withdrawn. Tapering can be difficult and should not be imposed on a patient against their will. A cluster randomised trial supports the effectiveness of a face-to-face educational intervention.[27] Continuing support can be required to prepare a patient for withdrawal and to support them through the process (e.g. psychological therapies or self-help groups).[28]

Dosage reduction (tapering)

Gradual reduction of benzodiazepine dose reduces the intensity of withdrawal symptoms by spreading them out over a longer time period (and giving time for neural adaptations to the drug to resolve).[22] Meta-analysis has confirmed that gradual dose reduction ('tapering') improves drug cessation rates compared with routine clinical care.[29] Most studies find that a gradual withdrawal over at least 10 weeks is most successful in achieving long-term abstinence,[30] although many patients will require considerably longer (sometimes several years). Sudden benzodiazepine withdrawal has potentially fatal consequences, so tapering is always advisable.

Direct taper or switching to diazepam?

Patients who take short- or intermediate-acting benzodiazepines can be tapered off these drugs directly but more than once a day dosing might be required.

An alternative approach is to switch to an equivalent dose of diazepam (which has a long half-life and therefore might provokes less severe withdrawal),[20,24] noting that some patients report withdrawal symptoms from abrupt switches to diazepam and so a step-wise switch is probably prudent. Cochrane is lukewarm about switching to diazepam.[30] Approximate 'diazepam equivalent'[31] doses are shown Table 3.29. Owing to

Table 3.29 Approximate 'diazepam equivalent'[31] doses

Chlordiazepoxide	25mg
Clonazepam	0.5mg
Diazepam	**10mg**
Lorazepam	1mg
Lormetazepam	1–2mg
Nitrazepam	10mg
Oxazepam	20mg
Temazepam	20mg

individual differences some patients may require more or less diazepam to control with-drawal symptoms.

The half-lives of benzodiazepines vary greatly. The degree of sedation that they induce also varies, making it difficult to determine exact equivalents. Table 3.28 is an approximate guide only. Extra precautions apply in patients with hepatic dysfunction, as diazepam and other longer-acting drugs may accumulate to toxic levels.

Pattern of tapering

The relationship between dose of benzodiazepine and their effect on their principal target, the GABA-A receptor, is hyperbolic, with the following implications:

- Reducing dose by fixed amounts (e.g. 12.5mg in Figure 3.6a) will give rise to increasingly large reductions in GABA-A occupancy.
- This is consistent with clinical observation that withdrawal symptoms are non-linearly related to dose reduction (e.g. a 1mg reduction of diazepam is tolerable from 20mg but intolerable from 5mg[32]).
- Reducing diazepam dose by 5mg from 50mg will cause a reduction of 2.3 percentage points of GABA-A occupancy, but a 5mg reduction from 5mg will cause a reduction of 18.3 percentage points.

In order to reduce the dose of benzodiazepine by equal amounts of effect at their major target, hyperbolically reducing doses are required (Figure 3.6b):

- This means that the size of dose reductions should be smaller and smaller as the total dose gets smaller.
- In practice, these reductions can be most easily calculated based on a proportion of the most recent dose (an exponential pattern).

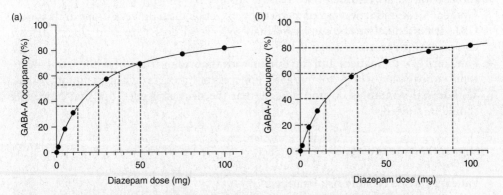

Figure 3.6 (a) Linear reductions of dose cause increasingly large reductions in effect on GABA-A receptor occupancy. (b) Reducing effect on GABA-A receptors by even amounts, requires hyperbolically reducing doses of diazepam. Note how small final doses will be required to be in order to prevent too large a final 'step down'. Adapted from Brouillet et al. (1991[33]).

CHAPTER 3

- Patients often report that 10% reductions (calculated on the last dose, so that they become increasingly small) every 2–4 weeks are tolerable, although some long-term users may need even slower reductions.
- Final doses before complete cessation will need to be very small (often much less than 1mg of diazepam equivalent)

Practical application of these principles

Before tapering

- All patients should be informed of the risk of withdrawal symptoms on stopping any benzodiazepine, z-drugs or gabapentinoid (high risk for alprazolam and lorazepam).
- Patient should be warned not to stop benzodiazepines abruptly, because this can cause seizures and can be fatal, and may be the method most likely to give rise to severe and long-lasting withdrawal symptoms.
- Although stopping benzodiazepines can cause unpleasant symptoms, if tapering is gradual and careful the process can be tolerable. Reassurance may be required for those that have rapidly tapered in the past.
- Most patients take months or years to taper. However, rate of reduction should be determined by what is tolerable for the patient, not externally imposed timetables.
- Past experience of reducing can help predict symptoms that may arise again on tapering.
- Preparation for benzodiazepine tapering may be required: e.g. lightening work or family duties or bolstering of non-pharmacological coping skills (including acceptance, breathing exercises, exercise, hobbies, diary keeping, and de-catastrophising).[28,34]
- People with insomnia may benefit from adjunctive treatment with melatonin, and those with panic disorder may benefit from CBT during the taper period.[24,35,36] Gradual dose reduction accompanied by psychological interventions (relaxation, CBT) is more likely to be successful than supervised dose reduction alone[29] or psychological interventions alone.[37]
- Familiarity of the patient and the doctor with the wide variety of withdrawal symptoms (above) may help to mitigate unnecessary anxiety when symptoms arise. Withdrawal symptoms do not indicate that the drug is needed but that taper rate should be slowed.

The process of tapering

- Patients may be broadly risk stratified:
  - For low-risk patients (<6 months use, long half-life benzodiazepine, no experience of significant withdrawal symptoms in the past), a test reduction could be made of 25%.
  - For high-risk patients (>6 months use, short half-life benzodiazepine, past history of withdrawal symptoms) a test reduction of 5–10% could be recommended.

- Reductions should be made according to a proportion (e.g. 10%) of the last dose. This means the reductions recommended will become smaller and smaller as the total dose is lowered. Most patients will be able to proceed between a rate of about 5–10% of their most recent dose per month.
- After reduction withdrawal symptoms should be monitored for 2–4 weeks, or until symptoms have resolved. Monitoring may take the form of simple measures of symptoms each day (e.g. out of 10) or using standardised benzodiazepine withdrawal scales.
- Further reduction should be titrated to the tolerability of this experience. If symptoms are intolerable, an increase in dose, a period of stabilisation and more gradual reduction is needed. Mild, tolerable symptoms mean the reduction can continue to reduce at the same rate.

Troubleshooting

- If significant withdrawal symptoms emerge at any point, either hold the current dose to allow them to resolve, or if intolerable increase to the last dose at which the symptoms were tolerable, and remain there until symptoms resolve. After stabilisation, tapering will need to be more gradual: with reduction in smaller amounts and/or longer periods in between reductions.
- The experience of distressing withdrawal symptoms does not indicate that a patient cannot stop benzodiazepines, but that they will need to taper more slowly, with smaller reductions than they have been undertaking (some need to taper at less than 5% of the most recent dose per month).
- At very small doses, liquid formulations may be required, which are available for drugs such as diazepam and lorazepam. Switching to these drugs may therefore be useful; other options include specially compounded liquids. Many patients report cutting up fragments of tablets and weighing them or making their own solutions from crushed tablets, but this approach cannot be recommended.
- Final doses before completely stopping the drug will need to be very small to avoid a larger reduction in effect on the brain. For example, for a patient reducing diazepam at 10% per month, the final dose will need to be 0.25mg.[33]

Reduction schedules

A simple guide to diazepam dose reductions:

- Reduce by 5–10mg/day every 2–4 weeks, down to a daily dose of 50mg
- Reduce by 2–5mg/day every 2–4 weeks, down to a daily dose of 20mg
- Reduce by 1–2mg/day every 2–4 weeks, down to a daily dose of 10mg
- Reduce by 0.5–1mg/day every 2–4 weeks, down to a daily dose of 5mg
- Reduce by 0.25–0.5mg/day every 2–4 weeks, down to a daily dose of 2.5mg
- Reduce by 0.1–0.25mg/day every 2–4 weeks until stopped

CHAPTER 3

Tapering other drug classes

The same principles apply to tapering z-drugs or gabapentinoids. Gabapentinoids can cause severe withdrawal effects, although there is wide inter-individual variation. Although z-drugs are used once daily, tolerance and withdrawal are reported, even after brief or intermittent use.[38,39] Tapering according to a similar exponential scheme (or sometimes cross-titration to diazepam) may be required for cessation. The main withdrawal symptoms are insomnia and anxiety. Ideally, they should be tapered at a rate that maintains sleep.

References

1. BNF Online. British national formulary. 2020; https://www.medicinescomplete.com/mc/bnf/current.
2. National Institute for Clinical Excellence. Guidance on the use of zaleplon, zolpidem and zopiclone for the short-term management of insomnia. Technical Appraisal [TA77]. 2004 (reviewed August 2010); https://www.nice.org.uk/guidance/ta77.
3. National Institute for Health and Clinical Excellence. Generalised anxiety disorder and panic disorder in adults: management. Clinical Guideline [CG113]. 2011 (last updated July 2019); https://www.nice.org.uk/guidance/cg113.
4. Davies J, et al. Long-term benzodiazepine and Z-drugs use in the UK: a survey of general practice. *Br J Gen Pract* 2017; 67:e609–e613.
5. National Institute for Health and Care Excellence. Benzodiazepine and z-drug withdrawal. 2019; https://cks.nice.org.uk/topics/benzodiazepine-z-drug-withdrawal/?_escaped_fragment_=topicsummary.
6. Schifano F, et al. An insight into Z-drug abuse and dependence: an examination of reports to the European Medicines Agency Database of Suspected Adverse Drug Reactions. *Int J Neuropsychopharmacol* 2019; 22:270–277.
7. Evoy KE, et al. Abuse and misuse of pregabalin and gabapentin. *Drugs* 2017; 77:403–426.
8. Public Health England. Advice for prescribers on the risk of the misuse of pregabalin and gabapentin. 2014; https://assets.publishing.service.gov.uk/government/uploads/system/uploads/attachment_data/file/385791/PHE-NHS_England_pregabalin_and_gabapentin_advice_Dec_2014.pdf.
9. Marsden J, et al. Medicines associated with dependence or withdrawal: a mixed-methods public health review and national database study in England. *Lancet Psychiatry* 2019; 6:935–950.
10. Gov.UK. Dependence and withdrawal associated with some prescribed medicines. An evidence review. 2020; https://www.gov.uk/government/publications/prescribed-medicines-review-report.
11. Crowe SF, et al. The residual medium and long-term cognitive effects of benzodiazepine use: an updated meta-analysis. *Arch Clin Neuropsychol* 2018; 33:901–911.
12. Brandt J, et al. Benzodiazepines and Z-drugs: an updated review of major adverse outcomes reported on in epidemiologic research. *Drugs in R&D* 2017; 17:493–507.
13. Donnelly K, et al. Benzodiazepines, Z-drugs and the risk of hip fracture: a systematic review and meta-analysis. *PLoS One* 2017; 12:e0174730.
14. Gutierrez MA, et al. Paradoxical reactions to benzodiazepines. *Am J Nurs* 2001; 101:34–39; quiz 39–40.
15. Guina J, et al. Benzodiazepines I: upping the care on downers: the evidence of risks, benefits and alternatives. *J Clin Med* 2018; 7:17.
16. Golombok S, et al. Cognitive impairment in long-term benzodiazepine users. *Psychol Med* 1988; 18:365–374.
17. Finkle WD, et al. Risk of fractures requiring hospitalization after an initial prescription for zolpidem, alprazolam, lorazepam, or diazepam in older adults. *J Am Geriatr Soc* 2011; 59:1883–1890.
18. Molero Y, et al. Associations between gabapentinoids and suicidal behaviour, unintentional overdoses, injuries, road traffic incidents, and violent crime: population based cohort study in Sweden. *BMJ* 2019; 365:l2147.
19. Schweizer E, et al. Long-term therapeutic use of benzodiazepines. II. Effects of gradual taper. *Arch Gen Psychiatry* 1990; 47:908–915.
20. Schweizer E, et al. Benzodiazepine dependence and withdrawal: a review of the syndrome and its clinical management. *Acta Psychiatr Scand* 1998; 98 Suppl 393:95–101.
21. Uhlenhuth EH, et al. International study of expert judgment on therapeutic use of benzodiazepines and other psychotherapeutic medications: IV. Therapeutic dose dependence and abuse liability of benzodiazepines in the long-term treatment of anxiety disorders. *J Clin Psychopharmacol* 1999; 19:23S–29S.
22. Ashton H. The diagnosis and management of benzodiazepine dependence. *Curr Opin Psychiatry* 2005; 18:249–255.
23. Ashton H. Benzodiazepine withdrawal: outcome in 50 patients. *Br J Addict* 1987; 82:665–671.
24. Soyka M. Treatment of benzodiazepine dependence. *N Engl J Med* 2017; 376:1147–1157.
25. Petursson H. The benzodiazepine withdrawal syndrome. *Addiction* 1994; 89:1455–1459.
26. Ashton H. Protracted Withdrawal From Benzodiazepines: The Post-Withdrawal Syndrome. *Psychiatr Ann* 1995; 1:174–179.
27. Tannenbaum C, et al. Reduction of inappropriate benzodiazepine prescriptions among older adults through direct patient education: the empower cluster randomized trial. *JAMA Int Med* 2014; 174:890–898.
28. Guy A, et al. *Guidance for psychological therapists: enabling conversations with clients taking or withdrawing from prescribed psychiatric drugs.* London: APPG for Prescribed Drug Dependence; 2019.

29. Parr JM, et al. Effectiveness of current treatment approaches for benzodiazepine discontinuation: a meta-analysis. *Addiction* 2009; 104:13–24.

30. Denis C, et al. Pharmacological interventions for benzodiazepine mono-dependence management in outpatient settings. *Cochrane Database Syst Rev* 2006; CD005194.

31. Ashton H. Benzodiazepines: how they work & how to withdraw, the Ashton Manual. 2002; http://www.benzo.org.uk/manual/bzcha01.htm.

32. Ashton H. Benzodiazepine dependence. *Adv Syndrom Psychiatric Drugs* 2004; 239–260.

33. Brouillet E, et al. In vivo bidirectional modulatory effect of benzodiazepine receptor ligands on GABAergic transmission evaluated by positron emission tomography in non-human primates. *Brain Res* 1991; 557:167–176.

34. Inner Compass Initiative Inc. The withdrawal project. 2019; https://withdrawal.theinnercompass.org.

35. Voshaar RCO, et al. Strategies for discontinuing long-term benzodiazepine use: meta-analysis. *Br J Psychiatry* 2006; 189:213–220.

36. Fluyau D, et al. Challenges of the pharmacological management of benzodiazepine withdrawal, dependence, and discontinuation. *Ther Adv Psychopharmacol* 2018; 8:147–168.

37. Gould RL, et al. Interventions for reducing benzodiazepine use in older people: meta-analysis of randomised controlled trials. *Br J Psychiatry* 2014; 204:98–107.

38. Pollmann AS, et al. Deprescribing benzodiazepines and Z-drugs in community-dwelling adults: a scoping review. *BMC Pharmacol & Toxicol* 2015; 16:19.

39. Kales A, et al. Rebound insomnia after only brief and intermittent use of rapidly eliminated benzodiazepines. *Clin Pharmacol Ther* 1991; 49:468–476.

CHAPTER 3

Benzodiazepines and disinhibition

Unexpected increases in aggressive or impulsive behaviour secondary to drug treatment are usually called disinhibitory or paradoxical reactions. These reactions may include acute excitement, hyperactivity, increased anxiety, vivid dreams, sexual disinhibition, aggression, hostility and rage. Examples of causative agents include amfetamines methylphenidate, benzodiazepines and alcohol. Paradoxical reactions are an important consideration with benzodiazepines because these drugs are used to sedate and tranquillise – a paradoxical reaction is thus the polar opposite of the desired effect. These reactions are also a major problem in general medicine where drugs such as midazolam are widely used for conscious sedation. In intensive care medicine, benzodiazepine-related disinhibition can be difficult to distinguish from hyperactive delirium.[1]

How common are disinhibitory reactions with benzodiazepines?

The incidence of disinhibitory reactions varies widely depending on the population studied (see the next section 'Who is at risk?'). For example, a meta-analysis of benzodiazepine RCTs that included many hundreds of patients with a wide range of diagnoses reported an incidence of less than 1% (the same as placebo).[2] Similarly, an analysis of behavioural disinhibition frequency in a psychiatric unit found no difference between those treated with benzodiazepines and those not.[3] However, a Norwegian study that reported on 415 cases of 'driving under the influence', in which flunitrazepam was the sole substance implicated, found that 6% of adverse effects could be described as disinhibitory reactions.[4] An RCT that recruited patients with panic disorder reported an incidence of disinhibition of 13%.[5] Authors of case series (often describing use in high-risk patients) reported rates of 10–20%,[2] and an RCT that included patients with borderline personality disorder reported a rate of 58%.[6]

Disinhibition is rather problematic to define, and so incident rates are correspondingly difficult to determine. Aggression may be considered to be a disinhibition reaction but not defined as disinhibition per se. Aggression is robustly linked to benzodiazepine use both in the long term and after exposure to a single dose.[7,8]

Other GABA agonists, particularly zolpidem, have also been linked to disinhibition associated with somnambulism, automatism, amnesia and mania.[9–12]

Who is at risk?

Those who have learning disability, neurological disorder or CNS degenerative disease,[13] are young (child or adolescent) or elderly,[13–16] or have a history of aggression or poor impulse control[6,17] are at increased risk of experiencing a disinhibitory reaction. The risk is further increased if the benzodiazepine is a high-potency drug, has a short half-life, is given in a high dose or is administered intravenously (so provoking high and rapidly fluctuating plasma levels).[13,18–20] Some people may be genetically predisposed to disinhibition reactions.[21]

Combinations of risk factors are clearly important: low-risk long-acting benzodiazepines may cause disinhibition in high-risk populations such as children,[16] higher risk, short-acting drugs given intravenously are extremely likely to cause disinhibition in personality disorder.

What is the mechanism?[18,22–24]

Various theories of the mechanism have been proposed. First, the anxiolytic and amnesic properties of benzodiazepines may lead to a loss of the restraint that governs normal social behaviour. Second, the sedative and amnesic properties of benzodiazepines may lead to a reduced ability to concentrate on the external social cues that guide appropriate behaviour. Lastly, benzodiazepine-mediated increases in GABA neurotransmission may lead to a reduction in the restraining influence of the cortex, resulting in untrammelled excitement, anxiety and hostility.

Flumazenil is usually used to reverse benzodiazepine sedation and respiratory depression, but it is also effective in treating disinhibition reactions.[25]

Subjective reports

People who take benzodiazepines rate themselves as being more tolerant and friendly, but respond more to provocation than placebo-treated patients.[26] People with impulse control problems who take benzodiazepines may self-report feelings of power and overwhelming self-esteem.[17] Psychology rating scales demonstrate increased suggestibility, failure to recognise anger in others and reduced ability to recognise social cues. The experience of this author (DT) (having once been given intravenous midazolam for a pre-surgical procedure) is that the patient may be completely unaware that their behaviour is bizarre or that it is the result of drug-induced disinhibition.

Clinical implications

Benzodiazepines are frequently used in rapid tranquillisation and the short-term management of disturbed behaviour. For the vast majority of treatment episodes, benzodiazepines produce sedation, and reductions in anxiety and aggression. It is important to be aware, nonetheless, of their propensity to cause paradoxical disinhibitory reactions.

Paradoxical disinhibitory/aggressive outbursts in the context of benzodiazepine use:

- are rare in the general population but more frequent in people with impulse control problems or CNS damage and in the very young or very old
- are most often associated with high doses of high-potency drugs that are administered parenterally
- usually occur in response to (often very mild) provocation, the exact nature of which is not always obvious to others
- are recognised by others but often not by the sufferer, who often believes that he is friendly and tolerant

Suspected paradoxical reactions should be clearly documented in the clinical notes. In extreme cases, flumazenil can be used to reverse the reaction. If the benzodiazepine was prescribed to control acute behavioural disturbance, future episodes should be managed with antipsychotic drugs[27] or other non-benzodiazepine sedatives.

CHAPTER 3

References

1. Schieveld JNM, et al. On benzodiazepines, paradoxical agitation, hyperactive delirium, and chloride homeostasis. *Crit Care Med* 2018; 46:1558–1559.

2. Dietch JT, et al. Aggressive dyscontrol in patients treated with benzodiazepines. *J Clin Psychiatry* 1988; 49:184–188.

3. Rothschild AJ, et al. Comparison of the frequency of behavioral disinhibition on alprazolam, clonazepam, or no benzodiazepine in hospital-ized psychiatric patients. *J Clin Psychopharmacol* 2000; 20:7–11.

4. Bramness JG, et al. Flunitrazepam: psychomotor impairment, agitation and paradoxical reactions. *Forensic Sci Int* 2006; 159:83–91.

5. O'Sullivan GH, et al. Safety and side-effects of alprazolam. Controlled study in agoraphobia with panic disorder. *Br J Psychiatry* 1994; 165:79–86.

6. Gardner DL, et al. Alprazolam-induced dyscontrol in borderline personality disorder. *Am J Psychiatry* 1985; 142:98–100.

7. Albrecht B, et al. Motivational drive and alprazolam misuse: a recipe for aggression? *Psychiatry Res* 2016; 240:381–389.

8. Albrecht B, et al. Benzodiazepine use and aggressive behaviour: a systematic review. *Aust N Z J Psychiatry* 2014; 48:1096–1114.

9. Sabe M, et al. Zolpidem stimulant effect: induced mania case report and systematic review of cases. *Prog Neuropsychopharmacol Biol Psychiatry* 2019; 94:109643.

10. Poceta JS. Zolpidem ingestion, automatisms, and sleep driving: a clinical and legal case series. *JClinSleep Med* 2011; 7:632–638.

11. Pressman MR. Sleep driving: sleepwalking variant or misuse of z-drugs? *Sleep MedRev* 2011; 15:285–292.

12. Daley C, et al. 'I did what?' Zolpidem and the courts. *J Am Acad Psychiatry Law* 2011; 39:535–542.

13. Bond AJ. Drug-induced behavioural disinhibition incidence, mechanisms and therapeutic implications. *CNS Drugs* 1998; 9:41–57.

14. Hakimi Y, et al. Paradoxical adverse drug reactions: descriptive analysis of French reports. *Eur J Clin Pharmacol* 2020; 76:1169–1174.

15. Hawkridge SM, et al. A risk-benefit assessment of pharmacotherapy for anxiety disorders in children and adolescents. *Drug Saf* 1998; 19:283–297.

16. Kandemir H, et al. Behavioral disinhibition, suicidal ideation, and self-mutilation related to clonazepam. *J Child Adolesc Psychopharmacol* 2008; 18:409.

17. Daderman AM, et al. Flunitrazepam (Rohypnol) abuse in combination with alcohol causes premeditated, grievous violence in male juvenile offenders. *J Am Acad Psychiatry Law* 1999; 27:83–99.

18. van der Bijl P, et al. Disinhibitory reactions to benzodiazepines: a review. *J Oral Maxillofac Surg* 1991; 49:519–523.

19. McKenzie WS, et al. Paradoxical reaction following administration of a benzodiazepine. *J Oral MaxillofacSurg* 2010; 68:3034–3036.

20. Wilson KE, et al. Complications associated with intravenous midazolam sedation in anxious dental patients. *Prim Dent Care* 2011; 18:161–166.

21. Short TG, et al. Paradoxical reactions to benzodiazepines–a genetically determined phenomenon? *Anaesth Intensive Care* 1987; 15:330–331.

22. Weisman AM, et al. Effects of clorazepate, diazepam, and oxazepam on a laboratory measurement of aggression in men. *Int Clin Psychopharmacol* 1998; 13:183–188.

23. Blair RJ, et al. Selective impairment in the recognition of anger induced by diazepam. *Psychopharmacology (Berl)* 1999; 147:335–338.

24. Wallace PS, et al. Reduction of appeasement-related affect as a concomitant of diazepam-induced aggression: evidence for a link between aggression and the expression of self-conscious emotions. *Aggress Behav* 2009; 35:203–212.

25. Tae CH, et al. Paradoxical reaction to midazolam in patients undergoing endoscopy under sedation: incidence, risk factors and the effect of flumazenil. *Dig Liver Dis* 2014; 46:710–715.

26. Bond AJ, et al. Behavioural aggression in panic disorder after 8 weeks' treatment with alprazolam. *J Affect Disord* 1995; 35:117–123.

27. Paton C. Benzodiazepines and disinhibition: a review. *Psychiatric Bull* 2002; 26:460–462.

Chapter 4

Addictions and substance misuse

Introduction

Mental and behavioural problems due to psychoactive substance use are common. The World Health Organisation (WHO) in the International Classification of Diseases 10 (ICD-10)[1] identifies acute intoxication, harmful use, dependence syndrome, withdrawal state, withdrawal state with delirium, psychotic disorder, amnesic syndrome, residual and late-onset psychotic disorder, other mental and behavioural disorders and unspecified mental and behavioural disorders as substance-related disorders. A wide range of psychoactive substances may be problematic, including alcohol, opioids, benzodiazepines, gamma-hydroxybutyrate (GHB)/gamma-butyrolactone (GBL), stimulants, new psychoactive substance (NPS) (including cathinones, synthetic cannabinoids and phenylethylamines), khat, nitrates, hallucinogens, anabolic steroids and tobacco.

Substance misuse is frequently seen in people with severe mental illness (so-called dual diagnosis) and personality disorder. In many adult psychiatry settings, dual diagnosis is the norm rather than the exception. In many parts of the world, substance misuse services may be provided separately from general psychiatric services. The model of care in most addiction services means that patients who are not motivated to engage will not be assertively treated and followed up. Dual diagnosis teams are not universally available, resulting in sub-optimal treatment of substance misuse for many patients with mental illness.[2]

According to ICD-10, dependence syndrome is 'a cluster of physiological, behavioural and cognitive phenomena in which the use of a substance or a class of substances takes on a much higher priority for a given individual than other behaviours that once had greater value'. A definite diagnosis of dependence should only be made if at least three of the following have been present together in the previous year:

- compulsion to take substance
- difficulties controlling substance-taking behaviour
- physiological withdrawal state
- evidence of tolerance

The Maudsley® Prescribing Guidelines in Psychiatry, Fourteenth Edition. David M. Taylor,
Thomas R. E. Barnes and Allan H. Young.
© 2021 David M. Taylor. Published 2021 by John Wiley & Sons Ltd.

- neglect of alternative interests
- persistent use despite harm

Substance-use disorders should generally be treated with a combination of psychosocial and pharmacological interventions. This chapter concentrates on pharmacological interventions for alcohol, opioids and nicotine use. Treatments for people misusing benzodiazepines, GHB/GBL, stimulants, NPS (including cathinones, synthetic cannabinoids and phenylethylamines), khat, nitrates, hallucinogens, anabolic steroids are discussed briefly. Note that various National Institute for Health and Clinical Excellence (NICE) guidelines and technology appraisals, Department of Health Substance Misuse Guidelines (the Orange Book)[3] and Public Health England[2] also provide a comprehensive overview of treatment approaches, as does a soon-to-be-updated British Association for Psychopharmacology (BAP) consensus guideline.[4]

References

1. World Health Organisation. International statistical classification of diseases and related health problems. Online version. 2016; http://apps.who.int/classifications/icd10/browse/2016/en.
2. Public Health England. Better care for people with co-occurring mental health and alcohol/drug use conditions. A guide for commissioners and service providers. 2017; https://www.gov.uk/government/uploads/system/uploads/attachment_data/file/625809/Co-occurring_mental_health_and_alcohol_drug_use_conditions.pdf.
3. Department of Health and Social Care. Drug misuse and dependence: UK guidelines on clinical management. 2017; https://www.gov.uk/government/publications/drug-misuse-and-dependence-uk-guidelines-on-clinical-management.
4. Lingford-Hughes AR, et al. Evidence-based guidelines for the pharmacological management of substance abuse, harmful use, addiction and comorbidity: recommendations from BAP. *J Psychopharmacol* 2012; 26:899–952.

Alcohol dependence

Alcohol

What is a unit of alcohol?

In the UK, one unit of alcohol is 10mL of ethanol or 1L of 1% alcohol. For example, 250mL of wine, that is, 10% alcohol contains 2.5 units.

How much alcohol is too much?

The UK Department of Health (DoH) has given the following advice and recommendations to minimise the health risks from alcohol consumption:[1]

- Not more than 14 units should be consumed per week on a regular basis. This applies to both men and women.
- Harm is minimised when these units are spread across 3 or more days.
- Heavy single occasion drinking is associated with the risk of harm, injury and accidents.
- The consumption of any volume of alcohol is still associated with a number of illnesses such as cancers of the throat, mouth and breast.
- There are no completely safe levels of drinking during pregnancy, and precautionary avoidance of alcohol is recommended to reduce the risk of harm to the baby.

Assessment and brief structured intervention

The UK NICE guideline on the diagnosis, assessment and management of harmful drinking and alcohol dependence recommends that staff working in services which might encounter problem drinkers should be competent in identifying and assessing harmful drinking and alcohol dependence.[2] The NICE public health guideline on reducing harmful drinking[3] recommends a session of brief structured advice based on FRAMES principles (feedback, responsibility, advice, menu, empathy, self-efficacy) as a useful intervention for everyone at increased risk of alcohol-related problems.

Where consumption above recommended levels has been identified, a more detailed clinical assessment is required. Depending on the context, this could include the following:

- history of alcohol use, including daily consumption and recent patterns of drinking
- history of previous episodes of alcohol withdrawal
- time of the most recent drink
- collateral history from a family member or carer
- other drug (illicit and prescribed) use
- severity of dependence and of withdrawal symptoms
- coexisting medical and psychiatric problems
- physical examination, including cognitive function
- breathalyser: absolute breath alcohol level and whether rising or falling (take at least 20 minutes after last drink to avoid falsely high readings from the mouth, and 1 hour later)

■ laboratory investigations: full blood count (FBC), urea and electrolytes (U&E), liver function tests (LFTs), international normalised ratio (INR), prothrombin time (PT) and urinary drug screen.

The following structured assessment tools are recommended:[2]

■ The Alcohol Use Disorders Identification Test (**AUDIT**)[4] questionnaire is a 10-item questionnaire which is useful as a screening tool in those identified as being at increasing risk. Questions 1–3 address the quantity of alcohol consumed, 4–6 the signs and symptoms of dependence and 7–10 the behaviours and symptoms associated with harmful alcohol use. Each question is scored 0–4, giving a maximum total score of 40. A score of 8 or more is suggestive of hazardous or harmful alcohol use. Hazardous drinking = consumption of alcohol likely to cause harm. Harmful drinking = consumption already causing mental or physical health problems.

■ The **Severity of Alcohol Dependence Questionnaire (SADQ)**[5] is a more detailed 20-item questionnaire with the score on each item ranging from 0 to 3, giving a maximum total score of 60.

Severity of alcohol dependence	
Mild	= SADQ score of 15 or less
Moderate	= SADQ score 15–30
Severe	= SADQ score >30

Alcohol withdrawal

In alcohol-dependent drinkers, the central nervous system has adjusted to the constant presence of alcohol in the body (neuro-adaptation). When the blood alcohol concentration (BAC) is suddenly lowered, the brain remains in a hyper-excited state, resulting in the withdrawal syndrome Table (4.1).

Table 4.1 Manifestations and complications of mild and severe alcohol withdrawal

Mild alcohol withdrawal – manifestations	Usual timing of onset after the last drink	Other information
■ Agitation/anxiety/irritability ■ Tremor of hands, tongue, eyelids ■ Sweating ■ Nausea/vomiting/diarrhoea ■ Fever ■ Tachycardia ■ Systolic hypertension ■ General malaise	Onset at 3–12 hours Peak at 24–48 hours Duration up to 14 days	■ Symptoms are non-specific ■ Absence does not exclude withdrawal ■ May commence before blood alcohol levels reach zero

Management

May be self-limiting, but mitigated with adequate benzodiazepine cover and supportive treatment. Monitor vital signs. Use a withdrawal assessment scale.

*See below for the various benzodiazepine regimes recommended.

Table 4.1 (*Continued*)

Severe alcohol withdrawal – complications	Usual timing of onset after the last drink	Other information
Generalised seizures	12–18 hours	■ May commence before blood alcohol levels reach zero

Management

■ The occurrence of a first seizure during medically assisted withdrawal requires investigation to rule out organic disease or idiopathic epilepsy.
■ A meta-analysis of trials assessing the efficacy of drugs preventing alcohol withdrawal seizures demonstrated that benzodiazepines, particularly long-acting preparations such as diazepam, significantly reduced seizures *de novo*.[6,7]
■ Long-acting benzodiazepine is recommended as prophylaxis in those with a previous history of seizures.[8]
■ Some antiseizure medications are as effective as benzodiazepines, with some units recommending carbamazepine loading in patients with untreated epilepsy, or where seizures have occurred despite adequate benzodiazepine loading.[6]
■ Phenytoin does not prevent alcohol withdrawal-related seizures when used on its own or in combination with benzodiazepines.[9] There is no need to continue antiseizure medications long term when used to prevent seizures in alcohol withdrawal.[9]

Severe alcohol withdrawal – complications	Usual timing of onset after the last drink	Other information and management
Delirium tremens (see specific section in this chapter) ■ Clouding of consciousness/confusion ■ Vivid hallucinations, particularly in visual and tactile modalities ■ Marked tremor Other clinical features also include autonomic hyperactivity (tachycardia, hypertension, sweating and fever), paranoid delusions, agitation and insomnia Prodromal symptoms include night-time insomnia, restlessness, fear and confusion Risk factors: Severe alcohol dependence, self-detoxification without medical input, multiple previous admissions for alcohol withdrawal, concurrent medical illness, previous history of delirium tremens and alcohol withdrawal seizures, low potassium, low magnesium, thiamine deficiency, inadequately treated withdrawal Recognition is important because treatment is different from delirium arising from other causes. DT **needs larger doses of benzodiazepines and more caution with antipsychotics**	3–4 days (72–96 hours)	■ Develops in 3–5% of those admitted to hospital for alcohol withdrawal ■ A medical emergency ■ Mortality 10–20% if untreated

Management

■ This is a medical emergency and requires prompt transfer to a general hospital,[9] and preferably to a high dependency setting.[10,11]
■ **The patient must be seen** (see section 'Delirium tremens' in this chapter).

Pharmacologically assisted withdrawal (alcohol detoxification)

Alcohol withdrawal is associated with significant morbidity and mortality when improperly managed.

Pharmacologically assisted withdrawal is likely to be needed when:

- regular consumption of >15 units/day
- AUDIT score >20
- there is a history of significant withdrawal symptoms.

Symptom scales can be helpful in determining the amount of pharmacological support required to manage withdrawal symptoms. The Clinical Institute Withdrawal Assessment of Alcohol Scale Revised (CIWA-Ar; Figure 4.1)[12] and Short Alcohol Withdrawal Scale (SAWS; Table 4.2)[13] are both 10-item scales that can be completed in around 5 minutes. The CIWA-Ar is an objective scale and the SAWS is a self-complete tool. A CIWA-Ar score >10 or a SAWS score >12 should prompt assisted withdrawal.

Community detoxification is usually possible when:

- There is a supervising carer, ideally 24 hours a day throughout the duration of detoxification process.
- The treatment plan has been agreed with the patient, their carer and their general practitioners (GP).
- A contingency plan has been agreed with the patient, their carer and their GP.
- The patient is able to pick up medication daily and be reviewed by professionals regularly throughout the process.
- Outpatient/community-based programmes including psychosocial support are available.

Community detoxification should be stopped if the patient resumes drinking or fails to engage with the agreed treatment plan.

Inpatient detoxification is likely to be required if:

- Regular consumption is >30 units/day.
- SADQ >30 (severe dependence).
- There is a history of seizures or delirium tremens.
- The patient is very young or old.
- There is current benzodiazepine use in combination with alcohol.
- Substances other than alcohol are also being misused/abused.
- There is co-morbid mental or physical illness, learning disability or cognitive impairment.
- The patient is pregnant.
- The patient is homeless or has no social support.
- There is a history of failed community detoxification.

In certain situations, there may be a clinical justification for undertaking a community detoxification in the above patients (Table 4.3); however, the reasons must be clear and the decision is made by an experienced clinician.

Patient:_____   Date: _____
Time: _____ (24 hours clock, midnight = 00:00)

Pulse or heart rate, taken for 1 minute:_____
Blood pressure:_____

NAUSEA AND VOMITING – Ask 'Do you feel sick to your stomach? Have you vomited?' Observation.
0 – no nausea and no vomiting
1 – mild nausea with no vomiting
2
3
4 – intermittent nausea with dry heaves
5
6
7 – constant nausea, frequent dry heaves and vomiting

TACTILE DISTURBANCES – Ask 'Have you any itching, pins and needles sensations, any burning, any numbness, or do you feel bugs crawling on or under your skin?' Observation.
0 – none
1 – very mild itching, pins and needles, burning or numbness
2 – mild itching, pins and needles, burning or numbness
3 – moderate itching, pins and needles, burning or numbness
4 – moderately severe hallucinations
5 – severe hallucinations
6 – extremely severe hallucinations
7 – continuous hallucinations

TREMOR – Arms extended and fingers spread apart. Observation.
0 – no tremor
1 – not visible, but can be felt fingertip to fingertip
2
3
4 – moderate, with patient's arms extended
5
6
7 – severe, even with arms not extended

AUDITORY DISTURBANCES – Ask 'Are you more aware of sounds around you? Are they harsh? Do they frighten you? Are you hearing anything that is disturbing to you? Are you hearing things you know are not there?' Observation.
0 – not present
1 – very mild harshness or ability to frighten
2 – mild harshness or ability to frighten
3 – moderate harshness or ability to frighten
4 – moderately severe hallucinations
5 – severe hallucinations
6 – extremely severe hallucinations
7 – continuous hallucinations

PAROXYSMAL SWEATS – Observation.
0 – no sweat visible
1 – barely perceptible sweating, palms moist
2
3
4 – beads of sweat obvious on forehead
5
6
7 – drenching sweats

VISUAL DISTURBANCES – Ask 'Does the light appear to be too bright? Is its colour different? Does it hurt your eyes? Are you seeing anything that is disturbing to you? Are you seeing things you know are not there?' Observation.
0 – not present
1 – very mild sensitivity
2 – mild sensitivity
3 – moderate sensitivity
4 – moderately severe hallucinations
5 – severe hallucinations
6 – extremely severe hallucinations
7 – continuous hallucinations

ANXIETY – Ask 'Do you feel nervous?' Observation.
0 – no anxiety, at ease
1 – mild anxious
2
3
4 – moderately anxious, or guarded, so anxiety is inferred
5
6
7 – equivalent to acute panic states as seen in severe delirium or acute schizophrenic reactions

HEADACHE, FULLNESS IN HEAD – Ask 'Does your head feel different? Does it feel like there is a band around your head?' Do not rate for dizziness or light-headedness. Otherwise, rate severity.
0 – not present
1 – very mild
2 – mild
3 – moderate
4 – moderately severe
5 – severe
6 – very severe
7 – extremely severe

AGITATION – Observation.
0 normal activity
1 – somewhat more than normal activity
2
3
4 – moderately fidgety and restless
5
6
7 – paces back and forth during most of the interview, or constantly thrashes about

ORIENTATION AND CLOUDING OF SENSORIUM – Ask 'What day is this? Where are you? Who am I?'
0 – oriented and can do serial additions
1 – cannot do serial additions or is uncertain about date
2 – disoriented for date by no more than 2 calendar days
3 – disoriented for date by more than 2 calendar days
4 – disoriented for place or person

Scores
≤10 – mild withdrawal (do not need additional medication)
≤15 – moderate withdrawal
>15 – severe withdrawal

Total **CIWA-Ar** score _____
Rater's initials _____
Maximum possible score 67

Figure 4.1 Clinical Institute Withdrawal Assessment of Alcohol Scale, Revised[12]
The **CIWA-Ar** is not copyrighted and may be reproduced freely.

CHAPTER 4

Table 4.2 Short Alcohol Withdrawal Scale (SAWS)[13]

	None(0)	Mild(1)	Moderate(2)	Severe(3)
Anxious				
Sleep disturbance				
Problems with memory				
Nausea				
Restless				
Tremor (shakes)				
Feeling confused				
Sweating				
Miserable				
Heart pounding				

Table 4.3 Alcohol withdrawal treatment interventions – summary

Severity	Supportive/ medical care	Pharmacotherapy for neuro-adaptation reversal	Thiamine supplementation	Setting
Mild CIWA-Ar ≤ 10	Moderate-to-high-level supportive care, little, if any medical care required	Little to none required Simple remedies only (see below)	Oral likely to be sufficient if patient is well nourished	Home
Moderate CIWA-Ar ≤ 15	Moderate-to-high-level supportive care, little medical care required	Little to none required Symptomatic treatment only	Intramuscular Pabrinex should be offered if the patient is malnourished followed by oral supplementation	Home or community team
Severe CIWA-Ar > 15	High-level supportive care plus medical monitoring	Symptomatic and substitution treatment (chlordiazepoxide) probably required	Intramuscular Pabrinex should be offered followed by oral supplementation	Community team or hospital
CIWA-Ar > 10 plus co-morbid alcohol-related medical problems	High-level supportive care plus specialist medical care	Symptomatic and substitution treatments usually required	Intramuscular Pabrinex followed by oral supplementation	Hospital

Benzodiazepines are the treatment of choice for alcohol withdrawal. They exhibit cross-tolerance with alcohol and have anticonvulsant properties. Use is supported by NICE guidelines;[2,14] a Cochrane systematic review;[7] and the BAP guidelines.[9] **Parenteral thiamine (vitamin B1)**, another vitamin replacement, is an important adjunctive treatment for the prophylaxis and/or treatment of Wernicke–Korsakoff syndrome and other vitamin-related neuropsychiatric conditions.

In the UK, chlordiazepoxide is the benzodiazepine used for most patients in most centres as it is considered to have a relatively low dependence-forming potential. Some centres use diazepam. A short-acting benzodiazepine such as oxazepam or lorazepam may be used in individuals with impaired liver function.

There are three types of assisted withdrawal regimens: **fixed-dose reduction** (the most common in non-specialist settings), **variable-dose reduction** (usually results in less benzodiazepine being administered but best reserved for settings where staff have specialist skills in managing alcohol withdrawal) and finally **front-loading** (infrequently used, and reserved for severe alcohol withdrawal).[2,9] Assisted withdrawal regimens should never be started if BAC is very high or is still rising. Monitor patients for oversedation/respiratory depression.

Fixed-dose reduction regimen

Fixed-dose regimens use can be used in community or non-specialist inpatient/residential settings for uncomplicated patients. Patients should be started on a dose of benzodiazepine selected after an assessment of the severity of alcohol dependence (clinical history, number of units per drinking day and score on the SADQ. With respect to chlordiazepoxide, a general rule of thumb is that the starting dose can be estimated from current alcohol consumption. For example, if 20 units/day are being consumed, the starting dose should be 20mg four times a day. The dose is then tapered to zero over 5–10 days. Alcohol withdrawal symptoms should be monitored using a validated instrument such as the CIWA-Ar[12] or the SAWS.[13]

Mild alcohol dependence usually requires very small doses of chlordiazepoxide or else may be managed without medication.

For **moderate alcohol dependence**, a typical regime might be 10–20mg chlordiazepoxide 4 times a day, reducing gradually over 5–7 days. Note that 5–7 days' treatment is adequate and longer treatment is rarely helpful or necessary. It is advisable to monitor withdrawal and BAC daily before providing the day's medication. This may mean that community pharmacologically assisted alcohol withdrawals should start on a Monday and last for 5 days.

Table 4.4 Moderate alcohol dependence: example of a fixed-dose chlordiazepoxide treatment regimen.

		Total daily dose (mg)
Day 1	20mg qds	80
Day 2	15mg qds	60
Day 3	10mg qds	40
Day 4	5mg qds	20
Day 5	5mg bd	10

bd, bis die (twice a day); qds, quarter die sumendum (four times a day).

CHAPTER 4

Severe alcohol dependence usually requires inpatient treatment for assisted withdrawal because of the significant risk of life-threatening complications. However, there are rare occasions where a pragmatic community approach is required. In such situations, the decision to undertake a community-assisted withdrawal must be made clear by an experienced clinician, to both patient and carer. Intensive daily monitoring is advised for the first 2–3 days. This may require special arrangements over a weekend.

Prescribing should not start if the patient is intoxicated. In such circumstances, they should be reviewed at the earliest opportunity when not intoxicated. The dose of benzodiazepine may need to be reduced over a 7–10-day period in this group (occasionally longer if dependence is very severe or there is a history of complications during previous detoxifications).

Symptom-triggered regimen

This should be reserved for managing assisted withdrawal in specialist alcohol inpatient or residential settings. Regular monitoring is required, e.g. pulse, BP, temperature and level of consciousness. Medication is only given when withdrawal symptoms are observed as determined using CIWA-Ar, SAWS or alternative validated measure. Symptom-triggered therapy is generally used in patients without a history of complications. A typical symptom-triggered regimen would be chlordiazepoxide 20–30mg hourly as needed. Note that the total dose given each day would be expected to decrease from day 2 onwards. It is common for symptom-triggered treatment to last only 24–48 hours before switching to an individualised fixed-dose reducing schedule. Occasionally (e.g. in DTs), the flexible regime may need to be prolonged beyond the first 24 hours.

Table 4.5 Severe alcohol dependence: example of a fixed-dose chlordiazepoxide regimen

		Total daily dose (mg)
Day 1 (first 24 hours)	40mg qds + 40mg PRN	200
Day 2	40mg qds	160
Day 3	30mg qds	120
Day 4	25mg qds	100
Day 5	20mg qds	80
Day 6	15mg qds	60
Day 7	10mg qds	40
Day 8	10mg tds	30
Day 9	5mg qds	20
Day 10	10mg nocte	10

nocte, at night; prn, pro re nata (as required); qds, quarter die sumendum (four times a day); tds, ter die sumendum (three times a day).

Example of a symptom-triggered chlordiazepoxide regime[2]

Days 1–5 : 20–30mg chlordiazepoxide as needed, up to hourly, based on symptoms.

Wernicke's encephalopathy

Wernicke's encephalopathy is an acute neuropsychiatric condition caused by thiamine deficiency. In alcohol dependence, thiamine deficiency is secondary to both reduced dietary intake and reduced absorption.

The following are the risk factors for Wernicke's encephalopathy in alcohol dependence:[14]

- Acute withdrawal
- Malnourishment
- Decompensated liver disease
- Emergency department (ED) attendance
- Hospitalisation for co-morbidity
- Homelessness

Presentation

The 'classical' triad of ophthalmoplegia, ataxia and confusion is rarely present in Wernicke's encephalopathy, and the syndrome is much more common than is recognised. A presumptive diagnosis of Wernicke's encephalopathy should therefore be made in any patient undergoing detoxification who experiences any of the following signs:

- Ataxia
- Hypothermia
- Hypotension
- Confusion
- Ophthalmoplegia/nystagmus
- Memory disturbance
- Unconsciousness/coma

Any history of malnutrition, recent weight loss, vomiting or diarrhoea or peripheral neuropathy should also be noted.[15]

Prophylactic thiamine

Low-risk drinkers without neuropsychiatric complications and with an adequate diet should be offered oral thiamine: a minimum of 300mg daily during assisted alcohol withdrawal and periods of continued alcohol intake.[9]

Caution: As thiamine is required to utilise glucose, a glucose load in a thiamine-deficient patient can precipitate Wernicke's encephalopathy.

Parenteral B-complex (in the UK – Pabrinex) must be administered <u>before glucose</u> is administered in all patients presenting with altered mental status

It is generally advised that patients undergoing inpatient detoxification should be given parenteral thiamine as prophylaxis,[2,9,14,16,17] although there is insufficient evidence from randomised controlled trials (RCTs) as to the best dose, frequency or duration of use.

Guidance is based on 'expert opinion'[9] and the standard advice is one pair of Pabrinex IM high potency daily (containing thiamine 250mg/dose) for 5 days, followed by oral thiamine and/or vitamin B compound for as long as needed (where diet is inadequate or alcohol consumption is resumed).[9] All inpatients should receive this regime as an absolute minimum.

Intramuscular (IM) thiamine preparations have a lower incidence of anaphylactic reactions than intravenous (IV) preparations, at 1 per 5 million pairs of ampoules of Pabrinex – far lower than many frequently used drugs that carry no special anaphylaxis warning. However, this risk has resulted in fears about using parenteral preparations and the inappropriate use of oral thiamine preparations (which do not offer adequate protection). Given the risks associated with Wernicke's encephalopathy, the benefit-to-risk ratio grossly favours parenteral thiamine.[9,16,18] Where parenteral thiamine is used, facilities for treating anaphylaxis should be available.[19]

If Wernicke's encephalopathy is suspected, the patient should be transferred to a medical unit where IV thiamine can be administered. If untreated, Wernicke's encephalopathy progresses to Korsakoff's syndrome (permanent memory impairment, confabulation, confusion and personality changes).

Treatment for patients with suspected/established Wernicke's encephalopathy (acute medical ward):

At least two pairs of Pabrinex IV high potency (i.e. 4 ampoules) *3 times daily* for 3–5 days, followed by one pair of ampoules once daily for a further 3–5 days or longer[2,9] (until no further response is seen).

Treatment of somatic symptoms

Somatic complaints are common during assisted withdrawal. The following simple remedies are recommended in Table 4.6:

Table 4.6 Treatment of somatic symptoms

Symptom	Recommended treatment
Dehydration	Ensure adequate fluid intake in order to maintain hydration and electrolyte balance. Dehydration can precipitate life-threatening cardiac arrhythmia
Pain	Paracetamol (acetaminophen)
Nausea and vomiting	Metoclopramide 10mg or prochlorperazine 5mg 4–6 hourly
Diarrhoea	Diphenoxylate and atropine (Lomotil) or loperamide
Skin itching	Occurs commonly and not only in individuals with alcoholic liver disease: use oral antihistamines

Relapse prevention

There is no place for the continued use of benzodiazepines beyond treatment of the acute alcohol withdrawal syndrome. Acamprosate and supervised disulfiram are licensed for treatment of alcohol dependence in the UK and may be offered in combination with psychosocial treatment.[2] Treatment should be initiated by a specialist service. After 12 weeks, transfer of the prescribing to the GP may be appropriate, although specialist care may continue (shared care). Naltrexone is also recommended as an adjunct in the treatment of moderate and severe alcohol dependence.[2] As it does not have marketing authorisation for the treatment of alcohol dependence in the UK, informed consent should be sought and documented prior to commencing treatment.

Acamprosate

Acamprosate is a synthetic taurine analogue that acts as a functional glutamatergic N-methyl-D-aspartate antagonist and also increases γ-aminobutyric acid (GABA)-ergic function. The number needed to treat (NNT) for the maintenance of abstinence has been calculated as 9–11.[9] The treatment effect is most pronounced at 6 months with the risk ratio (compared with placebo) of returning to drinking behaviour dropping to 0.83, though the effect has been shown to be significant for up to 12 months.[2,20,21] Acamprosate should be initiated as soon as possible after abstinence has been achieved (the BAP consensus guidelines[9] recommend that acamprosate should be started 'during detoxification' because of its potential neuroprotective effect). NICE[2] recommends that acamprosate should be continued for up to 6 months with regular (monthly) supervision. The SPC recommends that it is given for 1 year.

Acamprosate is relatively well tolerated; side effects include diarrhoea, abdominal pain, nausea, vomiting and pruritis.[2] It is contraindicated in severe renal or hepatic impairment, thus baseline liver and kidney function tests should be performed before commencing treatment. Acamprosate should be avoided in individuals who are pregnant or breastfeeding.

Acamprosate: NICE Clinical Guideline 115, 2011[2,20]

Acamprosate should be offered for relapse prevention in moderately to severely dependent drinkers, in combination with psychosocial treatment. It should be prescribed for up to 6 months, or longer for those who perceive benefit and wish to continue taking it. The dose is 1998mg daily (666mg three times per day) for individuals over 60kg. For those under 60kg, the dose is 1332mg daily. Treatment should be stopped in those who continue to drink for 4–6 weeks after starting the drug.

Naltrexone

Opioid blockade prevents increased dopaminergic activity after the consumption of alcohol, thus reducing its rewarding effects. Naltrexone, a non-selective opioid receptor antagonist, significantly reduces relapse to heavy drinking.[2,22] Although early trials used a dose of 50mg/day, more recent US studies have used 100mg/day. In the UK, the usual dose is 50mg/day with a trial dose of 25mg for 2 days to check for side effects.

Naltrexone is well tolerated but side effects include nausea (especially in the early stages of treatment), headache, abdominal pain, reduced appetite and tiredness. A comprehensive medical assessment should be carried out prior to commencing naltrexone, together with baseline renal function tests and LFTs. Naltrexone can be started when patients are still drinking or during medically assisted withdrawal. There is no clear evidence as to the optimal duration of treatment but 6 months appears to be an appropriate period with follow up, including monitoring liver function.[9]

Patients on naltrexone should not be given opioid agonist drugs for analgesia: non-opioid analgesics should be used instead. In the event that opioid analgesia is necessary, it can be instituted 48–72 hours after cessation of naltrexone. Hepatotoxicity has been described with high doses of naltrexone, so use should be avoided in acute liver failure.[23]

Naltrexone: NICE Clinical Guideline 115, 2011[2,22]

Naltrexone [50mg/day] should be offered for relapse prevention in moderately to severely dependent drinkers, in combination with psychosocial treatment. It should be prescribed for up to 6 months, or longer for those who perceive benefit and wish to continue taking it. Treatment should be stopped in those who continue to drink for 4–6 weeks after starting the drug or in those who feel unwell while taking it.

Long-acting injectable naltrexone has been developed to improve compliance. Side effects are similar to those seen with the oral preparation.[24] NICE concluded that the initial evidence was encouraging but not enough to support routine use.

Nalmefene

Nalmefene is also an opioid antagonist, recommended by NICE as an option for reducing alcohol consumption, for people with alcohol dependence.[2,22] It has been shown in one indirect meta-analysis to be superior to naltrexone in reducing heavy drinking.[25] However, use of nalmefene remains controversial, with another meta-analysis suggested that nalmefene had only limited efficacy in reducing alcohol consumption and that its value in treating alcohol addiction and relapse prevention is not fully established.[26]

Disulfiram (antabuse)

Disulfiram inhibits the enzyme aldehyde dehydrogenase, thus preventing complete metabolism of alcohol in the liver. This results in an accumulation of the toxic intermediate product acetaldehyde, which causes the alcohol–disulfiram reaction.

Mild alcohol–disulfiram reaction
- Facial flushing
- Sweating
- Nausea
- Hyperventilation
- Dyspnea
- Tachycardia
- Hypotension

Contraindications
- Ingestion of alcohol within the previous 24 hours
- Cardiac failure
- Coronary artery disease
- Hypertension
- Cerebrovascular disease
- Pregnancy
- Breastfeeding
- Liver disease
- Peripheral neuropathy
- Severe mental illness

Severe alcohol–disulfiram reaction
- Acute heart failure
- Myocardial infarction
- Arrhythmias
- Bradycardia
- Respiratory depression
- Severe hypotension

The therapeutic effect of disulfiram is thus mediated by its incompatibility with alcohol, resulting in alcohol aversion. Supervised medication optimises compliance and contributes to effectiveness.

The intensity of the intolerance reaction is dose dependent, both with regard to the amount of alcohol consumed and the dose of disulfiram. However, it is thought that much of the therapeutic effect is mediated by the mental anticipation of the aversive reaction, rather than the pharmacological action itself. Sudden death is more prevalent at doses above 1000mg.[27] With this in mind, the value of prescribing higher doses of disulfiram must be carefully considered.

Doses are 800mg for the first dose, reducing to 100–200mg daily for maintenance. In co-morbid alcohol and cocaine dependence, doses of 500mg daily have been given. Halitosis is a common side effect. If there is a sudden onset of jaundice (the rare complication of hepatotoxicity), the patient should stop the drug and seek urgent medical attention.

The evidence for disulfiram is weaker than for acamprosate and naltrexone.[2] In the UK, NICE recommends its use 'as a second-line option for moderate-to-severe alcohol dependence for patients who are not suitable for acamprosate or naltrexone or have a specified preference for disulfiram and who aim to stay abstinent from alcohol'.[2]

Disulfiram: NICE Clinical Guideline 115, 2011[2]

Disulfiram should be considered in combination with a psychological intervention for patients who wish to achieve abstinence, but for whom acamprosate or naltrexone is not suitable. Treatment should be started at least 24 hours after the last drink and should be overseen by a family member or a carer. Monitoring is recommended every 2 weeks for the first 2 months, then monthly for the following 4 months. Medical monitoring should be continued at 6 monthly intervals after the first 6 months. Patients must not consume any alcohol while taking disulfiram.

Baclofen

Baclofen is a GABA-B agonist that does not have a licence for use in alcohol dependence but is nevertheless used by some clinicians. A recent meta-analysis failed to find positive effects for baclofen and did not support its use as a first-line treatment for alcohol-use disorders.[28] Baclofen was associated with higher rates of adverse effects, including depression, vertigo, somnolence, numbness and muscle rigidity.

Antiseizure medications

There is currently insufficient evidence to support the clinical use of antiseizure medications in the treatment of alcohol dependence, although a significant association has been found for fewer drinks per drinking day and lower average heavy drinking compared with placebo.[29] Most research has been carried out on topiramate. There have been fewer studies on gabapentin[30] valproate and levetiracetam.

Pregnancy and alcohol use

Evidence indicates that alcohol consumption during pregnancy may cause harm to the foetus. The DoH advises that women should not drink any alcohol at all during pregnancy.[1] Drinking even 1–2 units/day during pregnancy can increase the risk of having a pre-term, low birthweight or small for gestational age baby. NICE guidelines changed in December 2018 to refer to the CMO guidelines.

For alcohol-dependent pregnant women who have withdrawal symptoms, pharmacological cover for detoxification should be offered, ideally in an inpatient setting. The timing of detoxification in relation to the trimester of pregnancy should be risk assessed against continued alcohol consumption and risks to the foetus.[9] Chlordiazepoxide has been suggested as being unlikely to pose a substantial risk; however, dose-dependent malformations have been observed.[9] The UK Teratology Information Service[31] provides national advice for healthcare professionals and likes to follow up on pregnancies that require alcohol detoxification. Specialist advice should always be sought (see also section 'Pregnancy' in Chapter 7). No relapse prevention medication has been evaluated in pregnancy.[9]

Children and adolescents

Children and young people (10–17 years) should be assessed as outlined in NICE Clinical Guideline 115, 2011.[2]

The number of young people who are dependent and needing pharmacotherapy is likely to be small, but for those who are dependent there should be a lower threshold for admission to hospital. Doses of chlordiazepoxide for medically assisted withdrawal may need to be adjusted, but the general principles of withdrawal management are the same as for adults. All young people should have a full health screen carried out routinely to allow identification of physical and mental health problems. The evidence base for acamprosate, naltrexone and disulfiram in 16–19-year-olds is evolving,[9] but naltrexone is best supported in this age group.[32,33]

Older adults

There should be a lower threshold for inpatient medically assisted alcohol withdrawal for older adults.[2] While benzodiazepines remain the treatment of choice, they may need to be prescribed in lower doses and in some situations shorter acting drugs may be preferred.[9] All older adults with alcohol-use disorders should have full routine health screens to identify physical and mental health problems. The evidence base for pharmacotherapy of alcohol-use disorders in older people is limited.

Concurrent alcohol and drug use disorders

Where alcohol and drug use disorders are co-morbid, treat both conditions actively.[2]

Co-existing alcohol and benzodiazepine dependence

This is best managed with one benzodiazepine, either chlordiazepoxide or diazepam. The starting dose should take into account the requirements for medically assisted alcohol withdrawal and the typical daily equivalent dose of the relevant benzodiazepine(s).[2] Inpatient treatment should be carried out over a 2–3-week period, possibly longer.[2]

Co-existing alcohol dependence and cocaine use

In co-morbid cocaine/alcohol dependence, naltrexone 150mg/day resulted in reduced cocaine and alcohol use in men but not in women.[34]

Co-existing alcohol and opioid dependence

Both conditions should be treated, and attention paid to the increased mortality of individuals withdrawing from both drugs.

Co-morbid alcohol and nicotine dependence

Encourage individuals to stop smoking. Refer for smoking cessation in primary care and other settings. In inpatient settings, offer nicotine patches/inhalator during assisted alcohol withdrawal. Always promote vaping as a safer alternative to tobacco smoking.

CHAPTER 4

Co-morbid mental health disorders

People with alcohol-use disorders often present with other mental health disorders, particularly anxiety and depression. Public Health England has described it as 'the norm rather than the exception' and encourage a collaborative, effective and flexible approach between frontline services, stating that it is 'everyone's job' and that there is 'no wrong door'.[35]

Substance-use disorders including alcohol *misuse* should never be a reason to exclude a patient from:

- **Crisis psychiatric services**
- **Mood/anxiety/personality services after completion of detoxification.**

Depression

Depressive and anxiety symptoms occur commonly during alcohol withdrawal, but usually diminish by the third or fourth week of abstinence. Meta-analyses suggest that antidepressants with mixed pharmacology (the tricyclics imipramine or trimipramine) perform better than selective serotonin reuptake inhibitors (SSRIs; fluoxetine or sertraline) in reducing depressive symptoms in individuals with an alcohol-use disorder, but the antidepressant effect is modest.[2,9,36,37] A greater antidepressant effect was seen if the diagnosis of depression was made after at least 1 week of abstinence, thus excluding those with affective symptoms caused by alcohol withdrawal. There is stronger evidence for depression categorised as independent, rather than substance induced.[36] As treatment effects are masked by comparatively large placebo effects, which conceal improvements that would otherwise be attributed to medication, there is a need for larger randomised placebo-controlled trials. Despite the evidence for tricyclics, they are not recommended in clinical practice because of their potential for cardiotoxicity and toxicity in overdose.

Relapse prevention medication should be considered in combination with antidepressants. Pettinati et al.[38] showed that the combination of sertraline (200mg/day) with naltrexone (100mg/day) had superior outcomes – improved drinking outcomes and better mood – compared with placebo and compared with each drug alone. In contrast, citalopram showed no benefit when added to naltrexone.[39]

Secondary analyses of acamprosate and naltrexone trials suggest that:

- acamprosate has an indirect modest beneficial effect on depression via increasing abstinence and
- in depressed alcohol-dependent patients, the combination of naltrexone and an antidepressant may be better than either drug alone,[9] but findings are not consistent.[39]

Bipolar affective disorder

Bipolar patients tend to use alcohol to reduce symptoms of anxiety. Where there is co-morbidity, it is important to treat the different phases as recommended in guidelines for bipolar disorder. It may be worth adding sodium valproate to lithium as two trials have shown that the combination was associated with better drinking outcomes than lithium alone. However, the combination did not confer any extra benefit than lithium alone in improving mood (see BAP consensus 2012).[9] Note that, in those who continue to drink, electrolyte imbalance may precipitate lithium toxicity. Lithium is best avoided completely in binge drinkers.

Naltrexone should be offered, in the first instance, to help bipolar patients reduce their alcohol consumption.[9] If naltrexone is not effective, then acamprosate should be offered. In the event that both naltrexone and acamprosate fail to promote abstinence, disulfiram should be considered, and the risks made known to the patient.

Anxiety

Anxiety is commonly observed in alcohol-dependent individuals during intoxication, withdrawal and in the early days of abstinence. Alcohol is typically used to self-medicate anxiety disorders, particularly social anxiety. In alcohol-dependent individuals who experience anxiety it is often difficult to determine the extent to which the anxiety is a symptom of the alcohol-use disorder or whether it is an independent disorder. Medically assisted withdrawal and supported abstinence for up to 8 weeks are required before a full assessment can be made. If a medically assisted withdrawal is not possible, then treatment of the anxiety disorder should still be attempted, following guidelines for the respective anxiety disorder.

The use of benzodiazepines is controversial[9] because of the increased risk of benzodiazepine misuse and dependence. Benzodiazepines should only be considered following assessment in a specialist addiction service.

One meta-analysis suggests that buspirone is effective in reducing symptoms of anxiety, but not alcohol consumption.[9,40] Studies have also shown that paroxetine (up to 60mg/day) was superior to placebo in reducing social anxiety in co-morbid patients: alcohol consumption was not affected.[9,40]

Either naltrexone or disulfiram, alone or combined, improved drinking outcomes compared with placebo in patients with post-traumatic stress disorder and alcohol dependence. Both acamprosate and baclofen have shown benefit in reducing anxiety in post hoc analyses of alcohol dependence trials (see BAP consensus for references[9]). It is therefore important to ensure that these patients are enabled to become abstinent and are prescribed relapse prevention medication. Anxiety should then be treated according to the appropriate NICE guidelines.

Schizophrenia

Patients with schizophrenia who also have an alcohol-use disorder should be assessed and alcohol-specific relapse prevention treatment considered, either naltrexone or acamprosate. Antipsychotic medication should be optimised,[9] and clozapine may be considered. However, there is insufficient evidence to recommend the use of any one antipsychotic medication over another.

CHAPTER 4

References

1. Department of Health and Social Care. UK chief medical officers' guidelines on how to keep health risks from drinking alcohol to a low level. 2016; https://www.gov.uk/government/publications/alcohol-consumption-advice-on-low-risk-drinking.

2. National Institute for Health and Clinical Excellence. Alcohol use disorders: diagnosis, assessment and management of harmful drinking and alcohol dependence. Clinical Guidance [CG115]. 2011 (last checked July 2019); https://www.nice.org.uk/guidance/cg115.

3. National Institute for Health and Care Excellence. Alcohol-use disorders: prevention. Public health guideline [PH24]. 2010; (last checked July 2019). https://www.nice.org.uk/guidance/ph24.

4. Babor T, et al. AUDIT: the alcohol use disorders identification test guidelines for use in primary care. 2nd edition. 2001; http://whqlibdoc.who.int/hq/2001/WHO_MSD_MSB_01.6a.pdf?ua=1.

5. Stockwell T, et al. The severity of alcohol dependence questionnaire: its use, reliability and validity. *Br J Addict* 1983; 78:145–155.

6. Minozzi S, et al. Anticonvulsants for alcohol withdrawal. *Cochrane Database Syst Rev* 2010; CD005064.

7. Amato L, et al. Efficacy and safety of pharmacological interventions for the treatment of the Alcohol Withdrawal Syndrome. *Cochrane Database Syst Rev* 2011; CD008537.

8. Brathen G, et al. EFNS guideline on the diagnosis and management of alcohol-related seizures: report of an EFNS task force. *Eur J Neurol* 2005; 12:575–581.

9. Lingford-Hughes AR, et al. Evidence-based guidelines for the pharmacological management of substance abuse, harmful use, addiction and comorbidity: recommendations from BAP. *J Psychopharmacol* 2012; 26:899–952.

10. NSW Government. Drug and alcohol withdrawal clinical practice guidelines. 2008; https://www1.health.nsw.gov.au/pds/ActivePDSDocuments/GL2008_011.pdf.

11. Schuckit MA. Recognition and management of withdrawal delirium (delirium tremens). *N Engl J Med* 2014; 371:2109–2113.

12. Sullivan JT, et al. Assessment of alcohol withdrawal: the revised clinical institute withdrawal assessment for alcohol scale (CIWA-Ar). *Br J Addict* 1989; 84:1353–1357.

13. Gossop M, et al. A Short Alcohol Withdrawal Scale (SAWS): development and psychometric properties. *Addict Biol* 2002; 7:37–43.

14. National Institute for Health and Clinical Excellence. Alcohol-use disorders: physical complications. Clinical Guidance [CG100] 2010 (last updated April 2017); https://www.nice.org.uk/guidance/cg100.

15. Thomson AD, et al. Time to act on the inadequate management of Wernicke's encephalopathy in the UK. *Alcohol Alcohol* 2013; 48:4–8.

16. Thomson AD, et al. The Royal College of Physicians report on alcohol: guidelines for managing Wernicke's encephalopathy in the accident and Emergency Department. *Alcohol Alcohol* 2002; 37:513–521.

17. Day E, et al. Thiamine for prevention and treatment of Wernicke-Korsakoff Syndrome in people who abuse alcohol. *Cochrane Database Syst Rev* 2013; 7:CD004033.

18. Thomson A, et al. Incidence of adverse reactions to parenteral thiamine in the treatment of Wernicke's encephalopathy, and recommendations. *Alcohol Alcohol* 2019; 54:609–614.

19. BNF Online. British national formulary. 2020; https://www.medicinescomplete.com/mc/bnf/current.

20. Rösner S, et al. Acamprosate for alcohol dependence. *Cochrane Database Syst Rev* 2010; Cd004332.

21. Donoghue K, et al. The efficacy of acamprosate and naltrexone in the treatment of alcohol dependence, Europe versus the rest of the world: a meta-analysis. *Addiction* 2015; 110:920–930.

22. Rösner S, et al. Opioid antagonists for alcohol dependence. *Cochrane Database Syst Rev* 2010; Cd001867.

23. Accord Healthcare Limited. Summary of Product Characteristics. Naltrexone Hydrochloride 50 mg Film-coated Tablets. 2014; https://www.medicines.org.uk/emc/medicine/25878.

24. Krupitsky E, et al. Injectable extended-release naltrexone (XR-NTX) for opioid dependence: long-term safety and effectiveness. *Addiction* 2013; 108:1628–1637.

25. Soyka M, et al. Comparing nalmefene and naltrexone in alcohol dependence: are there any differences? Results from an indirect meta-analysis. *Pharmacopsychiatry* 2016; 49:66–75.

26. Palpacuer C, et al. Risks and benefits of nalmefene in the treatment of adult alcohol dependence: a systematic literature review and meta-analysis of published and unpublished double-blind randomized controlled trials. *PLoS Med* 2015; 12:e1001924.

27. Mutschler J, et al. Current findings and mechanisms of action of disulfiram in the treatment of alcohol dependence. *Pharmacopsychiatry* 2016; 49:137–141.

28. Minozzi S, et al. Baclofen for alcohol use disorder. *Cochrane Database Syst Rev* 2018; 11:Cd012557.

29. Pani PP, et al. Anticonvulsants for alcohol dependence. *Cochrane Database Syst Rev* 2014; Cd008544.

30. Kranzler HR, et al. A meta-analysis of the efficacy of gabapentin for treating alcohol use disorder. *Addiction* 2019; 114:1547–1555.

31. UK Teratology Information Service (UKTIS). 2020; www.uktis.org.

32. O'Malley SS, et al. Reduction of alcohol drinking in young adults by naltrexone: a double-blind, placebo-controlled, randomized clinical trial of efficacy and safety. *J Clin Psychiatry* 2015; 76:e207–e213.

33. Miranda R, et al. Effects of naltrexone on adolescent alcohol cue reactivity and sensitivity: an initial randomized trial. *Addict Biol* 2014; 19:941–954.

34. Pettinati HM, et al. Gender differences with high-dose naltrexone in patients with co-occurring cocaine and alcohol dependence. *J Subst Abuse Treat* 2008; 34:378–390.

35. Public Health England. Better care for people with co-occurring mental health and alcohol/drug use conditions. A guide for commissioners and service providers. 2017; https://www.gov.uk/government/uploads/system/uploads/attachment_data/file/625809/Co-occurring_mental_health_and_alcohol_drug_use_conditions.pdf.

36. Agabio R, et al. Antidepressants for the treatment of people with co-occurring depression and alcohol dependence. *Cochrane Database Syst Rev* 2018; 4:Cd008581.

37. Stokes PRA, et al. Pharmacological treatment of mood disorders and comorbid addictions: a systematic review and meta-analysis: traitement pharmacologique des troubles de L'humeur et des Dépendances Comorbides: une Revue Systématique et une Méta-Analyse. *Can J Psychiatry* 2020; **65**:749–769.

38. Pettinati HM, et al. A double-blind, placebo-controlled trial combining sertraline and naltrexone for treating co-occurring depression and alcohol dependence. *Am J Psychiatry* 2010; **167**:668–675.

39. Adamson SJ, et al. A randomized trial of combined citalopram and naltrexone for nonabstinent outpatients with co-occurring alcohol dependence and major depression. *J Clin Psychopharmacol* 2015; 35:143–149.

40. Ipser JC, et al. Pharmacotherapy for anxiety and comorbid alcohol use disorders. *Cochrane Database Syst Rev* 2015; 1:Cd007505.

Further reading

Cheng HY, et al. Treatment interventions to maintain abstinence from alcohol in primary care: systematic review and network meta-analysis. BMJ 2020; **371**:m3934

CHAPTER 4

Alcohol withdrawal delirium – delirium tremens

Delirium tremens occurs in around 3–5% of those admitted to hospital for alcohol withdrawal, so it is likely to be encountered by those working in psychiatric liaison.[1] It is an agitated delirium that develops around 72 hours after the last drink. Previous seizures or delirium, low potassium, low magnesium, thiamine deficiency and systemic disease predispose to its development, as does under-treated alcohol withdrawal. Recognising delirium tremens is important because of its high mortality and because its treatment is different from delirium arising from other causes (larger doses of benzodiazepines, more caution with antipsychotics).

This is a prescribing guideline but it bears repeating that delirium tremens is a medical emergency and **you need to see the patient**. The patient should be nursed in a general hospital,[2] preferably in a high dependency unit[1,3] although in practice this can be difficult to arrange. Appropriate management requires joint work between psychiatric, medical and nursing teams, to identify and correct contributing physical factors such as electrolyte imbalance, thiamine deficiency and sepsis, while minimising behavioural disturbance via psychosocial measures (side room for a low stimulus environment, 1:1 nursing observations, frequent reorientation and reassurance) and pharmacological treatment. ITU outreach or on call should be informed early, and should be directly involved if the patient is not accepting oral medication and requires parenteral high-dose benzodiazepines.

The evidence base for treatment of delirium tremens is sparse and is mostly from before 1979.[1,4] Meta-analysis comparing sedative hypnotics (diazepam, pentobarbital and paraldehyde) and antipsychotics found a six-fold increased odds of mortality in patients treated with neuroleptics.[4] More recent studies comparing IV lorazepam with or without phenobarbital, or addition of dexmedetomidine,[5] were performed in the ICU environment, so have limited applicability to the general ward setting.

NICE guideline CG100 (update 2017) recommends nursing in a general hospital and use of lorazepam orally or IV, with little further elaboration.[2] The New South Wales guidance from Australia recommends diazepam and is more detailed (see Table 4.7). A recent *New England Journal of Medicine* (NEJM) review suggests to 'administer doses of benzodiazepines, preferably intravenously, in doses high enough to produce a lightly dozing, but still arousable, state, while monitoring vital signs, until delirium abates' and lists protocols for use of both lorazepam and diazepam, derived from earlier RCTs[1] (see Table 4.7).

The following points unite these approaches:

- Doses of diazepam or lorazepam are given close together in a 'loading fashion' with a maximum of an hour apart.
- High doses are permitted.
- Antipsychotics are not used, or are used only after large doses of benzodiazepines have failed.

Thus, available research evidence and more detailed government guidelines advocate treatment of delirium tremens, which differs from ordinarily rapid tranquillisation or other delirium protocols. This may need to be communicated explicitly to ITU teams, who may (unwisely) follow a standard rapid tranquillisation protocol with relatively low doses of benzodiazepines, including haloperidol.

CHAPTER 4

Table 4.7 Detailed administration schedules for delirium tremens

New South Wales Guidance[3]	NEJM diazepam[1]	NEJM lorazepam[1]
Regimen 1: 20mg diazepam orally hourly until light sedation achieved Max 80mg Sublingual olanzapine 10mg if continued agitation Regimen 2: If unable to accept diazepam, IV midazolam 5mg, then 2mg/hour in HDU setting 2mg lorazepam is an alternative to IV midazolam if it is not available	Regimen 1: 10–20mg diazepam orally or IV 1–4 hourly Regimen 2: 5mg IV bolus Then 10mg IV boluses every 10 minutes × 2 Then 20mg IV bolus if needed Then 5–20mg IV diazepam/hour	Regimen 1: 8mg lorazepam orally, IM or IV every 15 minutes (2 doses). If a third dose required, give 8mg IV When sedation achieved give 10–30mg/hour Regimen 2: 1–4mg lorazepam IM every 30–60 minutes until sedation achieved then hourly as needed Regimen 3: 1–4mg lorazepam IV every 5–15 minutes as needed

All patients with delirium tremens should have IV thiamine (as Pabrinex in the UK) at treatment dose, as malnutrition is a known predisposing cause of DTs. Sufficient sedation should be achieved to facilitate the giving of this treatment and IV rehydration.

Clinical experience indicates that medical and ITU teams are most comfortable with NSW Regime 1 (oral diazepam loading) or NEJM Regime 2 (IM lorazepam), in the first instance. NICE suggests that haloperidol can be used to manage behavioural disturbance in delirium tremens, but others urge caution in view of its cardiotoxicity and propensity to provoke seizures.[1,2] Both NICE and the New South Wales guidance suggest olanzapine as a possibility for behavioural disturbance refractory to benzodiazepines.[2,3]

Loading of benzodiazepines should not be done in patients with chronic obstructive pulmonary disease (COPD) or other respiratory compromise and it is more likely that these patients will require respiratory support in order to tolerate medically assisted detoxification, so early involvement of the ITU team is critical. Care should be taken to monitor respiratory rate (RR) and oxygenation particularly in those patients who are smokers and may have occult respiratory disease. Prescription of 'when necessary' flumazenil to reverse benzodiazepine toxicity is advisable.

References

1. Schuckit MA. Recognition and management of withdrawal delirium (delirium tremens). *N Engl J Med* 2014; 371:2109–2113.
2. National Institute for Health and Clinical Excellence. Alcohol-use disorders: physical complications. Clinical Guidance [CG100]. 2010 (last updated April 2017); https://www.nice.org.uk/guidance/cg100.
3. NSW Government. Drug and alcohol withdrawal clinical practice guidelines. 2008; https://www1.health.nsw.gov.au/pds/ActivePDSDocuments/GL2008_011.pdf.
4. Mayo-Smith MF, et al. Management of alcohol withdrawal delirium. An evidence-based practice guideline. *Arch Intern Med* 2004; 164:1405–1412.
5. Nguyen TA, et al. Phenobarbital and symptom-triggered lorazepam versus lorazepam alone for severe alcohol withdrawal in the intensive care unit. *Alcohol* 2020; 82:23–27.

CHAPTER 4

Opioid dependence

Prescribing for opioid dependence

> **Note**: Treatment of opioid dependence usually requires specialist intervention – generalists who do not have specialist experience should always contact substance misuse services before attempting to treat opioid dependence. It is strongly recommended that general adult psychiatrists *do not* initiate opioid substitute treatment without obtaining advice from specialist services. All opioids are respiratory depressants. Prescribed opioids such as methadone and buprenorphine have low lethal doses in drug-naïve individuals, and assessing tolerance is difficult.
>
> *Opioid toxicity can be fatal. Opioid withdrawal is not.*
>
> That having been said, self-discharge against medical advice from hospital because of intolerable opiate withdrawal also carries risks, and non-opiate medications should be used to treat opioid withdrawal until appropriate advice can be sought (see section pertaining to inpatient admission).

The pharmacological interventions used for opioid-dependent people in the UK range from harm minimisation measures such as provision of take-home naloxone (THN), maintenance treatment with opioid substitution treatment (OST) such as methadone or buprenorphine and naltrexone for relapse prevention. Pharmacological treatments form an integral part of recovery-orientated care alongside psychosocial treatment. The latter is not considered in this chapter and readers are referred to 'routes to recovery' and the psychosocial chapter of the 'Drug abuse and dependence: UK guidelines for clinical management' (or as it is more frequently called the 'Orange Guidelines') to understand more about these aspects of addiction treatment.[1,2]

Treatment of opioid overdose

Opioid overdose is a preventable cause of death in the opioid-using population. This includes overdose on illicit opioids such as heroin and more recently fentanyl and oxycodone, and overdose on prescribed opioids such as methadone or buprenorphine.

Opioid overdose is characterised clinically by:

- unconsciousness
- a low respiratory rate (RR < 12)
- pinpoint pupils
- cyanosis
- cold, clammy skin.

Naloxone is an opioid receptor antagonist that can reverse opioid overdose. It is available in pre-loaded syringes and should be administered intramuscularly after calling an ambulance and an initial round of chest compressions. An initial dose of 400µg is recommended, which can be repeated following three cycles of 30 chest compressions until the ambulance arrives or breathing resumes.[3] Higher doses of naloxone may be necessary to displace opioids of high affinity such as buprenorphine or fentanyl.[4]

Naloxone 400µg IM/IV should be prescribed 'as required' for any inpatient with suspected harmful opioid use or dependence and should be kept in the resuscitation bag on the ward. Anyone can give naloxone to prevent an overdose death. Patients discharged from inpatient wards should be warned about loss of tolerance and **they and their family members provided with naloxone training and THN.**[1] A summary of what to do in case of opioid overdose is captured in Figure 4.1, and training in THN covers these actions.

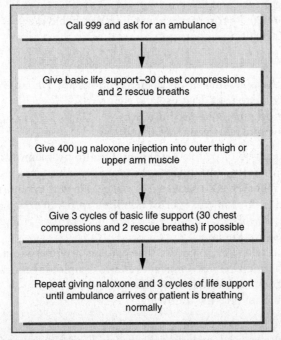

Figure 4.1 Flowchart for naloxone administration (adapted from WHO[3]).

Intranasal naloxone

Recently, concentrated intranasal (IN) naloxone has been developed as an alternative to IM naloxone.[5] Alternatives to injectable naloxone have been developed for THN because laypersons or bystanders may have difficulty administering injections because of fear or lack of knowledge of injecting procedures, and because of the risk of needle stick injury.[6]

The peak plasma concentration (C_{max}) of 1mg, 2mg and 4mg IN naloxone exceeds that of 400 μg IM naloxone[7] but time to attainment of peak concentrations (T_{max}) is delayed relative to IM administration (15–30 minutes vs 10 minutes). With respect to time to onset of action, 2mg IN is equivalent to 400 μg IM. IN administration results in more persistent naloxone plasma levels than IM or IV routes.[7]

Opioid substitution treatment (OST)

The mainstay of pharmacological management of opioid dependence is OST. OST can be prescribed for detoxification, that is, at a dose to control withdrawal symptoms followed by progressive reduction and discontinuation. Alternatively, OST can be

CHAPTER 4

prescribed as 'maintenance', which refers to a longer period of months to years on a stable dose of OST.

The goals of OST are as follows:

- To reduce or prevent withdrawal symptoms
- To reduce or eliminate non-prescribed drug use
- To stabilise drug intake and lifestyle
- To reduce drug-related harm (particularly injecting behaviour)
- To engage and provide an opportunity to work with the patient

Treatment will depend upon:

- what pharmacotherapies and/or other interventions are available
- patient's previous history of drug use and treatment
- patient's current drug use and circumstances
- location/service where treatment is initiated.

Most OST prescribing for people with mental health problems should be initiated by specialist addiction services, although they should continue to receive appropriate psychiatric care from mental health services.[8] Some people with co-morbid opioid dependence and mental health problems will be admitted to psychiatric inpatient wards and general psychiatrists will need to take over, or initiate prescribing in the immediate term[1] (see dedicated section later).

Clinicians should take care to ensure that patients are physiologically dependent on opioids before initiating OST, e.g. clinical evidence of opioid withdrawal, positive urine drug screens and documented ongoing OST.

Assessment should involve the following:

- What opioids the person is taking
- What other drugs are used, including alcohol and other depressants
- Frequency, quantity and route of administration of all substances used
- Time of last use
- Medical co-morbidity that may affect prescribing decisions, e.g. COPD
- Prescribed medication, which can interact with OST – respiratory depressants, those that prolong QT
- Previous experience of treatment
- Previous overdoses
- Whether they have Take Home Naloxone
- Whether there are objective signs of opioid withdrawal using a validated scale such as Objective Opiate Withdrawal Scale (OOWS) or Clinical Opiate Withdrawal Scale (COWS); see Table 4.8
- Examination of injection sites
- Collateral information from addiction services and pharmacy with respect to usual dose of OST and most recently dispensed dose

Untreated heroin withdrawal symptoms typically begin after 4–6 hours and reach their peak 32–72 hours after the last dose. Symptoms will have subsided substantially after 5 days. Untreated methadone withdrawal typically reaches its peak between 4 and 6 days after the last dose and symptoms do not subside for 10–12 days. Untreated

Table 4.8 Clinical Opiate Withdrawal Scale (COWS)

Resting pulse rate: _____beats/minute
Measured after patient is sitting or lying for 1
minute:
0 – pulse rate 80 or below
1 – pulse rate 81–100
2 – pulse rate 101–120
4 – pulse rate greater than 120

GI upset – *over last 1/2 hour*:
0 – no GI symptoms
1 – stomach cramps
2 – nausea or loose stool
3 – vomiting or diarrhoea
5 – multiple episodes of diarrhoea or vomiting

Sweating – *Over past 1/2 hour not accounted for*
by room temperature or patient activity:
0 – no report of chills or flushing
1 – subjective report of chills or flushing
2 – flushed or observable moistness on face
3 – beads of sweat on brow or face
4 – sweat streaming off face

Tremor – *Observation of outstretched hands*:
0 – no tremor
1 – tremor can be felt, but not observed
2 – slight tremor observable
4 – gross tremor or muscle twitching

Restlessness – *Observation during assessment*:
0 – able to sit still
1 – reports difficulty sitting still, but is able to do so
3 – frequent shifting or extraneous movements of
legs/arms
5 – unable to sit still for more than a few seconds

Yawning – *Observation during assessment*:
0 – no yawning
1 – yawning once or twice during assessment
2 – yawning 3 or more times during assessment
4 – yawning several times/minute

Pupil size:
0 – pupils pinned or normal size for room light
1 – pupils possibly larger than normal for room light
2 – pupils moderately dilated
5 – pupils so dilated that only the rim of the iris is
visible

Anxiety or irritability:
0 – none
1 – patient reports increasing irritability or anxiousness
2 – patient is obviously irritable or anxious
4 – patient is so irritable or anxious that participation in the
assessment is difficult

Bone or joint aches – *If patient was having pain*
previously, only the additional component attributed
to opiates withdrawal is scored:
0 – not present
1 – mild diffuse discomfort
2 – patient reports severe diffuse aching of joints/
muscles
4 – patient is rubbing joints or muscles and is unable
to sit still because of discomfort

Gooseflesh skin:
0 – skin is smooth
3 – piloerection of skin can be felt or hairs standing up on
arms
5 – prominent piloerection

Runny nose or tearing – *Not accounted for by*
cold – symptoms or allergies:
0 – not present
1 – nasal stuffiness or unusually moist eyes
2 – nose running or tearing
4 – nose constantly running or tears streaming
down cheeks

Total score_____
(The total score is the sum of all 11 items)

GI, gastrointestinal.
Score: 5–12 = mild; 13–24 = moderate; 25–36 = moderately severe; more than 36 = severe withdrawal.

CHAPTER 4

buprenorphine withdrawal typically lasts for up to 10 days. Specific opioid withdrawal scales are available, e.g. the COWS[9] or OOWS[10] which can be used to help assess levels of dependence and withdrawal.

Prescribing OST safely

- Use licensed medications for heroin dependence treatment (methadone and buprenorphine).
- Ensure that the patient is dependent on opioids.
- Give a safe initial dose (see further) and titrate cautiously.
- Use daily supervised consumption for the first few months of treatment or until stability is achieved (stability = abstinence from illicit opioids).
- Minimise take-away doses for first few months of treatment or until stability is achieved.

Induction and stabilisation of OST maintenance medication

Methadone and buprenorphine are the OST medications recommended by NICE for maintenance substitute prescribing. Both methadone and buprenorphine maintenance are effective in treating withdrawal symptoms and decreasing use of illicit opioids.[11] Recent guidelines and systematic reviews find that there is no evidence to support one over the other.[1] The pharmacology of methadone and buprenorphine differs. Methadone is a full agonist at μ-opioid receptors while buprenorphine is a partial agonist. This difference in pharmacology affords advantages and disadvantages of each drug tabulated in Table 4.9. The decision which to use is an individualised one based on the client's preference; their past experience of either; polysubstance use (especially co-morbid benzodiazepine or alcohol dependence); risk of diversion (medication not being taken by the person it was prescribed for and being sold/given to others); their long-term plans (including a preference for one or other as a detoxification regimen); and, in the case of buprenorphine, their ability to refrain from heroin use for long enough to avoid precipitated opioid withdrawal symptoms. Retention in treatment appears to be more easily achievable with methadone than buprenorphine, at least at low dose.[7]

The patient's physical health is also a significant factor to consider here; for example, there is some evidence to support that buprenorphine is less likely to cause respiratory depression than methadone for healthy opioid using patients.[12] Around a third of patients in drug services have spirometry consistent with COPD.[13] However, there is no published evidence that buprenorphine is better tolerated in this group.

In rare cases, patients may be allergic to methadone or buprenorphine or to some of the constituents within the formulations.

Methadone

Clinical effectiveness

Methadone is a long-acting opioid agonist. It has been shown to be an effective maintenance treatment of heroin dependence by retaining patients in treatment and decreasing

Table 4.9 Choosing between buprenorphine and methadone

	Methadone	Buprenorphine
Withdrawal syndrome	Appears to be more marked and prolonged – best for maintenance programmes	Appears to have a milder withdrawal syndrome than methadone and therefore may be preferred for detoxification programs[14,15]
Differences in initiation	Associated with increased mortality during the titration phase Need for gradual titration over a few weeks to reach therapeutic range (60–100mg/day)	Not associated with increased mortality during titration. Able to reach therapeutic dose (12–16mg od) over a few days Risk of precipitated withdrawal if patients are not already in withdrawal
Differences in retention	Methadone associated with greater retention in treatment than low-dose buprenorphine (<7mg)	Buprenorphine associated with greater drop-out from treatment only if prescribed at low and flexible doses (<7mg)[11]
Differences in adverse effects	Methadone may be associated with QTc prolongation and torsade de pointes which is a particular concern in patients prescribed QT lengthening antipsychotics or those with co-morbid cocaine use	Buprenorphine is often perceived as less sedating than methadone, which can be seen as undesirable by patients[1]
Chronic pain	Patients with chronic pain conditions that require additional opioid analgesia may have difficulties being treated with buprenorphine because of the 'blockade' effect although in practice this does not appear to be a major problem	Buprenorphine appears to provide greater 'blockade' effects than doses of methadone <60mg.[16–18] If a patient on buprenorphine requires treatment for acute pain, an additional opioid may be titrated against response[19]
Combining with other medications	Methadone plasma levels may alter with drugs that inhibit/induce CYP3A4 such as erythromycin, several SSRIs, ribavirin and some antiseizure medications and HIV medications. This may make dose assessment difficult, if a person is not consistent in their use of these CYP3A4-inhibiting/inducing drugs	Buprenorphine is less affected by drug interactions, and may be preferable for some patients
Pregnancy	Widely used in pregnancy	Buprenorphine is associated with less severe neonatal withdrawal symptoms.[20] However, buprenorphine should not be initiated in pregnancy or switched to from methadone because of the risk of inducing withdrawal in the foetus
Diversion	Patients at greater risk of diversion of medication (e.g. past history of this; treatment in a prison setting) may be better served with methadone treatment	Sublingual buprenorphine tablets can be more easily diverted with the risk of tablets being injected Available in combination with naloxone (Suboxone), which may prevent diversion for injection
Logistics		If daily supervised consumption is not feasible, buprenorphine may be preferable[1]

od, omni die (once a day).

CHAPTER 4

heroin use more than non-opioid-based replacement therapy.[11] Higher doses of methadone (60–100mg/day) are recommended in the DoH guidelines as they have been shown to be more effective than lower dosages in retaining patients in treatment and in reducing illicit heroin and cocaine use. According to the emerging small-scale open-label research, methadone is of equal efficacy to buprenorphine in reducing prescription opioid abuse in prescription opioid dependence and retaining people in treatment.[21] Methadone is also associated with a reduction in drug-taking behaviours related to HIV transmission. The 2017 POATS ($n = 653$) in the US found that buprenorphine–naloxone combination was an effective treatment of prescription opioid dependence, when this was prescribed as a maintenance (i.e. ongoing) rather than tapering prescription.[22]

Prescribing information: Methadone and buprenorphine are Controlled Drugs with high dependency potential. Methadone in particular has a low lethal dose. For these reasons, there are special documentation requirements, including specifying the patient's name, date of birth and address on prescriptions and writing the daily dose amount and total amount prescribed in both numbers and words. Instructions such as the requirement for consumption to be supervised should also be specified, e.g. 'Daily Supervised Consumption'.

Supervised daily consumption is recommended for new prescriptions, for a minimum of several months.[1] If this is not possible, instalment prescriptions for daily dispensing and collection should be used. No more than 1 week's supply should be dispensed at one time, except in exceptional circumstances.[1] During the COVID pandemic, a decision was taken by Public Health England that the risk of social contact during directly supervised consumption exceeded the risk of diversion and overdose so dispensing regimes were relaxed in most cases. It is currently unclear what the consequences of this change in practice have been and whether this change will persist or revert to old dispensing arrangements.

Methadone should only be prescribed as a 1mg in 1mL oral solution.[1] The patient's address and date of birth should be on the form, the amount prescribed per day and total prescribed written in figures and words. Directions for supervision should be written clearly. Tablets can be crushed and injected and therefore should not usually be prescribed.[1,23]

Important: All patients starting a methadone treatment programme must be informed of the risks of toxicity and overdose, and the necessity for safe storage of any take home medication.[1,24–26] Safe storage is vital, particularly if there are children in the household, as tragic deaths have occurred when children have ingested methadone. Prescribers should consider risks to children in all assessments and treatment plans of drug using patients.

In determining the **starting dose** for patients using heroin or other opioids not already on a prescription for methadone, consideration must be given to the potential for opioid toxicity, taking into account:

- Tolerance to opioids can be affected by a number of factors and significantly influences an individual's risk of toxicity.[27] Of particular importance in assessing this are the client's reported current quantity, frequency and route of administration, whilst being wary of possible over-reporting. A person's tolerance to methadone can be significantly reduced within 3–4 days of not using opioids, so caution must be exercised after this time, with careful re-titration from a starting dose.

- Use of other central nervous system depressant drugs, e.g. alcohol, benzodiazepines and psychiatric medications such as pregabalin, increases risks of toxicity.
- Age - risk of drug-related death is increased by a factor of 2.9 in patients over 45.[28]
- Co-morbid physical health problems, e.g. COPD, result in low baseline oxygen saturation.
- Long half-life of methadone, as cumulative toxicity, may develop over the course of 3–10 days.[29,30] For this reason, a patient should be reviewed regularly for signs of intoxication and the dose must be omitted if there is any sign of drowsiness or other evidence of toxicity.
- Inappropriate dosing can result in fatal overdose, particularly in the first few days.[24,25,31,32] Deaths have occurred following the commencement of a daily dose of less than 30mg methadone.[1]

It is safer to start with a low dose that can subsequently be increased at intervals if this dose later proves to be insufficient. Direct conversion tables for opioids and methadone should be viewed cautiously, as there are a number of factors influencing the values at any given time, e.g. changes in quality of street heroin. It is much safer to titrate the dose against presenting withdrawal symptoms.

The **initial total** daily dose for most cases will be in the range of **10–30mg** methadone depending on the level of tolerance.[1,33] If this level is uncertain, 10–20mg is recommended. In an acute medical or psychiatric ward, starting doses of up to 20mg daily are usually recommended, as patients in these settings are likely to be physically unwell in the former, or being treated with various other psychoactive drugs in the latter case.

Note: The onset of action should be evident within half an hour, with peak plasma levels being achieved after approximately 2–4 hours of dosing.

Methadone induction and stabilisation in the community

This applies to patients who have not been on a prescription in the previous 3 days (including those who have been on OST and not picked up their prescription for 3 days). The initial 2 weeks of treatment with methadone are associated with a substantially increased risk of overdose mortality.[1,23,34–36] It is important that appropriate assessment, titration of doses and monitoring are performed during this period. Induction is usually undertaken in specialist services by those with appropriate competencies and after a full assessment with urine toxicology and clear evidence of opioid use and withdrawal.

- **First week**

Outpatients should attend up to 3 times per week to enable assessment by the prescriber and any dose titration against withdrawal symptoms. Dose increases should not exceed 5–10mg on each occasion and not usually more than 30mg in the first week above the initial starting dose.[33] Note that steady-state plasma levels are only achieved approximately 5 days after the last dose increase. Once the patient has been stabilised on an adequate dose, methadone should be prescribed as a single regular daily dose. It should not be prescribed on a 'when necessary' basis or at variable dosage. It is good practice to supervise consumption for the first few months.

▪ Subsequent period

Subsequent increases of 5–10mg methadone can continue after the first week, but there should be at least a week between each successive increase.[1] It may take several weeks to reach the therapeutic daily dose of 60–120mg.[1] Stabilisation is usually achieved within 6 weeks but may take longer. However, it is important to consider that some patients may require more rapid stabilisation. This would need to be balanced by a high level of supervision and observation, thereby allowing the ability to increase doses more rapidly. A therapeutic dose is one that eliminates opioid withdrawal symptoms and is effective in stopping on top of use of heroin, without excess sedation.[37] Prescribers should take into account factors that may influence the choice of methadone dose, e.g. co-morbid cocaine use, as cocaine decreases methadone levels, and increased age as lower methadone doses appear to be associated with overdose risk in the population aged >45.[28]

Methadone cautions

▪ Intoxication

Methadone should not be given to any patient showing signs of intoxication, especially due to alcohol or other depressant drugs (e.g. benzodiazepines).[27,38] Risk of fatal overdose is greatly enhanced when methadone is taken concomitantly with alcohol and other respiratory depressant drugs, including benzodiazepines and pregabalin, which can increase the risk of overdose.[39,40] Concurrent alcohol and both prescribed and illicit drug consumption must be borne in mind when considering subsequent prescribing of methadone due to the increased risk of overdose associated with polysubstance misuse.[25,31,38,41]

▪ Severe hepatic/renal dysfunction

Metabolism and elimination of methadone may be affected in which case the dose or dosing interval should be adjusted accordingly against clinical presentation. Because of extended plasma half-life, the interval between assessments during initial dosing may need to be extended.

Methadone overdose

In the event of methadone overdose, **naloxone** should be administered as described in the section 'Opioid overdose'.

Methadone and risk of torsades de pointes/QT interval prolongation

Methadone, either alone or combined with other QT prolonging agents, may increase the likelihood of QT interval prolongation on the electrocardiogram, which is associated with torsades de pointes and can be fatal.[42–44]

Recommended ECG monitoring

In 2006, the MHRA recommended that patients with the following risk factors for QT interval prolongation are carefully monitored whilst taking methadone: heart or liver disease, electrolyte abnormalities, concomitant treatment with CYP3A4 inhibitors, or medicines with the potential to cause QT interval prolongation (e.g. some antipsychotics and erythromycin). Cocaine and synthetic cannabinoid receptor agonists (SCRAs), or 'Spice', may lengthen QT, so patients who also take cocaine or Spice should be monitored.[45,46] In addition, any patient requiring more than 100mg of methadone per day should be closely monitored[47] as the risk of QTc prolongation is dose related.[42] Other patient factors increasing the risk of QT prolongation include co-morbid eating disorder, history of heart disease or stroke, liver disease, metabolic derangements such as hypokalaemia, hypocalcaemia and HIV-positive status (irrespective of medications).[48]

Thus, in individuals with the risk factors listed earlier should have a baseline ECG and subsequent ECG monitoring. The timeframe for the latter is not yet subject to a rigorous evidence base; annual checks in the absence of cardiac symptomatology would be a reasonable minimum frequency. It is also important to check the actions of any medications being prescribed with methadone for CYP3A4 inhibitory activity, to inform the risk–benefit analysis when commencing methadone.[49] Buprenorphine appears to be associated with less QTc prolongation and therefore maybe a safer alternative in this respect,[50] although there are few studies in this area at present; and there are many other factors to take into account when choosing an appropriate opioid substitute.

Brief guidelines as to actions to take are documented in Table 4.10. Always seek specialist advice where there is any suspicion of prolongation of the QT interval. A review of ECG monitoring suggests that there is insufficient evidence for the efficacy of QTc screening strategies for preventing cardiac morbidity and mortality in methadone-maintained patients and there is concern that in some settings the procedures involved may be enough to deter patients from entering or staying in a methadone programme.[51] Patients on or about to start methadone in inpatient settings of both medical and psychiatric wards should always have an ECG. Patients on high doses or with other risk factors should, if possible, have ECGs, when treated in the community, although consideration should be taken of the risks and benefits if a community patient refuses to attend for ECG monitoring.

Buprenorphine

Buprenorphine (marketed as Subutex in most countries) is a synthetic partial opioid agonist with low intrinsic activity and high affinity at µ-opioid receptors. This means that it produces less euphoria even at receptor-saturating doses and simultaneously blocks the action of other opioids. It is an effective treatment for heroin addiction if prescribed at fixed doses, although not more effective than methadone at adequate dosages.[11] It is associated with lower likelihood retention in treatment than methadone, and clinical experience with buprenorphine suggests that it can be difficult to initiate because of the balancing act required to attain sufficient withdrawal to start, but in not so much withdrawal that prevents attendance at the treatment centre. It has also been found to be effective in reducing prescription opioid use and improving treatment

CHAPTER 4

Table 4.10 Recommended ECG monitoring

	Borderline prolonged QTc	Action	Prolonged QTc	Action	Very prolonged QTc	Action
Females	≥470ms	▪ Repeat ECG ▪ Electrolytes ▪ Try to modify QT risk factors, e.g. cocaine use, spice use, methadone dose, psychotropic medications ▪ Regular ECG until normal	≥500 ms	▪ Repeat ECG ▪ Electrolytes ▪ Try to modify QT risk factors ▪ Seek cardiology and addiction specialist advice ▪ Reduce methadone dose ▪ If persistent QTc despite reduction, plan switch to buprenorphine ▪ Regular ECGs until normal	≥550 ms	▪ Urgent cardiology and addiction specialist advice ▪ Repeat ECG ▪ Electrolytes ▪ Try to modify QT risk factors ▪ Reduce methadone and re-evaluate within the week. Plan switch to buprenorphine in inpatient setting
Males	≥440ms					

adherence in prescription opioid-dependent patients.[21] There is no significant difference between buprenorphine and methadone in terms of completion of detoxification treatment, but withdrawal symptoms may resolve more quickly with buprenorphine.[52]

Sublingual buprenorphine

The most commonly prescribed form of buprenorphine is absorbed via the sublingual route. Each tablet takes approximately 5–10 minutes to disintegrate and be absorbed. It is effective in treating opioid dependence because:

▪ It alleviates/prevents opioid withdrawal and craving.
▪ It reduces the effects of additional opioid use because of its high receptor affinity – what patients refer to as a 'blocking' effect.[16–18]
▪ It is long-acting allowing daily (or less frequent) dosing. The duration of action is related to the buprenorphine dose administered: low doses (e.g. 2mg) exert effects for up to 12 hours; higher doses (e.g. 16–32mg) exert effects for as long as 48–72 hours, allowing thrice weekly dosing.

Prolonged-release buprenorphine injection

A prolonged-release subcutaneous buprenorphine injection (trade name 'Buvidal' in the UK and EU, Sublocade and others in the US) is licenced in the UK in weekly and monthly injectable form (Table 4.11). Certain patients may have a preference for and/ or benefit from a weekly or monthly depot, for example, those with work or study

Table 4.11 Conventional sublingual buprenorphine daily treatment doses and recommended corresponding doses of weekly and monthly Buvidal®

Dose of daily sublingual buprenorphine	Dose of weekly Buvidal®	Dose of monthly Buvidal®
2–6mg	8mg	32mg
8–10mg	16mg	64mg
12–16mg	24mg	96mg
18–24mg	32mg	128mg

commitments, those who need to travel regularly (making daily medications pick-up difficult) and those struggling to adhere to a daily medication regime.

Prolonged-release buprenorphine injection offers the same benefits as sublingual buprenorphine, i.e. suppression of withdrawal symptoms and craving, alongside opioid blockade of additional opiates are taken. It has a sustained release and some patients find that it reduces the noticeable peaks and troughs experienced on sublingual buprenorphine. In turn, this may reduce 'on-top' use of opioids. Contraindications to prolonged-release buprenorphine injection are hypersensitivity or allergy to active substance or excipients, severe hepatic impairment, alcohol dependence and delirium tremens.

Different brands of oral buprenorphine and bioavailability

Espranor is a brand of buprenorphine which is increasingly used in the UK community addiction services. Espranor is placed on the tongue, not under it. The pharmacokinetics of buprenorphine show quite wide interindividual variation[53] and to some extent the variability in PK is accommodated by titrating people slowly against their personal therapeutic response. However, for conversion from buprenorphine or other brands of buprenorphine to Espranor, the following conversion table has been developed, based on clinical experience:

Buprenorphine sublingual	Espranor orodispersible
8mg	6mg
10mg	8mg
12mg	10mg
14/16mg	12mg
18mg	14mg
20/22mg	16mg
>26mg	18mg

Given the uncertainty regarding dose equivalence, it is prudent not to switch between brands without good cause.

Buprenorphine starting dose

The same principles as for methadone apply when starting treatment with buprenorphine. Doctors operating outside drug services should be aware that buprenorphine does not show up in standard multiple urine drug testing kits in the way that methadone, codeine or heroin do. It is commonly tested for using a separate UDS kit which is not usually available outside addiction services. Thus, to confirm use in a timely fashion, confirmation with pharmacy regarding observed consumption and potentially specific laboratory testing of a urine sample should be considered. However, of particular interest with buprenorphine is the phenomenon of *precipitated withdrawal*. Precipitated withdrawal occurs because buprenorphine is a partial agonist with a high receptor affinity. If it enters the brain when a full agonist, e.g. methadone or heroin, is still present, it competes for binding at the opioid receptors and replaces the full agonist. Therefore, some receptors that were previously fully stimulated become partially stimulated. The patient experiences this change as opioid withdrawal. If, however, the patient is already in withdrawal, they will experience the addition of a partial agonist that stimulates the receptors to a limited extent as relief of that withdrawal. Patient education is an important factor in reducing the problems during induction.

The first dose of buprenorphine should be administered when the patient is experiencing opioid withdrawal symptoms (a sign that agonist activity is decreasing) so as to reduce the risk of precipitated withdrawal. As with methadone, clear evidence of daily opioid use (including drug testing) and withdrawal symptoms is mandatory before commencing a prescription for buprenorphine.

The initial dose recommendations are as follows:

Patient in withdrawal and no risk factors	8mg buprenorphine
Patient not experiencing withdrawal and no risk factors	4mg buprenorphine
Patient has concomitant risk factors (e.g. medical condition, polydrug misuse, low or uncertain severity of dependence, on other psychiatric medications)	2–4mg buprenorphine

No more than 8mg buprenorphine should be given on the first day in a non-specialist setting. In some cases 8mg may be sufficient, but this may be increased to 12–16mg the following day if there is continuing evidence of withdrawal and no evidence of intoxication. The doses can be given in divided doses so that it can be reviewed promptly in the event of any intoxication, although in practice this is difficult in the absence of on-site dispensing. For maintenance, the 'Orange Guidelines'[1] recommend a dose between 12mg and 24mg a day. If there is concern that doses higher than 16mg may be required, specialist advice should be sought and the dose only increased under advice from addiction specialists.

If patients are on other respiratory sedatives such as benzodiazepines, the lower doses should be used and be monitored for intoxication and respiratory depression.

Transferring from methadone to buprenorphine

This should usually be under the supervision of a suitably experienced specialist pre-scriber. Patients transferring from methadone are at risk of experiencing precipitated withdrawal symptoms that may continue at a milder level for 1–2 weeks. Factors affect-ing precipitated withdrawal are listed in Table 4.12.

Table 4.12 Factors affecting risk of precipitated withdrawal with methadone to buprenorphine switch

Factor	Discussion	Recommended strategy
Dose of methadone	More likely with doses of methadone above 30mg. Generally, the higher the dose the more severe the precipitated withdrawal[54]	Attempt to transfer from doses of methadone <40mg (preferably ≤30mg). Transfer from >60mg should not be attempted
Time between last methadone dose and first buprenorphine dose	Interval should be at least 24 hours. Increasing the interval reduces the incidence and severity of withdrawal[55,56]	Cease methadone and delay first dose until patient is experiencing withdrawal from methadone
Dose of buprenorphine	Very low doses of buprenorphine (e.g. 2mg) are generally inadequate to substitute for methadone. High first doses of buprenorphine (e.g. 8mg) are more likely to precipitate withdrawal	First dose should generally be 4mg; review patient 2–3 hours later
Patient expectancy	Patients not prepared for precipitated withdrawal are more likely to become distressed and confused by the effect	Inform patients in advance. Have contingency plan for severe symptoms
Use of other medications	Symptomatic medication (e.g. lofexidine) can be useful to relieve symptoms	Prescribe in accordance to management plan

CHAPTER 4

Transferring from methadone dose <40mg (ideally ≤30mg) to buprenorphine

Methadone should be ceased abruptly, and the first dose of buprenorphine given at least 24 hours after the last methadone dose. The following conversion rates at the start of treatment are recommended but higher doses may be subsequently needed depend-ing on the clinical presentation:

Last methadone dose	Day 1: initial buprenorphine dose	Day 2: buprenorphine dose
20–40mg	4mg	6–8mg
10–20mg	4mg	4–8mg
1–10mg	2mg	2–4mg

Transferring from methadone 40–60mg dose to buprenorphine

- The methadone dose should be reduced as far as possible without the patient becoming unstable or chaotic, and then abruptly stopped.
- The first buprenorphine dose should be delayed until the patient displays clear signs of withdrawal, generally 48–96 hours after the last dose of methadone.
- An initial dose of 2–4mg should be given. The patient should then be reviewed 2–3 hours later.
- If withdrawal has been precipitated, further symptomatic medication can be prescribed.
- If there has been no precipitation or worsening of withdrawal, an additional 2–4mg of buprenorphine can be dispensed on the same day.
- The patient should be reviewed the following day at which point the dose should be increased to between 8mg and 12mg.

Transferring to buprenorphine from methadone doses >60mg

Such transfers should not be attempted in an outpatient setting except in exceptional circumstances by an experienced practitioner. Usually patients would be partially detoxified from methadone and transferred to buprenorphine when the methadone was at or below 30mg daily. However, if transfer from higher dose methadone to buprenorphine is required, a referral to a dedicated addiction's inpatient unit should be considered where possible.

Transferring from other prescribed opioids to buprenorphine

Evidence is accruing in the treatment of prescribed opioid dependence with buprenorphine and it has been found to improve adherence to drug treatment and reduce prescription opioid abuse.[21] In the UK, the Orange Guidelines recommend small divided doses given to establish the dose required for stabilisation.[1]

Starting buprenorphine from patient-controlled analgesia

Patient-controlled analgesia (PCA) is commonly used for management of severe acute pain. Patients can receive opioids (e.g. morphine or fentanyl) intravenously on demand, within predetermined limits.[57]

For patients who had been prescribed buprenorphine before being on a PCA, it is recommended that sublingual buprenorphine 0.4mg, **four times a day** be prescribed while the patient is still on their PCA as opioid substitution treatment initiation. Staggered dosing of buprenorphine is important to avoid the usual peak concentration, which would increase the risk of precipitated withdrawal.

On the first day when the PCA is no longer required (day 1 in Table 4.13), buprenorphine can be increased to 2mg sublingually, twice daily. The following day, the dose can be increased to 4mg, twice daily. By day 3, buprenorphine can be administered once daily at 8mg. **Dose adjustments may be necessary if withdrawal symptoms worsen**

Table 4.13 Patient-controlled analgesia to restarting*

Day	Patient on PCA?	Sublingual buprenorphine dose	Frequency
0	Yes	0.4mg	Four times a day
1	No	1mg	Twice daily
2	No	2mg	Twice daily
3	No	4mg	Once daily

*NB: Dose adjustments may be necessary if withdrawal symptoms worsen immediately following buprenorphine.

immediately following buprenorphine. In this case, do NOT give further buprenorphine and contact specialist addiction services for advice.

Stabilisation dose of buprenorphine

Outpatients should attend regularly for the first few days to enable assessment by the prescriber and any dose titration. Dose increases should be made in increments of 2–4mg at a time, daily if necessary, up to a maximum daily dose of 32mg. The recommended effective maintenance doses are in the range of 12–16mg daily,[1] and patients should generally be able to achieve maintenance levels within 1–2 weeks of starting buprenorphine – usually more quickly than with methadone.

Buprenorphine less than daily dosing

Buprenorphine is licensed in the UK as a medication to be taken daily. International evidence and experience indicate that many clients can be comfortably maintained on one dose every 2–3 days.[58–61] This may be pertinent for patients in buprenorphine treatment who are considered unsuitable for take-away medication because of the risk of diversion.

The following conversion rate is recommended:

2-day buprenorphine dose = 2 × daily dose of buprenorphine (to a max. 32mg)
3-day buprenorphine dose = 3× daily dose of buprenorphine (to a max. 32mg)

Note: In the event of patients being unable to stabilise comfortably on buprenorphine (often those transferring from methadone), the option of transferring to methadone should be available. Methadone can be commenced 24 hours after the last buprenorphine dose. Doses should be titrated cautiously according to the clinical response, being mindful of the residual 'blockade' effect of buprenorphine which may last for several days, meaning that methadone toxicity can occur in a delayed manner.

CHAPTER 4

Cautions with buprenorphine

- **Liver function:** There is some evidence suggesting that high-dose buprenorphine can cause changes in liver function in individuals with a history of liver disease.[62] Such patients should have LFTs measured before commencing with follow-up investigations conducted 6–12 weeks after commencing buprenorphine. More frequent testing should be considered in patients of particular concern, e.g. severe liver disease. Elevated liver enzymes in the absence of clinically significant liver disease, however, does not necessarily contraindicate treatment with buprenorphine.
- **Intoxication:** Buprenorphine should not be given to any patient showing signs of intoxication, especially due to alcohol or other depressant drugs (e.g. benzodiazepines, sedating antipsychotics and pregabalin[39]). Buprenorphine in combination with other sedative drugs can result in respiratory depression, sedation, coma and death. Concurrent alcohol and illicit drug consumption must be borne in mind when considering subsequent prescribing of buprenorphine due to the increased risk of overdose associated with polysubstance misuse.

Overdose with buprenorphine

Buprenorphine (as a single drug in overdose) is generally regarded as safer than methadone and heroin because it causes less respiratory depression and is less likely to be associated with overdose death.[63] However, in combination with other respiratory depressant drugs, the effects may be harder to manage. Very high doses of naloxone (e.g. 10–15mg) may be needed to reverse buprenorphine effects (although lower doses such as 0.8–2mg may be sufficient).[4] As a consequence, ventilator support is often required in cases where buprenorphine is contributing to respiratory depression (e.g. in polydrug overdose).

Buprenorphine with naloxone (Suboxone)

Consideration may be given by the prescriber to a buprenorphine/naloxone preparation which may reduce the risk of diversion. The different sublingual and parenteral absorption profiles of buprenorphine and naloxone are the key factors: if used sublingually, the naloxone will have negligible effects. However, if the combined preparation is injected, the naloxone will have a substantial effect and will attenuate the effects of buprenorphine in the short term and is also likely to precipitate withdrawal in opioid-dependent individuals on full opioid agonists.[64]

Alternative oral opioid preparations

Oral methadone and buprenorphine should continue to be the mainstay of treatment;[1] other oral options such as slow-release oral morphine (SROM) preparations and dihydrocodeine are not licensed in the UK for the treatment of opiate dependence.[1]

However, a specialised clinician may in very exceptional circumstances prescribe oral dihydrocodeine as maintenance therapy, where clients are unable to tolerate methadone or buprenorphine, or in other exceptional circumstances, taking into account the difficulties associated with its short half-life, supervision requirements and diversion potential.[1]

Slow release oral morphine preparations (SROM) preparations have been shown elsewhere in Europe to be useful as maintenance therapy in those who fail to tolerate methadone, again only for prescribing by specialised clinicians.[1] A review of studies on SROM suggested that there was insufficient evidence to assess the effectiveness of this treatment.[65]

Injectable diamorphine for maintenance prescribing

There is compelling evidence supporting the use of injectable diamorphine maintenance prescribing for treatment of patients who fail to benefit from first-line OST.[66] Contemporary injectable prescribing differs from the earlier practice of prescribing unsupervised injectable opioids in that the patient must:

- attend in person for their prescribed injectable opioid maintenance treatment – daily or more frequently, according to the treatment plan
- inject their dose under the direct supervision of a competent member of staff
- be given no take-away injectable medication.

In the UK, the prescribing doctor must have a licence from the Home Office to prescribe diamorphine for opioid dependence. Oral OST is prescribed for days when supervised injectable treatment is not available if the injectable clinic is not available daily. This treatment differs from 'injecting rooms', that is, safe places with sterile equipment for people who use IV drugs (usually not in treatment) in that it is part of a holistic package of care with adjunctive psychosocial interventions. Although its cost-effectiveness has been demonstrated,[67] its implementation has been limited by high set-up costs.

At present, clients should only be considered for injectable opioid prescribing in combination with psychosocial interventions, as part of a wider package of care. It is an option in cases where the individual has not responded adequately to oral OST, and in an area where it can be supported by the necessary provisions for supervised consumption.[1,68] Patients are generally seen for supervised injection in a specialist facility twice a day. Doctors caring for patients who are admitted to the acute hospital on diamorphine prescription will need to consult their local policies – ordinarily a documented conversation with the prescribing community addiction psychiatrist is sufficient to continue the prescription.

Treatment of opiate dependence on the psychiatric ward

Opiate overdose can occur in hospital settings. All inpatients with a history of opiate dependence should have naloxone prescribed as 'as necessary'.

In the inpatient setting, it is imperative to manage opiate withdrawal in order to allow the patient to remain on the ward and engage in interventions tailored to the reason for their psychiatric admission. The most effective prevention of opiate withdrawal during an acute psychiatric admission is continuation of their existing OST. In order to continue prescribing the same dose of OST, the following needs to be confirmed independently:

- Confirmation from addiction services regarding the prescribed dose.
- Confirmation from the pharmacy where this is dispensed with respect to most recent supervised dose and whether any take-away doses had been given. If the most recent

CHAPTER 4

supervised dose is more than 3 days ago, the patient will need to have their OST re-initiated to avoid overdose (see section regarding 'Initiation of treatment'). Patients admitted at weekends may have take-away doses and may not necessarily disclose these if they are not directly asked about them. If more than 3 days have passed since the patient's last dose of OST, they will have lost tolerance and will need to be re-initiated according to the advice of an addictions clinician.

Continuation at the reported dose of OST should only take place if the above information is confirmed and:

- The patient appears alert and comfortable on this dose.
- The patient does not appear to be intoxicated with other substances.

> IF THERE IS ANY DOUBT OR CONCERN REGARDING ANY FACTORS LISTED EARLIER, OST SHOULD NOT BE PRESCRIBED.

Junior doctors may find themselves looking after a patient in opioid withdrawal in circumstances where it is not immediately possible to establish all the above information and so safely prescribe OST. Opioid withdrawal, while not fatal, is highly aversive and carries risks if it is associated with a patient self-discharging when in need of inpatient care. Other medications can be helpful in managing opioid withdrawal until such help can be sought, though there is little place for them once OST is prescribed and their use during OST induction is discouraged because of the risks associated with polypharmacy and polysubstance use. The following are recommended by the current UK clinical guidelines for the treatment of drug dependence to target specific symptoms (Table 4.14):[1]

Table 4.14 Treatment of drug dependence to target specific symptoms (adapted from 'Drug misuse and dependence: UK guidelines for clinical management' 2017[1])

Symptom	Treatment
Diarrhoea	Loperamide 4mg then 2mg after each loose stool; maximum 16mg daily for up to 5 days
Nausea and vomiting	Metoclopramide 10mg tds for a maximum of 5 days or prochlorperazine 5mg tds or 12.5mg IM bd
Abdominal cramps	Mebeverine 135mg tds
Agitation, anxiety and insomnia	Diazepam up to 5–10mg tds when required or zopiclone 7.5mg nocte for patients with a history of benzodiazepine dependence
Muscular pains and headaches	Paracetamol, aspirin or non-steroidal anti-inflammatories. Topical rubefacients can be helpful in relieving muscle aches from methadone withdrawal

bd, bis die (twice a day); tds, ter die sumendum (three times a day).

Patients admitted for emergency psychiatric treatment should not be detoxified from their OST, and consideration should be given to the initiation of OST in opiate-dependent patients who are not yet in treatment (with the advice of local addiction specialists).

Methadone initiation on an acute ward (or by non-specialist in non-addiction setting)

Induction – day 1

The person must be exhibiting objective opioid withdrawal symptoms, as assessed on an opioid withdrawal scale such as COWS (see Table 4.3):

- Give a dose of 10mg of methadone mixture 1mg/1mL based on the severity of withdrawal. This should be given as a once only dose. Methadone will start to have an effect after 20–30 minutes with peak levels being reached at 4 hours.
- Continue to monitor for signs of withdrawal 4 hourly and give a further dose of 5–10mg as required – also observe for signs of intoxication.
- The initial daily dose (over 24 hours) will not usually be more than 30mg.
- Prescribe naloxone 'as required' in case of overdose. Beware of accumulation – small initial doses gradually become toxic when repeated.

Day 2:

- Prescribe the same dose as the patient required on day 1 as a single dose, or in divided doses.
- Continue to monitor withdrawal symptoms and sedation.

Ongoing prescribing

- Consider increasing the dose further in 5–10mg increments every 3–4 days until full relief of withdrawal symptoms achieved, in consultation with addiction specialists.
- Once stability has been achieved, continue to prescribe the required dose.

In the acute inpatient setting, it is usually advisable for the person to be maintained on a stable dose rather than attempt detoxification.

Swapping from twice-daily dosing to single dosing

Patients are often transferred from acute hospitals to psychiatric care with a split dose of methadone. Split dosing in the community carries with it the risk of diversion so is discouraged apart from in pregnancy. On the day prior to discharge, the dose should be converted to a single dose and sedation and respiratory depression should be monitored, as this tends to occur with the peak methadone concentration.

> All patients leaving the ward should be trained in the use of THN, issued with THN[1] and an appointment made in addiction services to continue prescribing prior to discharge.

Prescribing psychotropic medications in patients with opiate dependence

General psychiatrists often see patients with addictions with a view to treating psychiatric co-morbidity. General guidelines regarding treating co-morbid psychiatric conditions pharmacologically are found in the British Association of Psychopharmacology guidelines for Substance Misuse.[69] In general, prescribers should be cautious about

CHAPTER 4

prescribing medication licensed for co-morbid psychiatric disorders that is sedating, because of the increased risk of respiratory depression, e.g. pregabalin, which is associated with overdose death.[39] Pregabalin and olanzapine also appear to have an abuse liability in the opioid-dependent population.[70,71] Patients with opiate dependence suffer disproportionately from depression – about half of those entering treatment will meet criteria for depression. They may require 20–50% higher doses of methadone than non-depressed patients to stabilise[72] but stabilisation may precipitate remission in a majority of cases.[73] There is limited clinical trial evidence of low-to-moderate quality regarding antidepressant use in opioid dependence which suggests that it is of limited benefit for either mood or drug use.[69,73] Positive studies have largely been those using medication with mixed pharmacology such as tricyclic antidepressants;[74] however, TCAs are not recommended in people with co-morbid substance misuse because of their cardiotoxicity.[75] The recommended approach to treatment of depression based on the evidence includes stabilising the patient on OST first, then if depression persists trying an SSRI because of their relative safety, but considering mixed pharmacology antidepressants as a second line should the patient fail to respond.[74] Sertraline is the drug of choice in methadone-treated patients as it has limited interaction potential.

Opioid detoxification and reduction regimes

Opioid maintenance can be continued for a few weeks to almost indefinitely, depending on the clinical need. Some patients are keen to detoxify after short periods of stability and other patients may decide to detoxify after longer periods on maintenance prescriptions. All detoxification programmes should be part of a care programme. Given the risk of serious fatal overdose after detoxification, services providing such treatment should educate the patient about these risks and supply and train them with naloxone and overdose training for emergency use.

Regarding the length of detoxification, the NICE guidelines state that 'dose reduction can take place over anything from a few days to several months, with a higher initial stabilisation dose taking longer to taper', and indicate that 'up to 3 months is typical for methadone reduction, while buprenorphine reductions are typically carried out over 14 days to a few weeks'.[76] In practice, a detoxification in the community may extend over a longer period, if this facilitates the client's comfort during the process, compliance with the care plan, continued abstinence from illicit use during detoxification and subsequent abstinence following detoxification.

Detoxification in an inpatient setting, the NICE guidelines indicate, may take place over a shorter time than in the community (suggesting 14–21 days for methadone and 7–14 days for buprenorphine) 'as the supportive environment helps a service user to tolerate emerging withdrawal symptoms'.[77] As in the community, a stabilisation on the dose of a substitute opioid is first achieved, followed by gradual dose reduction, with additive medications judiciously prescribed for withdrawal symptoms if and as needed.

Detoxification carries a recognised risk of relapse and indeed fatal overdose. Therefore, if a patient is being detoxified there needs to be adequate aftercare in place, such as a rehabilitation programme and community support. For patients having emergency psychiatric or medical admissions, detoxification is not usually indicated unless with the support of specialist services and aftercare arrangements are in place.

Opioid withdrawal in a community setting

Methadone

Following a period of stabilisation with methadone or a longer period of mainte-nance, the patient and prescriber may agree a reduction programme as part of a care plan to reduce the daily methadone dose. The usual reduction would be by 5–10mg weekly or every 2 weeks although there can be much variation in the reduction and speed of reduction. In the community setting, patient preference is the most impor-tant variable in terms of dose reduction and rate of reduction. The detoxification programme should be reviewed regularly and remain flexible to adjustments and changes, such as relapse to illicit drug use or patient anxieties about speed of reduc-tion. Factors such as an increase in heroin or other drug use or worsening of the patient's physical, psychological or social well-being may warrant a temporary increase, or stabilisation of the dose or a slowing down of the reduction rate. Towards the end of the detoxification, the dose reduction may be slower: 1–2mg/week. Recent studies show that the length of stability on maintenance treatment and prolonged reduction schedules (up to a year) substantially improve the chances of achieving abstinence.[78]

Buprenorphine

The same principles as for methadone apply when planning a buprenorphine detoxifi-cation regime. Dose reduction should be gradual to minimise withdrawal discomfort. Suggested reduction regime:

Daily buprenorphine dose	Reduction rate
Above 16mg	4mg every 1–2 weeks
8–16mg	2–4mg every 1–2 weeks
2–8mg	2mg/week or fortnight
Below 2mg	Reduce by 0.4–0.8mg/week

Opioid withdrawal in a specialist addiction in-patient setting

Methadone

Patients should have a starting dose assessment of methadone, over 48 hours by a spe-cialist inpatient team. The dose may then be reduced following a linear regime over up to 4 weeks.[76]

Buprenorphine

Buprenorphine can be used effectively for short-term inpatient detoxifications follow-ing the same principles as for methadone.

Naltrexone in relapse prevention

Evidence for the effectiveness of naltrexone as a treatment for relapse prevention in opioid misusers has been inconclusive.[79] However, naltrexone has been found by NICE to be a cost-effective treatment strategy in aiding abstinence from opioid misuse for those who prefer an abstinence programme, are fully informed of the potential adverse effects and benefits of treatment, are highly motivated to remain on treatment and have a partner supporting concordance.[80] A naltrexone implant, not currently licensed in the UK, may also have a role to play in reducing opioid use in a motivated population of patients.[81]

Close monitoring is particularly important when naltrexone is initiated because of the higher risk of fatal overdose at this time. Discontinuation of naltrexone may also be associated with an increase in inadvertent overdose from illicit opioids. Thus, supervision of naltrexone administration and careful choice of who has prescribed it (those who are abstinence focused and motivated) is very important. Moreover, people taking naltrexone often experience adverse effects of unease (dysphoria), depression and insomnia, which can lead to relapse to illicit opioid use while on naltrexone treatment, or failure to continue on treatment. The dysphoria may be caused by either withdrawal from illicit drugs or by the naltrexone treatment itself, emphasising the importance of prescribing naltrexone as part of a care programme that includes psychosocial therapy and general support.[80]

Initiating naltrexone

Naltrexone has the propensity to cause a severe withdrawal reaction in patients who are either currently taking opioid drugs or who were previously taking opioid drugs and there has not been a sufficient 'wash-out' period before administering naltrexone.

The minimum recommended interval between stopping the opioid and starting naltrexone depends on the opioid used, duration of use and the amount taken as a last dose. Opioid agonists with long half-lives such as methadone will require a wash-out period of up to 10 days, whereas shorter acting opioids such as heroin, morphine or fentanyl may only require up to 7 days. Experience with buprenorphine indicates that a wash-out period of up to 7 days is sufficient if the final buprenorphine dose is >2mg, and duration of use >2 weeks. In some cases naltrexone may be started within 2–3 days of a patient stopping (e.g. if final buprenorphine dose <2mg and duration of use <2 weeks).

A test dose of naloxone (0.2–0.8mg, which has a much shorter half-life than naltrexone), may be given to the patient as an IM dose prior to starting naltrexone treatment. Any withdrawal symptoms precipitated will be of shorter duration than if precipitated by naltrexone.

Patients *must* be advised of the risk of withdrawal before giving the dose. It is worth thoroughly questioning the patient as to whether they have taken any opioid containing preparation unknowingly (e.g. over-the-counter analgesic).

Important points regarding prescribing naltrexone

- Ensure the client is fully informed of the increased risk of fatal opioid overdose.
- Following detoxification and any period of abstinence, an individual's tolerance to opioids will decrease markedly. At such a time, using opioids puts the individual at greatly increased risk of overdose.
- Discontinuation of naltrexone may also be associated with an increase in inadvertent overdose from illicit opioids, emphasising the need for close monitoring and support of the client at this time.

Dose of naltrexone

An initial dose of 25mg naltrexone should be administered after a suitable opioid-free interval (and naloxone challenge if appropriate). The patient should be monitored for 4 hours after the first dose for symptoms of opioid withdrawal. Symptomatic medication for withdrawal (e.g. lofexidine) should be available for use, if necessary, on the first day of naltrexone dosing (withdrawal symptoms may last up to 4–8 hours). Once the patient has tolerated this low naltrexone dose, subsequent doses can be increased to 50mg daily as a maintenance dose.

Naltrexone is contraindicated in patients with hepatic dysfunction, and LFTs should be monitored during treatment.

Pain control in patients on OST

Analgesia for methadone-prescribed patients

Non-opioid analgesics should be used in preference (e.g. paracetamol, NSAIDs) initially where appropriate. If opioid analgesia (e.g. codeine, dihydrocodeine and morphine) is indicated due to the type and severity of the pain, then this should be titrated accordingly for pain relief in line with usual analgesic protocols.

In the case of patients prescribed **methadone**, if an opioid analgesic is appropriate, a non-methadone opioid may be co-prescribed, i.e. it is not necessary to 'rationalise' the patient's entire opioid requirements to one drug.[82] Titrating the methadone dose to provide analgesia may be appropriate in certain circumstances but this should only be carried out by experienced specialists.

As outlined elsewhere in this chapter, patients taking **buprenorphine** or **naltrexone** may be relatively refractory to opioids prescribed for analgesia, although in practice if a patient on buprenorphine requires treatment for acute pain, an additional opioid may be titrated against response.[19] If naltrexone is stopped to allow for the prescribing of opioid analgesia, careful monitoring will be required because of the increased risk of both relapse and overdose.[35,82]

Patients with a history of substance misuse may also need acute pain management in hospital following surgery, trauma or other illness. The primary objectives during the period of acute pain are to manage the pain and avoid the consequences of withdrawal, so it is important to maintain sufficient background medication to achieve both. Liaison with both the inpatient pain team and the local addictions services, as well as collaborative discussion with the patient, is important. The patient may be known to the addiction services, who will be able to inform the treatment plan, assist in a reliable conversion from street drugs (if these are also being taken) to prescribed analgesics and help plan a smooth transition from acute pain intervention to ongoing management of the patient's substance misuse.[35] Further details can be found in a consensus document by the British Pain Society, Royal College of Psychiatrists, Royal College of GPs and the Advisory Council on the Misuse of Drugs.[82]

As advised in the consensus document, in palliative care, the principles of providing analgesia 'in substance misusers are fundamentally no different from those for other adult patients needing palliative care', although increased liaison with substance misuse services is essential. Those who are opioid dependent may receive maintenance therapy from a substance misuse service 'and this should be regarded as a separate prescription from that for analgesia when attending as a [pain clinic] outpatient', as also described in the context of chronic non-cancer pain above. During admission all medication would usually be received from the inpatient unit, but with 'a clear plan for separate follow-ups for substance misuse and symptom palliation … in place on discharge except during the terminal phase of an illness'.[82] Again, further details can be found in the consensus advice document.[82] Subsequent to the publication of this document, there have been concerns regarding the abuse potential of pregabalin, a non-opioid medication used for chronic pain,[70] and the potential for prescription of pregabalin and opioids to increase the potential for overdose.[39] Caution is advised when prescribing pregabalin for chronic pain.

Pregnancy and opioid use (also see section 'Substance misuse in pregnancy' in this chapter)

> Substitute prescribing can occur at any time in pregnancy and carries a lower risk than continuing illicit use. Treatment should strike a balance between stabilising drug use and minimising the dose of OST in order to prevent neonatal abstinence syndrome (NAS).[1]

Women can present with opioid dependency at any stage in pregnancy, and stabilisation on substitute methadone is the treatment of choice. Detoxification in the first trimester is contraindicated due to the risk of spontaneous abortion and in the third trimester it is associated with preterm delivery, foetal distress and stillbirth. If detoxification is requested, this is most safely achieved in the second trimester but should only be supervised by specialists with the appropriate competencies and with careful monitoring for any evidence of instability. Detoxification should be prescribed in small frequent decrements, e.g. 2–3mg of methadone every 3–5 days.[1] Enforcing detoxification is contraindicated as it is likely to deter some clients from seeking help, and the majority will then return to opioid use at some point during their pregnancy;[83] fluctuating opioid concentrations in the maternal blood from intermittent use of illicit opioids may then lead to foetal withdrawal or overdose.[84,85] Buprenorphine is associated with less severe neonatal withdrawal symptoms.[14] However, buprenorphine should not be initiated in pregnancy or switched to methadone because of the risk of inducing withdrawal in the foetus.

Substitute prescribing during pregnancy

This should take place within a multidisciplinary team (including obstetric team, anaesthetists, neonatologists and addiction specialists) delivering a holistic package of care. The body of evidence informing treatment is small.[86] Currently, methadone and buprenorphine do not seem to differ in terms of safety. Methadone is associated with superior treatment retention and buprenorphine with less severe NAS.[86] The most recent guidelines therefore suggest allowing the patient to choose either or to remain on whichever they are taking when they become pregnant.[1] Suboxone should be avoided in pregnancy. Changing from methadone to buprenorphine is not recommended, however, because of the risk of withdrawal for the foetus. Metabolism of methadone may increase during the third trimester requiring split dosing.

Neonatal abstinence syndrome (NAS)

The majority of neonates born to methadone-maintained others will require treatment for NAS.[83] NAS is characterised by a variety of signs and symptoms relating to the autonomic nervous system, gastrointestinal (GI) tract and respiratory system.[84] Infants may have a high-pitched cry, feed hungrily but ineffectively and be excessively wakeful. Severe NAS is associated with hypertonicity and seizures, but is uncommon. The NAS following methadone treatment usually commences after 48 hours[87] but can be delayed for 7–10 days.[1] In the case of any mother using drugs or in OST, it is important to have access to skilled neonatal paediatric care to monitor the neonate and treat as required. Breastfeeding may reduce the severity of NAS (see below).

It is useful to anticipate potential problems for women prescribed opioids during pregnancy with regard to opioid pain relief: such women should be managed in specialist antenatal clinics due to the increased associated risks. Antenatal assessment by anaesthetists may be recommended with regard to anticipating any anaesthetic risks, any analgesic requirements and problems with venous access.

Breastfeeding

Women prescribed methadone or buprenorphine should be encouraged to breastfeed even if they continue to use illicit opioids[1] for the following reasons:

- General health benefits to the mother and the infant
- Specific benefits in reducing admission length and need for intervention in NAS[88]
- Low concentrations of methadone and buprenorphine transferred to infant[88]

Patients should be warned to discontinue breastfeeding gradually as abrupt cessation can cause a delayed NAS.[88] Patients who take crack cocaine or high doses of benzodiazepines should not breastfeed.[1]

CHAPTER 4

References

1. Department of Health and Social Care. Drug misuse and dependence: UK guidelines on clinical management. 2017; https://www.gov.uk/government/publications/drug-misuse-and-dependence-uk-guidelines-on-clinical-management.

2. Ellis K, et al. Routes to recovery. 2007; http://americanradioworks.publicradio.org/features/nola/transcript.html.

3. World Health Organization. Community management of opioid overdose. 2014; http://www.who.int/substance_abuse/publications/management_opioid_overdose/en.

4. FDA. FDA advisory committee on the most appropriate dose or doses of naloxone to reverse the effects of life-threatening opioid overdose in the community settings. 2016; https://www.fda.gov/downloads/AdvisoryCommittees/CommitteesMeetingMaterials/Drugs/AnestheticAndAnalgesicDrugProductsAdvisoryCommittee/UCM522688.pdf.

5. Strang J, et al. Naloxone without the needle – systematic review of candidate routes for non-injectable naloxone for opioid overdose reversal. *Drug Alcohol Depend* 2016; **163**:16–23.

6. Beletsky L, et al. Prevention of fatal opioid overdose. *JAMA* 2012; **308**:1863–1864.

7. McDonald R, et al. Pharmacokinetics of concentrated naloxone nasal spray for opioid overdose reversal: phase I healthy volunteer study. *Addiction* 2018; **113**:484–493.

8. National Institute for Health and Care Excellence. Coexisting severe mental illness and substance misuse: community health and social care services. NICE Guidance NG58. 2016; https://www.nice.org.uk/guidance/ng58.

9. Wesson DR, et al. The Clinical Opiate Withdrawal Scale (COWS). *J Psychoactive Drugs* 2003; **35**:253–259.

10. Handelsman L, et al. Two new rating scales for opiate withdrawal. *Am J Drug Alcohol Abuse* 1987; **13**:293–308.

11. Mattick RP, et al. Buprenorphine maintenance versus placebo or methadone maintenance for opioid dependence. *Cochrane Database Syst Rev* 2014; **2**:CD002207.

12. Comer SD, et al. Abuse liability of prescription opioids compared to heroin in morphine-maintained heroin abusers. *Neuropsychopharmacology* 2008; **33**:1179–1191.

13. Jolley CJ, et al. P214 The prevalence of respiratory symptoms and lung disease in a South London 'lung health in addictions' service. *Thorax* 2016; **71**:A201.

14. Seifert J, et al. Detoxification of opiate addicts with multiple drug abuse: a comparison of buprenorphine vs. methadone. *Pharmacopsychiatry* 2002; **35**:159–164.

15. Jasinski DR, et al. Human pharmacology and abuse potential of the analgesic buprenorphine: a potential agent for treating narcotic addiction. *Arch Gen Psychiatry* 1978; **35**:501–516.

16. Bickel WK, et al. Buprenorphine: dose-related blockade of opioid challenge effects in opioid dependent humans. *J Pharmacol Exp Ther* 1988; **247**:47–53.

17. Walsh SL, et al. Acute administration of buprenorphine in humans: partial agonist and blockade effects. *J Pharmacol Exp Ther* 1995; **274**:361–372.

18. Comer SD, et al. Buprenorphine sublingual tablets: effects on IV heroin self-administration by humans. *Psychopharmacology* 2001; **154**:28–37.

19. Alford DP, et al. Acute pain management for patients receiving maintenance methadone or buprenorphine therapy. *Ann Intern Med* 2006; **144**:127–134.

20. Jones HE, et al. Neonatal abstinence syndrome after methadone or buprenorphine exposure. *N Engl J Med* 2010; **363**:2320–2331.

21. Nielsen S, et al. Opioid agonist treatment for pharmaceutical opioid dependent people. *Cochrane Database Syst Rev* 2016; Cd011117.

22. Weiss RD, et al. The prescription opioid addiction treatment study: what have we learned. *Drug Alcohol Depend* 2017; **173** Suppl 1:S48–S54.

23. Department of Health Task Force to Review Services for Drug Misusers. Report of an independent review of drug treatment services in England. 1996; http://www.dh.gov.uk.

24. Caplehorn JR. Deaths in the first two weeks of maintenance treatment in NSW in 1994: identifying cases of iatrogenic methadone toxicity. *Drug Alcohol Rev* 1998; **17**:9–17.

25. Zador D, et al. Deaths in methadone maintenance treatment in New South Wales, Australia 1990–1995. *Addiction* 2000; **95**:77–84.

26. Hall W. Reducing the toll of opioid overdose deaths in Australia. *Drug Alcohol Rev* 1999; **18**:213–220.

27. White JM, et al. Mechanisms of fatal opioid overdose. *Addiction* 1999; **94**:961–972.

28. Gao L, et al. Risk-factors for methadone-specific deaths in Scotland's methadone-prescription clients between 2009 and 2013. *Drug Alcohol Depend* 2016; **163**:214–223.

29. Wolff K, et al. The pharmacokinetics of methadone in healthy subjects and opiate users. *Br J Clin Pharmacol* 1997; **44**:325–334.

30. Rostami-Hodjegan A, et al. Population pharmacokinetics of methadone in opiate users: characterization of time-dependent changes. *Br J Clin Pharmacol* 1999; **48**:43–52.

31. Harding-Pink D. Methadone: one person's maintenance dose is another's poison. *Lancet* 1993; **341**:665–666.

32. Drummer OH, et al. Methadone toxicity causing death in ten subjects starting on a methadone maintenance program. *Am J Forensic Med Pathol* 1992; **13**:346–350.

33. National Institute for Clinical Excellence. Methadone and buprenorphine for the management of opioid dependence. Technology Appraisal guidance [TA114]. 2007 (last checked February 2016). https://www.nice.org.uk/guidance/ta114.

34. Amato L, et al. Methadone at tapered doses for the management of opioid withdrawal. *Cochrane Database Syst Rev* 2013; **2**:CD003409.

35. Cornish R, et al. Risk of death during and after opiate substitution treatment in primary care: prospective observational study in UK General Practice Research Database. *BMJ* 2010; **341**:c5475.

36. Strang J, et al. Loss of tolerance and overdose mortality after inpatient opiate detoxification: follow up study. *BMJ* 2003; **326**:959–960.

37. Bell J. Pharmacological maintenance treatments of opiate addiction. *Br J Clin Pharmacol* 2014; **77**:253–263.

38. Farrell M, et al. Suicide and overdose among opiate addicts. *Addiction* 1996; **91**:321–323.

39. Abrahamsson T, et al. Benzodiazepine, z-drug and pregabalin prescriptions and mortality among patients in opioid maintenance treatment-A nation-wide register-based open cohort study. *Drug Alcohol Depend* 2017; **174**:58–64.

40. Pierce M, et al. Impact of treatment for opioid dependence on fatal drug-related poisoning: a national cohort study in England. *Addiction* 2016; **111**:298–308.

41. Neale J. Methadone, methadone treatment and non-fatal overdose. *Drug Alcohol Depend* 2000; **58**:117–124.

42. Krantz MJ, et al. Torsade de pointes associated with very-high-dose methadone. *Ann Intern Med* 2002; **137**:501–504.

43. Kornick CA, et al. QTc interval prolongation associated with intravenous methadone. *Pain* 2003; **105**:499–506.

44. Martell BA, et al. The impact of methadone induction on cardiac conduction in opiate users. *Ann Intern Med* 2003; **139**:154–155.

45. Mayet S, et al. Methadone maintenance, QTc and torsade de pointes: who needs an electrocardiogram and what is the prevalence of QTc prolongation? *Drug Alcohol Rev* 2011; **30**:388–396.

46. Hancox JC, et al. Synthetic cannabinoids and potential cardiac arrhythmia risk: an important message for drug users. *Ther Adv Drug Saf* 2020; **11**:2042098620913416.

47. Medicines and Healthcare Products Regulatory Agency. Risk of QT interval prolongation with methadone. *Curr Prob Pharmacovigilance* 2006; **31**:6.

48. Isbister GK, et al. Drug induced QT prolongation: the measurement and assessment of the QT interval in clinical practice. *Br J Clin Pharmacol* 2013; **76**:48–57.

49. Cruciani RA. Methadone: to ECG or not to ECG ... that is still the question. *J Pain Symptom Manage* 2008; **36**:545–552.

50. Wedam EF, et al. QT-interval effects of methadone, levomethadyl, and buprenorphine in a randomized trial. *Arch Intern Med* 2007; **167**:2469–2475.

51. Pani PP, et al. QTc interval screening for cardiac risk in methadone treatment of opioid dependence. *Cochrane Database Syst Rev* 2013; **6**:CD008939.

52. Gowing L, et al. Buprenorphine for managing opioid withdrawal. *Cochrane Database Syst Rev* 2017; **2**:Cd002025.

53. Strain EC, et al. Relative bioavailability of different buprenorphine formulations under chronic dosing conditions. *Drug Alcohol Depend* 2004; **74**:37–43.

54. Walsh SL, et al. Effects of buprenorphine and methadone in methadone-maintained subjects. *Psychopharmacology* 1995; **119**:268–276.

55. Strain EC, et al. Acute effects of buprenorphine, hydromorphone and naloxone in methadone-maintained volunteers. *J Pharmacol Exp Ther* 1992; **261**:985–993.

56. Strain EC, et al. Buprenorphine effects in methadone-maintained volunteers: effects at two hours after methadone. *J Pharmacol Exp Ther* 1995; **272**:628–638.

57. Grass JA. Patient-controlled analgesia. *Anesth Analg* 2005; **101**:S44–S61.

58. Amass L, et al. Alternate-day buprenorphine dosing is preferred to daily dosing by opioid-dependent humans. *Psychopharmacology* 1998; **136**:217–225.

59. Amass L, et al. Alternate-day dosing during buprenorphine treatment of opioid dependence. *Life Sci* 1994; **54**:1215–1228.

60. Johnson RE, et al. Buprenorphine treatment of opioid dependence: clinical trial of daily versus alternate-day dosing. *Drug Alcohol Depend* 1995; **40**:27–35.

61. Eissenberg T, et al. Controlled opioid withdrawal evaluation during 72 h dose omission in buprenorphine-maintained patients. *Drug Alcohol Depend* 1997; **45**:81–91.

62. Berson A, et al. Hepatitis after intravenous buprenorphine misuse in heroin addicts. *J Hepatol* 2001; **34**:346–350.

63. Paone D, et al. Buprenorphine infrequently found in fatal overdose in New York City. *Drug Alcohol Depend* 2015; **155**:298–301.

64. Stoller KB, et al. Effects of buprenorphine/naloxone in opioid-dependent humans. *Psychopharmacology* 2001; **154**:230–242.

65. Ferri M, et al. Slow-release oral morphine as maintenance therapy for opioid dependence. *Cochrane Database Syst Rev* 2013; **6**:CD009879.

66. Strang J, et al. Heroin on trial: systematic review and meta-analysis of randomised trials of diamorphine-prescribing as treatment for refractory heroin addiction dagger. *Br J Psychiatry* 2015; **207**:5–14.

67. Byford S, et al. Cost-effectiveness of injectable opioid treatment v. oral methadone for chronic heroin addiction. *Br J Psychiatry* 2013; **203**:341–349.

68. Strang J, et al. Supervised injectable heroin or injectable methadone versus optimised oral methadone as treatment for chronic heroin addicts in England after persistent failure in orthodox treatment (RIOTT): a randomised trial. *Lancet* 2010; **375**:1885–1895.

69. Lingford-Hughes AR, et al. Evidence-based guidelines for the pharmacological management of substance abuse, harmful use, addiction and comorbidity: recommendations from BAP. *J Psychopharmacol* 2012; **26**:899–952.

70. Baird CR, et al. Gabapentinoid abuse in order to potentiate the effect of methadone: a survey among substance misusers. *Eur Addict Res* 2014; **20**:115–118.

71. James PD, et al. Non-medical use of olanzapine by people on methadone treatment. *B J Psych Bull* 2016; **40**:314–317.

72. Tenore PL. Psychotherapeutic benefits of opioid agonist therapy. *J Addict Dis* 2008; **27**:49–65.

73. Nunes EV, et al. Treatment of depression in patients with alcohol or other drug dependence: a meta-analysis. *JAMA* 2004; **291**:1887–1896.

74. Nunes EV, et al. Treatment of co-occurring depression and substance dependence: using meta-analysis to guide clinical recommendations. *Psychiatr Ann* 2008; **38**:nihpa128505.

CHAPTER 4

75. Lingford-Hughes AR, et al. BAP updated guidelines: evidence-based guidelines for the pharmacological management of substance abuse, harmful use, addiction and comorbidity: recommendations from BAP. *J Psychopharmacol* 2012; **26**:899–952.

76. National Institute for Clinical Excellence. Drug misuse in over 16s: opioid detoxification. Clinical Guidance 52. 2007; https://www.nice.org.uk/guidance/cg52.

77. National Institute for Clinical Excellence. Drug misuse in over 16s: psychosocial interventions. Clinical Guidance [CG51]. 2007; (last checked July 2016). https://www.nice.org.uk/guidance/cg51.

78. Nosyk B, et al. Defining dosing pattern characteristics of successful tapers following methadone maintenance treatment: results from a population-based retrospective cohort study. *Addiction* 2012; **107**:1621–1629.

79. Minozzi S, et al. Oral naltrexone maintenance treatment for opioid dependence. *Cochrane Database Syst Rev* 2011; **4**:CD001333.

80. National Institute for Clinical Excellence. Naltrexone for the management of opioid dependence. Technology Appraisal [TA115]. 2007 (reviewed November 2010); https://www.nice.org.uk/guidance/ta115.

81. Kunoe N, et al. Naltrexone implants after in-patient treatment for opioid dependence: randomised controlled trial. *Br J Psychiatry* 2009; **194**:541–546.

82. The British Pain Society, et al. Pain and substance misuse: improving the patient experience. A consensus statement prepared by The British Pain Society in collaboration with The Royal College of Psychiatrists, The Royal College of General Practitioners and The Advisory Council on the Misuse of Drugs. 2007; http://www.britishpainsociety.org/book_drug_misuse_main.pdf.

83. Winklbaur B, et al. Treating pregnant women dependent on opioids is not the same as treating pregnancy and opioid dependence: a knowledge synthesis for better treatment for women and neonates. *Addiction* 2008; **103**:1429–1440.

84. Finnegan LP. Neonatal abstinence syndrome. in RA Hoekelman, et al., ed. Primary pediatric care. St Louis: Mosby 1992; 1367–1378.

85. Winklbaur B, et al. Opioid dependence and pregnancy. *Curr Opin Psychiatry* 2008; **21**:255–259.

86. Minozzi S, et al. Maintenance agonist treatments for opiate-dependent pregnant women. *Cochrane Database Syst Rev* 2013; **12**:CD006318.

87. Fischer G, et al. Methadone versus buprenorphine in pregnant addicts: a double-blind, double-dummy comparison study. *Addiction* 2006; **101**:275–281.

88. Holmes AP, et al. Breastfeeding considerations for mothers of infants with neonatal abstinence syndrome. *Pharmacotherapy* 2017; **37**:861–869.

CHAPTER 4

Nicotine and smoking cessation

Tobacco smoking is the leading preventable cause of illness and premature death world-wide. Smoking cessation interventions are clinically and cost-effective for people with and without a mental illness.

In the UK, NICE recommends that every person who smokes, including those receiving community and inpatient mental health care, should be offered support to stop smoking; for people who are unable or are unwilling to give up, they should be provided with treatment to temporarily abstain from smoking whilst they are in a hospital setting.[1]

In those people wishing to make an attempt to give up smoking, there are three first-line stop smoking medications that are recommended by NICE: nicotine replacement therapy (NRT), varenicline and bupropion, all of which at least double the chance of successfully stopping. Quit rates can be increased further if the smoker is also provided with behavioural support from a trained tobacco dependence treatment advisor.[2]

Those people who are unwilling or feel unable to give up should be encouraged to minimise harm and substitute nicotine from tobacco cigarettes with either NRT or an electronic cigarette (e-cigarette)/vaping device.[3,4]

The effectiveness of smoking cessation treatments appears not to be reduced in patients with a variety of mental health problems.[5]

Nicotine replacement therapy (NRT)

NRT is licensed for smokers over the age of 12 to help those who want to stop smoking, reduce before quitting or during a temporary period of enforced abstinence when a person is unable to smoke. It is also indicated for pregnant and breastfeeding women attempting to stop smoking.

The aim of NRT in those stopping smoking is to assist the transition from cigarette smoking to complete abstinence. This is achieved by temporarily replacing some of the nicotine obtained from tobacco cigarettes with NRT products and minimising nicotine withdrawal symptoms and the motivation to smoke. People who have stopped smoking can safely use NRT if they wish to continue using nicotine recreationally or to prevent relapse back to smoking.

NRT is a versatile stop-smoking medicine. There are currently eight licensed NRT products in the UK: transdermal patches, lozenges, gum, sublingual tablets, inhalator, nasal spray, mouth spray and oral strips.

All products are all General Sales List medicines and can be bought over the counter (in the UK). NRT is formulated for systemic absorption either through the skin in the case of patches or the oral or nasal mucosa in the case of all the other products. This means that absorption of nicotine from NRT is much slower than nicotine from inhaling a tobacco cigarette and the risk of becoming addicted to NRT is lower.[6]

Clinical effectiveness

NRT is the most studied medication for smoking cessation. There have been over 150 trials, including over 50,000 smokers. The odds ratio (OR) of abstinence for any form of NRT compared with placebo is 1.84. **Combination NRT** (i.e. combining two

Table 4.15 Nicotine preparations and dose

	Smoking less than 20 cigarettes/day	Smoking more than 20 cigarettes/day or people who smoke within 30 minutes of waking up
Topical patch 24-hour formulation (21mg, 14mg and 7mg) 16-hour formulation (25mg, 15mg, 10mg)	If smoking >20 cigarettes/day use 21mg (24 hours) or 25mg (16 hours) patch There is no difference in efficacy between 16-hour and 24-hour formulations The 16-hour patch should be removed at bedtime	
Nasal spray (0.5mg/T)	One spray in each nostril when craving; not more than twice per hour; maximum 64 sprays/day	
Oral spray (1mg/T)	1–2 sprays when craving; not more than 2 sprays per episode; not more than 4 sprays/hour; maximum 64 sprays/day	
Lozenge (1mg, 2mg and 4mg)	One 1mg hourly to prevent craving	One 2mg or 4mg hourly to prevent craving. Usually not more than 15 lozenges/day
Gum (2mg, 4mg and 6mg)	One piece of 2mg hourly to prevent craving	One piece of 4mg or 6mg hourly to prevent craving. No more than 15 pieces 4mg/day
Inhalator (15mg)	No more than 6 cartridges of 15mg/day	
Sublingual tablet (2mg)	1–2 tablets hourly to prevent craving	2 tablets hourly to prevent craving; not more than 40 tablets/day
Mouth strips (2.5mg)	One strip of 2.5mg hourly to prevent craving	One strip hourly to prevent craving; not more than 15 strips/day

formulations such as a patch and an oral/nasal product) is more effective than using a single NRT product. The OR of abstinence for combination NRT compared to single NRT products is 1.43. Combination NRT has a similar efficacy to varenicline, and a greater efficacy than bupropion (Table 4.15).[7]

Studies with smokers from the general population suggest that each cigarette provides a smoker with approximately 1–2.9mg of nicotine, depending on the frequency and intensity of smoking.[8] Findings from studies in people with schizophrenia who smoke suggest that they take more frequent puffs over a shorter period of time and, as a result, extract more nicotine from cigarettes compared with those without a mental health condition.[9] It is therefore plausible that these smokers may require higher doses of nicotine replacement.

The nicotine from oral products has to be absorbed through the cheeks, gums and back of the lips. The correct technique is to chew the gum/suck the lozenge until the taste becomes strong and then rest it between the cheek and gum. When the taste starts to fade, it is advised to repeat this process for about 20–30 minutes. Many gum users press the gum down against the (buccal) gum to increase the surface area of contact and so the rate of nicotine absorption. Lozenges also allow sublingual absorption of nicotine but their physical size usually precludes this method unless the lozenge is broken into smaller pieces. Sublingual tablets are much smaller in size.

Drinking coffee and carbonated drinks may block the absorption of nicotine from oral nicotine products.[10]

Adverse effects

Adverse effects from using NRT are related to the type of product, and include skin irritation from patches and irritation to the inside of the mouth and coughs from oral products. Nausea may occur if the patient is still smoking. Some sleep disturbance can be expected in the early days of treatment, though this is also a symptom of nicotine withdrawal. NRT has no known interactions with psychotropic medication.

Varenicline

Varenicline is a selective nicotinic acetylcholine receptor partial agonist. It mimics the action of nicotine and causes a sustained release of dopamine in the mesolimbic pathway. It also blocks dopamine release resulting from subsequent nicotine intake. This means if taken as prescribed, any attempt to smoke a cigarette will be less pharmacologically rewarding and feel less satisfying to a smoker. Varenicline is indicated for smokers over the age of 18 who are motivated to stop smoking.

Clinical effectiveness

In the most recent Cochrane review, the OR of continuous abstinence for varenicline compared with placebo was 2.24. Varenicline was more effective when compared with bupropion (OR 1.39) and single-product NRT (OR 1.25), and was similarly effective compared with combination NRT.[11,12] In smokers with serious mental illness, varenicline improved the odds of stopping smoking by 4–5 times compared with placebo.[13,14]

Preparations and dose

People who smoke should set a target stopping date between 1 and 2 weeks after starting varenicline treatment. Those who are not willing or able to set a target date within 1–2 weeks can start treatment and then choose their own stopping date within 5 weeks. Dosage regimens can be found in the treatment algorithm for those people making an attempt to stop smoking at the end of this chapter. For people who have successfully stopped smoking at the end of 12 weeks, an additional course of 12-week treatment at 1mg twice daily may be considered for the maintenance of abstinence.[15]

Adverse effects

Common side effects include nausea, strange dreams and sleep disturbance, and headache, all occurring in greater than one in ten people. Varenicline has no known pharmacokinetic interaction with psychotropic medication.

Up until 2016, varenicline carried a black triangle symbol in the UK, indicating additional safety monitoring was required for people with a mental health condition. However, this was removed by the European Medicines Agency following the publication of the Evaluating Adverse Events in a Global Smoking Cessation Study (EAGLES) study; this found that neither varenicline nor bupropion significantly increased the risk of neuropsychiatric adverse events (including anxiety, depression, aggression, psychosis and suicidal behaviour) when compared with placebo or nicotine patch in patients with or without a history of psychiatric disorders.[16]

Bupropion

Bupropion is an antidepressant with dopaminergic and adrenergic actions and is additionally an antagonist at the nicotinic acetylcholine receptor. It is indicated for smokers over the age of 18 who are motivated to stop smoking.

Clinical effectiveness

In the most recent Cochrane review, the RR of abstinence for bupropion compared with placebo was 1.64.[12] Bupropion was of similar efficacy to single-product NRT (RR 0.99), and less effective for quitting compared with varenicline (although one trial suggested broad equality in outcome[17]), and combination NRT.[7] In smokers with serious mental illness, bupropion improved the odds of stopping by 3–4 times compared with placebo.[13,14]

Preparations and dose

People who smoke should set a target 'quit date' in the first 2 weeks of starting bupropion treatment. Dosage regimens can be found in the treatment algorithm for those people making an attempt to stop smoking at the end of this chapter.

Adverse effects

Bupropion is contraindicated in those with seizure disorders, eating disorders and alcohol dependence. Clinicians should be cautious of the potential for manic switch in patients with bipolar affective disorder (very low risk but can occur[18]). Common side effects include dizziness, taste changes, GI disturbance and insomnia, which can be reduced by avoiding a dose close to bedtime. Unlike NRT and varenicline, bupropion is known to interact with psychotropic medicines. It is metabolised by the cytochrome CYP2B6. Caution is advised when bupropion is co-administered with medicines known to induce (e.g. carbamazepine, phenytoin) or inhibit (e.g. valproate) cytochrome metabolism as clinical efficacy may be affected. Bupropion also inhibits the CYP2B6 pathway and therefore co-administration with medicines metabolised by this enzyme (e.g. risperidone and haloperidol) should be avoided.

Electronic cigarettes and vaping

E-cigarettes are nicotine delivery devices that do not contain tobacco and do not produce smoke. They are regulated under the European Union Tobacco Products Directive (i.e. there are controls on ingredients, packaging and advertising). E-cigarette manufacturers can apply to the Medicines and Healthcare Products Regulatory Agency (MHRA) for a medicinal licence. To date, the MHRA has licensed one e-cigarette but the manufacturers have not made this available; this means at the time of writing no e-cigarette can be prescribed in the EU. Public Health England, NHS England and the Care Quality Commission support the use of e-cigarettes and vaping devices in mental health inpatient settings.[19–21]

Clinical effectiveness

In the most recent Cochrane review of the effect of e-cigarettes for smoking cessation, quit rates were significantly higher for people who used e-cigarettes containing nicotine compared with those who either used an e-cigarette without nicotine (RR 1.71) or NRT (RR 1.69).[22] Since 2013, they have been the most popular quitting aid in England; it is estimated that in 2017, around 50,700 to 69,930 smokers had stopped smoking using an e-cigarette, who otherwise would have carried on smoking.[23] There is a small evidence base that they are also effective for helping people with a mental health condition reduce smoking.[24]

Preparations and dose

In Europe, disposable, prefilled cartridges or pods and bottles of e-liquids are labelled with the quantity of nicotine (in mg) present per millilitre (mL), or as the percentage weight per volume (0% w/v). Nicotine content ranges from zero (0%) to a maximum of 20mg/mL (or 2%). Nicotine salts (as an alternative to e-liquid) have recently become popular with e-cigarette users; salts have a lower pH level, enabling a smoother throat-hit and for some users, purportedly providing a sensation that is more similar to smoking. Additionally, nicotine salts allow vaporisation at a lower temperature and enable higher nicotine levels to be inhaled,[24] which may help with switching from smoking to vaping.

E-cigarettes come in various types and shapes. The following are some types of e-cigarettes:

- one-time disposable products (often referred to as 'cigalikes')
- reusable, rechargeable kits designed with replaceable cartridges or pods
- reusable, rechargeable kits designed to be refilled with liquid by the user (often referred to as tanks, but there are now also refillable pods available)
- reusable, rechargeable kits, often referred to as 'mods' (modifiables) that allow users to customise their product, e.g. by regulating the power delivery from the batteries to the heating element.

Adverse effects

Mouth, throat irritation, cough, headache and nausea are the most commonly reported symptoms of e-cigarette use, and these subside over time.[22] The Royal College of Physicians,[4] Public Health England[25] and the Committee on Toxicity of Chemicals in Food, Consumer Products and the Environment[26] advise that regulated e-cigarettes/ vaping devices are a much less harmful alternative to tobacco smoking for dependent smokers and bystanders. The Royal College of Physicians[4] hazard to health arising from long-term vapour inhalation from e-cigarettes is unlikely to exceed 5% of the harm from smoking tobacco. Concurrent smoking and vaping (dual use) may not reduce the risk of adverse health effects, and people who vape should be encouraged to stop smoking completely, whereas people who have never smoked should be encouraged not to smoke and not to vape.[24,26]

Table 4.16 Treatment algorithm for those people making an attempt to stop smoking

First-line quit attempt pharmacological treatment is **combination NRT** or **varenicline.**
All quit attempts should be supported at least weekly by a trained tobacco dependence treatment advisor.

Combination NRT quit attempt	Varenicline quit attempt
For people who smoke more than 20 cigarettes/day or who smoke within 30 minutes of waking up:	
Start 21mg (24 hours) or 25mg (16 hours) patch and an oral/nasal NRT product of the person's choice	Set target 'stopping date' between 1 and 2 weeks of varenicline treatment
Continue patch use for up to 12 weeks, aiming to reduce patch dosage every 4 weeks	Start 0.5mg PO varenicline once daily on days 1–3
Continue oral/nasal product use whilst experiencing craving	Increase to 0.5mg PO varenicline twice daily on days 4–7
For people who smoke less than 20 cigarettes/day and do not smoke within 30 minutes of waking up:	Increase to 1mg PO varenicline twice daily on days 8–84
Start 14mg (24 hours) or 15mg (16 hours) patch and/or an oral/nasal NRT product of the person's choice	Consider 1mg varenicline PO twice daily for an additional 12 weeks for the maintenance of abstinence in people who have successfully stopped smoking at the end of the initial 12 weeks course of varenicline
Continue patch use for up to 12 weeks, aiming to reduce patch dosage every 4 weeks	
Continue oral/nasal product use whilst experiencing craving	

Bupropion could be considered second line or where people who smoke express a preference for bupropion therapy.

Bupropion quit attempt

Set target 'stopping date' between 1 and 2 weeks of bupropion treatment
Start 150mg PO bupropion daily on days 1–6
Increase to 150mg PO bupropion twice daily on days 7–49 (with an interval of at least 8 hours between doses)
Maintain dose at 150mg PO bupropion on days 50–63 (otherwise, discontinue if person has not quit)

In patients with **serious mental illness**, both varenicline and bupropion have been shown to increase the odds of stopping smoking by greater than 4 times compared to placebo. In patients with stable psychiatric co-morbidity, an NRT patch was also found to double the abstinence rates compared to placebo. Both varenicline and bupropion did not significantly increase the risk of neuropsychiatric adverse events (including anxiety, depression, aggression, psychosis, and suicidal behaviour) when compared with placebo or NRT in patients with or without a history of psychiatric disorders
It is always advisable to monitor patient's mental health when undergoing a quit attempt

People who smoke wishing to use an **e-cigarette** to quit should generally set a quit date and use the e-cigarette to stop in one go by replacing all their tobacco cigarettes with an e-cigarette as soon as possible. Alternatively, they can gradually reduce the amount they smoke over several weeks and increase the use of the e-cigarette until they have completely switched. Similar to the use of NRT, advise the service user to start with a higher strength of nicotine

po, per os (by mouth)

Table 4.17 Treatment algorithm for those people not making an attempt to stop, i.e. those people temporarily abstaining or aiming to reduce their cigarette consumption

Those who are unwilling or feel unable to quit should be encouraged to minimise harm and substitute nicotine from tobacco cigarettes with either **combination NRT** or an **e-cigarette.**

Combination NRT	E-cigarettes/vaping devices
For people who smoke more than 20 cigarettes/day or who smoke within 30 minutes of waking up:	
Start 21mg (24 hours) or 25mg (16 hours) patch and an oral/nasal NRT product of the person's choice	The dose of nicotine a vaper extracts from an e-cigarette varies depending on the device, the volume of e-liquid, other ingredients in the liquid, the frequency, size and depth of inhalation. The more dependant a smoker is, the higher strength of nicotine is recommended
Continue to offer NRT products even if met with initial refusal	
Smokers should have fingertip control over NRT products at times of craving	A rough guide is that smokers of:
	20 tobacco cigarettes/day may require up to 20mg of nicotine/day
For people who smoke less than 20 cigarettes/day and do not smoke within 30 minutes of waking up:	
Start 14mg (24 hours) or 15mg (16 hours) patch and/or an oral/nasal NRT product of the person's choice	Smokers should have fingertip control over their e-cigarette at times of craving. Similar to NRT people who smoke should be encouraged to regularly use an e-cigarette between smoking episodes to promote smoke-free intervals
Continue to offer NRT products even if met with initial refusal	
Smokers should have fingertip control over NRT products at times of craving	

It is not currently possible to prescribe e-cigarettes in the NHS. Practitioners should consult local smoke-free policies to establish which type of e-cigarette is permitted in individual mental health inpatient settings and how to access them.

References

1. National Institute for Health and Care Excellence. Smoking cessation – acute, maternity and mental health services. Public Health Guidance 48. 2013 (last checked March 2017); http://guidance.nice.org.uk/PH48.
2. National Institute for Health and Clinical Excellence. Stop smoking interventions and services. NICE Guideline [NG92]. 2018; https://www.nice.org.uk/guidance/ng92.
3. National Institute for Health and Care Excellence. Smoking: harm reduction. Public Health Guidance [PH45]. 2013 (last checked March 2017); https://www.nice.org.uk/guidance/ph45.
4. Royal College of Physicians. Nicotine without smoke: tobacco harm reduction. A report by the Tobacco Advisory Group of the Royal College of Physicians. 2016; https://www.rcplondon.ac.uk/projects/outputs/nicotine-without-smoke-tobacco-harm-reduction-0.
5. Tidey JW, et al. Smoking cessation and reduction in people with chronic mental illness. *BMJ* 2015; 351:h4065.
6. Hajek P, et al. Dependence potential of nicotine replacement treatments: effects of product type, patient characteristics, and cost to user. *Prev Med* 2007; 44:230–234.
7. Cahill K, et al. Pharmacological interventions for smoking cessation: an overview and network meta-analysis. *Cochrane Database Syst Rev* 2013; Cd009329.
8. Henningfield JE, et al. Pharmacotherapy for nicotine dependence. *CA Cancer J Clin* 2005; 55:281–299; quiz 322–283, 325.
9. Williams JM, et al. Increased nicotine and cotinine levels in smokers with schizophrenia and schizoaffective disorder is not a metabolic effect. *Schizophr Res* 2005; 79:323–335.
10. Henningfield JE, et al. Drinking coffee and carbonated beverages blocks absorption of nicotine from nicotine polacrilex gum. *JAMA* 1990; 264:1560–1564.
11. Cahill K, et al. Nicotine receptor partial agonists for smoking cessation. *Cochrane Database Syst Rev* 2016; Cd006103.
12. Howes S, et al. Antidepressants for smoking cessation. *Cochrane Database Syst Rev* 2020; 4:Cd000031.
13. Roberts E, et al. Efficacy and tolerability of pharmacotherapy for smoking cessation in adults with serious mental illness: a systematic review and network meta-analysis. *Addiction* 2016; 111:599–612.
14. Siskind DJ, et al. Pharmacological interventions for smoking cessation among people with schizophrenia spectrum disorders: a systematic review, meta-analysis, and network meta-analysis. *Lancet Psychiatry* 2020; 7:762–774.

CHAPTER 4

15. Hajek P, et al. Varenicline in prevention of relapse to smoking: effect of quit pattern on response to extended treatment. *Addiction* 2009; **104**:1597–1602.

16. Anthenelli RM, et al. Neuropsychiatric safety and efficacy of varenicline, bupropion, and nicotine patch in smokers with and without psychiatric disorders (EAGLES): a double-blind, randomised, placebo-controlled clinical trial. *Lancet* 2016; **387**:2507–2520.

17. Benli AR, et al. A comparison of the efficacy of varenicline and bupropion and an evaluation of the effect of the medications in the context of the smoking cessation programme. *Tob Induc Dis* 2017; **15**:10.

18. Giasson-Gariepy K, et al. A case of hypomania during nicotine cessation treatment with bupropion. *Addict Sci Clin Pract* 2013; **8**:22.

19. Care Quality Commission. Brief guide: the use of 'blanket restrictions' in mental health wards. 2020; https://www.cqc.org.uk/sites/default/files/20191125_900767_briefguide-blanket_restrictions_mental_health_wards_v3.pdf.

20. Health and Social Care. Using electronic cigarettes in NHS mental health organisations. 2020; https://www.gov.uk/government/publications/e-cigarettes-use-by-patients-in-nhs-mental-health-organisations/using-electronic-cigarettes-in-nhs-mental-health-organisations.

21. NHS England. Long Term Plan. 2020; https://www.longtermplan.nhs.uk/wp-content/uploads/2019/08/nhs-long-term-plan-version-1.2.pdf.

22. Hartmann-Boyce J, et al. Electronic cigarettes for smoking cessation. *Cochrane Database Syst Rev* 2020; **10**:Cd010216.

23. Beard E, et al. Association of prevalence of electronic cigarette use with smoking cessation and cigarette consumption in England: a time-series analysis between 2006 and 2017. *Addiction* 2020; **115**:961–974.

24. McNeill A, et al. *Vaping in England: an evidence update including mental health and pregnancy, March 2020: a report commissioned by Public Health England*. London: Public Health England. 2020; https://assets.publishing.service.gov.uk/government/uploads/system/uploads/attachment_data/file/869401/Vaping_in_England_evidence_update_March_2020.pdf.

25. McNeill A, et al. *Evidence review of ecigarettes and heated tobacco products 2018. A report commissioned by Public Health England*. London: Public Health England. 2018; https://assets.publishing.service.gov.uk/government/uploads/system/uploads/attachment_data/file/684963/Evidence_review_of_e-cigarettes_and_heated_tobacco_products_2018.pdf.

26. Committee on Toxicity of Chemicals in Food Consumer Products and the Environment (COT). Statement on the potential toxicological risks from electronic nicotine (and non-nicotine) delivery systems (E(N)NDS – e-cigarettes). 2020; https://cot.food.gov.uk/sites/default/files/2020-09/COT%20E%28N%29NDS%20statement%202020-04.pdf.

Pharmacological treatment of dependence on stimulants

The most commonly misused stimulants are cocaine (as hydrochloride or free base) amfetamine sulphate and methamphetamine hydrochloride. These drugs are usually insufflated (snorted, e.g. cocaine HCl and amfetamine SO_4), smoked (cocaine base) or injected. Use, misuse and dependence of stimulants are relatively common in most of the world. They can be taken on their own or with other drugs such as a combination of heroin and crack cocaine, powder cocaine and alcohol, or methamphetamine and GBL.[1]

A wide variety of pharmacological agents have been assessed in the treatment of stimulant misuse and dependence. Although some have shown early promise, none has been found so far to show proven benefit.[2,3] Stimulant use for many will be self-limiting without treatment beyond the provision of harm minimisation advice and psychoeducation. For those that are used in combination with alcohol, heroin or GBL, effective treatment of the co-occurring dependency may deliver reductions in stimulant use. For those that are dependent on stimulants, research suggests that approaches that incorporate contingency management have been shown to have the greatest benefit. For many the route to abstinence is through mutual aid and peer support such as Cocaine Anonymous, Crystal Meth Anonymous or Rational Recovery. Further information on the effective treatment of cocaine dependence can be found in the UK clinical guidelines.[1]

Cocaine

Detoxification

Symptoms of withdrawal include depressed mood, agitation and insomnia. These are usually self-limiting. It should be noted that given cocaine's short half-life and the binge nature of cocaine use, many patients essentially detoxify themselves regularly with no pharmacological therapy. Symptomatic relief such as the short-term use of hypnotics may be helpful in some, but these agents may become agents of dependence themselves for some patients.[1]

Substitution treatment

There is little evidence for substitution therapy for the treatment of cocaine misuse and it should not usually be prescribed.[1-3]

Amfetamines

A wide variety of amfetamines are misused, including 'street' amfetamine, methamphetamine and pharmaceutical dexamfetamine. Any drug in this class is likely to have misuse potential.

Detoxification

A withdrawal syndrome is common in those who are dependent. Treatment should focus on symptomatic relief, although many symptoms of amfetamine withdrawal (low mood, listlessness, fatigue, etc.) are short-lived and may not be amenable to pharmacological treatment. Insomnia can be treated with short courses of hypnotics, again noting the risk of dependence on these agents.[1-3]

Maintenance

Dexamfetamine (or other stimulant medication) maintenance for the treatment of amfetamine dependence should not be initiated as there is no good evidence for this practice.[1-3]

Existing dexamfetamine patients

In the UK, there remain some patients who have been prescribed dexamfetamine as a maintenance treatment for drug dependence for many years. Ideally, such patients should be gradually detoxified over several months. For some, though, the consequences of enforced detoxification may be worse than continuing to prescribe dexamfetamine. In these cases, the best decision may be to continue to prescribe. A decision to continue prescribing dexamfetamine should only be made by an addiction specialist.[1]

Polysubstance abuse

In those who are dependent on opioids and cocaine, the provision of effective substitution therapy for treatment of the opioid dependence with either methadone or buprenorphine can lead to a reduction in cocaine use.[1]

Psychosis associated with stimulant drugs

Psychotic symptoms in association with methamphetamine are related to the frequency of use and severity of methamphetamine dependence.[4] In many, perhaps most cases, psychotic symptoms can resolve with the resolution of intoxication, i.e. over the course of a day or so. The majority of patients attending an emergency setting with acute psychotic symptoms in the context of very recent methamphetamine use can be managed with simple sedation,[5] e.g. diazepam 5–10mg as needed 4–6 hourly for agitation – and therapeutic rest. Some patients, however, may need more intensive treatment in line with the treatment of acute psychosis in Chapter 2.

It should be noted though that psychotic symptoms in the context of stimulant use are progressive with continued use; they tend to start earlier in each binge and to last longer. A median of 25% of patients report ongoing symptoms 1 month post methamphetamine consumption.[6] Psychosis in the context of intoxication is associated with persecutory delusions and tactile hallucinations, while more persistent methamphetamine-associated psychosis is characterised by delusions of persecution and auditory hallucinations and is largely indistinguishable from a primary psychotic disorder.[6] In the emergency department, it can be difficult to make a clear diagnosis. Between 16% and 38% of patients initially diagnosed with methamphetamine psychosis are later diagnosed as having schizophrenia.[6]

In the acute setting, another important differential in methamphetamine users presenting with agitated psychosis is GBL withdrawal delirium, where stimulant/GBL polysubstance-use pattern is prevalent. There is symptomatic overlap between stimulant intoxication – autonomic hyperactivity, agitation, hallucinations – and GBL withdrawal delirium. The latter requires higher doses of benzodiazepines and more prolonged treatment (see section 'GHB and GBL dependence', later in the chapter).

As stated earlier, in the emergency setting, simple sedation with benzodiazepines for agitation is often sufficient initially. If antipsychotics are indicated, the four-fold increased odds of developing extra-pyramidal side effects in patients who use methamphetamine should be borne in mind.[7] Agents with a low propensity to cause EPSEs should be used and there is evidence for efficacy of olanzapine. Aripiprazole may be preferred for rapid tranquillisation as olanzapine and benzodiazepines should not be co-administered. Haloperidol should not be used. Early and ongoing review regarding continuation is important, as for most patients symptoms resolve within 2 or 3 weeks and there is no evidence to support the benefit of prophylactic prescription of antipsychotics in methamphetamine-related psychosis.[8]

Stimulant-associated depression

Anhedonia for some patients can be profound in early abstinence from stimulants. For many, such low mood will resolve with duration of abstinence and supportive psychosocial interventions.[1] For those in whom it endures psychological treatments are effective[9] but may be difficult for addiction patients to access because of institutional barriers.

Antidepressants have primarily been evaluated as treatment for the substance dependence itself, with depression as a secondary outcome. There is some evidence, primarily regarding the tricyclic antidepressants, for a reduction in depressive symptoms;[10] however, tricyclic antidepressants are not recommended in those with co-morbid substance misuse because of their cardiotoxicity.[11] There is no evidence to support the use of SSRIs, and indeed these are associated with significant interactions with stimulants[1] and increased disengagement.[9]

References

1. Department of Health and Social Care. Drug misuse and dependence: UK guidelines on clinical management. 2017; https://www.gov.uk/government/publications/drug-misuse-and-dependence-uk-guidelines-on-clinical-management.
2. Siefried KJ, et al. Pharmacological treatment of methamphetamine/amphetamine dependence: a systematic review. *CNS Drugs* 2020; 1–29.
3. Ronsley C, et al. Treatment of stimulant use disorder: a systematic review of reviews. *PloS One* 2020; 15:e0234809.
4. Arunogiri S, et al. A systematic review of risk factors for methamphetamine-associated psychosis. *Aust N Z J Psychiatry* 2018; 52:514–529.
5. Isoardi KZ, et al. Methamphetamine presentations to an emergency department: management and complications. *Emerg Med Aust* 2019; 31:593–599.
6. Voce A, et al. A systematic review of the symptom profile and course of methamphetamine-associated psychosis: substance use and misuse. *Subst Use Misuse* 2019; 54:549–559.
7. Temmingh HS, et al. Methamphetamine use and antipsychotic-related extrapyramidal side-effects in patients with psychotic disorders. *J Dual Diag* 2020; 16:208–217.
8. Shoptaw SJ, et al. Treatment for amphetamine psychosis. *Cochrane Database Syst Rev* 2009; CD003026.
9. Farrell M, et al. Responding to global stimulant use: challenges and opportunities. *The Lancet* 2019; 394:1652–1667.
10. Pani PP, et al. Antidepressants for cocaine dependence and problematic cocaine use. *Cochrane Database Syst Rev* 2011.
11. Lingford-Hughes AR, et al. BAP updated guidelines: evidence-based guidelines for the pharmacological management of substance abuse, harmful use, addiction and comorbidity: recommendations from BAP. *J Psychopharmacol* 2012; 26:899–952.

CHAPTER 4

GHB and GBL dependence

GHB and GBL use is uncommon but medically important because, in dependent users, withdrawal can proceed rapidly to life-threatening agitated delirium. Complications include seizures, bradycardia, cardiac arrest and renal failure. Doctors in acute and psychiatric hospitals need to be able to recognise and manage acute withdrawal.

GHB (gamma-hydroxybutyrate) and GBL (gamma-butyrolactone, a pro-drug of GHB) are colloquially often referred to as 'G'. They reduce anxiety and produce disinhibition and sedation, primarily through actions at the GABA-B receptor. These drugs are used recreationally for socialising and occasionally to aid sleep. Among men who have sex with men, they can be used, often alongside stimulants such as mephedrone and crystal methamphetamine, to facilitate sex in the context of potential high-risk sexual behaviour ('chemsex'). Both GHB and GBL have a narrow therapeutic index, and overdose is not uncommon. Dependence is rare, but in dependent users withdrawal has rapid onset and can produce severe delirium with paranoid delusions and life-threatening complications.[1]

The withdrawal syndrome[1,2]

Dependent users take doses 'round the clock' (consuming doses day and night, every 1–3 hours or more frequently). Onset of withdrawal symptoms is typically a few hours following the last dose. The withdrawal syndrome is similar to alcohol withdrawal and may include symptoms such as tachycardia, insomnia, anxiety, sweating and fine tremors.[1] Untreated, this can progress to agitated delirium, often with psychotic features (including paranoid delusions and hallucinations) later followed by severe tremors, muscle rigidity and seizures.[1] Muscle rigidity may be so severe as to produce fever, rhabdomyolysis and acute renal failure. The requirement for medication to manage symptoms eases over 4–6 days, although there are case reports of more prolonged withdrawal.

Withdrawal management

The evidence base for detoxification is limited. The core principle of managing withdrawal is to treat early and so prevent the development of delirium and other complications. Once established, delirium can be difficult to control.[3] Early treatment with benzodiazepines is required, and baclofen (a GABA-B agonist) and phenobarbital have also been used effectively as adjunctive medications.[1,4] Baclofen is freely available online and may be obtained by users for unsupervised withdrawal,[5] something which, given the dangers involved in withdrawal, should be unequivocally discouraged.

GHB itself has also been successfully used to aid withdrawal[6] with reducing doses given every 3 hours over up to 2 weeks. Pharmaceutical GHB may be more effective than benzodiazepines in managing withdrawal.[7]

Existing alcohol withdrawal scales are unlikely to be helpful in evaluating withdrawal severity. For up-to-date guidance on the management of GHB/GBL withdrawal, it is recommended (in the UK) that information be sought from the National Poisons

Information Service (NPIS), specifically the NPIS 24-hour telephone service and the poisons information database TOXBASE®.

The two scenarios with which clinicians should be conversant are unplanned acute withdrawal and planned elective withdrawal in dependent users.

Table 4.18 Management of acute unplanned withdrawal

Setting	■ Acute unplanned withdrawal is a medical emergency and should be managed in the acute hospital inpatient setting ■ Severe withdrawal may require admission to an intensive care unit
Initial pharmacotherapy	■ Initiate diazepam 20mg PO when early withdrawal symptoms are observed ■ Diazepam can be repeated at 30 minutes to 4 hourly intervals until symptoms are controlled ■ Most cases of GBL withdrawal require 60–80mg diazepam in the first 24 hours ■ Higher daily dosages of up to 300mg PO diazepam may be necessary ■ If the patient becomes drowsy, withhold diazepam and review diagnosis ■ One-to-one nursing care may assist in managing severe cases ■ Have flumazenil to hand should reversal of effects be required
Adjunctive pharmacotherapy	■ Initiate baclofen 10mg PO tds in combination with benzodiazepine withdrawal regimen where benzodiazepines prove to be inadequate ■ This can be titrated to 20mg PO tds in cases of continued anxiety and agitation ■ In cases of severe withdrawal consider addition of phenobarbital in doses of 150–450mg/day IV* (ICU only) ■ In cases where severe withdrawal remains uncontrolled, IV anaesthetic such as propofol* may be required (ICU only). Thiopental* coma has also been used in severe resistant withdrawal[8]

*The respiratory depressant effects of phenobarbital, thiopental and propofol cannot be reversed, and facilities for mechanical ventilation should be available.
ICU, intensive care unit; IV, intravenous; po, per os (by mouth); tds, ter die sumendum (three times a day).

Table 4.19 Management of planned elective withdrawal

Setting	■ All patients undergoing planned withdrawal should be medically supervised ■ Ambulatory community detoxification should only be attempted where there is no history of delirium or psychosis. A third party should be at home who is able to monitor and support the withdrawal process. There should be the option of transferring the patient to an inpatient unit if symptoms are not well controlled
Pre-withdrawal	■ Discuss treatment plan with the patient and person who will be supporting them ■ Encourage the patient to keep a week-long diary of GBL use, including dose frequency and quantity ■ Encourage the patient to cease 'on-top' drug use such as mephedrone and crystal methamphetamine, prior to elective withdrawal ■ Start baclofen 10mg PO tds 3–7 days before target withdrawal date ■ Encourage patients to reduce GBL dose as much as tolerable either by reducing each dose by 0.1mL every 1–2 days or increasing the time period between doses

CHAPTER 4

Withdrawal	▪ On day 1 of planned ambulatory withdrawal, ask the patient to attend having used no GBL for a minimum of 2 hours, and advise to dispose of their remaining supplies of GBL
	▪ Advise patients who will need to stay at the clinic for up to 4 hours on day 1 that they cannot drive motor vehicles during withdrawal, and should not drink alcohol or take other sedatives during withdrawal
	▪ Increase baclofen to 20mg PO tds
	▪ Initiate benzodiazepine treatment once signs and symptoms of withdrawal develop – tachycardia, sweaty palms, fine tremor, anxiety. Start diazepam 20mg, review after 2 hours and monitor for anxiety/sedation/respiratory depression. Repeat up to 20mg PO diazepam if indicated
	▪ Once 6 hours have passed since the last GBL usage, the patient may be given up to a further 40mg diazepam, and then seen on the following 2 days
	▪ At each daily visit, review diazepam dosage and titrate to symptoms. Diazepam is seldom needed beyond 7 days. Typical initial daily doses of diazepam are around 40–60mg/day
Post-withdrawal	▪ Continue baclofen 20mg PO tds following benzodiazepine withdrawal reducing over 4–6 weeks. One of the few trials in this area successfully used 45–60mg a day for 3 months[9]
	▪ After withdrawal, persisting anxiety and insomnia are common, and there is a high risk of relapse. Before initiating elective withdrawal management, a plan should be in place to monitor and support patients for a minimum of 4 weeks to minimise the risk of relapse

po, per os (by mouth); tds, ter die sumendum (three times a day).

References

1. Kamal RM, et al. Pharmacological treatment in gamma-hydroxybutyrate (GHB) and gamma-butyrolactone (GBL) Dependence: detoxification and relapse prevention. *CNS Drugs* 2017; 31:51–64.
2. Bell J, et al. Gamma-butyrolactone (GBL) dependence and withdrawal. *Addiction* 2011; 106:442–447.
3. Novel Psychoactive Treatment UK Network (NEPTUNE). Guidance on the clinical management of acute and chronic harms of club drugs and novel psychoactive substances. 2015; http://neptune-clinical-guidance.co.uk/wp-content/uploads/2015/03/NEPTUNE-Guidance-March-2015.pdf.
4. LeTourneau JL, et al. Baclofen and gamma-hydroxybutyrate withdrawal. *Neurocrit Care* 2008; 8:430–433.
5. Floyd CN, et al. Baclofen in gamma-hydroxybutyrate withdrawal: patterns of use and online availability. *Eur J Clin Pharmacol* 2018; 74:349–356.
6. Dijkstra BA, et al. Detoxification with titration and tapering in gamma-hydroxybutyrate (GHB) dependent patients: the Dutch GHB monitor project. *Drug Alcohol Depend* 2017; 170:164–173.
7. Beurmanjer H, et al. Tapering with pharmaceutical GHB or benzodiazepines for detoxification in GHB-dependent patients: a matched-subject observational study of treatment-as-usual in Belgium and the Netherlands. *CNS Drugs* 2020; 34:651–659.
8. Vos CF, et al. Successful treatment of severe, treatment resistant GHB withdrawal through thiopental-coma. *Subst Abus* 2020; 1–6.
9. Beurmanjer H, et al. Baclofen to prevent relapse in gamma-hydroxybutyrate (GHB)-dependent patients: a multicentre, open-label, non-randomized, controlled trial. *CNS Drugs* 2018; 32:437–442.

CHAPTER 4

Benzodiazepine misuse

Benzodiazepine prescribing increased during the 1960s and 1970s, mainly because of their improved safety profile relative to barbiturates. However, it was soon noted that benzodiazepines have a high potential for causing dependence. Prescriptions originally started for other disorders were often continued long term and led to the development of dependence. This was and is particularly common in older patients and those with anxiety spectrum disorders or depression. In England, the prescribing of benzodiazepines has fallen to 14.9 million prescription items in 2018–2019, from 16.3 million in 2015–2016.

There are a number of novel or 'designer' benzodiazepines (e.g. etizolam, flualprazolam, flunitrazolam and norfludiazepam). There is limited information available about the health and social harms of these substances, but they are likely to be similar to or worse than the established benzodiazepines.[1] Some of these benzodiazepines (flualprazolam, flunitrazolam and norfludiazepam) are classified in Schedule 1 in the UK – pharmaceutical benzodiazepines are in Schedule 3 or 4. Outside being prescribed, benzodiazepines can be acquired via the illicit market, diversion of scripts and Internet purchasing (thought to be a rising trend).[2]

Benzodiazepine dependence can be thought of as either iatrogenic (low daily doses prescribed over many years) or non-iatrogenic (high doses, illicitly obtained, consumed intermittently).

Discontinuation

A previously published (now withdrawn) Cochrane review evaluated the evidence for pharmacological interventions for benzodiazepine mono-dependence, and concluded that a gradual reduction of benzodiazepine dose was preferable to an abrupt discontinuation.[3] A more recent review confirmed that withdrawal over a period of less than 6 months is appropriate for most patients[4] and the UK drug misuse and dependence guidelines suggest a reduction of about one-eighth of the daily dose every 2 weeks.[5] The Australian GP guidelines comment that the evidence for the 'optimal rate of tapering is lacking' and 'the exact rate of reduction should be individualised according to the drug, dose and duration of treatment'.[6]

A meta-analysis supports the effectiveness of multi-faceted prescribing interventions (usually including psychological interventions/support) in reducing benzodiazepine use in older patients,[7] and one RCT has demonstrated that a simple educational approach based on self-efficacy theory resulted in about a quarter of long-term elderly benzodiazepine users engaging voluntarily in reducing and discontinuing use.[8] A 2018 Cochrane review could find no pharmaceutical add-on that could help facilitate the withdrawal process. Some drugs seemed to be associated with some beneficial effects, but the evidence quality was too low for any clinical recommendations to be made.[9]

A large number of patients presenting to addiction services may be using illicit benzodiazepines in addition to their primary substance of abuse. People with non-iatrogenic benzodiazepine dependence often consume doses greater than 100mg diazepam a day. Although some services provide prescriptions for benzodiazepines, there is no evidence that substitute prescribing of benzodiazepines ultimately reduces benzodiazepine misuse. If benzodiazepines are prescribed, this should ideally be for a short-term, time-limited (2–3 weeks) prescription and with a view to detoxification.

CHAPTER 4

If patients have been prescribed benzodiazepines for a substantial period of time, it may be preferable to convert to equivalents of diazepam as this is longer acting and so less likely to be associated with withdrawal symptoms. Benzodiazepine dependence as part of polysubstance dependence should also be treated by a gradual withdrawal of the medication. Benzodiazepines prescribed at greater than 30mg diazepam equivalent per day may cause harm[5] and so this should be avoided if at all possible (such doses are rare in iatrogenic dependence[10]). Psychosocial interventions including contingency management have had some success at reducing benzodiazepine use. A Cochrane review found that 'there is evidence to support the use of CBT plus taper to reduce BZD use in the short term. There is currently no evidence to support the use of MI. In addition, there is some emerging evidence that simple interventions, such as structured consultation and individually tailored GP letters, may be worth exploring further.'[11]

Pregnancy and benzodiazepine misuse

Benzodiazepines are not major human teratogens but should ideally be gradually discontinued before a planned pregnancy. If a woman is prescribed benzodiazepines and found to be pregnant, the prescription should be gradually withdrawn over as short a time as possible, being mindful of the risk of withdrawal seizures and the potential consequences for the pregnant woman and foetus. A risk–benefit analysis should be undertaken and specialist advice sought (see section 'Pregnancy' in Chapter 7). As for all patients, it may be appropriate for a woman dependent on benzodiazepines to be stabilised on diazepam, prior to dose reduction.[5]

Summary

- Benzodiazepines should be withdrawn at a rate of around one-eighth of the dose every 2 weeks.
- Discontinuation should usually be completed within 6 months.
- Switching to an equivalent dose of diazepam before withdrawal is commonplace.
- Benzodiazepine misuse is frequently seen in multi-substance misuse where opioids may be the primary drug of dependence.

Typical diazepam withdrawal schedule for iatrogenic dependence	
Baseline	30mg/day
Week 2	25mg/day
Week 4	20mg/day
Week 6	18mg/day
Week 8	16mg/day
Week 10	14mg/day
Week 12	12mg/day
Week 14	10mg/day

Then reduce by 2mg/day every 2 weeks if tolerated.

References

1. Advisory Council on the Misuse of Drugs (ACMD). *A review of the evidence of use and harms of Novel Benzodiazepines.* London: Home Office. 2020; https://assets.publishing.service.gov.uk/government/uploads/system/uploads/attachment_data/file/881969/ACMD_report_-_a_review_of_the_evidence_of_use_and_harms_of_novel_benzodiazepines.pdf.

2. Manchester KR, et al. The emergence of new psychoactive substance (NPS) benzodiazepines: A review. *Drug Test Anal* 2018; **10**:392–393.

3. Denis C, et al. Pharmacological interventions for benzodiazepine mono-dependence management in outpatient settings. *Cochrane Database Syst Rev* 2006; CD005194.

4. Lader M, et al. Withdrawing benzodiazepines in primary care. *CNS Drugs* 2009; **23**:19–34.

5. Department of Health (DoH). *Drug misuse and dependence: UK guidelines on clinical management.* London: Department of Health. 2017; https://assets.publishing.service.gov.uk/government/uploads/system/uploads/attachment_data/file/673978/clinical_guidelines_2017.pdf.

6. Royal Australian College of General Practitioners (RACGP). Prescribing drugs of dependence in general practice, Part B – benzodiazepines. Melbourne, Australia. 2015; https://www.racgp.org.au/FSDEDEV/media/documents/Clinical%20Resources/Guidelines/Drugs%20of%20dependence/Prescribing-drugs-of-dependence-in-general-practice-Part-B-Benzodiazepines.pdf.

7. Gould RL, et al. Interventions for reducing benzodiazepine use in older people: meta-analysis of randomised controlled trials. *Br J Psychiatry* 2014; **204**:98–107.

8. Tannenbaum C, et al. Reduction of inappropriate benzodiazepine prescriptions among older adults through direct patient education: the EMPOWER cluster randomized trial. *JAMA Inter Med* 2014; **174**:890–898.

9. Baandrup L, et al. Pharmacological interventions for benzodiazepine discontinuation in chronic benzodiazepine users. *Cochrane Database Syst Rev* 2018; 3:Cd011481.

10. Vicens C, et al. Comparative efficacy of two interventions to discontinue long-term benzodiazepine use: cluster randomised controlled trial in primary care. *Br J Psychiatry* 2014; **204**:471–479.

11. Darker CD, et al. Psychosocial interventions for benzodiazepine harmful use, abuse or dependence. *Cochrane Database Syst Rev* 2015; Cd009652.

CHAPTER 4

Synthetic cannabinoid receptor agonists (SCRAs)

> The clinical importance of SCRAs relates to their acute toxicity (which is potentially life-threatening), their relationship to psychosis and their propensity to induce dependence. Doctors working in Emergency Departments, psychiatric settings and addiction services should be able to recognise and manage acute intoxication with synthetic cannabinoids.

SCRAs are a structurally diverse group of chemicals that act as an agonist at the CB1 receptor. Nomenclature is complex and the vast array of chemical structures is difficult to classify.[1] New classes of SCRAs frequently emerge.[2]

In the UK, SCRAs were used predominantly by vulnerable groups such as the homeless and prisoners. However, recent post-mortem toxicological evidence suggests that a majority of descendants lived in stable accommodation and took SCRAs as part of a more general pattern of polysubstance use.[3]

Most commonly, SCRAs are dissolved in alcohol and sprayed on plant material, then smoked. More than one SCRA compound may be present in a single herbal pack and at the time of writing, there are more than 700 street names for SCRAs, the most common of which are 'Spice' and 'K2'.[4] Many patients may not admit to SCRA use despite their recent use.[5] SCRAs are more potent in their action at the CB1 receptor and can be longer lasting than tetrahydracannabinol (THC), the main psychoactive ingredient in cannabis. They also have diverse non-CB1 actions, which can influence their clinical effects.[6]

Acute intoxication is distinct from and more severe than THC intoxication and is associated with physical harms that can be life-threatening.[7,8] In the UK, deaths associated with SCRAs are rising, albeit overwhelmingly with polysubstance ingestion[3] – in contrast with deaths reported worldwide, where SCRAs are usually the single substance.[9]

SCRA deaths in the UK:

- Occur via sudden collapse with cardiac or respiratory arrest
- Majority are unwitnessed
- Majority occur in those without pre-existing physical health problems
- Over 40% have opioids detected post-mortem

SCRAs are associated with cardiotoxicity and at least some precipitate QT prolongation.[10] Therefore, consider offering ECGs to those who use SCRAs, particularly those who are prescribed methadone. A case report exists of successful reversal of SCRA overdose with naloxone, which some have hypothesised relates to the interplay between opioid and cannabinoid systems.[11]

It is estimated that the risk of requiring emergency treatment is 30 times higher than that associated with the use of cannabis.[12] SCRAs can precipitate psychosis that persists after intoxication. Around 15% of users report symptoms of dependence and a withdrawal syndrome similar to cannabis withdrawal.

Acute SCRA intoxication

Acute SCRA intoxication needs to be recognised clinically as urine drug testing for SCRAs is not possible in the acute setting because of their structural diversity.[13] Laboratory testing can be helpful but may not give results within a clinically meaningful timeframe. Features of SCRA intoxication are detailed on Table 4.20 and are based on case series of presentations to emergency units.[5,7,8,14] Presentations and incidence of particular symptoms vary widely, which may reflect their chemical diversity. The most common features appear to be agitation, nausea and tachycardia. Intoxication is usually short-lived with 78% resolving within 8 hours.[5] A psychotic episode is commonly precipitated – 41% of presentations of acutely intoxicated patients to A&E were associated with psychotic symptoms.[14]

Table 4.20 Features of acute SCRA intoxication

System affected	
Cardiovascular system	Tachycardia
	Hypertension
	Bradycardia
	Hypotension
	Chest pain – can precipitate myocardial ischaemia
	Cardiac arrest
Gastrointestinal system and abdominal organs	Nausea
	Vomiting – often profuse
	Abdominal pain
	Hepatotoxicity
	Acute renal injury – acute tubular necrosis and acute interstitial nephritis
Nervous system	Agitation
	Anxiety
	Aggression
	Confusion
	Psychotic symptoms – can persist after intoxication
	Seizures
	Coma
	Catatonia with posturing
Other	Conjunctival injection
	Rhabdomyolysis

CHAPTER 4

Management of acute SCRA intoxication

- Patients should be cared for in an appropriate setting
- ECG cardiac monitoring to detect ischaemia and arrhythmias
- Blood tests – blood gas, U&Es, creatine kinase and LFTs
- Supportive treatment with benzodiazepines
- IV fluids, supplemental oxygen and anti-emetics
- Rarely antipsychotics or anaesthesia.

Reassuringly, neither antipsychotic nor benzodiazepine use in SCRA intoxication has been associated with adverse cardiovascular effects and antipsychotics have not been associated with increased incidence of seizures.[15]

Management of SCRA-related psychosis

Psychotic symptoms are common aspects of SCRA intoxication and can outlast the acute intoxication phase in 30%.[16]

SCRA-associated psychosis:

- has more prominent positive symptoms than cannabis-related psychosis
- has less prominent negative symptoms than cannabis-related psychosis
- is less likely to have manic features
- is commonly associated with suicidal thinking
- psychiatric admission may be necessary to manage behavioural disturbance
- requires higher doses of antipsychotic than cannabis-related psychosis (mean dose equivalent to 11mg haloperidol, whereas in cannabis users mean dose was 6mg/day and those without either co-morbidity 3mg/day)[17]
- requires longer treatment than cannabis-related psychosis.

For the treatment of acute behavioural disturbance (ABD) caused by SCRAs, see section 'Acute Behavioural Disturbance (ABD) in acute admissions' in this chapter.

Management of SCRA dependence and withdrawal

SCRA dependence is reported in case studies and surveys and may be expected to occur at higher rates than dependence on cannabis given the higher potency of SCRA. Generic psychosocial addiction treatment approaches to SCRA dependence using motivational interviewing techniques and drug diaries with the aim to cut down slowly are recommended. Advising patients to switch to cannabis as a lower potency (and hence less harmful) alternative should be undertaken with caution given reports that cannabis does not alleviate SCRA withdrawal[18] and with the patient having a full understanding of the legal implications – possession of cannabis is an offence, whereas possession of most SCRAs is not.

Patients with months of daily use experience a physiological withdrawal syndrome, lasting several days, including the following:

- Disturbed sleep
- Strange dreams
- Restlessness
- Anxiety
- Craving
- Shivering
- Muscle twitching
- Increased heart rate and blood pressure

Treatment with benzodiazepines has been reported both to be effective and ineffective. Low-dose quetiapine (50mg) was effective in the case of benzodiazepine failure.[19]

References

1. Potts AJ, et al. Synthetic cannabinoid receptor agonists: classification and nomenclature. *Clin Toxicol (Phila)* 2020; **58**:82–98.

2. Alam RM, et al. Adding more 'spice' to the pot: A review of the chemistry and pharmacology of newly emerging heterocyclic synthetic cannabinoid receptor agonists. *Drug Test Anal* 2020; **12**:297–315.

3. Yoganathan P, et al. Synthetic cannabinoid-related deaths in England, 2012–2019. *OSF* 2020.

4. European Monitoring Centre for Drugs and Drug Addiction. Synthetic cannabinoids. 2020; https://www.emcdda.europa.eu/topics/synthetic-cannabinoids_en.

5. Abouchedid R, et al. Analytical confirmation of synthetic cannabinoids in a cohort of 179 presentations with acute recreational drug toxicity to an Emergency Department in London, UK in the first half of 2015. *Clin Toxicol (Phila)* 2017; **55**:338–345.

6. Fattore L. Synthetic cannabinoids – further evidence supporting the relationship between cannabinoids and psychosis. *Biol Psychiatry* 2016; **79**:539–548.

7. Tait RJ, et al. A systematic review of adverse events arising from the use of synthetic cannabinoids and their associated treatment. *Clin Toxicol (Phila)* 2016; **54**:1–13.

8. Hoyte CO, et al. A characterization of synthetic cannabinoid exposures reported to the National Poison Data System in 2010. *Ann Emerg Med* 2012; **60**:435–438.

9. Giorgetti A, et al. Post-mortem toxicology: a systematic review of death cases involving synthetic cannabinoid receptor agonists. *Front Psychiatry* 2020; **11**:464.

10. Hancox JC, et al. Synthetic cannabinoids and potential cardiac arrhythmia risk: an important message for drug users. *Ther Adv Drug Saf* 2020; **11**:2042098620913416.

11. Jones JD, et al. Can naloxone be used to treat synthetic cannabinoid overdose? *Biol Psychiatry* 2017; **81**:e51–e52.

12. Winstock A, et al. Risk of emergency medical treatment following consumption of cannabis or synthetic cannabinoids in a large global sample. *J Psychopharmacol* 2015; **29**:698–703.

13. Novel Psychoactive Treatment UK Network (NEPTUNE). Guidance on the clinical management of acute and chronic harms of club drugs and novel psychoactive substances 2015; http://neptune-clinical-guidance.co.uk/wp-content/uploads/2015/03/NEPTUNE-Guidance-March-2015.pdf.

14. Monte AA, et al. Characteristics and treatment of patients with clinical illness due to synthetic cannabinoid inhalation reported by medical toxicologists: a toxic database study. *J Med Toxicol* 2017; **13**:146–152.

15. Gurney SM, et al. Pharmacology, toxicology, and adverse effects of synthetic cannabinoid drugs. *Forensic Sci Rev* 2014; **26**:53–78.

16. Hobbs M, et al. Spicing it up – synthetic cannabinoid receptor agonists and psychosis - a systematic review. *Eur Neuropsychopharmacol* 2018; **28**:1289–1304.

17. Bassir Nia A, et al. Psychiatric comorbidity associated with synthetic cannabinoid use compared to cannabis. *J Psychopharmacol* 2016; **30**:1321–1330.

18. Nacca N, et al. The synthetic cannabinoid withdrawal syndrome. *J Addict Med* 2013; **7**:296–298.

19. Castaneto MS, et al. Synthetic cannabinoids: epidemiology, pharmacodynamics, and clinical implications. *Drug Alcohol Depend* 2014; **144**:12–41.

CHAPTER 4

Drug-induced acute behavioural disturbance (ABD) in acute admissions

ABD or 'excited delirium' is an under-recognised and potentially life-threatening syndrome of delirium, aggression and dysregulated physiological responses.[1] Illicit drugs are the most common cause, notably cocaine and new psychoactive stimulants (NPS) including synthetic cannabinoids ('spice') and stimulants such as mephedrone. Substance withdrawal and medical causes of delirium can also produce ABD.[2]

The aim of this section is to draw attention to the approach required for people whose behaviour presents a danger to themselves or others because of the acute effect of illicit substances. Neither 'acute behavioural disturbance' nor 'excited delirium' are recognised diagnoses, both terms are highly controversial, and their use in this section does not imply that there is an expected course to the conditions and situations potentially included under these terms. Specifically, physiological deterioration may or may not occur, but such deterioration is not definitively linked to behavioural change resulting from acute use of illicit substances or to the use of the substances themselves. Early intervention and de-escalation are crucial to effective and safe treatment. Physical restraint should be avoided where possible because of the substantial risk to life presented by such procedures in these patients.

Pathophysiology

Delirium produces disorientation and a 'fight or flight' response, and the physical exertion to 'escape' results in hyperthermia and catecholamine release.[3] Hyperthermia in turn leads to rhabdomyolysis (with raised creatine kinase),[4] as well as worsening delirium.[5] Excess sympathetic catecholamines prolong the cardiac QT interval and may 'stun' the myocardium.[6] Excess muscle activity, raised catecholamines, hyperthermia and dehydration contribute to a metabolic acidosis and the production of carbon dioxide. This manifests with tachypnoea and may herald pending cardiovascular collapse.

Identification

No symptoms are pathognomonic, but a prospective study found that the most common symptoms were violent behaviour, increased pain tolerance and constant activity.[7] Rapid breathing, a lack of fatigue, hyperpyrexia and tactile hyperthermia are also frequently reported.[8]

Management

Verbally de-escalate and try to ensure environmental safety for the individuals and others – standard delirium orientation cues may help. **Minimise physical contact** and be aware that restraint may exacerbate hyperthermia and catecholamine release, worsening outcomes.[9] Sedation is important to calm aggression and reduce perpetuating heat generation and catecholamine release. There is evidence to support IM use of: benzodiazepines, including diazepam, lorazepam, midazolam;[10] antipsychotics, including haloperidol, droperidol, olanzapine and chlorpromazine;[10,11,] and their combination.[12] Caution is required because of the risk of neuroleptic malignant syndrome.

Record pulse, blood pressure and temperature, where safe to do so. Urinary drug screens typically have limited validity for NPS but many clinical laboratories can identify causative compounds. An ECG is unlikely to be viable until individuals have been sedated. Full assessment and treatment requires urgent ambulance transfer to an emergency department (ED).[13] Psychiatric nursing might be required to contain and support the individual. In the ED, IM ketamine is the preferred sedative, with a predictable dose–response effect at 2–4mg/kg.[14] Antipyretics are ineffective cooling agents, and cooled IV fluids, water sprays and ice to the whole body may be required.

Outcomes

Mortality rates are not known with the only source of data available being non-scientific observations[15]. Physiological deterioration associated with NPS use is sometimes missed or not anticipated. Risk of death is related to the duration of hyperthermia and peak temperature reached: temperatures over 42°C usually have very poor outcomes. Body mass index >25kg/m^2 is associated with worse outcomes. In non-fatal instances, most cases are brief, and fully resolve within 48 hours, but longer term cardiac, renal and hepatic damage can occur.

References

1. Tracy DK, et al. Acute behavioural disturbance: a physical emergency psychiatrists need to understand. *B J Psych Advances* 2020:1–10

2. Kennedy DB, et al. Delayed in-custody death involving excited delirium. *J Correct Health Care* 2018; 24:43–51.

3. Bunai Y, et al. Fatal hyperthermia associated with excited delirium during an arrest. *Leg Med (Tokyo)* 2008; 10:306–309.

4. Borek HA, et al. Hyperthermia and multiorgan failure after abuse of 'bath salts' containing 3,4-methylenedioxypyrovalerone. *Ann Emerg Med* 2012; 60:103–105.

5. Otahbachi M, et al. Excited delirium, restraints, and unexpected death: a review of pathogenesis. *Am J Forensic Med Pathol* 2010; 31:107–112.

6. Wittstein IS, et al. Neurohumoral features of myocardial stunning due to sudden emotional stress. *N Engl J Med* 2005; 352:539–548.

7. Hall CA, et al. Frequency of signs of excited delirium syndrome in subjects undergoing police use of force: descriptive evaluation of a prospective, consecutive cohort. *J Forensic Leg Med* 2013; 20:102–107.

8. Baldwin S, et al. Distinguishing features of excited delirium syndrome in non-fatal use of force encounters. *J Forensic Leg Med* 2016; 41:21–27.

9. Stratton SJ, et al. Factors associated with sudden death of individuals requiring restraint for excited delirium. *Am J Emerg Med* 2001; 19:187–191.

10. Isbister GK, et al. Randomized controlled trial of intramuscular droperidol versus midazolam for violence and acute behavioral disturbance: the DORM study. *Ann Emerg Med* 2010; 56:392–401 e391.

11. Page CB, et al. A prospective study of the safety and effectiveness of droperidol in children for prehospital acute behavioral disturbance. *Prehosp Emerg Care* 2019; 23:519–526.

12. O'Connor N, et al. Pharmacological management of acute severe behavioural disturbance: a survey of current protocols. *Aust Psychiatry* 2017; 25:395–398.

13. Wetli CV, et al. Cocaine-associated agitated delirium and the neuroleptic malignant syndrome. *Am J Emerg Med* 1996; 14:425–428.

14. Li M, et al. Evaluation of ketamine for excited delirium syndrome in the adult emergency department. *J Emerg Med* 2019.

15. Baldwin S, et al. Excited delirium syndrome (ExDS): situational factors and risks to officer safety in non-fatal use of force encounters. *Int J Law Psychiatry* 2018; 60:26–34.

CHAPTER 4

Interactions between 'street drugs' and prescribed psychotropic drugs

Potential interactions between drugs of misuse and prescribed psychotropics are common, not least because of the high rates of psychotropic prescribing in such patients.[1] Information on adverse interactions is derived largely from case reports and theoretical assumptions and rarely from systematic investigation. A summary of major interactions can be found in Table 4.21.

In all patients who misuse street drugs:

- Infection with hepatitis B and C is common. The associated liver damage may lead to a reduced ability to metabolise other drugs and increased sensitivity to adverse effects.
- Infection with HIV is common.[2,3] Antiretroviral drugs are involved in pharmacokinetic interactions with a number of prescribed and non-prescribed drugs.[4] For example, ritonavir can decrease the metabolism of ecstasy and precipitate toxicity, and a number of antiretrovirals can increase or decrease methadone metabolism.[5]
- Prescribed drugs may be used in the same way as illicit drugs (i.e. erratically and not as intended). Large quantities of prescribed drugs should not be given to outpatients.
- Additive or synergistic effects of respiratory depressants may play a contributory role in deaths from overdose with methadone or other opioid agonists.[6] Caution is needed in prescribing sedative medicines such as benzodiazepines.

Table 4.21 Interactions between 'street drugs' and psychotropics

	Cannabis	Heroin/methadone[6]	Cocaine, amfetamine, ecstasy, MDA, 6-APD	Alcohol	Ketamine[7]
General considerations	■ Usually smoked in cigarettes (induces CYP1A2) ■ Can be sedative ■ Dose-related tachycardia ■ THC/CBD inhibit CYP3A4 and CYP2C19 and CYP2D6[8,9]	■ Can produce sedation/respiratory depression ■ QTc prolongation with methadone (see section 'Methadone')	■ Stimulants (cocaine can be sedative in higher doses) ■ Arrhythmia possible ■ Cerebral/cardiac ischaemia with cocaine – may be fatal ■ MDMA (3,4-methylenedioxymethamphetamine) inhibits CYPs 2D6/3A4 ■ Hyperthermia/dehydration with ecstasy[10]	■ Sedative ■ Liver damage possible ■ Induces various enzymes	■ Sedative readily causes unconsciousness ■ Onset of effects may be rapid if snorted or injected
Older antipsychotics	■ Antipsychotics reduce the psychotropic effects of almost all drugs of abuse by blocking dopamine receptors (dopamine is the neurotransmitter responsible for 'reward', e.g. haloperidol and MDMA[11]) ■ Patients prescribed antipsychotics may increase their consumption of illicit substances to compensate ■ Patients who have taken ecstasy may be more prone to EPS ■ Cardiotoxic or very sedative antipsychotics are best avoided, at least initially. Sulpiride is a reasonably safe first choice ■ Methamphetamines increase the risk of EPS with haloperidol[12]				
Second-generation antipsychotics	■ Risk of additive sedation ■ Cannabis smoking in tobacco can reduce plasma levels of olanzapine and clozapine via induction of CYP1A2[13] ■ Clozapine might reduce cannabis and alcohol consumption[14] ■ Outcome of THC/CBD inhibition of CYP1A2 unknown	■ Risk of additive sedation ■ Case report of methadone withdrawal being precipitated by risperidone[15] ■ Isolated report of quetiapine increasing methadone levels, especially in those with slowed CYP2D6 hepatic metabolism[16]	■ Antipsychotics may reduce craving and cocaine-induced euphoria[17-21] ■ Olanzapine may worsen cocaine dependency[22] ■ Clozapine may increase cocaine levels but diminish subjective response[23]	■ Increased risk of hypotension with olanzapine (and possibly other β-blockers)	■ Increased sedation

(Continued)

Table 4.21 (Continued)

	Cannabis	Heroin/methadone[6]	Cocaine, amfetamine, ecstasy, MDA, 6-APD	Alcohol	Ketamine[7]
Antidepressants	■ Tachycardia has been reported (monitor pulse and take care with TCAs)[24] ■ Complex, unpredictable effects of CYP induction (tobacco) and CYP inhibition (THC/CBD)	■ Avoid very sedative antidepressants ■ Some SSRIs can increase methadone plasma levels[25] (citalopram is SSRI of choice but note the small risk of additive QTc prolongation) ■ Case report of serotonin syndrome occurring when sertraline prescribed with methadone for a palliative care patient[26]	■ Avoid TCAs (arrhythmia risk) ■ MAOIs contraindicated (hypertension) ■ Combining moclobemide and MDMA can be fatal[27] ■ SSRIs may increase plasma concentrations of MDMA[28] but reduce subjective effects[29] ■ Risk of SSRIs increasing cocaine levels, especially fluoxetine[30] ■ Concomitant use of SSRIs or aripiprazole and lamotrigine with cocaine or other stimulants (especially MDA and 6-APD) could precipitate a serotonin syndrome[31,32] ■ SSRIs may enhance subjective reaction to cocaine[33]	■ Avoid very sedative antidepressants ■ Avoid antidepressants that are toxic in OD ■ Impaired psychomotor skills (not SSRIs)	■ Inhibitors of CYP3A4 (e.g. fluoxetine/paroxetine) will lengthen ketamine half-life ■ Beware of hypertension with SNRIs and reboxetine
Anticholinergics	■ Misuse is likely. Try to avoid if at all possible (by using a second-generation drug if an antipsychotic is required) ■ Can cause hallucinations, elation and cognitive impairment				
Lithium	■ Very toxic if taken erratically ■ Always consider the effects of dehydration (particularly problematic with alcohol or ecstasy)				
Carbamazepine (CBZ)/valproate	■ CBZ may decrease THC concentrations via induction of CYP3A4[34]	■ CBZ decreases methadone levels[35] (danger if CBZ stopped suddenly) ■ Valproate seems less likely to interact	■ CBZ induces CYP3A4, which leads to more rapid formation of norcocaine (hepatotoxic and more cardiotoxic than cocaine)[36]	■ Monitor LFTs	■ CBZ decreases ketamine plasma concentrations via CYP3A4 induction
Benzodiazepines	■ Monitor level of sedation	■ Oversedation (and respiratory depression possible) ■ Concomitant use can lead to accidental overdose ■ Possible pharmacokinetic interaction (increased methadone levels)	■ Oversedation (if high doses of cocaine have been taken) ■ Widely used after cocaine intoxication ■ Future misuse possible detoxification	■ Oversedation (and respiratory depression) possible ■ Widely used in alcohol detoxification	■ Oversedation and respiratory depression

References

1. Zapelini Do Nascimento D, et al. Potential psychotropic drug interactions among drug-dependent people. *J Psychoactive Drugs* 2020; 1–9.

2. Vocci FJ, et al. Medication development for addictive disorders: the state of the science. *Am J Psychiatry* 2005; **162**:1432–1440.

3. Tsuang J, et al. Pharmacological treatment of patients with schizophrenia and substance abuse disorders. *Addict Disord Their Treatment* 2005; **4**:127–137.

4. Bracchi M, et al. Increasing use of 'party drugs' in people living with HIV on antiretrovirals: a concern for patient safety. *AIDS* 2015; **29**:1585–1592.

5. Gruber VA, et al. Methadone, buprenorphine, and street drug interactions with antiretroviral medications. *Curr HIV/AIDS Rep* 2010; **7**:152–160.

6. Department of Health and Social Care. Drug misuse and dependence: UK guidelines on clinical management. 2017; https://www.gov.uk/government/publications/drug-misuse-and-dependence-uk-guidelines-on-clinical-management.

7. Pfizer Limited. Summary of product characteristics. Ketalar 10 mg/ml Injection. 2020; https://www.medicines.org.uk/emc/medicine/12939.

8. Arellano AL, et al. Neuropsychiatric and general interactions of natural and synthetic cannabinoids with drugs of abuse and medicines. *CNS Neurol Disord Drug Targets* 2017; **16**:554–566.

9. Abbott KL, et al. Adverse pharmacokinetic interactions between illicit substances and clinical drugs. *Drug Metab Rev* 2020; **52**:44–65.

10. Gowing LR, et al. The health effects of ecstasy: a literature review. *Drug Alcohol Rev* 2002; **21**:53–63.

11. Liechti ME, et al. Acute psychological and physiological effects of MDMA ("Ecstasy") after haloperidol pretreatment in healthy humans. *Eur Neuropsychopharmacol* 2000; **10**:289–295.

12. Matthew BJ, et al. Drug-induced parkinsonism following chronic methamphetamine use by a patient on haloperidol decanoate. *Int J Psychiatry Med* 2015; **50**:405–411.

13. Zullino DF, et al. Tobacco and cannabis smoking cessation can lead to intoxication with clozapine or olanzapine. *Int Clin Psychopharmacol* 2002; **17**:141–143.

14. Green AI, et al. Alcohol and cannabis use in schizophrenia: effects of clozapine vs. risperidone. *Schizophr Res* 2003; **60**:81–85.

15. Wines JD, Jr., et al. Opioid withdrawal during risperidone treatment. *J Clin Psychopharmacol* 1999; **19**:265–267.

16. Uehlinger C, et al. Increased (R)-methadone plasma concentrations by quetiapine in cytochrome P450s and ABCB1 genotyped patients. *J Clin Psychopharmacol* 2007; **27**:273–278.

17. Poling J, et al. Risperidone for substance dependent psychotic patients. *Addict Disord Treat* 2005; **4**:1–3.

18. Albanese MJ, et al. Risperidone in cocaine-dependent patients with comorbid psychiatric disorders. *J Psychiatr Pract* 2006; **12**:306–311.

19. Sattar SP, et al. Potential benefits of quetiapine in the treatment of substance dependence disorders. *J Psychiatry Neurosci* 2004; **29**:452–457.

20. Grabowski J, et al. Risperidone for the treatment of cocaine dependence: randomized, double-blind trial. *J Clin Psychopharmacol* 2000; **20**:305–310.

21. Kishi T, et al. Antipsychotics for cocaine or psychostimulant dependence: systematic review and meta-analysis of randomized, placebo-controlled trials. *J Clin Psychiatry* 2013; **74**:e1169–e1180.

22. Kampman KM, et al. A pilot trial of olanzapine for the treatment of cocaine dependence. *Drug Alcohol Depend* 2003; **70**:265–273.

23. Farren CK, et al. Significant interaction between clozapine and cocaine in cocaine addicts. *Drug Alcohol Depend* 2000; **59**:153–163.

24. Benowitz NL, et al. Effects of delta-9-tetrahydrocannabinol on drug distribution and metabolism. Antipyrine, pentobarbital, and ethanol. *Clin Pharmacol Ther* 1977; **22**:259–268.

25. Hemeryck A, et al. Selective serotonin reuptake inhibitors and cytochrome P-450 mediated drug-drug interactions: an update. *Curr Drug Metabol* 2002; **3**:13–37.

26. Bush E, et al. A case of serotonin syndrome and mutism associated with methadone. *J Palliat Med* 2006; **9**:1257–1259.

27. Vuori E, et al. Death following ingestion of MDMA (ecstasy) and moclobemide. *Addiction* 2003; **98**:365–368.

28. Rietjens SJ, et al. Pharmacokinetics and pharmacodynamics of 3,4-methylenedioxymethamphetamine (MDMA): interindividual differences due to polymorphisms and drug-drug interactions. *Crit Rev Toxicol* 2012; **42**:854–876.

29. Papaseit E, et al. MDMA interactions with pharmaceuticals and drugs of abuse. *Expert Opin Drug Metab Toxicol* 2020; **16**:357–369.

30. Fletcher PJ, et al. Fluoxetine, but not sertraline or citalopram, potentiates the locomotor stimulant effect of cocaine: possible pharmacokinetic effects. *Psychopharmacology* 2004; **174**:406–413.

31. Silins E, et al. Qualitative review of serotonin syndrome, ecstasy (MDMA) and the use of other serotonergic substances: hierarchy of risk. *Aust N Z J Psychiatry* 2007; **41**:649–655.

32. Kotwal A, et al. Serotonin syndrome in the setting of lamotrigine, aripiprazole, and cocaine use. *Case Rep Med* 2015; **2015**:769531.

33. Soto PL, et al. Citalopram enhances cocaine's subjective effects in rats. *Behav Pharmacol* 2009; **20**:759–762.

34. GW Pharma Ltd. Summary of product characteristics. Sativex oromucosal spray. 2020; https://www.medicines.org.uk/emc/product/602.

35. Miller BL, et al. Neuropsychiatric effects of cocaine: SPECT measurements. in A Paredes, Gorelick, eds. Cocaine: physiological and physiopathological effects. 1st edition. New York: Haworth Press 1993; 47–58.

36. Roldan CJ, et al. Toxicity, cocaine. 2004. http://www.emedicine.com/med/topic400.htm.

CHAPTER 4

Drugs of misuse – a summary

Urine testing for illicit drugs is routine on many psychiatric wards and in outpatients and doctors' offices. It is important to be aware of the duration of detection of drugs in urine and of other commonly used substances and drugs that can give a false-positive result. Some false positives are unpredictable (i.e. not related to chemical similarity), for example, amisulpride can give a false positive for buprenorphine.[1] False positive results are most likely with point-of-care immunoassay kits. If a positive result has implications for a patient's liberty, and the patient denies use of substances, a second sample should be sent to the laboratory for definitive testing by liquid chromatography and mass spectrometry (LC-MS).

Table 4.22 Basic summary of drugs of misuse

Drug	Physical signs/ symptoms of intoxication	Most common mental state changes[2]	Withdrawal symptoms	Duration of withdrawal	Duration of detection in the urine[3,4]	Other substances that give a positive urine test result[5-7]
Amfetamine type stimulants[8]	Tachycardia, increased BP, anorexia, tremor, restlessness	Visual/tactile/ olfactory auditory hallucinations, paranoia, elation	Fatigue, hunger, depression, irritability, craving, social withdrawal	Peaks 7–34 hours; lasts maximum of 5 days	Depends on half-life, mostly 48–72 hours	Cough and decongestant preparations, bupropion, chloroquine, chlorpromazine, labetalol, promethazine, ranitidine, selegiline, large quantities of tyramine, tranylcypromine, trazodone and many others Desvenlafaxine may give a positive result for phencyclidine[9]
GHB/GBL	Drowsiness, coma, disinhibition	Sociability, confidence	Tremor, tachycardia, paranoia, delirium, psychosis, visual/ tactile/olfactory/ auditory hallucinations	3–4 days	Difficult to detect, not routinely screened for	Not known Usually (and reliably) measured by LC-MS[10]
Benzodiazepines	Sedation, disinhibition	Relaxation, visual hallucinations, disorientation, sleep disturbance	Anxiety, insomnia, delirium, seizures, visual/tactile/ olfactory auditory hallucinations, psychosis	Usually short-lived but may last weeks to months	Up to 28 days: depending on half-life of drug taken	Nefopam, sertraline, zopiclone, efavirenz
Cannabis[11-17]	Tachycardia, lack of co-ordination, red eyes, postural hypotension	Elation, psychosis, perceptual distortions, disturbance of memory/judgement, twofold increase in risk of developing schizophrenia	Restlessness, irritability, insomnia, anxiety	Uncertain Probably less than 1 month (longer in heavy users)	Single use: 3 days; chronic heavy use: up to 30 days	Passive 'smoking' of cannabis Efavirenz, ibuprofen, naproxen

(Continued)

Table 4.22 (Continued)

Drug	Physical signs/symptoms of intoxication	Most common mental state changes[2]	Withdrawal symptoms	Duration of withdrawal	Duration of detection in the urine[3,4]	Other substances that give a positive urine test result[5-7]
Synthetic cannabinoid receptor agonists (SCRAs)	Tachycardia, hypertension, red eyes, agitation	Anxiety, agitation, aggression, psychotic symptoms, clouded consciousness	Anxiety, sleep disturbance, headache	Uncertain	Difficult to detect using conventional screening methods because of chemical heterogeneity	Too chemically diverse for urine screens, e.g. AB-fubinaca, ADB-fubinaca AB-chminaca 3-methylbutanoic acid, ADB-chminaca and 5-fluoro-PB-22 are all grouped as SCRAs. Best detected and measured by LC-MS[18]
Cocaine	Tachycardia/tachypnoea, increased BP/headache, respiratory, depression, chest pain	Euphoria, paranoid psychosis, panic attacks/anxiety, insomnia/excitement	Fatigue, hunger, depression, irritability, craving, social withdrawal	12–18 hours	Up to 96 hours	Food/tea containing coca leaves Codeine Ephedrine/pseudoepledrine
Heroin	Pinpoint pupils, clammy skin, respiratory depression	Drowsiness, euphoria, hallucinations	Dilated pupils, nausea, diarrhoea, generalised pains, gooseflesh, runny nose/eyes	Peaks after 36–72 hours	Up to 72 hours	Diphenoxylate, naltrexone, naloxone, opiate analgesics, food/tea containing poppy seed, amisulpride, diphenhydramine, 4-quinolones, tramadol
Methadone	Pinpoint pupils, respiratory depression, pulmonary oedema	As above	As above but milder and longer lasting	Peaks after 4–6 days, can last 6 weeks	Up to 7 days with chronic use	Quetiapine

Table 4.22 (Continued)

Ketamine[19-22]	Increased heart rate, increased BP, palpitations, dizziness, abdominal discomfort, lower urinary tract symptoms, ataxia	Impaired consciousness, dissociation, hallucinations, ego diffusion	Fatigue, poor appetite, drowsiness, craving, anxiety, dysphoria, restlessness, palpitations, tremor, sweating	48 hours	Ketamine – up to 2 days Norketamine – up to 14 days	Quetiapine
LSD[23]	Variable Dilated pupils Moderate increase in HR and BP, flushing, sweating, hypersalivation, increased tendon reflexes	Euphoria, introspection, illusions, pseudo-hallucinations, altered sense of time, altered thought processes, altered perception of body, vivid recollections of significant memories	None	N/A	Up to 4 days	Ambroxol, amitriptyline, brompheniramine, bupropion, buspirone, cephadrine, chlorpromazine, desipramine, diltiazem, doxepin, ergonovine, fentanyl, fluoxetine, haloperidol, imipramine, labetalol, lysergol, methylphenidate, metoclopramide, prochlorperaxine, risperidone, sertraline, thioridazine, trazodone, verapamil

This table is a basic summary.
For more detail on cross-reacting substances in urine testing, see Moeller et al.[24]
BP, blood pressure; GHB/GBL, gamma-hydroxybutyrate/gamma-butyrolactone; HR, heart rate; LSD, lysergic acid diethylamide; N/A, not applicable

References

1. Couchman L, et al. Amisulpride and sulpiride interfere in the C&DIA DAU buprenorphine test. *Ann Clin Psychiatry* 2008; 45 Suppl 1.
2. Truven Health Analytics. Micromedex 2.0. 2017; https://www.micromedexsolutions.com/home/dispatch.
3. Substance Abuse and Mental Health Services Administration (US). Substance abuse: clinical issues in intensive outpatient treatment. Treatment Improvement Protocol (TIP) Series, No. 47. 2006.
4. Mayo Medical Laboratories. Approximate Detection Times. 2016; http://www.mayomedicallaboratories.com/test-info/drug-book/viewall.html.
5. Brahm NC, et al. Commonly prescribed medications and potential false-positive urine drug screens. *Am J Health Syst Pharm* 2010; 67:1344–1350.
6. Saitman A, et al. False-positive interferences of common urine drug screen immunoassays: a review. *J Anal Toxicol* 2014; 38:387–396.
7. Liu CH, et al. False positive ketamine urine immunoassay screen result induced by quetiapine: A case report. *J Formos Med Assoc* 2017; 116:720–722.
8. Shoptaw SJ, et al. Treatment for amphetamine psychosis. *Cochrane Database Syst Rev* 2009; CD003026.
9. Farley TM, et al. False-positive phencyclidine (PCP) on urine drug screen attributed to desvenlafaxine (Pristiq) use. *BMJ Case Rep* 2017; 2017:bcr-2017-222106.
10. Busardò FP, et al. Ultra-high performance liquid chromatography tandem mass spectrometry (UHPLC-MS/MS) for determination of GHB, precursors and metabolites in different specimens: application to clinical and forensic cases. *J Pharm Biomed Anal* 2017; 137:123–131.
11. Johns A. Psychiatric effects of cannabis. *Br J Psychiatry* 2001; 178:116–122.
12. Hall W, et al. Long-term cannabis use and mental health. *Br J Psychiatry* 1997; 171:107–108.
13. Murray RM, et al. Traditional marijuana, high-potency cannabis and synthetic cannabinoids: increasing risk for psychosis. *World Psychiatry* 2016; 15:195–204.
14. Marconi A, et al. Meta-analysis of the association between the level of cannabis use and risk of psychosis. *Schizophr Bull* 2016; 42:1262–1269.
15. Arseneault L, et al. Causal association between cannabis and psychosis: examination of the evidence. *Br J Psychiatry* 2004; 184:110–117.
16. Budney AJ, et al. Review of the validity and significance of cannabis withdrawal syndrome. *Am J Psychiatry* 2004; 161:1967–1977.
17. Bonnet U, et al. The cannabis withdrawal syndrome: current insights. *Subst Abuse Rehabil* 2017; 8:9–37.
18. Tebo C, et al. Suspected synthetic cannabinoid receptor agonist intoxication: does analysis of samples reflect the presence of suspected agents? *Am J Emerg Med* 2019; 37:1846–1849.
19. Novel Psychoactive Treatment UK Network (NEPTUNE). Guidance on the clinical management of acute and chronic harms of club drugs and novel psychoactive substances. 2015; http://neptune-clinical-guidance.co.uk/wp-content/uploads/2015/03/NEPTUNE-Guidance-March-2015.pdf.
20. Chen WY, et al. Gender differences in subjective discontinuation symptoms associated with ketamine use. *Subst Abuse Treatment Prev Policy* 2014; 9:39.
21. Critchlow DG. A case of ketamine dependence with discontinuation symptoms. *Addiction* 2006; 101:1212–1213.
22. Adamowicz P, et al. Urinary excretion rates of ketamine and norketamine following therapeutic ketamine administration: method and detection window considerations. *J Anal Toxicol* 2005; 29:376–382.
23. Passie T, et al. The pharmacology of lysergic acid diethylamide: a review. *CNS Neurosci Ther* 2008; 14:295–314.
24. Moeller KE, et al. Clinical interpretation of urine drug tests: what clinicians need to know about urine drug screens. *Mayo Clin Proc* 2017; 92:774–796.

Substance misuse in pregnancy[1]

Substance misuse during pregnancy has numerous adverse effects. These include low birthweight and prematurity,[2] various neonatal withdrawal syndromes and a range of developmental, emotional and behavioural problems in offspring.[3]

Alcohol

Consumption of alcohol during pregnancy is well known to have profound consequences on offspring. Pregnant women who misuse alcohol should be encouraged to cease alcohol intake and to have withdrawal symptoms managed with benzodiazepines, preferably as inpatients.[4]

Acamprosate, disulfiram and naltrexone are not proven to be safe in pregnancy but their use may be preferred to the higher risk of relapse in untreated individuals (also see section 'Alcohol dependence' in this chapter).

Tobacco

Patients should be encouraged to cease smoking completely as continuing to smoke increases the risk of miscarriage, prematurity and stillbirth.[5] Vaping may be preferred but its safety is not established. NICE recommends NRT.[6] Bupropion and varenicline are not recommended.

Opioids (see longer pregnancy in section 'Opioid dependence' in this chapter).

Use of opioids during pregnancy may not be directly teratogenic but the risk of NAS exceeds 70% in regular users.[7]

The use of prescribed methadone or buprenorphine is preferred to illicit opioid misuse because it offers the possibility of dose decrease and reduces the harms associated with illicit use. Even when dose decreases are not possible the use of these replacements reduces the risk of premature birth.

Methadone requirements may increase in the third trimester, presumably because of an increased volume of distribution. There is mounting evidence that buprenorphine use produces less severe NAS than methadone.[8,9]

Most authorities recommend that withdrawal from opiates should not normally be attempted in pregnant women.[4,10] Women on stable opioid replacement treatment should generally be encouraged to breast feed and to carefully wean off their babies after several weeks.

Cannabis and synthetic cannabinoid receptor agonists

Use of cannabis during pregnancy is linked to a wide range of adverse outcomes in pregnancy and in the offspring.[11] Abstinence should be encouraged. There are no pharmacological treatments currently available.

Benzodiazepines

The safety of benzodiazepines in pregnancy is not clearly established (see Chapter 7). Third trimester use is well known to cause 'floppy baby syndrome'.

CHAPTER 4

Most guidelines[3,9] recommend that benzodiazepines be slowly withdrawn using long-acting drugs such as diazepam and that inpatient detoxification be considered.

Stimulants

Use of cocaine and amfetamines is associated with a range of congenital abnormalities and both prematurity and low birthweight. There are no effective pharmacological interventions, and detoxification is the primary aim, possibly as an inpatient.[4]

References

1. Wilson CA, et al. Alcohol, smoking, and other substance use in the perinatal period. *BMJ* 2020; 369:m1627–m1627.
2. Mayet S, et al. Drugs and pregnancy – outcomes of women engaged with a specialist perinatal outreach addictions service. *Drug Alcohol Rev* 2008; 27:497–503.
3. Kaltenbach K, et al. Neonatal abstinence syndrome, pharmacotherapy and developmental outcome. *Neurobehav Toxicol Teratol* 1986; 8:353–355.
4. World Health Organisation. WHO guidelines approved by the guidelines review committee. Guidelines for the identification and management of substance use and substance use disorders in pregnancy. Geneva. 2014.
5. Cohen A, et al. Substance misuse in pregnancy. *Obstetr Gynaecol Reprod Med* 2017; 27:316–321.
6. National Institute for Clinical Excellence. Pregnancy and complex social factors: a model for service provision for pregnant women with complex social factors. Clinical guideline [CG110]. 2010 (last checked August 2018); https://www.nice.org.uk/Guidance/CG110.
7. Winklbaur B, et al. Treating pregnant women dependent on opioids is not the same as treating pregnancy and opioid dependence: a knowledge synthesis for better treatment for women and neonates. *Addiction* 2008; 103:1429–1440.
8. Jones HE, et al. Maternal Opioid Treatment: Human Experimental Research (MOTHER)–approach, issues and lessons learned. *Addiction* 2012; 107 Suppl 1:28–35.
9. U.S. Department of Health & Human Services. Substance Abuse and Mental Health Services Administration (SAMHSA). 2020; https://www.samhsa.gov.
10. McAllister-Williams RH, et al. British Association for Psychopharmacology consensus guidance on the use of psychotropic medication preconception, in pregnancy and postpartum 2017. *J Psychopharmacol* 2017; 31:519–552.
11. Jansson LM, et al. Perinatal marijuana use and the developing child. *JAMA* 2018; 320:545–546.

Part 2

Drug treatment of special patient groups

Children and adolescents

Principles of prescribing practice in childhood and adolescence

- **Target symptoms, not diagnoses**
  Diagnosis can be difficult in children and co-morbidity is very common. Treatment should target key symptoms. While a working diagnosis is beneficial to frame expectations and help communication with patients and parents, it should be kept in mind that it could take some time for the illness to evolve.
- **Technical aspects of paediatric prescribing**
  The Medicines Act 1968 and European legislation make provision for doctors to use medicines in an off-label or out-of-licence capacity or to use unlicensed medicines. However, individual prescribers are always responsible for ensuring that there is adequate information to support the quality, efficacy, safety and intended use of a drug before prescribing it. It is recognised that the informed use of unlicensed medicines, or of licensed medicines for unlicensed applications ('off-label' use), is often necessary in paediatric practice.
  - Prescription writing in the UK: Inclusion of age is a legal requirement in the case of prescription-only medicines for children under 12 years of age, but it is preferable to state the age for all prescriptions for children.
- **Begin with less, go slow and monitor efficacy and adverse reactions**
  In outpatient care, dosage will usually commence lower in mg/kg per day terms than adults. Gradually increase dose as needed, and finish at a dose that produces adequate symptom control with minimum adverse reactions (adverse reactions are more common in children and adolescents). In routine clinical care, regular monitoring of efficacy and adverse reactions is essential, in order to ensure that treatment is necessary and that it should continue.
- **Multiple medications are often required in the severely ill**
  Monotherapy is ideal. However, childhood-onset illness can be severe and may require treatment with psychosocial approaches in combination with more than one medication. Co-pharmacy is using different medications for different disorders or

The Maudsley® Prescribing Guidelines in Psychiatry, Fourteenth Edition. David M. Taylor,
Thomas R. E. Barnes and Allan H. Young.
© 2021 David M. Taylor. Published 2021 by John Wiley & Sons Ltd.

symptoms, while poly-pharmacy is the use of multiple medications to manage the same problem. As children often have multiple co-occurring conditions, co-pharmacy is common.

- **Allow time for an adequate trial of treatment**
  Children are generally more ill than their adult counterparts and will often require longer periods of treatment before responding. An adequate trial of treatment for those who have required in-patient care may well be 8 weeks for depression or schizophrenia.

- **Where possible, change one drug at a time**
  Make changes to one drug at a time and attempt to remove a drug when adding a new drug, if possible.

- **Monitor outcome in more than one setting**
  For symptomatic treatments (such as stimulants for attention deficit hyperactivity disorder [ADHD]), bear in mind that the expression of problems may be different across settings (e.g. home and school); a dose titrated against parent reports may be too high for the daytime at school.

- **Patient and family medication education is essential**
  For some child and adolescent psychiatric patients the need for medication will be life-long. The first experiences with medications are therefore crucial to long-term outcomes and adherence. Education regarding the problems, medication, adverse reactions and medication adherence should be addressed. Patients and their guardians should be encouraged to ask for changes to their treatment regimen.

Detailed sources

For detailed description of prescribing and adverse effects of CNS Drugs in Children and Adolescents, see:

British Medical Association et al. *British National Formulary for Children 2020/2021* (September 2020). London: Pharmaceutical Press; 2020.

Elbe D, et al. *Clinical Handbook of Psychotropic Drugs for Children and Adolescents*. 4th revised edn. Oxford, UK: Hogrefe Publishing; 2019.

Gerlach M, et al. *Psychiatric Drugs in Children and Adolescents. Basic Pharmacology and Practical Applications*. Vienna: Springer-Verlag Wien; 2014.

Martin A, et al. *Pediatric Psychopharmacology: Principles and Practice*. Second Edition. New York, USA: Oxford University Press; 2011.

Depression in children and adolescents

Diagnostic issues

Approximately 15% of young people experience depression by age 18 and these young people often have significant functional impairment and risk of harm.[1] Compared to depressed adults, young people with depression tend to experience more irritability, loss of energy, insomnia and weight change, and less anhedonia and concentration problems.[2] These symptoms can overlap with and appear similar to other disorders, or can be minimised and incorrectly attributed to typical teenage development, making diagnosis challenging. Assessments should therefore be undertaken by clinicians who understand developmental variations and can accurately identify depression in young people.[3]

Clinical guidance

For mild depression in children and adolescents, the UK National Institute for Health and Care Excellence (NICE) guidelines[4] and American Academy of Child and Adolescent Psychiatry (AACAP) practice parameter[3] recommend that supportive care or psychological intervention should be considered as first-line treatment, and that antidepressant medication should not be prescribed.

For moderate to severe depression in young people, these guidelines recommend offering psychological therapy, either alone or in combination with antidepressant medication. In addition, the ACAPP practice parameter recommends that antidepressant medication alone could be considered, particularly if the presentation is severe and the patient is unable to engage in talking therapy, if psychological interventions are not available, or if this is the patient's and family's preference.

These guidelines relating to antidepressant medications were mainly informed by three large randomised controlled trials, which found evidence for the effectiveness of selective serotonin reuptake inhibitors (SSRIs) in treating depression in young people: the Treatment of Adolescents with Depression Study (TADS),[5] Treatment of Resistant Depression in Adolescents (TORDIA),[6] and Adolescent Depression Antidepressants and Psychotherapy Trial (ADAPT).[7] For example, TADS found a fluoxetine response rate of 61% over the acute (12-week) phase, which was significantly higher than the placebo response rate of 35%, giving a number needed to treat (NNT) of 4.[5] Subsequent systematic reviews and meta-analyses, which include these trials and others, have provided further evidence demonstrating that SSRIs are effective and largely acceptable treatments for depression in young people.[8,9] Most studies found relatively modest effects, giving an NNT of 10 in a meta-analysis,[10] possibly because of high placebo response rates.[11]

The current evidence base is unclear about whether SSRI medications alone, psychological therapy alone, or combined treatment is most effective for treating depression in children and adolescents. TADS found that fluoxetine alone or in combination CBT might accelerate treatment response, and that adding CBT might decrease adverse effects including suicidality, so enhancing the safety of fluoxetine.[5,12] However, other studies have not replicated this finding,[7] and meta-analyses have found only limited evidence that combination therapy is more effective than antidepressant medication alone for the young people included in the trials.[13,14]

CHAPTER 5

Prescribing for depression in children and adolescents

Before prescribing

- Undertake a comprehensive assessment: Establish a clinical diagnosis of depression. Exclude differential diagnoses, including psychiatric disorders (such as bipolar affective disorder) medical disorders (such as endocrine disorders) and medication-related effects (such as steroid adverse effects). Identify any comorbid psychiatric or medical conditions. Consider contraindications to SSRIs and potential interactions. Assess the risk of harm to self and others. Formulate considering factors that could predispose, precipitate and perpetuate depression, such as family history of psychiatric disorders (including depression and bipolar affective disorder) and environmental stressors (including victimisation and other adverse experiences). If any co-occurring problems are identified, these should be addressed and prioritised based on a comprehensive formulation.
- Measure baseline severity: Measures of depression symptoms include the clinician-administered Children's Depression Rating Scale-Revised (CDRS-R)[15,16] and the child and parent-reported Mood and Feelings Questionnaire (MFQ)[17] or Revised Children's Anxiety and Depression Scale (RCADS).[18] Measures of functional impairment include the Children's Global Assessment Scale (CGAS).[19]
- Obtain informed consent: Discuss the nature, course and treatment of depression, potential adverse effects of medication, delay in onset of treatment effects, plan for monitoring and maintenance of medication and potential discontinuation effects.
- Develop a safety plan: In all but exceptional circumstances, a parent or carer should be responsible for the secure storage of medication for a child or adolescent. Advise the young person and their parent/carer of professionals or services they should contact if they experience significant adverse effects, risk of harm, or worsening symptoms.

What to prescribe

- Fluoxetine is the recommended first-line medication for depression in children and adolescents.[3,4] It has the strongest current evidence for efficacy,[8,20–22] and UK NICE states that it is the only antidepressant for which clinical trial evidence shows that benefits outweigh risks.[4] Fluoxetine should be started at a low dose of 10mg daily which can be increased after one week to the minimum therapeutic dose of 20mg daily. Higher doses (up to 40–60mg daily) may be considered, particularly in older children of higher body weight and/or when, in severe illness, an early clinical response is considered a priority.[4–7] The long half-life of fluoxetine may be beneficial for adolescents, as they would be less likely to experience discontinuation effects if a dose is delayed or missed.[23] Fluoxetine is approved by the USA Food and Drug Administration (FDA) for treatment of depression in patients aged 8 years and over.
- Sertraline and escitalopram have also been found to be more effective for treating depression in young people than placebo,[8,21] and could be considered as alternatives if fluoxetine is not tolerated. Sertraline and escitalopram should also be

started at low doses (25–50mg daily and 5–10mg daily, respectively) and titrated to therapeutic doses (50–200mg daily and 10–20mg daily, respectively). The half-lives of sertraline, escitalopram, and some other antidepressants may be shorter in young people than adults, so twice-daily dosing may be considered, particularly at low doses, to prevent discontinuation symptoms.[24] Escitalopram is approved by the FDA for treatment of depression in patients aged 12 years and over.

- Partial or non-response to SSRI alone: For children and adolescents who have significant depressive symptoms resulting in distress or impairment despite an adequate trial of an SSRI alone, consider combination SSRI and psychological therapy.[21,25]
- Medication for treatment-resistant depression (partial or non-response to SSRI and psychological therapy): For children and adolescents who have significant depressive symptoms resulting in distress or impairment despite adequate trials of an SSRI (fluoxetine) and psychological therapy, consider a switch to a different SSRI (sertraline, citalopram[4] or escitalopram).[25] This guidance is based on the TORDIA trial, the only randomised controlled trial that has examined the comparative efficacy of different treatment strategies for SSRI-resistant depression in young people.[6] This trial found that many participants improved when switched to another SSRI or venlafaxine, and improved even more when this medication switch was combined with concurrent CBT. A switch to an SSRI was just as efficacious as a switch to venlafaxine but had less severe side effects, so an SSRI switch is preferred.
- If limited response despite adequate trials of the above medications, consider augmenting SSRI treatment with another medication such as a second-generation antipsychotic or lithium – in particular, consider augmentation if there has been partial response to an SSRI. Alternatively, consider switching to an antidepressant from a different class, for example mirtazapine (particularly consider mirtazapine if sleep is poor).
  Finally, if still no response to these medications and the young person's depression is very severe, interventional treatments could be considered, such as repetitive transcranial magnetic stimulation, electroconvulsive therapy or esketamine. These interventional treatments are not recommended for young children. Owing to a lack of research in children and adolescents, all recommendations beyond switching to a different SSRI are based on evidence from adult studies.[25]
- NICE recommends against prescribing paroxetine, venlafaxine, tricyclic antidepressants, or St. John's Wort for depression in young people, because of potential side effects and interactions.[4]
- Omega-3 fatty acid supplementation has minimal-to-no benefit in adults with depression,[25] and although an initial randomised controlled trial in young people suggested a benefit,[26] a subsequent larger trial did not demonstrate effectiveness.[27] Therefore, omega-3 fatty acid supplementation is not recommended for depression in young people.
- Box 5.1 summarises medication treatment for depression in children and adolescents.

CHAPTER 5

Box 5.1 Summary of pharmacotherapy for depression in children and adolescents[3,4,21,25]

	Medication	Starting dose	Therapeutic dose range
First line	Fluoxetine (FDA approved for 8 years and over)	10mg/day	20–60mg/day
Second line	Sertraline or	25–50mg/day	50–200mg/day
	Citalopram*	5–10mg/day	10–40mg/day
Third line	Escitalopram (FDA approved for 12 years and over)	5–10mg/day	10–20mg/day
Fourth line	Consider augmentation of antidepressant with second-generation antipsychotic or lithium** Consider mirtazapine** (where sedation required)		

*Caution advised in cardiac or hepatic disease.
**No RCTs available in young people (but evidence from adult trials).

After prescribing

Acute phase

- Monitor for adverse effects regularly, for example weekly for the first four weeks. Children and adolescents generally tolerate SSRIs well. Potential adverse effects include those experienced by adults, described in Chapter 3. Additionally, young people taking SSRIs have a small increased risk of suicidality and switch to mania (see 'specific issues' below). Therefore risk of harm, mood, and behaviour should be monitored closely and addressed.[3,4,21,25]
- After four weeks of SSRI treatment at a therapeutic dose, assess response including depression severity using the measures completed at baseline. Most therapeutic effects appear by four weeks.[9]
- If partial or non-response, consider the possibility of poor treatment adherence, inaccurate diagnosis, comorbidity, or modifiable maintaining factors.
- If none of these factors explain the continued depressive symptoms and the young person does not have adverse effects, consider increasing the dose. Reassess four weekly.[3,25]
- If adverse effects develop, consider reducing the dose to the highest tolerated dose.
- If partial or non-response after eight weeks of the maximum recommended (or highest tolerated) therapeutic dose of an SSRI, consider the medication changes outlined above.

Maintenance phase

- Continue medication for 6–12 months after remission to reduce the risk of relapse. Consider a longer maintenance phase if depressive episodes were recurrent or chronic.[3,4,21,25]

Discontinuation phase

- Discontinuation may be considered after the maintenance phase. This is best undertaken during a period of low stress. Taper medications slowly (see section in Chapter 3) to minimise the risk of discontinuation symptoms.[3,4,21,25]

Specific issues

- Age: The evidence base for the above recommendations is stronger for adolescents than for children, so caution should be higher when considering prescribing for children. There has been no research investigating antidepressant medication use in pre-school children, and medications are not recommended for this age group.[4,8]
- Suicidality: Antidepressant medication has been linked to an increased risk of suicidality in young people, which led to Black Box warnings issued by the USA FDA, UK Medicines and Healthcare Products Regulatory Agency, and the European Medicines Agency in 2003. Several meta-analyses have found evidence of this association with suicidality,[8,10] particularly for venlafaxine,[20,22] as well as a link with aggression.[28] However, the risk of suicidal ideation or attempts is small, for example a meta-analysis found a pooled absolute rate in antidepressant-treated participants of 2% and in those receiving placebo of 1%, giving a number needed to harm (NNH) of 112.[10] In addition, there has been no link between antidepressant use and completed suicides. Importantly, untreated depression is a significant risk factor for suicidality. After the FDA warning on antidepressant use in children, antidepressant use declined, untreated depression increased, and suicide rates increased.[29,30] Given the risks of untreated depression, including completed suicide and impaired functioning, and that many more patients benefit from SSRIs than those who experience these serious adverse events, it is thought that the benefits of antidepressants, particularly fluoxetine, are likely to outweigh these risks in moderate to severe depression. Nonetheless, risk of harm should be carefully monitored.[3,4,21,25]
- Manic switch: Conversion to mania occurs in an estimated 6% of young people taking antidepressants per year, and the risk seems to be higher in children than in adults.[31] However, there is no clear evidence that this switch is caused by antidepressants. These symptoms should be differentiated from activation adverse effects, a transient disinhibitory response to starting antidepressant medication or increasing dose, characterised by impulsivity, restlessness and irritability.[3]

CHAPTER 5

References

1. Avenevoli S, et al. Major depression in the national comorbidity survey-adolescent supplement: prevalence, correlates, and treatment. *J Am Acad Child Adolesc Psychiatry* 2015; 54:37–44.e32.
2. Rice F, et al. Adolescent and adult differences in major depression symptom profiles. *J Affect Disord* 2019; 243:175–181.
3. Birmaher B, et al. Practice parameter for the assessment and treatment of children and adolescents with depressive disorders. *J Am Acad Child Adolesc Psychiatry* 2007; 46:1503–1526.
4. National Institute for Health and Care Excellence (NICE). Depression in children and young people: identification and management. NICE Guideline [NG134]. 2019; www.nice.org.uk/guidance/ng134.
5. March J, et al. Fluoxetine, cognitive-behavioral therapy, and their combination for adolescents with depression: Treatment for Adolescents with Depression Study (TADS) randomized controlled trial. *JAMA* 2004; 292:807–820.
6. Brent D, et al. Switching to another SSRI or to venlafaxine with or without cognitive behavioral therapy for adolescents with SSRI-resistant depression: the TORDIA Randomized Controlled Trial. *JAMA: The Journal of the American Medical Association* 2008; 299:901–913.

7. Goodyer I, et al. Selective Serotonin Reuptake Inhibitors (SSRIs) and routine specialist care with and without cognitive behaviour therapy in adolescents with major depression: randomised controlled trial. *BMJ* 2007; **335**:142.

8. Hetrick SE, et al. Newer generation antidepressants for depressive disorders in children and adolescents. *Cochrane Database Syst Rev* 2012; **11**:CD004851.

9. Varigonda AL, et al. Systematic review and meta-analysis: early treatment responses of selective serotonin reuptake inhibitors in pediatric major depressive disorder. *J Am Acad Child Adolesc Psychiatry* 2015; **54**:557–564.

10. Bridge JA, et al. Clinical response and risk for reported suicidal ideation and suicide attempts in pediatric antidepressant treatment: a meta-analysis of randomized controlled trials. *JAMA* 2007; **297**:1683–1696.

11. Walkup JT Antidepressant efficacy for depression in children and adolescents: industry- and NIMH-funded studies. *Am J Psychiatry* 2017; **174**:430–437.

12. Treatment for Adolescents With Depression Study (TADS) Team. The Treatment for Adolescents With Depression Study (TADS): long-term effectiveness and safety outcomes. *Arch Gen Psychiatry* 2007; **64**:1132–1143.

13. Cox GR, et al. Psychological therapies versus antidepressant medication, alone and in combination for depression in children and adolescents. *Cochrane Database Syst Rev* 2014; Cd008324.

14. Dubicka B, et al. Combined treatment with cognitive-behavioural therapy in adolescent depression: meta-analysis. *Br J Psychiatry* 2010; **197**:433–440.

15. Poznanski EO, et al. *Children's Depression Rating Scale, Revised (CDRS-R)*. Los Angeles, Calif.: Western Psychological Services 1996.

16. Mayes TL, et al. Psychometric properties of the Children's Depression Rating Scale-Revised in adolescents. *J Child Adolesc Psychopharmacol* 2010; **20**:513–516.

17. Angold A, et al. Development of a short questionnaire for use in epidemiological studies of depression in children and adolescents. *Int J Methods Psychiatr Res* 1995; **5**:237–249.

18. Chorpita BF, et al. Assessment of symptoms of DSM-IV anxiety and depression in children: a revised child anxiety and depression scale. *Behav Res Ther* 2000; **38**:835–855.

19. Shaffer D, et al. A children's global assessment scale (CGAS). *Arch Gen Psychiatry* 1983; **40**:1228–1231.

20. Cipriani A, et al. Comparative efficacy and tolerability of antidepressants for major depressive disorder in children and adolescents: a network meta-analysis. *Lancet* 2016; **388**:881–890.

21. Goodyer IM, et al. Practitioner review: therapeutics of unipolar major depressions in adolescents. *J Child Psychol Psychiatry* 2019; **60**:232–243.

22. Zhou X, et al. Comparative efficacy and acceptability of antidepressants, psychotherapies, and their combination for acute treatment of children and adolescents with depressive disorder: a systematic review and network meta-analysis. *Lancet Psychiatry* 2020; **7**:581–601.

23. Wilens TE, et al. Fluoxetine pharmacokinetics in pediatric patients. *J Clin Psychopharmacol* 2002; **22**:568–575.

24. Findling RL, et al. The relevance of pharmacokinetic studies in designing efficacy trials in juvenile major depression. *J Child Adolesc Psychopharmacol* 2006; **16**:131–145.

25. Dwyer JB, et al. Annual research review: defining and treating pediatric treatment-resistant depression. *J Child Psychol Psychiatry* 2020; **61**:312–332.

26. Nemets H, et al. Omega-3 treatment of childhood depression: a controlled, double-blind pilot study. *Am J Psychiatry* 2006; **163**:1098–1100.

27. Marangell LB, et al. A double-blind, placebo-controlled study of the omega-3 fatty acid docosahexaenoic acid in the treatment of major depression. *Am J Psychiatry* 2003; **160**:996–998.

28. Sharma T, et al. Suicidality and aggression during antidepressant treatment: systematic review and meta-analyses based on clinical study reports. *BMJ* 2016; **352**:i65.

29. Gibbons RD, et al. Early evidence on the effects of regulators' suicidality warnings on SSRI prescriptions and suicide in children and adolescents. *Am J Psychiatry* 2007; **164**:1356–1363.

30. Libby AM, et al. Decline in treatment of pediatric depression after FDA advisory on risk of suicidality with SSRIs. *Am J Psychiatry* 2007; **164**:884–891.

31. Baldessarini RJ, et al. Antidepressant-associated mood-switching and transition from unipolar major depression to bipolar disorder: a review. *J Affect Disord* 2013; **148**:129–135.

Bipolar illness in children and adolescents

Clinical guidance

Before prescribing

- Establish clinical diagnosis informed by structured instrument assessment if possible. Try to monitor symptom patterns prospectively with mood or sleep diaries. If in doubt, seek specialist advice early on.
- Explain diagnosis to the patient and family and invest time and effort in psycho-education. This is likely to improve adherence and there is evidence that it reduces relapse rates, at least in adults.[1]
- Measure baseline symptoms of mania (e.g. Young Mania Rating Scale,[2] YMRS), depression (e.g. Children's Depression Rating Scale,[3] CDRS) and impairment (e.g. Clinical Global Impression – BD version[4]). Use these to set clear and realistic treatment goals.
- Measure baseline height, weight, waist circumference, pulse, ECG, blood pressure and obtain baseline bloods as appropriate (fasting blood glucose, HbA1c, fasting lipid profile, full blood count (FBC), urea and electrolytes (U&E), creatine kinase, liver function tests (LFTs), prolactin).

What to prescribe?

- For the treatment of mania and hypomania in youth, NICE guidelines suggest following the same recommendations as adults: second-generation antipsychotics (SGAs) may be used as first-line treatment, and mood stabilisers (MS) can be added after failure of two trials of SGA.[5]
- SGAs seem to show greater short-term efficacy (effect size [ES] = 0.65 compared with placebo) than MS (ES = 0.20 compared with placebo) in youth, according to a meta-analysis.[6]
- SGAs seem to produce significantly greater weight gain and somnolence in youth compared with adults,[6] although weight gain assessment is made complicated by normal anticipated growth at this time of life.
- Valproate should be completely avoided in girls.
- Adherence to lithium and blood level testing may be difficult in adolescents.
- Overall, we recommend the use of SGAs as first line for the acute treatment of mania in children and adolescents (see Table 5.1), similar to recommendations in adults.

After prescribing

- Assess and measure symptoms on a regular basis to establish effectiveness.
- Monitor weight and height at each visit and repeat all fasting bloods at 3 months (then every 6 months). Offer advice on a healthy lifestyle and exercise.

CHAPTER 5

- The duration of most medication trials is between 3 and 5 weeks. This should guide decisions about how long to try a single drug in a patient. A complete absence of response at 1–2 weeks should prompt a switch to another SGA.
- If non-response, check compliance, measure levels (where possible) and consider increasing dose. Consider concurrent use of SGA and MS.
- Judicious extrapolation of the evidence from adults[7] is required because of the very limited evidence base in youth with BP. This includes treatment duration and prophylaxis.[5,6,8]
- Maintenance treatment should follow adult guidelines. Consider the use of lithium early in the course of treatment, either by switching to lithium monotherapy prophylaxis or as an adjunct to a successful acute medication.

Specific issues

- Bipolar depression is a common clinical challenge and its treatment has been studied much less in youth compared than in adults (see Table 5.2). Antidepressants should be used with care and only in presence of an antimanic agent.[5] There is limited evidence for the benefit of antidepressants in bipolar depression in adults.[9] Because of the dearth of trials in youth, we are compelled to extrapolate from adult studies[5] and recommend use of the olanzapine/fluoxetine combination or quetiapine as first-line treatment, along with lurasidone which is supported by evidence from trials in children aged 10–17.[10–12]
- The exact relationship between ADHD and BD is still debated. Some evidence suggests that stimulants in children with ADHD and manic symptoms may be well tolerated[13] and that they may be safe and effective to use after mood stabilisation.[13] Caution and experience with prescribing these drugs are required (see Tables 5.3 and 5.4).
- The DSM-5 has introduced the new category of Disruptive Mood Dysregulation Disorder (DMDD) to capture severely irritable children (who were commonly misdiagnosed as having BD in the United States). There is as yet no established treatment for DMDD; lithium is ineffective,[14] but SSRIs and psychological treatment options, such as parenting interventions, may be considered.[15]

Other treatments

- There is evidence for adults and children that adjunct treatments including psychoeducation, CBT and especially family-focused interventions, can enhance treatment and reduce depression relapse rates in bipolar disorder.[16]
- The use of high-frequency repetitive transcranial magnetic stimulation (rTMS) in adolescents with treatment-resistant unipolar depression is only supported by open-label studies[17] and no RCT has been done in youth with either unipolar or bipolar depression. Therefore, its use is still considered experimental. One randomised sham-controlled study of rTMS in the right prefrontal cortex was ineffective in treating acute mania in youth, as an add-on to standard pharmacotherapy (N = 26).[18]
- One small trial supports the adjunctive use of melatonin (6mg/day) in adults with mania.[19] Evidence is not sufficient to recommend the use of melatonin in children but it is enough to allow an assumption of safety in this age group during manic episodes.

Table 5.1 Summary of RCT evidence on medication used in youth with bipolar mania

Medication	Comments
Lithium	Lithium is cleared relatively quickly in children so twice daily dosing will be required, especially when using liquid or non-modified release preparations.[20] One double-blind placebo-controlled randomised trial[21] showed *significant* reductions in substance use and clinical ratings after 6 weeks, in 25 adolescents with BD and comorbid substance misuse. In a double-blind placebo-controlled discontinuation trial (N = 40) over 2 weeks, *no significant difference* in relapse rates were found between lithium and placebo[22]
	A later double-blind placebo-controlled study (N = 81), over 8 weeks, demonstrated a *significantly larger* change in YMRS score in lithium-treated youth, but with a differentiation from the placebo group only appearing after 6 weeks of treatment. There was a significant increase in thyrotropin with lithium, but no difference in weight gain[23]
	Lithium and divalproex *did not differ* in an 18-month maintenance trial in youths (N = 60), who initially stabilised on the combination pharmacotherapy of lithium and divalproex.[24] However, given the compelling evidence for lithium maintenance and prophylaxis in adults, we recommend that clinicians consider its use in adolescents in preference to valproate
	A meta analysis[25] found lithium to be 'clearly inferior' to risperidone in mania. One small 6-month study found higher relapse rates in those who discontinued lithium compared with those who continued.[26] Another naturalistic 8-month study showed lithium to be effective and well tolerated[27]
Valproate	In an RCT (N = 150)[28] divalproex ER (titrated to clinical response or 80–125mg/L) *did not lead to significant differences* in mean YMRS compared with placebo at 4 weeks (also see risperidone and quetiapine sections below)
Oxcarbazepine	A double-blind placebo-controlled study (N = 116) *did not show significant differences* between placebo and oxcarbazepine (mean dose 1,515mg/day) in reducing mania rating at 7 weeks[29]
Olanzapine	A double-blind, placebo-controlled study (N = 161)[30] showed olanzapine (5–20mg/day) to be *significantly more effective* than placebo in YMRS mean score reduction over a period of 3 weeks. Note the higher weight gain in the treatment group (weight gain was 3.7kg for olanzapine versus 0.3kg for placebo) and the associated significantly increased fasting glucose, total cholesterol, AST, ALT and uric acid
Risperidone	A double-blind, placebo-controlled study (N = 169) showed risperidone (at doses 0.5–2.5 or 3–6mg) to be *significantly more effective* than placebo in YMRS mean score reduction in a 3-week follow up.[31] The lower dose seems to lead to same benefits at a lower risk of side effects. Sleepiness and fatigue were common in the treatment arms. Note, mean weight increase in treatment groups (0.7kg versus 1.7kg for the low and 1.4 for the high dose arm)
	In the Treatment of Early Age Mania (TEAM) study, *higher response rates* (and metabolic side effects) occurred with risperidone (mean dose of 2.57mg) versus lithium (mean level of 1.09mmol/L) and divalproex sodium (mean level of 113.6mg/L).[32] A randomised follow-up of this study, showed again the superiority of risperidone as an alternative treatment for non-responders to lithium and divalproex sodium, and as an add-on treatment to partially responders to the two MS.[33] However, these results need to be interpreted with caution as the definition of mania was broad and different to how bipolar disorder is defined by most UK clinicians. Similar reasons provoke caution when considering another placebo-controlled double-blind trial showing significantly better results for risperidone (mean dose 0.5mg) versus valproic acid (mean level 81mg/L) in 3–7 years old children supposedly diagnosed with mania[34]

(Continued)

CHAPTER 5

Table 5.1 (Continued)

Medication	Comments
Quetiapine	A double-blind, placebo-controlled study (N = 277)[35] showed quetiapine (at doses of 400mg/day or 600mg/day) to be *significantly better* than placebo in reducing mean YMRS scores at 3 weeks. The most common side effects included somnolence and sedation. Weight gain was 1.7kg in the quetiapine group versus 0.4kg for placebo
	Quetiapine is *effective* as an adjunct to valproate compared with valproate alone (N = 30, 6 weeks)[36] and was *as effective* as valproate in a double-blind trial (N = 50, 4 weeks)[37]
Aripiprazole	A double-blind placebo-controlled study[38,39] showed aripiprazole (at doses 10mg/day or 30mg/day) to be *significantly better* than placebo in reducing mean YMRS scores at both 4 weeks (N = 296)[38] and 30 weeks (N = 210).[39] Note the significantly higher incidence of extrapyramidal side effects in the treatment groups (especially the higher dose). Weight gain was *significantly higher* in the treatment groups compared to placebo (3.0kg versus 6.5kg for the low and 6.6kg for the high dose arm) at week 30 but not at week 4
Ziprasidone	A double-blind, placebo-controlled trial (N = 237)[40] showed ziprasidone (at flexible doses 40–160mg) to be *significantly more effective* than placebo in reducing mean YMRS scores at 4 weeks. Sedation and somnolence were the most common side effects, while it demonstrated a neutral metabolic profile and no QTc prolongation
Asenapine	A 3 weeks double-blind, placebo-controlled study (N = 350) demonstrated statistical superiority of asenapine over placebo for each of the doses used (2.5, 5 or 10mg b.i.d.), with significant difference as early as day 4. However, many side effects were reported, including weight gain of more than 7% from baseline (8–12% incidence in asenapine group vs 1.1% in placebo group), metabolic changes (increase in fasting insulin, lipids, glucose), as well as somnolence, sedation, oral hypoaesthesia and paraesthesia[41]

ALT, alanine transaminase; AST, aspartate aminotransferase; ER, extended release; MS, mood stabilisers; RCT, randomised controlled trial; YMRS, Young Mania Rating Scale.

Table 5.2 Summary of RCT evidence on medication used in youth with bipolar depression

Medication	Comments
Quetiapine	In adults, there is considerably better evidence for efficacious treatments (see the section on bipolar depression), such as quetiapine.[42,43] Surprisingly, however, a small study in 32 adolescents,[44] followed by a larger RCT (N = 193)[45] failed to show effectiveness. This latest study had a high placebo response, which is not present in adult quetiapine studies[46] and which may reflect issues that have been noted before about phenotyping of mood disorders and multi-site studies[47]
Olanzapine/fluoxetine combination	The only double-blind randomised placebo-controlled trial with positive results for the treatment of bipolar depression in youth is a large study (N = 255) of the olanzapine/fluoxetine combination (either 6/25mg or 12/50mg daily) for 8 weeks.[48] Between-group differences were significant at week 1 and all subsequent visits. Most frequent side effects were weight gain (4.4kg for the olanzapine/fluoxetine combination vs 0.5kg for placebo), somnolence and hyperlipidaemia. The olanzapine/fluoxetine combination is recommended by NICE guidelines,[5] along with quetiapine, as first-line treatment for bipolar depression in youth, as in adults. Although the olanzapine/fluoxetine combination is not currently available as a single preparation in the UK, its effects can be achieved by combining olanzapine and fluoxetine (e.g. 5/20mg or 10/40mg)

Table 5.2 (Continued)

Medication	Comments
Lurasidone	Lurasidone has been shown to be effective in bipolar depression in adults[49–51] and it does not seem to cause weight gain and other metabolic disturbances. It is safe and effective in treating schizophrenia in adolescents[52] and has been shown to be effective in children (10–17 years) both acutely[10] and in a 2-year follow-up.[12] Dose ranged from 18.5(20)mg to 74(80)mg but a small majority received the lowest dose. Lurasidone may be the preferred antipsychotic in children on account of its good tolerability[53]
Lamotrigine	Lamotrigine has only modest, if any, effects in adult bipolar depression;[54] it has not been studied in RCTs for the treatment of acute bipolar depression in children and adolescents and is, therefore, not recommended as a first line. Moreover, a placebo-controlled randomised withdrawal study of adjunctive lamotrigine for bipolar disorder in youth, lasting over 36 weeks, failed to show any benefit in preventing time to occurrence of a bipolar event[55]

RCT, randomised controlled trial.

Table 5.3 Recommended first-line treatments for acute mania*

Aripiprazole	10mg daily
Risperidone	0.5–2.5mg daily
Olanzapine	5–20mg daily
Quetiapine	Up to 400mg daily
Asenapine	2.5–10mg twice daily

*Continue acutely effective dosing regimen as prophylaxis, and consider need for lithium.

Table 5.4 Recommended first-line treatments for bipolar depression*

Lurasidone	18.5(20)mg–74(80)mg a day
Olanzapine/fluoxetine	6/25–12/50mg daily
Quetiapine	Up to 300mg daily

*Continue acutely effective dosing regimen as prophylaxis, and consider need for lithium.

CHAPTER 5

CHAPTER 5

References

1. Colom F, et al. A randomized trial on the efficacy of group psychoeducation in the prophylaxis of recurrences in bipolar patients whose disease is in remission. *Arch Gen Psychiatry* 2003; 60:402–407.
2. Young RC, et al. A rating scale for mania: reliability, validity and sensitivity. *Br J Psychiatry* 1978; 133:429–435.
3. Poznanski EO, et al. Preliminary studies of the reliability and validity of the children's depression rating scale. *J Am Acad Child Psychiatry* 1984; 23:191–197.
4. Spearing MK, et al. Modification of the Clinical Global Impressions (CGI) Scale for use in bipolar illness (BP): the CGI-BP. *Psychiatry Res* 1997; 73:159–171.
5. National Institute for Health and Care Excellence. Bipolar disorder: assessment and management: Clinical Guidance [CG185] 2014 (last updated February 2020); https://www.nice.org.uk/guidance/cg185.
6. Correll CU, et al. Antipsychotic and mood stabilizer efficacy and tolerability in pediatric and adult patients with bipolar I mania: a comparative analysis of acute, randomized, placebo-controlled trials. *Bipolar disorders* 2010; 12:116–141.
7. Geddes JR, et al. Treatment of bipolar disorder. *Lancet* 2013; 381:1672–1682.
8. Diaz-Caneja CM, et al. Practitioner review: Long-term pharmacological treatment of pediatric bipolar disorder. *J Child Psychol Psychiatry* 2014; 55:959–980.
9. Pacchiarotti I, et al. The International Society for Bipolar Disorders (ISBD) task force report on antidepressant use in bipolar disorders. *AmJPsychiatry* 2013; 170:1249–1262.
10. DelBello MP, et al. Efficacy and Safety of Lurasidone in Children and Adolescents With Bipolar I Depression: A Double-Blind, Placebo-Controlled Study. *J Am Acad Child Adolesc Psychiatry* 2017; 56:1015–1025.
11. Singh MK, et al. Lurasidone in children and adolescents with bipolar depression presenting with mixed (subsyndromal hypomanic) features: post hoc analysis of a randomized placebo–controlled trial. *J Child Adolesc Psychopharmacol* 2020; 30:590–598.
12. DelBello MP, et al. 159 Safety and efficacy of lurasidone in children and adolescents with bipolar depression: results from a 2-year open-label extension study. *CNS Spectr* 2020; 25:301–302.
13. Goldsmith M, et al. Antidepressants and psychostimulants in pediatric populations: is there an association with mania? *PaediatrDrugs* 2011; 13:225–243.
14. Dickstein DP, et al. Randomized double-blind placebo-controlled trial of lithium in youths with severe mood dysregulation. *J Child Adolesc Psychopharmacol* 2009; 19:61–73.
15. Vidal-Ribas P, et al. The status of irritability in psychiatry: a conceptual and quantitative review. *J Am Acad Child Adolesc Psychiatry* 2016; 55:556–570.
16. Miklowitz DJ. Evidence-based family interventions for adolescents and young adults with bipolar disorder. *J Clin Psychiatry* 2016; 77 Suppl E1:e5.
17. Wall CA, et al. Magnetic resonance imaging-guided, open-label, high-frequency repetitive transcranial magnetic stimulation for adolescents with major depressive disorder. *J Child Adolesc Psychopharmacol* 2016; 26:582–589.
18. Pathak V, et al. Efficacy of adjunctive high frequency repetitive transcranial magnetic stimulation of right prefrontal cortex in adolescent mania: a randomized sham-controlled study. *Clinical psychopharmacology and neuroscience : the official scientific journal of the Korean College of Neuropsychopharmacology* 2015; 13:245–249.
19. Moghaddam HS, et al. Efficacy of melatonin as an adjunct in the treatment of acute mania: a double-blind and placebo-controlled trial. *Int Clin Psychopharmacol* 2020; 35:81–88.
20. Grant B, et al. Using Lithium in Children and adolescents with bipolar disorder: efficacy, tolerability, and practical considerations. *Paediatr Drugs* 2018; 20:303–314.
21. Geller B, et al. Double-blind and placebo-controlled study of lithium for adolescent bipolar disorders with secondary substance dependency. *J Am Acad Child Adolesc Psychiatry* 1998; 37:171–178.
22. Kafantaris V, et al. Lithium treatment of acute mania in adolescents: a placebo-controlled discontinuation study. *J Am Acad Child Adolesc Psychiatry* 2004; 43:984–993.
23. Findling RL, et al. Lithium in the acute treatment of bipolar I disorder: a double-blind, placebo-controlled study. *Pediatrics* 2015; 136:885–894.
24. Findling RL, et al. Double-blind 18-month trial of lithium versus divalproex maintenance treatment in pediatric bipolar disorder. *J Am Acad Child Adolesc Psychiatry* 2005; 44:409–417.
25. Duffy A, et al. Efficacy and tolerability of lithium for the treatment of acute mania in children with bipolar disorder: a systematic review: a report from the ISBD-IGSLi joint task force on lithium treatment. *Bipolar disorders* 2018; 20:583–593.
26. Findling RL, et al. Lithium for the maintenance treatment of bipolar I disorder: a double-blind, placebo-controlled discontinuation study. *J Am Acad Child Adolesc Psychiatry* 2019; 58:287–296.e284.
27. Masi G, et al. Lithium treatment in bipolar adolescents: a follow-up naturalistic study. *Neuropsychiatr Dis Treat* 2018; 14:2749.
28. Wagner KD, et al. A double-blind, randomized, placebo-controlled trial of divalproex extended-release in the treatment of bipolar disorder in children and adolescents. *J Am Acad Child Adolesc Psychiatry* 2009; 48:519–532.
29. Wagner KD, et al. A double-blind, randomized, placebo-controlled trial of oxcarbazepine in the treatment of bipolar disorder in children and adolescents. *Am J Psychiatry* 2006; 163:1179–1186.
30. Tohen M, et al. Olanzapine versus placebo in the treatment of adolescents with bipolar mania. *Am J Psychiatry* 2007; 164:1547–1556.
31. Haas M, et al. Risperidone for the treatment of acute mania in children and adolescents with bipolar disorder: a randomized, double-blind, placebo-controlled study. *Bipolar Disorders* 2009; 11:687–700.

32. Geller B, et al. A randomized controlled trial of risperidone, lithium, or divalproex sodium for initial treatment of bipolar I disorder, manic or mixed phase, in children and adolescents. *Arch Gen Psychiatry* 2012; **69**:515–528.

33. Walkup JT, et al. Treatment of early-age mania: outcomes for partial and nonresponders to initial treatment. *J Am Acad Child Adolesc Psychiatry* 2015; **54**:1008–1019.

34. Kowatch RA, et al. Placebo-controlled trial of valproic acid versus risperidone in children 3–7 years of age with bipolar I disorder. *J Child Adolesc Psychopharmacol* 2015; **25**:306–313.

35. Pathak S, et al. Efficacy and safety of quetiapine in children and adolescents with mania associated with bipolar I disorder: a 3-week, double-blind, placebo-controlled trial. *JClinPsychiatry* 2013; **74**:e100–e109.

36. Delbello MP, et al. A double-blind, randomized, placebo-controlled study of quetiapine as adjunctive treatment for adolescent mania. *J Am Acad Child Adolesc Psychiatry* 2002; **41**:1216–1223.

37. Delbello MP, et al. A double-blind randomized pilot study comparing quetiapine and divalproex for adolescent mania. *J Am Acad Child Adolesc Psychiatry* 2006; **45**:305–313.

38. Findling RL, et al. Acute treatment of pediatric bipolar I disorder, manic or mixed episode, with aripiprazole: a randomized, double-blind, placebo-controlled study. *J Clin Psychiatry* 2009; **70**:1441–1451.

39. Findling RL, et al. Aripiprazole for the treatment of pediatric bipolar I disorder: a 30–week, randomized, placebo-controlled study. *BipolarDisord* 2013; **15**:138–149.

40. Findling RL, et al. Ziprasidone in adolescents with schizophrenia: results from a placebo-controlled efficacy and long-term open-extension study. *J Child Adolesc Psychopharmacol* 2013; **23**:531–544.

41. Findling RL, et al. Asenapine for the acute treatment of pediatric manic or mixed episode of bipolar I disorder. *J Am Acad Child Adolesc Psychiatry* 2015; **54**:1032–1041.

42. Calabrese JR, et al. A randomized, double-blind, placebo-controlled trial of quetiapine in the treatment of bipolar I or II depression. *Am J Psychiatry* 2005; **162**:1351–1360.

43. Thase ME, et al. Efficacy of quetiapine monotherapy in bipolar I and II depression: a double-blind, placebo-controlled study (the BOLDER II study). *J Clin Psychopharmacol* 2006; **26**:600–609.

44. Delbello MP, et al. A double-blind, placebo-controlled pilot study of quetiapine for depressed adolescents with bipolar disorder. *Bipolar disorders* 2009; **11**:483–493.

45. Findling RL, et al. Efficacy and safety of extended-release quetiapine fumarate in youth with bipolar depression: an 8 week, double-blind, placebo-controlled trial. *J Child Adolesc Psychopharmacol* 2014; **24**:325–335.

46. Suttajit S, et al. Quetiapine for acute bipolar depression: a systematic review and meta-analysis. *Drug Des Devel Ther* 2014; **8**:827–838.

47. Bridge JA, et al. Clinical response and risk for reported suicidal ideation and suicide attempts in pediatric antidepressant treatment: a meta-analysis of randomized controlled trials. *JAMA* 2007; **297**:1683–1696.

48. Detke HC, et al. Olanzapine/fluoxetine combination in children and adolescents with bipolar I depression: a randomized, double-blind, placebo-controlled trial. *J Am Acad Child Adolesc Psychiatry* 2015; **54**:217–224.

49. Loebel A, et al. Lurasidone monotherapy in the treatment of bipolar I depression: a randomized, double-blind, placebo-controlled study. *AmJPsychiatry* 2014; **171**:160–168.

50. Suppes T, et al. Lurasidone adjunctive with lithium or valproate for bipolar depression: A placebo-controlled trial utilizing prospective and retrospective enrolment cohorts. *J Psychiatr Res* 2016; **78**:86–93.

51. Suppes T, et al. Lurasidone for the treatment of major depressive disorder with mixed features: a randomized, double-blind, placebo-controlled study. *Am J Psychiatry* 2016; **173**:400–407.

52. Goldman R, et al. Efficacy and safety of lurasidone in adolescents with schizophrenia: a 6–week, randomized placebo-controlled study. *J Child Adolesc Psychopharmacol* 2017:516–525.

53. Solmi M, et al. Safety of 80 antidepressants, antipsychotics, anti-attention-deficit/hyperactivity medications and mood stabilizers in children and adolescents with psychiatric disorders: a large scale systematic meta-review of 78 adverse effects. *World psychiatry* 2020; **19**:214–232.

54. Calabrese JR, et al. Lamotrigine in the acute treatment of bipolar depression: results of five double-blind, placebo-controlled clinical trials. *Bipolar disorders* 2008; **10**:323–333.

55. Findling RL, et al. Adjunctive Maintenance Lamotrigine for Pediatric Bipolar I Disorder: A Placebo-Controlled, Randomized Withdrawal Study. *J Am Acad Child Adolesc Psychiatry* 2015; **54**:1020-1031.e1023.

CHAPTER 5

Psychosis in children and adolescents

Schizophrenia is rare in children but the incidence increases rapidly in adolescence. A detailed developmental and physical assessment is often needed before the diagnosis is made.[1,2] Early-onset schizophrenia-spectrum (EOSS) disorder is often chronic and in the majority of cases requires long-term treatment with antipsychotic medication.[3]

There have been several RCTs of first-generation antipsychotics, many of them using very high doses, and all of them showing high rates of EPSEs and significant sedation.[4] Treatment-emergent dyskinesias can also be problematic[5] even when smaller doses are used.[6] First-generation antipsychotics (FGAs) should be avoided in children and adolescents.

There have also been a number of randomised controlled trials of second-generation antipsychotics in EOSS disorder. Olanzapine,[7-9] risperidone,[7,8,10,11] aripiprazole,[12,13] quetiapine,[13,14] paliperidone,[15] asenapine,[16] ziprasidone[17] and lurasidone[18] have all been shown to be effective in the treatment of psychosis. There is evidence from a systematic review and network meta-analysis to suggest comparable efficacy for most second-generation antipsychotics with the exception of ziprasidone (inferior efficacy) and asenapine (unclear efficacy).[19] Concerns have been raised about the cardiac safety of ziprasidone[20,21] because of its facility for increasing the QT interval. Aripiprazole does not seem to have effect on QT in adolescents.[22]

Children and adolescents are at greater risk than adults for side effects such as extrapyramidal symptoms, raised prolactin, sedation (even with aripiprazole[13]), weight gain and metabolic effects.[23]

There is evidence that clozapine is effective in treatment-resistant psychosis in adolescents, although this population may be more prone to neutropenia and seizures than adults.[24-27] Based on data obtained from the treatment of younger adults, olanzapine should probably be tried before moving to clozapine[28] because there is a palpable chance that it will be effective, although clozapine is clearly more effective than olanzapine in adolescents.[25,26]

Overall, algorithms for treating psychosis in children and adolescents are the same as those for adult patients (see chapter on schizophrenia). NICE[29] recommends oral antipsychotics in conjunction with family interventions and individual CBT. Starting doses should be at the lower end of, or below the adult range.

When prescribing antipsychotics in children and adolescents always measure baseline parameters and monitor as per guidance in chapter on schizophrenia. For children and adolescents also include waist and hip circumference, assessment of any movement disorders and assessment of nutritional status, diet and level of physical activity.[29]

References

1. Pina-Camacho L, et al. Autism spectrum disorder and schizophrenia: boundaries and uncertainties. *Br J Psych Adv* 2016; **22**:316–324.

2. Hayes D, et al. Dilemmas in the treatment of early-onset first-episode psychosis. *Ther Adv Psychopharmacol* 2018; **8**:231–239.

3. Kumra S, et al. Efficacy and tolerability of second-generation antipsychotics in children and adolescents with schizophrenia. *Schizophr Bull* 2008; **34**:60–71.

4. Lee ES, et al. Psychopharmacologic treatment of schizophrenia in adolescents and children. *Child Adolesc Psychiatr Clin N Am* 2020; **29**:183–210.

5. Connor DF, et al. Neuroleptic-related dyskinesias in children and adolescents. *J Clin Psychiatry* 2001; **62**:967–974.

6. Campbell M, et al. Neuroleptic-related dyskinesias in autistic children: a prospective, longitudinal study. *J Am Acad Child Adolesc Psychiatry* 1997; **36**:835–843.

7. Sikich L, et al. A pilot study of risperidone, olanzapine, and haloperidol in psychotic youth: a double-blind, randomized, 8-week trial. *Neuropsychopharmacology* 2004; **29**:133–145.

8. Sikich L, et al. Double-blind comparison of first- and second-generation antipsychotics in early-onset schizophrenia and schizo-affective disorder: findings from the treatment of early-onset schizophrenia spectrum disorders (TEOSS) study. *Am J Psychiatry* 2008; **165**:1420–1431.

9. Kryzhanovskaya L, et al. Olanzapine versus placebo in adolescents with schizophrenia: a 6-week, randomized, double-blind, placebo-controlled trial. *J Am Acad Child Adolesc Psychiatry* 2009; **48**:60–70.

10. Haas M, et al. A 6-week, randomized, double-blind, placebo-controlled study of the efficacy and safety of risperidone in adolescents with schizophrenia. *J Child Adolesc Psychopharmacol* 2009; **19**:611–621.

11. Haas M, et al. Efficacy, safety and tolerability of two dosing regimens in adolescent schizophrenia: double-blind study. *Br J Psychiatry* 2009; **194**:158–164.

12. Findling RL, et al. A multiple-center, randomized, double-blind, placebo-controlled study of oral aripiprazole for treatment of adolescents with schizophrenia. *Am J Psychiatry* 2008; **165**:1432–1441.

13. Pagsberg AK, et al. Quetiapine extended release versus aripiprazole in children and adolescents with first-episode psychosis: the multicentre, double-blind, randomised tolerability and efficacy of antipsychotics (TEA) trial. *Lancet Psychiatry* 2017; **4**:605–618.

14. Findling RL, et al. Efficacy and safety of quetiapine in adolescents with schizophrenia investigated in a 6-week, double-blind, placebo-controlled trial. *J Child Adolesc Psychopharmacol* 2012; **22**:327–342.

15. Singh J, et al. A randomized, double-blind study of paliperidone extended-release in treatment of acute schizophrenia in adolescents. *Biol Psychiatry* 2011; **70**:1179–1187.

16. Findling RL, et al. Safety and efficacy from an 8 week double-blind trial and a 26 week open-label extension of asenapine in adolescents with schizophrenia. *J Child Adolesc Psychopharmacol* 2015; **25**:384–396.

17. Findling RL, et al. Ziprasidone in adolescents with schizophrenia: results from a placebo-controlled efficacy and long-term open-extension study. *J Child Adolesc Psychopharmacol* 2013; **23**:531–544.

18. Arango C, et al. Lurasidone compared to other atypical antipsychotic monotherapies for adolescent schizophrenia: a systematic literature review and network meta-analysis. *Eur Child Adolesc Psychiatry* 2020; **29**:1195–1205.

19. Pagsberg AK, et al. Acute antipsychotic treatment of children and adolescents with schizophrenia-spectrum disorders: a systematic review and network meta-analysis. *J Am Acad Child Adolesc Psychiatry* 2017; **56**:191–202.

20. Scahill L, et al. Sudden death in a patient with Tourette syndrome during a clinical trial of ziprasidone. *J Psychopharmacol* 2005; **19**:205–206.

21. Blair J, et al. Electrocardiographic changes in children and adolescents treated with ziprasidone: a prospective study. *J Am Acad Child Adolesc Psychiatry* 2005; **44**:73–79.

22. Jensen KG, et al. Change and dispersion of QT interval during treatment with quetiapine extended release versus aripiprazole in children and adolescents with first-episode psychosis: results from the TEA trial. *Psychopharmacology (Berl)* 2018; **235**:681–693.

23. Correll CU Addressing adverse effects of antipsychotic treatment in young patients with schizophrenia. *J Clin Psychiatry* 2011; **72**:e01.

24. Kumra S, et al. Childhood-onset schizophrenia. A double-blind clozapine-haloperidol comparison. *Arch Gen Psychiatry* 1996; **53**:1090–1097.

25. Shaw P, et al. Childhood-onset schizophrenia: a double-blind, randomized clozapine-olanzapine comparison. *Arch Gen Psychiatry* 2006; **63**:721–730.

26. Kumra S, et al. Clozapine and "high-dose" olanzapine in refractory early-onset schizophrenia: a 12-week randomized and double-blind comparison. *Biol Psychiatry* 2008; **63**:524–529.

27. Schneider C, et al. Systematic review of the efficacy and tolerability of clozapine in the treatment of youth with early onset schizophrenia. *Eur Psychiatry* 2014; **29**:1–10.

28. Agid O, et al. An algorithm-based approach to first-episode schizophrenia: response rates over 3 prospective antipsychotic trials with a retrospective data analysis. *J Clin Psychiatry* 2011; **72**:1439–1444.

29. National Institute for Health and Care Excellence. Psychosis and schizophrenia in children and young people: recognition and management. Clinical Guidance 155 [CG155]. 2013 (last updated October 2016). https://www.nice.org.uk/guidance/cg155.

CHAPTER 5

Anxiety disorders in children and adolescents

Diagnostic issues

Fear and worry are common in children and they are part of normal development. At the same time, anxiety disorders often begin in childhood and adolescence[1] and they are the most common psychiatric disorders in this age group, with overall prevalence between 8% and 30% depending on the impairment cut-offs used.[2] Anxiety disorders may be even more common in children with neurodevelopment disorders.[3]

In children, the more obvious clinical presentation with distress and avoidance may be masked by prominent behavioural symptoms (e.g. irritability and angry outbursts linked to avoidance). Therefore, the assessment and treatment of anxiety disorders in children needs to be undertaken by clinicians who can discriminate normal, developmentally appropriate worries, fears and shyness from anxiety disorders that significantly impair a child's functioning, and who can appreciate developmental variations in the presentation of symptoms.

Clinical guidance

Anxiety symptoms in children and adolescents often improve with age, presumably in parallel to the development of the prefrontal cortex and, in particular, executive function. However, anxiety disorders are distressing and impairing conditions that need to be treated promptly. Chronic stress mediators may have significant impact on brain development[4] and functional impairment linked to anxiety symptoms may prevent young people from accessing normative experiences that are critical for social, emotional and cognitive development. Finally, early and effective treatment may prevent continuity of psychopathology into adulthood, for example, young people with anxiety disorders are three times more likely to have anxiety and depression in adult life compared to non-anxious youths.[5]

Guidelines for treatment of anxiety disorders in children and adolescents have been made available in the UK and the United States. NICE guidelines focus on the treatment of social anxiety disorder in children and adolescents, suggesting the use of cognitive behavioural therapy (CBT) and cautioning against the routine use of pharmacological treatment for social anxiety in this age group.[6] Guidelines from the American Academy of Child and Adolescent Psychiatry (AACAP) cover the treatment of all non-OCD, non-PTSD anxiety disorders.[7] AACAP guidelines suggest multimodal treatment including psychoeducation, psychotherapy (e.g. a 12-session course of exposure-based CBT), and pharmacotherapy. Drug treatment is endorsed for moderate-to-severe anxiety symptoms, when impairment makes participation in psychotherapy difficult or when psychotherapy leads to only partial response.

Prescribing for anxiety disorders in children and adolescents

Before prescribing

- **Exclude other diagnoses.** Anxiety symptoms can be mimicked by a range of psychiatric disorders including depression (inattention, sleep problems), bipolar disorder (irritability, sleep problems, restlessness), oppositional-defiant disorder

(irritability, oppositional behaviour), psychotic disorders (social withdrawal, restlessness), ADHD (inattention, restlessness), Asperger syndrome (social withdrawal, poor social skills, repetitive behaviours and routines) and learning disabilities. They may also be mimicked by a range of endocrine (hyperthyroidism, hypoglycemia, pheochromocytoma), neurological (migraine, seizures, delirium, brain tumours), cardiovascular (cardiac arrhythmias) and respiratory (asthma) conditions and lead intoxication. Anxiety-like symptoms can be observed in response to several drugs and substances including anti-asthma medications, sympathomimetics, steroids, SSRIs, antipsychotics (akathisia), diet pills, cold medicines, caffeine and energy drinks.
- **Beware of contraindications to SSRIs and potential interactions.**
- **Measure baseline severity.** Structured interviews including the Anxiety Disorders Interview Schedule (ADIS) and the Kiddie-Schedule for Affective Disorders and Schizophrenia (Kiddie-SADS). Questionnaires, including the Revised Children's Anxiety and Depression Scale (RCADS), Screen for Child Anxiety and Related Emotional Disorders (SCARED) or the Multidimensional Anxiety Scale for Children (MASC). Measures of functional impairment including the Children's Global Assessment Scale (CGAS).
- **Obtain consent.** Discuss treatment with the young person and the family (e.g. name of medication, starting/estimated ending dose, titration timeline, possible side effects and strategies to monitor/minimise them, strategies to monitor progress, interventions for treatment-resistant cases). Document consent in writing.

What to prescribe

- **Selective serotonin reuptake inhibitors (SSRIs)** are the medications of choice for the treatment of anxiety disorders in children and adolescents. A meta-analysis identified seven short-term RCTs (<16 weeks; n treatment = 446, n control = 386) testing the efficacy of SSRIs (fluoxetine, fluvoxamine, paroxetine, sertraline) on changes in impairment for anxiety disorders in young people (CGI-I). The overall odds ratio of treatment response was 4.6 (95% CI = 3.1–7.5) and mean improvement in anxiety symptoms was 5.2 (95% CI = 2.8–8.8) over placebo.[8] The Childhood Anxiety Multimodal Study (CAMS) showed that monotherapy with sertraline (55% response) is as effective as CBT for anxiety (60% response) compared with placebo (24% response), and that combined therapy with sertraline and CBT is most likely to be successful (81% response).[9] A network meta-analysis found that SSRIs significantly reduce clinician-reported and parent-reported (but not child-reported) anxiety symptoms and increased remission.[10] A network meta-analysis found that the likelihood of treatment response was higher for SSRI compared to other medications below[8] and a standard meta-analysis showed that clinically significant treatment effects typically emerge by week 6 of treatment, and that SSRIs are associated with more rapid and greater improvement than other medications below.[11] With regard to tolerability, SSRIs are the most tolerable class of medications, particularly escitalopram and fluoxetine.[12]

  Sertraline, fluoxetine and fluvoxamine have been approved by the US Food and Drug Administration (FDA) for treatment of paediatric OCD, and fluoxetine and

CHAPTER 5

escitalopram have been approved for treatment of paediatric depression. The US FDA issued in 2004 a Black Box warning for concerns related to worsening of depression, agitation, and suicidal ideation linked to SSRIs. These concerns were based on a review of studies of adolescents with depression rather than young people with anxiety.

- **Serotonin–norepinephrine reuptake inhibitors (SNRIs).** Venlafaxine was tested in two short-term RCTs (n treatment = 294, n control = 311), duloxetine was tested in one short-term RCT (n treatment = 135, n control = 137), and atomoxetine was tested in one short-term RCT. The overall odds ratio of treatment response for SNRIs was 2.4 (95% CI = 1.7–3.6) over placebo.[8] However, SNRIs did show statistically significant effects on improvement in anxiety symptoms over placebo, with mean difference of 2.5 (95% CI =0.1–5.1).[8] The network meta-analysis mentioned earlier found that SNRIs significantly reduce clinician-reported (but not parent-reported or child-reported) anxiety symptoms.[10] SSRIs are more effective and better tolerated[8] so SNRIs could be considered a third-line treatment for anxiety disorders when two trials with different SSRIs prove ineffective.

- The $5HT_{1A}$ agonist, buspirone has been examined in one short-term RCT (n treatment = 334, n control = 225) and found not to be associated with significant odds ratio for treatment response (1.3 (95% CI = 0.7–3.4)) or mean improvement in anxiety symptoms (0.8 (95% CI = –3.1 to 4.8)) over placebo.[13]

- The $alpha_2$ agonist, guanfacine, was evaluated in one short-term RCT (n treatment = 62, n control = 21) and found to be associated with significant odds ratio for treatment response (5.6 (95% CI = 1.4–26.8)) but not in mean improvement in anxiety symptoms (3.4 (95% CI = –3.2 to 10)) over placebo.[14]

- Neither benzodiazepine nor tricyclic antidepressant use is supported by controlled trials in children.[8] Benzodiazepine may also lead to paradoxical disinhibition in some children. Nevertheless, use of longer-acting benzodiazepines is at times considered in clinical practice to alleviate disabling anxiety during initial titration of SSRIs and for rapid tranquillisation (see Table 5.5).

After prescribing

- Acute phase
  - Start at lowest available dose
  - Monitor side effects. SSRIs are generally well tolerated during treatment for anxiety disorders in young people. Psychological side effects include worsening of anxiety symptoms, agitation and disinhibition. Physical side effects including gastrointestinal symptoms (e.g. nausea, vomiting, dyspepsia, abdominal pain, diarrhoea, constipation), headache, increased motor activity, and insomnia may occur, often in mild and transient form.
  - After 1 week of treatment with SSRIs (2 weeks for SNRIs) when the child is compliant with medications and does not manifest more than minimal side effects, titrate incrementally with weekly intervals to the minimal therapeutic dose.
  - Monitor side effects (see the list point above) and response (e.g. RCADS, SCARED, MASC, CGAS, CGI-I) frequently and systematically.

Table 5.5 Typical dosage of medications for treatment of anxiety disorders in children and adolescents

Medication	Starting dose (mg)	Dose range (mg/day)
SSRI		
Sertraline	12.5–25	25–200
Fluoxetine	5–10	10–60
Fluvoxamine	12.5–25	50–200 (BD if >50)
Paroxetine	5–10	10–40
Citalopram*	5–10	10–40
SNRI		
Venlafaxine XR	37.5	37.5–225
Duloxetine	30	30–120
Alpha$_2$ agonist		
Guanfacine	1	1–6
5-HT$_{1A}$ partial agonist		
Buspirone*	5 TDS	15–60
Benzodiazepine (PRN)		
Clonazepam*	0.25–0.5	–
Lorazepam*	0.5–1	–

*Treatments not supported by RCT evidence.
Note: Always check dose with latest formal guidance, for example British National Formulary for Children (in the UK).
BD - twice daily
TDS - three times daily

- Dosage for treatment with SSRIs is often similar to dosage in adults because of faster metabolism in children.
- Therapeutic effect should appear by 6–8 weeks of treatment. It is important to communicate this to families.
- If partial or non-response, consider accuracy of diagnosis, adequacy of medication trial, and compliance of patient.
- To improve response, consider: adding CBT, changing medication (e.g. switch SSRIs, other classes), or combining medications (e.g. for co-morbidities, to treat side effects, to potentiate action). Augmentation strategies with buspirone, benzodiazepines, atypical antipsychotics, and stimulant medications have been proposed but lack empirical support.[7]
- Maintenance phase
  - Continue maintenance treatment for at least 1 year of stable improvement.
  - Monitor response and side effects regularly.
- Discontinuation phase

- Because of lack of information on long-term safety and possible improvement in symptoms with age and learning, consider discontinuing treatment after a period of stable improvement. A trial of medication should be started at a period of low stress/demands. Discontinuation should also be considered if the medication is no longer working or the side effects are too severe. Taper SSRIs slowly (e.g. 25–50% weekly) to minimize risk of discontinuation symptoms. Monitor closely for recurrence of symptoms/relapse and, if deterioration is noted, promptly restart medication.

Specific issues

Treatment of anxiety disorders in pre-school children must routinely focus on psychotherapy. In rare cases when a very young child has extreme ongoing symptoms and impairment, clinicians should reconsider diagnosis and case formulation, and reassess the adequacy of the psychotherapy trial. There are no RCTs of pharmacological interventions for anxiety in pre-school children, but case reports suggest potential benefit of fluoxetine and buspirone.[15] Therefore, any prescription in pre-school children is off-label.[16]

References

1. Kessler RC, et al. Lifetime prevalence and age-of-onset distributions of DSM-IV disorders in the National Comorbidity Survey Replication. *Arch Gen Psychiatry* 2005; **62**:593–602.
2. Merikangas KR, et al. Lifetime prevalence of mental disorders in U.S. adolescents: results from the National Comorbidity Survey Replication–Adolescent Supplement (NCS-A). *J Am Acad Child Adolesc Psychiatry* 2010; **49**:980–989.
3. Simonoff E, et al. Psychiatric disorders in children with autism spectrum disorders: prevalence, comorbidity, and associated factors in a population-derived sample. *J Am Acad Child Adolesc Psychiatry* 2008; **47**:921–929.
4. Danese A, et al. Adverse childhood experiences, allostasis, allostatic load, and age-related disease. *Physiol Behav* 2012; **106**:29–39.
5. Pine DS, et al. The risk for early-adulthood anxiety and depressive disorders in adolescents with anxiety and depressive disorders. *Arch Gen Psychiatry* 1998; **55**:56–64.
6. National Institute for Health and Clinical Excellence. Social anxiety disorder: recognition, assessment and treatment. Clinical Guidance 159 2013 (last checked June 2017); https://www.nice.org.uk/guidance/cg159.
7. Connolly SD, et al. Practice parameter for the assessment and treatment of children and adolescents with anxiety disorders. *J Am Acad Child Adolesc Psychiatry* 2007; **46**:267–283.
8. Dobson ET, et al. Efficacy and tolerability of pharmacotherapy for pediatric anxiety disorders: a network meta-analysis. *J Clin Psychiatry* 2019; **80**:17r12064.
9. Walkup JT, et al. Cognitive behavioral therapy, sertraline, or a combination in childhood anxiety. *N Engl J Med* 2008; **359**:2753–2766.
10. Wang Z, et al. Comparative effectiveness and safety of cognitive behavioral therapy and pharmacotherapy for childhood anxiety disorders: a systematic review and meta-analysis. *JAMA Pediatrics* 2017; **171**:1049–1056.
11. Strawn JR, et al. The impact of antidepressant dose and class on treatment response in pediatric anxiety disorders: a meta-analysis. *J Am Acad Child Adolesc Psychiatry* 2018; **57**:235–244.e232.
12. Solmi M, et al. Safety of 80 antidepressants, antipsychotics, anti-attention-deficit/hyperactivity medications and mood stabilizers in children and adolescents with psychiatric disorders: a large scale systematic meta-review of 78 adverse effects. *World Psychiatry Off J World Psychiatric Assoc (WPA)* 2020; **19**:214–232.
13. Strawn JR, et al. Buspirone in children and adolescents with anxiety: a review and Bayesian analysis of abandoned randomized controlled trials. *J Child Adolesc Psychopharmacol* 2018; **28**:2–9.
14. Strawn JR, et al. Extended release guanfacine in pediatric anxiety disorders: a pilot, randomized, placebo-controlled trial. *J Child Adolesc Psychopharmacol* 2017; **27**:29–37.
15. Gleason MM, et al. Psychopharmacological treatment for very young children: contexts and guidelines. *J Am Acad Child Adolesc Psychiatry* 2007; **46**:1532–1572.
16. Mohatt J, et al. Treatment of separation, generalized, and social anxiety disorders in youths. *Am J Psychiatry* 2014; **171**:741–748.

Obsessive compulsive disorder (OCD) and body dysmorphic disorder (BDD) in children and adolescents

The treatment of OCD and BDD in children and adolescents follows the same principles as in adults (see Chapter 3). BDD is now recognised by both DSM-V and ICD-11 as one of the OCD spectrum of disorders. CBT is effective in both conditions and is recommended by NICE as the treatment of first choice[1,2] although it may be combined with medication.[3] At least 2% of adolescent age group have BDD but it remains consistently underdiagnosed.[4] NICE recommends routine screening questions for BDD in high risks groups, such as individuals who attempt suicide or self-harm, or those with symptoms of depression, social phobia, alcohol or substance misuse, OCD or an eating disorder; or for those with mild disfigurements or blemishes who are seeking a cosmetic or dermatological procedure.[5]

Drug treatment

Sertraline[6-8] (from age 6 years) and **fluvoxamine** (from age 8 years) are the selective serotonin reuptake inhibitors (SSRIs) licensed in the UK for the treatment of OCD in young people. Studies spanning 20 years have established the efficacy of SSRIs in the paediatric population in placebo-controlled trials. A meta-analysis of 12 RCTs of pharmacotherapy against control in young people showed that medication is consistently significantly more effective than placebo.[9] Sertraline and fluoxetine are equally effective, but fluvoxamine may be somewhat less so.[9] While an initial meta-analysis suggested SSRIs have a medium to large effect size in the treatment of OCD in young people,[7] the most recent analysis suggests an effect size of around 0.43 (somewhere between 'small' and 'moderate').[9] Paroxetine is not recommended for use in children and young people.

Clomipramine remains a useful drug for some individuals, although its side-effect profile (sedation, dry mouth, constipation, potential for cardiac side-effects) tend to limit its use in this age group. There is on-going debate as to whether clomipramine is more efficacious than SSRIs in treating OCD in young people. SSRIs generally remain the recommended first choice medication for young people with OCD. For BDD, no treatment is licensed in the UK for either adults or children. However, the available evidence show significant improvements with SSRIs, both in terms of BDD symptoms and the often co-morbid depressive symptoms.[10] NICE recommends fluoxetine for treating BDD in children and adolescents.

Although 50% of BDD cases have beliefs of delusional intensity about their appearance, anti-psychotics are not beneficial. Research in adults show that patients with such beliefs are just as likely to respond to SSRI monotherapy as are non-delusional patients.[10]

Initiation of treatment with medication

SSRIs show a similar slow and incremental effect on symptoms from as early as 1–2 weeks after initiation and placebo-referenced improvements continue for at least 24 weeks. In some cases, positive impact on mood may be noted before changes in OCD or BDD symptoms.[11] The effects on core OCD or BDD schema may take some weeks to months to become noticeable. In the UK, NICE therefore recommend treatment trials of SSRIs for OCD or BDD of three months and increasing towards the maximum tolerated effective dosage. Carefully explaining these temporal effects to patients can be important in sustaining compliance. In addition, the earliest signs of improvement may be apparent to an informant before the patient. Use of an observer-rated quantitative measure such as the CY-BOCS[12] or BDD-YBOCS,[13] may therefore be helpful to monitor progress in clinical settings. The British Association of Psychopharmacology suggest starting at the lowest dose known to be effective and waiting for up to 12 weeks before evaluating effectiveness.[14] Thereafter dosage titration is recommended if there is insufficient clinical response.

Prescribing SSRIs in children

In 2004, the British Medicines and Healthcare Products Regulatory Authority Agency (MHRA) cautioned against the use of SSRIs in young people, owing to a possible increased risk of suicidal ideation.[15] The risk–benefit ratio in children is markedly different in OCD/BDD than depression. Careful re-analysis of treatment data highlights that SSRIs are clearly more efficacious in childhood OCD than they are in the treatment of moderate depressive episodes in children and young people.[16] Investigators concluded that in the paediatric OCD group, the pooled risk for suicidal ideation and attempts was less than 1% across all studies. This of course is an important risk and should be explained and carefully monitored. Nonetheless, the naturalistic course of untreated OCD and BDD is that it tends not to spontaneously remit and has tremendous morbidity. It is also now known that untreated OCD and BDD is associated with very significant morbidity including a ten-fold increased risk of completed suicide compared with the general population.[10,17] These factors need to be carefully considered and discussed with the patient and their carers or family in making informed choices about treatment.

On occasion, medications other than sertraline and fluvoxamine may be used as 'off-label' preparations with the appropriate and suitable caution. NICE guidance[5] for the treatment of OCD recommends the use of SSRIs before use of clomipramine, because of the latter drug's greater propensity for side effects and need for cardiac monitoring. Factors guiding the choice of other medications may include issues such as the presence of other disorders (NICE recommends fluoxetine for OCD with co-morbid depression); a good treatment response to a certain drug in other family members; and the presence of other disorders, as well as cost and availability. Compliance with medication can be a problem with some young people, which can guide the choice of preparation in some instances. For instance, young people with patchy compliance may be better suited to treatment with fluoxetine considering its long half-life, when compared with other SSRIs. Some children find tablets or capsules hard to swallow and the availability of licensed liquid formulations is limited in most countries.

Some young people are very reluctant to engage in CBT as part of the treatment. Whilst CBT is the mainstay of treatment packages for OCD and BDD, in some instances medication alone may be the only viable therapeutic option. Some children have very poor insight or find accessing CBT particularly difficult. This very often includes patients with learning problems or autism spectrum disorders. Insight in BDD can often be poorer than is seen with OCD. This in turn can affect motivation to engage with psychological therapy. Where medication is being used as the only evidence-based treatment, it is essential that this remains under review so that motivation and ability to engage with CBT is regularly revisited.

NICE guidelines for the assessment and treatment of OCD and BDD

NICE published guidelines in 2005 on the evidence-based treatment options for OCD and BDD for young people and adults. NICE recommends a 'stepped care' model, with increasing intensity of treatment according to clinical severity and complexity.[5] The assessment of the severity and impact can be aided by the use of the CY-BOCS or BDD-YBOCS questionnaire or other quantitative measures, both at baseline and as a helpful monitoring tool.[12]

The summary treatment algorithm from the NICE guideline is shown in Figure 5.1.

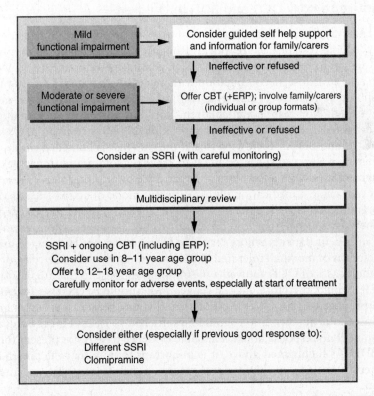

Figure 5.1 Treatment options for children and young people with OCD or BDD. CBT = cognitive behaviour therapy; ERP = exposure and response prevention; SSRI = selective serotonin reuptake inhibitor. (adapted from NICE guidance).[5] Reprinted with permission.[18]

CBT and medication in the treatment of childhood OCD and BDD

Studies now show convincingly that CBT is superior to placebo and that efforts should be made to try and ensure access to a suitably experienced CBT practitioner.

The principle study that directly compared the efficacy of CBT, sertraline, and their combination, in children and adolescents, led NICE to conclude that children with OCD should begin treatment with CBT alone or CBT plus an SSRI.[2] There is ongoing debate as to whether CBT should be recommended as initial monotherapy or whether combination therapy should be offered from the outset. Internationally there is a growing trend to offer a combination of psychological therapy and medication, most particularly for patients with BDD. The addition of an SSRI to a CBT treatment package has been shown to significantly address the differential response to CBT treatment alone, seen between experienced and less experienced therapists.[6]

Some children, particularly those with developmental disabilities can find CBT extremely challenging. Efforts to tailor treatment protocols can be efficacious in many instances. For some children, however the experience of anxiety during exposure tasks can be overwhelming. On occasions to use of beta blocker such as propranolol can moderate the physical concomitants of anxiety to a degree such that CBT can continue.

Treatment-refractory OCD and BDD in children

Evidence from randomised trials suggest that up to three quarters of medicated patients make an adequate response to treatment. Roughly one quarter of children with OCD will therefore fail to respond to an initial SSRI, administered for at least 12 weeks at the maximum tolerated dose, in combination with an adequate trial of CBT and ERP. These children should be reassessed, clarifying compliance, and ensuring that co-morbidity is not being missed. Non-responding children should usually have additional trials of at least one other SSRI. Research suggests approximately 40% respond to a second SSRI in both OCD[19] and BDD.[10] Following this, if the response is limited, a child should usually be referred to a specialist centre. In OCD, trials of clomipramine may be considered and/or augmentation with a low dose of risperidone or aripiprazole.[18,20] Research hints at the fact that using a medication with a different mode of action such as risperidone or clomipramine may benefit patients who have failed to respond to two adequate SSRI trials.[11] There is evidence that low dose antipsychotic augmentation, as an 'off-label' therapy, can benefit patients whose response to treatment has been inadequate despite at least 3 months of maximal tolerated SSRI. Unfortunately, only one-third of treatment resistant adult cases of OCD showed a meaningful response to this augmentation strategy. The data would, therefore, suggest that caution should be exercised when augmenting treatment packages for OCD in children and young people. A six-week trial of low dose anti-psychotic augmentation should be sufficient to assess efficacy. It is important to discontinue if no response noted. The same evidence base is not present for the treatment of BDD. As highlighted above, it is important to note that the presence of delusional intensity beliefs in BDD does predict a better response to antipsychotic medication.

Often children whose OCD or BDD has been difficult to treat have co-morbidities such as autism spectrum disorder (ASD), ADHD, or tic disorders. The response to medication can be differentially affected by these co-morbidities. For instance, cases with tic disorders may be benefitted somewhat more from augmentation with second-generation anti-psychotics. Untreated ADHD can also commonly interfere with engagement with CBT due to poor focus. Very often efforts to address ADHD with appropriate treatments including medication can dramatically improve engagement with CBT. Careful clinical review and reformulation is important in OCD or BDD treatment resistance. The impact of co-morbidities and wider psychosocial factors need to be considered on the treatment response overall. Very often clinical experience shows that it can be vital to extensively support families and carers during treatment. This often requires helping families drop well-established patterns of accommodation around OCD or BDD.

Duration of treatment and long-term follow-up

Untreated OCD runs a chronic course. A series of adult studies have shown that discontinuation of medication tends to result in symptomatic relapse. Some authors have suggested that those with co-morbidities are at the greatest risk of relapse. Given that studies frequently exclude cases with additional comorbidities, it is likely that the relapse rates have been underestimated. In the UK, NICE Guidelines recommend that if a young person has responded to medication for BDD or OCD, treatment should continue for at least 6 months after remission. Clinical experience would suggest that when discontinuation of treatment is attempted it should be done slowly, cautiously and in a transparent manner with the patient and their family. Once again, the careful use of clinical outcome measures should be considered when stopping medication.

Discontinuing medication is very typically associated with a deterioration in symptoms of OCD or BDD. Increasingly adult and young people are being counselled to consider whether they wish to remain on SSRI medication long-term to mitigate the substantial risk of relapse. Individuals with developmental disabilities often struggle to generalise the lessons taken from successful CBT. Therefore, this population benefits from concerted and close review in follow up after treatment. It is important that throughout childhood, adolescence and into adult life, the individual with OCD or BDD should have access to healthcare professionals, treatment opportunities and other support as needed. NICE recommends that if relapse occurs, people with OCD or BDD should be seen as soon as possible rather than placed on a routine waiting list.

References

1. O'Kearney RT, et al. Behavioural and cognitive behavioural therapy for obsessive compulsive disorder in children and adolescents. *Cochrane Database Syst Rev* 2006:CD004856.

2. Freeman JB, et al. Cognitive behavioral treatment for young children with obsessive-compulsive disorder. *Biol Psychiatry* 2007; 61:337–343.

3. Mancuso E, et al. Treatment of pediatric obsessive-compulsive disorder: a review. *J Child Adolesc Psychopharmacol* 2010; 20:299–308.

4. National & Specialist OCD BDD and Related Disorders Service for Young People Maudsley Hospital. *Appearance Anxiety: A book on BDD for Young People, Families and Professionals.* Jessica Kingsley Publications; 2019.

5. National Institute for Clinical Excellence. Obsessive-compulsive disorder: core interventions in the treatment of obsessive-compulsive disorder and body dysmorphic disorder. *Clinical Guidance* 2005; 31 [CG31]. https://www.nice.org.uk/guidance/cg31.

6. The Pediatric OCD Treatment Study Team (POTS). Cognitive-behavior therapy, sertraline, and their combination for children and adolescents with obsessive-compulsive disorder: the Pediatric OCD Treatment Study (POTS) randomized controlled trial. *JAMA* 2004; 292:1969–1976.

7. Geller DA, et al. Which SSRI? A meta-analysis of pharmacotherapy trials in pediatric obsessive-compulsive disorder. *Am J Psychiatry* 2003; 160:1919–1928.

8. March JS, et al. Treatment benefit and the risk of suicidality in multicenter, randomized, controlled trials of sertraline in children and adolescents. *J Child Adolesc Psychopharmacol* 2006; 16:91–102.

9. Kotapati VP, et al. The effectiveness of selective serotonin reuptake inhibitors for treatment of obsessive-compulsive disorder in adolescents and children: a systematic review and meta-analysis. *Frontiers Psychiatry* 2019; 10:523.

10. Phillips KA, et al. Treating body dysmorphic disorder with medication: evidence, misconceptions, and a suggested approach. *Body Image* 2008; 5:13–27.

11. Bloch MH, et al. Assessment and management of treatment-refractory obsessive-compulsive disorder in children. *J Am Acad Child Adolesc Psychiatry* 2015; 54:251–262.

12. Scahill L, et al. Children's Yale-Brown Obsessive Compulsive Scale: reliability and validity. *J Am Acad Child Adolesc Psychiatry* 1997; 36:844–852.

13. Phillips KA, et al. A severity rating scale for body dysmorphic disorder: development, reliability, and validity of a modified version of the Yale-Brown Obsessive Compulsive Scale. *Psychopharmacol Bull* 1997; 33:17–22.

14. Baldwin DS, et al. Evidence-based pharmacological treatment of anxiety disorders, post-traumatic stress disorder and obsessive-compulsive disorder: a revision of the 2005 guidelines from the British Association for Psychopharmacology. *J Psychopharmacol* 2014; 28:403–439.

15. Medicines and Healthcare Products Regulatory Agency. Report of the CSM expert working group on the safety of selective serotonin reuptake inhibitor antidepressants. 2005; https://www.neuroscience.ox.ac.uk/publications/474047.

16. Garland J, et al. Update on the use of SSRIs and SNRIs with children and adolescents in clinical practice. *J Can Acad Child Adolesc Psychiatry* 2016; 25:4–10.

17. Fernandez de la Cruz L, et al. Suicide in obsessive-compulsive disorder: a population-based study of 36 788 Swedish patients. *Mol Psychiatry* 2017; 22:1626–1632.

18. Heyman I, et al. Obsessive-compulsive disorder. *BMJ* 2006; 333:424–429.

19. Grados M, et al. Pharmacotherapy in children and adolescents with obsessive-compulsive disorder. *Child Adolesc Psychiatr Clin N Am* 1999; 8:617–634, x.

20. Bloch MH, et al. A systematic review: antipsychotic augmentation with treatment refractory obsessive-compulsive disorder. *Mol Psychiatry* 2006; 11:622–632.

Further reading

Nazeer A, et al. Obsessive-compulsive disorder in children and adolescents: epidemiology, diagnosis and management. *Translational Pediatrics* 2020; 9:S76–S93.

Post-traumatic stress disorder in children and adolescents

Diagnostic issues

Traumatic events and PTSD are common in young people. One in three children experiences traumatic events[1] and about 1 in 13 children develops PTSD before age 18.[1] The prevalence of PTSD in adolescents can be much higher in at-risk groups, for example those attending emergency departments, in forensic settings, or among refugee/asylum seekers. Young people with PTSD are at high risk of self-harm (nearly 50%) and suicide attempt (20%) and are often functionally impaired, for example not being in education, employment or education (NEET) (more than 25%).[1] Of note, more than three out of four young people with PTSD have comorbid psychiatric diagnoses, most commonly depression, conduct disorder, alcohol dependence or generalised anxiety disorder.[1] Furthermore, PTSD is not the most common diagnosis in trauma-exposed young people - disorders that are most prevalent in the general population (e.g. depression, conduct disorder and alcohol dependence) are also more prevalent in trauma-exposed young people.[1]

A diagnosis of PTSD is based on the triad of intrusive re-experiencing, avoidance of stimuli associated with the trauma, and hyper-arousal after trauma exposure. Because of the abnormal processing of traumatic memories, young people with PTSD persistent *re-experiencing* of the traumatic event(s) through nightmares or unwanted and distressing memories, which are often experienced as if they were happening in the 'here and now' but often in young people do not appear as frank dissociative symptoms or flashbacks. In order to minimise *re-experiencing* symptoms, young people with PTSD often develop overt or covert *avoidance* strategies, keeping themselves busy or distracted or staying away from people or places that remind them of the traumatic event. As a result of the above symptoms, young people with PTSD often feel under continued threat and, therefore, display *physiological hyper-arousal*, appearing alert and vigilant for danger, irritable and struggling to concentrate on daily tasks. Because of the varied clinical manifestations, the assessment and treatment of PTSD in children and adolescents should be undertaken by clinicians who have expertise in the clinical presentations seen in trauma-exposed children and can appreciate developmental variations in the manifestation of symptoms.

Clinical guidance

The NICE guidelines[2] advise that treatment of PTSD in young people should focus on psychotherapy with 12-sessions of trauma-focused CBT (TF-CBT) for PTSD resulting from a single traumatic event or longer for chronic or recurrent events. If TF-CBT is not effective or based on the young person's preference, treatment may also include eye movement desensitization and reprocessing (EMDR).

Based on the current evidence in the NICE guidelines,[2] the American Academy of Child & Adolescent Psychiatry[3] and the International Society for Traumatic Stress Studies (ISTSS),[4] pharmacotherapy is not recommended for treatment of PTSD in young people. The evidence for efficacy of pharmacotherapy (SSRIs and SGAs) in adults is also somewhat limited at present.[5,6] However, because of the high rates of comorbidity,[1] pharmacotherapy may be needed to target co-occurring psychiatric disorders. In adult PTSD, the best supported treatments are fluoxetine, paroxetine and venlafaxine.[7] MDMA[8] and psychedelic drugs[9] also show promise. None of these agents is currently used to any extent in children and adolescents.

References

1. Lewis SJ, et al. The epidemiology of trauma and post-traumatic stress disorder in a representative cohort of young people in England and Wales. *Lancet Psychiatry* 2019; 6:247–256.
2. National Institute for Clinical Excellence. Post-traumatic stress disorder. NICE guideline [NG116] 2018; https://www.nice.org.uk/guidance/NG116.
3. Cohen JA, et al. Practice parameter for the assessment and treatment of children and adolescents with posttraumatic stress disorder. *J Am Acad Child Adolesc Psychiatry* 2010; 49:414–430.
4. International Society for Traumatic Stress Studies (ISTSS). Posttraumatic stress disorder prevention and treatment guidelines: methodology and recommendations 2019; https://istss.org/getattachment/Treating-Trauma/New-ISTSS-Prevention-and-Treatment-Guidelines/ISTSS_PreventionTreatmentGuidelines_FNL-March-19-2019.pdf.aspx.
5. Cipriani A, et al. Comparative efficacy and acceptability of pharmacological treatments for post-traumatic stress disorder in adults: a network meta-analysis. *Psychol Med* 2018; 48:1975–1984.
6. Huang ZD, et al. Comparative efficacy and acceptability of pharmaceutical management for adults with post-traumatic stress disorder: a systematic review and meta-analysis. *Front Pharmacol* 2020; 11:559.
7. Ehret M. Treatment of posttraumatic stress disorder: focus on pharmacotherapy. *Ment Health Clin* 2019; 9:373–382.
8. Jerome L, et al. Long-term follow-up outcomes of MDMA-assisted psychotherapy for treatment of PTSD: a longitudinal pooled analysis of six phase 2 trials. *Psychopharmacology (Berl)* 2020; 237:2485–2497.
9. Krediet E, et al. Reviewing the potential of psychedelics for the treatment of PTSD. *Int J Neuropsychopharmacol* 2020; 23:385–400.

Attention deficit hyperactivity disorder

Attention deficit hyperactivity disorder (ADHD) in children

- A diagnosis of ADHD should be made only after a comprehensive assessment by a specialist with expertise in ADHD.[1] Appropriate psychological, psychosocial and behavioural interventions should be put in place. Drug treatments should be only a part of the overall treatment plan.
- The indication for drug treatment is the presence of impairment resulting from ADHD despite environmental modifications, parent training (if appropriate), advice on parenting strategies, and liaison with school.
- **Methylphenidate** is the first line treatment when medication is indicated. It is a central nervous system (CNS) stimulant with a large evidence base from trials. Most common adverse effects include insomnia, appetite suppression, raised blood pressure and pulse rate and growth deceleration – which can usually be managed by symptomatic management, treatment breaks, and/or dose reduction depending on the side effect. In the UK, there are several modified release preparations with different release profiles available, including generic options (see Box 5.2).
- **Dexamfetamine** is an alternative CNS stimulant. Effects and adverse reactions are broadly similar to methylphenidate, but there is much less evidence on efficacy and safety than exists for methylphenidate and is probably more likely to be diverted and misused. Both methylphenidate and dexamfetamine are Schedule 2 Controlled Drugs and prescriptions should be written appropriately (total amount in words and figures) and for a maximum supply of 30 days (in the UK).
- **Lisdexamfetamine** is a prodrug – the dexamfetamine is complexed with the amino acid lysine and in this form is inactive. It is broken down in red blood cells so that dexamfetamine is gradually made available. It, therefore, has a similar practical role to extended-release preparations of methylphenidate and, like them, is unlikely to be abused for recreational or dependency-driven purposes. Several randomised controlled trials have established it as superior to placebo in children[2,3] and adolescents.[4] Effect size from preliminary research appears to be at least as great as that of Oros-methylphenidate[3] and it seems to have a similar range of adverse effects.[5,6] Recent network meta-analyses found lisdexamfetamine to be more effective than methylphenidate[7,8] and long-term data suggest that it can be considered as an alternative to extended-release methylphenidate.[9]
- **Atomoxetine**[10–13] is a non-stimulant alternative. It may be particularly useful for children who do not respond to stimulants, where stimulant diversion is a problem or when 'dopaminergic' adverse effects (such as tics, anxiety and stereotypies) become problematic on stimulants. Parents should be warned of the possibilities of suicidal thinking and liver disease emerging and advised of the possible features that they might notice. It is less effective than stimulants.[7,8,11,14,15]
- Other medications include the alpha-2 agonists **clonidine**[16] and **guanfacine**. A licensed modified-release preparation of guanfacine was approved in the UK in January 2016[17] for use in children with ADHD and can be considered as an alternative non-stimulant medication to atomoxetine.

CHAPTER 5

Box 5.2 Summary of NICE guidance for ADHD in children[1]

- Drug treatment should only be initiated by a specialist and only after a comprehensive assessment of mental and physical health and social influences. In children under 5 years, medication should be initiated after a second specialist opinion from an ADHD service with expertise in managing ADHD in younger children (ideally a tertiary service).
- An ADHD-focused group parent-training programme should be offered for parents or carers of children under 5 years with ADHD. Environmental modifications need to be implemented in all cases. If ADHD symptoms are still causing a persistent significant impairment in at least one domain despite environmental modifications, medication can be offered following a baseline assessment.
- Methylphenidate, lisdexamfetamine, dexamfetamine, atomoxetine and guanfacine are recommended within their licensed indications.
- Methylphenidate (either short or long acting) is the first choice of medication.
- Consider switching to lisdexamfetamine for children aged 5 years and over and young people who have had a 6-week trial of methylphenidate at an adequate dose and not derived enough benefit in terms of reduced ADHD symptoms and associated impairment.
- Consider dexamfetamine for children aged 5 years and over and young people whose ADHD symptoms are responding to lisdexamfetamine but who cannot tolerate the longer effect profile.
- Offer atomoxetine or guanfacine to children aged 5 years and over and young people if they cannot tolerate methylphenidate or lisdexamfetamine or their symptoms have not responded to separate 6-week trials of lisdexamfetamine and methylphenidate, having considered alternative preparations and adequate doses.
- Monitoring should include measurement of height and weight (with entry on growth charts) and recording of blood pressure and heart rate. An electrocardiogram (ECG) is not needed before starting stimulants, atomoxetine or guanfacine, unless the person has any of the following:
  - history of congenital heart disease or previous cardiac surgery
  - history of sudden death in a first-degree relative under 40 years suggesting a cardiac disease
  - shortness of breath on exertion compared with peers
  - fainting on exertion or in response to fright or noise
  - palpitations that are rapid, regular and start and stop suddenly
  - chest pain suggesting cardiac origin
  - signs of heart failure
  - a murmur heard on cardiac examination
  - blood pressure that is classified as hypertensive for adults
  - a co-existing condition that is being treated with a medicine that may pose an increased cardiac risk.

A cardiology opinion should be sought if any of the above apply.

- There is some evidence supporting the efficacy of **tricyclic antidepressants**[18,19] but these are not recommended in clinical practice.
- **Bupropion**[8,20,21] seems to be efficacious and well-tolerated. **Modafinil** also appears to have useful activity in children but not in adults with ADHD.[8,22,23] Evidence supporting the use of these drugs is somewhat limited compared with standard treatments.[8]

- The use of **second-generation antipsychotics**[24,25] for ADHD is not recommended.[24,25] These may reduce hyperactivity in ASD[26] but should not be prescribed for this indication.
- Co-morbid psychiatric illness is common in children with ADHD. Stimulants are often helpful overall but are unlikely to be appropriate for children who have a psychotic illness. Problems with substance misuse should be managed in their own right alongside ADHD treatment[27] and treatments need to be chosen carefully.
- Combinations of stimulants and atomoxetine have been used, but there are few trials and no clear evidence for improved efficacy.[28]
- Once stimulant treatment has been established, it is appropriate for repeat prescriptions to be supplied through general practitioners.[1]

ADHD in adults

ADHD first diagnosed in adult life is compatible with both ICD-11 and DSM-5. NICE guidance regards the first line of treatment as medication, following the same principles as for drug treatment in children (see Table 5.6).

- Around 65% of patients with ADHD continue to meet full criteria or have achieved only partial remission by adulthood.[29] It is appropriate to **continue treatment started in childhood** in adults whose symptoms remain disabling.
- A first-time diagnosis of ADHD in an adult should only be made after a comprehensive assessment. Whenever possible this should include information from other informants and from adults who knew the patient as a child. It is recommended to establish the symptoms and impairments of ADHD using a validated diagnostic interview assessment such as the Diagnostic Interview for DSM-IV ADHD (DIVA).[30]
- The prevalence of substance misuse and antisocial personality disorder are high in adults whose ADHD was not recognised in childhood.[31] Methylphenidate can be effective in this population,[32] but caution is appropriate in prescribing and monitoring.
- For adults with ADHD and drug or alcohol addiction disorders, there should be close liaison between the professional treating the ADHD and an addiction specialist.
- **Methylphenidate** or **lisdexamfetamine** are considered first-line choices of medication in adults.[1]
- **Dexamfetamine** can be used for adults whose ADHD symptoms are responding to lisdexamfetamine but who cannot tolerate the longer effect profile.
- For **atomoxetine,** monitoring for symptoms of liver dysfunction and suicidal thinking is advised.
- **Atomoxetine, lisdexamfetamine and two modified release formulations of methylphenidate (Medikinet XL, Ritalin XL)** are licensed for first-time use in adults with ADHD. Concerta XL (another modified-release formulation of methylphenidate) is licensed for continued treatment when initiated before the age of 18 years.

CHAPTER 5

Summary of NICE guidance for ADHD in adults[1]

- Drug treatment should only be initiated by a specialist and only after a comprehensive assessment of mental and physical health and social influences.
- Medication for ADHD should be offered to adults if their ADHD symptoms are still causing a significant impairment in at least one domain after environmental modifications have been implemented and reviewed.
- Non-pharmacological options (supportive therapy, CBT, regular reviews) can be considered depending on choice, difficulties with adherence or intolerable side effects. Combination of medication with non-pharmacological options can also be considered in partial response to medication treatment.
- Methylphenidate or lisdexamfetamine are recommended for use in adults with ADHD as first-line treatments. Switching between the two could be considered after a 6-week trial of an adequate dose with suboptimal response.
- Dexamfetamine can be used for adults whose ADHD symptoms are responding to lisdexamfetamine but who cannot tolerate the longer effect profile.
- Atomoxetine could be offered to adults if:
  - they cannot tolerate lisdexamfetamine or methylphenidate or
  - their symptoms have not responded to separate 6-week trials of lisdexamfetamine and methylphenidate, having considered alternative preparations and adequate doses.
- Monitoring should include measurement of weight, blood pressure and heart rate. A cardiology opinion and ECG should be organised as in the case of children and adolescents mentioned above.

Table 5.6 Prescribing in attention deficit hyperactivity disorder.

Medication	Onset and duration of action	Dose	Notes	Recommended monitoring/general notes
Methylphenidate immediate release Branded products (Ritalin, Medikinet, Tranquilyn) and various generic preparations available[33-35]	Onset: 20–60 minutes Duration: 2–4 hours	Initially 5–10mg daily titrated up in weekly increments of 5–10mg, to a maximum of 2.1mg/kg/day in divided doses. Licensed maximum dose 60mg daily (or after specialist review up to 90mg daily N.B. unlicensed)[1]	Methylphenidate usually first-line treatment in ADHD. Generally well tolerated[36]	For methylphenidate, dexamfetamine and lisdexamfetamine:[37] ■ Blood pressure ■ Pulse ■ Height ■ Weight
Methylphenidate modified release*			An afternoon dose of immediate release methylphenidate may be necessary in some children to optimise treatment	Monitor for insomnia, mood and appetite change and the development of tics,[38] although some evidence suggests tics are not associated with psychostimulants[39]
Concerta XL[33,34,40-42] Bioequivalent versions of Concerta XL: Matoride XL, Xenidate XL, Xenidate XL, Delmosart modified release	Onset: 30 minutes–2 hours Duration: 12 hours	Initially 18mg in the morning, titrated up to a licensed maximum dose of 54mg daily (or after specialist review up to 108mg daily N.B. unlicensed) 18mg = 15mg methylphenidate immediate release	Consists of an immediate-release component (22% of the dose) and a modified-release component (78% of the dose)	Discontinue if no benefits seen in 1 month Controlled Drug
Equasym XL[43,44]	Onset: 20–60 minutes Duration: 8 hours	Initially 10mg in the morning, titrated up to a licensed maximum dose of 60mg daily	Consists of an immediate-release component (30% of the dose) and a modified-release component (70% of the dose). Capsules can be opened and sprinkled	
Medikinet XL	Onset: 20–60 minutes Duration: up to 8 hours	Dose as for Equasym XL	Consists of an immediate-release component (50% of the dose) and a modified-release component (50% of the dose). Capsules can be opened and sprinkled[45]	

(Continued)

Table 5.6 (Continued)

Medication	Onset and duration of action	Dose	Notes	Recommended monitoring/general notes
Ritalin XL (refs SPC, public assessment report)	Onset: 60 minutes Duration: 8–12 hours	Dose as for Equasym XL	Consists of an immediate-release component (50% of the dose) and a modified-release component (50% of the dose)	
Dexamfetamine immediate release[36,46]	Onset: 20–60 minutes Duration: 3–6 hours	Initially 2.5–10mg daily, titrated up in weekly increments of 2.5–5mg, to a maximum of 20mg daily in divided doses (occasionally up to 40mg daily necessary)	Considered to be less well tolerated than methylphenidate[36]	
Lisdexamfetamine (Elvanse)[2–4]	Onset: 20–60 minutes Duration: 13+ hours	Initially 20 or 30mg in the morning, titrated up to a licensed maximum dose of 70mg daily	Prodrug, gradually hydrolysed to dexamfetamine Capsules can be opened and sprinkled[47] Licensed in adults	
Atomoxetine[48,49]	Approximately 4–6 weeks (atomoxetine is a noradrenaline reuptake inhibitor)	When switching from a stimulant, continue stimulant for first 4 weeks of therapy For children <70kg: Initially 0.5mg/kg/day for 7 days, then increase according to response. Recommended maintenance dose 1.2mg/kg/day (in single or divided doses) and up to 1.8mg/kg/day, to a maximum of 120mg daily if necessary[1] For children >70kg: Initially 40mg daily for 7 days, then increase according to response. Recommended maintenance dose 80mg daily	Less effective than stimulants (see main ADHD text)[11,15] May be useful where stimulant diversion is a problem[50] Licensed in adults	Blood pressure[51] Pulse Height Weight Monitor for insomnia, mood and appetite change and the development of tics Monitor young people and adults with ADHD for sexual dysfunction (that is, erectile and ejaculatory dysfunction) as potential adverse effects of atomoxetine. Not a Controlled Drug

Table 5.6 (*Continued*)

Guanfacine modified-release[8,52]	Approximately 1–5 weeks[53] (Guanfacine is a central alpha2A-adrenergic receptor agonist)	For Child 6–12 years (body-weight 25kg and above) Initially 1mg once daily; adjusted in steps of 1mg every week if necessary and if tolerated; maintenance 0.05–0.12mg/kg once daily (max. per dose 4mg)	Efficacy and tolerability data should be interpreted with caution[8]	Similar monitoring to other medication for ADHD.
		For Child 13–17 years (body weight 34–41.4kg) Initially 1mg once daily; adjusted in steps of 1mg every week if necessary and if tolerated; maintenance 0.05–0.12mg/kg once daily (max. per dose 4mg)		
		For Child 13–17 years (body weight 41.5–49.4kg) Initially 1 mg once daily; adjusted in steps of 1 mg every week if necessary and if tolerated; maintenance 0.05–0.12 mg/kg once daily (max. per dose 5 mg)		
		For Child 13–17 years (body-weight 49.5–58.4kg) Initially 1mg once daily; adjusted in steps of 1mg every week if necessary and if tolerated; maintenance 0.05–0.12mg/kg once daily (max. per dose 6mg)		
		For Child 13–17 years (body weight 58.5kg and above) Initially 1mg once daily; adjusted in steps of 1mg every week if necessary and if tolerated; maintenance 0.05–0.12mg/kg once daily (max. per dose 7mg)		

*For details of other preparations available outside the UK, see Cortese et al. (2017).[54]

References

1. National Institute for Health and Clinical Excellence. Attention deficit hyperactivity disorder: diagnosis and management. NICE guideline [NG87] 2018 (Last updated September 2019); https://www.nice.org.uk/guidance/NG87.

2. Biederman J, et al. Lisdexamfetamine dimesylate and mixed amphetamine salts extended-release in children with ADHD: a double-blind, placebo-controlled, crossover analog classroom study. *Biol Psychiatry* 2007; 62:970–976.

3. Coghill D, et al. European, randomized, phase 3 study of lisdexamfetamine dimesylate in children and adolescents with attention-deficit/hyperactivity disorder. *Eur Neuropsychopharmacol* 2013; 23:1208–1218.

4. Findling RL, et al. Efficacy and safety of lisdexamfetamine dimesylate in adolescents with attention-deficit/hyperactivity disorder. *J Am Acad Child Adolesc Psychiatry* 2011; 50:395–405.

5. Heal DJ, et al. Amphetamine, past and present – a pharmacological and clinical perspective. *J Psychopharmacol* 2013; 27:479–496.

6. Coghill DR, et al. Long-term safety and efficacy of lisdexamfetamine dimesylate in children and adolescents with ADHD: a phase IV, 2-year, open-label study in Europe. *CNS Drugs* 2017; 31:625–638.

7. Joseph A, et al. Comparative efficacy and safety of attention-deficit/hyperactivity disorder pharmacotherapies, including guanfacine extended release: a mixed treatment comparison. *Eur Child Adolesc Psychiatry* 2017; 26:875–897.

8. Cortese S, et al. Comparative efficacy and tolerability of medications for attention-deficit hyperactivity disorder in children, adolescents, and adults: a systematic review and network meta-analysis. *Lancet Psychiatry* 2018; 5:727–738.

9. Findling RL, et al. Long-term effectiveness and safety of lisdexamfetamine dimesylate in school-aged children with attention-deficit/hyperactivity disorder. *CNS Spectr* 2008; 13:614–620.

10. Michelson D, et al. Once-daily atomoxetine treatment for children and adolescents with attention deficit hyperactivity disorder: a randomized, placebo-controlled study. *Am J Psychiatry* 2002; 159:1896–1901.

11. Kratochvil CJ, et al. Atomoxetine and methylphenidate treatment in children with ADHD: a prospective, randomized, open-label trial. *J Am Acad Child Adolesc Psychiatry* 2002; 41:776–784.

12. Weiss M, et al. A randomized, placebo-controlled study of once-daily atomoxetine in the school setting in children with ADHD. *J Am Acad Child Adolesc Psychiatry* 2005; 44:647–655.

13. Kratochvil CJ, et al. A double-blind, placebo-controlled study of atomoxetine in young children with ADHD. *Pediatrics* 2011; 127:e862–e868.

14. Catala-Lopez F, et al. The pharmacological and non-pharmacological treatment of attention deficit hyperactivity disorder in children and adolescents: a systematic review with network meta-analyses of randomised trials. *PLoS One* 2017; 12:e0180355.

15. Liu Q, et al. Comparative efficacy and safety of methylphenidate and atomoxetine for attention-deficit hyperactivity disorder in children and adolescents: meta-analysis based on head-to-head trials. *J Clin Exp Neuropsychol* 2017; 39:854–865.

16. Connor DF, et al. A meta-analysis of clonidine for symptoms of attention-deficit hyperactivity disorder. *J Am Acad Child Adolesc Psychiatry* 1999; 38:1551–1559.

17. National Institute for Health and Care Excellence. Attention deficit hyperactivity disorder in children and young people: guanfacine prolonged-release. Evidence summary [ESNM70] 2016; https://www.nice.org.uk/advice/esnm70/chapter/Key-points-from-the-evidence.

18. Hazell P. Tricyclic antidepressants in children: is there a rationale for use? *CNS Drugs* 1996; 5:233–239.

19. Otasowie J, et al. Tricyclic antidepressants for attention deficit hyperactivity disorder (ADHD) in children and adolescents. *Cochrane Database Syst Rev* 2014:Cd006997.

20. Gorman DA, et al. Canadian guidelines on pharmacotherapy for disruptive and aggressive behaviour in children and adolescents with attention-deficit hyperactivity disorder, oppositional defiant disorder, or conduct disorder. *Can J Psychiatry* 2015; 60:62–76.

21. Ng QX. A systematic review of the use of bupropion for attention-deficit/hyperactivity disorder in children and adolescents. *J Child Adolesc Psychopharmacol* 2017; 27:112–116.

22. Biederman J, et al. A comparison of once-daily and divided doses of modafinil in children with attention-deficit/hyperactivity disorder: a randomized, double-blind, and placebo-controlled study. *J Clin Psychiatry* 2006; 67:727–735.

23. Wang SM, et al. Modafinil for the treatment of attention-deficit/hyperactivity disorder: a meta-analysis. *J Psychiatr Res* 2017; 84:292–300.

24. Einarson TR, et al. *Novel antipsychotics for patients with attention-deficit hyperactivity disorder: a systematic review*. Ottawa: Canadian Coordinating Office for Health Technology Assessment (CCOHTA) 2001: Technology Report No 17.

25. Pringsheim T, et al. The pharmacological management of oppositional behaviour, conduct problems, and aggression in children and adolescents with attention-deficit hyperactivity disorder, oppositional defiant disorder, and conduct disorder: a systematic review and meta-analysis. Part 2: antipsychotics and traditional mood stabilizers. *Can J Psychiatry* 2015; 60:52–61.

26. Ji N, et al. An update on pharmacotherapy for autism spectrum disorder in children and adolescents. *Current Opinion Psychiatry* 2015; 28:91–101.

27. Humphreys KL, et al. Stimulant medication and substance use outcomes: a meta-analysis. *JAMA Psychiatry* 2013; 70:740–749.

28. Treuer T, et al. A systematic review of combination therapy with stimulants and atomoxetine for attention-deficit/hyperactivity disorder, including patient characteristics, treatment strategies, effectiveness, and tolerability. *J Child Adolesc Psychopharmacol* 2013; 23:179–193.

29. Thapar A, et al. Attention deficit hyperactivity disorder. *Lancet* 2016; 387:1240–1250.

30. DIVA Foundation. DIVA-5: diagnostic interview for ADHD in adults (DIVA) 2019; https://www.divacenter.eu/DIVA.aspx?id=461.

31. Cosgrove PVF. Attention deficit hyperactivity disorder. *Primary Care Psychiatry* 1997; 3:101–114.

32. Spencer T, et al. A double-blind, crossover comparison of methylphenidate and placebo in adults with childhood-onset attention-deficit hyperactivity disorder. *Arch Gen Psychiatry* 1995; 52:434–443.

33. Wolraich ML, et al. Pharmacokinetic considerations in the treatment of attention-deficit hyperactivity disorder with methylphenidate. *CNS Drugs* 2004; 18:243–250.

34. BNF Online. British National Formulary 2020; https://www.medicinescomplete.com/mc/bnf/current.

35. Janssen-Cilag Ltd. Summary of product characteristics. Concerta XL 18 mg 27 mg 36 mg and 54 mg prolonged-release tablets. 2020; https://www.medicines.org.uk/emc/product/6872/smpc.

36. Efron D, et al. Side effects of methylphenidate and dexamphetamine in children with attention deficit hyperactivity disorder: a double-blind, crossover trial. *Pediatrics* 1997; **100**:662–666.

37. Hennissen L, et al. Cardiovascular effects of stimulant and non-stimulant medication for children and adolescents with ADHD: a systematic review and meta-analysis of trials of methylphenidate, amphetamines and atomoxetine. *CNS Drugs* 2017; **31**:199–215.

38. Gadow KD, et al. Efficacy of methylphenidate for attention-deficit hyperactivity disorder in children with tic disorder. *Arch Gen Psychiatry* 1995; **52**:444–455.

39. Cohen SC, et al. Meta-analysis: risk of tics associated with psychostimulant use in randomized, placebo-controlled trials. *J Am Acad Child Adolesc Psychiatry* 2015; **54**:728–736.

40. Hoare P, et al. 12-month efficacy and safety of OROS MPH in children and adolescents with attention-deficit/hyperactivity disorder switched from MPH. *Eur Child Adolesc Psychiatry* 2005; **14**:305–309.

41. Remschmidt H, et al. Symptom control in children and adolescents with attention-deficit/hyperactivity disorder on switching from immediate-release MPH to OROS MPH results of a 3-week open-label study. *Eur Child Adolesc Psychiatry* 2005; **14**:297–304.

42. Wolraich ML, et al. Randomized, controlled trial of OROS methylphenidate once a day in children with attention-deficit/hyperactivity disorder. *Pediatrics* 2001; **108**:883–892.

43. Findling RL, et al. Comparison of the clinical efficacy of twice-daily ritalin and once-daily equasym XL with placebo in children with attention deficit/hyperactivity disorder. *Eur Child Adolesc Psychiatry* 2006; **15**:450–459.

44. Anderson VR, et al. Spotlight on methylphenidate controlled-delivery capsules (equasym XL™) in the treatment of children and adolescents with attention-deficit hyperactivity disorder. *CNS Drugs* 2007; **21**:173–175.

45. Flynn Pharma Ltd. Summary of Product Characteristics. Medikinet XL 5 mg 10 mg 20 mg 30 mg 40 mg 50 mg 60 mg modified release capsules 2019; https://www.medicines.org.uk/emc/product/313/smpc.

46. Cyr M, et al. Current drug therapy recommendations for the treatment of attention deficit hyperactivity disorder. *Drugs* 1998; **56**:215–223.

47. Shire Pharmaceuticals Limited. Summary of Product Characteristics. Elvanse 20 mg, 30 mg, 40 mg, 50 mg, 60 mg & 70 mg capsules, hard (lisdexamfetamine) 2019; https://www.medicines.org.uk/emc/medicine/27442.

48. Kelsey DK, et al. Once-daily atomoxetine treatment for children with attention-deficit/hyperactivity disorder, including an assessment of evening and morning behavior: a double-blind, placebo-controlled trial. *Pediatrics* 2004; **114**:e1-e8.

49. Wernicke JF, et al. Cardiovascular effects of atomoxetine in children, adolescents, and adults. *Drug Saf* 2003; **26**:729–740.

50. Heil SH, et al. Comparison of the subjective, physiological, and psychomotor effects of atomoxetine and methylphenidate in light drug users. *Drug Alcohol Depend* 2002; **67**:149–156.

51. Reed VA, et al. The safety of atomoxetine for the treatment of children and adolescents with attention-deficit/hyperactivity disorder: a comprehensive review of over a decade of research. *CNS Drugs* 2016; **30**:603–628.

52. Childress A, et al. Evaluation of the current data on guanfacine extended release for the treatment of ADHD in children and adolescents. *Expert Opin Pharmacother* 2020; **21**:417–426.

53. Takeda UK ltd. Guanfacine modified-release. Personal Communication, 2020.

54. Cortese S, et al. New formulations of methylphenidate for the treatment of attention-deficit/hyperactivity disorder: pharmacokinetics, efficacy, and tolerability. *CNS Drugs* 2017; **31**:149–160.

CHAPTER 5

Autism Spectrum Disorder

ASD is a complex condition characterised by core deficits in social communication development and behaviour (stereotypies and/or restricted and unusual patterns of interests) as well as sensory difficulties. The ASDs (autism, Asperger's syndrome and PDD-NOS) in ICD-10 are found under pervasive developmental disorders (PDD) and DSM-V defines ASD in one single category.

The heterogeneity of ASD poses assessment and treatment challenges. Co-occurring mental health conditions are highly prevalent in ASD[1] with 69–79% of individuals experiencing at least one in their lifetime.[2,3] These include attention deficit hyperactivity disorder (ADHD), disruptive behavioural disorders, anxiety, obsessive-compulsive and mood disorders. Other associated problems include intellectual disability, epilepsy, sleep disturbance, self-harm, irritability and aggression towards others. Associated neurodevelopmental, medical and psychiatric disorders complicate the symptom profile and affect overall outcome. Evaluating and optimally treating co-occurring conditions and/or associated problem behaviours is, therefore, essential.

Currently there are no validated or licensed pharmacological treatments that alleviate core ASD symptoms.[4,5] Targeting problem behaviours and comorbid psychiatric conditions with pharmacological interventions is, however, common practice.

Pharmacotherapies are commonly used in individuals with ASD as adjuncts to psychological interventions. The evidence to date[4,6] shows reasonable efficacy of risperidone, aripiprazole for irritability and aggression, supports use of methylphenidate, atomoxetine and guanfacine for ADHD, and melatonin for sleep problems but shows limited efficacy of SSIRs for anxiety, depression and repetitive behaviours. The evidence for antiepileptics remains inconsistent. There is a potential role for α2 agonists, cholinergic agonists, glutamatergic, (GABA)ergic agents and oxytocin but these require further investigation.[4,6]

Individuals with ASD are likely to experience more severe adverse effects than typically developing individuals.[4–6] Therefore, achieving an effective dose with minimum adverse effects can be a challenging task. Treatment should be initiated in small doses, and increased about every five half-lives of the drug, and it may take 4–6 weeks of titration to determine the therapeutic dose for every individual case.[7] Excluding any medical conditions, the presence of pain or any other physical discomfort such as gastro-esophageal reflux must be a priority before managing problem behaviour with psychotropic drugs. A comprehensive physical examination should be part of standard practice.

The efficacy and adverse effects associated with pharmacotherapy in individuals with ASD should be systematically monitored, in view of their impaired communication and the increased propensity for more adverse effects. Standardised behaviour ratings scales and adverse effect checklists are an essential tool in monitoring progress.[8]

Pharmacological treatment of core ASD symptoms

Evidence from clinical trials to date has not demonstrated clear efficacy of any of the psychotropic agents in routinely treating core symptoms of ASD.[4,6]

Restricted repetitive behaviours and interests (RRBI)

RRBIs are distressing and disruptive to functioning and therefore an important treatment target to improve overall outcomes in ASD.[9] Behavioural therapies should be used as first line. When RRBIs are severe with significant impact on functioning and/or pose risks to others or self then pharmacotherapy can be considered.

A Cochrane review (last updated in 2013) found 'no evidence of effect of SSRIs on reducing RRBIs in children and emerging evidence of harm' although there are data that support their use in adults.[10] Research with risperidone indicates that it is effective in reducing RRBIs in children who have high levels of irritability or aggression,[11] thus making doubtful any specific efficacy for repetitive behaviours. Reductions in stereotypical behaviours have also been reported[12–15] albeit in studies with methodological limitations.[6] A 2020 meta-analysis of studies on a wide range of currently available pharmacological agents showed evidence supporting only antipsychotic medication[16] whereas another recent meta-analysis of nine studies found no evidence for any pharmacological agent in reducing RRBIs.[17] Overall, given the profile of adverse effects of dopamine blocking agents, the recent consensus guidance from the British Association for Psychopharmacology[6] cautions against their routine use for the treatment of RRBIs. If they are used, they should be prescribed in small doses and as part of a carefully considered, time-limited and monitored overall treatment plan.

Social and communication impairment

Currently, no drug has been consistently shown to improve the core social and communication impairments in ASD.[7] **Risperidone** may have a secondary effect through improvement in irritability.[18] Analysis of data from two multi-centre trials suggested that risperidone was effective for the treatment of social disability in children with ASD.[19] Glutamatergic drugs and oxytocin are currently the most promising.[20] However, a recent meta-analysis of 12 RCTs suggested that **oxytocin** had no significant effect on social communication even though individual RCTs had reported improvements from oxytocin.[21] Larger studies with better methodology are needed.[22] **Sulforaphane,**[23] **insulin growth factor 1** (IGF-1)[24] await further work to prove their efficacy in modifying ASD core symptoms, as do **glutamatergic agents.**[25] **Acetylcysteine**[26] is probably not effective.

There is growing albeit inconsistent evidence for dietary interventions reducing ASD core symptoms.[27,28] Targeting the gut microbiome, including probiotic treatment and faecal microbiota transplants as novel and potential therapeutics for ASD conditions has also drawn much interest recently.[29] However, there is little evidence to support the use of nutritional supplements or dietary therapies for children with ASD[27] or indeed any relationship between maternal food intake and child's diet and the development of ASD/symptoms severity.[28]

CHAPTER 5

Pharmacological treatment of co-occurring disorders and problem behaviours in ASD

Inattention, overactivity and impulsiveness in ASD (symptoms of ADHD)

Individuals with ASD have high rates of inattention, overactivity and impulsiveness and in an around one-third these symptoms merit the diagnosis of ADHD.[1,30]

The largest controlled trial to date has been with **methylphenidate** and conducted by the Research Units on Paediatric Psychopharmacology (RUPP) Autism Network.[31,32] In a previous retrospective and prospective study of children with ASD, Santosh and colleagues[33] reported positive benefits of treatment with methylphenidate. In general, methylphenidate produces highly variable responses in children with ASD and ADHD symptoms, ranging from marked improvement with few adverse effects to poor response with or without problematic adverse effects. A large double-blind, placebo-controlled trial of methylphenidate in children with intellectual disability and ADHD showed that optimal dosing with methylphenidate was effective in some.[34] Adverse effects are more commonly reported than in children with ADHD alone.[35-37] However, where ADHD symptoms are severe and/or disabling, it is reasonable to proceed with a treatment trial of methylphenidate. It is advisable to warn parents of the lower likelihood of response and the potential adverse effects and to proceed with low initial does (around 0.125mg/kg three times daily, depending on the preparation) increasing with small increments. Treatment should be stopped immediately if behaviour deteriorates or there are unacceptable adverse effects. A recent systematic review[6] confirms that although effective, the efficacy of methylphenidate for the treatment of ADHD in ASD is less than in ADHD alone and that more adverse effects (decreased appetite, sleeping difficulties, abdominal discomfort, social withdrawal, irritability and emotional outbursts) should be expected in ASD.

There are no published data on the efficacy of **amfetamines** in children with ASD even though they have been used to treat ADHD in these patients as well as typically developed children. **Lisdexamfetamine** (pro-drug containing d-amphetamine bound to amino acid lysine) has been found to have efficacy and tolerability in treating ADHD in children and young people[38] but with no specific data about those with ASD.

Atomoxetine is a noradrenergic reuptake inhibitor licensed to treat ADHD with similar efficacy to methylphenidate.[6] Preliminary evidence from small open-label trials and a handful randomised double-blind trials[39,40] that it may be useful in children with ASD, with the most common side effects being nausea, fatigue and sleep difficulties were followed by a larger trial which confirmed that atomoxetine (alone and combined with parent training) significantly reduced ADHD symptoms.[41] At 24-week extension of the same study, atomoxetine combined with parent training was superior at reducing ADHD symptoms to atomoxetine alone.[42]

There is evidence that α2 **agonists** (clonidine and guanfacine) can be used as alternative treatments. A recent multisite RCT of extended-release guanfacine compared with placebo in children with ASD (mean age 8.5 years) over a period of 8 weeks showed that it is safe and effective in managing hyperactivity in this group.[43] No serious adverse events except for drowsiness, fatigue, and decreased appetite were reported.

There are reports from controlled studies supporting the use of **risperidone** or **aripiprazole** for ADHD symptoms. However, these were not primary outcomes of the studies and therefore need further investigation.

Irritability (aggression, self-injurious behaviour, severe disruptive behaviours)

Aggression towards others and the self, frequently underlined by irritability, are common problems in ASD. Although behavioural and environment approaches should be first-line treatments, more severe and dangerous behaviours usually necessitate pharmacotherapy.[44] Duration of recommended treatment is difficult to derive from published evidence but treatment appears to be beneficial for up to 6–12 months.[45] Efforts to reduce and possibly discontinue such treatment at the end of this period should be strongly considered.[44,45]

Second-generation antipsychotics are the first-line pharmacological treatment for children and adolescents with ASD and associated irritability.[45–48] **Risperidone**[49,50] and **aripiprazole**[51] have been reliably shown to help with irritability and associated disruptive behaviours[5] in ASD and have been approved for this use by the US FDA. In a meta-analysis of data from 46 RCTs[52] comparing efficacy of risperidone, aripiprazole and other compounds with placebo, risperidone and aripiprazole were the most effective, with moderate to large effect sizes. Another meta-analysis of short-term (8 weeks) aripiprazole in the treatment of irritability in ASD children aged 6–17 years[53] found similar results when compared with placebo. The most recent Cochrane review[54] which is an update of the previous one[55] concluded that aripiprazole may be beneficial in managing irritability, hyperactivity and stereotypes in children with ASD. The usual recommended clinical dose of aripiprazole for maintenance is between 5 and 15mg daily.[45] The starting dose of aripiprazole is 2mg/day. The dosing of risperidone is rather more complicated; FDA recommended dosages for risperidone are outlined in Box 5.3.

Despite their promising efficacy adverse effects such as weight gain and metabolic changes, increased appetite and somnolence (even with aripiprazole) can be problematic.[15,56–59] One long-term, placebo discontinuation study found that relapse rates did not differ between those who stayed on aripiprazole versus those randomised to switch to only placebo, suggesting that re-evaluation of aripiprazole use after a period of stabilisation in irritability symptoms is warranted.[54] There is only one study that makes a direct head-to-head comparison[60] showing similar tolerability and efficacy profiles for risperidone and aripiprazole. Risperidone usually causes hyperprolactinaemia which although may be asymptomatic, it may have longer term effects therefore necessitating close monitoring whereas aripiprazole does not which makes it a preferred option. Aripiprazole may on the other hand be ineffective for self-injurious behaviours.[6]

The effectiveness of other SGAs, such as **olanzapine**,[61] **quetiapine**, **ziprasidone** and **clozapine**, has not been tested in adequately powered RCTs. Whilst controlled studies support the use of mood stabilizers, such as **lithium**[62,63] and **sodium valproate**,[64] in the treatment of persistent aggression in children they are not as effective as SGAs for the treatment of irritability in ASD.[65] Limited data support the combination of **risperidone** and **topiramate** being better than risperidone alone.[66] Further RCTs are warranted of BDNF stimulators such as loxapine and amitriptyline.[67]

Use of risperidone in children and adolescents

Risperidone is indicated for the treatment of irritability associated with autistic disorder in children (aged 5 and over) and adolescents in the UK/EU and the United States

The dosage of risperidone should be individualised according to the response of the patient.

Box 5.3 FDA Guidance for risperidone dosing in children and adolescents[68]

Doses of Risperidone in Paediatric Patients with Autism Spectrum Disorders (by total mg/day)

Weight categories	Days 1–3	Days 4–18	Increments if dose increases are needed	Dose range
<20kg*	0.25mg	0.5mg	+0.25mg at ≥2 week intervals	0.5mg–3mg**
≥20kg	0.5mg	1.0mg	+0.5mg at ≥2 week intervals	1.0mg–3mg***

*Caution should be exercised for children <15kg – no dosing data available
**Therapeutic effect plateaus at 1mg/day
***Those weighing >45kg may require higher doses – therapeutic effect plateaus at 3mg

General considerations

- Risperidone can be administered once daily or twice daily.
- Patients experiencing somnolence may benefit from taking the whole daily dose at bedtime.
- Once sufficient clinical response has been achieved and maintained, consideration may be given to gradually lowering the dose to achieve the optimal balance of efficacy and safety.
- There is insufficient evidence from controlled trials to indicate how long treatment should continue.

Adverse effects

Weight gain, somnolence and hyperglycaemia require monitoring, and the long-term safety of risperidone in children and adolescents with ASD remains to be fully determined

---

Using **benzodiazepines** (BZ) to manage irritability and aggression in ASD is not recommended. However, it may be necessary to manage acute aggression with a BZ. The possibility of behavioural disinhibition which may worsen aggression must be born in mind.

Recent guidance from BAP does not recommend the use of **minocycline, arbaclofen** or **amantadine** for irritability before better evidence from randomised double-blind controlled trials is available.[6]

Sleep disturbance

Children with ASD have significant sleep problems[69] with sleep-onset insomnia, sleep-maintenance insomnia and irregularities of the sleep–wake cycle being the typical problems encountered. It is essential to understand the aetiology of the sleep problem before embarking on a course of treatment. Abnormalities in the melatonin system have received some attention.[70]

Melatonin, has been shown in 17 studies to be beneficial in children with ASD.[71] A meta-analysis of five studies showed good efficacy with doses ranging from 1mg to 10mg and treatment lasting from 14 days to over 4 years.[72] Melatonin is usually very well tolerated.[72,73] One RCT showed that, whilst melatonin improved sleep onset, child's behaviour during the day did not improve.[74]

There is also evidence that melatonin combined with CBT is superior to melatonin only, CBT only and placebo in reducing symptoms of insomnia.[75]

Risperidone may benefit sleep difficulties in those with extreme irritability. In the anxious or depressed child, antidepressants may be beneficial. Insomnia due to hyperarousal may benefit from clonidine or clonazepam.[76]

Anxiety, OCD and depression

SSRIs have yet to show specific efficacy in ASD. Recent preliminary data from a randomised placebo-blind clinical trial showed beneficial effects of fluoxetine in reducing OCD symptoms in children with ASD, although confounding factors precluded firm conclusions.[77] In a recent systematic review,[6] although risperidone was reported by several studies to reduce OCD and anxiety symptoms in young people with ASD, the primary selection of participants for high levels of irritability did not allow firm conclusions about specific effects of risperidone on OCD and anxiety. The review concluded that overall, there is little or no evidence for treating anxiety or OCD symptoms with risperidone, clomipramine or an SSRI. The recent BAP guidance[6] is to cautiously follow the existing BAP guidelines for treating anxiety and OCD.[78] There are some data on **buspirone** effectively targeting anxiety in ASD[79] and propranolol showing positive cognitive effects in ASD.[80] However, further evaluation is needed. Guidance on doses of fluoxetine can be found in Box 5.4.

Fluoxetine in children and adolescents

When using fluoxetine to treat repetitive behaviours in ASD patients, doses much lower than those used to treat depression are normally required. It is advisable to use a liquid preparation and begin at the lowest possible dose, monitoring for adverse effects. A suitable regime is outlined in Box 5.4.

Box 5.4   Use of fluoxetine in children and adolescents

Liquid fluoxetine: (as hydrochloride) 20mg/5mL
2.5mg/day a day for 1 week; note that 2.5mg = 0.625mL which is difficult to measure accurately.

Follow with flexible titration schedule based on weight, tolerability and adverse-effects up to a maximum dose of 0.8mg/kg/day (0.3mg/kg for week 2, 0.5mg/kg/day for week 3, and 0.8mg/kg/day subsequently). Reduction may be indicated if adverse effects are problematic.

Adverse effects

- Monitor for treatment emergent **suicidal** behaviour, self-harm and hostility, particularly at the beginning of treatment.
- Hyponatraemia is also possible – see section in Chapter 3.

References

1. Lai MC, et al. Prevalence of co-occurring mental health diagnoses in the autism population: a systematic review and meta-analysis. *Lancet Psychiatry* 2019; 6:819–829.
2. Lever AG, et al. Psychiatric co-occurring symptoms and disorders in young, middle-aged, and older adults with autism spectrum disorder. *J Autism Dev Disord* 2016; 46:1916–1930.
3. Buck TR, et al. Psychiatric comorbidity and medication use in adults with autism spectrum disorder. *J Autism Dev Disord* 2014; 44:3063–3071.
4. Goel R, et al. An update on pharmacotherapy of autism spectrum disorder in children and adolescents. *Int Rev Psychiatry (Abingdon, England)* 2018; 30:78–95.
5. Accordino RE, et al. Psychopharmacological interventions in autism spectrum disorder. *Expert Opin Pharmacother* 2016; 17:937–952.
6. Howes OD, et al. Autism spectrum disorder: consensus guidelines on assessment, treatment and research from the British Association for Psychopharmacology. *J Psychopharmacol* 2018; 32:3–29.
7. Santosh P. Medication in autism spectrum disorder. *Cut Edge Psychiatry Pract* 2014; 1:143–155.
8. Greenhill LL. Assessment of safety in pediatric psychopharmacology. *J Am Acad Child Adolesc Psychiatry* 2003; 42:625–626.
9. Leekam SR, et al. Restricted and repetitive behaviors in autism spectrum disorders: a review of research in the last decade. *Psychol Bull* 2011; 137:562–593.
10. Williams K, et al. Selective serotonin reuptake inhibitors (SSRIs) for autism spectrum disorders (ASD). *Cochrane Database Syst Rev* 2013; 8:CD004677.
11. McDougle CJ, et al. A double-blind, placebo-controlled study of risperidone addition in serotonin reuptake inhibitor-refractory obsessive-compulsive disorder. *Arch Gen Psychiatry* 2000; 57:794–801.
12. McDougle CJ, et al. Risperidone for the core symptom domains of autism: results from the study by the autism network of the research units on pediatric psychopharmacology. *Am J Psychiatry* 2005; 162:1142–1148.
13. McCracken JT, et al. Risperidone in children with autism and serious behavioral problems. *N Engl J Med* 2002; 347:314–321.
14. Arnold LE, et al. Parent-defined target symptoms respond to risperidone in RUPP autism study: customer approach to clinical trials. *J Am Acad Child Adolesc Psychiatry* 2003; 42:1443–1450.
15. Dinnissen M, et al. Clinical and pharmacokinetic evaluation of risperidone for the management of autism spectrum disorder. *Expert Opin Drug Metab Toxicol* 2015; 11:111–124.
16. Zhou MS, et al. Meta-analysis: pharmacologic treatment of restricted and repetitive behaviors in autism spectrum disorders. *J Am Acad Child Adolesc Psychiatry* 2020:Epub ahead of print.
17. Yu Y, et al. Pharmacotherapy of restricted/repetitive behavior in autism spectrum disorder: a systematic review and meta-analysis. *BMC Psychiatry* 2020; 20:121.
18. Canitano R, et al. Risperidone in the treatment of behavioral disorders associated with autism in children and adolescents. *Neuropsychiatr Dis Treat* 2008; 4:723–730.
19. Scahill L, et al. Brief report: social disability in autism spectrum disorder: results from Research Units on Pediatric Psychopharmacology (RUPP) Autism Network trials. *J Autism Dev Disord* 2013; 43:739–746.
20. Posey DJ, et al. Developing drugs for core social and communication impairment in autism. *Child Adolesc Psychiatr Clin N Am* 2008; 17:787–801.
21. Ooi YP, et al. Oxytocin and autism spectrum disorders: a systematic review and meta-analysis of randomized controlled trials. *Pharmacopsychiatry* 2017; 50:5–13.
22. Alvares GA, et al. Beyond the hype and hope: critical considerations for intranasal oxytocin research in autism spectrum disorder. *Autism Res Off Int Soc Autism Res* 2017; 10:25–41.
23. Singh K, et al. Sulforaphane treatment of autism spectrum disorder (ASD). *Proc Natl Acad Sci USA* 2014; 111:15550–15555.
24. Riikonen R. Treatment of autistic spectrum disorder with insulin-like growth factors. *Eur J Paediatr Neurol* 2016; 20:816–823.
25. Fung LK, et al. Developing medications targeting glutamatergic dysfunction in autism: progress to date. *CNS Drugs* 2015; 29:453–463.
26. Dean OM, et al. A randomised, double blind, placebo-controlled trial of a fixed dose of N-acetyl cysteine in children with autistic disorder. *Aust N Z J Psychiatry* 2017; 51:241–249.
27. Sathe N, et al. Nutritional and dietary interventions for autism spectrum disorder: a systematic review. *Pediatrics* 2017; 139:e20170346.
28. Peretti S, et al. Diet: the keystone of autism spectrum disorder? *Nutr Neurosci* 2019; 22:825–839.
29. Yang Y, et al. Targeting gut microbiome: a novel and potential therapy for autism. *Life Sci* 2018; 194:111–119.
30. Lee YJ, et al. Advanced pharmacotherapy evidenced by pathogenesis of autism spectrum disorder. *Clin Psychopharmacol Neurosci Off Sci J Korean College Neuropsychopharmacol* 2014; 12:19–30.
31. Research Units on Pediatric Psychopharmacology (RUPP) Autism Network. Randomized, controlled, crossover trial of methylphenidate in pervasive developmental disorders with hyperactivity. *Arch Gen Psychiatry* 2005; 62:1266–1274.
32. Posey DJ, et al. Positive effects of methylphenidate on inattention and hyperactivity in pervasive developmental disorders: an analysis of secondary measures. *Biol Psychiatry* 2007; 61:538–544.
33. Santosh PJ, et al. Impact of comorbid autism spectrum disorders on stimulant response in children with attention deficit hyperactivity disorder: a retrospective and prospective effectiveness study. *Child Care Health Dev* 2006; 32:575–583.
34. Simonoff E, et al. Randomized controlled double-blind trial of optimal dose methylphenidate in children and adolescents with severe attention deficit hyperactivity disorder and intellectual disability. *J Child Psychol Psychiatry* 2013; 54:527–535.
35. Sung M, et al. What's in the pipeline? Drugs in development for autism spectrum disorder. *Neuropsychiatr Dis Treat* 2014; 10:371–381.

36. Siegel M, et al. Psychotropic medications in children with autism spectrum disorders: a systematic review and synthesis for evidence-based practice. *J Autism Dev Disord* 2012; **42**:1592–1605.

37. Williamson ED, et al. Psychotropic medications in autism: practical considerations for parents. *J Autism Dev Disord* 2012; **42**:1249–1255.

38. Coghill D, et al. European, randomized, phase 3 study of lisdexamfetamine dimesylate in children and adolescents with attention-deficit/hyperactivity disorder. *Eur Neuropsychopharmacol* 2013; **23**:1208–1218.

39. Arnold LE, et al. Atomoxetine for hyperactivity in autism spectrum disorders: placebo-controlled crossover pilot trial. *J Am Acad Child Adolesc Psychiatry* 2006; **45**:1196–1205.

40. Harfterkamp M, et al. A randomized double-blind study of atomoxetine versus placebo for attention-deficit/hyperactivity disorder symptoms in children with autism spectrum disorder. *J Am Acad Child Adolesc Psychiatry* 2012; **51**:733–741.

41. Handen BL, et al. Atomoxetine, parent training, and their combination in children with autism spectrum disorder and attention-deficit/hyperactivity disorder. *J Am Acad Child Adolesc Psychiatry* 2015; **54**:905–915.

42. Smith T, et al. Atomoxetine and parent training for children with autism and attention-deficit/hyperactivity disorder: a 24-week extension study. *J Am Acad Child Adolesc Psychiatry* 2016; **55**:868–876.e862.

43. Scahill L, et al. Extended-release guanfacine for hyperactivity in children with autism spectrum disorder. *Am J Psychiatry* 2015; **172**:1197–1206.

44. National Institute for Health and Care Excellence. Autism spectrum disorder in under 19s: support and management. Clinical Guidance 170 [CG170] 2013 (Reviewed September 2016); https://www.nice.org.uk/Guidance/CG170.

45. Kaplan G, et al. Psychopharmacology of autism spectrum disorders. *Pediatr Clin North Am* 2012; **59**:175–187, xii.

46. McDougle CJ, et al. Atypical antipsychotics in children and adolescents with autistic and other pervasive developmental disorders. *J Clin Psychiatry* 2008; **69** Suppl 4:15–20.

47. Parikh MS, et al. Psychopharmacology of aggression in children and adolescents with autism: a critical review of efficacy and tolerability. *J Child Adolesc Psychopharmacol* 2008; **18**:157–178.

48. DeVane CL, et al. Pharmacotherapy of autism spectrum disorder: results from the randomized BAART clinical trial. *Pharmacotherapy* 2019; **39**:626–635.

49. Jesner OS, et al. Risperidone for autism spectrum disorder. *Cochrane Database Syst Rev* 2007:CD005040.

50. Scahill L, et al. Risperidone approved for the treatment of serious behavioral problems in children with autism. *J Child Adolesc Psychiatr Nurs* 2007; **20**:188–190.

51. Curran MP. Aripiprazole: in the treatment of irritability associated with autistic disorder in pediatric patients. *Paediatr Drugs* 2011; **13**:197–204.

52. Fung LK, et al. Pharmacologic treatment of severe irritability and problem behaviors in autism: a systematic review and meta-analysis. *Pediatrics* 2016; **137** Suppl 2:S124–135.

53. Douglas-Hall P, et al. Aripiprazole: a review of its use in the treatment of irritability associated with autistic disorder patients aged 6-17. *J Cent Nerv Syst Dis* 2011; **3**:1–11.

54. Hirsch LE, et al. Aripiprazole for autism spectrum disorders (ASD). *Cochrane Database Syst Rev* 2016:Cd009043.

55. Ching H, et al. Aripiprazole for autism spectrum disorders (ASD). *Cochrane Database Syst Rev* 2012; **5**:CD009043.

56. Caccia S. Safety and pharmacokinetics of atypical antipsychotics in children and adolescents. *Paediatr Drugs* 2013; **15**:217–233.

57. Sharma A, et al. Efficacy of risperidone in managing maladaptive behaviors for children with autistic spectrum disorder: a meta-analysis. *J Pediatr Health Care* 2012; **26**:291–299.

58. Kent JM, et al. Risperidone dosing in children and adolescents with autistic disorder: a double-blind, placebo-controlled study. *J Autism Dev Disord* 2013; **43**:1773–1783.

59. Maayan L, et al. Weight gain and metabolic risks associated with antipsychotic medications in children and adolescents. *J Child Adolesc Psychopharmacol* 2011; **21**:517–535.

60. Ghanizadeh A, et al. A head-to-head comparison of aripiprazole and risperidone for safety and treating autistic disorders, a randomized double blind clinical trial. *Child Psychiatry Hum Dev* 2014; **45**:185–192.

61. Hollander E, et al. A double-blind placebo-controlled pilot study of olanzapine in childhood/adolescent pervasive developmental disorder. *J Child Adolesc Psychopharmacol* 2006; **16**:541–548.

62. Campbell M, et al. Lithium in hospitalized aggressive children with conduct disorder: a double-blind and placebo-controlled study. *J Am Acad Child Adolesc Psychiatry* 1995; **34**:445–453.

63. Malone RP, et al. A double-blind placebo-controlled study of lithium in hospitalized aggressive children and adolescents with conduct disorder. *Arch Gen Psychiatry* 2000; **57**:649–654.

64. Donovan SJ, et al. Divalproex treatment for youth with explosive temper and mood lability: a double-blind, placebo-controlled crossover design. *Am J Psychiatry* 2000; **157**:818–820.

65. Stigler KA, et al. Pharmacotherapy of irritability in pervasive developmental disorders. *Child Adolesc Psychiatr Clin N Am* 2008; **17**:739–752.

66. Rezaei V, et al. Double-blind, placebo-controlled trial of risperidone plus topiramate in children with autistic disorder. *Prog Neuropsychopharmacol Biol Psychiatry* 2010; **34**:1269–1272.

67. Hellings JA, et al. Dopamine antagonists for treatment resistance in autism spectrum disorders: review and focus on BDNF stimulators loxapine and amitriptyline. *Expert Opin Pharmacother* 2017; **18**:581–588.

68. Janssen Pharmaceutical Companies. Highlights of Prescribing Information: RISPERDAL® (risperidone) tablets, RISPERDAL® (risperidone) oral solution, RISPERDAL® M-TAB® (risperidone) orally disintegrating tablets 2019; https://www.accessdata.fda.gov/drugsatfda_docs/label/2019/020272s082,020588s070,021444s056lbl.pdf.

CHAPTER 5

69. Krakowiak P, et al. Sleep problems in children with autism spectrum disorders, developmental delays, and typical development: a population-based study. *J Sleep Res* 2008; **17**:197–206.

70. Sanchez-Barcelo EJ, et al. Clinical uses of melatonin in pediatrics. *Int J Pediatr* 2011; **2011**:892624.

71. Doyen C, et al. Melatonin in children with autistic spectrum disorders: recent and practical data. *Eur Child Adolesc Psychiatry* 2011; **20**:231–239.

72. Rossignol DA, et al. Melatonin in autism spectrum disorders: a systematic review and meta-analysis. *Dev Med Child Neurol* 2011; **53**:783–792.

73. Andersen IM, et al. Melatonin for insomnia in children with autism spectrum disorders. *J Child Neurol* 2008; **23**:482–485.

74. Gringras P, et al. Melatonin for sleep problems in children with neurodevelopmental disorders: randomised double masked placebo controlled trial. *BMJ* 2012; **345**:e6664.

75. Cortesi F, et al. Controlled-release melatonin, singly and combined with cognitive behavioural therapy, for persistent insomnia in children with autism spectrum disorders: a randomized placebo-controlled trial. *J Sleep Res* 2012; **21**:700–709.

76. Johnson KP, et al. Sleep in children with autism spectrum disorders. *Curr Treat Options Neurol* 2008; **10**:350–359.

77. Reddihough DS, et al. Effect of fluoxetine on obsessive-compulsive behaviors in children and adolescents with autism spectrum disorders: a randomized clinical trial. *JAMA* 2019; **322**:1561–1569.

78. Baldwin DS, et al. Evidence-based guidelines for the pharmacological treatment of anxiety disorders: recommendations from the British Association for Psychopharmacology. *J Psychopharm* 2005; **19**:567–596.

79. Buitelaar JK, et al. Buspirone in the management of anxiety and irritability in children with pervasive developmental disorders: results of an open-label study. *J Clin Psychiatry* 1998; **59**:56–59.

80. Narayanan A, et al. Effect of propranolol on functional connectivity in autism spectrum disorder–a pilot study. *Brain Imaging and Behavior* 2010; **4**:189–197.

Tics and Tourette syndrome

Transient tics occur in 5–20% of children. Tourette syndrome (TS) occurs in about 1% of children and is defined by persistent motor and vocal tics. As many as 65% of individuals with TS will have no tics or only very mild tics by adult life. Tics wax and wane over time and are variably exacerbated by external factors such as stress, inactivity and fatigue, depending on the individual. Tics are about two to three times more common in boys than girls.[1]

Detection and treatment of comorbidity

Co-morbid OCD, attention deficit hyperactivity disorder, depression, anxiety and behavioural problems are more prevalent than would be expected by chance, and often cause the major impairment in people with tic disorders.[2] These comorbid conditions are usually treated first before assessing the level of disability caused by the tics.[3]

Education and behavioural treatments

Most people with tics do not require pharmacological treatment but education for the individual with tics, their family and the people they interact with, especially schools, is crucial. Treatment aimed primarily at reducing tics is warranted if they cause distress to the patient or are functionally disabling. Behavioural interventions have been found to be effective with similar effect sizes to antipsychotic medication.[4,5] Habit Reversal, comprehensive behavioural interventions, and Exposure and Response Prevention are the behavioural treatments of choice.[6]

Pharmacological treatments

Studies of pharmacological interventions in TS are difficult to interpret for several reasons:

- There is a large inter-individual variation in tic frequency and severity. Small, randomised studies may include patients that are very different at baseline.
- The severity of tics in a given individual varies markedly over time, making it difficult to separate drug effect from natural variation.
- The bulk of the literature consists of case reports, case series, open studies and underpowered, randomised studies. Publication bias is also likely to be an issue.
- A high proportion of patients have co-morbid psychiatric illness. It can be difficult to disentangle any direct effect on tics from an effect on the co-morbid illness. This makes it difficult to interpret studies that report improvements in global functioning rather than specific reductions in tics.
- Large numbers of individuals attending clinics with TS appear to use complementary or alternative therapies with the majority reporting benefits and up to half finding these more helpful compared to medication.[7] However, robust research about the use of complementary or alternative therapies, their efficacy, and potential side effects is lacking.[8]

The placebo effect in clinical trials of tic disorders is not as large as previously thought.[9]

CHAPTER 5

Adrenergic α2 agonists

Clonidine has been shown in open studies to reduce the severity and frequency of tics but in one study this effect did not seem to be convincingly larger than placebo.[10] Other studies have shown more substantial reductions in tics.[11-14] Therapeutic doses of clonidine are in the order or 3–5µg/kg, and the dose should be built up gradually. A transdermal patch has also shown effectiveness.[15] Main side-effects are sedation, postural hypotension and depression. Patients and their families should be informed not to stop clonidine suddenly because of the risk of rebound hypertension. **Guanfacine** has also been shown to be effective in the treatment of tics[16,17] and would merit a therapeutic trial in specific individuals (e.g. those with comorbid ADHD).

Antipsychotics

Adverse effects of antipsychotics may outweigh beneficial effects in the treatment of tics and so it is recommended that clonidine or guanfacine are always tried first. Antipsychotics may, however, be more effective than adrenergic α2 agonists in alleviating tics in some individuals.

A number of first-generation antipsychotics have been used in TS.[18] In a Cochrane review, **pimozide** demonstrated robust efficacy in a meta-analysis of 6 trials.[19] In these trials, pimozide was compared with haloperidol (one trial), placebo (one trial), haloperidol and placebo (two trials) and risperidone (two trials) and was found to be more effective than placebo, as effective as risperidone and slightly less effective than haloperidol in reducing tics. It was associated with fewer adverse reactions compared with haloperidol but did not differ from risperidone in that respect. ECG monitoring is essential for pimozide and haloperidol. **Haloperidol** is often poorly tolerated. Given their side effect profile, most authors recommend the use of second-generation rather than first-generation antipsychotics in the treatment of TS.[18]

More recent studies suggest that **aripiprazole** is an effective and well-tolerated treatment of children with TS (and also tics[20]). A 10-week multicentre double-blind randomised placebo-controlled trial (N = 61) demonstrated the efficacy of aripiprazole in tic reduction in TS. Treatment was associated with significantly decreased serum prolactin concentration, increased mean body weight (by 1.6kg), body mass index, and waist circumference.[21] Aripiprazole was also found to be effective in another randomized, double-blind, placebo-controlled trial (N = 133) comparing low-dose aripiprazole (5mg/day if <50kg; 10mg/day if ≥50kg), high-dose aripiprazole (10mg/day if <50kg; 20mg/day if ≥50kg), or placebo for 8 weeks.[22] At week 8, tics as measured by the Yale Global Tic Severity Scale Total Tic Score were reduced in both the high dose group (–9.9; 95% CI: –13.8 to –5.9) and the low dose group (–6.3; 95% CI: –10.2 to –2.3) with 69% (29/42) of patients in the low-dose and 74% (26/35) in the high-dose group being very much improved or much improved compared with 38% (16/42) in the placebo group. Surprisingly, a higher proportion of children in the low dose group (18.2%) compared to the high dose group (9.3%) and placebo group (9.1%) gained clinically significant weight (≥7%) which may have been related to a lower average baseline weight in this group by >3kg compared to the other two groups. Several case series also support the use of aripiprazole.[23-26] A study evaluating the metabolic side effects of aripiprazole (N = 25) and pimozide (N = 25) in TS over a 24-month period demonstrated that treatment was not associated with significant increase in body mass index. However, pimozide treatment was associated with increases in blood glucose which did not plateau from 12 to 24 months, aripiprazole treatment was associated with increased cholesterol and both medications were associated with increased triglycerides.[27] Two meta-analyses support the efficacy of aripiprazole.[28,29] One study[30] suggests twice weekly administration may be better tolerated than daily dosing. A small randomised controlled trial (N = 24) comparing aripiprazole with sodium valproate in children with TS demonstrated a statistically significant difference in tic reduction favouring aripiprazole.[31]

Risperidone has in addition to the studies mentioned above also been shown to be more effective than placebo in a small (N = 34), randomised study.[32] Fatigue and increased appetite were problematic in the risperidone arm and a mean weight gain of 2.8kg over 8 weeks was reported. One small randomised, controlled trial found risperidone and clonidine to be equally effective.[33] A small double-blind crossover study suggested that **olanzapine**[34] may be more effective than pimozide. **Sulpiride** has been shown to be effective and relatively well tolerated,[35] as has **ziprasidone**.[36] Open studies support the efficacy of **quetiapine**[37] and **olanzapine**.[38,39] One very small crossover study (N = 7) found no effect for **clozapine**.[40]

Overall, metabolic side-effects and weight gain are common with second generation antipsychotics, even aripiprazole, so benefit/risk ratios need careful discussion.[18]

Other drugs

A small, double-blind, placebo-controlled, crossover trial of **baclofen** was suggestive of beneficial effects in overall impairment rather than a specific effect on tics.[41] The numerical benefits shown in this study did not reach statistical significance. Similarly, a double-blind, placebo-controlled trial of **nicotine** augmentation of haloperidol found beneficial effects in overall impairment rather than a specific effect on tics.[42] These benefits persisted for several weeks after nicotine (in the form of patches) was withdrawn. Nicotine patches were associated with a high prevalence of nausea and vomiting (71% and 40%, respectively). The authors suggest that PRN use may be appropriate. **Pergolide** (a D_1–D_2–D_3 agonist) given in low dose significantly reduced tics in a double-blind, placebo-controlled, crossover study in children and adolescents.[43] Side-effects included sedation, dizziness, nausea and irritability. Pergolide was also evaluated in a randomised trial in children and adolescents with chronic tics and TS, and showed significant tic reduction compared with placebo.[44] **Flutamide**, an antiandrogen, has been the subject of a small RCT in adults with TS. Modest, short-lived effects were seen in motor but not phonic tics.[45] A small randomised controlled trial has shown significant advantages for **metoclopramide** over placebo[46] and for **topiramate** over placebo.[47] A meta-analysis identified 14 randomised controlled trials (all from China) comparing topiramate with haloperidol or **tiapride**. It concluded that owing to the overall low quality of the study designs, there is not enough evidence to support the routine use of topiramate in clinical practice.[48] More recently the use of the monoamine depleting agent **deutetrabenazine** has been shown to be effective.[49] **Tetrabenazine** may also be useful as an add-on treatment.[50] **Ecopipam**, a D1 receptor antagonist, was also found to be effective in the treatment of tics in a recent randomised placebo-controlled crossover study including children and adolescents with TS.[51]

Case reports or case series describing positive effects for **ondansetron**,[52] **clomiphene**[53] **tramadol**,[54] **ketanserin**,[55] **cyproterone**,[56] **levetiracetam**,[57] **pregabalin**[58] and **cannabis**[59] have been published. A Cochrane Review of cannabinoids concluded that there was little if any current evidence for efficacy[60] and, despite a strong biological rationale for use, their overall efficacy and safety remain largely unknown.[61] Many other drugs have been reported to be effective in single case reports. Patients in these reports all had co-morbid psychiatric illness, making it difficult to determine the effect of these drugs on TS alone.

Botulinum toxin has been used to treat bothersome or painful focal motor tics, particularly those affecting neck muscles.[18] However, a recent Cochrane review expressed uncertainty about its place in the treatment of tics owing to the low quality of available evidence.[62]

There may be a sub-group of children who develop tics and/or obsessive-compulsive disorder in association with streptococcal or other infections or triggers. This group has been given (in the case of streptococcus) the acronym PANDAS (Paediatric Autoimmune Neuropsychiatric Disorder Associated with Streptococcus)[63] or, more broadly, PANS (Paediatric Acute-onset Neuropsychiatric Syndrome).[64] This is thought to be an autoimmune-mediated effect, and there have been trials of immune-modulatory therapy in these children as well as treatment with antibiotics for active infections and also as preventative treatment. More research in this area is warranted (Figure 5.2).

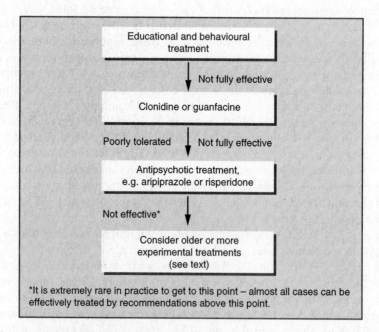

Figure 5.2 Summary of recommendations.

References

1. Murphy TK, et al. Practice parameter for the assessment and treatment of children and adolescents with tic disorders. *J Am Acad Child Adolesc Psychiatry* 2013; 52:1341–1359.
2. Cath DC, et al. European clinical guidelines for Tourette syndrome and other tic disorders. Part I: Assessment. *Eur Child Adolesc Psychiatry* 2011; 20:155–171.
3. Singer HS Treatment of tics and Tourette syndrome. *Curr Treat Options Neurol* 2010; 12:539–561.
4. McGuire JF, et al. A meta-analysis of behavior therapy for Tourette syndrome. *J Psychiatr Res* 2014; 50:106–112.
5. Rizzo R, et al. A randomized controlled trial comparing behavioral, educational, and pharmacological treatments in youths with chronic tic disorder or Tourette syndrome. *Frontiers Psychiatry* 2018; 9:100.
6. Fründt O, et al. Behavioral therapy for Tourette syndrome and chronic tic disorders. *Neurol Clin Practice* 2017; 7:148–156.
7. Patel H, et al. Use of complementary and alternative medicine in children with Tourette syndrome. *J Child Neurol* 2020; 35:512–516.
8. Kumar A, et al. A comprehensive review of Tourette syndrome and complementary alternative medicine. *Current Dev Disorders Rep* 2018; 5:95–100.
9. Cubo E, et al. Impact of placebo assignment in clinical trials of tic disorders. *Mov Disord* 2013; 28:1288–1292.
10. Goetz CG, et al. Clonidine and Gilles de la Tourette's syndrome: double-blind study using objective rating methods. *Ann Neurol* 1987; 21:307–310.
11. Leckman JF, et al. Clonidine treatment of Gilles de la Tourette's syndrome. *Arch Gen Psychiatry* 1991; 48:324–328.
12. Group TsSS. Treatment of ADHD in children with tics: a randomized controlled trial. *Neurology* 2002; 58:527–536.
13. Du YS, et al. Randomized double-blind multicentre placebo-controlled clinical trial of the clonidine adhesive patch for the treatment of tic disorders. *Aust N Z J Psychiatry* 2008; 42:807–813.
14. Hedderick EF, et al. Double-blind, crossover study of clonidine and levetiracetam in Tourette syndrome. *Pediatr Neurol* 2009; 40:420–425.
15. Song PP, et al. The efficacy and tolerability of the clonidine transdermal patch in the treatment for children with tic disorders: a prospective, open, single-group, self-controlled study. *Front Neurol* 2017; 8:32.
16. Scahill L, et al. A placebo-controlled study of guanfacine in the treatment of children with tic disorders and attention deficit hyperactivity disorder. *Am J Psychiatry* 2001; 158:1067–1074.
17. Cummings DD, et al. Neuropsychiatric effects of guanfacine in children with mild Tourette syndrome: a pilot study. *Clin Neuropharmacol* 2002; 25:325–332.
18. Roessner V, et al. Pharmacological treatment of tic disorders and Tourette syndrome. *Neuropharmacology* 2013; 68:143–149.
19. Pringsheim T, et al. Pimozide for tics in Tourette's syndrome. *Cochrane Database Syst Rev* 2009:CD006996.
20. Yoo HK, et al. An open-label study of the efficacy and tolerability of aripiprazole for children and adolescents with tic disorders. *J Clin Psychiatry* 2007; 68:1088–1093.
21. Yoo HK, et al. A multicenter, randomized, double-blind, placebo-controlled study of aripiprazole in children and adolescents with Tourette's disorder. *J Clin Psychiatry* 2013; 74:e772–e780.
22. Sallee F, et al. Randomized, double-blind, placebo-controlled trial demonstrates the efficacy and safety of oral aripiprazole for the treatment of Tourette's disorder in children and adolescents. *J Child Adolesc Psychopharmacol* 2017; 27:771–781.
23. Davies L, et al. A case series of patients with Tourette's syndrome in the United Kingdom treated with aripiprazole. *Human Psychopharmacol* 2006; 21:447–453.
24. Seo WS, et al. Aripiprazole treatment of children and adolescents with Tourette disorder or chronic tic disorder. *J Child Adolesc Psychopharmacol* 2008; 18:197–205.
25. Murphy TK, et al. Open label aripiprazole in the treatment of youth with tic disorders. *J Child Adolesc Psychopharmacol* 2009; 19:441–447.
26. Wenzel C, et al. Aripiprazole for the treatment of Tourette syndrome: a case series of 100 patients. *J Clin Psychopharmacol* 2012; 32:548–550.
27. Rizzo R, et al. Metabolic effects of aripiprazole and pimozide in children with Tourette syndrome. *Pediatr Neurol* 2012; 47:419–422.
28. Liu Y, et al. Effectiveness and tolerability of aripiprazole in children and adolescents with Tourette's disorder: a meta-Analysis. *J Child Adolesc Psychopharmacol* 2016; 26:436–441.
29. Wang S, et al. The efficacy and safety of aripiprazole for tic disorders in children and adolescents: a systematic review and meta-analysis. *Psychiatry Res* 2017; 254:24–32.
30. Ghanizadeh A Twice-weekly aripiprazole for treating children and adolescents with tic disorder, a randomized controlled clinical trial. *Ann General Psychiatry* 2016; 15:21.
31. Tao D, et al. Randomized controlled clinical trial comparing the efficacy and tolerability of aripiprazole and sodium valproate in the treatment of Tourette syndrome. *Ann General Psychiatry* 2019; 18:24.
32. Scahill L, et al. A placebo-controlled trial of risperidone in Tourette syndrome. *Neurology* 2003; 60:1130–1135.
33. Gaffney GR, et al. Risperidone versus clonidine in the treatment of children and adolescents with Tourette's syndrome. *J Am Acad Child Adolesc Psychiatry* 2002; 41:330–336.
34. Onofrj M, et al. Olanzapine in severe Gilles de la Tourette syndrome: a 52-week double-blind cross-over study vs. low-dose pimozide. *J Neurol* 2000; 247:443–446.
35. Robertson MM, et al. Management of Gilles de la Tourette syndrome using sulpiride. *Clin Neuropharmacol* 1990; 13:229–235.
36. Sallee FR, et al. Ziprasidone treatment of children and adolescents with Tourette's syndrome: a pilot study. *J Am Acad Child Adolesc Psychiatry* 2000; 39:292–299.

CHAPTER 5

37. Mukaddes NM, et al. Quetiapine treatment of children and adolescents with Tourette's disorder. *J Child Adolesc Psychopharmacol* 2003; **13**:295–299.

38. Budman CL, et al. An open-label study of the treatment efficacy of olanzapine for Tourette's disorder. *J Clin Psychiatry* 2001; **62**:290–294.

39. McCracken JT, et al. Effectiveness and tolerability of open label olanzapine in children and adolescents with Tourette syndrome. *J Child Adolesc Psychopharmacol* 2008; **18**:501–508.

40. Caine ED, et al. The trial use of clozapine for abnormal involuntary movement disorders. *Am J Psychiatry* 1979; **136**:317–320.

41. Singer HS, et al. Baclofen treatment in Tourette syndrome: a double-blind, placebo-controlled, crossover trial. *Neurology* 2001; **56**:599–604.

42. Silver AA, et al. Transdermal nicotine and haloperidol in Tourette's disorder: a double-blind placebo-controlled study. *J Clin Psychiatry* 2001; **62**:707–714.

43. Gilbert DL, et al. Tourette's syndrome improvement with pergolide in a randomized, double-blind, crossover trial. *Neurology* 2000; **54**:1310–1315.

44. Gilbert DL, et al. Tic reduction with pergolide in a randomized controlled trial in children. *Neurology* 2003; **60**:606–611.

45. Peterson BS, et al. A double-blind, placebo-controlled, crossover trial of an antiandrogen in the treatment of Tourette's syndrome. *J Clin Psychopharmacol* 1998; **18**:324–331.

46. Nicolson R, et al. A randomized, double-blind, placebo-controlled trial of metoclopramide for the treatment of Tourette's disorder. *J Am Acad Child Adolesc Psychiatry* 2005; **44**:640–646.

47. Jankovic J, et al. A randomised, double-blind, placebo-controlled study of topiramate in the treatment of Tourette syndrome. *J Neurol Neurosurg Psychiatry* 2010; **81**:70–73.

48. Yang CS, et al. Topiramate for Tourette's syndrome in children: a meta-analysis. *Pediatr Neurol* 2013; **49**:344–350.

49. Jankovic J, et al. 152 development of deutetrabenazine as a potential new non-antipsychotic treatment for Tourette syndrome in children and adolescents. *CNS Spectr* 2020; **25**:297.

50. Porta M, et al. Tourette's syndrome and role of tetrabenazine: review and personal experience. *Clin Drug Invest* 2008; **28**:443–459.

51. Gilbert DL, et al. Ecopipam, a D1 receptor antagonist, for treatment of Tourette syndrome in children: a randomized, placebo-controlled crossover study. *Mov Disord* 2018; **33**:1272–1280.

52. Toren P, et al. Ondansetron treatment in patients with Tourette's syndrome. *Int Clin Psychopharmacol* 1999; **14**:373–376.

53. Sandyk R Clomiphene citrate in Tourette's syndrome. *Int J Neurosci* 1988; **43**:103–106.

54. Shapira NA, et al. Novel use of tramadol hydrochloride in the treatment of Tourette's syndrome. *J Clin Psychiatry* 1997; **58**:174–175.

55. Bonnier C, et al. Ketanserin treatment of Tourette's syndrome in children. *Am J Psychiatry* 1999; **156**:1122–1123.

56. Izmir M, et al. Cyproterone acetate treatment of Tourette's syndrome. *Can J Psychiatry* 1999; **44**:710–711.

57. Awaad Y, et al. Use of levetiracetam to treat tics in children and adolescents with Tourette syndrome. *Mov Disord* 2005; **20**:714–718.

58. Hienert M, et al. Pregabalin in Tourette's syndrome: a case series. *Am J Psychiatry* 2016; **173**:1242–1243.

59. Sandyk R, et al. Marijuana and Tourette's syndrome. *J Clin Psychopharmacol* 1988; **8**:444–445.

60. Curtis A, et al. Cannabinoids for Tourette's syndrome. *Cochrane Database Syst Rev* 2009:CD006565.

61. Artukoglu BB, et al. The potential of cannabinoid-based treatments in Tourette syndrome. *CNS Drugs* 2019; **33**:417–430.

62. Pandey S, et al. Botulinum toxin for motor and phonic tics in Tourette's syndrome. *Cochrane Database Syst Rev* 2018; **1**:Cd012285.

63. Martino D, et al. The PANDAS subgroup of tic disorders and childhood-onset obsessive-compulsive disorder. *J Psychosom Res* 2009; **67**:547–557.

64. Chang K, et al. Clinical evaluation of youth with pediatric acute-onset neuropsychiatric syndrome (PANS): recommendations from the 2013 PANS Consensus Conference. *J Child Adolesc Psychopharmacol* 2015; **25**:3–13.

CHAPTER 5

Melatonin in the treatment of insomnia in children and adolescents

Insomnia is a common symptom in childhood. Underlying causes may be behavioural (inappropriate sleep associations or bedtime resistance), physiological (delayed sleep phase syndrome) or related to underlying mood disorders (anxiety, depression and bipolar disorder). All forms of insomnia are more common in children with learning difficulties, autism, ADHD and sensory impairments (particularly visual). Although behavioural interventions should be the primary intervention and have a robust evidence base, exogenous melatonin is now the 'first-line' medication prescribed for childhood insomnia.[1]

Melatonin is a hormone that is produced by the pineal gland in a circadian manner. The evening rise in melatonin, enabled by darkness, precedes the onset of natural sleep by about 2 hours.[2] Melatonin is involved in the induction of sleep and in synchronisation of the circadian system.

There is a wide variety of unlicensed fast-release, slow-release and liquid preparations of melatonin. Many products rely on food-grade rather than pharmaceutical grade melatonin and some are expensive. A prolonged-release formulation of melatonin (Circadin) was licensed in the UK in April 2008 as a short term treatment of insomnia in patients over 55 years of age. Many children are unable to swallow these tablets, and although they can be crushed (and become immediate release) the Product Licence limited children's access to a pharmaceutical-grade prolonged release preparation. However, in the UK, a prolonged-release melatonin minitablet 'Slenyto' mimicking the endogenous release profile of the hormone at night has now been licensed for children with autism. It was evaluated in a phase III multicentre randomized, placebo-controlled study of children with autism. The study began with a 13-week double-blind treatment period followed by an extended open-label period with continued efficacy and safety monitoring. Results included clinically significant improvement in caregivers' diary-reported sleep initiation and maintenance (sleep latency, total sleep time, longest sleep period).[3] Effects were maintained in the long-term period. The medication was well tolerated and no unexpected safety issues were reported. The study was the only 'Class 1' rated study in a recent Practice Guideline publication on the treatment for insomnia and disrupted sleep behaviour in children and adolescents with ASD by the American Academy of Neurology.[4] Secondary outcomes showed improvements in child's social functioning and behaviour, and caregivers' well-being.

Lack of any 'head to head' studies means that there are still no good data on whether, or when, immediate-release melatonin preparations should be used. There are additionally a number of melatonin analogues already produced, or in development[5] although they are virtually never used in the paediatric population. There is no evidence from equivalence studies of any superiority over melatonin itself.

Efficacy

A meta-analysis that included adult and paediatric studies of melatonin used for the treatment of primary sleep disorders demonstrated that melatonin decreases sleep

CHAPTER 5

onset latency, increases total sleep time and improves overall sleep quality. The effects of melatonin on sleep are modest but do not appear to dissipate with continued melatonin use.[6]

Adverse effects

Many of the children who have received melatonin in RCTs and published case series had developmental problems and/or sensory deficits. The scope for detecting subtle adverse effects in this population is limited. Screening for adverse effects was not routine in all studies. Early reports included a very small case series cases where melatonin was been reported to worsen seizures[7] and exacerbate asthma[8,9] in the short term. Other reported adverse effects include headache, depression, restlessness, confusion, nausea, tachycardia and pruritis.[10,11] In the more recent largest placebo-controlled studies to date involving children with learning difficulty, autism and epilepsy,[12–14] and the most recent minitablet study (PedPRM) there were no excess adverse effects in the treatment group over that recorded for placebo, and in particular seizures were not worsened. A Cochrane review found no worsening of seizure frequency in patients with epilepsy given melatonin.[15] There was no detectable impact on puberty in a recent paper.[16]

Dose

The cut-off point between physiological and pharmacological doses in children is less than 500µg. Physiological doses of melatonin may result in very high receptor occupancy. The doses used in RCTs and published case series vary hugely with between 500µg and 5mg being the most common doses although much lower and higher doses have been used. The optimal dose is unknown and there is no evidence to support a direct relationship between dose and response.[17] In one large RCT 18% of children seemed to respond to a 500µg dose but others seemed to require much higher doses (12mg).[14] Increasing doses above 5mg is likely to provoke the direct sedative effects on melatonin, rather than its sleep phase-shifting properties. This might be necessary and helpful for some children with severe and bilateral brain injury.

The use of salivary melatonin measurements is an expensive but effective way to identify those children with the most delayed sleep phase (likely to have the best response to exogenous melatonin) and those children who are slow metabolisers of melatonin in whom serum levels accumulate during the daytime (particularly on higher doses) and in whom efficacy will eventually be lost (Figure 5.3).

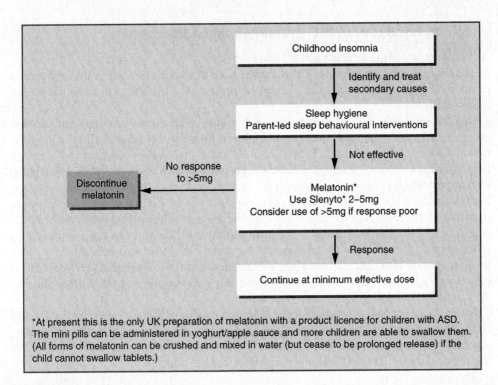

*At present this is the only UK preparation of melatonin with a product licence for children with ASD. The mini pills can be administered in yoghurt/apple sauce and more children are able to swallow them. (All forms of melatonin can be crushed and mixed in water (but cease to be prolonged release) if the child cannot swallow tablets.)

Figure 5.3 Summary of recommendations.

References

1. Gringras P. When to use drugs to help sleep. *Arch Dis Child* 2008; **93**:976–981.
2. Macchi MM, et al. Human pineal physiology and functional significance of melatonin. *Front Neuroendocrinol* 2004; **25**:177–195.
3. Gringras P, et al. Efficacy and safety of pediatric prolonged-release melatonin for insomnia in children with autism spectrum disorder. *J Am Acad Child Adolescent Psychiatry* 2017; **56**:948–957.e944.
4. Williams Buckley A, et al. Practice guideline: treatment for insomnia and disrupted sleep behavior in children and adolescents with autism spectrum disorder: report of the Guideline Development, Dissemination, and Implementation Subcommittee of the American Academy of Neurology. *Neurology* 2020; **94**:392–404.
5. Arendt J, et al. Melatonin and its agonists: an update. *Br J Psychiatry* 2008; **193**:267–269.
6. Ferracioli-Oda E, et al. Meta-analysis: melatonin for the treatment of primary sleep disorders. *PLoS One* 2013; **8**:e63773.
7. Sheldon SH Pro-convulsant effects of oral melatonin in neurologically disabled children. *Lancet* 1998; **351**:1254.
8. Maestroni GJ The immunoneuroendocrine role of melatonin. *J Pineal Res* 1993; **14**:1–10.
9. Sutherland ER, et al. Elevated serum melatonin is associated with the nocturnal worsening of asthma. *J Allergy Clin Immunol* 2003; **112**:513–517.
10. Chase JE, et al. Melatonin: therapeutic use in sleep disorders. *Ann Pharmacother* 1997; **31**:1218–1226.
11. Jan JE, et al. Melatonin treatment of sleep-wake cycle disorders in children and adolescents. *Dev Med Child Neurol* 1999; **41**:491–500.
12. Coppola G, et al. Melatonin in wake-sleep disorders in children, adolescents and young adults with mental retardation with or without epilepsy: a double-blind, cross-over, placebo-controlled trial. *Brain Dev* 2004; **26**:373–376.
13. Garstang J, et al. Randomized controlled trial of melatonin for children with autistic spectrum disorders and sleep problems. *Child Care Health Dev* 2006; **32**:585–589.
14. Gringras P, et al. Melatonin for sleep problems in children with neurodevelopmental disorders: randomised double masked placebo controlled trial. *BMJ* 2012; **345**:e6664.
15. Brigo F, et al. Melatonin as add-on treatment for epilepsy. *Cochrane Database Syst Rev* 2016:Cd006967.
16. Malow BA, et al. Sleep, growth, and puberty after 2 years of prolonged-release melatonin in children with autism spectrum disorder. *J Am Acad Child Adolesc Psychiatry* 2020:S0890-8567(0820)30034-30034.
17. Sack RL, et al. Sleep-promoting effects of melatonin: at what dose, in whom, under what conditions, and by what mechanisms? *Sleep* 1997; **20**:908–915.

Rapid tranquillisation (RT) in children and adolescents

As in adults, a comprehensive mental state assessment and appropriately implemented treatment plan along with staff skilled in the use of de-escalation techniques and appropriate placement of the patient are key to minimising the need for enforced parenteral medication.

Healthcare professionals undertaking RT and/or restraint in children and adolescents should be trained and competent in undertaking these procedures in this population and should be clear about the legal context for any restrictive practices they employ. Be particularly cautious when considering high-potency antipsychotic medication (such as haloperidol) especially those who have not taken antipsychotic medication before, because of the increased risk of acute dystonic reactions in this age group.[1] Children are particularly prone to acute extrapyramidal effects of psychotropic and physical medicine drugs.[2] NICE recommends using intramuscular lorazepam (and recommends no other drug).[3] A recent review of practice suggested that lorazepam is effective (at a median dose of 1mg) and rarely causes oxygen desaturation.[4] In severe cases parenteral olanzapine and oral aripiprazole have been safely used but more than half of patients may require a second drug to achieve sedation.[5]

A wide dose range is given here for medication used in RT. Caution is required, especially for younger children, but in older adolescents consider the use of adult doses, especially in those who are not drug naïve and where doses in the lower end of the quoted dose range have proved ineffective (see Table 5.7).

Table 5.7 Recommended drugs for RT if the oral route is refused or has proven ineffective

Medication	Dose	Onset of action	Comment
Olanzapine IM[6,7]	2.5–10mg	15–30 minutes	Possibly increased risk of respiratory depression when administered with benzodiazepines, particularly if alcohol has been consumed. Separate administration by at least 1 hour
Haloperidol IM[8]	0.025–0.075mg/kg/dose (max 2.5mg) IM Adolescents >12 years can receive the adult dose (2.5–5mg)	20–30 minutes	Must have parenteral anticholinergics present in case of laryngeal spasm or other dystonia (young people more vulnerable to severe dystonia) Adult data suggest co-administration of promethazine may reduce EPS risk[9] **ECG essential**
Lorazepam* IM[10,11]	<12 years: 0.5–1mg; >12 years: 0.5–2mg	20–40 minutes	Slower onset of action than midazolam Only treatment recommended by NICE Flumazenil is the reversing agent for all benzodiazepines

(Continued)

Table 5.7 (Continued)

Medication	Dose	Onset of action	Comment
Midazolam* IM, IV or buccal[11,12]	0.1–0.15mg/kg (IM) Buccal midazolam 300–500µg/kg or 6–10 years = 7.5mg >10 years = 10mg	10–20 minutes IM (1–3 minutes IV)	Quicker onset and shorter duration of action than lorazepam or diazepam. IV administration should only be used (usually as a last resort) with extreme caution and where resuscitation facilities are available. Shorter onset and duration of action than haloperidol When given as buccal liquid, onset of action is 15–30 minutes.[13] Some published data in mental health but only in adults.[14] Buccal liquid is unlicensed for this use.
Diazepam* IV (not for IM administration)[15]	0.1mg/kg/dose by slow IV injection. Max 40mg total daily dose <12 years and 60mg >12 years	1–3 minutes	Long half-life that does not correlate with length of sedation. Possibility of accumulation **Never give as IM injection**
Ziprasidone IM[16–19] (not UK)	10–20mg	15–30 minutes IM	Apparently effective. QT prolongation is of concern in this patient group **ECG essential**
Aripiprazole IM[20,21]	9.75mg	15–30 minutes	Evidence of effectiveness in adults but no clinical trial data for children and adolescents
Promethazine IM	<12 years: 5–25mg (max 50mg/day) >12 years: 25–50mg (max 100mg/day)	Up to 60 minutes	An effective sedative, although has a slow onset of action. Useful if the cause of behavioural disturbance is unknown and there is concern about the use of antipsychotic medication in a child or young person

*Note that young people are particularly vulnerable to disinhibitory reactions with benzodiazepines.

Oral medication should always be offered (and repeated if necessary if the young person is willing to take it), before resorting to parenteral treatment. Buccal midazolam[14] and inhaled loxapine[22] have not been widely investigated in children in RT at the time of writing and have limited availability. Buccal midazolam is commonly used for seizures in children. Monitoring after RT is the same as in adults (see section on RT, Chapter 3).

References

1. National Institute for Health and Care Excellence. Psychosis and schizophrenia in children and young people: recognition and management. Clinical Guidance 155 2013 (last updated October 2016); https://www.nice.org.uk/guidance/cg155.
2. Chang MY, et al. Drug-induced extrapyramidal symptoms at the pediatric emergency department. *Pediatr Emerg Care* 2020; 36:468–472.
3. National Institute for Health and Care Excellence. Violence and aggression: short-term management in mental health, health and community settings. *Clinical Guidance* 10 [CG10]. 2015 (Last checked December 2019); https://www.nice.org.uk/guidance/ng10.
4. Kendrick JG, et al. Pharmacologic management of agitation and aggression in a pediatric emergency department – a retrospective cohort study. *J Pediatric Pharmacol Therapeutics* 2018; 23:455–459.
5. Rudolf F, et al. A retrospective review of antipsychotic medications administered to psychiatric patients in a tertiary care pediatric emergency department. *J Pediatric Pharmacol Therapeutics* 2019; 24:234–237.
6. Breier A, et al. A double-blind, placebo-controlled dose-response comparison of intramuscular olanzapine and haloperidol in the treatment of acute agitation in schizophrenia. *Arch Gen Psychiatry* 2002; 59:441–448.
7. Lindborg SR, et al. Effects of intramuscular olanzapine vs. haloperidol and placebo on QTc intervals in acutely agitated patients. *Psychiatry Res* 2003; 119:113–123.
8. Powney MJ, et al. Haloperidol for psychosis-induced aggression or agitation (rapid tranquillisation). *Cochrane Database Syst Rev* 2012; 11:CD009377.
9. TREC Collaborative Group. Rapid tranquillisation for agitated patients in emergency psychiatric rooms: a randomised trial of midazolam versus haloperidol plus promethazine. *BMJ* 2003; 327:708–713.
10. Sorrentino A Chemical restraints for the agitated, violent, or psychotic pediatric patient in the emergency department: controversies and recommendations. *Curr Opin Pediatr* 2004; 16:201–205.
11. Nobay F, et al. A prospective, double-blind, randomized trial of midazolam versus haloperidol versus lorazepam in the chemical restraint of violent and severely agitated patients. *Acad Emerg Med* 2004; 11:744–749.
12. Kennedy RM, et al. The "ouchless emergency department". Getting closer: advances in decreasing distress during painful procedures in the emergency department. *Pediatr Clin North Am* 1999; 46:1215–1247.
13. Schwagmeier R, et al. Midazolam pharmacokinetics following intravenous and buccal administration. *Br J Clin Pharmacol* 1998; 46:203–206.
14. Taylor D, et al. Buccal midazolam for agitation on psychiatric intensive care wards. *Int J Psychiatry Clin Pract* 2008; 12:309–311.
15. Nunn K, et al. Medication Table. in K N, C D, ed. *The Clinician's Guide to Psychotropic Prescribing in Children and Adolescents*. 1. Sydney: Glad Publishing 2003:383–452.
16. Khan SS, et al. A naturalistic evaluation of intramuscular ziprasidone versus intramuscular olanzapine for the management of acute agitation and aggression in children and adolescents. *J Child Adolesc Psychopharmacol* 2006; 16:671–677.
17. Staller JA Intramuscular ziprasidone in youth: a retrospective chart review. *J Child Adolesc Psychopharmacol* 2004; 14:590–592.
18. Hazaray E, et al. Intramuscular ziprasidone for acute agitation in adolescents. *J Child Adolesc Psychopharmacol* 2004; 14:464–470.
19. Barzman DH, et al. A retrospective chart review of intramuscular ziprasidone for agitation in children and adolescents on psychiatric units: prospective studies are needed. *J Child Adolesc Psychopharmacol* 2007; 17:503–509.
20. Sanford M, et al. Intramuscular aripiprazole: a review of its use in the management of agitation in schizophrenia and bipolar I disorder. *CNS Drugs* 2008; 22:335–352.
21. National Institute for Health and Clinical Excellence. Aripiprazole for schizophrenia in people aged 15 to 17 years. Technology Appraisal 13 [TA213] 2011; https://www.nice.org.uk/guidance/ta213.
22. Lesem MD, et al. Rapid acute treatment of agitation in individuals with schizophrenia: multicentre, randomised, placebo-controlled study of inhaled loxapine. *Br J Psychiatry* 2011; 198:51–58.

Doses of commonly used psychotropic drugs in children and adolescents

The doses of commonly used drugs are presented in Table 5.8.

Table 5.8 Starting doses of commonly used psychotropic drugs in children and adolescents[1,2]*

Drug	Starting dose**	Comment
Antipsychotics		
Aripiprazole	2mg	Adjust dose according to response and adverse effects
Clozapine	6.25–12.5mg	Use plasma levels to determine maintenance dose
Olanzapine	2.5–5mg	Adjust dose according to response and adverse effects
Quetiapine	25mg	Effective dose usually in the range 150–200mg daily
Risperidone	0.25–2mg	Adjust dose according to response and adverse effects
Antidepressants		
Fluoxetine	5–10mg/day	Adjust dose according to response and adverse effects
Sertraline	25–50mg daily	Effective dose usually in the range 50–100mg daily
Citalopram	10mg daily	Effective dose 10–40mg (note QT effects)
Other Drugs		
Lithium	100–200mg/day lithium carbonate	Use plasma levels to determine maintenance dose
Valproate	10–20mg/kg/day in divided doses	Use plasma levels to determine maintenance dose. Do not offer valproate to girls or young women of child bearing potential unless there is a pregnancy prevention programme (PPP) in place[3]
Melatonin	2mg at night	Effective dose 2–10mg

*We have removed haloperidol, amitriptyline, escitalopram and carbamazepine from this table as none of these are recommended in children.
**Suggested approximate oral starting doses (see primary literature for doses in individual indications). Lower dose in suggested range is for children weighing less than 25kg.

References

1. BNF Online. British National Formulary 2020; https://www.medicinescomplete.com/mc/bnf/current.
2. BNFC Online. British National Formulary for Children 2020; https://www.medicinescomplete.com/#/browse/bnfc.
3. GOV.UK Guidance. Valproate use by women and girls 2020; https://www.gov.uk/guidance/valproate-use-by-women-and-girls.

Chapter 6

Prescribing in older people

General principles

The pharmacokinetics and pharmacodynamics of most drugs are altered to an important extent in older people. These changes in drug handling and action must be taken into account if treatment is to be effective and adverse effects minimised. Older people often have a number of concurrent illnesses and may require treatment with several drugs. This leads to a greater chance of problems arising because of drug interactions and to a higher rate of drug-induced problems, in general.[1] It is reasonable to assume that all drugs are more likely to cause adverse effects in older patients than in younger patients.

How drugs affect the ageing body (altered pharmacodynamics)

As we age, control over reflex actions such as blood pressure and temperature regulation is reduced. Receptors may become more sensitive. This results in an increased incidence and severity of adverse effects. For example, drugs that decrease gut motility are more likely to cause constipation (e.g. anticholinergics and opioids) and drugs that affect blood pressure are more likely to cause falls (e.g. tricyclic antidepressants (TCAs) and diuretics). Older people demonstrate an exaggerated response to central nervous system (CNS)-active drugs such as benzodiazepines and opioids. This is partly due to an age-related decline in CNS function and partly due to increased pharmacodynamics sensitivity to these drugs.[2] Therapeutic response to medication can also be delayed; for example, older adults may take longer to respond to antidepressants than younger adults.[3]

Older people may be more prone to develop serious adverse effects such as agranulocytosis[4] and neutropenia[5] with clozapine, stroke with antipsychotic drugs[6] and bleeding with selective serotonin reuptake inhibitors (SSRIs).

The Maudsley® Prescribing Guidelines in Psychiatry, Fourteenth Edition. David M. Taylor, Thomas R. E. Barnes and Allan H. Young.
© 2021 David M. Taylor. Published 2021 by John Wiley & Sons Ltd.

How ageing affects drug therapy (altered pharmacokinetics)[7]

Absorption

Gut motility decreases with age as does secretion of gastric acid. This leads to drugs being absorbed more slowly, resulting in a slower onset of action. The same *amount* of drug is absorbed as in a younger adult, but rate of absorption is slower.

Distribution

Older adults have more body fat, less body water and less albumin than younger adults. This leads to an increased volume of distribution and a longer duration of action for some fat-soluble drugs (e.g. diazepam), higher concentrations of some drugs at the site of action (e.g. digoxin) and a reduction in the amount of drug bound to albumin (increased amounts of active 'free drug'; e.g. warfarin and phenytoin).

Metabolism

The majority of drugs are hepatically metabolised. Liver size is reduced in the elderly, but in the absence of hepatic disease or significantly reduced hepatic blood flow, there is no significant reduction in metabolic capacity. The magnitude of pharmacokinetic interactions is unlikely to be altered but the pharmacodynamic consequences of these interactions may be amplified.

Excretion

Renal function declines with age: 35% of function is lost by the age of 65 years and 50% by the age of 80 years.

More functions are lost if there are concurrent medical problems such as heart disease, diabetes or hypertension. Measurement of serum creatinine or urea can be misleading in the elderly because muscle mass is reduced, so less creatinine is produced. It is particularly important that estimated glomerular filtration rate (eGFR)[8] is used as a measure of renal function in this age group. It is best to assume that all elderly patients have at most two-thirds of normal renal function.

Most drugs are eventually (after metabolism) excreted by the kidney. A few do not undergo biotransformation first. Lithium and sulpiride are important examples. Drugs primarily excreted via the kidney will accumulate in the elderly, leading to toxicity and adverse effects. Dosage reduction is likely to be required (see section on renal failure and psychotropics).

Drug interactions

Some drugs have a narrow therapeutic index (a small increase in dose can cause toxicity and a small reduction in dose can cause a loss of therapeutic action). The most commonly prescribed ones are digoxin, warfarin, theophylline, phenytoin and lithium. Changes in the way these drugs are handled in older people and the greater chance of interaction with other drugs mean that toxicity and therapeutic failure are more likely. These drugs can be used safely but extra care must be taken and blood concentrations should be measured where possible.

Some drugs inhibit or induce hepatic metabolising enzymes. Important examples include some SSRIs, erythromycin and carbamazepine. This may lead to the metabolism of another drug being altered. Many drug interactions occur through this mechanism. Details of individual interactions and their consequences can be found in the *BNF online* for individual drugs.[9] Most can be predicted by a sound knowledge of pharmacology.

Reducing drug-related risk in older people

Adherence to the following principles will reduce drug-related morbidity and mortality:

- Use drugs only when absolutely necessary.
- Avoid, if possible, drugs that block α_1 adrenoceptors, have anticholinergic adverse effects, are very sedative, have a long half-life or are potent inhibitors of hepatic metabolising enzymes.
- Start with a low dose and increase slowly but do not undertreat. Some drugs still require the full adult dose.
- Try not to treat the adverse effects of one drug with another drug. Find a better-tolerated alternative.
- Keep therapy simple; that is, once daily administration whenever possible.

Administering medicines in foodstuffs[10–12]

Sometimes patients may refuse treatment with medicines, even when such treatment is thought to be in their best interests. In the UK, where the patient has a mental illness or has capacity, the Mental Health Act (MHA) should be used, but if the patient lacks capacity, this option may not be desirable. Medicines should never be administered covertly to elderly patients with dementia without a full discussion with the Multi-Disciplinary Team (MDT) and the patient's relatives. The outcome of this discussion should be clearly documented in the patient's clinical notes. Medicines should be administered covertly only if the clear and express purpose is to reduce suffering for the patient. (For further information, see section 'Covert administration of medicines within food and drink' in this chapter.)

For advice on dosing of psychotropics in the elderly, see section 'A guide to medication doses of commonly used psychotropics in older adults' in this chapter.

References

1. Royal College of Physicians. Medication for older people. Summary and recommendations of a report of a working party of The Royal College of Physicians. *J R Coll Physicians Lond* 1997; 31:254–257.
2. Bowie MW, et al. Pharmacodynamics in older adults: a review. *Am J Geriatr Pharmacother* 2007; 5:263–303.
3. Baldwin R, et al. Management of depression in later life. *Adv Psychiatr Treatment* 2004; 10:131–139.
4. Munro J, et al. Active monitoring of 12,760 clozapine recipients in the UK and Ireland. Beyond Pharmacovigilance. *Br J Psychiatry* 1999; 175:576–580.
5. O'Connor DW, et al. The safety and tolerability of clozapine in aged patients: a retrospective clinical file review. *World J Biol Psychiatry* 2010; 11:788–791.
6. Douglas IJ, et al. Exposure to antipsychotics and risk of stroke: self-controlled case series study. *BMJ* 2008; 337:a1227.
7. Mayersohn M. Special pharmacokinetic considerations in the elderly. In W Evans, J Schentage, J Jusko, eds. *Applied pharmacokinetics: principles of therapeutic drug monitoring.* Vancouver, WA: Applied Therapeutics Inc, 1992.
8. Morriss R, et al. Lithium and eGFR: a new routinely available tool for the prevention of chronic kidney disease. *Br J Psychiatry* 2008; 193:93–95.
9. National Institute for Health and Care Excellence. British National Formulary (BNF). 2020; https://bnf.nice.org.uk
10. Royal College of Psychiatrists. College statement on covert administration of medicines. *Psychiatric Bulletin* 2004; 28:385–386.
11. Haw C, et al. Administration of medicines in food and drink: a study of older inpatients with severe mental illness. *Int Psychogeriatr* 2010; 22:409–416.
12. Haw C, et al. Covert administration of medication to older adults: a review of the literature and published studies. *J Psychiatr Ment Health Nurs* 2010; 17:761–768.

CHAPTER 6

Dementia

Dementia is a progressive syndrome affecting around 5% of those aged over 65 years, and increases to 20% in those aged over 80 years. This disorder is characterised by cognitive decline, impaired memory and thinking and a gradual loss of skills needed to carry out activities of daily living. Changes in mood, personality and social behaviour are frequent.[1]

The various types of dementia are classified according to the different disease processes affecting the brain. The most common cause of dementia is Alzheimer's disease (AD), accounting for around 60% of all cases. Vascular dementia and dementia with Lewy bodies (DLB) are responsible for most other cases. AD and vascular dementia may coexist and are often difficult to separate clinically. Dementia is also encountered in about 30–70% of patients with Parkinson's disease[1] (see separate section on Parkinson's disease).

Alzheimer's disease

Mechanism of action of cognitive enhancers used in AD

Acetylcholinesterase (AChE) inhibitors

The cholinergic hypothesis of AD is predicated on the observation that the cognitive deterioration associated with the disease results from progressive loss of cholinergic neurons and decreasing levels of acetylcholine (ACh) in the brain.[2] However, it is no longer widely believed that cholinergic depletion alone is responsible for the symptoms of AD.[3]

Three inhibitors of AChE are currently licensed in the UK and elsewhere for the treatment of mild-to-moderate dementia in AD: donepezil, rivastigmine and galantamine. These three drugs are now also recommended in severe AD. In addition, rivastigmine is licensed in the treatment of mild-to-moderate dementia associated with Parkinson's disease.

Both acetylcholinesterase (AChE) and butyrylcholinesterase (BuChE) have been found to play an important role in the degradation of ACh.[4] Cholinesterase inhibitors differ in pharmacological action: donepezil selectively inhibits AChE, rivastigmine affects both AChE and BuChE and galantamine selectively inhibits AChE and also has nicotinic receptor agonist properties.[5] To date, these differences have not been shown to result in important differences in efficacy or tolerability. (See Table 6.1 for comparison of AChE inhibitors (AChE-Is).)

Memantine

Memantine is licensed in the UK and elsewhere for the treatment of moderate-to-severe dementia in AD. It is believed to exert its therapeutic effect by acting as a low-to-moderate affinity, non-competitive N-methyl-D-aspartate (NMDA) receptor antagonist that binds preferentially to open NMDA receptor-operated calcium channels. This activity-dependent binding blocks NMDA-mediated ion flux and is thought to mitigate the effects of sustained and pathologically elevated levels of glutamate (and this excitotoxicity) that may lead to neuronal dysfunction.[6] (See Table 6.1.)

Table 6.1 Characteristics of cognitive enhancers[7-14]

Characteristic	Donepezil	Rivastigmine	Galantamine	Memantine
Primary mechanism	AChE-I (selective + reversible)	AChE-I (reversible, non-competitive inhibitor)	AChE-I (competitive + reversible)	Glutamate receptor antagonist
Other mechanism	None	BuChE-I	Nicotine receptor agonist	5-HT3 receptor antagonist
Starting dose	5mg daily	1.5mg bd (oral) (or 4.6mg/24 hours patch)	8mg XL daily (or 4mg bd solution) (instant release tablets have been discontinued in some countries)	5mg daily
Usual treatment dose (and max dose)	10mg daily	3–6mg bd (oral) or 9.5mg/24 hours patch	16–24mg XL daily (or 8–12mg bd solution)	20mg daily or (10mg bd)
Recommended minimum interval between dose increases	4 weeks (increase by 5mg daily)	2 weeks for oral (increase by 1.5mg twice a day) 4 weeks for patch (increase to 9.5mg/24 hours) (can consider increase to 13.3mg/24 hours after 6 months if tolerated and meaningful cognitive/functional decline occurs on 9.5mg/24 hours)	4 weeks (increase by 8mg XL daily or by 4mg bd for solution)	1 week (increase by 5mg weekly)
Adverse effects[7-13] *Very common: ≥1/10 and common: ≥1/100	Diarrhoea*, nausea*, headache*, common cold, anorexia, hallucinations, agitation, aggressive behaviour, abnormal dreams and nightmares, syncope, dizziness, insomnia, vomiting, abdominal disturbance, rash, pruritus, muscle cramps, urinary incontinence, fatigue, pain	Anorexia*, dizziness*, nausea*, vomiting* diarrhoea*, decreased appetite, nightmares, agitation, confusion, anxiety, headache, somnolence, tremor, abdominal pain and dyspepsia, sweating, fatigue and asthenia, malaise, weight loss (frequency of adverse effects with the patch may differ from capsules)	Nausea*, vomiting*, decreased appetite, hallucination, depression, syncope, dizziness; tremor, headache, somnolence, lethargy, bradycardia, hypertension, abdominal pain and discomfort, diarrhoea, dyspepsia, muscle spasms, fatigue, asthenia, malaise, weight loss, fall	Drug hypersensitivity, somnolence, dizziness, balance disorders, hypertension, dyspnoea, constipation, elevated liver function test, headache

(Continued)

Table 6.1 (Continued)

Characteristic	Donepezil	Rivastigmine	Galantamine	Memantine
Half life (hours)	~70	~1 (oral) 3.4 (patch)	7–8 (oral solution) 8–10 (XL capsules)	60–100
Metabolism	CYP 3A4 CYP 2D6 (minor)	Minimal involvement of CYP isoenzymes	CYP 3A4 CYP 2D6	Primarily non-hepatic
Drug–drug interactions	Yes (see separate table)	Interactions unlikely	Yes (see separate table)	Yes (see separate table)
Effect of food on absorption	None	Delays rate and extent of absorption	Delays rate but not extent of absorption	None
Cost of preparations[7,14] (for 1-month treatment at usual, i.e. max dose in the UK)	Tablets: £1.52 Orodispersible tablets: £10.43 Oral solution (1mg/mL): £100.22	Capsules: £66.10 Oral solution (2mg/mL): £135.55 Patches 9.5mg: £19.97 4.6mg and 13.3mg: £77.97	Capsules m/r: £79.80 Oral solution (4mg/mL): £201.60	Tablets: £8.46 Orodispersible tablets: £49.98 Oral solution (10mg/mL): £61.77 NB: Bottles supplied with a dosing pump dispensing 5mg in 0.5mL per actuation
Relative cost	$	$$	$$	$
Patent status	Generics available	Generics available	Generics available	Generics available

Efficacy of cognitive enhancers used in dementia

Currently, no treatment exists to modify or reverse disease progression in dementia. Therapeutic interventions are therefore targeted at specific symptoms or improving or slowing the decline in cognitive function. AChE-Is may provide some modest cognitive, functional and global benefits in mild-to-moderate AD.[15]

The three AChE-Is seem to have broadly similar clinical effects, as measured with the Mini Mental State Examination (MMSE), a 30-point basic evaluation of cognitive function and the Alzheimer's Disease Assessment Scale – cognitive subscale (ADAS-cog), a 70-point evaluation largely of cognitive dysfunction. Estimates of the number needed to treat (NNT) (for an improvement of >4 points ADAS-cog) range from 4 to 12.[16]

Memantine

An analysis of memantine studies found NNT ranged from 3 to 8[17] for improved cognitive function. A Cochrane review of memantine concluded that it had a small beneficial effect at 6 months in moderate-to-severe AD. In patients with mild-to-moderate dementia, the small beneficial effect on cognition was not clinically detectable in those with vascular dementia and barely detectable in those with AD.[17]

A 2020 study[18] investigated the 'real-world' effectiveness of cholinesterase inhibitors and memantine. The study found that in general, the initial decline in MMSE and Montreal Cognitive Assessment scores occurs approximately 2 years before medication is initiated. Medication prescription stabilises cognitive performance for the ensuing 2–5 months. The effect is enhanced in more cognitively impaired cases at the point of medication prescription and attenuated in those taking antipsychotics. Importantly, patients who are switched at least once tended to continue to decline at their pre-medication rate, thus apparently not benefiting from pharmacological interventions. Overall, 68% of individuals responded to treatment with a period of cognitive stabilisation before continuing their decline at the pre-treatment rate.

Switching between drugs used in dementia

The benefits of treatment with AChE-Is are rapidly lost when drug administration is interrupted[19] and may not be fully regained when drug treatment is re-initiated.[20] Poor tolerability with one agent does not rule out good tolerability with another.[21] The recently revised British Association for Psychopharmacology Guidelines for Dementia confirm that previous comparative trials have failed to consistently demonstrate any significant differences in efficacy between the three AChE-Is, the main differences found being in frequency and type of adverse events. As a result, their recommendation that a significant proportion of patients (up to 50%) appear to both tolerate and benefit from switching between AChE-Is if they cannot tolerate one remains valid.[22]

Several cases of discontinuation syndrome upon stopping donepezil have been published,[23,24] suggesting that a gradual withdrawal should be carried out where possible. However, a study comparing abrupt versus stepwise switching from donepezil to memantine found no clinically relevant differences in adverse effects despite patients in the abrupt group experiencing more frequent adverse effects than the stepwise discontinuation group (46% vs 32%, respectively).[25] (For switching to rivastigmine patch see under tolerability section)

Following a systematic review of the literature,[26] a practical approach to switching between AChE-Is has been proposed: in the case of intolerance, switching to another agent should be done only after complete resolution of side effects following discontinuation of the initial agent. In the case of lack of efficacy, switching can be done overnight, with a quicker titration scheme thereafter. Switching to another AChE-I is not recommended in individuals who show loss of benefit several years after initiation of therapy.

Other effects

AChE-Is may also affect non-cognitive aspects of AD and other dementias. Several studies have investigated their safety and efficacy in managing the non-cognitive symptoms of dementia. For more information about the management of these symptoms, see section 'Management of behavioural and psychological symptoms of dementia (BPSD)'.

Dosing and formulations

For dosing information, see Table 6.1.

Rivastigmine transdermal patch (9.5mg/24 hours) has been shown to be as effective as the highest doses of capsules but with a superior tolerability profile in a 6-month double-blind, placebo-controlled randomised controlled trial (RCT),[27] and confirmed in a Chinese study.[28] A nasal spray has also been developed.[29]

The FDA has approved a higher daily dose of **donepezil sustained release (23mg)** for moderate-to-severe AD on the basis of positive phase III trial results. Donepezil, 23mg/day is currently marketed in the USA and parts of Asia. In the global phase III study in patients with moderate-to-severe AD, donepezil 23mg/day demonstrated significantly greater cognitive benefits than donepezil 10mg/day, with a between-treatment difference in mean change in the Severe Impairment Battery score of 2.2 points in the overall study population and 3.1 points in patients with advanced AD. Dose escalation was somewhat challenging, given the increased incidence of gastrointestinal (GI) side effects observed when increasing the dose of donepezil from 10mg to 23mg daily. These side effects seldom persist beyond a 1-month period. Using stepwise titration strategies may address these GI side effects and could potentially involve increasing the dose of donepezil from 10 to 23mg over a 1–2-month period by taking one 10mg tablet plus one 5mg tablet once daily for 1 month followed by a 23mg once daily or a 10mg tablet and 23mg tablet on alternate days. A study in South Korea has been designed to determine the optimal dose escalation strategy for successful titration to 23mg/day.[30] Clinical recommendations emphasise the importance of patient selection (AD severity, tolerability of lower doses of donepezil and absence of contraindications), a stepwise titration strategy for dose escalation and appropriate monitoring and counselling of patients and caregivers in the management of patients with AD.[30]

Memantine extended release (ER) 28mg once-daily capsule formulation was approved in the USA in 2010 is now fairly widely available. Its efficacy was demonstrated in a large, multinational, phase III trial which showed that the addition of memantine ER to ongoing cholinesterase inhibitors improved key outcomes compared with cholinesterase inhibitor monotherapy, including measures of cognition and global status. The most common adverse events were headache, diarrhoea and dizziness.[31]

Note that these high doses of donepezil and memantine have not yet been approved in the UK and many other countries. In addition, most older people seen in practice with AD are likely to be frailer and have more co-morbidities than patients in clinical trials and may therefore be less likely to tolerate the higher doses.

Combination treatment

Although studies investigating the benefits of combining AChE-Is and memantine have found conflicting results, both the European Academy of Neurology (EAN) Guidelines and the UK's National Institute for Health and Care Excellence (NICE)[1] recommend the use of a combination of AChE-I plus memantine rather than AChE-I alone in patients with moderate-to-severe AD. The strength of the evidence supporting this recommendation is rather weak.[32] Studies have confirmed that there are no pharmacokinetic or pharmacodynamic interactions between AChE-Is and memantine.[33,34]

Tolerability

Drug tolerability may differ between AChE-Is, but, again, in the absence of sufficient direct comparisons, it is difficult to draw conclusions. Overall tolerability can be broadly evaluated by reference to the numbers withdrawing from clinical trials. Withdrawal rates in trials of donepezil[35,36] ranged from 4% to 16% (placebo 1–7%). With rivastigmine,[37,38] rates ranged from 7% to 29% (placebo 7%) and with galantamine[39–41] from 7% to 23% (placebo 7–9%). These figures relate to withdrawals specifically associated with adverse effects. The number needed to harm (NNH) has been reported to be 12.[16] A study of the French pharmacovigilance database identified age, the use of antipsychotic drugs, antihypertensives and drugs targeting the alimentary tract and metabolism as factors associated with serious reactions to AChE-Is.[42]

Tolerability seems to be affected by speed of titration and, perhaps less clearly, by dose. Most adverse effects occurred in trials during titration, and slower titration schedules are recommended in clinical use. This may mean that these drugs are equally well tolerated in practice.

Rivastigmine patches offer convenience and a superior tolerability profile to rivastigmine capsules.[27,28] Data from three trials found that rivastigmine patch was better tolerated than the capsules with fewer GI adverse effects and fewer discontinuations due to these adverse effects.[43] Data support recommendations for patients on high doses of rivastigmine capsules (>6mg/day) to switch directly to the 9.5mg/24 hours patch, while those on lower doses (≤6mg/day) should start on 4.6mg/hour patch for 4 weeks before increasing to the 9.5mg/hour patch. This latter switch is also recommended for patients switching from other oral cholinesterase inhibitors to the rivastigmine patch (with a 1 week washout period in patients who are sensitive to adverse effects or who have very low body weight or a history of bradycardia).[44] It is possible to consider increasing the dose to 13.3mg/24 hours after 6 months on 9.5mg/24 hours if tolerated, and meaningful cognitive or functional decline occurs. A 48-week RCT found the higher strength patch (13.3mg) to significantly reduce deterioration in Instrumental Activities of Daily Living (IADL) compared with the 9.5mg/24 hours patch and it was well tolerated.[45]

Patients and caregivers should be instructed on important administration details for the rivastigmine patch:[9]

- The transdermal patch should not be applied to the skin that is red, irritated or cut.
- Reapplication to the exact same skin location within 14 days should be avoided to minimise the potential **risk of skin irritation**
- The previous day's patch must be removed before applying a new one every day.
- Only one patch should be worn at a time.
- The patch should not be cut into pieces.

The following cautions exist while using AChE-Is: asthma, chronic obstructive pulmonary disease (COPD), sick sinus syndrome, supraventricular conduction abnormalities, susceptibility to peptic ulcers, history of seizures and bladder outflow obstruction; and while using rivastigmine patch, there is risk of fatal overdose with patch administration errors.[46]

Memantine appears to be well tolerated[47,48] and the only conditions associated with warnings include severe hepatic impairment and epilepsy/seizures[49] (see BNF or equivalent for required dosage adjustments in renal impairment). Isolated cases of international normalised ratio (INR) increases have been reported when memantine is co-administered with warfarin.

Adverse effects

Cholinesterase inhibitors

When adverse effects occur with AChE-Is, they are largely predictable: excess cholinergic stimulation leads to nausea, vomiting, dizziness, insomnia and diarrhoea.[50] Such effects are most likely to occur at the start of therapy or when the dose is increased. They are dose related and tend to be transient. Urinary incontinence has also been reported.[51] There appear to be no important differences between drugs with respect to the type or frequency of adverse events, although clinical trials generally suggest a relatively lower frequency of adverse events for donepezil. This may simply be a reflection of the aggressive titration schedules used in trials of other drugs. GI effects appeared to be more common with oral rivastigmine in clinical trials than with other cholinesterase inhibitors, however slower titration, ensuring oral rivastigmine is taken with food or using the patch reduces the risk of GI effects.

An analysis of 16 years of Individual Case Safety Reports from VigiBase found that the most common adverse effects reported with AChE-Is were neuropsychiatric symptoms (31.4%), GI disorders (15.9%) and general disorders and administration site conditions (11.9%). Cardiovascular adverse drug reactions (ADRs) accounted for 11.7%.[52]

In view of their pharmacological action, AChE-Is can be expected to have vagotonic effects on heart rate (i.e. bradycardia) (See figure 6.1). The potential for this action may be of particular importance in patients with 'sick sinus syndrome' or other supraventricular cardiac conduction disturbances, such as sinoatrial or atrioventricular block.[7-12]

Concerns over the potential cardiac adverse effects associated with AChE-Is were raised following findings from controlled trials of galantamine in mild cognitive impairment (MCI) in which increased mortality was associated with galantamine

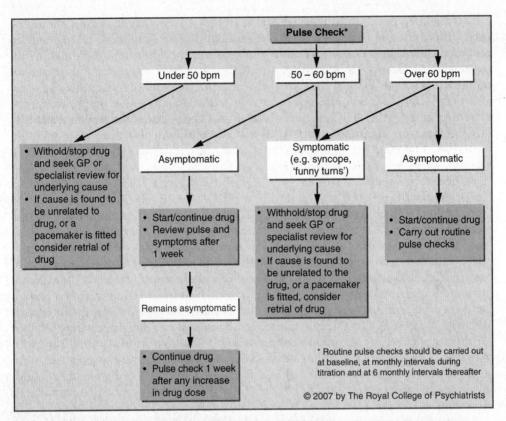

Figure 6.1 Suggested guidelines for managing cardiovascular risk prior to and during treatment with AChEIs in AD[53,54].
bpm, heartbeats per minute; the 'drug' means the chosen AChE inhibitors.
Reproduced with permission

compared with placebo (1.5% vs 0.5%, respectively).[55] Although no specific cause of death was dominant, half of the deaths reported were due to cardiovascular disorders. As a result, the FDA issued a warning restricting galantamine in patients with MCI. The relevance to AD remains unclear.[56] A Cochrane review of pooled data from RCTs of the AChE-Is revealed that there was a significantly higher incidence of syncope amongst the AChE-I groups compared with the placebo groups (3.43% vs 1.87%). A population-based study using a case–time–control design examined health records for 1.4 million older adults in Ontario and found that treatment with AChE-Is was associated with a doubled risk of hospitalisation for bradycardia. (The drugs were resumed at discharge in over half the cases suggesting that cardiovascular toxicity of AChE-Is is underappreciated by clinicians.[57]) It seems that patients with Lewy body dementia are more susceptible to the bradyarrhythmic adverse effects of these drugs, owing to the autonomic insufficiency associated with the disease.[58] A similar study found that hospital visits for syncope were also more frequent in people receiving AChE-Is than in controls: 31.5 vs 18.6 events per 1000 person-years (adjusted hazard ratio 1.76).[59]

The manufacturers of all three agents therefore advise that the drugs should be used with caution in patients with cardiovascular disease or in those taking concurrent medicines that reduce heart rate, e.g. digoxin or beta blockers. Although a pre-treatment mandatory electrocardiogram (ECG) has been suggested,[56] a review of published evidence showed that the incidence of cardiovascular side effects is low and that serious adverse effects are rare. In addition, the value of pre-treatment screening and routine ECGs is questionable and is not currently recommended by NICE. However, in patients with a history of cardiovascular disease or who are prescribed concomitant negative chronotropic drugs with AChE-Is, an ECG is advised. (See Yorkshire and the Humber Clinical Networks Guidelines – The Assessment of Cardiac Status Before Prescribing Acetyl Cholinesterase Inhibitors for Dementia 2016.[53])

In a study of 204 elderly patients with AD, each had their ECG and blood pressure assessed before and after starting AChE-I therapy. It was noted that none of the AChE-Is was associated with increased negative chronotropic, arrhythmogenic or hypotensive effects and therefore a preferred drug could not be established with regard to vagotonic effects.[60] Similarly, a Danish retrospective cohort study[61] found no substantial differences in the risk of myocardial infarction (MI) or heart failure between participants on donepezil and those using the other AChE-Is. Memantine was in fact associated with greatest risk of all-cause mortality, although sicker individuals were selected for memantine therapy. A Swedish cohort study[62] found that AChE-Is were associated with a 35% reduced risk of MI or death in patients with AD. These associations were stronger with increasing doses of AChE-Is. RCTs are required in order to confirm findings from this observational study, but they fit well with other observations of reduced mortality.

A review of the cardiovascular effects of dementia drugs[63] found that although such events with AChE-Is are very uncommon, there was evidence that they are associated with small but significant increase in the risk of syncope and bradycardia. There are also a few reports that they may occasionally be associated with QT prolongation and *torsades de pointes*.

Memantine

Although little is known about the cardiovascular effects of memantine, there have been reports of bradycardia and reduced cardiovascular survival associated with its use.[63]

An analysis of pooled prospective data for **memantine** revealed that the most frequently reported adverse effects in placebo-controlled trials included agitation (7.5% memantine vs 12% placebo), falls (6.8% vs 7.1%), dizziness (6.3% vs 5.7%), accidental injury (6.0% vs 7.2%), influenza-like symptoms (6.0% vs 5.8%), headache (5.2% vs 3.7%) and diarrhoea (5.0% vs 5.6%).[64]

An analysis of the French Pharmacovigilance Database compared adverse effects reported with **donepezil** with **memantine**. The most frequent ADRs with donepezil alone and memantine alone were, respectively, bradycardia (10% vs 7%), weakness (5% vs 6%) and convulsions (4% vs 3%). Although it is well known that donepezil is often associated with bradycardia and memantine associated with seizures, this analysis suggests that memantine can also induce bradycardia and donepezil seizures, thus highlighting the care required when treating patients with dementia who have a history of bradycardia or epilepsy.[65]

Interactions

Potential for interaction may also differentiate currently available cholinesterase inhibitors. Donepezil[66] and galantamine[67] are metabolised by cytochromes 2D6 and 3A4 and so drug levels may be altered by other drugs affecting the function of these enzymes. Cholinesterase inhibitors themselves may also interfere with the metabolism of other drugs, although this is perhaps a theoretical consideration. Rivastigmine has almost no potential for interaction since it is metabolised at the site of action and does not affect hepatic cytochromes. A prospective pharmacodynamic analysis of potential drug interactions between rivastigmine and other medications (22 different therapeutic classes) commonly prescribed in the elderly population compared adverse effects' odds ratios between rivastigmine and placebo. Rivastigmine was not associated with any significant pattern of increase in adverse effects that would indicate a drug interaction compared with placebo.[68] Rivastigmine thus appears to be least likely to cause problematic drug interactions, a factor that may be important in an elderly population subject to polypharmacy (see Table 6.2).

Analysis of the French pharmacovigilance database found that the majority of reported drug interactions concerning AChE-Is were found to be pharmacodynamic in nature and most frequently involved the combination of AChE-I and bradycardic drugs (beta blockers, digoxin, amiodarone and calcium channel antagonists). Almost a third of these interactions resulted in cardiovascular ADRs such as bradycardia, atrioventricular block and arterial hypotension. The second most frequent drug interaction reported was the combination of AChE-I with anticholinergic drugs leading to pharmacological antagonism.[69]

The pharmacodynamic, pharmacokinetic and pharmacogenetic aspects of drugs used in dementia have recently been summarised in two comprehensive reviews.[70,71]

When to stop treatment

A large multicentre study[72] of community-dwelling patients with moderate or severe AD investigated the long-term effects of donepezil over 12 months compared with stopping donepezil after 3 months, switching to memantine or combining donepezil with memantine. Continued treatment with donepezil was associated with continued cognitive benefits, and patients with a Mini Mental State (MMSE) score as low as 3 also benefitted from treatment. This suggests that patients should continue treatment with AChE-Is for as long as possible and there should not be a cut-off MMSE score where treatment is stopped automatically. Moreover, secondary and post-hoc analyses of this study found that withdrawal of donepezil in patients with moderate-to-severe AD increased the risk of nursing home placement during 12 months of treatment but made no difference during the following 3 years of follow-up. This highlights the point that decisions to stop or continue treatment should be informed by potential risks of withdrawal, even if the perceived benefits of continued treatment are not clear.[73]

CHAPTER 6

Table 6.2 Drug–drug interactions[8–12,74,75]

Drug	Metabolism	Plasma levels increased by	Plasma levels decreased by	Pharmacodynamic interactions
Donepezil (Aricept®)	Substrate at 3A4 and 2D6	Ketoconazole Itraconazole Erythromycin Quinidine Fluoxetine Paroxetine	Rifampicin Phenytoin Carbamazepine Alcohol	Antagonistic with **anticholinergic drugs** and **competitive neuromuscular blockers (e.g. tubocurarine)**. Potential for synergistic activity with **cholinomimetics** such as **depolarising neuro-muscular blocking agents (e.g. succinylcholine)**, cholinergic agonists and peripherally acting cholinesterase inhibitors, **e.g. neostigmine**. Beta blockers, amiodarone or calcium channel blockers may have additive effects on cardiac conduction. Caution with concomitant use of **drugs known to induce QT prolongation and/or torsade de pointes**. Movement disorders and neuroleptic malignant syndrome have occurred with concomitant use of **antipsychotics** and cholinesterase inhibitors. Concurrent use with **seizure lowering agents** may result in reduced seizure threshold.
Rivastigmine (Exelon®)	Non-hepatic metabolism	Metabolic interactions appear unlikely. Rivastigmine may inhibit the butyrylcholinesterase-mediated metabolism of other substances, e.g. **cocaine**. Smoking **tobacco** increases the clearance of rivastigmine		Antagonistic effects with **anticholinergic** and **competitive neuromuscular blockers (e.g. tubocurarine)**. Potential for synergistic activity with **cholinomimetics** such as **depolarising neuro-muscular blocking agents (e.g. succinylcholine) – cholinergic agonists**, e.g. **bethanechol or peripherally acting cholinesterase inhibitors, e.g. neostigmine**. Synergistic effects on cardiac conduction with **beta blockers, amiodarone, calcium channel blockers**. Caution with concomitant use of **drugs known to induce QT prolongation and/or torsade de pointes**. Movement disorders and neuroleptic malignant syndrome have occurred with concomitant use of **antipsychotics** and cholinesterase inhibitors. Concurrent use with **metoclopramide** may result in increased risk of extrapyramidal symptoms
Galantamine (Reminyl®)	Substrate at 3A4 and 2D6	Ketoconazole Erythromycin Ritonavir Quinidine Paroxetine Fluoxetine Fluvoxamine Amitriptyline	None known	Antagonistic effects with **anticholinergic** and **competitive neuromuscular blockers (e.g. tubocurarine)**. Potential for synergistic activity with **cholinomimetics** such as **depolarising neuro-muscular blocking agents (e.g. succinylcholine)**, cholinergic agonists and peripherally acting cholinesterase inhibitors, **e.g. neostigmine**. Possible interaction with agents that significantly reduce heart rate, e.g. **digoxin, beta blockers, certain calcium-channel blockers** and **amiodarone**. Caution with concomitant use of drugs known to induce QT prolongation and/or torsade de pointes (manufacturer recommends ECG in such cases). Movement disorders and neuroleptic malignant syndrome have occurred with concomitant use of **antipsychotics** and cholinesterase inhibitors

| Memantine (Exiba®) | Primarily non-hepatic metabolism Renally eliminated | **Cimetidine Ranitidine Procainamide Quinidine Quinine Nicotine Trimethoprim**

Isolated cases of INR increases reported with concomitant warfarin (close monitoring of prothrombin time or INR advisable).

Drugs that alkalinise urine (pH ~ 8) may reduce renal elimination of memantine, e.g. **carbonic anhydrase inhibitors, sodium bicarbonate** | None known (Possibility of reduced serum level of **hydrochlorothiazide** when co-administered with memantine). | Effects of **L-dopa, dopaminergic agonists, selegiline** and **anticholinergics** may be enhanced. Effects of **barbiturates** and **antipsychotics** may be reduced. Avoid concomitant use with **amantadine, ketamine** and **dextromethorphan** – increased risk of CNS toxicity. One published case report on possible risk for **phenytoin** and memantine combination.

Dosage adjustment may be necessary for **antispasmodic agents, dantrolene** or **baclofen** when administered with memantine.

A single case report of myoclonus and confusion when co-administered with **co-trimoxazole** or **trimethoprim** |

NB: This list is not exhaustive – caution with other drugs that are also inhibitors or enhancers of CYP 3A4 and 2D6 enzymes.

The efficacy of AChE-Is over the time course of a dementing illness is not fully understood. On the one hand, there is evidence that the drugs, when initially prescribed, may achieve stabilisation of cognitive function for 2–5 months[18] but the study referenced earlier suggests that stopping the drugs even late in the course of the illness may have detrimental effects. The reality is that there are probably individual variations in treatment response which as yet are not well understood and cannot be predicted. Hence, decisions on whether to stop an AChE-I should be made on a patient-by-patient basis, taking into account views of family and carers. However, the consensus of opinion is that if the drug is well tolerated and the patient's physical health is stable, then it is probably best to continue the drug. The risks of discontinuation of dementia medication should be balanced against side effects and costs of continuing treatment.[95]

In addition to this, a meta-analysis evaluating the efficacy of the three AChE-Is and memantine in relation to the severity of AD found that the efficacy of all drugs except memantine was independent of dementia severity in all domains. The effect of memantine on functional impairment was actually better in more severe patients. Results clearly demonstrated that patients in differing stages of AD retain the ability to respond to treatment with AChE-Is and memantine. Medication effects are therefore substantially independent from disease severity, and patients with a wide range of severities can benefit from drug therapy. This suggests that the severity of a patient's illness should not preclude treatment with these drugs.[76]

Guidance for discontinuation of dementia medication in clinical practice has been summarised in the following section.[77]

Reasons for stopping treatment

- When the patient/caregiver decides to stop (after being advised on the risks and benefits of stopping treatment)
- When the patient refuses to take the medication (but see section on covert administration)
- When there are problems with patient compliance which cannot be reasonably resolved
- When the patient's cognitive, functional or behavioural decline is worsened by treatment
- When there are intolerable side effects
- When co-morbidities make treatment risky or futile (e.g. terminal illness)
- Where there is no clinically meaningful benefit to continuing therapy (clinical judgement should be used here rather than ceasing treatment when a patient reaches a certain score on a cognitive outcome or when they are institutionalised)
- When dementia has progressed to a severely impaired stage (Global Deterioration Scale stage 7: development of swallowing difficulties)

When a decision is made to stop therapy (for reasons other than lack of tolerability), tapering of the dose and monitoring the patient for evidence of significant decline during the next 1–3 months are advised. If such decline occurs, reinstatement of therapy should be considered.

NICE recommendations

NICE Guidance on Dementia[78] was last updated in June 2018.

Summary of NICE guidance for the treatment of Alzheimer's disease[78,79]

- The three AChE-Is donepezil, galantamine and rivastigmine are recommended for managing mild-to-moderate AD.
- Memantine is recommended for managing moderate AD for people who are intolerant of or have a contrain-dication to AChE-Is, or for managing severe AD.
- For people with an established diagnosis of AD who are already taking an AChE-I:
  - consider memantine in addition to an AChE-I if they have moderate disease;
  - offer memantine in addition to an AChE-I if they have severe disease.
- Treatment should be under the following conditions:
  For people who are not taking an AChE-I or memantine, prescribers should only start treatment with these on the advice of a clinician who has the necessary knowledge and skills.
  This could include:
  - secondary care medical specialists such as psychiatrists, geriatricians and neurologists; and
  - other healthcare professionals (such as GPs, nurse consultants and advanced nurse practitioners), if they have specialist expertise in diagnosing and treating AD.
- Once a decision has been made to start an AChE-I or memantine, the first prescription may be made in primary care.
- For people with an established diagnosis of AD who are already taking an AChE-I, primary care prescribers may start treatment with memantine without taking advice from a specialist clinician.
- Ensure that local arrangements for prescribing, supply and treatment review follow the NICE guideline on medicines optimisation.[80]
- Do not stop AChE-Is in people with AD because of disease severity alone.
- Therapy with AChE-I should be initiated with a drug with the lowest acquisition cost (taking into account required daily dose and the price per dose once shared care has started). An alternative may be considered on the basis of adverse effects profile, expectations about adherence, medical co-morbidity, possibility of drug interactions and dosing profiles.

Summary of NICE guidance for the treatment of non-AD dementia[78,79]

- Offer donepezil or rivastigmine to people with mild-to-moderate DLB.
- Only consider galantamine for people with mild-to-moderate DLB if donepezil and rivastigmine are not tolerated.
- Consider donepezil or rivastigmine for people with severe DLB.
- Consider memantine for people with DLB if AChE-Is are not tolerated or are contraindicated.
- Only consider AChE-Is or memantine for people with vascular dementia if they have suspected co-morbid AD, Parkinson's disease dementia or DLB.
- Do not offer AChE-Is or memantine to people with frontotemporal dementia.
- Do not offer AChE-Is or memantine to people with cognitive impairment caused by multiple sclerosis.
- For guidance on pharmacological management of Parkinson's disease dementia, see Parkinson's disease dementia in the NICE guideline on Parkinson's disease.

Medicines that may cause cognitive impairment[1]

- Be aware that some commonly prescribed medicines are associated with increased anticholinergic burden, and therefore cognitive impairment.
- Consider minimising the use of medicines associated with increased anticholinergic burden, and if possible look for alternatives:
  - when assessing whether to refer a person with suspected dementia for diagnosis
  - during medication reviews with people living with dementia.
- Be aware that there are validated tools for assessing anticholinergic burden but there is insufficient evidence to recommend one over the others (see section 'Safer prescribing for physical health conditions in dementia').
- For guidance on carrying out medication reviews, see medication review in the NICE guideline on medicines optimisation.

NB: The Anticholinergic Effect on Cognition (AEC) scale can be accessed at www.medichec.com

CHAPTER 6

Other treatments (where the evidence remains less certain)

A Cochrane review found that although **Ginkgo biloba** appears to be safe with no excess side effects compared with placebo, there was no convincing evidence that it is efficacious for dementia and cognitive impairment. Many of the trials were too small and used unsatisfactory methods, and publication bias could not be excluded. The review concluded that ginkgo's clinical benefit in dementia or cognitive impairment is somewhat inconsistent and unconvincing.[81] An overview of systematic reviews found that it has potentially beneficial effects when it is administered at doses greater than 200mg/day (usually 240mg/day) for at least 5 months. Given the lower quality of the evidence, further rigorously designed, multicentre, large-scale RCTs are warranted.[82] Several reports have noted that ginkgo may increase the risk of bleeding.[83] The drug is widely used in Germany but less so elsewhere.

A Cochrane review of **Vitamin E** for AD and mild cognitive impairment (MCI) examined three studies. The authors' conclusions were that there is no evidence of efficacy of vitamin E in prevention or treatment of people with AD or MCI and that further research is required in order to identify its role in this area.[84] However, the TEAM-AD trial, an RCT of vitamin E 2000IU/day in 613 patients with mild-to-moderate AD, showed a 19% decrease in the primary outcome, annual rate of decline in activities of daily living, in the vitamin E arm; the authors note that this was equivalent to a 6-month delay in progression. For secondary outcomes, the increase in caregiving time required was 2 hours higher in the placebo group than in the vitamin E group; there was no benefit on cognition or any of the other secondary outcomes.[85] Trials of vitamin E in AD have used α-tocopherol at doses much higher than the recommended daily allowance of 22.4IU, which have been associated with adverse effects such as increased risks of haemorrhagic stroke, prostate cancer, heart failure and higher mortality. As evidence for the efficacy of vitamin E in AD is limited, its utility must be weighed against these potential adverse effects before its recommendation.[86]

A Cochrane review found no evidence that **folic acid** with or without **vitamin B$_{12}$** improves cognitive function of unselected elderly people with or without dementia.[87] Although, according to data from a recent review, it seems that **folic acid** supplementation could improve cognitive function by decreasing homocysteine (Hcy), vascular care, attenuating inflammatory status, modification of cerebral folic acid deficiency and antioxidant responses, specifically, people with high levels of Hcy have a better response to folic acid supplementation, which may arise from low serum folate concentration. The optimal dose of folic acid required to possible improvement in cognitive function is currently unknown.[88]

Increase in serum Hcy is shown to be a potential risk factor for cognitive impairment. Some evidence suggests that vitamin B supplementation may reduce cognitive decline by lowering the Hcy levels. A recent meta-analysis evaluated the efficacy of folic acid along with vitamin **B12 and/or B6** in lowering Hcy, thereby attenuating cognitive decline in elderly patients with AD or dementia. Vitamin B supplementation was effective in reducing serum Hcy levels; however, this did not translate into cognitive improvement, indicating that the existing data on vitamin B-induced improvement in cognition by lowering Hcy levels are conflicting.[89]

A Cochrane review of **Omega-3 fatty acids** for the treatment of dementia included three trials that investigated 632 people with mild-to-moderate AD. The review found that taking omega-3 PUFA supplements for 6 months had no effect on cognition (learning and understanding), everyday functioning, quality of life or mental health. It also had no effect on ratings of the overall severity of the illness. The trials did not report side effects very well, but none of the studies described significant harmful effects on health.[90]

A prospective open-label study of **ginseng** in AD measured cognitive performance in 97 patients randomly assigned ginseng or placebo for 12 weeks and then 12 weeks after the ginseng had been discontinued. After ginseng treatment, the cognitive subscales of ADAS and MMSE scores began to show improvement continued up to 12 weeks but scores declined to levels of the control group following discontinuation of ginseng.[91] A recent systematic review and meta-analysis, including four RCTs involving 259 participants, showed that the effects of ginseng on AD remain unproven. The main limitations of the available studies were small sample sizes, poor methodological qualities and no placebo controls. Larger, well-designed studies are needed to test the effect of ginseng on AD in the future.[92]

Dimebon (also known as latrepirdine), a non-selective antihistamine previously approved in Russia but later discontinued for commercial reasons, has been assessed for safety, tolerability and efficacy in the treatment of patients with mild-to-moderate AD. It acts as a weak inhibitor of BuChE and AChE, weakly blocks the NMDA-receptor signalling pathway and inhibits the mitochondrial permeability transition pore opening.[93] A recent Cochrane review concluded that there was no beneficial effect of dimebon on cognition and function in mild-to-moderate AD, though there appeared to be modest benefit for behaviour.[94]

Natural **hirudin**, isolated from salivary gland of medicinal leech, is a direct thrombin inhibitor and has been used for many years in China. A small 20-week open-label RCT of 84 patients receiving donepezil or donepezil plus hirudin (3g/day) found that patients on the combination showed significant decrease in ADAS-Cog scores and significant increase in ADL scores when compared with donepezil alone. However, haemorrhage and hypersensitivity reactions were more common in the combination group compared with donepezil group (11.9% and 7.1% vs 2.4% and 2.4%, respectively).[95] The potential haemorrhagic effects of hirudin need further exploration before it can be considered for clinical use.

Huperzine A, an alkaloid isolated from the Chinese herb *Huperzia serrata*, is a potent, highly selective, reversible AChE-I used for treating AD since 1994 in China and available as a nutraceutical in the USA. A meta-analysis found that huperzine A 300–500µg daily for 8–24 weeks in AD led to significant improvements in MMSE (mean change 3.5) and ADL with effect size shown to increase over treatment time. Most adverse effects were cholinergic in nature and no serious adverse effects occurred.[96] A later meta-analysis produced similarly positive, if uncertain, results.[97] A Cochrane review of huperzine A in vascular dementia, however, found no convincing evidence for its value in vascular dementia.[98] Similarly, a Cochrane review of huperzine A for MCI concluded that the current evidence is insufficient for this indication as no eligible trials were identified at the time.[99] However, in a recent network meta-analysis, huperzine A achieved good efficacy in the mild and moderate cognitive function decline groups.[100]

CHAPTER 6

There is increasing evidence to suggest possible efficacy of *Crocus sativus* (**saffron**) in the management of AD. A recent systematic review and meta-analysis of RCTs revealed that saffron significantly improves cognitive function measured by the ADAS-cog and Clinical Dementia Rating Scale-Sums of Boxes, compared to placebo groups. In addition, there was no significant difference between saffron and conventional medicines (donepezil and memantine). Saffron improved the daily living function, but the changes were not statistically significant. No serious adverse events were reported in the included studies. Saffron may be beneficial to improve cognitive function in patients with MCI and AD. No evidence was found to support the effects of saffron on other types of dementia. More high-quality randomised placebo-controlled trials are needed to further confirm the efficacy and safety of saffron for MCI and dementia.[101]

Cerebrolysin is a parenterally administered, porcine brain-derived peptide preparation that has pharmacodynamic properties similar to those of endogenous neurotrophic factors. A meta-analysis included six RCTs comparing cerebrolysin 30mg/day with placebo in mild-to-moderate AD. Cerebrolysin was significantly more effective than placebo at 4 weeks regarding cognitive function and at 4 weeks and 6 months regarding global clinical change and 'global benefit'. The safety of cerebrolysin was comparable to placebo. In addition, a large 28-week RCT comparing cerebrolysin, donepezil or combination therapy showed significantly higher improvements in global outcome for cerebrolysin and the combination therapy than for donepezil at study endpoint; lack of significant group differences in cognitive, functional and behavioural domains at the endpoint; and best scores of cognitive improvement in the combination therapy group at all study visits.[102]

The Cochrane review assessing cerebrolysin in vascular dementia was updated in 2019. Courses of intravenous cerebrolysin improved cognition and general function in people living with vascular dementia, with no suggestion of adverse effects. However, these data are not definitive. The analyses were limited by heterogeneity, and the included papers had high risk of bias. If there are benefits of cerebrolysin, the effects may be too small to be clinically meaningful. Cerebrolysin continues to be used and promoted as a treatment for vascular dementia, but the supporting evidence base is weak. The most commonly reported non-serious adverse events were headache, asthenia, dizziness, hypertension and hypotension.[103]

In AD, amyloid protein is deposited in the form of extracellular plaques, and studies have determined that amyloid protein generation is cholesterol dependent. Hypercholesterolaemia has also been implicated in the pathogenesis of vascular dementia. Because of the role of **statins** in cholesterol reduction, they have been explored as a means to treat dementia. A Cochrane review, however, found that there is still insufficient evidence to recommend statins for the treatment of dementia. Analyses from available studies indicate that they have no benefit on the outcome measures such as ADAS-Cog or MMSE.[104] A further Cochrane review examined whether statins could prevent dementia. Only two randomised trials were suitable for inclusion in this review with 26,340 participants; neither showed any reduction in occurrence of AD or dementia in people treated with statins compared to people given placebo.[105] A subsequent systematic review and meta-analysis, including 25 studies which met eligibility criteria, found that the use of statins may reduce the risk of all-type dementia, AD and MCI, but not of incident vascular dementia.[106] Similarly, a meta-analysis of observational studies

(30 studies, including 9,162,509 participants) suggested that the use of statin is significantly associated with a decreased risk of dementia. The overall pooled reduction of AD in patients with statin use was risk ratio (RR) 0.69 (95% CI 0.60–0.80, $p < 0.0001$), and the overall pooled RR of statin use and vascular dementia risk was RR 0.93 (95% CI 0.74–1.16, $p = 0.54$). However, until further evidence is established, clinicians need to make sure that statin use should remain restricted to the treatment of cardiovascular disease.[107]

A longitudinal prospective study examined the relationship between **chocolate** consumption and cognitive decline in an elderly cognitively healthy population. A total of 531 participants aged ≥65 years with normal MMSE scores were followed for a median of 48 months. Dietary habits were evaluated at baseline and the MMSE was used to assess global cognitive function at baseline and at follow-up. After adjustment for confounders, chocolate intake was associated with a lower risk of cognitive decline (RR = 0.59, 95%CI 0.38–0.92). This protective effect was observed only among subjects with an average daily consumption of caffeine lower than 75mg.[108]

Souvenaid is a medical food for the dietary management of early AD. The mix of nutrients in this drink is suggested to have a beneficial effect on cognitive function; however, health claims for medical foods are not evaluated by government agencies. In a 24-week trial of 259 patients with mild AD, there was a statistically significant benefit in favour of Souvenaid on the primary outcome, a memory composite score, but a 24-month trial in participants with biomarkers for AD, and episodic memory impairment did not show a benefit on the primary outcome. Although these medical foods are likely to be safe, overall, the evidence for their efficacy in AD is weak.[86]

Idalopirdine is a 5-HT$_6$ receptor antagonist. Given that 5-HT$_6$ receptor is expressed in areas of the CNS involved with memory and that there is evidence suggesting that blocking of these receptors induces ACh release, it has become a promising approach that 5-HT$_6$ antagonism could restore ACh levels in a deteriorated cholinergic system.[109] A recent systematic review and meta-analysis analysed four RCTs with 2,803 patients with AD. Idalopirdine was not shown to be effective for AD patients and is associated with a risk of elevated liver enzymes and vomiting. Although idalopirdine might be more effective at high doses and in moderate AD subgroups, the effect size is small and may be limited.[110]

Anti-inflammatory drugs: A large number of RCTs of anti-inflammatory agents in AD have failed to reach primary outcomes. Large-scale studies of non-steroidal anti-inflammatory drugs (NSAIDs), including indomethacin, naproxen and rofecoxib in AD, have been unsuccessful. RCTs with a range of other anti-inflammatory drugs, including prednisolone, hydroxychloroquine, simvastatin, atorvastatin, aspirin and rosiglitazone, have also shown no clinically significant changes in primary cognitive outcomes in patients with AD.[22] A 2020 Cochrane review evaluated aspirin and other NSAIDs for the prevention of dementia and found no evidence to support the use of low-dose aspirin or other NSAIDs of any class (celecoxib, rofecoxib or naproxen) for the prevention of dementia. There was, however, evidence of harm, including higher rates of death and major bleeding compared to placebo with aspirin, and in one of the studies, more people developed dementia in the NSAID group. More stomach bleeding and other stomach problems, such as pain, nausea and gastritis, were also reported with NSAIDs.[111]

Trazodone and dibenzoylmethane

Two existing compounds have been found to be markedly neuroprotective in mouse models of neurodegeneration, using clinically relevant doses over a prolonged period of time, without systemic toxicity. **Trazodone** is an antidepressant in the serotonin antagonist and reuptake inhibitor class, which has additional anxiolytic and hypnotic effects, has been shown to reduce behavioural and psychological symptoms of dementia (BPSD) in AD. A recent small retrospective study examined whether long-term use of trazodone, a slow-wave-sleep enhancer, was associated with delayed cognitive decline. Trazodone non-users had 2.6-fold faster decline MMSE (primary outcome) than trazodone users. The observed effects were especially associated with subjective improvement of sleep complaints in post-hoc analyses. Results suggested an association between trazodone use and delayed cognitive decline although whether the observed relationship of trazodone to cognitive function is causal or an indirect marker of other effects, such as treated sleep disruption (mediated through slow-wave-sleep enhancement), requires confirmation through prospective studies.[112]

Dibenzoylmethane (DBM) is a minor constituent of liquorice that has been found to have antineoplastic effects, with efficacy against prostate and mammary tumours. In prion-diseased mice, both trazodone and DBM treatment restored memory deficits, abrogated development of neurological signs, prevented neurodegeneration and significantly prolonged survival. In tauopathy-frontotemporal dementia mice, both drugs were neuroprotective, rescued memory deficits and reduced hippocampal atrophy. Further, trazodone reduced p-tau burden. These compounds represent potential new disease-modifying treatments for dementia.[113] There are no available observational data suggesting that trazodone reduces the risk of dementia but some data are available that suggest important adverse outcomes in older people.[114]

Novel treatments

Several new drugs have failed to improve clinical outcomes in phase III trials for AD, including the following:

- **Semagacestat** is a γ-secretase inhibitor;[115] the trials including 3,000 patients were discontinued in 2010 because of the absence of improvement in cognition in the study group and worsening cognition at higher doses compared to controls. Incidence of skin cancer was also higher in the study group.[116]
- **Solanezumab** is a humanised monoclonal antibody that binds soluble forms of amyloid and promotes its clearance from the brain.[117] An RCT (EXPEDITION3) of 2,129 patients with mild AD found that solanezumab at a dose of 400mg administered every 4 weeks did not significantly affect cognitive decline.[118]
- **Bapineuzumab** is a humanised anti-amyloid-β monoclonal antibody.[119] A 2017 meta-analysis of RCTs with bapineuzumab confirmed its lack of clinical efficacy and its associations with serious adverse effects (vasogenic oedema). The doses of bapineuzumab used in these studies were limited because of higher rates of amyloid-related imaging abnormalities with effusion or oedema at higher doses. Its use is not recommended in patients with mild-to-moderate AD.[120]

Aducanumab is an antibody and works by targeting Aβ. It preferentially binds to the aggregated Aβ. Through this interaction, aducanumab could reduce the build-up of β-amyloid and therefore the number of amyloid plaques present in the brain thus potentially slows neurodegeneration and disease progression. Although in early 2019, the manufacturers (Biogen) announced that aducanumab failed futility analyses in two identically designed phase 3 AD trials and discontinued its development, later in the year they made the announcement that they were applying for US FDA marketing approval. They explained that they had reanalysed data from the trials to include patients who had continued in the studies after the cut-off date for the futility analyses and stated that one trial showed significant findings and a subset from the second trial supports these positive findings.[121] Whilst a recent review of the data by a panel of external experts was not promising, the FDA is set to announce its final decision on whether to approve aducanumab by March 2021.

Therapies targeting β-amyloid have been the focus of research for almost 30 years. However, highly promising drugs have failed to show clinical benefits in phase III trials. Even the positive findings presented by Biogen on aducanumab are not entirely clear, and further data are necessary to confirm its validity. Therefore, researchers are turning their efforts around to tau-targeting therapies, since tau protein appears to be better correlated with the severity of cognitive decline than amyloid β. Currently, most anti-tau agents in clinical trials are immunotherapies and they are in the early stages of clinical research. Four **monoclonal antibodies anti-tau** (**gosuranemab, tilavonemab, semorinemab** and **zagotenemab**) and one **anti-tau vaccine (AADvac1)** have reached phase II, so far.[122]

Vascular dementia (VaD)

Vascular dementia has been reported to comprise 10–50% of dementia cases and is the second most common type of dementia after AD. It is caused by ischaemic damage to the brain and is associated with cognitive impairment and behavioural disturbances. The management options are currently very limited and focus on controlling the underlying risk factors for cerebrovascular disease.[123]

Note that it is impossible to diagnose with certainty vascular or Alzheimer's dementia and much dementia has mixed causation. This might explain why certain AChE-Is do not always provide consistent results in probable vascular dementia, and the data indicating efficacy in cognitive outcomes were derived from older patients, who were therefore likely to have concomitant AD pathology.[124]

None of the currently available drugs is formally licensed in the UK for vascular dementia. The management of vascular dementia has been summarised.[125,126] Unlike the situation with stroke, there is no conclusive evidence that treatment of hyperlipidaemia with statins or treatment of blood clotting abnormalities with acetylsalicylic acid do have an effect on vascular dementia incidence or disease progression.[127] Similarly, a Cochrane review found that there were no studies supporting the role of statins in the treatment of VaD.[105] The Cochrane review for donepezil in vascular cognitive impairment found evidence to support its benefit in improving cognition function, clinical global impression and activities of daily living after 6 months treatment.[128] In a Cochrane review for galantamine for vascular cognitive impairment,[129,130] there were limited data suggesting some advantage over placebo in areas of cognition and global clinical state. Trials of galantamine reported high rates of GI side effects. The Cochrane review for rivastigmine in vascular cognitive impairment found some evidence of benefit; however, the conclusion was based on one large study, and side effects with rivastigmine lead to withdrawal in a significant proportion of patients.[105,131] Furthermore, a meta-analysis of RCTs found that cholinesterase inhibitors and memantine produce small benefits in cognition of uncertain clinical significance and concluded that data were insufficient to support widespread use of these agents in vascular dementia.[123] Recently, a systematic review and Bayesian network meta-analysis comparing the efficacy and safety of cognitive enhancers for treating vascular cognitive impairment found significant efficacy for donepezil, galantamine and memantine on cognition. Memantine was found to provide significant efficacy in global status. They were all safe and well tolerated.[132] A new Cochrane review of systematic reviews of cholinesterase inhibitors for vascular dementia and other vascular cognitive impairments is underway.

Dementia with Lewy bodies (DLB)

It has been suggested that DLB may account for 15–25% of cases of dementia (although autopsy suggests much lower rates). Characteristic symptoms are dementia with fluctuation of cognitive ability, early and persistent visual hallucinations and spontaneous motor features of parkinsonism. Falls, syncope, transient disturbances of consciousness, neuroleptic sensitivity and hallucinations in other modalities are also common.[133]

The 2018 update of the NICE guidelines[1] recommends the use of cholinesterase inhibitors and memantine in DLB (see table of summary of NICE guidance).

Meta-analyses of clinical trials of rivastigmine and donepezil support the use of cholinesterase inhibitors in DLB for improving cognition, global function and activities of living, with evidence that even if patients do not improve with AChE-Is they are less likely to deteriorate while taking them. The efficacy of memantine in DLB is less clear, but it is well tolerated and may have benefits, either as monotherapy or adjunctive to an AChE-I.[134]

There are significant complexities in managing an individual with DLB. Presentation varies between patients and can vary over time within an individual. Treatments can address one symptom but worsen another, which makes disease management difficult. Symptoms are often managed in isolation and by different specialists, which makes high-quality care difficult to accomplish. Clinical trials and meta-analyses now provide an evidence base for the treatment of cognitive, neuropsychiatric and motor symptoms in patients with Lewy body dementia. Furthermore, consensus opinion from experts supports the application of treatments for related conditions, such as Parkinson's disease, for the management of common symptoms (e.g. autonomic dysfunction) in patients with Lewy body dementia. However, evidence gaps remain and future clinical trials need to focus on the treatment of symptoms specific to patients with Lewy body dementia.[135] For a helpful guide on management of specific symptoms in DLB, see 'Management of Lewy body dementia Summary sheets – Diamond Lewy'.[136]

Mild cognitive impairment (MCI)

MCI is hypothesised to represent a pre-clinical stage of dementia but forms a heterogeneous group with variable prognosis. A Cochrane review assessing the safety and efficacy of AChE-Is in MCI found there was very little evidence that they affect progression to dementia or cognitive test scores. This weak evidence was countered by the increased risk of adverse effects particularly GI effects meaning that AChE-Is could not be recommended in MCI.[137] A systematic review[138] found that there was no replicated evidence that any intervention was effective for MCI, including AChE-Is and the NSAID rofecoxib. A further systematic review and meta-analysis found that although AChE-Is have a slight efficacy in the treatment of MCI, there are many safety issues; therefore, they are difficult to recommend for MCI.[139] Experts from several different countries recently reviewed the available evidence for the pharmacological and non-pharmacological treatment for MCI.[140]

Other dementias

A systemic review of RCTs for **frontotemporal dementias** showed that certain drugs may be effective in reducing behavioural symptoms (e.g. SSRIs and trazodone) but none of these had an effect on cognition.[141]

A Cochrane review assessed the efficacy and safety of AChE-Is for **rare dementias associated with neurological conditions.** The sample sizes of most trials were very small, and efficacy on cognitive function and ASL was found to be unclear, although AChE-Is were associated with more GI side effects compared with placebo.[142]

Summary of clinical practice guidance with anti-dementia drugs from BAP[22]

AChE-Is and memantine are effective in AD of a broad range of severity. Other drugs, including statins, anti-inflammatory drugs, vitamin E, nutritional supplements and ginkgo, cannot be recommended either for the treatment or prevention of AD. Neither AChE-Is nor memantine are effective in MCI. AChE-Is are not effective in frontotemporal dementia and may cause agitation. AChE-Is may be used for people with LBDs (both Parkinson's disease dementia and DLB), and memantine may be helpful. No drugs are clearly effective in vascular dementia, though AChE-Is are beneficial in mixed dementia. Early evidence suggests multifactorial interventions may have potential to prevent or delay the onset of dementia. Many novel pharmacological approaches involving strategies to reduce amyloid and/or tau deposition in those with or at high risk of AD are in progress. Though results of pivotal studies in early (prodromal/mild) AD are awaited, results to date in more established (mild-to-moderate) AD have been equivocal and no disease-modifying agents are either licensed or can be currently recommended for clinical use.

Table 6.3 Summary of BAP recommendations

	First choice	Second choice
Alzheimer's disease	AChE-Is	Memantine
Vascular dementia	None	None
Mixed dementia	AChE-Is	Memantine
Dementia with Lewy bodies	AChE-Is	Memantine
Mild cognitive impairment	None	None
Dementia with Parkinson's disease	AChE-Is	Memantine
Frontotemporal dementia	None	None

References

1. National Institute for Clinical Excellence. Dementia: assessment, management and support for people living with dementia and their carers. NICE guideline [NG97] 2018; www.nice.org.uk/guidance/ng97.
2. Francis PT, et al. The cholinergic hypothesis of Alzheimer's disease: a review of progress. *J Neurol Neurosurg Psychiatry* 1999; 66:137–147.
3. Craig LA, et al. Revisiting the cholinergic hypothesis in the development of Alzheimer's disease. *Neurosci Biobehav Rev* 2011; 35:1397–1409.
4. Mesulam M, et al. Widely spread butyrylcholinesterase can hydrolyze acetylcholine in the normal and Alzheimer brain. *Neurobiol Dis* 2002; 9:88–93.
5. Weinstock M. Selectivity of cholinesterase inhibition: clinical implications for the treatment of Alzheimer's disease. *CNS Drugs* 1999; 12:307–323.
6. Matsunaga S, et al. Memantine monotherapy for Alzheimer's disease: a systematic review and meta-analysis. *PLoS One* 2015; 10:e0123289.
7. BNF Online. British National Formulary. 2020; https://www.medicinescomplete.com/mc/bnf/current.
8. Eisai Ltd. Summary of product characteristics. Aricept tablets (donepezil hydrochloride). 2018; https://www.medicines.org.uk/emc/product/3776/smpc.
9. Novartis Pharmaceuticals UK Limited. Summary of product characteristics. Exelon 4.6 mg/24h, 9.5 mg/24h, 13.3 mg/24h transdermal patch. 2020; https://www.medicines.org.uk/emc/product/7764/smpc.
10. Sandoz Limited. Summary of product characteristics. Rivastigmine Sandoz 1.5 mg, 3 mg, 4.5 mg, 6 mg hard capsules. 2016; https://www.medicines.org.uk/emc/product/8407/smpc.
11. Shire Pharmaceuticals Limited. Summary of product characteristics. Reminyl XL 8mg, 16mg and 24mg prolonged release capsules. 2019; https://www.medicines.org.uk/emc/product/3934/smpc.
12. Shire Pharmaceuticals Limited. Summary of product characteristics. Reminyl Oral Solution. 2020; https://www.medicines.org.uk/emc/medicine/10337.
13. Lundbeck Limited. Summary of product characteristics. Ebixa 5mg/pump actuation oral solution, 20mg and 10 mg Tablets and Treatment Initiation Pack. 2019; https://www.medicines.org.uk/emc/product/8222/smpc.
14. NHS Prescription Services. Drug tariff. 2020; http://www.drugtariff.nhsbsa.nhs.uk/#/00791628-DD/DD00791615/Home.
15. Buckley JS, et al. A risk-benefit assessment of dementia medications: systematic review of the evidence. *Drugs Aging* 2015; 32:453–467.
16. Lanctot KL, et al. Efficacy and safety of cholinesterase inhibitors in Alzheimer's disease: a meta-analysis. *CMAJ* 2003; 169:557–564.
17. McShane R, et al. Memantine for dementia. *Cochrane Database Syst Rev* 2006; CD003154.
18. Vaci N, et al. Real-world effectiveness, its predictors and onset of action of cholinesterase inhibitors and memantine in dementia: retrospective health record study. *Br J Psychiatry* 2020:1–7. [Epub ahead of print].
19. Burns A, et al. Efficacy and safety of donepezil over 3 years: an open-label, multicentre study in patients with Alzheimer's disease. *Int J Geriatr Psychiatry* 2007; 22:806–812.
20. Doody RS, et al. Open-label, multicenter, phase 3 extension study of the safety and efficacy of donepezil in patients with Alzheimer disease. *Arch Neurol* 2001; 58:427–433.
21. Farlow MR, et al. Effective pharmacologic management of Alzheimer's disease. *Am J Med* 2007; 120:388–397.
22. O'Brien JT, et al. Clinical practice with anti-dementia drugs: A revised (third) consensus statement from the British Association for Psychopharmacology. *J Psychopharmacol* 2017; 31:147–168.
23. Singh S, et al. Discontinuation syndrome following donepezil cessation. *Int J Geriatr Psychiatry* 2003; 18:282–284.
24. Bidzan L, et al. Withdrawal syndrome after donepezil cessation in a patient with dementia. *Neurol Sci* 2012; 33:1459–1461.
25. Waldemar G, et al. Tolerability of switching from donepezil to memantine treatment in patients with moderate to severe Alzheimer's disease. *Int J Geriatr Psychiatry* 2008; 23:979–981.

26. Massoud F, et al. Switching cholinesterase inhibitors in older adults with dementia. *Int Psychogeriatr* 2011; 23:372–378.

27. Winblad B, et al. A six-month double-blind, randomized, placebo-controlled study of a transdermal patch in Alzheimer's disease–rivastigmine patch versus capsule. *Int J Geriatr Psychiatry* 2007; 22:456–467.

28. Zhang ZX, et al. Rivastigmine patch in Chinese Patients with Probable Alzheimer's disease: A 24-week, randomized, double-blind parallel-group study comparing rivastigmine patch (9.5 mg/24 h) with Capsule (6 mg Twice Daily). *CNS Neurosci Ther* 2016; 22:488–496.

29. Morgan TM, et al. Absolute bioavailability and safety of a novel rivastigmine nasal spray in healthy elderly individuals. *Br J Clin Pharmacol* 2017; 83:510–516.

30. Sabbagh M, et al. Clinical recommendations for the use of donepezil 23 mg in moderate-to-severe Alzheimer's disease in the Asia-Pacific region. *Dementia Geriatr Cogn Disord Extra* 2016; 6:382–395.

31. Plosker GL. Memantine extended release (28 mg once daily): a review of its use in Alzheimer's disease. *Drugs* 2015; 75:887–897.

32. Schmidt R, et al. EFNS-ENS/EAN guideline on concomitant use of cholinesterase inhibitors and memantine in moderate to severe Alzheimer's disease. *Eur J Neurol* 2015; 22:889–898.

33. Periclou AP, et al. Lack of pharmacokinetic or pharmacodynamic interaction between memantine and donepezil. *Ann Pharmacother* 2004; 38:1389–1394.

34. Grossberg GT, et al. Rationale for combination therapy with galantamine and memantine in Alzheimer's disease. *J Clin Pharmacol* 2006; 46:17S-26S.

35. Rogers SL, et al. Donepezil improves cognition and global function in Alzheimer disease: a 15-week, double-blind, placebo-controlled study. Donepezil Study Group. *Arch Intern Med* 1998; 158:1021–1031.

36. Rogers SL, et al. A 24-week, double-blind, placebo-controlled trial of donepezil in patients with Alzheimer's disease. Donepezil Study Group. *Neurology* 1998; 50:136–145.

37. Corey-Bloom J, et al. A randomized trial evaluating the efficacy and safety of ENA 713 (rivastigmine tartrate), a new acetylcholinesterase inhibitor, in patients with mild to moderately severe Alzheimer's disease. *International Journal of Geriatric Psychopharmacology* 1998; 1:55–64.

38. Rosler M, et al. Efficacy and safety of rivastigmine in patients with Alzheimer's disease: international randomised controlled trial. *BMJ* 1999; 318:633–638.

39. Tariot PN, et al. A 5-month, randomized, placebo-controlled trial of galantamine in AD. The Galantamine USA-10 Study Group. *Neurology* 2000; 54:2269–2276.

40. Raskind MA, et al. Galantamine in AD: A 6-month randomized, placebo-controlled trial with a 6-month extension. The Galantamine USA-1 Study Group. *Neurology* 2000; 54:2261–2268.

41. Wilcock GK, et al. Efficacy and safety of galantamine in patients with mild to moderate Alzheimer's disease: multicentre randomised controlled trial. Galantamine International-1 Study Group. *BMJ* 2000; 321:1445–1449.

42. Pariente A, et al. Factors associated with serious adverse reactions to cholinesterase inhibitors: a study of spontaneous reporting. *CNS Drugs* 2010; 24:55–63.

43. Sadowsky CH, et al. Safety and tolerability of rivastigmine transdermal patch compared with rivastigmine capsules in patients switched from donepezil: data from three clinical trials. *Int J Clin Pract* 2010; 64:188–193.

44. Sadowsky C, et al. Switching from oral cholinesterase inhibitors to the rivastigmine transdermal patch. *CNS Neurosci Ther* 2010; 16:51–60.

45. Cummings J, et al. Randomized, double-blind, parallel-group, 48-week study for efficacy and safety of a higher-dose rivastigmine patch (15 vs. 10 cm(2)) in Alzheimer's disease. *Dement Geriatr Cogn Disord* 2012; 33:341–353.

46. National Institute for Health and Care Excellence. British National Formulary (BNF). 2020; https://bnf.nice.org.uk.

47. Parsons CG, et al. Memantine is a clinically well tolerated N-methyl-D-aspartate (NMDA) receptor antagonist–a review of preclinical data. *Neuropharmacology* 1999; 38:735–767.

48. Reisberg B, et al. Memantine in moderate-to-severe Alzheimer's disease. *N Engl J Med* 2003; 348:1333–1341.

49. Jones RW. A review comparing the safety and tolerability of memantine with the acetylcholinesterase inhibitors. *Int J Geriatr Psychiatry* 2010; 25:547–553.

50. Dunn NR, et al. Adverse effects associated with the use of donepezil in general practice in England. *J Psychopharmacol* 2000; 14:406–408.

51. Hashimoto M, et al. Urinary incontinence: an unrecognised adverse effect with donepezil. *Lancet* 2000; 356:568.

52. Kroger E, et al. Adverse drug reactions reported with cholinesterase inhibitors: an analysis of 16 years of individual case safety reports from VigiBase. *Ann Pharmacother* 2015; 49:1197–1206.

53. NHS Yorkshire and Humber Clinical Networks. The assessment of cardiac status before prescribing acetyl cholinesterase inhibitors for dementia. Version 1. 2016; http://www.yhscn.nhs.uk/media/PDFs/mhdn/Dementia/ECG%20Documents/ACHEIGuidance%20V1_Final.pdf.

54. Rowland JP, et al. Cardiovascular monitoring with acetylcholinesterase inhibitors: a clinical protocol. *Adv Psychiatr Treatment* 2007; 13:178–184.

55. FDA Alert for Healthcare Professionals. Galantamine hydrobromide (marketed as Razadyne, formerly Reminyl). 2005; https://www.fda.gov/Drugs/DrugSafety/ucm109350.htm.

56. Malone DM, et al. Cholinesterase inhibitors and cardiovascular disease: a survey of old age psychiatrists' practice. *Age Ageing* 2007; 36:331–333.

57. Park-Wyllie LY, et al. Cholinesterase inhibitors and hospitalization for bradycardia: a population-based study. *PLoS Med* 2009; 6:e1000157.

58. Rosenbloom MH, et al. Donepezil-associated bradyarrhythmia in a patient with dementia with Lewy bodies (DLB). *Alzheimer Dis Assoc Disord* 2010; 24:209–211.

59. Gill SS, et al. Syncope and its consequences in patients with dementia receiving cholinesterase inhibitors: a population-based cohort study. *Arch Intern Med* 2009; 169:867–873.

CHAPTER 6

60. Isik AT, et al. Which cholinesterase inhibitor is the safest for the heart in elderly patients with Alzheimer's disease? *Am J Alzheimers Dis Other Demen* 2012; **27**:171–174.

61. Fosbol EL, et al. Comparative cardiovascular safety of dementia medications: a cross-national study. *J Am Geriatr Soc* 2012; **60**:2283–2289.

62. Nordstrom P, et al. The use of cholinesterase inhibitors and the risk of myocardial infarction and death: a nationwide cohort study in subjects with Alzheimer's disease. *Eur Heart J* 2013; **34**:2585–2591.

63. Howes LG. Cardiovascular effects of drugs used to treat Alzheimer's disease. *Drug Saf* 2014; **37**:391–395.

64. Farlow MR, et al. Memantine for the treatment of Alzheimer's disease: tolerability and safety data from clinical trials. *Drug Saf* 2008; **31**:577–585.

65. Babai S, et al. Comparison of adverse drug reactions with donepezil versus memantine: analysis of the French Pharmacovigilance Database. *Therapie* 2010; **65**:255–259.

66. Dooley M, et al. Donepezil: a review of its use in Alzheimer's disease. *Drugs Aging* 2000; **16**:199–226.

67. Scott LJ, et al. Galantamine: a review of its use in Alzheimer's disease. *Drugs* 2000; **60**:1095–1122.

68. Grossberg GT, et al. Lack of adverse pharmacodynamic drug interactions with rivastigmine and twenty-two classes of medications. *Int J Geriatr Psychiatry* 2000; **15**:242–247.

69. Tavassoli N, et al. Drug interactions with cholinesterase inhibitors: an analysis of the French pharmacovigilance database and a comparison of two national drug formularies (Vidal, British National Formulary). *Drug Saf* 2007; **30**:1063–1071.

70. Noetzli M, et al. Pharmacodynamic, pharmacokinetic and pharmacogenetic aspects of drugs used in the treatment of Alzheimer's disease. *Clin Pharmacokinet* 2013; **52**:225–241.

71. Pasqualetti G, et al. Potential drug-drug interactions in Alzheimer patients with behavioral symptoms. *Clin Interv Aging* 2015; **10**:1457–1466.

72. Howard R, et al. Donepezil and memantine for moderate-to-severe Alzheimer's disease. *N Engl J Med* 2012; **366**:893–903.

73. Howard R, et al. Nursing home placement in the Donepezil and Memantine in Moderate to Severe Alzheimer's Disease (DOMINO-AD) trial: secondary and post-hoc analyses. *Lancet Neurol* 2015; **14**:1171–1181.

74. Medicines Complete. Stockley's drug interactions. 2020; https://www.medicinescomplete.com.

75. Truven Health Analytics. Micromedex 2.0. 2017; https://www.micromedexsolutions.com/home/dispatch.

76. Di Santo SG, et al. A meta-analysis of the efficacy of donepezil, rivastigmine, galantamine, and memantine in relation to severity of Alzheimer's disease. *J Alzheimers Dis* 2013; **35**:349–361.

77. Parsons C. Withdrawal of antidementia drugs in older people: who, when and how? *Drugs Aging* 2016; **33**:545–556.

78. National Institute for Health and Clinical Excellence. Dementia: assessment, management and support for people living with dementia and their carers. NICE Guideline [NG97]. 2018; https://www.nice.org.uk/guidance/ng97.

79. National Institute for Health and Clinical Excellence. Donepezil, galantamine, rivastigmine and memantine for the treatment of Alzheimer's disease. Technology Appraisal Guidance TA217. 2011 (last updated June 2018); https://www.nice.org.uk/Guidance/TA217.

80. National Institute for Health and Clinical Excellence. Medicines optimisation: the safe and effective use of medicines to enable the best possible outcomes. National Guidance [NG5]. 2015 (last checked March 2019); https://www.nice.org.uk/guidance/ng5.

81. Birks J, et al. Ginkgo biloba for cognitive impairment and dementia. *Cochrane Database Syst Rev* 2009; CD003120.

82. Yuan Q, et al. Effects of Ginkgo biloba on dementia: an overview of systematic reviews. *J Ethnopharmacol* 2017; **195**:1–9.

83. Bent S, et al. Spontaneous bleeding associated with ginkgo biloba: a case report and systematic review of the literature: a case report and systematic review of the literature. *J Gen Intern Med* 2005; **20**:657–661.

84. Farina N, et al. Vitamin E for Alzheimer's dementia and mild cognitive impairment. *Cochrane Database Syst Rev* 2017; **1**:Cd002854.

85. Dysken MW, et al. Effect of vitamin E and memantine on functional decline in Alzheimer disease: the TEAM-AD VA cooperative randomized trial. *JAMA* 2014; **311**:33–44.

86. Joe E, et al. Cognitive symptoms of Alzheimer's disease: clinical management and prevention. *BMJ* 2019; **367**:l6217.

87. Malouf R, et al. Folic acid with or without vitamin B12 for the prevention and treatment of healthy elderly and demented people. *Cochrane Database Syst Rev* 2008; CD004514.

88. Enderami A, et al. The effects and potential mechanisms of folic acid on cognitive function: a comprehensive review. *Neurol Sci* 2018; **39**:1667–1675.

89. Zhang DM, et al. Efficacy of Vitamin B supplementation on cognition in elderly patients with cognitive-related diseases. *J Geriatr Psychiatry Neurol* 2017; **30**:50–59.

90. Burckhardt M, et al. Omega-3 fatty acids for the treatment of dementia. *Cochrane Database Syst Rev* 2016; **4**:Cd009002.

91. Lee ST, et al. Panax ginseng enhances cognitive performance in Alzheimer disease. *Alzheimer Dis Assoc Disord* 2008; **22**:222–226.

92. Wang Y, et al. Ginseng for Alzheimer's disease: a systematic review and meta-analysis of randomized controlled trials. *Curr Top Med Chem* 2016; **16**:529–536.

93. Doody RS, et al. Effect of dimebon on cognition, activities of daily living, behaviour, and global function in patients with mild-to-moderate Alzheimer's disease: a randomised, double-blind, placebo-controlled study. *Lancet* 2008; **372**:207–215.

94. Chau S, et al. Latrepirdine for Alzheimer's disease (Dimebon). *Cochrane Database Syst Rev* 2015; Cd009524.

95. Li DQ, et al. Donepezil combined with natural hirudin improves the clinical symptoms of patients with mild-to-moderate Alzheimer's disease: a 20-week open-label pilot study. *Int J Med Sci* 2012; **9**:248–255.

96. Wang BS, et al. Efficacy and safety of natural acetylcholinesterase inhibitor huperzine A in the treatment of Alzheimer's disease: an updated meta-analysis. *J Neural Transm* 2009; **116**:457–465.

97. Yang G, et al. Huperzine A for Alzheimer's disease: a systematic review and meta-analysis of randomized clinical trials. *PLoS One* 2013; 8:e74916.

98. Hao Z, et al. Huperzine A for vascular dementia. *Cochrane Database Syst Rev* 2009; CD007365.

99. Yue J, et al. Huperzine A for mild cognitive impairment. *Cochrane Database Syst Rev* 2012; 12:CD008827.

100. Cui CC, et al. The effect of anti-dementia drugs on Alzheimer disease-induced cognitive impairment: a network meta-analysis. *Medicine (Baltimore)* 2019; 98:e16091.

101. Ayati Z, et al. Saffron for mild cognitive impairment and dementia: a systematic review and meta-analysis of randomised clinical trials. *BMC Complement Med Ther* 2020; 20:333.

102. Gavrilova SI, et al. Cerebrolysin in the therapy of mild cognitive impairment and dementia due to Alzheimer's disease: 30 years of clinical use. *Med Res Rev* 2020. [Epub ahead of print].

103. Cui S, et al. Cerebrolysin for vascular dementia. *Cochrane Database Syst Rev* 2019; CD008900

104. McGuinness B, et al. Cochrane review on 'Statins for the treatment of dementia'. *Int J Geriatr Psychiatry* 2013; 28:119–126.

105. McGuinness B, et al. Statins for the prevention of dementia. *Cochrane Database Syst Rev* 2016; Cd003160.

106. Chu CS, et al. Use of statins and the risk of dementia and mild cognitive impairment: A systematic review and meta-analysis. *Sci Rep* 2018; 8:5804.

107. Poly TN, et al. Association between use of statin and risk of dementia: a meta-analysis of observational studies. *Neuroepidemiology* 2020; 54:214–226.

108. Moreira A, et al. Chocolate consumption is associated with a lower risk of cognitive decline. *J Alzheimers Dis* 2016; 53:85–93.

109. Galimberti D, et al. Idalopirdine as a treatment for Alzheimer's disease. *Exp Opinion Invest Drugs* 2015; 24:981–987.

110. Matsunaga S, et al. Efficacy and safety of idalopirdine for Alzheimer's disease: a systematic review and meta-analysis. *Int Psychogeriatr* 2019; 31:1627–1633.

111. Jordan F, et al. Aspirin and other non-steroidal anti-inflammatory drugs for the prevention of dementia. *Cochrane Database Syst Rev* 2020; 4:Cd011459.

112. La AL, et al. Long-term trazodone use and cognition: a potential therapeutic role for slow-wave sleep enhancers. *J Alzheimers Dis* 2019; 67:911–921.

113. Halliday M, et al. Repurposed drugs targeting eIF2alpha-P-mediated translational repression prevent neurodegeneration in mice. *Brain* 2017; 140:1768–1783.

114. Coupland C, et al. Antidepressant use and risk of adverse outcomes in older people: population based cohort study. *BMJ* 2011; 343:d4551.

115. Doody RS, et al. A phase 3 trial of semagacestat for treatment of Alzheimer's disease. *N Engl J Med* 2013; 369:341–350.

116. Briggs R, et al. Drug treatments in Alzheimer's disease. *Clin Med (Lond)* 2016; 16:247–253.

117. Doody RS, et al. Phase 3 trials of solanezumab for mild-to-moderate Alzheimer's disease. *N Engl J Med* 2014; 370:311–321.

118. Honig LS, et al. Trial of solanezumab for mild dementia due to Alzheimer's disease. *N Engl J Med* 2018; 378:321–330.

119. Salloway S, et al. Two phase 3 trials of bapineuzumab in mild-to-moderate Alzheimer's disease. *N Engl J Med* 2014; 370:322–333.

120. Abushouk AI, et al. Bapineuzumab for mild to moderate Alzheimer's disease: a meta-analysis of randomized controlled trials. *BMC Neurol* 2017; 17:66.

121. Schneider L. A resurrection of aducanumab for Alzheimer's disease. *Lancet Neurol* 2020; 19:111–112.

122. Vaz M, et al. Alzheimer's disease: recent treatment strategies. *Eur J Pharmacol* 2020; 887:173554.

123. Kavirajan H, et al. Efficacy and adverse effects of cholinesterase inhibitors and memantine in vascular dementia: a meta-analysis of randomised controlled trials. *Lancet Neurol* 2007; 6:782–792.

124. Wang J, et al. Cholinergic deficiency involved in vascular dementia: possible mechanism and strategy of treatment. *Acta Pharmacol Sin* 2009; 30:879–888.

125. Bocti C, et al. Management of dementia with a cerebrovascular component. *Alzheimer's Dementia* 2007; 3:398–403.

126. Demaerschalk BM, et al. Treatment of vascular dementia and vascular cognitive impairment. *Neurologist* 2007; 13:37–41.

127. Baskys A, et al. Pharmacological prevention and treatment of vascular dementia: approaches and perspectives. *Exp Gerontol* 2012; 47:887–891.

128. Malouf R, et al. Donepezil for vascular cognitive impairment. *Cochrane Database Syst Rev* 2004; CD004395.

129. Birks J. Cholinesterase inhibitors for Alzheimer's disease. *Cochrane Database Syst Rev* 2006; CD005593.

130. Craig D, et al. Galantamine for vascular cognitive impairment. *Cochrane Database Syst Rev* 2006; CD004746.

131. Birks J, et al. Rivastigmine for vascular cognitive impairment. *Cochrane Database Syst Rev* 2013; 5:CD004744.

132. Jin BR, et al. Comparative efficacy and safety of cognitive enhancers for treating vascular cognitive impairment: systematic review and Bayesian network meta-analysis. *Neural Regen Res* 2019; 14:805–816.

133. Wild R, et al. Cholinesterase inhibitors for dementia with Lewy bodies. *Cochrane Database Syst Rev* 2003; CD003672.

134. McKeith IG, et al. Diagnosis and management of dementia with Lewy bodies: fourth consensus report of the DLB consortium. *Neurology* 2017; 89:88–100.

135. Taylor JP, et al. New evidence on the management of Lewy body dementia. *Lancet Neurol* 2020; 19:157–169.

136. Newcastle University. Management of Lewy body dementia summary sheet Diamond Lewy. 2019; https://research.ncl.ac.uk/media/sites/researchwebsites/diamond-lewy/One%20page%20symptom%20LBD%20management%20summaries.pdf.

137. Russ TC, et al. Cholinesterase inhibitors for mild cognitive impairment. *Cochrane Database Syst Rev* 2012; 9:CD009132.

138. Cooper C, et al. Treatment for mild cognitive impairment: systematic review. *Br J Psychiatry* 2013; 203:255–264.

CHAPTER 6

139. Matsunaga S, et al. Efficacy and safety of cholinesterase inhibitors for mild cognitive impairment: asystematic review and meta-analysis. *J Alzheimers Dis* 2019; 71:513–523.

140. Kasper S, et al. Management of mild cognitive impairment (MCI): the need for national and international guidelines. *World J Biol Psychiatry* 2020; 21:579–594.

141. Nardell M, et al. Pharmacological treatments for frontotemporal dementias: a systematic review of randomized controlled trials. *Am J Alzheimers Dis Other Demen* 2014; 29:123–132.

142. Li Y, et al. Cholinesterase inhibitors for rarer dementias associated with neurological conditions. *Cochrane Database Syst Rev* 2015; Cd009444.

Safer prescribing for physical conditions in dementia

People with dementia are more susceptible to cognitive side effects of drugs. Drugs may affect cognition through their action on cholinergic, histaminergic or opioid neuro-transmitter pathways or through more complex actions. Medications prescribed for physical disorders may also interact with cognitive-enhancing medication.

Anticholinergic drugs

Anticholinergic drugs reduce the efficacy of AChE-Is[1] and also cause sedation, cognitive impairment, delirium and falls.[2] These effects are more severe in older patients with dementia.[3] Table 6.4 summarises the Anticholinergic Effect on Cognition (AEC) of drugs commonly prescribed for older adults in the UK.[4] Combining several drugs with anticholinergic activity increases the anticholinergic burden for an individual. Studies have shown that a high anticholinergic burden total score was associated with a greater decline in MMSE score[5] and a higher mortality.[5,6]

It is good practice to keep the anticholinergic burden to a minimum (preferably zero) in older people, especially if they have cognitive impairment.

Where possible, drugs with no anticholinergic action and an equivalent therapeutic effect should be used. If this is not possible, the prescription of a drug with low anticholinergic activity or high specificity to the site of action (and thus minimal central activity) should be encouraged. Anticholinergic drugs that do not cross the blood–brain barrier (BBB) have less profound effects on cognitive function.[7] The AEC scale takes all of these factors into account.

The following are recommendations for using the AEC scores:[4]

- All individual drugs with an AEC score of 2 or 3 in older people presenting with symptoms of cognitive impairment, dementia or delirium should either be:
  - stopped, or
  - switched to an alternative drug with a lower AEC score (preferably 0).
- In patients who are not receiving any individual drug with AEC score of 2 or 3 but have a *total* AEC score of 3 or above 3, a similar patient–clinician review should take place.
- If withdrawal of drug is deemed appropriate, this should be gradual (where possible) to avoid rebound (nausea, sweating, urinary frequency, diarrhoea).

Safety of physical health medication prescribed in dementia

Anticholinergic drugs used in urinary incontinence

Oxybutynin easily penetrates the CNS and has consistently been associated with dete-rioration in cognitive function. Although studies of **tolterodine** found no adverse CNS effects,[8] case reports have described adverse effects, including memory loss, hallucina-tions and delirium.[9–11] In contrast, **darifenacin**, an M_3-selective receptor antagonist, has been investigated in healthy older people for its effects on cognitive function and had no effects on cognitive tests compared with placebo,[12,13] although studies in dementia are lacking. **Solifenacin** may cause impairment of working memory[14] although it was investigated in stroke patients and was found not to affect their short-term cognitive performance.[15] While some cases of CNS adverse effects have been reported with

Table 6.4 Anticholinergic effect on cognition (AEC) scores[a] (updated October 2020)

Adcal – 0	Clarithromycin – NK	Gabapentin – 0	Naproxen – 0	Sitagliptin – 0
Alendronic acid (Alendronate) – 0	Clemastine – 3	Galantamine – 0	Nifedipine – 0	Solifenacin – 1
Alfuzosin – 0	Clomipramine – 3	Gaviscon – 0	Nimodipine – 0	Sotalol – 0
Alimemazine (trimeprazine) – 3	Clonazepam – NK	Gliclazide – 0	Nitrofurantoin – NK	Spironolactone – NK
Allopurinol – NK	Clonidine – NK	Granisetron – 0	Nortriptyline – 3	Sulphasalazine – 0
Alprazolam – 0	Clopidogrel – 0	Haloperidol – 0	Olanzapine – 2	Sulpiride – 0
Alverine – 0	Clozapine – 3	Heparin – 0	Omeprazole – 0	Tamoxifen – NK
Amantadine – 2	Co-beneldopa – 0	Hydrochlorothiazide – 0	Ondansetron – 0	Tamsulosin – 0
Amiloride – 0	Co-careldopa – 0	Hydrocodone – NK	Orlistat – 0	Temazepam – 1
Aminophylline – 0	Codeine – NK	Hydrocortisone – NK	Orphenadrine – 3	Tetracycline – 0
Amiodarone – 1	Colchicine – NK	Hydroxyzine – 1	Oxcarbazepine – NK	Theophylline – 0
Amisulpride – 0	Co-tenidone – 0	Hyoscine hydrobromide – 3	Oxybutynin – 3	Thiamine – 0
Amitriptyline – 3	Cyclizine – 1	Hysoscine butylbromide (buscopan) – 1	Oxycodone – NK	Tiotropium bromide (inhalation) – 0
Amlodipine – 0	Cyproheptadine – 3	Ibuprofen – 0	Paliperidone – 1	Tizanidine – NK
Amoxicillin – 0	Dabigatran – NK	Iloperidone – 1	Pantoprazole – 0	Tolcapone – 0
Anastrozole – NK	Darifenacin – 0	Imipramine – 3	Paracetamol – 0	Tolterodine – 2
Apixaban – NK	Desipramine – 2	Indapamide – 0	Paroxetine – 2	Topiramate – NK
Apomorphine – 0	Dexamethasone – NK	Insulin – 0	Penicillin – 0	Tramadol – 0
Aripiprazole – 1	Dexamfetamine (dexamphetamine) – 0	Ipratropium bromide – 0	Peppermint oil – 0	Trazodone – 0

Aspirin – 0	Dextropropoxyphene – NK	Irbesartan – NK	Pergolide – 0	Trifluoperazine – 2
Atenolol – 0	Diazepam – 1	Isocarboxazid – 1	Perindopril – 0	Trihexyphenidyl (benzhexol) – 3
Atomoxetine – 0	Diclofenac – 0	Isosorbide dinitrate – 0	Perphenazine – 1	Trimethoprim – 0
Atorvastatin – 0	Dicycloverine (dicyclomine) – 2	Isosorbide mononitrate – 0	Pethidine – 2	Trimipramine – 3
Atropine – 3	Digoxin – NK	Ketorolac – 0	Phenelzine – 1	Trospium – 0
Atropine eye drops – 1	Dihydrocodeine – NK	Labetalol – 0	Phenytoin – NK	Valproate – 0
Azathioprine – 0	Diltiazem – 0	Lactulose – 0	Pimozide – 2	Venlafaxine – 0
Baclofen – NK	Dimenhydrinate – 2	Lamotrigine – 0	Pirenzepine – 1	Verapamil – NK
Beclometasone dipropionate (inhaler) – 0	Diphenhydramine – 2	Lansoprazole – NK	Pravastatin – 0	Vitamin B12 – 0
Bendroflumethiazide – 0	Dipyridamole – 0	Lercanidipine – 0	Prazosin – 0	Vitamins – 0
Benzatropine – 3	Disopyramide – 2	Levetiracetam – NK	Prednisolone – 1	Vortioxetine – 0
Betahistine – 0	Docusate sodium – 0	Levodopa – 0	Pregabalin – NK	Warfarin – 0
Bezafibrate – 0	Domperidone – 1	Levomepromazine (methotrimeprazine) – 2	Prochlorperazine – 2	Ziprasidone – 0
Bisacodyl – 0	Donepezil – 0	Levothyroxine (Thyroxine) – 0	Procyclidine – 3	Zolpidem – 0
Bisoprolol – NK	Dothiepin (Dosulepin) – 3	Liraglutide – 0	Promazine – 2	Zopiclone – NK
Bromocriptine – 1	Doxazosin – 0	Lisinopril – 0	Promethazine – 3	Zotepine – 2
Budesonide (inhaler) – 0	Doxepin – 3	Lithium – 1	Propantheline – 2	Zuclopentixol (zuclopenthixol) – 1
Bumetanide – NK	Doxycycline – 0	Lofepramine – 3	Propranolol – 0	
Buprenorphine – 0	Dulaglutide – 0	Loperamide – 0	Quetiapine – 2	
Bupropion – 0	Duloxetine – 0	Loratadine – 0	Quinidine – 1	
Buspirone – 1	Enalapril – 0	Lorazepam – 0	Quinine – 1	
Cabergoline – 0	Enoxaparin – 0	Losartan – 0	Rabeprazole – 0	

(Continued)

Table 6.4 (*Continued*)

Calcium – 0	Entacapone – 0	Lovastatin – 0	Ramipril – NK
Calcium and Vitamin D – 0	Erythromycin – NK	Lurasidone – 0	Ranitidine – 0
Candersartan – 0	Exanatide – 0	Macrogol – 0	Rasagiline – 0
Captopril – NK	Ezetimibe – 0	Magnesium – 0	Reboxetine – 0
Carbachol – 0	Felodipine – 0	Mebeverine – 0	Risedronate – 0
Carbamazepine – 1	Fentanyl – 1	Melatonin – 0	Risperidone – 0
Carbimazole – NK	Ferrous sulphate – 0	Meloxicam – 0	Rivaroxaban – NK
Carbocisteine – 0	Fesoterodine – 0	Memantine – 0	Rivastigmine – 0
Carvedilol – NK	Fexofenadine – 0	Mesalazine – 0	Ropinirole – 0
Cefalexin (Cephalexin) – 0	Finasteride – 0	Metformin – NK	Rosiglitazone – 0
Cetirizine – 0	Flavoxate* – NK	Methocarbamol – NK	Rosuvastatin – NK
Chloral hydrate – NK	Flecainide – 0	Methotrexate – NK	**Salbutamol** – 0
Chlordiazepoxide – 0	Flucloxacillin – 0	Metoclopramide – 0	
Chlorphenamine – 2	Fludrocortisone – NK	Metoprolol – 0	Salmeterol (inhaler) – 0
Chlorpromazine – 3	Fluoxetine – 1	Midazolam – 1	Selegiline – 0
Chlortalidone – NK	Flupentixol (flupenthixol) – 1	Minocycline – 0	Senna – 0
Cimetidine – 0	Fluphenazine – 1	Mirabegron – 0	Sertindole – 1
Cinnarizine – 1	Fluvoxamine – 0	Mirtazapine – 1	Sertraline – 1
Ciprofloxacin – 0	Folic acid – 0	Moclobemide – 0	Sildenafil – 0
Citalopram – 1	Furosemide – 0	Morphine – 0	Simvastatin – 0

The AEC scale is available as a regularly updated web-based app. Please visit www.medichec.com. This site has recently been updated to include the identification of medications that are reported to cause dizziness and drowsiness since these adverse effects can add to cognitive impairment and confusion in older people and can increase the risk of falls.

trospium,[16] studies found no significant change in cognitive function.[17,18] Studies investigating whether or not **fesoterodine** causes cognitive impairment found no detectable impairment of cognition in a variety of cognitive measurements (Table 6.5).[19,20]

All tertiary amine drugs, i.e. oxybutynin, tolterodine, solifenacin, fesoterodine and darifenacin, are metabolised by cytochrome P450 (CYP450) enzymes. Increasing age or co-administration of drugs that inhibit these enzymes (e.g. erythromycin and fluoxetine) can lead to higher serum levels and therefore increased adverse effects. The metabolism of **trospium** is unknown, although metabolism via CYP450 system does not occur, meaning that pharmacokinetic drug interactions are unlikely with this drug.[8]

Alpha-blockers for urinary retention

Alpha-blockers such as **tamsulosin, alfuzosin** and **prazosin** cause drowsiness, dizziness and depression.[21] There is no published literature reporting their effects on cognition, but alpha-blockers do not feature on any anticholinergic cognitive burden list.

Drugs used in GI disorders

Loperamide
Although loperamide may have some anticholinergic activity, there are no data to suggest that it can worsen cognitive function in patients with dementia. It may add to the anticholinergic cognitive burden if used in conjunction with other anticholinergic drugs.

Laxatives
There is no evidence to suggest that laxatives have any negative impact on cognitive function. In fact, since constipation can lead to delirium and BPSD, treating it may improve these symptoms.

Antiemetics
Cyclizine is a first-generation histamine antagonist and can impair cognitive and psychomotor performance (see antihistamines section).[22]

Metoclopramide has little anticholinergic action, but the D_2 receptor antagonism of both metoclopramide and prochlorperazine can produce movement disorders and so these drugs must be used with caution in people with dementia.

Domperidone is a dopamine D_2 receptor antagonist that does not usually cross the BBB. However, since BBB alterations can occur in dementia, CNS penetration of domperidone and resulting adverse effects can occur.[23] Recent reports have highlighted a small increased risk of serious cardiac adverse effects with domperidone, especially in older people. The maximum dose has been reduced to 30mg/day and the maximum treatment duration should not exceed 1 week. Domperidone is now contraindicated in those with underlying cardiac conditions or severe hepatic impairment and in patients receiving other medications known to prolong QT interval or potent CYP3A4 inhibitors.[24]

Serotonin 5-HT$_3$ receptor antagonists, used for treating chemotherapy-induced nausea and vomiting, do not have adverse effects on cognition, and they may have some

Table 6.5 Physicochemical properties of anticholinergic drugs in urinary incontinence[14,25] (adapted with permission[26])

Drug	Muscarinic receptor (M3:M1 affinity ratio)	Polarity	Lipophilicity	Molecular weight (kDa)	P-gp substrate	Theoretical ability to cross BBB	Effect on cognition
Darifenacin	Mainly M_3 (9.3:1)	Neutral	High	507.5 (relatively large)	Yes	High (but bladder selective and P-gp substrate)	–
Fesoterodine	Non-selective	Neutral	Very low	411.6	Yes	Very low	–
Oxybutynin	Non-selective	Neutral	Moderate	357 (relatively small)	No	Moderate/high	+++
Solifenacin	Mainly M_3 (2.5:1)	Neutral	Moderate	480.6	No	Moderate	–/+
Tolterodine	Non-selective	Neutral	Low	475.6	No	Low	+
Trospium chloride	Non-selective	Positively charged	Not lipophilic	428	Yes	Almost none	–

– represents no reports of adverse effects on cognition.
+ represents some adverse effects on cognition reported.
+++ represents consistent reports of adverse effects on cognition.

cognitive-enhancing action.[27] These drugs carry cardiovascular warnings and should be used cautiously in patients with cardiac co-morbidities or taking concomitant arrhythmogenic drugs or drugs known to prolong QT interval. **Granisetron** can be administered once daily, which is preferable in elderly patients with memory problems or swallowing difficulties. Granisetron is metabolised exclusively via a single CYP family (CYP3A4), and thus has a lower propensity for drug interactions.[28] All 5HT$_3$ antagonists cause constipation.

Antispasmodics

Hyoscine hydrobromide (scopolamine) is a centrally acting anticholinergic which is lipophilic and penetrates the BBB easily. It impairs memory, speed of processing and attention. Older patients suffer these symptoms at lower doses and are more vulnerable to confusion and hallucinations.[29] People with AD have experienced clinically significant cognitive impairment at lower doses compared with healthy, age-matched controls.[3] The effect that hyoscine has on cognition is so significant that it is used in trials to produce memory deficits similar to those seen in dementia (the scopolamine challenge test).[30] There is rarely a good reason to use this drug in people with dementia.

Hyoscine butylbromide (Buscopan) exerts topical spasmolytic action on the smooth muscle of the GI tract. Hyoscine butylbromide is not thought to enter the CNS, so central anticholinergic adverse effects are extremely rare.[31]

Alverine, mebeverine and **peppermint oil** are relaxants of intestinal smooth muscle and do not have an effect on cognition.

Bronchodilators

Beta-agonists

In patients with coexisting Parkinson's disease or essential tremor, tremor induced by beta-agonists may result in misdiagnosis and over-treatment of Parkinson's disease.[32] Tremor is a common adverse effect of cholinesterase inhibitors, so caution should be exercised when used with beta-agonists.

Anticholinergic bronchodilators

Inhaled anticholinergic drugs have few systemic side effects compared with oral medication.[32] A randomised, double-blind placebo-controlled comparison of ipratropium and theophylline treatment was unable to detect a negative effect with either drug on the psychometric test performance of older patients. This suggests that treatment with inhaled ipratropium is not associated with significant cognitive impairment in older people.[33]

Theophylline

As with cholinesterase inhibitors, nausea and vomiting are common adverse effects of theophylline. Neurological effects such as headaches, anxiety, behavioural disturbances, depression and seizures can occur in 50% of patients on theophylline. Although seizures are rare, they are much more likely in older people. Theophylline does not cause significant cognitive impairment.[33]

CHAPTER 6

Hypersalivation

Oral anticholinergic agents used for hypersalivation (e.g. hyoscine hydrobromide) should be avoided in the elderly because of the risk of cognitive impairment, delirium and constipation (see section on anticholinergic and antispasmodic drugs). Pirenzepine is a relatively selective M_1 and M_4 muscarinic receptor antagonist which is not thought to cross the BBB and therefore has little CNS penetration.[34]

Atropine solution given sublingually or used as a mouthwash is sometimes used to manage hypersalivation. There are no data available on the extent of penetration through the BBB when atropine is administered by this route.

Myasthenia gravis (MG)

Unlike AChE-Is used in AD (donepezil, rivastigmine and galantamine), those used in myasthenia gravis (**pyridostigmine** and **neostigmine**) act peripherally and do not cross the BBB (so as to minimise unwanted central effects).[35] It is possible that combining peripheral and central AChE-Is may add to the cholinomimetic adverse effect burden (e.g. nausea, vomiting diarrhoea, abdominal cramps and increased salivation). Memantine may be an alternative to cholinesterase inhibitors in cases where the combined cholinomimetic effects of drugs used for MG and AD are not tolerated.

Analgesics

NSAIDs and paracetamol

Paracetamol (acetaminophen) is a safe drug and there is no evidence that it causes cognitive impairment other than in overdose when it may cause delirium.[36] There is some evidence that chronic use of aspirin can cause confusional states.[37] Case reports implicate NSAIDs in causing delirium and psychosis,[38] although clinical trials have not demonstrated significant adverse effects on cognition with naproxen[39] or indomethacin.[40] NSAIDs are difficult to use in older people due to their cardiovascular risk and risk of GI bleeding.[41] It is good practice to prescribe gastroprotection with these drugs or consider using topical NSAIDs (if clinically appropriate), to reduce the risk of GI bleeding.

Opiates

Sedation is a potential problem with all opiates.[42] Delirium induced by opioids may be associated with agitation, hallucinations or delusions.[42] **Pethidine** is associated with a high risk of cognitive impairment, as its metabolites have anti-cholinergic properties and accumulate rapidly if renal function is impaired.[43] **Codeine** may increase the risk of falls, and both tramadol and codeine have a high risk of drug–drug interactions, as well as considerable variation in response and adverse effects.[44] **Fentanyl patches,** useful as they can be, should not be used to initiate opioid analgesia in frail older people[45] because of their long duration of action even after the patch is removed, making the treatment of side effects more difficult.[44] **Morphine** is a very effective analgesic but is likely to cause cognitive problems and other adverse effects in older patients.[46] **Oxycodone** has a short half-life, few drug–drug interactions and more predictable dose–response relationships than other opiates. It is therefore, theoretically at least, a good candidate for oral analgesia in dementia.[44] Caution, however, should be used in addictive behaviours due to considerable problems with addiction and misuse. **Buprenorphine** transdermal patches probably have fewer side effects than many other opiates.

Antihistamines

First-generation H_1 antihistamines include **chlorpheniramine, hydroxyzine, cyclizine** and **promethazine.** They are non-selective, have anticholinergic activity and readily penetrate the BBB, which can lead to unwanted cognitive side effects. They can impair cognitive and psychomotor performance and can trigger seizures, dyskinesia, dystonia and hallucinations. The second-generation H_1 antihistamines (such as **loratadine, cetirizine** and **fexofenadine**) penetrate poorly into the CNS and are considerably less likely to cause these adverse effects. Moreover, they lack any anticholinergic effects.[22]

Statins

A Cochrane review assessed the clinical efficacy and tolerability of statins in the treatment of dementia[47] and showed that there was no significant benefit from statins in terms of cognitive function, but equally no evidence that statins were detrimental to cognition. Earlier case reports had highlighted subjective complaints of memory loss associated with the use of statins.[48] These tended to occur within 2 months of starting the drug and were most commonly associated with simvastatin. In the event of a patient experiencing cognitive problems on simvastatin, it may be worth first stopping the drug, and if the complaint resolves, try atorvastatin or pravastatin instead, as these drugs are less likely to cross the BBB. A more recent Cochrane review[49] assessed the efficacy of statins in the prevention of dementia and concluded that there was no evidence that statins given in late life to people at risk of vascular disease prevented cognitive decline or dementia.

Antihypertensives

Mid-life hypertension has negative effects on cognition and increases the risk of a person developing dementia.[50] There is no evidence that antihypertensive treatment worsens cognition. It appears to have a positive effect on global cognition, and long-term treatment of hypertension can reduce the risk of dementia.[51,52]

Other cardiac drugs

Digoxin has been associated with acute confusional states at therapeutic drug concentrations.[53] It has also been reported to cause nightmares.[54] However, one study showed that the treatment of cardiac failure with digoxin improved cognitive performance in 25% of the patients treated (and in 23% of the patients treated who did not have cardiac failure).[55] There are some case reports of amiodarone being associated with delirium.[56,57]

H_2 antagonists and proton pump inhibitors (PPIs)

Histamine-2 receptor antagonists (e.g. cimetidine, ranitidine and famotidine) are rarely used nowadays. Cimetidine causes several pharmacokinetic interactions, and ranitidine products have been recalled due to possible contamination with NDMA (N-nitrosodimethylamine). NDMA has been identified as a potential risk factor in the development of certain cancers. Famotidine remains in use. CNS reactions to these drugs have been reported, especially with cimetidine.[58] A study looking at observational data on PPIs found an association between PPI use and incident dementia. This is supported by pharmacoepidemiological analyses on primary data and is in line with animal studies in which the use of PPIs increased the levels of β-amyloid in the brains of mice.[59] Randomised, prospective clinical trials are needed to confirm this association. Many patients on PPIs have *Helicobacter pylori*–infected gastric mucosa. As *Helicobacter* has been reported to be associated with cognitive deterioration, this could be the mechanism behind the apparent link between PPI drugs and dementia. Furthermore, this association was not replicated in other studies.[60,61]

Antibiotics

There are reports of many antibiotics being associated with delirium[62,63] but there is no consistent pattern of them causing cognitive impairment. Given the importance of treating infection in dementia, the most appropriate antibiotic for the infection being treated should be used. Antituberculous therapy, particularly isoniazid, has attracted some case reports of adverse psychiatric reactions (Table 6.6).[64]

Table 6.6 Recommended drugs and drugs to avoid in dementia (adapted with permission[26])

Condition	Drug class or drug name	Drugs to avoid in dementia	Recommended drugs in dementia
Allergic conditions	Antihistamines	Chlorphenamine Promethazine Hydroxyzine Cyproheptadine Cyclizine (and other first-generation antihistamines)	Cetirizine Loratadine Fexofenadine (and other second-generation antihistamines)
Asthma/COPD	Bronchodilators		Beta-agonists Inhaled anticholinergics (have not been reported to affect cognition) Theophylline
Constipation	Laxatives	No evidence to suggest that laxatives have any negative impact on cognitive function Constipation itself may worsen cognition	
Diarrhoea	Loperamide	Low-potency anticholinergic. Not known to have effects on cognitive function; however, may add to the anticholinergic cognitive burden if used in combination to other anticholinergics	

Condition	Drug class or drug name	Drugs to avoid in dementia	Recommended drugs in dementia
Hyperlipidaemia	Statins		All are safe but atorvastatin and pravastatin are less likely to cross blood–brain barrier
Hypersalivation	Anticholinergics	Hyoscine hydrobromide	Pirenzepine Atropine (sublingually)
Hypertension	Antihypertensives	Beta-blockers (avoidance may not always be possible)	Calcium channel blockers, angiotensin-converting enzyme inhibitors and angiotensin receptor blockers may all improve cognitive function
Infections	Antibiotics	Delirium reported mostly with quinolone and macrolide antibiotics But given the importance of treating infections, the most appropriate antibiotic for the infections should be used	
Myasthenia gravis	Peripheral acetylcholinesterase inhibitors, e.g. neostigmine and pyridostigmine	May add to the cholinergic adverse effects of central acetylcholinesterase inhibitors (e.g. donepezil, etc.) in patients with dementia, i.e. increased risk of nausea/vomiting, etc.	
Nausea/vomiting	Antiemetics	Cyclizine Metoclopramide Prochlorperazine	Domperidone (see main text for restrictions) Serotonin 5HT3 receptor antagonists
Other GI conditions	Antispasmodics	Atropine sulphate Dicycloverine Hydrochloride	Alverine, mebeverine, peppermint oil Hyoscine-*n*-butylbromide Propantheline bromide
Pain	Analgesics	Pethidine Pentazocine Dextropropoxyphene Codeine Tramadol Methadone	Paracetamol Oxycodone Buprenorphine Topical NSAIDs (where appropriate)
		Fentanyl patches (caution in opioid-naive patients) Morphine (may be indicated in treatment-resistant pain or palliative care – use cautiously due to associated cognitive and other adverse effects)	
Urinary frequency	Anticholinergic drugs used in overactive bladder	Oxybutynin Tolterodine	Darifenacin Trospium Solifenacin (use if others not available – some reports of cognitive adverse effects)
		Data for fesoterodine are still lacking – it is non-selective, has high central anticholinergic activity but theoretically has very low ability to cross the BBB	
Urinary retention	Alpha-blockers	Not known to have effects on cognitive function	

CHAPTER 6

References

1. Sink KM, et al. Dual use of bladder anticholinergics and cholinesterase inhibitors: long-term functional and cognitive outcomes. *J Am Geriatr Soc* 2008; 56:847–853.
2. Ruxton K, et al. Drugs with anticholinergic effects and cognitive impairment, falls and all-cause mortality in older adults: A systematic review and meta-analysis. *Br J Clin Pharmacol* 2015; 80:209–220.
3. Sunderland T, et al. Anticholinergic sensitivity in patients with dementia of the Alzheimer type and age-matched controls. A dose-response study. *Arch Gen Psychiatry* 1987; 44:418–426.
4. Bishara D, et al. Anticholinergic effect on cognition (AEC) of drugs commonly used in older people. *Int J Geriatr Psychiatry* 2017; 32:650–656.
5. Fox C, et al. Anticholinergic medication use and cognitive impairment in the older population: the medical research council cognitive function and ageing study. *J Am Geriatr Soc* 2011; 59:1477–1483.
6. Bishara D, et al. The anticholinergic effect on cognition (AEC) scale-Associations with mortality, hospitalisation and cognitive decline following dementia diagnosis. *Int J Geriatr Psychiatry* 2020; 35:1069–1077.
7. Wagg A. The cognitive burden of anticholinergics in the elderly – implications for the treatment of overactive bladder. *Eur Urological Rev* 2012; 7:42–49.
8. Pagoria D, et al. Antimuscarinic drugs: review of the cognitive impact when used to treat overactive bladder in elderly patients. *Curr Urol Rep* 2011; 12:351–357.
9. Womack KB, et al. Tolterodine and memory: dry but forgetful. *Arch Neurol* 2003; 60:771–773.
10. Tsao JW, et al. Transient memory impairment and hallucinations associated with tolterodine use. *N Engl J Med* 2003; 349:2274–2275.
11. Edwards KR, et al. Risk of delirium with concomitant use of tolterodine and acetylcholinesterase inhibitors. *J Am Geriatr Soc* 2002; 50:1165–1166.
12. Kay G, et al. Differential effects of the antimuscarinic agents darifenacin and oxybutynin ER on memory in older subjects. *Eur Urol* 2006; 50:317–326.
13. Lipton RB, et al. Assessment of cognitive function of the elderly population: effects of darifenacin. *J Urol* 2005; 173:493–498.
14. Chancellor MB, et al. Blood-brain barrier permeation and efflux exclusion of anticholinergics used in the treatment of overactive bladder. *Drugs Aging* 2012; 29:259–273.
15. Park JW. The effect of solifenacin on cognitive function following stroke. *Dement Geriatr Cogn Dis Extra* 2013; 3:143–147.
16. Liabeuf S, et al. Trospium chloride for overactive bladder may induce central nervous system adverse events. *Eur Geriatr Med* 2014; 5:220–224.
17. Isik AT, et al. Trospium and cognition in patients with late onset Alzheimer disease. *J Nutr Health Aging* 2009; 13:672–676.
18. Geller EJ, et al. Effect of trospium chloride on cognitive function in women aged 50 and older: a randomized trial. *Female Pelvic Med Reconstr Surg* 2017; 23:118–123.
19. Wagg A. Fesoterodine fumarate for the treatment of overactive bladder in the elderly – a review of the latest clinical data. *Clin Investig (Lond)* 2012; 2:825–833.
20. Yonguc T, et al. Randomized, controlled trial of fesoterodine fumarate for overactive bladder in Parkinson's disease. *World J Urol* 2020; 38:2013–2019.
21. BNF Online. British National Formulary. 2020; https://www.medicinescomplete.com/mc/bnf/current.
22. Mahdy AM, et al. Histamine and antihistamines. *Anaesthesia Intensive Care Med* 2011; 12:324–329.
23. Roy-Desruisseaux J, et al. Domperidone-induced tardive dyskinesia and withdrawal psychosis in an elderly woman with dementia. *Ann Pharmacother* 2011; 45:e51.
24. Medicines and Healthcare Products Regulatory Agency. Domperidone: risks of cardiac side effects – indication restricted to nausea and vomiting, new contraindications, and reduced dose and duration of use. 2014; http://www.mhra.gov.uk/Safetyinformation/DrugSafetyUpdate/CON418518.
25. Kay GG, et al. Preserving cognitive function for patients with overactive bladder: evidence for a differential effect with darifenacin. *Int J Clin Pract* 2008; 62:1792–1800.
26. Bishara D, et al. Safe prescribing of physical health medication in patients with dementia. *Int J Geriatr Psychiatry* 2014; 29:1230–1241.
27. Bentley KR, et al. Therapeutic potential of serotonin 5-HT3 antagonists in neuropsychiatric disorders. *CNS Drugs* 1995; 3:363–392.
28. Gridelli C. Same old story? Do we need to modify our supportive care treatment of elderly cancer patients? Focus on antiemetics. *Drugs Aging* 2004; 21:825–832.
29. Flicker C, et al. Hypersensitivity to scopolamine in the elderly. *Psychopharmacology* 1992; 107:437–441.
30. Ebert U, et al. Scopolamine model of dementia: electroencephalogram findings and cognitive performance. *Eur J Clin Invest* 1998; 28:944–949.
31. Sanofi. Summary of product characteristics. Buscopan 10 mg Tablets. 2020; https://www.medicines.org.uk/emc/medicine/30089.
32. Gupta P, et al. Potential adverse effects of bronchodilators in the treatment of airways obstruction in older people: recommendations for prescribing. *Drugs Aging* 2008; 25:415–443.
33. Ramsdell JW, et al. Effects of theophylline and ipratropium on cognition in elderly patients with chronic obstructive pulmonary disease. *Ann Allergy Asthma Immunol* 1996; 76:335–340.
34. Fritze J, et al. Pirenzepine for clozapine-induced hypersalivation. *Lancet* 1995; 346:1034.
35. Pohanka M. Acetylcholinesterase inhibitors: a patent review. *Expert Opin Ther Pat* 2012; 22:871–886.
36. Gray SL, et al. Drug-induced cognition disorders in the elderly: incidence, prevention and management. *Drug Saf* 1999; 21:101–122.

37. Bailey RB, et al. Chronic salicylate intoxication. A common cause of morbidity in the elderly. *J Am Geriatr Soc* 1989; **37**:556–561.

38. Hoppmann RA, et al. Central nervous system side effects of nonsteroidal anti-inflammatory drugs. Aseptic meningitis, psychosis, and cognitive dysfunction. *Arch Intern Med* 1991; **151**:1309–1313.

39. Wysenbeek AJ, et al. Assessment of cognitive function in elderly patients treated with naproxen. A prospective study. *Clin Exp Rheumatol* 1988; **6**:399–400.

40. Bruce-Jones PN, et al. Indomethacin and cognitive function in healthy elderly volunteers. *Br J Clin Pharmacol* 1994; **38**:45–51.

41. Barber JB, et al. Treatment of chronic non-malignant pain in the elderly: safety considerations. *Drug Saf* 2009; **32**:457–474.

42. Ripamonti C, et al. CNS adverse effects of opioids in cancer patients. *CNS Drugs* 1997; **8**:21–37.

43. Alagiakrishnan K, et al. An approach to drug induced delirium in the elderly. *Postgrad Med J* 2004; **80**:388–393.

44. McLachlan AJ, et al. Clinical pharmacology of analgesic medicines in older people: impact of frailty and cognitive impairment. *Br J Clin Pharmacol* 2011; **71**:351–364.

45. Dosa DM, et al. Frequency of long-acting opioid analgesic initiation in opioid-naive nursing home residents. *J Pain Symptom Manage* 2009; **38**:515–521.

46. Tannenbaum C, et al. A systematic review of amnestic and non-amnestic mild cognitive impairment induced by anticholinergic, antihistamine, GABAergic and opioid drugs. *Drugs Aging* 2012; **29**:639–658.

47. McGuinness B, et al. Statins for the treatment of dementia. *Cochrane Database Syst Rev* 2014; Cd007514.

48. Wagstaff LR, et al. Statin-associated memory loss: analysis of 60 case reports and review of the literature. *Pharmacotherapy* 2003; **23**:871–880.

49. McGuinness B, et al. Statins for the prevention of dementia. *Cochrane Database Syst Rev* 2016; Cd003160.

50. Qiu C, et al. The age-dependent relation of blood pressure to cognitive function and dementia. *Lancet Neurol* 2005; **4**:487–499.

51. Wändell P, et al. Antihypertensive drugs and relevant cardiovascular pharmacotherapies and the risk of incident dementia in patients with atrial fibrillation. *Int J Cardiol* 2018; **272**:149–154.

52. Levi MN, et al. Antihypertensive classes, cognitive decline and incidence of dementia: a network meta-analysis. *J Hypertens* 2013; **31**:1073–1082.

53. Eisendrath SJ, et al. Toxic neuropsychiatric effects of digoxin at therapeutic serum concentrations. *Am J Psychiatry* 1987; **144**:506–507.

54. Brezis M, et al. Nightmares from digoxin. *Ann Intern Med* 1980; **93**:639–640.

55. Laudisio A, et al. Digoxin and cognitive performance in patients with heart failure: a cohort, pharmacoepidemiological survey. *Drugs Aging* 2009; **26**:103–112.

56. Athwal H, et al. Amiodarone-induced delirium. *Am J Geriatr Psychiatry* 2003; **11**:696–697.

57. Foley KT, et al. Separate episodes of delirium associated with levetiracetam and amiodarone treatment in an elderly woman. *Am J Geriatr Pharmacother* 2010; **8**:170–174.

58. Cantu TG, et al. Central nervous system reactions to histamine-2 receptor blockers. *Ann Intern Med* 1991; **114**:1027–1034.

59. Gomm W, et al. Association of proton pump inhibitors with risk of dementia: a pharmacoepidemiological claims data analysis. *JAMA Neurol* 2016; **73**:410–416.

60. Goldstein FC, et al. Proton pump inhibitors and risk of mild cognitive impairment and dementia. *J Am Geriatr Soc* 2017; **65**:1969–1974.

61. Lochhead P, et al. Association between proton pump inhibitor use and cognitive function in women. *Gastroenterology* 2017; **153**:971–979. e974.

62. Grahl JJ, et al. Antimicrobial exposure and the risk of delirium in critically ill patients. *Crit Care* 2018; **22**:337.

63. Bhattacharyya S, et al. Antibiotic-associated encephalopathy. *Neurology* 2016; **86**:963–971.

64. Kass JS, et al. Nervous system effects of antituberculosis therapy. *CNS Drugs* 2010; **24**:655–667.

CHAPTER 6

Management of behavioural and psychological symptoms of dementia (BPSD)

BPSD include a wide range of difficulties, including aggression, agitation, vocalisation, distress during care, disinhibition, hallucinations, delusions, apathy, low mood and anxiety.[1] Such symptoms occur in over 90% of patients to varying degrees.[2] The fact that several of these occur simultaneously in individuals makes it difficult to target specific symptoms. The drug treatment of these symptoms is not supported by a robust body of scientific evidence[3] and many available agents have serious adverse effects.

Non-drug measures

Since the publication in the UK of the report *Time for Action*, which detailed the risks associated with antipsychotic use in dementia,[4] there has been a drive to review evidence for antipsychotics and to formulate non-pharmacological treatment pathways for BPSD. Systematic reviews have been completed,[5] new models of care have been developed[6,7] and guidance documents have been written.[8] The key themes include the following:

1. An individualised and pragmatic approach to treatment rather than the application of 'off-the-shelf' therapies.
2. Ensuring contributory physical factors are addressed as a first step. These include pain (see section later), acute physical illness, constipation and medication side effects (see safer prescribing in dementia section).
3. The importance of understanding 'problem behaviours' as an expression of distress and unmet need.[6,7]
4. Use of life history, direct observation of care and data collection (e.g. sleep, pain and ABC charts) to understand what the unmet needs might be and to inform treatment changes.[8]
5. Formulation meetings to develop a model of the factors leading to and perpetuating the behaviour, which can be modified in light of new evidence.
6. Clear and pragmatic care plans developed with carers to address unmet needs identified through the above processes.
7. Care plans reviewed and adjusted according to effectiveness of the interventions tried.

Some more structured psychosocial interventions for BPSD[9] are reasonably well supported by research.[10] These interventions can be useful to consider as part of an individualised care plan and are better if implemented by supporting care givers and developing their skills. Behavioural management techniques and caregiver psychoeducation centred on individual patient's behaviour have been found to be generally successful and the effects can last for months.[11]

A systematic review of systematic reviews[12] provided an overview of the evidence for these interventions. Among sensory simulation interventions, the only convincingly effective intervention (reducing agitation and aggressive behaviour) was **music therapy**. Whilst a well-conducted study[13] ($n = 71$) reported a favourable treatment effect on measures of agitation and behavioural symptoms with **Melissa balm**, this has not been replicated due to methodological limitations.[12] The efficacy of **aromatherapy** and massage therapy remains unproven. **Light therapy** and **Snoezelen multisensory stimulation therapy** did not show any significant benefit. There was inadequate evidence for the efficacy of cognitive/emotion-oriented interventions, such as **reminiscence therapy, simulated presence therapy** and **validation therapy. Multicomponent interventions** that use a comprehensive, integrated multidisciplinary approach combining medical, psychiatric and nursing interventions may be more effective at reducing severe behavioural problems in nursing home patients. Other interventions such as **animal-assisted** and **exercise therapy** did not show any convincing effect on any BPSD.[12]

In summary, multicomponent interventions that are tailored to individual unmet needs are more likely to be of benefit than the routine use of 'off-the-shelf' interventions.

> *Recommendation: Evidence-based, multicomponent non-drug measures, which are personalised and involve working closely with care-givers are first-line treatments for BPSD. There is some evidence for music therapy in the reduction of agitation.*

Pharmacological measures

Analgesics

Pain in people with cognitive impairment may manifest as agitation; therefore, treatment of undiagnosed pain may help in the management of agitation.[14] An RCT investigating the effects of a stepwise protocol of treatment with analgesics in patients with moderate-to-severe dementia and agitation noted significant improvement in agitation, overall neuropsychiatric symptoms and pain. The majority of patients in the study received only paracetamol (acetaminophen).

A Cochrane review investigated the clinical efficacy and safety of opioids for agitation in people with dementia.[15] RCTs of opioids compared with placebo were assessed; however, there was insufficient evidence to establish their clinical efficacy or safety in this patient group.

> *Recommendation: The assessment and effective treatment of pain is important. Even in people without overt pain, a trial of analgesics (usually paracetamol) is worthwhile.*

Antipsychotics in behavioural and psychological symptoms of dementia

Antipsychotic drugs were once widely used in dementia-related behaviour disturbance[16] but their use is now highly controversial.[17,18] There are three reasons for this: effect size is small,[19–22] tolerability is poor[22–24] and there is an association with increased mortality.[25] Despite this, antipsychotic medications have been the subject of the largest number of studies of any intervention for BPSD.

Typical antipsychotics show no clear efficacy in BPSD (with the exception of haloperidol), but atypical antipsychotics do have some efficacy. A Comparative Effectiveness Review found that the most effective antipsychotics include risperidone (psychosis, agitation, overall BPSD), olanzapine (agitation) and aripiprazole (overall BPSD). Though commonly used, quetiapine has failed to show effectiveness for BPSD, except at higher doses (100–200mg/day) that may not be well tolerated. The CATIE-AD study comparing risperidone, olanzapine and quetiapine with placebo in persons with BPSD demonstrated efficacy for risperidone and olanzapine but a large percentage of participants discontinued medication due to adverse effects.[26]

A 2006 Cochrane review[27] of atypical antipsychotics for aggression and psychosis in AD concluded that risperidone and olanzapine are useful in diminishing aggression, and risperidone reduces psychotic symptoms. However, the authors concluded that because of modest efficacy and significant increase in adverse effects, neither risperidone nor olanzapine should be routinely used to treat dementia patients unless there is severe distress or a serious risk of physical harm to those living or working with the patient.

Increased mortality with antipsychotics in dementia

Following analysis of published and unpublished data in 2004, warnings were issued in the UK and USA regarding increased mortality in patients with dementia with certain SGAs (mainly risperidone and olanzapine).[28–30] These warnings have been extended to include all SGAs as well as conventional antipsychotics,[30,31] and a warning about a possible risk of cerebrovascular events (CVAEs) has now been added to product labelling for all FGAs and SGAs.

Some studies suggested that the risk of CVAEs in elderly users of antipsychotics may not be cumulative.[32,33] The risk was elevated during the first weeks of treatment but then decreased over time, returning to base level after 3 months. In contrast, a long-term study (24–54 months) deduced that mortality was progressively increased over time for antipsychotic-treated (risperidone and FGAs) patients compared with those receiving placebo.[34] At present this is not a widely held view.

Whether the risk of mortality differs from one antipsychotic to another has been investigated in several studies.[35–38] In general, haloperidol users had an increased risk of mortality, whereas quetiapine users had a decreased risk. No clinically meaningful differences were observed for olanzapine, aripiprazole and ziprasidone[35] (or valproic acid[36]). The effects were strongest shortly after the start of treatment and remained after adjustment for dose. There was a dose–response relation for all drugs except quetiapine.[35] Another study[37] investigated adjusted hazard ratios of death of 14 individual antipsychotics compared with risperidone in new users of antipsychotics. A higher mortality was found for haloperidol, levomepromazine and zuclopenthixol, and to a lesser extent for melperone compared with risperidone. Lower risks were observed for quetiapine, olanzapine, clozapine and flupentixol. No statistically significant difference was found for amisulpride.

In a 2019 network meta-analysis of 17 studies (5,373 patients), no significant differences were found across measures of effectiveness and safety among aripiprazole, olanzapine, quetiapine and risperidone, although differences were found for some of these drugs and outcomes when compared with placebo.[39]

Several mechanisms have been postulated for the causes of CVAEs with antipsychotics.[40] Orthostatic hypotension may impair cerebral perfusion in people with cerebrovascular insufficiency or atherosclerosis. Tachycardia may decrease cerebral perfusion or dislodge a thrombus in a patient with atrial fibrillation (see section on psychotropics in AF).

Following an episode of orthostatic hypotension, there could be a rebound excess of catecholamines with vasoconstriction, thus aggravating cerebral insufficiency. In addition, hyperprolactinaemia could in theory accelerate atherosclerosis, and sedation might cause dehydration and haemoconcentration.[40] A study[32] suggests affinity for M_1, and alpha-2 receptors predict effects on stroke.

Risperidone clinical trial data were recently examined to look for individual patient characteristics associated with CVAEs and death and for treatment-emergent risk factors.[41] Baseline complications of depression and delusions were associated with a lower relative risk of CVAEs in risperidone-treated patients. For mortality, the only significant baseline predictor in patients treated with risperidone was depression which was associated with a lower relative risk. The relative risk of death was higher in risperidone-taking patients treated with anti-inflammatory medications.

Both typical[42] and atypical antipsychotics[43] may also hasten cognitive decline in dementia, although there is some evidence to rebut this.[44–46]

Recommendation: Use of risperidone (licensed for persistent aggression in AD) and olanzapine may be justified in some cases of severe aggression and/or psychosis. Effect is modest at best. When prescribed, regular review is recommended.

Clinical information for antipsychotic use in dementia

Antipsychotics should not be used routinely to treat agitation and aggression in people with dementia.[47]

Risperidone (and haloperidol) are the only drugs licensed in the UK for the management of non-cognitive symptoms associated with dementia. Due to the serious adverse effects of haloperidol, risperidone is the agent of choice. It is specifically indicated for short-term treatment (up to 6 weeks) of persistent aggression in patients with moderate-to-severe AD unresponsive to non-pharmacological approaches and when there is a risk of harm to self or others.[48] Risperidone is licensed up to 1mg twice a day,[49] although optimal dose in dementia has been found to be 500µg twice a day (1mg daily).[50]

Alternative antipsychotic drugs may be used (off-licence) if risperidone is contraindicated or not tolerated. Olanzapine has some positive efficacy data for reducing aggression in dementia[27] (work is underway, investigating the efficacy and tolerability of amisulpride in dementia),[51,52] and quetiapine (although not as effective as risperidone and olanzapine) may be considered in patients with Parkinson's disease, or Lewy body dementia (at very small doses) because of its low propensity for causing movement disorders.

Only prescribe antipsychotics after:

- careful risk assessment, balancing the cerebrovascular risk (taking into account hypertension, diabetes, smoking, atrial fibrillation and previous stroke);
- discussion of possible risks and benefits with carer (and patient if she/he has capacity);
- clear documentation of the above.[47]

CHAPTER 6

It is recommended that all patients prescribed antipsychotics should have the following tests at **baseline**, at **3 months** and **annually**:

1. Blood pressure and pulse
2. Weight (ideally also monitor monthly for the first 3 months)
3. Blood tests
   a. fasting glucose or HbA1c
   b. urea and electrolytes (U&Es), including eGFR
   c. full blood count (FBC)
   d. lipids (if possible fasting)
   e. liver function tests (LFTs)
   f. prolactin levels
4. ECG (repeat at between 4 weeks and 3 months or when clinically indicated)

- In-patients or physically frail patients may need more frequent physical health monitoring.
- Review of the antipsychotic drug needs to be done at 4–6 weeks (maybe earlier for in-patients), then at 3 months and then every 6 months if physically stable and there are no adverse effects. Consider stopping the antipsychotic at each review, where appropriate.
- It may sometimes be difficult to get the recommended investigations, for example due to high levels of patient agitation and resistance, or due to the urgency of the situation. In these cases, a risk benefit analysis should again be carried out, recognising that by not having the investigations, the risk of prescribing an antipsychotic is even higher and an antipsychotic should only be prescribed if the risks of not giving it are even higher still.

Table 6.7 Reduction or discontinuation regimen for antipsychotic drugs in BPSD – a guide[53]

Antipsychotic	Usual dose range in dementia	Suggested regimen for reduction/discontinuation (generally reduce over 2–4 weeks, ideally over 4 weeks if possible)
Amisulpride	25–50mg/day	Reduce by 12.5–25mg every 1–2 weeks (depending on dose), then stop
Aripiprazole	5–15mg/day	Reduce by 5mg every 1–2 weeks (depending on dose), then stop (if patient is on 5mg daily, reduce to 2.5mg for 2 weeks; however, note that tablets are not scored and liquid is expensive – contact local pharmacist for advice)
Haloperidol	Not recommended in older people with dementia (except in delirium) Reduce by 0.25–0.5mg every 1–2 weeks (depending on the dose), then stop	
Olanzapine	2.5–10mg/day	Reduce by 2.5mg every 1–2 weeks (depending on dose), then stop
Quetiapine	12.5–300mg/day	For doses 12.5–100mg/day: reduce by 12.5–25mg every 1–2 weeks (depending on the dose) and then stop For doses >100mg to 300mg/day: reduce by 25–50mg every 1–2 weeks (depending on the dose), then stop If dose is 300mg/day, reduce to 150–200mg/day for 1 week, then by 50mg per week
Risperidone	0.25–2mg/day	Reduce by 0.25–0.5mg every 1–2 weeks (depending on dose), then stop

For higher doses, reduce gradually over 4 weeks.
NB: If serious adverse effects occur, stop antipsychotic drug immediately.

The Halting Antipsychotic Use in Long-Term Care study was a single-arm longitudinal study conducted in Australian long-term care facilities among patients taking antipsychotics, 98.5% of whom had dementia. Of the 93 patients who completed the study, 69 (74%) had antipsychotics successfully de-prescribed without re-initiation or experiencing increase in BPSD. Here, the de-prescribing protocol followed Australian guidelines: a dose reduction of 50% every 2 weeks and ceasing after 2 weeks on the minimum dose, withdrawing one antipsychotic at a time, with risperidone (if prescribed) withdrawn last.[54]

Other pharmacological agents in BPSD

Cognitive enhancers

AChE-Is and memantine have only a mild effect on BPSD. According to a meta-analysis, the effect of AChE-I on BPSD is statistically significant; however, the clinical benefit remains unclear.[55] Overall, studies suggest cholinesterase inhibitors are more effective for depression, dysphoria, apathy and anxiety symptoms than for agitation or aggression. Memantine has been shown to improve agitation, aggression and delusions. Because the benefit of cognitive enhancers may not be seen until 3–6 months after initiation, these medications will not have clinical utility in acute treatment of BPSD. However, since clinicians prescribe cholinesterase inhibitors and memantine to help slow cognitive decline, eventually these medications may also assist with reducing distressing behaviours.[56]

> *Recommendation: Use of AChE-Is or memantine can be justified in situations described above and may be worth considering if a patient is not on one of these drugs and they fall within the licenced indications. Effect is modest at best.*

Benzodiazepines

Benzodiazepines[57,58] are widely used but their use is poorly supported. Benzodiazepines have been associated with cognitive decline,[57] risk of dementia,[59] risk of pneumonia,[60] *increase in all-cause mortality*[61] and may contribute to increased frequency of falls and hip fractures[58,62] in older people.

> *Recommendation: Avoid benzodiazepines other than for emergency sedation.*

Antidepressants

Substantial evidence suggests that depression is both a risk factor and consequence of AD. The prevalence of depression and AD co-morbidity is estimated to be 30–50%.[63] Two potential mechanisms by which antidepressants affect cognition in depression have been postulated: a direct effect caused by the pharmacological action of the drugs on specific neurotransmitters and a secondary effect caused by improvement of depression.[64]

The evidence for efficacy of antidepressants in BPSD is mixed and limited showing that antidepressants are most helpful for treating agitation and less so for depression, apathy, anxiety or psychosis in dementia.[26] **Citalopram** has the strongest evidence for efficacy in agitation with the CitAD trial,[65] showing that 30mg of citalopram daily had a positive effect on agitation in dementia; unfortunately, this study also confirmed the risk of QT prolongation with citalopram at this dose. The maximum dose of citalopram in older people is 20mg a day because of the drug's effect on cardiac QT interval. Although there is less evidence, **escitalopram** may also be effective in BPSD. The evidence for efficacy of **sertraline** is mixed, though its cardiac safety is a strong point.[26]

Whilst a previous Cochrane review of **trazodone** for agitation in dementia[66] found insufficient evidence from RCTs to support its use in dementia, in a recent Cochrane review, trazodone 50mg at bedtime was noted to be well tolerated and improved sleep for people with dementia and insomnia. Additionally, trazodone 150–300mg/day was found to be effective in reducing BPSD in frontotemporal dementia. Although **mirtazapine** plays an important role in treatment of older adults with depression, a recent pilot study showed no significant therapeutic effect of 15mg mirtazapine on Alzheimer's patients with sleep disorders and in fact found worsening of daytime sleep patterns. **Bupropion** has not been studied in controlled trials in dementia.[26]

TCAs are best avoided in patients with dementia. They can cause falls, possibly via orthostatic hypotension, and can worsen cognition due to their anticholinergic adverse effect.[67]

Findings suggest that in AD patients treated with cholinesterase inhibitors, SSRIs may exert some degree of protection against the negative effects of depression on cognition. To date, literature analysis does not clarify if the combined effect of SSRIs and AChE-Is is synergistic, additive or independent.[64] In addition, it is still unclear whether SSRIs have beneficial effects on cognition in AD patients who are not actively manifesting mood or behavioural problems.[68]

Whilst some emerging studies have found that antidepressant use in older people may be associated with an increased risk of dementia, it is important to keep in mind that previous studies have shown that late-life depression is associated with an increased risk for dementia. Hence, any comparisons of antidepressant users with non-depressed non-users are subject to indication bias as the increased dementia risk could be due to depression, and not the medication.

A Swedish study[69] included 20,050 memory clinic patients diagnosed with incident dementia and collected data on antidepressant use at the time of dementia diagnosis and over the 3-year period before a dementia diagnosis. Use of antidepressant treatment for 3 consecutive years before a dementia diagnosis was associated with a lower mortality risk for all dementia disorders and in AD.

> *Recommendation: Although evidence is weak, use of antidepressants is justified in people with dementia who have clear symptoms of moderate or severe depression, especially if non-pharmacological approaches have been ineffective.*

Mood stabilisers/antiseizure medications

RCTs of mood stabilisers in non-cognitive symptoms of dementia have been completed for **oxcarbazepine**,[70] **carbamazepine**[71] and **valproate**.[72] Gabapentin, lamotrigine and topiramate have also been used.[73] Of the mood stabilisers, carbamazepine has the most robust evidence of efficacy in non-cognitive symptoms.[74] However, its serious adverse effects (especially Stevens–Johnson syndrome) and its potential for drug interactions limit its use.

One RCT of valproate that included an open-label extension found it to be ineffective in controlling symptoms. Seven of the 39 patients enrolled died during the 12-week extension phase study period, although the deaths could not be attributed to the drug.[75] A study investigating the optimal dose of valproic acid in dementia found that whilst serum levels between 40µg/L and 60µg/L and relatively low doses (7–12mg/kg/day) are associated with improvements in agitation in some patients, similar levels produced no significant improvements in others and led to substantial side effects.[76] A 2009 Cochrane review of valproate for the treatment of agitation in dementia found no evidence of efficacy but advocated the need for further research into its use in dementia.[77] Valproate does not delay emergence of agitation in dementia.[78] Literature reviews of antiseizure medication in non-cognitive symptoms of dementia found that valproate, oxcarbazepine and lithium showed low or no evidence of efficacy and that more RCTs are needed to strengthen the evidence for gabapentin, topiramate and lamotrigine.[74]

Preliminary low-grade evidence based on case series and case reviews suggests a possible benefit of **gabapentin** and **pregabalin** in patients with BPSD in AD. Evidence in frontotemporal dementia is lacking.[79] In a small case series, gabapentin reduced aggression among seven patients with vascular dementia or mixed vascular/AD, using daily doses ranging from 200mg to 600mg daily. Three of the seven patients were able to discontinue antipsychotics after gabapentin initiation; thus, it may be useful in patients with cardiac conditions where antipsychotics are inappropriate. Caution should be noted about the use of gabapentin in Lewy body dementia; dramatic worsening of neuropsychiatric symptoms has been reported after its use to treat behavioural symptoms.[80]

Although clearly beneficial in some patients, antiseizure medications/mood stabilisers cannot be recommended for routine use in the treatment of the neuropsychiatric symptoms in dementia at present.[73]

> *Recommendation: Limited evidence to support its use – use may be justified where other treatments are contraindicated or ineffective. Valproate is best avoided.*

Melatonin and sleep disturbances in AD

Evidence regarding the effectiveness of melatonin supplementation on sleep in patients with AD is limited. Six double-blind randomised placebo-controlled trials, mostly of limited sample size have been published. Although it is clear that melatonin has no significant side effects, even at high doses, the results of studies have been equivocal. Some studies showed beneficial effects, mainly improvement of day/night-time sleep ratio and decrease of nocturnal activity whilst other studies failed to demonstrate objective effectiveness.[81] Non-pharmacological management of sleep disturbances using established sleep hygiene methods should be the first-line treatment for insomnia in dementia.[82]

A 2016 Cochrane review[83] of pharmacotherapies for sleep disturbances in dementia found no RCTs of many drugs that are widely prescribed for sleep problems in dementia, including the benzodiazepine and non-benzodiazepine hypnotics, although there is considerable uncertainty about the balance of benefits and risks associated with these common treatments. From the studies identified, there was no evidence that melatonin (up to 10mg) helped sleep problems in patients with moderate-to-severe dementia due to AD. There was

CHAPTER 6

some evidence to support the use of a low dose (50mg) of trazodone, although a larger trial is needed to allow a more definitive conclusion to be reached on the balance of risks and benefits. There was no evidence of any effect of ramelteon on sleep in patients with mild-to-moderate dementia due to AD. This is an area with a high need for pragmatic trials, particularly of those drugs that are in common clinical use for sleep problems in dementia.

> **Recommendation: Limited evidence to support the use of melatonin – but safe to use and may be justified in some cases where benefits are seen. Non-pharmacological management of sleep disturbances should be tried first.**

Sedating antihistamines, e.g. promethazine

Promethazine is frequently used in BPSD for its sedative effects. It has strong anticholinergic effects and readily penetrates the BBB, therefore, potentially causing significant cognitive impairment.[84]

> **Recommendation: Promethazine may be used for short-term use only but evidence is minimal.**

Miscellaneous agents

A pooled analysis provided evidence of efficacy of **Ginkgo biloba** at a daily dose of 240mg in the treatment of out-patients suffering from Alzheimer's, vascular or mixed dementia with BPSD.[85]

Newer antipsychotic agents are being explored for the management of BPSD, including **brexpiprazole, lumateperone** (a potent antagonist at 5-HT_{2A} receptors and a serotonin reuptake inhibitor) and **pimavanserin** (an inverse agonist and antagonist at 5-HT_{2A} receptors). Other agents currently being investigated for BPSD include **dextromethorphan/quinidine, bupropion/dextromethorphan** and **methylphenidate.**[86]

Recently, **nabilone**, a synthetic **cannabinoid**, significantly improved agitation and aggression in patients with AD in a randomised, placebo-controlled, crossover trial with 39 participants. Nabilone was well tolerated and although sedation was a more common adverse effect, it was not significantly different between the treatment groups.[87] Nabilone appears to be a promising therapeutic cannabinoid for treating agitation and aggressive symptoms due to AD.[86]

Electroconvulsive therapy (ECT)

ECT may benefit individuals with BPSD by enhancing the central transmission of neurochemicals, including GABA, glutamate, dopamine and noradrenaline/norepinephrine. Case reports, case series, retrospective chart reviews, retrospective case–control studies and an open-label prospective study on ECT have demonstrated promising results in decreasing agitation in patients with dementia. A systematic review reported that clinically significant improvement was observed in 88% of the 122 individuals in these studies, and the effect was often noted early in the treatment course. Additionally, the adverse effects were most often mild, transient or not reported (although reports of significant cognitive adverse effects have been documented in some studies).[88] Patients who relapsed were found to benefit from maintenance of ECT. ECT may be a promising option for the treatment of aggression and agitation in patients with severe dementia who are refractory to other treatment options, who have tolerability issues to pharmacotherapy and in those individuals in whom there is a need for the quick resolution of symptoms for their safety and well-being. However, the limitations of available studies suggest that a cautious approach is warranted.[88,89]

Overall, ECT would not be recommended as a common intervention given limited evidence practical aspects of transporting patients to the ECT clinic and difficulty with obtaining consent.

> **Recommendation: Insufficient evidence to recommend ECT use in BPSD. Caution: can cause significant cognitive adverse effects.**

Summary

The evidence base available to guide treatment in this area is insufficient to allow specific recommendations on appropriate management and drug choice. The basic approach is to try non-drug measures and analgesia before resorting to the use of psychotropics. Whichever drug is chosen, the following approach should be noted:

- Exclude physical illness potentially precipitating non-cognitive symptoms of dementia, e.g. constipation, infection and pain
- Target the symptoms requiring treatment
- Consider non-pharmacological methods
- Carry out a risk–benefit analysis tailored to individual patient needs when selecting a drug
- Make evidence-based decisions when choosing a drug
- Discuss treatment options and explain the risks to patient (if they have capacity) and family/ carers
- Titrate drug from a low starting dose and maintain the lowest dose possible for the shortest period necessary
- Review appropriateness of treatment regularly so that ineffective drug is not continued unnecessarily
- Monitor for adverse effects
- Document clearly treatment choices and discussions with patient, family or carers

References

1. National Institute for Health and Care Excellence. Dementia: assessment, management and support for people living with dementia and their carers [NG97]. 2018; https://www.nice.org.uk/guidance/ng97.

2. Steinberg M, et al. Point and 5-year period prevalence of neuropsychiatric symptoms in dementia: the Cache County Study. *Int J Geriatr Psychiatry* 2008; 23:170–177.

3. Salzman C, et al. Elderly patients with dementia-related symptoms of severe agitation and aggression: consensus statement on treatment options, clinical trials methodology, and policy. *J Clin Psychiatry* 2008; 69:889–898.

4. Department of Health. The use of antipsychotic medication for people with dementia: time for action. A report for the Minister of State for Care Services by Professor Sube Banerjee. 2009; https://www.rcpsych.ac.uk/pdf/Antipsychotic%20Bannerjee%20Report.pdf.

5. Livingston G, et al. A systematic review of the clinical effectiveness and cost-effectiveness of sensory, psychological and behavioural interventions for managing agitation in older adults with dementia. *Health Technol Assess* 2014; 18:1–226, v–vi.

6. Kales HC, et al. Assessment and management of behavioral and psychological symptoms of dementia. *BMJ* 2015; 350:h369.

7. James IA. *Understanding behaviour in dementia that challenges: a guide to assessment and treatment.* London, UK: Jessica Kingsley Publishers, 2011.

8. Brechin D, et al. British Psychological Society. Briefing paper. Alternatives to antipsychotic medication: psychological approaches in managing psychological and behavioural distress in people with dementia. 2013: http://www.bps.org.uk/system/files/Public%20files/antipsychotic.pdf.

9. Douglas S, et al. Non-pharmacological interventions in dementia. *Adv Psychiatr Treatment* 2004; 10:171–177.

10. Ayalon L, et al. Effectiveness of nonpharmacological interventions for the management of neuropsychiatric symptoms in patients with dementia: a systematic review. *Arch Intern Med* 2006; 166:2182–2188.

11. Livingston G, et al. Systematic review of psychological approaches to the management of neuropsychiatric symptoms of dementia. *Am J Psychiatry* 2005; 162:1996–2021.

12. Abraha I, et al. Systematic review of systematic reviews of non-pharmacological interventions to treat behavioural disturbances in older patients with dementia. The SENATOR-OnTop Series. *BMJ Open* 2017; 7:e012759.

13. Ballard CG, et al. Aromatherapy as a safe and effective treatment for the management of agitation in severe dementia: the results of a double-blind, placebo-controlled trial with Melissa. *J Clin Psychiatry* 2002; 63:553–558.

14. Husebo BS, et al. Efficacy of treating pain to reduce behavioural disturbances in residents of nursing homes with dementia: cluster randomised clinical trial. *BMJ* 2011; 343:d4065.

15. Brown R, et al. Opioids for agitation in dementia. *Cochrane Database Syst Rev* 2015:Cd009705.

16. Lee PE, et al. Atypical antipsychotic drugs in the treatment of behavioural and psychological symptoms of dementia: systematic review. *BMJ* 2004; 329:75.

17. Jeste DV, et al. Atypical antipsychotics in elderly patients with dementia or schizophrenia: review of recent literature. *Harv Rev Psychiatry* 2005; 13:340–351.

18. Jeste DV, et al. ACNP White Paper: update on use of antipsychotic drugs in elderly persons with dementia. *Neuropsychopharmacology* 2008; 33:957–970.

19. Aupperle P. Management of aggression, agitation, and psychosis in dementia: focus on atypical antipsychotics. *Am J Alzheimers Dis Other Demen* 2006; 21:101–108.

20. Yury CA, et al. Meta-analysis of the effectiveness of atypical antipsychotics for the treatment of behavioural problems in persons with dementia. *Psychother Psychosom* 2007; 76:213–218.

21. Deberdt WG, et al. Comparison of olanzapine and risperidone in the treatment of psychosis and associated behavioral disturbances in patients with dementia. *Am J Geriatr Psychiatry* 2005; 13:722–730.

22. Schneider LS, et al. Efficacy and adverse effects of atypical antipsychotics for dementia: meta-analysis of randomized, placebo-controlled trials. *Am J Geriatr Psychiatry* 2006; 14:191–210.

23. Anon. How safe are antipsychotics in dementia? *Drug Ther Bull* 2007; 45:81–86.

24. Rosack J. Side-effect risk often tempers antipsychotic use for dementia. *Psychiatr News* 2006; 41:1–38.

25. Schneider LS, et al. Risk of death with atypical antipsychotic drug treatment for dementia: meta-analysis of randomized placebo-controlled trials. *JAMA* 2005; 294:1934–1943.

26. Bessey LJ, et al. Management of behavioral and psychological symptoms of dementia. *Current Psychiatry Rep* 2019; 21:66.

27. Ballard C, et al. Atypical antipsychotics for aggression and psychosis in Alzheimer's disease (review). *Cochrane Database Syst Rev* 2006; CD14003476.

28. Pharmacovigilance Working Party. Antipsychotics and cerebrovascular accident. SPC wording for antipsychotics. 2005.

29. Duff G. Atypical antipsychotic drugs and stroke – committee on safety of medicines. 2004; https://webarchive.nationalarchives.gov.uk/20141206131857/http://www.mhra.gov.uk/home/groups/pl-p/documents/websiteresources/con019488.pdf.

30. FDA. Information on conventional antipsychotics – FDA alert [6/16/2008]. 2008; http://www.fda.gov.

31. European Medicines Agency. CHMP assessment report on conventional antipsychotics. 2008; http://www.emea.europa.eu.

32. Wu CS, et al. Association of stroke with the receptor-binding profiles of antipsychotics-a case-crossover study. *Biol Psychiatry* 2013; 73:414–421.

33. Kleijer BC, et al. Risk of cerebrovascular events in elderly users of antipsychotics. *J Psychopharmacol* 2009; 23:909–14.

34. Ballard C, et al. The dementia antipsychotic withdrawal trial (DART-AD): long-term follow-up of a randomised placebo-controlled trial. *Lancet Neurol* 2009; 8:151–157.

35. Huybrechts KF, et al. Differential risk of death in older residents in nursing homes prescribed specific antipsychotic drugs: population based cohort study. *BMJ* 2012; 344:e977.

36. Kales HC, et al. Risk of mortality among individual antipsychotics in patients with dementia. *Am J Psychiatry* 2012; 169:71–79.

37. Schmedt N, et al. Comparative risk of death in older adults treated with antipsychotics: a population-based cohort study. *Eur Neuropsychopharmacol* 2016; 26:1390–1400.

38. Maust DT, et al. Antipsychotics, other psychotropics, and the risk of death in patients with dementia: number needed to harm. *JAMA Psychiatry* 2015; 72:438–445.

39. Yunusa I, et al. Assessment of reported comparative effectiveness and safety of atypical antipsychotics in the treatment of behavioral and psychological symptoms of dementia: a network meta-analysis. *JAMA Network Open* 2019; 2:e190828.

40. Smith DA, et al. Association between risperidone treatment and cerebrovascular adverse events: examining the evidence and postulating hypotheses for an underlying mechanism. *J Am Med Dir Assoc* 2004; 5:129–132.

41. Howard R, et al. Baseline characteristics and treatment-emergent risk factors associated with cerebrovascular event and death with risperidone in dementia patients. *Br J Psychiatry* 2016; 209:378–384.

42. McShane R, et al. Do neuroleptic drugs hasten cognitive decline in dementia? Prospective study with necropsy follow up. *BMJ* 1997; 314:266–270.

43. Ballard C, et al. Quetiapine and rivastigmine and cognitive decline in Alzheimer's disease: randomised double blind placebo controlled trial. *BMJ* 2005; 330:874.

44. Livingston G, et al. Antipsychotics and cognitive decline in Alzheimer's disease: the LASER-Alzheimer's disease longitudinal study. *J Neurol Neurosurg Psychiatry* 2007; 78:25–29.

45. Rainer M, et al. Quetiapine versus risperidone in elderly patients with behavioural and psychological symptoms of dementia: efficacy, safety and cognitive function. *Eur Psychiatry* 2007; 22:395–403.

46. Paleacu D, et al. Quetiapine treatment for behavioural and psychological symptoms of dementia in Alzheimer's disease patients: a 6-week, double-blind, placebo-controlled study. *Int J Geriatr Psychiatry* 2008; 23:393–400.

47. Corbett A, et al. Don't use antipsychotics routinely to treat agitation and aggression in people with dementia. *BMJ* 2014; 349:g6420.

48. Janssen-Cilag Ltd. Summary of product characteristics. Risperdal film-coated tablets, oral solution and powder and solvent for prolonged-release suspension for injection. 2018; https://www.medicines.org.uk/emc/product/6856/smpc.

49. BNF Online. British National Formulary. 2020; https://www.medicinescomplete.com/mc/bnf/current.

50. Katz IR, et al. Comparison of risperidone and placebo for psychosis and behavioral disturbances associated with dementia: a randomized, double-blind trial. Risperidone Study Group. *J Clin Psychiatry* 1999; 60:107–115.

51. NHS Health Research Authority. Optimisation of amisulpride prescribing in older people. 2012; https://www.hra.nhs.uk/planning-and-improving-research/application-summaries/research-summaries/optimisation-of-amisulpride-prescribing-in-older-people.

52. Reeves S, et al. A population approach to characterise amisulpride pharmacokinetics in older people and Alzheimer's disease. *Psychopharmacology* 2016; 233:3371–3381.

53. NHS PrescQIPP. Reducing antipsychotic prescribing in dementia toolkit. 2014; https://www.prescqipp.info/our-resources/bulletins/t7-reducing-antipsychotic-prescribing-in-dementia/#:~:text=The%20PrescQIPP%20reducing%20antipsychotic%20prescribing%20in%20dementia%20toolkit,prescribing%20in%20those%20already%20being%20prescribed%20these%20drugs.

54. Brodaty H, et al. Antipsychotic deprescription for older adults in long-term care: the HALT study. *J Am Med Dir Assoc* 2018; 19:592–600. e597.

55. Campbell N, et al. Impact of cholinesterase inhibitors on behavioral and psychological symptoms of Alzheimer's disease: a meta-analysis. *Clin Interv Aging* 2008; 3:719–728.

56. Mathys M. Pharmacologic management of behavioral and psychological symptoms of major neurocognitive disorder. *Ment Health Clin* 2018; 8:284–293.

57. Verdoux H, et al. Is benzodiazepine use a risk factor for cognitive decline and dementia? A literature review of epidemiological studies. *Psychol Med* 2005; 35:307–315.

58. Lagnaoui R, et al. Benzodiazepine utilization patterns in Alzheimer's disease patients. *Pharmacoepidemiol Drug Saf* 2003; 12:511–515.

59. Billioti de Gage S, et al. Benzodiazepine use and risk of dementia: prospective population based study. *BMJ* 2012; 345:e6231.

60. Taipale H, et al. Risk of pneumonia associated with incident benzodiazepine use among community-dwelling adults with Alzheimer disease. *CMAJ* 2017; 189:E519–e529.

61. Palmaro A, et al. Benzodiazepines and risk of death: results from two large cohort studies in France and UK. *Eur Neuropsychopharmacol* 2015; 25:1566–1577.

62. Chang CM, et al. Benzodiazepine and risk of hip fractures in older people: a nested case-control study in Taiwan. *Am J Geriatr Psychiatry* 2008; 16:686–692.

63. Aboukhatwa M, et al. Antidepressants are a rational complementary therapy for the treatment of Alzheimer's disease. *Mol Neurodegener* 2010; 5:10.

64. Rozzini L, et al. Efficacy of SSRIs on cognition of Alzheimer's disease patients treated with cholinesterase inhibitors. *Int Psychogeriatr* 2010; 22:114–119.

65. Porsteinsson AP, et al. Effect of citalopram on agitation in Alzheimer disease: the CitAD randomized clinical trial. *JAMA* 2014; 311:682–691.

66. Martinon-Torres G, et al. Trazodone for agitation in dementia. *Cochrane Database Syst Rev* 2004; CD004990.

67. Ballard C, et al. Management of neuropsychiatric symptoms in people with dementia. *CNS Drugs* 2010; 24:729–739.

CHAPTER 6

68. Chow TW, et al. Potential cognitive enhancing and disease modification effects of SSRIs for Alzheimer's disease. *Neuropsychiatr Dis Treat* 2007; 3:627–636.

69. Enache D, et al. Antidepressants and mortality risk in a dementia cohort: data from SveDem, the Swedish Dementia Registry. *Acta Psychiatr Scand* 2016; 134:430–440.

70. Sommer OH, et al. Effect of oxcarbazepine in the treatment of agitation and aggression in severe dementia. *Dement Geriatr Cogn Disord* 2009; 27:155–163.

71. Tariot PN, et al. Efficacy and tolerability of carbamazepine for agitation and aggression in dementia. *Am J Psychiatry* 1998; 155:54–61.

72. Lonergan E, et al. Valproate preparations for agitation in dementia. *Cochrane Database Syst Rev* 2009; CD003945.

73. Konovalov S, et al. Anticonvulsants for the treatment of behavioral and psychological symptoms of dementia: a literature review. *Int Psychogeriatr* 2008; 20:293–308.

74. Yeh YC, et al. Mood stabilizers for the treatment of behavioral and psychological symptoms of dementia: an update review. *Kaohsiung J Med Sci* 2012; 28:185–193.

75. Sival RC, et al. Sodium valproate in aggressive behaviour in dementia: a twelve-week open label follow-up study. *Int J Geriatr Psychiatry* 2004; 19:305–312.

76. Dolder CR, et al. Valproic acid in dementia: does an optimal dose exist? *J Pharm Pract* 2012; 25:142–150.

77. Lonergan E, et al. Valproate preparations for agitation in dementia. *Cochrane Database Syst Rev* 2009; CD003945.

78. Tariot PN, et al. Chronic divalproex sodium to attenuate agitation and clinical progression of Alzheimer disease. *Arch Gen Psychiatry* 2011; 68:853–861.

79. Supasitthumrong T, et al. Gabapentin and pregabalin to treat aggressivity in dementia: a systematic review and illustrative case report. *Br J Clin Pharmacol* 2019; 85:690–703.

80. Cooney C, et al. Use of low-dose gabapentin for aggressive behavior in vascular and Mixed Vascular/Alzheimer Dementia. *J Neuropsychiatry Clin Neurosci* 2013; 25:120–125.

81. Peter-Derex L, et al. Sleep and Alzheimer's disease. *Sleep Med Rev* 2015; 19:29–38.

82. David R, et al. Non-pharmacologic management of sleep disturbance in Alzheimer's disease. *J Nutr Health Aging* 2010; 14:203–206.

83. McCleery J, et al. Pharmacotherapies for sleep disturbances in dementia. *Cochrane Database Syst Rev* 2016; 11:Cd009178.

84. Bishara D, et al. Anticholinergic effect on cognition (AEC) of drugs commonly used in older people. *Int J Geriatr Psychiatry* 2017; 32:650–656.

85. von Gunten A, et al. Efficacy of Ginkgo biloba extract EGb 761(®) in dementia with behavioural and psychological symptoms: A systematic review. *World J Biol Psychiatry* 2016; 17:622–633.

86. Ahmed M, et al. Current agents in development for treating behavioral and psychological symptoms associated with dementia. *Drugs Aging* 2019; 36:589–605.

87. Herrmann N, et al. Randomized placebo-controlled trial of nabilone for agitation in Alzheimer's disease. *Am J Geriatr Psychiatry* 2019; 27:1161–1173.

88. Tampi RR, et al. The place for electroconvulsive therapy in the management of behavioral and psychological symptoms of dementia. *Neurodegener Dis Manag*, 2019. [Epub ahead of print].

89. Glass OM, et al. Electroconvulsive therapy (ECT) for treating agitation in dementia (major neurocognitive disorder) – a promising option. *Int Psychogeriatr* 2017; 29:717–726.

CHAPTER 6

A guide to medication doses of commonly used psychotropics in older adults

Drug	Specific indication/ additional notes	Starting dose	Usual maintenance dose	Maximum dose in elderly
Antidepressants				
Agomelatine	Depression Monitor LFTs; data suggest that agomelatine is not effective in patients >75 years	25mg nocte	25–50mg daily	50mg nocte
Citalopram	Depression/anxiety disorder	10mg mane	10–20mg mane	20mg mane
Clomipramine	Depression/phobic and obsessional states	10mg nocte (dose increases should be cautious)	30–75mg daily[1] should be reached after about 10 days	75mg daily[1]
Desvenlafaxine	No formal recommendations are available for dosing in older adults[2] Reduced doses may be advisable in geriatric patients due to decreased clearance; every other day dosing may be considered in geriatric patients with poor tolerability to the drug For older adults, possible reduced renal clearance of desvenlafaxine should be considered when determining an appropriate dose Dosage in renal impairment: CrCl 50–80mL/minute: no dosage adjustment needed CrCl 30–50mL/minute: 50mg daily is the recommended daily and maximum dose CrCl <30mL/minute or end-stage renal disease: 50mg every other day is the recommended daily and maximum dose Older adults are also at greater risk for developing clinically significant hyponatremia[2]			400mg daily[2]
Duloxetine	Depression/anxiety disorder	30mg daily*	60mg daily	120mg daily[3] (caution as limited data in elderly for this dose)
Escitalopram	Depression/anxiety disorder	5mg mane	5–10mg mane	10mg mane

(Continued)

(Continued)

Drug	Specific indication/ additional notes	Starting dose	Usual maintenance dose	Maximum dose in elderly
Fluoxetine	Depression/anxiety disorder Caution as long half-life and inhibitor of several CYP enzymes	20mg mane	20mg mane	40mg mane usually (but 60mg can be used)
Lofepramine	Depression	35mg nocte*	70mg nocte*	140mg nocte or in divided doses* (occasionally 210mg nocte required)
Mirtazapine	Depression	7.5mg nocte or usually 15mg nocte*	15–30mg nocte	45mg nocte
Sertraline	Depression/anxiety disorder	25–50mg mane (25mg can be increased to 50mg mane after 1 week)	50–100mg mane*	100mg (occasionally up to 150mg mane)*
Trazodone	Depression	100mg daily in divided doses or as a single night-time dose[4]	100–200mg daily*	300mg daily[4]
	Agitation in dementia Avoid single doses >100mg	25mg bd*	25–100mg daily*	200mg daily* (in divided doses)
Venlafaxine	Depression/anxiety disorder Monitor BP on initiation	37.5mg mane (increased to 75mg XL mane after 1 week)*	75–150mg (XL) mane*	150mg daily (occasionally 225mg daily necessary)*
Vortioxetine	Major depressive disorder	5–10mg daily[5]	5–20mg daily[5]	20mg daily[5] Max for CYP2D6 poor metabolisers: 10mg/day. Co-administration of certain drugs may need to be avoided or dosage adjustments may be necessary; review drug interactions

Antipsychotics

Amisulpride	Chronic schizophrenia	50mg daily*	100–200mg daily*	400mg daily[6] (caution > 200mg daily)*
	Late life psychosis	25–50mg daily*	50–100mg daily* (increase in 25mg steps)	200mg daily[7] (caution > 100mg daily)*
	Agitation/psychosis in dementia Caution: QTc prolongation	25mg nocte[8]	25–50mg daily[8]	50mg daily[8]
Aripiprazole	Schizophrenia, mania (oral)	5mg mane*	5–15mg daily*	20mg mane*
	Control of agitation (IM injection)	5.25mg*	5.25–9.75mg*	15mg daily* (combined oral + IM)
Brexpiprazole	Dosage not established in older adults[9]			
Cariprazine	Dosage not established in older adults[10]			
Clozapine	Schizophrenia	6.25–12.5mg daily[11,12] increased by not more than 6.25–12.5mg once or twice a week[11]	50–100mg daily[11,12]	100mg daily[11,12]
	Parkinson's related psychosis	6.25mg daily[13]	25–37.5mg daily[13]	50mg daily[13]
	IM injection	The oral bioavailability of clozapine is about half that of the intramuscular injection. E.g. 50mg daily of the IM injection is roughly equivalent to 100mg daily of the tablets/oral solution. After each injection has been given, the patient must be observed every 15 minutes for the first 2 hours to check for excess sedation. NB: If IM lorazepam is required, leave at least ONE HOUR between administration of IM clozapine and IM lorazepam		
Iloperidone	No formal recommendations are available for dosing in older adults			

(Continued)

Drug	Specific indication/additional notes	Starting dose	Usual maintenance dose	Maximum dose in elderly
Lumateperone[14]	Schizophrenia	42mg daily (equivalent to 60mg lumateperone tosylate) Dose titration not required	42mg daily	42mg daily
Lurasidone	Schizophrenia	37mg once daily (or 18.5mg daily when given with concomitant moderate CYP3A4 inhibitors (max. dose 74 mg once daily). Dosing for elderly with normal renal function (CrCl ≥80mL/minute) are the same as for adults with normal renal function. However, because elderly may have diminished renal function, dose adjustments may be required according to their renal function status[15]	18.5–111mg daily[16]	Limited data on higher doses used in older adults. No data are available in elderly people treated with 148mg. Caution should be exercised when treating patients ≥65 years of age with higher doses[15]
Olanzapine	Schizophrenia	2.5mg nocte*	5–10mg daily*	15mg nocte[12]
	Agitation/psychosis in dementia	2.5mg nocte*	2.5–10mg daily*	10mg nocte* (optimal dose is 5mg daily)[12]
Pimavanserin[17]	Schizophrenia	34mg daily (or 10mg daily if co-administered with strong CYP3A4 inhibitors) Dose titration not required	34mg daily (or 10mg daily if co-administered with strong CYP3A4 inhibitors)	34mg daily (or 10mg daily if co-administered with strong CYP3A4 inhibitors) Monitor patients for reduced efficacy if used concomitantly with strong CYP3A4 inducers
Quetiapine	Schizophrenia	12.5–25mg daily[12]	75–125mg daily[11]	200–300mg daily[12]
	Agitation/psychosis in dementia	12.5–25mg daily*	50–100mg daily*	100–300mg daily[12]

Drug	Specific indication/additional notes	Starting dose	Usual maintenance dose	Maximum dose in elderly
Risperidone	Psychosis	0.5mg bd (0.25–0.5mg daily in some cases)[12]	1–2.5mg daily[11]	4mg daily
	Late onset psychosis	0.5mg daily*	1mg daily*	2mg daily* (optimal dose is 1mg daily)
	Agitation/psychosis in dementia	0.25mg daily* or bd	0.5mg bd	2mg daily (optimal dose is 1mg daily)[12]
Haloperidol	Psychosis	0.25–0.5mg daily[11]	1–3.5mg daily[11]	Caution >3.5mg- assess tolerability and ECG
	Agitation Avoid in older adults (except in delirium) owing to the risk of QTc prolongation	0.25–0.5mg daily*	0.5–1.5mg daily or bd	Max 5mg/day (oral) Max 5mg/day (IM) Doses >5mg/day should only be considered in patients who have tolerated higher doses and after reassessment of the patient's individual benefit–risk profile

NB: All antipsychotic drugs contain warnings for increased mortality in elderly patients with dementia.

Drug	Specific indication/additional notes	Starting dose	Usual maintenance dose	Maximum dose in elderly
Long-acting conventional antipsychotic drugs				
Flupentixol decanoate		Test dose: 5–10mg	After at least 7 days of test dose: 10–20mg every 2–4 weeks* Dose increased gradually according to response and tolerability in steps of 5–10mg every 2 weeks*	40mg every 2 weeks* (extend frequency to every 3–4 weeks if EPS develops) (occasionally up to 50 or 60mg every 2 weeks* may be used if tolerated)

(Continued)

(Continued)

Drug	Specific indication/additional notes	Starting dose	Usual maintenance dose	Maximum dose in elderly
Fluphenazine decanoate	Caution: high risk of EPSE	Test dose 6.25mg	After 4–7 days of test dose: 12.5–25mg every 2–4 weeks Dose increased gradually according to response and tolerability in steps of 12.5mg every 2–4 weeks*	50mg every 4 weeks*
Haloperidol decanoate	Risk of EPSE and QTc prolongation	(No test dose) 12.5–25mg every 4 weeks	12.5–25mg every 4 weeks	50mg every 4 weeks*
Pipotiazine palmitate[18]		Test dose 5–10mg	25–100mg every 4 weeks	100mg every 4 weeks*
Zuclopenthixol decanoate		Test dose: 25–50mg	After at least 7 days of test dose: 50–200mg every 2–4 weeks*	200mg every 2 weeks*

Long-acting atypical antipsychotic drugs

Drug	Specific indication/additional notes	Starting dose	Usual maintenance dose	Maximum dose in elderly
Aripiprazole Long-acting injection	No formal recommendations are available for dosing in older adults However, there is no detectable effect of age on pharmacokinetics[19]			
Olanzapine pamoate[20]	Has not been systematically studied in elderly patients (>65 years). Not recommended for treatment in the elderly population unless a well-tolerated and effective dose regimen using oral olanzapine has been established. A lower starting dose (150mg/4 weeks) is not routinely indicated but should be considered for those 65 and above when clinical factors warrant. Not recommended to be started in patients >75 years old			
Paliperidone palmitate	Dose based on renal function: Because elderly patients may have diminished renal function, they are dosed as in mild renal impairment even if tests show normal renal function*	Loading doses: Day 1: 100mg Day 8: 75mg (lower loading doses may be appropriate in some)*	25–100mg monthly*	100mg monthly*

Drug	Specific indication/Additional notes	Starting dose	Usual maintenance dose	Maximum dose in elderly
Paliperidone palmitate 3-monthly injection	Dose based on renal function: Because elderly patients may have diminished renal function, they are dosed as in mild renal impairment even if tests show normal renal function*	If the last dose of 1-monthly paliperidone palmitate injectable is: 50mg 75mg 100mg	Initiate the 3-monthly injection at the following doses: 175mg 263mg 350mg (There is no equivalent dose for the 25mg dose of 1-monthly paliperidone palmitate injection)[21]	350mg 3 monthly*
Risperidone Long-acting injection	Monitor renal function	25mg every 2 weeks	25mg every 2 weeks	25mg every 2 weeks Consider 37.5mg every 2 weeks in patients treated with oral risperidone doses >4mg/day[22]

NB: All antipsychotic drugs contain warnings for increased mortality in elderly patients with dementia.

Drug	Specific indication/Additional notes	Starting dose	Usual maintenance dose	Maximum dose in elderly
Mood stabilisers				
Carbamazepine	Bipolar disorder Caution: drug interactions Check LFTs, FBC and U&Es Consider checking plasma levels	50mg bd or 100mg bd*	200–400mg/day*	600–800mg/day*
Lamotrigine	Bipolar disorder (titration as in young adults) Check for interactions and make appropriate dose alterations (see BNF)	25mg daily (monotherapy)	Increase by 25mg steps every 14 days	200mg/day*
		25mg on alternate days (if with valproate)	Increase by 25mg steps every 14 days	100mg/day*
		50mg daily (if with carbamazepine)	Increase by 50mg steps every 14 days	100mg bd*

(Continued)

Drug	Specific indication/Additional notes	Starting dose	Usual maintenance dose	Maximum dose in elderly
Lithium carbonate M/R	Bipolar disorder Mania/depression Caution: drug interactions Check renal and thyroid function and regularly monitor plasma levels	100*–200mg nocte	200–600mg daily*	600–1200mg daily (aim for plasma levels 0.4–0.7 mmol/L in elderly)[23]
Sodium valproate	Bipolar disorder Check LFTs and consider checking plasma levels	Sodium valproate: 100–200mg bd* Semi-sodium valproate: 250mg daily or bd*	Sodium valproate: 200–400mg bd* Semi-sodium valproate: 500mg to 1g daily*	Sodium valproate: 400mg bd* Semi-sodium valproate: 1g daily*
	Agitation in dementia (not licensed and not recommended) Check response, tolerability and plasma levels for guide	Sodium valproate: 50mg bd (liquid) or 100mg bd*	Sodium valproate: 100–200mg bd*	Sodium valproate: 200mg bd*

Drug	Specific indication/additional notes	Starting dose	Usual maintenance dose	Maximum dose in elderly
Anxiolytics/hypnotics				
Clonazepam	Agitation	0.5mg daily	1–2mg/day*	4mg/day*
Diazepam	Agitation	1mg tds	1mg tds*	7.5–15mg/day in divided doses (for anxiety)
Lemborexant[24]	Insomnia	5mg nocte (take no more than once per night, immediately before bed)	5–10mg nocte	10mg nocte Elderly are at a higher risk of falls. Caution when using doses >5mg in patients ≥65 years old

Drug	Indication / notes			
Lorazepam	PRN only – avoid regular use due to short half-life and risk of dependence	0.5mg daily	0.5–2mg daily*	2mg/day
Melatonin	Insomnia – short-term use (up to 13 weeks)	2mg (modified release) once daily (1–2 hours before bedtime)		
Pregabalin	Generalised anxiety disorder Dose adjustment based on renal function (see product information)[25]	Usually 25mg bd (increase by 25mg bd weekly) Up to 75mg bd (if healthy and normal renal function)	Usually 150mg daily* Up to 150mg bd (if healthy and normal renal function)	150–300mg/day*
Zolpidem	Insomnia (short-term use – up to 4 weeks)	5mg nocte	5mg nocte	5mg nocte
Zopiclone	Insomnia (short-term use – up to 4 weeks)	3.75mg nocte	3.75–7.5mg nocte	7.5mg nocte

*There is no specific information available in the literature for these drug doses in elderly patients – the doses stated are a guide only. Where there are no data, the maximum doses are conservative and may be exceeded if the drug is well tolerated and following clinician's assessment.
bs, bis die (twice a day); mane, morning; nocte, at night; prn, pro re nata (as required); tds, ter die sumendum (three times a day).

References

1. Mylan. Summary of product characteristics. Clomipramine 25 mg Capsules, Hard. 2017; https://www.medicines.org.uk/emc/medicine/33260

2. Prescribers' Digital Reference. Desvenlafaxine – drug summary. 2017 (Last accessed September 2020); http://www.pdr.net/drug-summary/Khedezla-desvenlafaxine-3333.8274.

3. Eli Lilly and Company Limited. Summary of product characteristics. Cymbalta 30mg hard gastro-resistant capsules, Cymbalta 60mg hard gastro-resistant capsules. 2020; https://www.medicines.org.uk/emc/medicine/15694.

4. Zentiva. Summary of product characteristics. Molipaxin 100mg/Trazodone 100mg Capsules. 2020; https://www.medicines.org.uk/emc/medicine/26734.

5. Prescribers' Digital Reference. Trintellix (vortioxetine) – drug information. 2017 (Last accessed September 2020); http://www.pdr.net/drug-information/trintellix?druglabelid=3348

6. Muller MJ, et al. Amisulpride doses and plasma levels in different age groups of patients with schizophrenia or schizoaffective disorder. *J Psychopharmacol* 2009; 23:278–286.

7. Psarros C, et al. Amisulpride for the treatment of very-late-onset schizophrenia-like psychosis. *Int J Geriatr Psychiatry* 2009; 24:518–522.

8. Clark-Papasavas C, et al. Towards a therapeutic window of D2/3 occupancy for treatment of psychosis in Alzheimer's disease, with [F]fallypride positron emission tomography. *Int J Geriatr Psychiatry* 2014; 29:1001–1009.

9. Prescribers' digital reference. Brexpiprazole – Drug Summary. 2017 (Last accessed September 2020); http://www.pdr.net/drug-summary/Rexulti-brexpiprazole-3759

10. Prescribers' Digital Reference. Vraylar (cariprazine) – drug information. 2017 (Last accessed September 2020); http://www.pdr.net/drug-information/vraylar?druglabelid=3792.

11. Jeste DV, et al. Conventional vs. newer antipsychotics in elderly patients. *Am J Geriatr Psychiatry* 1999; 7:70–76.

12. Karim S, et al. Treatment of psychosis in elderly people. *Adv Psychiatr Treatment* 2005; 11:286–296.

13. Group TPS. Low-dose clozapine for the treatment of drug-induced psychosis in Parkinson's disease. *N Engl J Med* 1999; 340: 757–763.

14. Intra-Cellular Therapies Inc. Highlights of prescribing information. Caplyta (lumateperone) capsules for oral use. 2019; https://www.accessdata.fda.gov/drugsatfda_docs/label/2019/209500s000lbl.pdf.

15. Sunovion Pharmaceuticals Europe Ltd. Summary of product characteristics. Latuda 18.5mg, 37mg and 74mg film-coated tablets. 2020; https://www.medicines.org.uk/emc/medicine/29125.

16. Sajatovic M, et al. Efficacy and tolerability of lurasidone in older adults with bipolar depression: analysis of two 6-week double-blind, placebo-controlled studies. *Eur Psychiatry* 2015; 30:1136.

17. ACADIA Pharmaceuticals Inc. Highlights of prescribing information. Nuplazid (pimavanserin) tablets for oral use. 2016; https://www.accessdata.fda.gov/drugsatfda_docs/label/2016/207318lbl.pdf.

18. Drugs.com. Piportil depot 50 mg/ml solution for injection. 2020 (Last accessed September 2020); https://www.drugs.com/uk/piportil-depot-50-mg-ml-solution-for-injection-leaflet.html#.

19. Otsuka Pharmaceutical (UK) Ltd. Summary of product characteristics. Abilify Maintena 300mg & 400mg powder and solvent for prolonged-release suspension for injection and suspension for injection in pre filled syringe. 2020; https://www.medicines.org.uk/emc/medicine/31386.

20. Eli Lily and Company Limited. Summary of product characteristics. Zypadhera 210mg powder and solvent for prolonged release suspension for injection. 2020; https://www.medicines.org.uk/emc/product/6429/smpc.

21. Janssen-Cilag Limited. Summary of product characteristics. TREVICTA 175mg, 263mg, 350mg, 525mg prolonged release suspension for injection. 2019; https://www.medicines.org.uk/emc/medicine/32050.

22. Janssen-Cilag Limited. Summary of product characteristics. RISPERDAL CONSTA 25 mg powder and solvent for prolonged-release suspension for intramuscular injection. 2018; https://www.medicines.org.uk/emc/medicine/9939.

23. Essential Pharma Ltd. Summary of product characteristics. Camcolit 400mg controlled release Lithium Carbonate. 2020; https://www.medicines.org.uk/emc/product/10829/smpc.

24. Eisai Inc. Highlights of prescribing information. DAYVIGO (lemborexant) tablets for oral use [controlled substance schedule pending]. 2019; https://www.accessdata.fda.gov/drugsatfda_docs/label/2019/212028s000lbl.pdf#page=21.

25. Upjohn UK Limited. Summary of product characteristics. Lyrica Capsules. 2020; https://www.medicines.org.uk/emc/medicine/14651.

Covert administration of medicines within food and drink

This section deals with covert medication provision within UK law only.

In mental health settings it is common for patients to refuse medication. Some patients with cognitive disorders may lack capacity to make an informed choice about whether medication will be beneficial to them or not. In these cases, the clinical team may consider whether it would be in the patient's best interests to conceal medication in food or drink. This practice is known as covert administration of medicines. Guidance from the Royal Pharmaceutical Society and Royal College of Nursing,[1] and the Royal College of Psychiatrists[2] has been published in order to protect patients from the unlawful and inappropriate administration of medication in this way. In the UK, the legal framework for such interventions is either the Mental Capacity Act (MCA)[3] or, more rarely, the MHA.[4]

Assessment of mental capacity[3,5,6]

When it applies to the covert administration of medicines, the assessment of capacity regarding treatment is primarily a matter for the prescriber, usually a doctor treating the patient,[3,5] or less commonly a pharmacist or a nurse prescriber. Nurses and allied health professionals who are not prescribers will also have to be mindful of their own codes of professional practice and should be satisfied that the doctor's assessment is reasonable. In assessing capacity, the assessment must be made in relation to the particular treatment proposed. Capacity can vary over time and the assessment should be made at the time of the proposed treatment. The assessment should be documented in the patient's notes and recorded in the care plan.

A patient is presumed to have the capacity to make treatment decisions unless he/she is felt to have some form of mental illness or disturbance of mind *and* is unable to do one or more of the following:

- understand the information relevant to the decision
- retain that information
- use or weigh that information as part of the process of making the decision, or
- communicate his/her decision (whether by talking, using sign language or any other means).

Guidance on covert administration

If a patient has the capacity to give a valid refusal to medication and is not detainable under the MHA, their refusal should be respected.

If a patient has the capacity to give a valid refusal and is either being treated under the MHA or is legally detainable under the Act, the provisions of the MHA with regard to treatment will apply (which are outside the scope of this chapter).

The administration of medicines to patients who lack the capacity to consent and who are unable to appreciate that they are taking medication (e.g. unconscious patients) should not need to be carried out covertly. However, some patients who lack the capacity to consent would be aware of receiving medication, if they were not deceived into thinking otherwise.[7] For example, a patient with moderate dementia who has no insight and does not believe he/she needs to take medication, but will take liquid medication if this is mixed with his/her tea without him/her being aware of this. It is this group to whom the rest of this guidance applies.

Treatment may be given to people who lack capacity if it has been concluded that treatment is in the patient's best interests (Section 5 MCA[3]) and is proportionate to the harm to be avoided (Chapter 6.41, MCA Code of Practice[6]). So, there should be a clear expectation that the patient will benefit from covert administration, and that this will avoid significant harm (either mental or physical) to the patient or others. The treatment must be necessary to save the patient's life, to prevent deterioration in health or to ensure an improvement in physical or mental health.[3,6]

Covert administration must be the least restrictive option after trying all other options. A functional assessment should be carried out to try to understand why the person is refusing to take their medicines. Alternative methods of administration (e.g. liquid formulation), and trial of different approaches in nursing care (e.g. spending time with the patient to explain about the medicines at the time they are administered or changing the time of administration to a time of day when the patient is more alert or less distressed) should also be considered.[8]

The decision to administer medication covertly should not be made by a single individual but should involve discussion with the multidisciplinary team caring for the patient and the patient's relatives or informal carers. It is good practice to hold a 'Best Interests Meeting'. If it were determined at the Best Interests Meeting that the provision of covert medication would amount to a deprivation of liberty (where previously there was none), then an application for Deprivation of Liberty Safeguards (DoLS) authorisation should be made. Decisions regarding covert administration of medication should be carefully documented in the patient's medical records with a clear management plan, including details of how the covert medication plan will be reviewed. This documentation must be easily accessible on viewing the person's records and the decision should be subject to regular review.

It is not necessary to have a new Best Interests Meeting each time there is a change in medication. However, when covert medication is first considered, healthcare professionals should consider what types of changes in medication may be anticipated in future and should agree on the thresholds of what changes may require a new Best Interests Meeting. This management plan should be recorded in the patient's notes. If significant changes that could cause adverse effects are envisaged, then a new Best Interests Meeting should be held before these changes are made.

In deciding how often capacity assessments should be repeated, clinicians should follow the guidance within the Practical Guide to the MCA.[5] If there is any evidence that the patient has re-gained capacity, an immediate capacity assessment must be done. Decisions in the patient's best interests can no longer be made, their DoLS authorisation will no longer be valid and covert administration of medication must cease immediately.

Recent Case Law[9,10] has dealt with the relationship between the use of covert medication and the need for a DoLS authorisation. Patients are deprived of their liberty when they are under continuous supervision and control and are not free to leave. The administration of covert medication will only in itself lead to a deprivation of liberty where that covert medication affects the patients' behaviour, mental health or it acts as a sedative to such an extent that it will deprive the patients of their liberty. The use of covert medication within a care plan must be clearly identified within the DoLS assessment and authorisation.

When considering covert use of psychiatric medication:[11]

1. If the patient meets the criteria for the MHA, this must be used in preference to the MCA.
2. The MCA can be used as authority for covert use of psychiatric medication in patients who are not under the MHA if the medication is necessary to prevent deterioration or ensure an improvement in the patient's mental health and it is in the person's best interest to receive the drug. The usual procedures for covert medication, including documentation of capacity assessment, best interests meeting and pharmacist's review, should be followed.
3. Caution is needed in the use of medication, which may sedate or reduce a patient's physical mobility (see the earlier paragraph), as use of such drugs may constitute a Deprivation of Liberty and require the patient to be under the DoLS framework. Documentation of whether the proposed use of a covert psychiatric drug constitutes a Deprivation of Liberty is important. NB: if a patient is found to lack capacity to consent to the admission and does not meet the criteria for detention under the MHA, DoLS should be used, so most inpatients who lack capacity to consent to medication will already be under the MHA or DoLS, although there may be some who can consent to admission but not to medication.

Summary of process

The process for covert administration of medicines should include the following:

- The assurance that all efforts have been made to give medication openly in its normal form before considering covert administration.
- Assessment of capacity of the patient to make a decision regarding their treatment with medication. If the patient has capacity, their wishes should be respected and covert medication not administered.
- A record of the examination of the patient's capacity must be made in the clinical notes, and evidence for incapacity documented.
- If the patient lacks capacity, there should be a Best Interests Meeting which should be attended by relevant health professionals and a person who can communicate the views and interests of the patient (family member, friend or independent mental capacity advocate). These meetings can be held virtually. If the patient has an attorney appointed under the MCA for health and welfare decisions, then this person should be present at the meeting.

- Those attending the meeting should ascertain whether the patient has made an Advance Decision refusing a particular medication or treatment which can be used to guide decision-making.
- The Best Interests Meeting should consider whether a formal legal procedure such as the MHA or DoLS is appropriate. Discussion of the indications and use of this legislation in the context of covert medication is outside the scope of this guidance but specialist psychiatric and/or legal opinion should be sought in individual circumstances if necessary.
- Medication should not be administered covertly until a Best Interests Meeting has been held. If the situation is urgent it is acceptable for a less formal discussion to occur between carer/nursing staff, prescriber and family/advocate in order to make an urgent decision, but a formal meeting should be arranged as soon as possible.
- After the meeting, there should be clear documentation of the outcome of the meeting. If the decision is to use covert administration of medication, a check should be made with the pharmacy to determine whether the properties of the medications are likely to be affected by crushing and/or being mixed with food or drink. The medication chart should be amended to describe how the medication is to be administered.
- When the medication is administered in foodstuffs, it is the responsibility of the dispensing nurse to ensure that the medication is taken. This can be facilitated by direct observation or by nominating another member of the clinical team to observe the patient taking the medication.
- A plan should be made to review on a regular basis the need for continued covert administration of medicines.

Additional information

- For patients in Care Homes, the NICE Guidelines – Managing medicines in care homes – March 2014 should be referred to.[12,13] The basic principles of this NICE guidance are the same as this policy. Mental health practitioners have a duty to inform the Care Home manager if they suspect the correct procedures are not being followed as regards covert medication, and to discuss with their team leader possible safeguarding referral if the home manager does not act on their advice. The role of mental health teams supporting care homes is to support the care homes and prescriber (usually GP) in carrying out this guidance. For patients with complex mental health needs, it may be appropriate that they attend or contribute to the Best Interests Meeting. However, it should be the prescriber (usually the GP), care home staff and care home pharmacist who manage the process.
- There are no specific restrictions to state that relatives or other informal carers cannot give medication covertly and in certain cases it may be acceptable as long as they have been advised to do so by a health professional (e.g. GP), and all standards of the policy have been met.

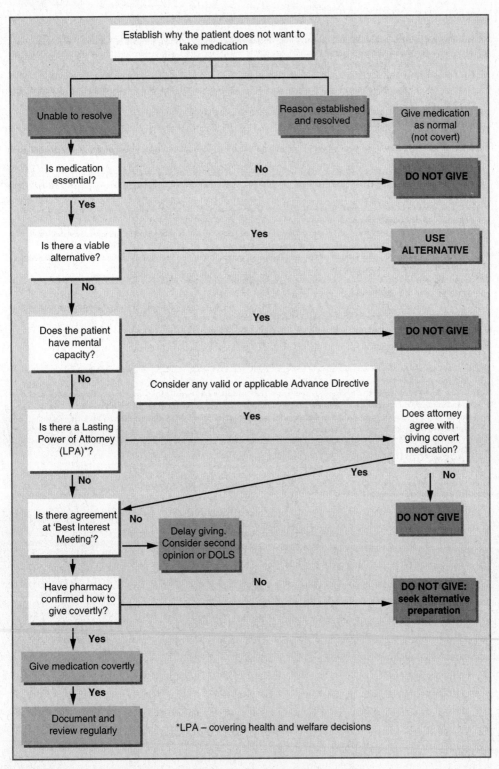

Figure 6.2 Algorithm for determining whether or not to administer medicines covertly

References

1. Royal Pharmaceutical Society and Royal College of Nursing. Professional guidance on the administration of medicines in healthcare settings. 2019; https://www.rpharms.com/Portals/0/RPS%20document%20library/Open%20access/Professional%20standards/SSHM%20and%20 Admin/Admin%20of%20Meds%20prof%20guidance.pdf?ver=2019-01-23-145026-567.

2. Royal College of Psychiatrists. College statement on covert administration of medicines. *Psychiatric Bulletin* 2004; 28:385–386.

3. Office of Public Sector Information. Mental capacity act 2005 – Chapter 9. 2005; http://www.legislation.gov.uk/ukpga/2005/9/pdfs/ukpga_20050009_en.pdf.

4. The National Archives. Mental health act 2007; http://www.legislation.gov.uk/ukpga/2007/12/contents.

5. British Medical Association and the Law Society. *Assessment of mental capacity. a practical guide for doctors and lawyer*, 4th ed. London: Law Society Publishing, 2015.

6. Office of the Public Guardian. Mental capacity act code of practice (updated 2016). https://www.gov.uk/government/publications/mental-capacity-act-code-of-practice.

7. Department for Constitutional Affairs. Mental capacity act 2005 – code of practice. 2005; http://www.justice.gov.uk.

8. Care Quality Commission. Covert administration of medicines. 2020; https://www.cqc.org.uk/guidance-providers/adult-social-care/covert-administration-medicines.

9. Hempsons. Newsflash: covert medication and DOLS – new court guidance. 2016; http://www.hempsons.co.uk/news/newsflash-covert-medication-dols-new-court-guidance.

10. The Prescription Training Company Ltd. Covert administration of medicines. Recent court of protection ruling on covert medication – 6th July 2016. https://medicationtraining.co.uk/covert-administration-medicines.

11. Care Quality Commission. Brief guide: covert medication in mental health services. 2016; https://www.cqc.org.uk/sites/default/files/20161122_briefguide-covert_medication.pdf.

12. National Institute for Health and Care Excellence. Managing medicines in care homes. Social Care Guideline [SC1] 2014 (updated 2020); https://www.nice.org.uk/guidance/sc1.

13. PrescQIPP. Bulletin 101 – Best practice guidance in covert administration of medication. 2015; https://www.prescqipp.info/umbraco/surface/authorisedmediasurface/index?url=%2fmedia%2f1174%2fb101-covert-administration-21.pdf.

Further reading

Quality Care Commission. Covert administration of medicines 2020; https://www.cqc.org.uk/guidance-providers/adult-social-care/covert-administration-medicines

Kelly Fatemi. Covert administration of medicines in care homes The Pharmaceutical Journal 2016. https://www.pharmaceutical-journal.com/cpd-and-learning/learning-article/covert-administration-of-medicines-in-care-homes/20201536.fullarticle?firstPass=false

National Institute for Health and Care Excellence. Medicines Management in care Homes. NICE Quality Standard 2015; https://www.nice.org.uk/guidance/qs85/resources/medicines-management-in-care-homes-pdf-2098910254021

For Scotland

Mental Welfare Commission for Scotland. Good Practice Guide: Covert administration 2013 (reviewed 2017); https://www.mwcscot.org.uk/sites/default/files/2019-06/covert_medication.pdf

Treatment of depression in older people

The prevalence of most physical illnesses increases with age. Many physical problems such as cardiovascular disease, chronic pain, diabetes and Parkinson's disease are associated with a high risk of depressive illness.[1,2] The morbidity and mortality associated with depression are increased in older adults[3] as they are more likely to be physically frail and therefore vulnerable to serious consequences from self-neglect (e.g. life-threatening dehydration or hypothermia) and immobility (e.g. venous stasis). Almost 20% of completed suicides occur in older people.[4] Mortality is reduced by effective treatment of depression.[5]

Meta-analysis of placebo-controlled and antidepressant-controlled studies has found a response rate of 51% in older patients,[6] similar to that for the adult population (Table 6.8).[7] There is a common perception that older patients do not respond as well to antidepressants as their younger counterparts,[8] perhaps because of structural brain changes or higher rates of physical co-morbidity.[9] It may be that biological age is more relevant than chronological age;[10] presence of physical illness, as well as baseline anxiety and reduced executive functioning are associated with poorer treatment outcomes.[11]

Nonetheless, even in older people, it may still be possible to identify non-responders as early as 4 weeks into treatment.[12,13]

A Cochrane review examined the efficacy, and associated withdrawal rates of different classes of antidepressants in older people found that SSRIs and tricyclics are of the same efficacy; however, TCAs are associated with higher withdrawal rates.[14] NICE guidance for Depression in adults recommends starting with an SSRI in the first instance (sertraline is the commonly used first line in older people). When switching to another antidepressant, NICE recommend switching initially to a different SSRI or a better tolerated newer generation antidepressant (often mirtazapine), and subsequently an antidepressant of a different pharmacological class that may be less well tolerated, for example venlafaxine, a TCA or an Monoamine oxidase inhibitor (MAOI)[15] (note that caution should be used when using TCAs and MAOIs in older people due to associated adverse effects and drug interactions).

Network meta-analysis suggests that quetiapine, duloxetine, agomelatine, imipramine and vortioxetine are superior for efficacy in major depressive disorder in older people, although individual data are somewhat inconsistent.[16] Two studies have found that older people who had recovered from an episode of depression and had received antidepressants for 2 years, 60% relapsed within 2 years if antidepressant treatment was withdrawn.[17,18] This finding held true for first episode patients. Lower doses of antidepressants may be effective as prophylaxis. Dothiepin (dosulepin) 75mg/day has been shown to be effective in this regard.[19] Note that NICE recommend that dosulepin should not be used as it is particularly cardiotoxic in overdose.[15]

There is no ideal antidepressant in older people. All are associated with problems. TCAs are broadly considered less desirable due to the increased risk of cardiac conduction abnormalities and anticholinergic effects. SSRIs are generally better tolerated than TCAs;[14] they do, however, increase the risk of GI bleeds, particularly in the very old and those with established risk factors such as a history of bleeds or treatment with a NSAID, steroid or warfarin. The risk of other types of bleed such as haemorrhagic

Table 6.8 Antidepressants and older people

	Anticholinergic side effects (urinary retention, dry mouth, blurred vision, constipation)	Postural hypotension	Sedation	Weight gain	Safety in overdose	Other side effects	Drug interactions
Older tricyclics[20]	Variable: moderate with nortriptyline, imipramine and dosulepin (dothiepin) Marked with others All can also cause central anticholinergic effects (confusion)	All can cause postural hypotension Dosage titration is required	Variable: from minimal with imipramine to profound with trimipramine	All tricyclics can cause weight gain	Dothiepin and amitriptyline are the most toxic (seizures and cardiac arrhythmia)	Seizures, anticholinergic-induced cognitive impairment Increased risk of bleeds with serotonergic drugs	Mainly pharmacodynamic: increased sedation with benzodiazepines, increased hypotension with diuretics, increased constipation with other anticholinergic drugs, etc.
Lofepramine	Moderate, although constipation/sweating can be severe	Can be a problem but generally better tolerated than the older tricyclics	Minimal	Few data, but lack of spontaneous reports may indicate less potential than the older tricyclics	Relatively safe	Raised LFTs Less likely to cause hyponatraemia than other TCAs and SSRIs	

Table 6.8 (Continued)

SSRIs[20,21]	Dry mouth can be a problem with paroxetine	Much less of a problem, but an increased risk of falls is documented with SSRIs	Can be a problem with paroxetine and fluvoxamine. Unlikely with the other SSRIs	Paroxetine and possibly citalopram may cause weight gain. Others are weight neutral	Safe with the possible exception of citalopram; one minor metabolite can cause QTc prolongation. Significance unknown	GI effects and headaches, hyponatraemia, increased risk of bleeds in the older person (add gastroprotection if also on an NSAID or aspirin), orofacial dyskinesia with paroxetine, cognitive impairment,[22] interstitial lung disease[23,24]	Fluvoxamine, fluoxetine and paroxetine are potent inhibitors of several hepatic cytochrome enzymes (see section on antidepressant drug interactions). Sertraline is safer and citalopram, escitalopram and vortioxetine are safest
Others[25,26]	Minimal with mirtazapine and venlafaxine*. Can be rarely a problem with reboxetine*. Duloxetine* – few effects. Very low incidence with agomelatine	Venlafaxine can cause hypotension at lower doses, but it can increase BP at higher doses, as can duloxetine. Dizziness common with agomelatine	Mirtazapine, mianserin and trazodone are sedatives. Venlafaxine, duloxetine – neutral effects. Agomelatine aids sleep	Greatest problem is with mirtazapine, although older people are not particularly prone to weight gain. Low incidence with agomelatine	Venlafaxine is more toxic in overdose than SSRIs, but safer than TCAs. Others are relatively safe	Insomnia and hypokalaemia with reboxetine. Nausea with venlafaxine, duloxetine. Weight loss and nausea with duloxetine. Possibly hepatotoxicity with agomelatine. Monitor LFTs. Cognitive impairment with trazodone[22]. Interstitial lung disease with serotonin and norepinephrine reuptake inhibitors[24]	Duloxetine inhibits CYP2D6. Moclobemide and venlafaxine inhibit CYP450 enzymes. Check for potential interactions. Reboxetine is safe. Agomelatine should be avoided in patients who take potent CYP1A2 inhibitors

*Noradrenergic drugs may produce 'anticholinergic' effects via norepinephrine re-uptake inhibition.

stroke may also be increased[27,28] (see section 'SSRIs and bleeding'). Older people are also particularly prone to develop hyponatraemia[29] with SSRIs (see section 'Hyponatraemia', Chapter 3), as well as postural hypotension and falls (the clinical consequences of which may be increased by SSRI-induced osteopenia;[30] TCAs may also increase fracture risk.[31]

Agomelatine is effective in older patients, is well tolerated and has not been linked to hyponatraemia.[32,33] Its use is limited by the need for frequent blood sampling to check LFTs. Vortioxetine and duloxetine have also been shown to be effective and reasonably well tolerated in the older person[34] but caveats related to SSRIs, above, are relevant here. A general practice database study found that, compared with SSRIs, 'other antidepressants' (venlafaxine, mirtazapine, etc.) were associated with a greater risk of a number of potentially serious side effects in the older people (stroke/TIA, fracture, seizures, attempted suicide/self-harm) as well as increased all-cause mortality;[29] the study was observational and so could not separate the effect of antidepressants from any increased risk inherent in the group of patients treated with these antidepressants. Polysaturated fatty acids (fish oils) may be helpful in mild-to-moderate depression (compared with placebo).[35]

The effect of antidepressants on cognition in later life is still debated – some studies found antidepressants to worsen cognitive outcomes,[22,36,37] others found no effect.[38] The choice of antidepressant may affect the risk; highly anticholinergic medicines are known to increase the likelihood of developing dementia.[39]

Ultimately, choice is determined by the individual clinical circumstances of each patient, particularly physical co-morbidity and concomitant medication (both prescribed and 'over the counter'; (See section on antidepressant interactions with physical drugs).

References

1. Katona C, et al. Impact of screening old people with physical illness for depression? *Lancet* 2000; **356**:91–92.
2. Lyketsos CG. Depression and diabetes: more on what the relationship might be. *Am J Psychiatry* 2010; **167**:496–497.
3. Gallo JJ, et al. Long term effect of depression care management on mortality in older adults: follow-up of cluster randomized clinical trial in primary care. *BMJ* 2013; **346**:f2570.
4. Cattell H, et al. One hundred cases of suicide in elderly people. *Br J Psychiatry* 1995; **166**:451–457.
5. Ryan J, et al. Late-life depression and mortality: influence of gender and antidepressant use. *Br J Psychiatry* 2008; **192**:12–18.
6. Gutsmiedl K, et al. How well do elderly patients with major depressive disorder respond to antidepressants: a systematic review and single-group meta-analysis. *BMC Psychiatry* 2020; **20**:102.
7. Cipriani A, et al. Comparative efficacy and acceptability of 21 antidepressant drugs for the acute treatment of adults with major depressive disorder: a systematic review and network meta-analysis. *Lancet* 2018; **391**:1357–1366.
8. Paykel ES, et al. Residual symptoms after partial remission: an important outcome in depression. *Psychol Med* 1995; **25**:1171–1180.
9. Iosifescu DV, et al. Brain white-matter hyperintensities and treatment outcome in major depressive disorder. *Br J Psychiatry* 2006; **188**:180–185.
10. Brown PJ, et al. Biological age, not chronological age, is associated with late-life depression. *J Gerontol A Biol Sci Med Sci* 2018; **73**:1370–1376.
11. Tunvirachaisakul C, et al. Predictors of treatment outcome in depression in later life: A systematic review and meta-analysis. *J Affect Disord* 2018; **227**:164–182.
12. Zilcha-Mano S, et al. Early symptom trajectories as predictors of treatment outcome for citalopram versus placebo. *Am J Geriatr Psychiatry* 2017; **25**:654–661.
13. Mulsant BH, et al. What is the optimal duration of a short-term antidepressant trial when treating geriatric depression? *J Clin Psychopharmacol* 2006; **26**:113–120.
14. Mottram P, et al. Antidepressants for depressed elderly. *Cochrane Database Syst Rev* 2006; CD003491.
15. National Institute for Health and Care Excellence. Depression in adults: recognition and management. Clinical guideline [CG90]. 2009 (Last updated December 2013); https://www.nice.org.uk/Guidance/cg90.

16. Krause M, et al. Efficacy and tolerability of pharmacological and non-pharmacological interventions in older patients with major depressive disorder: A systematic review, pairwise and network meta-analysis. *Eur Neuropsychopharmacol* 2019; **29**:1003–1022.

17. Flint AJ, et al. Recurrence of first-episode geriatric depression after discontinuation of maintenance antidepressants. *Am J Psychiatry* 1999; **156**:943–945.

18. Reynolds CF, III, et al. Maintenance treatment of major depression in old age. *N Engl J Med* 2006; **354**:1130–1138.

19. Old Age Depression Interest Group. How long should the elderly take antidepressants? A double-blind placebo-controlled study of continuation/prophylaxis therapy with dothiepin. *Br J Psychiatry* 1993; **162**:175–182.

20. Draper B, et al. Tolerability of selective serotonin reuptake inhibitors: issues relevant to the elderly. *Drugs Aging* 2008; **25**:501–519.

21. Bose A, et al. Escitalopram in the acute treatment of depressed patients aged 60 years or older. *Am J Geriatr Psychiatry* 2008; **16**:14–20.

22. Leng Y, et al. Antidepressant use and cognitive outcomes in very old women. *J Gerontol A Biol Sci Med Sci* 2018; **73**:1390–1395.

23. Deidda A, et al. Interstitial lung disease induced by fluoxetine: systematic review of literature and analysis of Vigiaccess, Eudravigilance and a national pharmacovigilance database. *Pharmacol Res* 2017; **120**:294–301.

24. Rosenberg T, et al. The relationship of SSRI and SNRI usage with interstitial lung disease and bronchiectasis in an elderly population: a case-control study. *Clin Interv Aging* 2017; **12**:1977–1984.

25. Raskin J, et al. Safety and tolerability of duloxetine at 60 mg once daily in elderly patients with major depressive disorder. *J Clin Psychopharmacol* 2008; **28**:32–38.

26. Johnson EM, et al. Cardiovascular changes associated with venlafaxine in the treatment of late-life depression. *Am J Geriatr Psychiatry* 2006; **14**:796–802.

27. Smoller JW, et al. Antidepressant use and risk of incident cardiovascular morbidity and mortality among postmenopausal women in the Women's Health Initiative study. *Arch Intern Med* 2009; **169**:2128–2139.

28. Laporte S, et al. Bleeding risk under selective serotonin reuptake inhibitor (SSRI) antidepressants: A meta-analysis of observational studies. *Pharmacol Res* 2017; **118**:19–32.

29. Coupland C, et al. Antidepressant use and risk of adverse outcomes in older people: population based cohort study. *BMJ* 2011; **343**:d4551.

30. Williams LJ, et al. Selective serotonin reuptake inhibitor use and bone mineral density in women with a history of depression. *Int Clin Psychopharmacol* 2008; **23**:84–87.

31. Power C, et al. Bones of contention: a comprehensive literature review of Non-SSRI antidepressant use and bone health. *J Geriatr Psychiatry Neurol* 2019; **33**:340–352.

32. Heun R, et al. The efficacy of agomelatine in elderly patients with recurrent Major Depressive Disorder: a placebo-controlled study. *J Clin Psychiatry* 2013; **74**:587–594.

33. Laux G. The antidepressant efficacy of agomelatine in daily practice: results of the non-interventional study VIVALDI. *Eur Psychiatry* 2011; **26** Suppl 1:647.

34. Katona C, et al. A randomized, double-blind, placebo-controlled, duloxetine-referenced, fixed-dose study comparing the efficacy and safety of Lu AA21004 in elderly patients with major depressive disorder. *Int Clin Psychopharmacol* 2012; **27**:215–223.

35. Bae JH, et al. Systematic review and meta-analysis of omega-3-fatty acids in elderly patients with depression. *Nutr Res* 2018; **50**:1–9.

36. Moraros J, et al. The association of antidepressant drug usage with cognitive impairment or dementia, including Alzheimer disease: A systematic review and meta-analysis. *Depress Anxiety* 2017; **34**:217–226.

37. Chan JYC, et al. Depression and antidepressants as potential risk factors in dementia: a systematic review and meta-analysis of 18 longitudinal studies. *J Am Med Dir Assoc* 2019; **20**:279–286.e271.

38. Carriere I, et al. Antidepressant use and cognitive decline in community-dwelling elderly people – the three-city cohort. *BMC Med* 2017; **15**:81.

39. Wang YC, et al. Increased risk of dementia in patients with antidepressants: a meta-analysis of observational studies. *Behav Neurol* 2018; **2018**:5315098.

Further reading

Kok RM, et al. Management of depression in older adults: a review. *JAMA* 2017; **317**:2114–2122.

Pruckner N, et al. Antidepressant pharmacotherapy in old-age depression – a review and clinical approach. *Eur J Clin Pharmacol* 2017; **73**:661–667.

Wilkinson P, et al. Continuation and maintenance treatments for depression in older people. *Cochrane Database of Sys Rev* 2016; **9**:Cd006727.

Chapter 7

Pregnancy and breastfeeding

Drug choice in pregnancy

A 'normal' outcome to pregnancy can never be guaranteed. The spontaneous abortion rate in confirmed early pregnancy is 10–20% and the risk of spontaneous major malformation is 2–3% (approximately 1 in 40 pregnancies).[1]

Lifestyle factors have an important influence on pregnancy outcome. It is well established that smoking cigarettes, eating a poor diet and drinking alcohol during pregnancy can have adverse consequences for the foetus. Pre-pregnancy obesity increases the risk of neural tube defects (obese women seem to require higher doses of folate supplementation than women who have a BMI in the healthy range[2]).

In addition, psychiatric illness during pregnancy is an independent risk factor for congenital malformations, stillbirths and neonatal deaths.[3] Perinatal mental disorders are associated with risks for a broad range of negative child outcomes, many of which can persist into late adolescence.[4] Affective illness, anxiety disorders, eating disorders and other mental disorders increase the risk of preterm delivery.[5,6] Note that preterm delivery is also associated with an increased risk of depression, bipolar disorder and schizophrenia spectrum disorders in subsequent adult life.[7]

The safety of psychotropics in pregnancy cannot be clearly established because robust, prospective trials are obviously unethical and long-term observational studies are obviously challenging to undertake. Individual decisions on psychotropic use in pregnancy are therefore based on database studies that have many limitations (e.g. failure to control for the effects of illness, smoking, obesity, other medications and other confounders, multiple statistical tests increasing the risk of Type 2 error and exposure status based on pharmacy data), limited prospective data from teratology information centres, and published case reports which are known to be biased towards selective reporting of adverse outcomes. At worst there may be no human data at all, but only animal data from early preclinical studies. With new drugs early reports of adverse outcomes may or may not be replicated and a 'best guess' assessment must be made of the risks and benefits associated with withdrawal or continuation of drug treatment. Even with established drugs, data related to long-term outcomes are rare.

The Maudsley® Prescribing Guidelines in Psychiatry, Fourteenth Edition. David M. Taylor,
Thomas R. E. Barnes and Allan H. Young.
© 2021 David M. Taylor. Published 2021 by John Wiley & Sons Ltd.

It is also important to note that pregnancy does not protect against mental illness and may even elevate overall risk if medication is stopped. In late pregnancy and early post-partum there is an increased risk of relapse, irrespective of medication use.

The patient's view of risks and benefits have paramount importance and needs to be informed by up to date evidence provided by their clinician. Clinicians should be aware of the importance of prescribing medication to women with a severe mental illness. Perinatal suicides are notable for being associated with lack of active treatment, specifically treatment with psychotropic medication.[8]

This section provides a brief summary of the relevant issues and evidence to date. Box 7.1 summarises the general principles of prescribing in pregnancy.

Box 7.1 General principles of prescribing in pregnancy

In all women of child-bearing potential

- Always discuss the possibility of pregnancy – half of all pregnancies are unplanned.[9]
- Avoid using drugs that are contra-indicated during pregnancy in women of reproductive age (notably valproate and carbamazepine). If these drugs are prescribed, women should be made fully aware of their teratogenic properties even if not planning pregnancy. Consider prescribing folate. Valproate should be reserved for post-menopausal women only. Its use in younger women should be treatment of last resort.[10]

If mental illness is newly diagnosed in a pregnant woman

- Try to avoid all drugs in the first trimester (when major organs are being formed) unless benefits outweigh risks, that is, if non-drug treatments are not effective/appropriate, and then use an established drug at the lowest effective dose

If a woman taking psychotropic drugs is planning a pregnancy

- Consideration should be given to discontinuing treatment if the woman is well and at low risk of relapse.
- Discontinuation of treatment for women with SMI and at a high risk of relapse is unwise, but consideration should be given to switching to a low-risk drug. However, be aware that switching drugs may increase the risk of relapse and consider changes in the context of the woman's illness history and previous response to treatment

If a woman taking psychotropic medication discovers that she is pregnant

- Abrupt discontinuation of treatment post-conception for women with SMI and at a high risk of relapse is unwise; relapse may ultimately be more harmful to the mother and child than continued, effective drug therapy.
- Consider remaining with current (effective) medication rather than switching, to minimise the risk of relapse and hence the number of drugs to which the foetus is exposed.
- Valproate (if prescribed as a mood stabiliser) should be stopped.

If the patient smokes (smoking is more common in pregnant women with psychiatric illness[11])

- Smoking has been associated with the greatest proportion of excess risk associated with poor pregnancy outcomes.[12]
- Always encourage switching to nicotine replacement therapy – smoking has numerous adverse outcomes, NRT does not.[13] Referral to smoking cessation services is mandated by NICE and engagement should therefore be encouraged and supported where possible.
- Stopping smoking can increase plasma levels of certain drugs, for example, clozapine.

In all pregnant women

- Ensure that the parents are as involved as possible in all decisions.
  - Use the lowest effective dose.
  - Use the drug with the lowest known risk to mother and foetus.
- Prescribe as few drugs as possible both simultaneously and in sequence.
- Be prepared to adjust doses as pregnancy progresses and drug handling is altered. Dose increases are frequently required in the third trimester[14] when blood volume expands by around 30%. Plasma level monitoring may be helpful, where available. Note that hepatic enzyme activity changes markedly during pregnancy; CYP2D6 activity is increased by almost 50% by the end of pregnancy while the activity of CYP1A2 is reduced by up to 70%.[15]
- Consider referral to specialist perinatal services.
- Ensure adequate foetal screening.
- Be aware of potential problems with individual drugs around the time of delivery.
- Inform the obstetric team of psychotropic use and possible complications.
- Monitor the neonate for withdrawal effects after birth.
- Document all decisions.

What to include in discussions with pregnant women[16]

Discussions should include:
- The woman's ability to be treated with non-pharmacological interventions. This should include previous response to non-pharmacological interventions.
- The potential impact of an untreated mental disorder on the foetus or infant.
- The risks from stopping medication abruptly.
- Severity of previous episodes, response to treatment and the woman's preference.
- The background risk of foetal malformations for pregnant women without a mental disorder.
- The increased risk of harm associated with drug treatments during pregnancy and the postnatal period, including the risk of overdose (and acknowledge uncertainty surrounding risks).
- The possibility that stopping a drug with known teratogenic risk after pregnancy is confirmed may not remove the risk of malformations.
- Breastfeeding.

Where possible, written material should be provided to explain the risks (preferably individualised). Absolute and relative risks should be discussed. Risks should be described using natural frequencies rather than percentages (e.g., 1 in 10 rather than 10%) and common denominators (e.g., 1 in 100 and 25 in 100, rather than 1 in 100 and 1 in 4).

Psychosis during pregnancy and postpartum

- Pregnancy does not protect against relapse.
- Psychosis during pregnancy predicts postpartum psychosis.[17]
- The incidence of postpartum psychosis is 0.1–0.25% in the general population (around 1–2 psychiatric hospitalisations per 1000 births).
- Women with bipolar disorder have an increased risk of postpartum psychosis with around one in five experiencing a psychotic relapse postpartum.[18]

- There is a high risk of relapse in women with a family history of postpartum psychosis or a personal history of postpartum psychosis.[19]
- The mental health of the mother in the perinatal period influences foetal well-being, obstetric outcome and child development.

The risks of not treating psychosis include:

- Harm to the mother through poor self-care or judgement, lack of obstetric care or impulsive acts including suicide.
- Harm to the foetus or neonate (ranging from neglect to infanticide).

It has long been established that people with schizophrenia are more likely to have minor physical anomalies than the general population. Some of these anomalies may be apparent at birth, while others are more subtle and may not be obvious until later in life. This background risk complicates assessment of the effects of antipsychotic drugs. (Psychiatric illness itself during pregnancy is an independent risk factor for congenital malformations and perinatal mortality.)

Treatment with antipsychotics

First generation antipsychotics

- Are generally considered to have minimal risk of teratogenicity,[20,21] although data are less than convincing, as might be expected.
- Most initial data originated from studies that included primarily women with hyperemesis gravidarum (a condition associated with an increased risk of congenital malformations) treated with low doses of phenothiazines. The modest increase in risk identified in some of these studies, along with no clear clustering of congenital abnormalities, suggests that the condition being treated may be responsible rather than drug treatment.
- A prospective study that included 284 women who took an FGA (mostly haloperidol, promethazine or flupentixol) during pregnancy concluded that preterm birth and low birth weight were more common with FGAs than SGAs (or no antipsychotic exposure).[22] In total, 20% of neonates exposed to an FGA in the last week of gestation experienced early somnolence and jitteriness.
- In a recent large American study including over a million women, no meaningful increase in the risk of major malformations or cardiac malformations was seen in 733 women prescribed an FGA.[23]
- There may be an association between haloperidol and limb defects (based on a small number of cases), but if real, the risk is likely to be extremely low.
- Neonatal dyskinesia has been reported with FGAs.[24]
- Neonatal jaundice has been reported with phenothiazines.[20]

It remains uncertain whether FGAs are entirely without risk to the foetus or to later development.[20,21] However, this continued uncertainty and the wide use of these drugs over several decades suggest that any risk is small – an assumption borne out by most studies.[25]

Second-generation antipsychotics

- Are unlikely to be major teratogens.
- A prospective study that included 561 women who took an SGA (mostly olanzapine, quetiapine, clozapine, risperidone or aripiprazole) during pregnancy concluded that SGA exposure was associated with increased birth weight, a modestly increased risk of cardiac septal defects (possibly due to screening bias or co-exposure to SSRIs), and, as with FGAs, withdrawal effects in 15% neonates.[20]
- However, in a large American study including over a million women, no meaningful increase in the risk of major malformations or cardiac malformations was seen in 9258 women prescribed an SGA. A small increase in absolute risk was seen with risperidone. The authors suggest that this particular finding should be interpreted with caution and be seen as an initial safety signal which requires further investigation.[23] In a separate study of 214 women taking an SGA the absolute risk of major malformation was estimated to be 1.4% compared with 1.1% in the control group.[23]
- A separate American study which analysed data from the National Birth Defects Prevention Study reported an increased association between SGA use in early pregnancy and conotruncal heart defects, tetralogy of fallot, anorectal atresia/stenosis and gastroschisis. The study included over 22,000 cases and over 11,000 controls. Women exposed to SGAs were more likely to report pre-pregnancy obesity, illicit drug use, smoking and alcohol use and use of other psychiatric medications during pregnancy.[26]
- In a population-based study of over a million women an increased risk of gestational diabetes, caesarean section, large for gestational age and preterm birth were reported in women prescribed an SGA compared with no antipsychotic. The risks of caesarean section and large for gestational age were reported to be higher with SGAs compared with FGAs.[27] Maternal mental illness may also be an important factor in the risk for gestational diabetes.[28,29] Aripiprazole may not be associated with an increased risk.[30]
- There are most data for olanzapine, which has been associated with both lower birth weight and increased risk of intensive care admission,[31] a large head circumference[32] and with macrosomia;[33] the last of these is consistent with the reported increase in the risk of gestational diabetes.[20,32,34,35] Olanzapine seems to be relatively safe with respect to congenital malformations; the prevalence being consistent with population norms in a study that reported on 610 prospectively followed pregnancies.[36] Olanzapine has however been associated with a range of problems including hip dysplasia,[37] meningocele, ankyloblepharon,[38] and neural tube defects[20] (an effect that could be related to pre-pregnancy obesity rather than drug exposure[39]). Importantly there is no clustering of congenital malformations.
- The use of clozapine appears to present no increased risk of malformation, although gestational diabetes and neonatal seizures may be more likely to occur.[34] There is a single case report of maternal overdose resulting in foetal death[20] and there are theoretical concerns about the risk of agranulocytosis in the foetus/neonate.[20] Pharmacovigilance data do not indicate clozapine to be less safe in pregnancy than other antipsychotics.[40] Clozapine is now included by NICE in medications that may be prescribed in pregnancy. Lower mean adaptive behaviour scores have been reported in infants exposed to clozapine in-utero compared with risperidone, quetiapine or olanzapine. A higher rate of disturbed sleep and liability was reported in clozapine-exposed infants in the same study.[41] On the balance of evidence available,

clozapine should usually be continued. Clozapine plasma level monitoring may be beneficial[42] and especially if there are changes in smoking habits.
- No congenital malformations at birth or development abnormalities were observed at five months in an infant exposed to aripiprazole long-acting injection in utero.[43]
- The manufacturers of cariprazine have advised against its use in pregnancy because of an increased risk of malformations noted in animal studies.
- Antipsychotic exposure in pregnancy increases the risk of gestational diabetes mellitus.[44] Maternal mental illness and associated risk factors are also important factors.[29]
- The effect of SGAs on long-term neurodevelopment remains unclear.[45] A small prospective case-control study reported that babies who were exposed to antipsychotics in-utero, had delayed cognitive, motor and social-emotional development at 2 and 6 months old but not at 12 months.[46] The clinical significance of this finding, if any, is unclear.

Overall, these data do not allow an assessment of relative risks associated with different agents and certainly do not confirm absolutely the safety of any particular drug. At least two studies have suggested a small increased risk of malformation[22,31]; however, a more recent study including over a million women found no meaningful increase in the risk of malformations with FGAs or SGAs after correcting for key confounders.[23] Antipsychotic use during pregnancy may be associated with an increased risk of gestational diabetes, caesarean section[31] and stillbirth,[47] though this may be due to confounders. As with other drugs, decisions must be based on the latest available information and an individualised assessment of probable risks and benefits. If possible, specialist advice should be sought, and primary reference sources consulted. Recommendations for the psychosis in pregnancy are outlined in Box 7.2.

Box 7.2 Recommendations – psychosis in pregnancy

- Patients with a history of psychosis who are maintained on antipsychotic medication should be advised to discuss a planned pregnancy as early as possible.
- Women should be supported to minimise the risks in pregnancy from smoking and alcohol and drug misuse. Women should be referred to appropriate services, such as smoking cessation clinics and addictions services.
- Be aware that drug-induced hyperprolactinaemia may prevent pregnancy. Consider switching to alternative drug if hyperprolactinaemia occurs and pregnancy is planned.
- If a pregnant woman is stable on an antipsychotic and likely to relapse without medication, advise her to continue the antipsychotic.[16] Switching medication is generally not advised owing to the risk of relapse. Consider using the antipsychotic that has worked best for the woman after discussion of benefits and risks.[48] This may minimise foetal exposure by avoiding the need for higher doses if woman relapses, and/or multiple drugs should relapse occur.
- Most reproductive safety data are available for quetiapine, olanzapine, risperidone, and haloperidol with more limited data for clozapine, aripiprazole and ziprasidone. Quetiapine has a relative low rate of placental passage.[48,49]
- Advise pregnant women taking antipsychotic medication about diet and monitor for excessive weight gain.
- Women taking an antipsychotic during pregnancy should be monitored for gestational diabetes. NICE recommends women be offered an oral glucose tolerance test.
- NICE recommends avoiding depot preparations in a woman planning a pregnancy, pregnant or considering breastfeeding, unless she is responding well to a depot and has a previous history of non-adherence with oral medication.[16]

- Antipsychotic discontinuation symptoms can occur in the neonate (e.g. crying, agitation, increased suckling). This is thought to be a class effect.[50] When antipsychotics are taken in pregnancy it is recommended that the woman gives birth in a unit that has access to paediatric intensive care facilities.[22] Some centres used mixed (breast/bottle) feeding to minimise withdrawal symptoms.

Depression during pregnancy and postpartum[51-53]

- Approximately 10% of pregnant women develop or have a preexisting depressive illness. Around a third of cases of postpartum depression begin before birth.
- There is a significant increase in new psychiatric episodes in the first 3 months after delivery. At least 80% are mood disorders, particularly severe depression.
- Women who have had a previous episode of depressive illness (postpartum or not) are at higher risk of further episodes during pregnancy and postpartum. The risk is highest in women with bipolar illness who are also at risk of mania or mixed affective episodes.
- There is some evidence that depression increases the risk of spontaneous abortion, having a low birth weight or small for gestational age baby, or of preterm delivery, though effects are small.[4,54,55] The mental health of the mother influences foetal well-being, obstetric outcome and child development.

The risks of not treating depression include:

- Harm to the mother through poor self-care, lack of obstetric care or self-harm.
- Harm to the foetus or neonate (ranging from neglect to infanticide).

Treatment with antidepressants

Relapse rates are higher in those with a history of depression who discontinue medication compared to those who continue. One study found that 68% of women who were well on antidepressant treatment and stopped during pregnancy relapsed, compared with 26% who continued antidepressants.[51] Risk is likely to be highest for women with a history of severe and/or recurrent depression.[56]

Some data suggest that antidepressants may increase the risk of spontaneous abortion (but note that confounding factors were not controlled for), preterm delivery, low birth weight, respiratory distress in the neonate, a low APGAR score at birth and admission to a special care baby unit.[57] Most studies are observational and do not control for maternal depression. In a large cohort study the presence of depressive symptoms but not antidepressant use[58] was associated with preterm birth and babies small for gestational age. Interestingly, a large Finnish study found SSRI use to be associated with a lower risk of preterm birth and caesarean delivery compared with unexposed women diagnosed with a psychiatric illness[59] and untreated maternal depression itself is associated with an increased risk of both low birth weight and preterm birth[60]. SSRIs do not appear to increase the risk of stillbirth or neonatal mortality.[61,62]

While it is reasonably certain that commonly used antidepressants are not major teratogens,[63] some antidepressants have been associated with specific congenital malformations,[64] many of which are rare. Most of these potential associations remain unreplicated[54] and it is not possible to exclude confounding by indication.[65] There are conflicting data on the issue of the influence of duration of antidepressant use.[66,67]

The effects on early growth and neurodevelopment are poorly studied; the limited data that do exist, are reassuring.[68-70] One small study reported abnormal general movements in neonates exposed to SSRIs in utero.[71] A small increase in the risk of childhood autism has also been suggested[72,73] but not confirmed by several large studies[74-76] and a meta-analysis which found that preconception exposure was more consistently associated with autism spectrum disorders than any trimester exposure, suggesting confounding by indication.[77] SSRIs may be associated with a higher risk of poor neonatal adaptation syndrome than SNRIs.[78] Increased levels of anxiety symptoms have been reported in exposed children.[79]

Women who take antidepressants during pregnancy may be at increased risk of developing hypertension,[80,81] preeclampsia[82] and postpartum haemorrhage.[83-85] It has been suggested that SSRIs may cause the last of these by reducing serotonin mediated uterine contraction as well as interfering with hemostasis.[86] A subsequent smaller study did not confirm this association; possibly because it was underpowered to do so.[87] Depression itself may increase the risk of preeclampsia.[88]

There is also some evidence that successful antidepressant use can be beneficial for child behavioural outcomes, for example, a Danish study on antidepressant exposure found that adverse outcomes were more likely in depressed women not taking antidepressants.[85]

Tricyclic antidepressants

- Foetal exposure to tricyclics (via umbilicus and amniotic fluid) is high.[89,90]
- TCAs have been widely used throughout pregnancy without apparent detriment to the foetus.[63,91,92]
- A weak association between clomipramine use and cardiovascular defects cannot be excluded[93] and the European SPC for Anafranil states: 'Neonates whose mothers had taken tricyclic antidepressants until delivery have developed dyspnoea, lethargy, colic, irritability, hypotension or hypertension, tremor or spasms, during the first few hours or days. Studies in animals have shown reproductive toxicity. Anafranil is not recommended during pregnancy and in women of childbearing potential not using contraception.' One case of neonatal QT prolongation and Torsades de Pointes has been reported following maternal clomipramine use[94] and one case of Timothy Syndrome 1, a disorder characterised by severe QT prolongation in a newborn whose mother took amitriptyline in early pregnancy.[95]
- Some authorities recommend the use of nortriptyline and desipramine (not available in the UK) if using tricyclics because these drugs are less anticholinergic and hypotensive than amitriptyline and imipramine (respectively, their tertiary amine parent molecules).
- TCA use during pregnancy increases the risk of preterm delivery.[91,92,96]
- Use of TCAs in the third trimester is well known to produce neonatal withdrawal effects; agitation, irritability, seizures, respiratory distress and endocrine and metabolic disturbances.[91] These are usually mild and self-limiting.
- Little is known of the developmental effects of prenatal exposure to tricyclics, although one small study detected no adverse consequences.[97] Limited data suggest in utero exposure to tricyclics has no effects on later development.[97,98]

Selective serotonin reuptake inhibitors

- Sertraline appears to result in the least placental exposure.[99]
- SSRIs appear not to be major teratogens,[63,67,91,100] with most data supporting the safety of fluoxetine.[97,101–104] Note though that one study revealed a slight overall increase in rate of malformation with SSRIs.[105,106] Database and case–control studies have reported an association between SSRIs and anencephaly, craniosynostosis, omphalocele, clubfoot and increased umbilical cord length[107] in the newborn.[108–110] A population study which aimed to examine the risk of specific birth defects with individual antidepressants reported an elevated risk for specific SSRIs and non-heart defects.[111] However, the study only partially accounted for the underlying condition.[111]
- Paroxetine has been specifically associated with cardiac malformations[112–114] particularly after high dose (>25mg/day), first trimester exposure.[115] However some studies have failed to replicate this finding for paroxetine,[91,116] and have implicated other SSRIs.[117–119] A higher risk of some cardiac birth defects has been reported to be associated with paroxetine and fluoxetine compared with other SSRIs.[120] Other studies have found no association between any SSRI and an increased risk of cardiac septal defects[109,121,122] and other heart defects.[111,123–126] Note that one database study reported that foetal alcohol disorders were 10 times more common in those exposed to SSRIs in utero than controls,[127] and that alcohol use during pregnancy (which may be used as self-medication for depression) is associated with an increased risk of cardiac defects in the foetus.[93]
- SSRIs have also been associated with decreased gestational age[128] (usually a few days which is of questionable clinical significance[129]), spontaneous abortion[130] gestational hypertension and pre-eclampsia,[131] decreased birth weight (mean 175g)[101,102,132] and suboptimal foetal growth.[133] It is possible that these effects are primarily associated with maternal depression rather than specifically with antidepressant treatment.[129] The longer the duration of in utero exposure, the greater the chance of low birth weight and respiratory distress.[66] Three groups of symptoms are seen in neonates exposed to antidepressants in late pregnancy; those associated with serotonergic toxicity, those associated with antidepressant discontinuation symptoms and those related to early birth.[134] Neonatal discontinuation syndrome may be associated with prematurity.[135] Third-trimester exposure to sertraline has been associated with reduced early APGAR scores.[101] Third-trimester use of paroxetine may give rise to neonatal complications, presumably related to abrupt withdrawal.[136,137] Other SSRIs have similar, possibly less severe effects.[137,138] Body temperature instability, poor feeding, respiratory distress, cardiac rhythm disturbance, lethargy, muscle tone anomalies, jitteriness, jerky movements and seizures have been reported.[93] A case of transient neonatal long QT syndrome has been reported after in utero exposure to paroxetine.[139]
- Data relating to neurodevelopmental outcome of foetal exposure to SSRIs are less than conclusive.[97,98,140–143] Depression itself may have more obvious adverse effects on development.[97] Maternal SSRI use has been associated with autism spectrum disorders.[144–146] However, large studies have either failed to show this association after accounting for maternal illness[74–76] or have found it to be no longer significant.[147,148] Authors of a study which reported a small increased risk of ADHD in children whose

fathers used an SSRI before conception proposed this may be due to the underlying indications related to SSRI use.[149]

- Poorer cognitive and gross motor development[150] and problems with speech and language,[151–153] behaviour[154,155] and fine motor control and have been reported[156] but it is not clear whether or not this is due to confounding.

- Exposure to selective serotonin reuptake inhibitors or serotonin norepinephrine reuptake inhibitors during pregnancy is associated with an increased risk for persistent pulmonary hypertension of the newborn. The risk with sertraline may be lower than with other SSRIs.[157] The absolute risk appears to be small and more modest than previously estimated[158] and may exist only in late pregnancy exposure.[159]

- An association between SSRIs and an increased the risk of postpartum haemorrhage has been reported.[84,160] However, SSRIs have also been shown not to significantly increase the risk of blood loss at delivery.[161] Obstetricians and midwives need to be aware of this possible increase in risk and monitor for blood loss after labour.

Other antidepressants

- Duloxetine is unlikely to be a major teratogen. A large cohort study using propensity scores and several sensitivity analyses found that use in pregnancy may be associated with a small increase in the risk of postpartum hemorrhage.[162] No specific risks were identified with duloxetine in a study that prospectively followed 233 women through pregnancy and delivery.[163] However, a case of suspected withdrawal syndrome, requiring hospitalisation has been reported.[164]

- Rather more scarce data suggest the absence of teratogenic potential with moclobemide[165] and reboxetine.[166] Venlafaxine has been associated with cardiac defects, anencephaly and cleft palate,[167] neonatal withdrawal and poor neonatal adaptation syndrome[102] and PPH.[162] However, newer data suggests that first trimester use appears not to be associated with an increased risk of major congenital malformations.[168] Second trimester exposure to venlafaxine has been associated with babies being born small for gestational age.[169] An observational study of 281 venlafaxine exposed pregnancies did not find conclusive evidence that venlafaxine increases the risk of adverse pregnancy or foetal outcomes.[170] A population study which aimed to examine the risk of specific birth defects with individual antidepressants reported venlafaxine use to be associated with a higher risk. However, the study only partially accounted for the underlying condition.[111] Trazodone, bupropion (amfebutamone) and mirtazapine have few data supporting their safety.[102,171,172] Data suggest that both bupropion and mirtazapine are not associated with malformations but, like SSRIs, may be linked to an increased rate of spontaneous abortion.[173–175] First trimester exposure to bupropion may be associated with a slightly elevated risk of ventricular septal defects.[176] Bupropion exposure in-utero has been associated with an increased risk of ADHD in young children.[177,178]

- MAOIs should be avoided in pregnancy because of a suspected increased risk of congenital malformations and because of the risk of hypertensive crisis.[179]

- There is no evidence to suggest that ECT causes harm to either the mother or foetus during pregnancy[180] although general anaesthesia is of course not without risks.

NICE recommends ECT for pregnant women with severe depression, severe mixed affective states or mania, or catatonia, whose physical health or that of the fetus is at serious risk. Box 7.3 summarises recommendations for treating depression in pregnancy.

Box 7.3 Recommendations – depression in pregnancy

- Patients who are already receiving antidepressants and are at high risk of relapse are best maintained on the same antidepressant during and after pregnancy.
- Those who develop a moderate–severe or severe depressive illness during pregnancy should be treated with antidepressant drugs.
- If initiating an antidepressant during pregnancy or for a woman considering pregnancy previous response to treatment must be taken into account. The antidepressant which has previously proved to be effective should be considered. For previously untreated patients, sertraline may be considered.
- Screen for alcohol use and be vigilant for the development of hypertension and preeclampsia. Women who take SSRIs may be at increased risk of postpartum haemorrhage.
- When taken in late pregnancy, SSRIs may increase the risk of persistent pulmonary hypertension of the new-born. The absolute risk is very low.
- The neonate may experience discontinuation symptoms, which are usually mild, such as agitation and irritability, or rarely respiratory distress and convulsions (with SSRIs). The risk is assumed to be particularly high with short half-life drugs such as paroxetine and venlafaxine. Continuing to breastfeed and then 'weaning' by switching to mixed (breast/bottle) feeding may help reduce the severity of reactions.

Bipolar illness during pregnancy and postpartum

- The risk of relapse during pregnancy if mood stabilising medication is discontinued is high; one study found that bipolar women who were euthymic at conception and discontinued mood stabilisers were twice as likely to relapse and spent five times as long in relapse ill than women who continued mood stabilisers.[181] However, others have found illness severity rather than medication changes in pregnancy to predict pregnancy relapse.[182]
- The risk of relapse after delivery is hugely increased.
- The mental health of the mother influences foetal well-being, obstetric outcome and child development.
- Women with bipolar illness are 50% more likely than controls to have their labour induced or a caesarean delivery, a preterm delivery, and a neonate that is small for gestational age; the neonate is also more likely to have hypoglycaemia and micro-cephaly.[6] These associations hold true in both treated and untreated women.
- Bipolar illness itself does not seem to significantly increase the malformation rate; any such association is with mood stabilising drugs.[6]

The risks of not stabilising mood include:

- Harm to the mother through poor self-care, lack of obstetric care or self-harm.
- Harm to the foetus or neonate (ranging from neglect to infanticide).

Treatment with mood stabilisers

- **Lithium** completely equilibrates across the placenta.[183]
- Lithium exposure during pregnancy has been associated with an increased risk of congenital anomalies.[184] The risk is higher in the first trimester[185] and maybe be higher at higher doses.[184] Although the overall risk of major malformations in infants exposed in utero has probably been overestimated in the past lithium should be avoided in pregnancy if possible. However, if lithium is the best drug for the woman and the drug most likely to keep her well the woman should be advised of the increased risk but supported to stay on lithium.
- If discontinuation is planned slow discontinuation before conception is the preferred course of action[34,186] because abrupt discontinuation is suspected of worsening the risk of relapse. The relapse rate postpartum may be as high as 70% in women who discontinued lithium before conception.[187] If discontinuation is unsuccessful during pregnancy restart and continue.
- Lithium use during pregnancy has a well-known association with the cardiac malformation Ebstein's anomaly. However, more recent data suggest that the magnitude of the effect is much smaller than previously estimated.[188,189] Furthermore, a large surveillance study of 5.6 million births found an association with maternal mental health problems generally rather than specifically with lithium.[190]
- The period of maximum risk to the foetus is 2–6 weeks after conception,[191] before many women know that they are pregnant. The risk of atrial and ventricular septal defects may also be increased.[31]
- If lithium is continued during pregnancy, high-resolution ultrasound and echocardiography should be performed in liaison with foetal medicine obstetric services.
- In the third trimester, the use of lithium may be problematic because of changing pharmacokinetics: an increasing dose of lithium is required to maintain the lithium level during pregnancy as total body water increases, but the requirements return abruptly to pre-pregnancy levels immediately after delivery.[192] NICE recommends lithium plasma be adjusted to maintain the plasma level within the woman's therapeutic range and that lithium should be stopped during active labour and the plasma level checked 12 hours after her last dose.[16,193] Women taking lithium should deliver in hospital where fluid balance can be monitored and maintained.
- A large cohort study reported that lithium was not associated with placenta-mediated complications or preterm birth.[194]
- Lithium use may increase the risk of neonatal readmission within 4 weeks postpartum.[185]
- Neonatal goitre, hypotonia, lethargy and cardiac arrhythmia can occur.
- Most data relating to **carbamazepine, valproate** and lamotrigine come from studies in epilepsy, a condition associated with increased neonatal malformation. These data may not be precisely relevant to use in mental illness.
- Both carbamazepine and valproate have a clear causal link with increased risk of a variety of foetal abnormalities, particularly neural tube defects including spina bifida.[195] Both drugs should be avoided, if possible, and an antipsychotic prescribed instead. Valproate confers a higher risk (around 10% for major malformations) than carbamazapine[196–198] and should not be used in women of child-bearing age except

where all other treatment has failed. Although 1 in 20 women of childbearing age who are in long term contact with mental health services are prescribed mood stabilising drugs, awareness of the teratogenic potential of these drugs amongst psychiatrists is low.[195]

- There is no evidence that folate protects against anticonvulsant-induced neural tube defects if given during pregnancy,[199] but may do so if given prior to conception (the neural tube is essentially formed by 8 weeks of pregnancy[200] before many women realise they are pregnant). However, folate supplementation may be beneficial with regard to early neurodevelopment and so should always be offered.[199]

- Valproate monotherapy has also been associated with an increased relative risk of atrial septal defects, cleft palate, hypospadias, polydactyly and craniosynostosis, although absolute risks are low.[201] Valproate is also associated with a reduced head circumference in the neonate.[202]

- There appears to be clear causal association between valproate use in pregnancy and motor and neurodevelopmental problems in exposed children. A review of studies by the European Medicines Agency showed that up to 40% of pre-school children exposed to valproate in utero experienced some form of developmental delay, including delayed walking and talking, memory problems, difficulty with speech and language and a lower intellectual ability. Poorer outcomes have been shown in language functioning, attention, memory, executive functioning and adaptive behaviour compared with carbamazepine and lamotrigine exposure. Lower IQs and an increased diagnosis rate of autistic spectrum disorder are also reported.[203,204] Processing, working memory, and learning deficits appear to be dose-related.[205] Decreased school performance has been associated with valproate use compared with children unexposed to anticonvulsants and children exposed to lamotrigine.[206]

- Valproate use may increase risk of pre-eclampsia.[207]

- Where continued use of carbamazepine is deemed essential, low-dose (but effective) monotherapy is strongly recommended, as the teratogenic effect is probably dose-related.[208,209] Use of carbamazepine in the third trimester may necessitate maternal vitamin K.

- There is growing evidence that **lamotrigine** is safer in pregnancy than carbamazepine or valproate across a range of outcomes.[199,203,210-212] The risk of major malformations appears to be in the range reported for children not exposed to anticonvulsants.[213] Clearance of lamotrigine seems to increase radically during pregnancy[214,215] and then reduces postpartum[216] so frequent lamotrigine levels are necessary.

- Behaviour problems have been reported by parents of children exposed to lamotrigine in pregnancy.[217] Lamotrigine may be associated with an increased risk of autism.[218]

- Lower APGAR scores at birth have been reported with carbamazepine, valproate and topiramate. If an association exists the absolute risk is low.[219]

- Major malformations, specifically orofacial clefts, have been reported with topiramate.[220] The risk of oral clefts may be higher in women with epilepsy who use higher doses.[221]

- A large cohort study reported that anticonvulsant mood stabilisers were not associated with placenta-mediated complications or preterm birth.[205]

Recommendations for the treatment of bipolar disorder in pregnancy are outlined in Box 7.4.

Box 7.4   Recommendations – bipolar disorder in pregnancy

- For women who have had a long period without relapse, the possibility of switching to a safer drug (antipsychotic) or withdrawing treatment completely before conception and for at least the first trimester should be considered.
- The risk of relapse both pre- and postpartum is very high if medication is discontinued abruptly.
- No mood stabiliser is clearly safe. NICE recommends the use of mood stabilising antipsychotics as a preferable alternative to continuation with a mood stabiliser.
- Women with severe illness or who are known to relapse quickly after discontinuation of a mood stabiliser should be advised to continue their medication following discussion of the risks.
- NICE recommends that if lithium is considered essential in a woman planning pregnancy the woman be informed of the risk of foetal heart malformations when lithium is taken in the first trimester and the risk of toxicity in the baby if lithium is continued during breastfeeding. Lithium plasma levels should be monitored more frequently throughout pregnancy and the postnatal period and lithium should be stopped during active labour. Women prescribed lithium should undergo appropriate monitoring of the foetus in liaison with foetal medicine obstetric services to screen for Ebstein's anomaly.
- NICE advises against the use of valproate in pregnancy. Valproate should be discontinued before a woman becomes pregnant. Women taking valproate who are planning a pregnancy should be advised to gradually stop the drug because of the high risk of foetal malformations and adverse neurodevelopment outcomes after any exposure in pregnancy. If valproate is the only drug that works for a particular woman, and this is seen as the only option for her during pregnancy, then she needs to be given a clear briefing of the risks and to sign a consent form confirming that she understands the risk of malformations and developmental delays.
- NICE advises discussing the possibility of stopping carbamazepine if a woman is planning a pregnancy or becomes pregnant. If carbamazepine is used, prophylactic vitamin K should be administered to the mother and neonate after delivery.
- NICE advises if a woman is taking lamotrigine to check lamotrigine levels frequently during pregnancy and into the postnatal period because they vary substantially at these times.
- In acute mania in pregnancy use an antipsychotic and if ineffective consider ECT.
- In bipolar depression during pregnancy use CBT for moderate depression and an SSRI for more severe depression. Lamotrigine is also an option.

Sedatives

Anxiety disorders and insomnia are commonly seen in pregnancy.[222] Preferred treatments are CBT and sleep-hygiene measures, respectively.

- First-trimester exposure to **benzodiazepines** has been associated with an increased risk of oral clefts in newborns,[223] although subsequent studies have failed to confirm this association.[224-226] A recent meta-analysis concluded that first trimester exposure is not associated with an increased risk of major malformations.[227] However, benzodiazepine use in pregnancy may be a marker for cardiac and total malformation risk.[228]
- Benzodiazepines have been associated with pylorostenosis and alimentary tract atresia.[224] A large Swedish cohort study (n = 1,406 women who took a benzodiazepine

during pregnancy) did not confirm these associations, nor suggest others.[225] Note that data on elective terminations were not available.

- Benzodiazepine use in pregnancy, has been associated with caesarean delivery, spontaneous abortion, neonatal intensive care admission, neonatal ventilatory support, low birth weight, preterm delivery small head circumference, and small for gestational age babies.[224,229–233]
- Third-trimester use is commonly associated with neonatal difficulties (floppy baby syndrome).[234]
- **Promethazine** has been used in hyperemesis gravidarum and appears not to be teratogenic, although data are limited.
- Data on Z drugs are limited. However, available data suggest that Z drugs are not associated with an increased risk of congenital malformations.[235]
- Zolpidem may be associated with an increased risk of preterm delivery, low birthweight, increased likelihood of caesarean section.[236]

Rapid tranquillisation

There is almost no published information on the use of rapid tranquillisation in pregnant women. The acute use of short-acting benzodiazepines such as lorazepam and of the sedative antihistamine promethazine is unlikely to be harmful. Presumably, the use of either drug will be problematic immediately before birth. NICE also recommends the use of an antipsychotic but do not specify a particular drug.[16] Involvement of an anaesthetist if rapid tranquillisation is needed during labour is strongly advised. Note that antipsychotics are not generally recommended as a first line treatment for managing acute behavioural disturbance (see section on acute behavioural disturbance). Where sedative drugs have been given during labour an anaesthetist and neonatologist should be present for resuscitation of the baby in cases of respiratory depression.

ADHD

Limited data suggest that methylphenidate is not a major teratogen.[237] A small increased risk of cardiac malformations has been reported. The risk was not reported with amphetamines.[238] Modafinil may be associated with an increased risk of congenital malformations (including congenital heart defects, hypospadias and orofacial clefts).[239, 240] Modafinil should not be initiated in pregnancy.[239] Women of childbearing age must understand the risk of taking modafinil in pregnancy and should be advised to use effective contraception during treatment with modafinil and for 2 months after discontinuing treatment.[239]

Table 7.1 outlines recommendations for the treatment of psychotropics in pregnancy.

CHAPTER 7

Table 7.1 Recommendations[*] – psychotropic drugs in pregnancy.
Minimise the number of drugs the foetus is exposed to

Psychotropic	Recommendations
Antidepressants	Women who are at a high risk of relapse are best maintained on the same antidepressant during and after pregnancy.
	When initiating an antidepressant in a woman planning pregnancy, previous response must be taken in to account. Sertraline is an option.
Antipsychotics	No clear evidence that any antipsychotic is a major teratogen. Consider using/continuing drug mother has previously responded to rather than switching prior to/during pregnancy.
	Screen for adverse metabolic effects. Offer women an oral glucose tolerance test. Arrange for the woman to give birth in a unit with access to neonatal intensive care facilities.
	When initiating an antipsychotic in a woman planning pregnancy previous response must be taken in to account. Quetiapine has relative low rate of placental passage.
Mood stabilisers	Valproate should be stopped if a woman becomes pregnant. Where medication history clearly shows that no other agent has been effective and that if valproate is stopped the woman will relapse a careful risk benefit analysis must be conducted. The woman must understand the risks of valproate use in pregnancy. Avoid other anticonvulsants unless risks and consequences of relapse outweigh the known risk of teratogenesis. Consider using a mood stabilising antipsychotic.
	Lamotrigine is also an option (bipolar depression only).
Sedatives	Non drug measures are preferred.
	Benzodiazepines, zopiclone and zolpidem are probably not teratogenic but are best avoided in late pregnancy. Promethazine is widely used but supporting safety data are scarce.

[*]It cannot be overstated that treatment needs to be individualised for each patient. This summary box is not intended to suggest that all patients should be switched to a recommended drug. For each patient, take into account their current prescription, response to treatment, history of response to other treatments and the risks known to apply in pregnancy (both for current treatment and for switching).

References

1. McElhatton PR. Pregnancy: (2) General principles of drug use in pregnancy. *Pharm J* 2003; **270**:232–234.
2. Rasmussen SA, et al. Maternal obesity and risk of neural tube defects: a metaanalysis. *Am J Obstet Gynecol* 2008; **198**:611–619.
3. Schneid-Kofman N, et al. Psychiatric illness and adverse pregnancy outcome. *Int J Gynaecol Obstet* 2008; **101**:53–56.
4. Stein A, et al. Effects of perinatal mental disorders on the fetus and child. *Lancet* 2014; **384**:1800–1819.
5. MacCabe JH, et al. Adverse pregnancy outcomes in mothers with affective psychosis. *Bipolar Disorders* 2007; **9**:305–309.
6. Boden R, et al. Risks of adverse pregnancy and birth outcomes in women treated or not treated with mood stabilisers for bipolar disorder: population based cohort study. *BMJ* 2012; **345**:e7085.
7. Nosarti C, et al. Preterm birth and psychiatric disorders in young adult life. *Arch Gen Psychiatry* 2012; **69**:E1–E8.
8. Khalifeh H, et al. Suicide in perinatal and non-perinatal women in contact with psychiatric services: 15 year findings from a UK national inquiry. *Lancet Psychiatry* 2016; **3**:233–242.
9. de La Rochebrochard E, et al. Children born after unplanned pregnancies and cognitive development at 3 years: social differentials in the United Kingdom Millennium Cohort. *Am J Epidemiol* 2013; **178**:910–920.
10. Gov.uk Guidance. Valproate (Epilim▼, Depakote▼) pregnancy prevention programme: updated educational materials 2020; https://www.gov.uk/drug-safety-update/valproate-epilim-depakote-pregnancy-prevention-programme-updated-educational-materials

11. Goodwin RD, et al. Mental disorders and nicotine dependence among pregnant women in the United States. *Obstet Gynecol* 2007; **109**:875–883.
12. Vigod SN, et al. Maternal schizophrenia and adverse birth outcomes: what mediates the risk? *Soc Psychiatry Psychiatr Epidemiol* 2020; **55**:561–570.
13. Royal College of Physicians. Nicotine without smoke: tobacco harm reduction. A report by the Tobacco Advisory Group of the Royal College of Physicians 2016; https://www.rcplondon.ac.uk/projects/outputs/nicotine-without-smoke-tobacco-harm-reduction-0
14. Sit DK, et al. Changes in antidepressant metabolism and dosing across pregnancy and early postpartum. *J Clin Psychiatry* 2008; **69**:652–658.
15. Ter Horst PG, et al. Pharmacological aspects of neonatal antidepressant withdrawal. *Obstet Gynecol Surv* 2008; **63**:267–279.
16. National Institute for Health and Care Excellence. Antenatal and postnatal mental health: clinical management and service guidance. Clinical Guidance [CG192] 2014 Last updated: February 2020. https://www.nice.org.uk/guidance/cg192
17. Harlow BL, et al. Incidence of hospitalization for postpartum psychotic and bipolar episodes in women with and without prior prepregnancy or prenatal psychiatric hospitalizations. *Arch Gen Psychiatry* 2007; **64**:42–48.
18. Wesseloo R, et al. Risk of postpartum relapse in bipolar disorder and postpartum psychosis: a systematic review and meta-analysis. *Am J Psychiatry* 2016; **173**:117–127.
19. Jones I, et al. Bipolar disorder, affective psychosis, and schizophrenia in pregnancy and the post-partum period. *Lancet* 2014; **384**:1789–1799.
20. Gentile S. Antipsychotic therapy during early and late pregnancy. A systematic review. *Schizophr Bull* 2010; **36**:518–544.
21. Diav-Citrin O, et al. Safety of haloperidol and penfluridol in pregnancy: a multicenter, prospective, controlled study. *J Clin Psychiatry* 2005; **66**:317–322.
22. Habermann F, et al. Atypical antipsychotic drugs and pregnancy outcome: a prospective, cohort study. *J Clin Psychopharmacol* 2013; **33**:453–462.
23. Huybrechts KF, et al. Antipsychotic use in pregnancy and the risk for congenital malformations. *JAMA Psychiatry* 2016; **73**:938–946.
24. Collins KO, et al. Maternal haloperidol therapy associated with dyskinesia in a newborn. *Am J Health Syst Pharm* 2003; **60**:2253–2255.
25. Trixler M, et al. Use of antipsychotics in the management of schizophrenia during pregnancy. *Drugs* 2005; **65**:1193–1206.
26. Anderson KN, et al. Atypical antipsychotic use during pregnancy and birth defect risk: National Birth Defects Prevention Study, 1997–2011. *Schizophr Res* 2020; **215**:81–88.
27. Ellfolk M, et al. Second-generation antipsychotics and pregnancy complications. *Eur J Clin Pharmacol* 2020; **76**:107–115.
28. Galbally M, et al. The association between gestational diabetes mellitus, antipsychotics and severe mental illness in pregnancy: a multicentre study. *Aust N Z J Obstet Gynaecol* 2020; **60**:63–69.
29. Uguz F. Antipsychotic use during pregnancy and the risk of gestational diabetes mellitus: a systematic review. *J Clin Psychopharmacol* 2019; **39**:162–167.
30. Galbally M, et al. Aripiprazole and pregnancy: a retrospective, multicentre study. *J Affect Disord* 2018; **238**:593–596.
31. Reis M, et al. Maternal use of antipsychotics in early pregnancy and delivery outcome. *J Clin Psychopharmacol* 2008; **28**:279–288.
32. Boden R, et al. Antipsychotics during pregnancy: relation to fetal and maternal metabolic effects. *Arch Gen Psychiatry* 2012; **69**:715–721.
33. Newham JJ, et al. Birth weight of infants after maternal exposure to typical and atypical antipsychotics: prospective comparison study. *Br J Psychiatry* 2008; **192**:333–337.
34. Ernst CL, et al. The reproductive safety profile of mood stabilizers, atypical antipsychotics, and broad-spectrum psychotropics. *J Clin Psychiatry* 2002; **63 Suppl** 4:42–55.
35. McKenna K, et al. Pregnancy outcome of women using atypical antipsychotic drugs: a prospective comparative study. *J Clin Psychiatry* 2005; **66**:444–449.
36. Brunner E, et al. Olanzapine in pregnancy and breastfeeding: a review of data from global safety surveillance. *BMC Pharmacol Toxicol* 2013; **14**:38.
37. Spyropoulou AC, et al. Hip dysplasia following a case of olanzapine exposed pregnancy: a questionable association. *Arch Women's Mental Health* 2006; **9**:219–222.
38. Arora M, et al. Meningocele and ankyloblepharon following in utero exposure to olanzapine. *Eur Psychiatry* 2006; **21**:345–346.
39. CARE Study Group. Maternal caffeine intake during pregnancy and risk of fetal growth restriction: a large prospective observational study. *BMJ* 2008; **337**:a2332.
40. Beex-Oosterhuis MM, et al. Safety of clozapine use during pregnancy: analysis of international pharmacovigilance data. *Pharmacoepidemiol Drug Saf* 2020; **29**:725–735.
41. Shao P, et al. Effects of clozapine and other atypical antipsychotics on infants development who were exposed to as fetus: a post-hoc analysis. *PLoS One* 2015; **10**:e0123373.
42. Nguyen T, et al. Obstetric and neonatal outcomes of clozapine exposure in pregnancy: a consecutive case series. *Arch Women's Mental Health* 2020; **23**:441–445.
43. Ballester-Gracia I, et al. Use of long acting injectable aripiprazole before and through pregnancy in bipolar disorder: a case report. *BMC Pharmacol Toxicol* 2019; **20**:52.
44. Kucukgoncu S, et al. Antipsychotic exposure in pregnancy and the risk of gestational diabetes: a systematic review and meta-analysis. *Schizophr Bull* 2020; **46**:311–318.
45. Gentile S, et al. Neurodevelopmental outcomes in infants exposed in utero to antipsychotics: a systematic review of published data. *CNS Spectr* 2017; **22**:273–281.
46. Peng M, et al. Effects of prenatal exposure to atypical antipsychotics on postnatal development and growth of infants: a case-controlled, prospective study. *Psychopharmacology (Berl)* 2013; **228**:577–584.

47. Sorensen MJ, et al. Risk of fetal death after treatment with antipsychotic medications during pregnancy. *PLoS One* 2015; 10:e0132280.

48. McAllister-Williams RH, et al. British Association for Psychopharmacology consensus guidance on the use of psychotropic medication preconception, in pregnancy and postpartum 2017. *J Psychopharmacol (Oxford, England)* 2017; 31:519–552.

49. Schoretsanitis G, et al. Excretion of antipsychotics into the amniotic fluid, umbilical cord blood, and breast milk: a systematic critical review and combined analysis. *Ther Drug Monit* 2020; 42:245–254.

50. European Medicines Agency. Antipsychotics - Risk of extrapyramidal effects and withdrawal symptoms in newborns after exposure during pregnancy. Pharmacovigilance Working Party, July 2011 plenary meeting. Issue 1107. http://www.ema.europa.eu/docs/en_GB/document_library/Report/2011/07/WC500109581.pdf

51. Cohen LS, et al. Relapse of major depression during pregnancy in women who maintain or discontinue antidepressant treatment. *JAMA* 2006; 295:499–507.

52. Munk-Olsen T, et al. New parents and mental disorders: a population-based register study. *JAMA* 2006; 296:2582–2589.

53. Mahon PB, et al. Genome-wide linkage and follow-up association study of postpartum mood symptoms. *Am J Psychiatry* 2009; 166:1229–1237.

54. Yonkers KA, et al. The management of depression during pregnancy: a report from the American Psychiatric Association and the American College of Obstetricians and Gynecologists. *Gen Hosp Psychiatry* 2009; 31:403–413.

55. Engelstad HJ, et al. Perinatal outcomes of pregnancies complicated by maternal depression with or without selective serotonin reuptake inhibitor therapy. *Neonatology* 2014; 105:149–154.

56. Yonkers KA, et al. Does antidepressant use attenuate the risk of a major depressive episode in pregnancy? *Epidemiology* 2011; 22:848–854.

57. Chang Q, et al. Antidepressant use in depressed women during pregnancy and the risk of preterm birth: a systematic review and meta-analysis of 23 cohort studies. *Front Pharmacol* 2020; 11:659.

58. Venkatesh KK, et al. Association of antenatal depression symptoms and antidepressant treatment with preterm birth. *Obstet Gynecol* 2016; 127:926–933.

59. Malm H, et al. Pregnancy complications following prenatal exposure to SSRIs or maternal psychiatric disorders: results from population-based national register data. *Am J Psychiatry* 2015; 172:1224–1232.

60. Jarde A, et al. Neonatal outcomes in women with untreated antenatal depression compared with women without depression: a systematic review and meta-analysis. *JAMA Psychiatry* 2016; 73:826–837.

61. Jimenez-Solem E, et al. SSRI use during pregnancy and risk of stillbirth and neonatal mortality. *Am J Psychiatry* 2013; 170:299–304.

62. Stephansson O, et al. Selective serotonin reuptake inhibitors during pregnancy and risk of stillbirth and infant mortality. *JAMA* 2013; 309:48–54.

63. Ban L, et al. Maternal depression, antidepressant prescriptions, and congenital anomaly risk in offspring: a population-based cohort study. *BJOG* 2014; 121:1471–1481.

64. Berard A, et al. Antidepressant use during pregnancy and the risk of major congenital malformations in a cohort of depressed pregnant women: an updated analysis of the Quebec Pregnancy Cohort. *BMJ Open* 2017; 7:e013372.

65. Gao SY, et al. Selective serotonin reuptake inhibitor use during early pregnancy and congenital malformations: a systematic review and meta-analysis of cohort studies of more than 9 million births. *BMC Med* 2018; 16:205.

66. Oberlander TF, et al. Effects of timing and duration of gestational exposure to serotonin reuptake inhibitor antidepressants: population-based study. *Br J Psychiatry* 2008; 192:338–343.

67. Ramos E, et al. Duration of antidepressant use during pregnancy and risk of major congenital malformations. *Br J Psychiatry* 2008; 192:344–350.

68. Nulman I, et al. Neurodevelopment of children following prenatal exposure to venlafaxine, selective serotonin reuptake inhibitors, or untreated maternal depression. *Am J Psychiatry* 2012; 169:1165–1174.

69. Wisner KL, et al. Does fetal exposure to SSRIs or maternal depression impact infant growth? *Am J Psychiatry* 2013; 170:485–493.

70. Suri R, et al. A prospective, naturalistic, blinded study of early neurobehavioral outcomes for infants following prenatal antidepressant exposure. *J Clin Psychiatry* 2011; 72:1002–1007.

71. de Vries NK, et al. Early neurological outcome of young infants exposed to selective serotonin reuptake inhibitors during pregnancy: results from the observational SMOK study. *PLoS One* 2013; 8:e64654.

72. Hviid A, et al. Use of selective serotonin reuptake inhibitors during pregnancy and risk of autism. *N Engl J Med* 2013; 369:2406–2415.

73. Rai D, et al. Parental depression, maternal antidepressant use during pregnancy, and risk of autism spectrum disorders: population based case-control study. *BMJ* 2013; 346:f2059.

74. Brown HK, et al. Association between serotonergic antidepressant use during pregnancy and autism spectrum disorder in children. *JAMA* 2017; 317:1544–1552.

75. Sujan AC, et al. Associations of maternal antidepressant use during the first trimester of pregnancy with preterm birth, small for gestational age, autism spectrum disorder, and attention-deficit/hyperactivity disorder in offspring. *JAMA* 2017; 317:1553–1562.

76. Castro VM, et al. Absence of evidence for increase in risk for autism or attention-deficit hyperactivity disorder following antidepressant exposure during pregnancy: a replication study. *Trans Psychiatry* 2016; 6:e708.

77. Mezzacappa A, et al. Risk for autism spectrum disorders according to period of prenatal antidepressant exposure: a systematic review and meta-analysis. *JAMA Pediatrics* 2017; 171:555–563.

78. Kieviet N, et al. Risk factors for poor neonatal adaptation after exposure to antidepressants in utero. *Acta Paediatr* 2015; 104:384–391.

79. Brandlistuen RE, et al. Behavioural effects of fetal antidepressant exposure in a Norwegian cohort of discordant siblings. *Int J Epidemiol* 2015; 44:1397–1407.

80. De Vera MA, et al. Antidepressant use during pregnancy and the risk of pregnancy-induced hypertension. *Br J Clin Pharmacol* 2012; **74**:362–369.

81. Zakiyah N, et al. Antidepressant use during pregnancy and the risk of developing gestational hypertension: a retrospective cohort study. *BMC Pregnancy Childbirth* 2018; **18**:187.

82. Palmsten K, et al. Antidepressant use and risk for preeclampsia. *Epidemiology* 2013; **24**:682–691.

83. Bruning AH, et al. Antidepressants during pregnancy and postpartum hemorrhage: a systematic review. *Eur J Obstet Gynecol Reprod Biol* 2015; **189**:38–47.

84. Hanley GE, et al. Postpartum hemorrhage and use of serotonin reuptake inhibitor antidepressants in pregnancy. *Obstet Gynecol* 2016; **127**:53–61.

85. Grzeskowiak LE, et al. Antidepressant use in late gestation and risk of postpartum haemorrhage: a retrospective cohort study. *BJOG* 2016; **123**:1929–1936.

86. Palmsten K, et al. Use of antidepressants near delivery and risk of postpartum hemorrhage: cohort study of low income women in the United States. *BMJ* 2013; **347**:f4877.

87. Lupattelli A, et al. Risk of vaginal bleeding and postpartum hemorrhage after use of antidepressants in pregnancy: a study from the Norwegian Mother and Child Cohort Study. *J Clin Psychopharmacol* 2014; **34**:143–148.

88. Uguz F. Is there any association between use of antidepressants and preeclampsia or gestational hypertension? A systematic review of current studies. *J Clin Psychopharmacol* 2017; **37**:72–77.

89. Loughhead AM, et al. Placental passage of tricyclic antidepressants. *Biol Psychiatry* 2006; **59**:287–290.

90. Loughhead AM, et al. Antidepressants in amniotic fluid: another route of fetal exposure. *Am J Psychiatry* 2006; **163**:145–147.

91. Davis RL, et al. Risks of congenital malformations and perinatal events among infants exposed to antidepressant medications during pregnancy. *Pharmacoepidemiol Drug Saf* 2007; **16**:1086–1094.

92. Kallen B. Neonate characteristics after maternal use of antidepressants in late pregnancy. *Arch Pediatr Adolesc Med* 2004; **158**:312–316.

93. Gentile S. Tricyclic antidepressants in pregnancy and puerperium. *Exp Opinion Drug Saf* 2014; **13**:207–225.

94. Fukushima N, et al. A neonatal prolonged QT syndrome due to maternal use of oral tricyclic antidepressants. *Eur J Pediatr* 2016; **175**:1129–1132.

95. Corona-Rivera JR, et al. Unusual retrospective prenatal findings in a male newborn with Timothy syndrome type 1. *Eur J Med Genet* 2015; **58**:332–335.

96. Maschi S, et al. Neonatal outcome following pregnancy exposure to antidepressants: a prospective controlled cohort study. *BJOG* 2008; **115**:283–289.

97. Nulman I, et al. Child development following exposure to tricyclic antidepressants or fluoxetine throughout fetal life: a prospective, controlled study. *Am J Psychiatry* 2002; **159**:1889–1895.

98. Nulman I, et al. Neurodevelopment of children exposed in utero to antidepressant drugs. *N Engl J Med* 1997; **336**:258–262.

99. Hendrick V, et al. Placental passage of antidepressant medications. *Am J Psychiatry* 2003; **160**:993–996.

100. Gentile S. Selective serotonin reuptake inhibitor exposure during early pregnancy and the risk of birth defects. *Acta Psychiatr Scand* 2011; **123**:266–275.

101. Hallberg P, et al. The use of selective serotonin reuptake inhibitors during pregnancy and breast-feeding: a review and clinical aspects. *J Clin Psychopharmacol* 2005; **25**:59–73.

102. Gentile S. The safety of newer antidepressants in pregnancy and breastfeeding. *Drug Saf* 2005; **28**:137–152.

103. Kallen BA, et al. Maternal use of selective serotonin re-uptake inhibitors in early pregnancy and infant congenital malformations. *Birth Defects Res A Clin Mol Teratol* 2007; **79**:301–308.

104. Einarson TR, et al. Newer antidepressants in pregnancy and rates of major malformations: a meta-analysis of prospective comparative studies. *Pharmacoepidemiol Drug Saf* 2005; **14**:823–827.

105. Wogelius P, et al. Maternal use of selective serotonin reuptake inhibitors and risk of congenital malformations. *Epidemiology* 2006; **17**:701–704.

106. Jordan S, et al. Selective Serotonin Reuptake Inhibitor (SSRI) antidepressants in pregnancy and congenital anomalies: analysis of linked databases in Wales, Norway and Funen, Denmark. *PLoS One* 2016; **11**:e0165122.

107. Kivisto J, et al. Maternal use of selective serotonin reuptake inhibitors and lengthening of the umbilical cord: indirect evidence of increased foetal activity – a retrospective cohort study. *PLoS One* 2016; **11**:e0154628.

108. Chambers CD, et al. Selective serotonin-reuptake inhibitors and risk of persistent pulmonary hypertension of the newborn. *N Engl J Med* 2006; **354**:579–587.

109. Alwan S, et al. Use of selective serotonin-reuptake inhibitors in pregnancy and the risk of birth defects. *N Engl J Med* 2007; **356**:2684–2692.

110. Yazdy MM, et al. Use of selective serotonin-reuptake inhibitors during pregnancy and the risk of clubfoot. *Epidemiology* 2014; **25**:859–865.

111. Anderson KN, et al. Maternal use of specific antidepressant medications during early pregnancy and the risk of selected birth defects. *JAMA Psychiatry* 2020; e202453.

112. Thormahlen GM. Paroxetine use during pregnancy: is it safe? *Ann Pharmacother* 2006; **40**:1834–1837.

113. Myles N, et al. Systematic meta-analysis of individual selective serotonin reuptake inhibitor medications and congenital malformations. *Aust NZJ Psychiatry* 2013; **47**:1002–1012.

114. Berard A, et al. The risk of major cardiac malformations associated with paroxetine use during the first trimester of pregnancy: a systematic review and meta-analysis. *Br J Clin Pharmacol* 2016; **81**:589–604.

115. Berard A, et al. First trimester exposure to paroxetine and risk of cardiac malformations in infants: the importance of dosage. *Birth Defects Res B Dev Reprod Toxicol* 2007; **80**:18–27.

116. Einarson A, et al. Evaluation of the risk of congenital cardiovascular defects associated with use of paroxetine during pregnancy. *Am J Psychiatry* 2008; 165:749–752.

117. Diav-Citrin O, et al. Paroxetine and fluoxetine in pregnancy: a prospective, multicentre, controlled, observational study. *Br J Clin Pharmacol* 2008; 66:695–705.

118. Louik C, et al. First-trimester use of selective serotonin-reuptake inhibitors and the risk of birth defects. *N Engl J Med* 2007; 356:2675–2683.

119. Berard A, et al. Sertraline use during pregnancy and the risk of major malformations. *Am J Obstet Gynecol* 2015; 212:795.e791–795.e712.

120. Reefhuis J, et al. Specific SSRIs and birth defects: Bayesian analysis to interpret new data in the context of previous reports. *BMJ* 2015; 351:h3190.

121. Margulis AV, et al. Use of selective serotonin reuptake inhibitors in pregnancy and cardiac malformations: a propensity-score matched cohort in CPRD. *Pharmacoepidemiol Drug Saf* 2013; 22:942–951.

122. Riggin L, et al. The fetal safety of fluoxetine: a systematic review and meta-analysis. *J Obstet Gynaecol Can* 2013; 35:362–369.

123. Furu K, et al. Selective serotonin reuptake inhibitors and venlafaxine in early pregnancy and risk of birth defects: population based cohort study and sibling design. *BMJ* 2015; 350:h1798.

124. Petersen I, et al. Selective serotonin reuptake inhibitors and congenital heart anomalies: comparative cohort studies of women treated before and during pregnancy and their children. *J Clin Psychiatry* 2016; 77:e36–e42.

125. Wang S, et al. Selective Serotonin Reuptake Inhibitors (SSRIs) and the risk of congenital heart defects: a meta-analysis of prospective cohort studies. *J Am Heart Assoc* 2015; 4:e001681.

126. Ansah DA, et al. A prospective study evaluating the effects of SSRI exposure on cardiac size and function in newborns. *Neonatology* 2019; 115:320–327.

127. Malm H, et al. Selective serotonin reuptake inhibitors and risk for major congenital anomalies. *Obstet Gynecol* 2011; 118:111–120.

128. Ross LE, et al. Selected pregnancy and delivery outcomes after exposure to antidepressant medication: a systematic review and meta-analysis. *JAMA Psychiatry* 2013; 70:436–443.

129. Andrade C. Antenatal exposure to selective serotonin reuptake inhibitors and duration of gestation. *J Clin Psychiatry* 2013; 74:e633–e635.

130. Hemels ME, et al. Antidepressant use during pregnancy and the rates of spontaneous abortions: a meta-analysis. *Ann Pharmacother* 2005; 39:803–809.

131. Guan HB, et al. Prenatal selective serotonin reuptake inhibitor use and associated risk for gestational hypertension and preeclampsia: a meta-analysis of cohort studies. *J Women's Health (2002)* 2018; 27:791–800.

132. Oberlander TF, et al. Neonatal outcomes after prenatal exposure to selective serotonin reuptake inhibitor antidepressants and maternal depression using population-based linked health data. *Arch Gen Psychiatry* 2006; 63:898–906.

133. Zhao X, et al. A meta-analysis of selective serotonin reuptake inhibitors (SSRIs) use during prenatal depression and risk of low birth weight and small for gestational age. *J Affect Disord* 2018; 241:563–570.

134. Boucher N, et al. A new look at the neonate's clinical presentation after in utero exposure to antidepressants in late pregnancy. *J Clin Psychopharmacol* 2008; 28:334–339.

135. Yang A, et al. Neonatal discontinuation syndrome in serotonergic antidepressant-exposed neonates. *J Clin Psychiatry* 2017; 78:605–611.

136. Haddad PM, et al. Neonatal symptoms following maternal paroxetine treatment: Serotonin Toxicity or Paroxetine Discontinuation Syndrome? *J Psychopharmacol (Oxford, England)* 2005; 19:554–557.

137. Sanz EJ, et al. Selective serotonin reuptake inhibitors in pregnant women and neonatal withdrawal syndrome: a database analysis. *Lancet* 2005; 365:482–487.

138. Koren G. Discontinuation syndrome following late pregnancy exposure to antidepressants. *Arch Pediatr Adolesc Med* 2004; 158:307–308.

139. Leerssen ECM, et al. Severe transient neonatal long QT syndrome due to maternal paroxetine usage: a case report. *Cardiol Young* 2019; 29:1300–1301.

140. Gentile S. SSRIs in pregnancy and lactation: emphasis on neurodevelopmental outcome. *CNS Drugs* 2005; 19:623–633.

141. Casper RC, et al. Follow-up of children of depressed mothers exposed or not exposed to antidepressant drugs during pregnancy. *J Pediatr* 2003; 142:402–408.

142. Hermansen TK, et al. Prenatal SSRI exposure: effects on later child development. *Child Neuropsychol* 2015; 21:543–569.

143. Kaplan YC, et al. Maternal SSRI discontinuation, use, psychiatric disorder and the risk of autism in children: a meta-analysis of cohort studies. *Br J Clin Pharmacol* 2017; 83:2798–2806.

144. Boukhris T, et al. Antidepressant use in pregnancy and the risk of attention deficit with or without hyperactivity disorder in children. *Paediatr Perinat Epidemiol* 2017; 31:363–373.

145. Croen LA, et al. Antidepressant use during pregnancy and childhood autism spectrum disorders. *Arch Gen Psychiatry* 2011; 68:1104–1112.

146. Healy D, et al. Links between serotonin reuptake inhibition during pregnancy and neurodevelopmental delay/spectrum disorders: a systematic review of epidemiological and physiological evidence. *Int J Risk Saf Med* 2016; 28:125–141.

147. Clements CC, et al. Prenatal antidepressant exposure is associated with risk for attention-deficit hyperactivity disorder but not autism spectrum disorder in a large health system. *Mol Psychiatry* 2015; 20:727–734.

148. Brown HK, et al. The association between antenatal exposure to selective serotonin reuptake inhibitors and autism: a systematic review and meta-analysis. *J Clin Psychiatry* 2017; 78:e48–e58.

149. Yang F, et al. Preconceptional paternal antiepileptic drugs use and risk of congenital anomalies in offspring: a nationwide cohort study. *Eur J Epidemiol* 2019; 34:651–660.

150. van der Veere CN, et al. Intra-uterine exposure to selective serotonin reuptake inhibitors (SSRIs), maternal psychopathology, and neurodevelopment at age 2.5years – results from the prospective cohort SMOK study. *Early Hum Dev* 2020; **147**:105075.

151. Brown AS, et al. Association of selective serotonin reuptake inhibitor exposure during pregnancy with speech, scholastic, and motor disorders in offspring. *JAMA Psychiatry* 2016; **73**:1163–1170.

152. Skurtveit S, et al. Prenatal exposure to antidepressants and language competence at age three: results from a large population-based pregnancy cohort in Norway. *BJOG* 2014; **121**:1621–1631.

153. Handal M, et al. Prenatal exposure to folic acid and antidepressants and language development: a population-based cohort study. *J Clin Psychopharmacol* 2016; **36**:333–339.

154. Hanley GE, et al. Prenatal exposure to serotonin reuptake inhibitor antidepressants and childhood behavior. *Pediatr Res* 2015; **78**:174–180.

155. Johnson KC, et al. Preschool outcomes following prenatal serotonin reuptake inhibitor exposure: differences in language and behavior, but not cognitive function. *J Clin Psychiatry* 2016; **77**:e176–e182.

156. Partridge MC, et al. Fine motor differences and prenatal serotonin reuptake inhibitors exposure. *J Pediatr* 2016; **175**:144–149.e141.

157. Masarwa R, et al. Prenatal exposure to selective serotonin reuptake inhibitors and serotonin norepinephrine reuptake inhibitors and risk for persistent pulmonary hypertension of the newborn: a systematic review, meta-analysis, and network meta-analysis. *Am J Obstet Gynecol* 2019; **220**:57.e51–57.e13.

158. Huybrechts KF, et al. Antidepressant use late in pregnancy and risk of persistent pulmonary hypertension of the newborn. *JAMA* 2015; **313**:2142–2151.

159. Byatt N, et al. Exposure to selective serotonin reuptake inhibitors in late pregnancy increases the risk of persistent pulmonary hypertension of the newborn, but the absolute risk is low. *Evid Based Nurs* 2015; **18**:15–16.

160. Skalkidou A, et al. SSRI use during pregnancy and risk for postpartum haemorrhage: a national register-based cohort study in Sweden. *BJOG* 2020: **127**:1366–1373.

161. Kim DR, et al. Is third trimester serotonin reuptake inhibitor use associated with postpartum hemorrhage? *J Psychiatr Res* 2016; **73**:79–85.

162. Huybrechts KF, et al. Maternal and fetal outcomes following exposure to duloxetine in pregnancy: cohort study. *BMJ* 2020; **368**:m237.

163. Hoog SL, et al. Duloxetine and pregnancy outcomes: safety surveillance findings. *Int J Med Sci* 2013; **10**:413–419.

164. Abdy NA, et al. Duloxetine withdrawal syndrome in a newborn. *Clin Pediatr (Phila)* 2013; **52**:976–977.

165. Rybakowski JK. Moclobemide in pregnancy. *Pharmacopsychiatry* 2001; **34**:82–83.

166. Pharmacia Ltd. Erdronax: use on pregnancy, renally and hepatically impaired patients. Personal Communication, 2003.

167. Polen KN, et al. Association between reported venlafaxine use in early pregnancy and birth defects, national birth defects prevention study, 1997–2007. *Birth Defects ResA Clin Mol Teratol* 2013; **97**:28–35.

168. Lassen D, et al. First-trimester pregnancy exposure to venlafaxine or duloxetine and risk of major congenital malformations: a systematic review. *Basic Clin Pharmacol Toxicol* 2016; **118**:32–36.

169. Ramos E, et al. Association between antidepressant use during pregnancy and infants born small for gestational age. *Can J Psychiatry* 2010; **55**:643–652.

170. Richardson JL, et al. Pregnancy outcomes following maternal venlafaxine use: a prospective observational comparative cohort study. *Reprod Toxicol* 2019; **84**:108–113.

171. Einarson A, et al. A multicentre prospective controlled study to determine the safety of trazodone and nefazodone use during pregnancy. *Can J Psychiatry* 2003; **48**:106–110.

172. Rohde A, et al. Mirtazapine (Remergil) for treatment resistant hyperemesis gravidarum: rescue of a twin pregnancy. *Arch Gynecol Obstet* 2003; **268**:219–221.

173. Djulus J, et al. Exposure to mirtazapine during pregnancy: a prospective, comparative study of birth outcomes. *J Clin Psychiatry* 2006; **67**:1280–1284.

174. Cole JA, et al. Bupropion in pregnancy and the prevalence of congenital malformations. *Pharmacoepidemiol Drug Saf* 2007; **16**:474–484.

175. Smit M, et al. Mirtazapine in pregnancy and lactation – a systematic review. *Eur Neuropsychopharmacol* 2016; **26**:126–135.

176. Louik C, et al. First-trimester exposure to bupropion and risk of cardiac malformations. *Pharmacoepidemiol Drug Saf* 2014; **23**:1066–1075.

177. Figueroa R. Use of antidepressants during pregnancy and risk of attention-deficit/hyperactivity disorder in the offspring. *J Dev Behav Pediatr* 2010; **31**:641–648.

178. Forsberg L, et al. School performance at age 16 in children exposed to antiepileptic drugs in utero – a population-based study. *Epilepsia* 2010; **52**:364–369.

179. Hendrick V, et al. Management of major depression during pregnancy. *Am J Psychiatry* 2002; **159**:1667–1673.

180. Miller LJ. Use of electroconvulsive therapy during pregnancy. *Hosp Community Psychiatry* 1994; **45**:444–450.

181. Viguera AC, et al. Risk of recurrence in women with bipolar disorder during pregnancy: prospective study of mood stabilizer discontinuation. *Am J Psychiatry* 2007; **164**:1817–1824.

182. Taylor CL, et al. Predictors of severe relapse in pregnant women with psychotic or bipolar disorders. *J Psychiatr Res* 2018; **104**:100–107.

183. Newport DJ, et al. Lithium placental passage and obstetrical outcome: implications for clinical management during late pregnancy. *Am J Psychiatry* 2005; **162**:2162–2170.

184. Fornaro M, et al. Lithium exposure during pregnancy and the postpartum period: a systematic review and meta-analysis of safety and efficacy outcomes. *Am J Psychiatry* 2020; **177**:76–92.

CHAPTER 7

185. Munk-Olsen T, et al. Maternal and infant outcomes associated with lithium use in pregnancy: an international collaborative meta-analysis of six cohort studies. *Lancet Psychiatry* 2018; 5:644–652.

186. Dodd S, et al. The pharmacology of bipolar disorder during pregnancy and breastfeeding. *Exp Opinion Drug Saf* 2004; 3:221–229.

187. Viguera AC, et al. Risk of recurrence of bipolar disorder in pregnant and nonpregnant women after discontinuing lithium maintenance. *Am J Psychiatry* 2000; 157:179–184.

188. Diav-Citrin O, et al. Pregnancy outcome following in utero exposure to lithium: a prospective, comparative, observational study. *Am J Psychiatry* 2014; 171:785–794.

189. McKnight RF, et al. Lithium toxicity profile: a systematic review and meta-analysis. *Lancet* 2012; 379:721–728.

190. Boyle B, et al. The changing epidemiology of Ebstein's anomaly and its relationship with maternal mental health conditions: a European registry-based study. *Cardiol Young* 2017; 27:677–685.

191. Yonkers KA, et al. Lithium during pregnancy: drug effects and therapeutic implications. *CNS Drugs* 1998; 4:269.

192. Blake LD, et al. Lithium toxicity and the parturient: case report and literature review. *Int J Obstet Anesth* 2008; 17:164–169.

193. Molenaar NM, et al. Management of lithium dosing around delivery: an observational study. *Bipolar Disorders* 2021; 23:49–54.

194. Cohen JM, et al. Anticonvulsant mood stabilizer and lithium use and risk of adverse pregnancy outcomes. *J Clin Psychiatry* 2019; 80:18m12572.

195. James L, et al. Informing patients of the teratogenic potential of mood stabilising drugs; a case notes review of the practice of psychiatrists. *J Psychopharmacol* 2007; 21:815–819.

196. Wide K, et al. Major malformations in infants exposed to antiepileptic drugs in utero, with emphasis on carbamazepine and valproic acid: a nation-wide, population-based register study. *Acta Paediatr* 2004; 93:174–176.

197. Wyszynski DF, et al. Increased rate of major malformations in offspring exposed to valproate during pregnancy. *Neurology* 2005; 64:961–965.

198. Weston J, et al. Monotherapy treatment of epilepsy in pregnancy: congenital malformation outcomes in the child. *Cochrane Database Syst Rev* 2016; 11:Cd010224.

199. Campbell E, et al. Malformation risks of antiepileptic drug monotherapies in pregnancy: updated results from the UK and Ireland Epilepsy and Pregnancy Registers. *J Neurol Neurosurg Psychiatry* 2014; 85:1029–1034.

200. Bestwick JP, et al. Prevention of neural tube defects: a cross-sectional study of the uptake of folic acid supplementation in nearly half a million women. *PLoS One* 2014; 9:e89354.

201. Jentink J, et al. Valproic acid monotherapy in pregnancy and major congenital malformations. *N Engl J Med* 2010; 362:2185–2193.

202. Tomson T, et al. Teratogenic effects of antiepileptic drugs. *Lancet Neurol* 2012; 11:803–813.

203. Bromley R, et al. Treatment for epilepsy in pregnancy: neurodevelopmental outcomes in the child. *Cochrane Database Syst Rev* 2014; Cd010236.

204. Bromley RL, et al. Fetal antiepileptic drug exposure and cognitive outcomes. *Seizure* 2017; 44:225–231.

205. Cohen MJ, et al. Fetal antiepileptic drug exposure and learning and memory functioning at 6 years of age: the NEAD prospective observational study. *Epilepsy Behav* 2019; 92:154–164.

206. Elkjær LS, et al. Association between prenatal valproate exposure and performance on standardized language and mathematics tests in school-aged children. *JAMA Neurol* 2018; 75:663–671.

207. Danielsson KC, et al. Hypertensive pregnancy complications in women with epilepsy and antiepileptic drugs: a population-based cohort study of first pregnancies in Norway. *BMJ Open* 2018; 8:e020998.

208. Vajda FJ, et al. Critical relationship between sodium valproate dose and human teratogenicity: results of the Australian register of antiepileptic drugs in pregnancy. *J Clin Neurosci* 2004; 11:854–858.

209. Vajda FJ, et al. Maternal valproate dosage and foetal malformations. *Acta Neurol Scand* 2005; 112:137–143.

210. Tomson T, et al. Dose-dependent risk of malformations with antiepileptic drugs: an analysis of data from the EURAP epilepsy and pregnancy registry. *Lancet Neurol* 2011; 10:609–617.

211. Molgaard-Nielsen D, et al. Newer-generation antiepileptic drugs and the risk of major birth defects. *JAMA* 2011; 305:1996–2002.

212. Vajda FJE, et al. Antiepileptic drugs and foetal malformation: analysis of 20 years of data in a pregnancy register. *Seizure* 2019; 65:6–11.

213. Tomson T, et al. Comparative risk of major congenital malformations with eight different antiepileptic drugs: a prospective cohort study of the EURAP registry. *Lancet Neurol* 2018; 17:530–538.

214. de Haan GJ, et al. Gestation-induced changes in lamotrigine pharmacokinetics: a monotherapy study. *Neurology* 2004; 63:571–573.

215. Karanam A, et al. Lamotrigine clearance increases by 5 weeks gestational age: relationship to estradiol concentrations and gestational age. *Ann Neurol* 2018; 84:556–563.

216. Clark CT, et al. Lamotrigine dosing for pregnant patients with bipolar disorder. *Am J Psychiatry* 2013; 170:1240–1247.

217. Huber-Mollema Y, et al. Neurocognition after prenatal levetiracetam, lamotrigine, carbamazepine or valproate exposure. *J Neurol* 2020; 267:1724–1736.

218. Veroniki AA, et al. Comparative safety of antiepileptic drugs for neurological development in children exposed during pregnancy and breast feeding: a systematic review and network meta-analysis. *BMJ Open* 2017; 7:e017248.

219. Christensen J, et al. Apgar-score in children prenatally exposed to antiepileptic drugs: a population-based cohort study. *BMJ Open* 2015; 5:e007425.

220. Bromley RL, et al. Cognition in school-age children exposed to levetiracetam, topiramate, or sodium valproate. *Neurology* 2016; 87:1943–1953.

221. Hernandez-Diaz S, et al. Topiramate use early in pregnancy and the risk of oral clefts: a pregnancy cohort study. *Neurology* 2018; 90:e342–e351.

222. Ross LE, et al. Anxiety disorders during pregnancy and the postpartum period: a systematic review. *J Clin Psychiatry* 2006; 67:1285–1298.

223. Dolovich LR, et al. Benzodiazepine use in pregnancy and major malformations or oral cleft: meta-analysis of cohort and case-control studies. *BMJ* 1998; 317:839–843.

224. Wikner BN, et al. Use of benzodiazepines and benzodiazepine receptor agonists during pregnancy: neonatal outcome and congenital malformations. *Pharmacoepidemiol Drug Saf* 2007; 16:1203–1210.

225. Reis M, et al. Combined use of selective serotonin reuptake inhibitors and sedatives/hypnotics during pregnancy: risk of relatively severe congenital malformations or cardiac defects. A Register Study. *BMJ Open* 2013; 3:e002166.

226. Tinker SC, et al. Use of benzodiazepine medications during pregnancy and potential risk for birth defects, National Birth Defects Prevention Study, 1997–2011. *Birth Defects Res* 2019; 111:613–620.

227. Grigoriadis S, et al. Benzodiazepine use during pregnancy alone or in combination with an antidepressant and congenital malformations: systematic review and meta-analysis. *J Clin Psychiatry* 2019; 80:18r12412.

228. Andrade C. Gestational Exposure to Benzodiazepines, 2: The Risk of Congenital Malformations Examined Through the Prism of Compatibility Intervals. *J Clin Psychiatry* 2019; 80:19f13081.

229. Calderon-Margalit R, et al. Risk of preterm delivery and other adverse perinatal outcomes in relation to maternal use of psychotropic medications during pregnancy. *Am J Obstet Gynecol* 2009; 201:579–578.

230. Okun ML, et al. A review of sleep-promoting medications used in pregnancy. *Am J Obstet Gynecol* 2015; 212:428–441.

231. Yonkers KA, et al. Maternal antidepressant use and pregnancy outcomes. *JAMA* 2017; 318:665–666.

232. Freeman MP, et al. Obstetrical and neonatal outcomes after benzodiazepine exposure during pregnancy: results from a prospective registry of women with psychiatric disorders. *Gen Hosp Psychiatry* 2018; 53:73–79.

233. Sheehy O, et al. Association between incident exposure to benzodiazepines in early pregnancy and risk of spontaneous abortion. *JAMA Psychiatry* 2019; 76:948–957.

234. McElhatton PR. The effects of benzodiazepine use during pregnancy and lactation. *Reprod Toxicol* 1994; 8:461–475.

235. Wikner BN, et al. Are hypnotic benzodiazepine receptor agonists teratogenic in humans? *J Clin Psychopharmacol* 2011; 31:356–359.

236. Wang LH, et al. Increased risk of adverse pregnancy outcomes in women receiving zolpidem during pregnancy. *Clin Pharmacol Ther* 2010; 88:369–374.

237. Pottegard A, et al. First-trimester exposure to methylphenidate: a population-based cohort study. *J Clin Psychiatry* 2014; 75:e88–e93.

238. Huybrechts KF, et al. Association between methylphenidate and amphetamine use in pregnancy and risk of congenital malformations: a cohort study from the international pregnancy safety study consortium. *JAMA Psychiatry* 2018; 75:167–175.

239. Gov.UK. Modafinil (Provigil): increased risk of congenital malformations if used during pregnancy. 2020; https://www.gov.uk/drug-safety-update/modafinil-provigil-increased-risk-of-congenital-malformations-if-used-during-pregnancy?utm_source=e-shot&utm_medium=email&utm_campaign=DSU_November2020split1.

240. Damkier P, et al. First-Trimester Pregnancy Exposure to Modafinil and Risk of Congenital Malformations. *JAMA* 2020; 323:374-376.

Further reading

National Institute for Health Care and Excellence. Antenatal and postnatal mental health: clinical management and service guidance. Clinical guideline [CG192] 2014 (Last updated February 2020); https://www.nice.org.uk/guidance/cg192

Other sources of information

National Teratology Information Service. http://www.hpa.org.uk

CHAPTER 7

Breastfeeding

The long-term benefits of breastfeeding on child physical health and cognitive development are well known. Women are generally encouraged to breastfeed for at least 6 months. One factor that may influence a mother's decision to breastfeed is the safety of a drug taken whilst breastfeeding. With some notable exceptions most psychotropic drugs should be continued in breastfeeding women because of the benefits of breastfeeding and the lack of evidence of harm for most drugs. However current evidence suggests that for a few drugs (see below) the woman should be advised not to breastfeed if such medications are the best option for her care.

Data on the safety of psychotropic medication in breast-feeding are largely derived from small studies or case reports and case series. Reported infant and neonatal outcomes in most cases are limited to short term acute adverse effects. Long-term safety cannot, therefore, be guaranteed for the psychotropics mentioned here. The information presented must be interpreted with caution with respect to the limits of the data from which it is derived and the need for such information to be regularly updated.

Infant exposure

All psychotropics are excreted in breast milk to varying degrees. The most direct measure of infant exposure is, of course, infant plasma levels but these data are rarely available. Instead, many publications report only drug concentrations in breast milk and in maternal plasma. Maternal plasma levels of antipsychotics may be a useful estimate of infant exposure.[1] Breast milk drug concentrations can be used to estimate the daily infant dose (by assuming a milk intake of 150mL/kg/day). The infant weight-adjusted dose when expressed as a proportion of the maternal weight-adjusted dose is known as the Relative Infant Dose (RID). The RID should be used as a guide only, as values are estimates and these estimates vary widely in the literature for individual drugs.

Drugs with a RID below 10% are usually regarded as safe in breastfeeding. Where measured, infant plasma levels below 10% of average maternal plasma levels have also been proposed as safe in breastfeeding.[2]

General principles of prescribing psychotropics in breastfeeding

- The safety of individual drugs in breastfeeding should be taken into account when prescribing psychotropic medication for women considering pregnancy.
- Discussions about the safety of drugs in breastfeeding should be held as early as possible ideally before conception or early in pregnancy. Decisions about the use of drugs in pregnancy should include the discussion about breastfeeding. Switching drugs at the end of pregnancy or in the days after birth is not advisable because of the high risk of relapse.
- Where a mother has taken a particular psychotropic during pregnancy and until delivery, continuation with the drug while breastfeeding will usually be appropriate (see notable exceptions below), as this may minimise withdrawal symptoms in the infant.
- In each case the benefits of breastfeeding to the mother and infant must be weighed against the risk of drug exposure in the infant.

- It is usually inappropriate to stop breastfeeding except when the currently prescribed drug is contraindicated in breastfeeding. As treatment of maternal mental illness is the priority, in such cases treatment should not be withheld but the mother should be advised to bottle feed with formula milk.
- When initiating a drug postpartum it is:
  - important to consider the mother's previous response to treatment.
  - Best to avoid a psychotropic with high reported infant plasma levels or a high RID.
  - Important to consider the half-lives of the drugs: drugs with a long half-life can accumulate in breast milk and infant serum.
- Neonates and infants do not have the same capacity for drug clearance as adults. Premature infants and infants with renal, hepatic, cardiac or neurological impairment are at a greater risk from exposure to drugs.
- Infants should be monitored for any specific adverse effects of the drugs as well as for abnormalities in feeding patterns and growth and development.
- Infant plasma levels should be monitored if adverse effects are noted or toxicity is suspected.
- Women receiving sedating medication should be strongly advised to not breastfeed in bed as they may fall asleep and roll onto the baby, with a potential risk of hypoxia to the baby.
- Sedation may affect a woman's ability to interact with their children. Women receiving sedating drugs should be monitored for this effect.
- Wherever possible:
  - Use the lowest effective dose.
  - Avoid polypharmacy.
  - Continue the regimen prescribed during pregnancy.

Table 7.2 provides summary recommendations for drug choice in breast feeding. Information on individual drugs is contained in Tables 7.3–7.7.

Table 7.2 Summary of recommendations
It is usually advisable to continue the drug which has been used during pregnancy. When initiating a drug postpartum previous response and tolerability should be considered

Drug group	Recommended drugs
Antidepressants	When initiating an antidepressant postpartum sertraline and mirtazapine may be considered. Other drugs may be used. See Table 7.3.
Antipsychotics	Women taking clozapine should be advised against breastfeeding and clozapine should be continued. When initiating an antipsychotic postpartum olanzapine or quetiapine may be considered. Other drugs may be used. See Table 7.4.
Mood stabilisers	Women taking lithium should be advised against breastfeeding and lithium should be continued. When initiating a mood stabiliser postpartum a mood-stabilising antipsychotic, such as olanzapine or quetiapine may be considered. Other drugs may be used. See Table 7.4.
Sedatives	Best avoided. Use drug with short half-life. Lorazepam may be considered.

CHAPTER 7

Antidepressants in breastfeeding

Table 7.3 provides information on individual drugs in breastfeeding based on available published data in mid-2020. Manufacturers' formal advice on drugs in breastfeeding is available in the Summary of Product Characteristics or European Public Assessment Report for individual drugs. Table 7.3 does not include this advice (which is often uninformative), but instead uses primary reference sources.

It is usually advisable to continue the antidepressant prescribed during pregnancy. Switching drugs postpartum for the purpose of breastfeeding is usually not sensible. Table 7.3 should be used as a guide when initiating treatment postpartum. In each case previous response (and lack of response) to treatment must be considered.

Antipsychotics in breastfeeding

Table 7.4 provides information on individual drugs in breastfeeding based on available published data in mid-2020. Manufacturers' formal advice on drugs in breastfeeding is available in the Summary of Product Characteristics or European Public Assessment Report for individual drugs. Table 7.4 does not include this advice (which is often uninformative), but instead uses primary reference sources. It is usually advisable to continue the antipsychotic prescribed during pregnancy. Switching drugs postpartum for the purpose of breastfeeding is usually not sensible. The exception to this is clozapine – clozapine should continue but breastfeeding should be avoided. Table 7.4 should be used as a guide when initiating treatment postpartum. In each case the previous response (and lack of response) to treatment must be considered.

Mood stabilisers in breastfeeding

Table 7.5 provides information on individual drugs in breastfeeding based on available published data in mid-2020. Manufacturers' formal advice on drugs in breastfeeding is available in the Summary of Product Characteristics or European Public Assessment Report for individual drugs. Table 7.5 does not include this advice (which is often uninformative), but instead uses primary reference sources. It is usually advisable to continue the mood stabiliser prescribed during pregnancy. Switching drugs postpartum for the purpose of breastfeeding is usually not sensible. The exception to this is lithium. Lithium should be continued but breastfeeding should not be permitted. Table 7.5 should be used as a guide when initiating treatment postpartum. In each case the previous response (and lack of response) to treatment must be considered.

Hypnotics in breastfeeding

Table 7.6 provides information on individual drugs in breastfeeding based on available published data in mid-2020. Manufacturers' formal advice on drugs in breastfeeding is available in the Summary of Product Characteristics or European Public Assessment Report for individual drugs. Table 7.6 does not include this advice (which is often uninformative), but instead uses primary reference sources.

Stimulants in breastfeeding

Table 7.7 provides information on individual drugs in breastfeeding based on available published data in mid-2020. Manufacturers' formal advice on drugs in breastfeeding is available in the Summary of Product Characteristics or European Public Assessment

Table 7.3 Antidepressants in breastfeeding

Drug	Infant plasma concentrations	Relative infant dose (RID)	Reported acute adverse effects in infant	Reported developmental effects in infant
Agomelatine[3,4]	Not assessed	Not available	None reported but not studied	None reported but not studied
Brexanolone[5]	Not assessed	1–2%	None reported but not studied	None reported but not studied
Bupropion[4,6–13]	Undetectable or low	0.2–2%	Two reports of seizure-like activity in 6-month olds. In one of the cases the infant experienced sleep disturbance, severe emesis and somnolence. The infant plasma levels were below the level required for quantification. The mother was also taking escitalopram.	None reported but not studied
Citalopram[2,4,11,14–23]	Undetectable to up to 10% of maternal plasma levels. Higher than for fluvoxamine, sertraline, paroxetine and escitalopram, but lower than for fluoxetine.	3–10%	Sleep disturbance (which resolved on halving maternal dose), colic, decreased feeding, and irritability and restlessness. One case of irregular breathing, sleep disorder and hypo- and hypertonia Infant exposed to citalopram *in utero*. Symptoms attributed to withdrawal syndrome despite the mother continuing citalopram postpartum.	None reported. In a study of 78 infants of mothers taking an SSRI or venlafaxine no difference in weight was noted at 6 months compared with the 'normative' weight. In a study of 11 infants normal neurodevelopment was observed up to 1 year. One of the children was unable to walk at 1-year, However, neurological status of the child was deemed normal 6 months later.

(Continued)

Table 7.3 (Continued)

Drug	Infant plasma concentrations	Relative infant dose (RID)	Reported acute adverse effects in infant	Reported developmental effects in infant
Duloxetine[4,11,24–27]	<1% of maternal plasma levels.	<1%	Dizziness, nausea, fatigue	None reported but not assessed
Escitalopram[4,11,13,28–33]	Undetectable or low	3–8.3%	Necrotising enterocolitis in 5-day infant (necessitating intensive care admission and intravenous antibiotic treatment).Infant was exposed to escitalopram *in utero*. Symptoms were lethargy, decreased oral intake and blood in the stools. Seizure-like activity, sleep disturbance, severe emesis and somnolence in 6-month old. Mother was also taking bupropion.	None reported but not studied
Fluoxetine[2,4,11,14,23,34–45]	Variable: can be > 10% of maternal plasma levels. Highest reported levels of SSRIs.	1.6–14.6%	Colic, excessive crying, decreased sleep, diarrhoea, vomiting, somnolence, decreased feeding, hypotonia, moaning, grunting and hyperactivity. One case of seizure activity at 3 weeks, 4 months and then 5 months. Mother was also taking carbamazepine. One case of tachypnoea, jitteriness, irritability, fever and compensated metabolic acidosis. Infant plasma levels were in the adult therapeutic range. The authors diagnosed serotonin syndrome. Mother was taking fluoxetine 60mg.	Normal weight gain and neurological development has been reported for many infants. One retrospective study found lower growth curves compared with non-exposed infants. One case of a reduction in platelet serotonin.

(Continued)

Table 7.3 (Continued)

Drug	Infant plasma concentrations	Relative infant dose (RID)	Reported acute adverse effects in infant	Reported developmental effects in infant
Fluvoxamine[4,11,14,46-53]	Undetectable to up to half the maternal plasma level.	1–2%	Neonatal jaundice, severe diarrhoea, mild vomiting, decreased sleep and agitation.	None reported In a study of 78 infants of mothers taking an SSRI or venlafaxine no difference in weight was noted at 6 months compared with the 'normative' weight.
MAOIs[54,55]	No published data available at the time of writing.	Isoniazid = 1.2–18%.	None reported	None reported but not assessed
Mianserin[4,56]	Not assessed.	Not assessed.	None reported	None reported but not studied
Mirtazapine[4,11,57,58]	Undetectable or low. There is one case of higher mirtazapine plasma levels. The authors suggest there may be a large difference in mirtazapine elimination rates between individual infants.	0.5–4.4%	In a study of 54 infants exposed to mirtazapine *in utero* the incidence of poor neonatal adaptation syndrome was significantly diminished in those who were breastfed.	No abnormalities reported: In a study of eight infants weights for three were observed to be between the 10th to 25th percentiles. All three were noted to also have a low birth weight.
Moclobemide[4,59,60]	Low.	3.4%	None reported	None reported but not studied
Paroxetine[2,4,11,14,23,38,46,61-70]	Undetectable or low.	0.5–2.8%	Vomiting and irritability which were attributed to severe hyponatraemia. In a study of 72 infants adverse effects were noted in 9 infants. Insomnia, restlessness and constant crying were most commonly reported.	None reported. In a study of 78 infants of mothers taking an SSRI or venlafaxine no difference in weight was noted at 6 months compared with the 'normative' weight. Breast-fed infants of 27 women taking paroxetine reached the usual developmental milestones at 3, 6 and 12 months, similar to a control group.

(Continued)

Table 7.3 (Continued)

Drug	Infant plasma concentrations	Relative infant dose (RID)	Reported acute adverse effects in infant	Reported developmental effects in infant
Reboxetine[4,11,71]	Undetectable or low.	1–3%	None reported	In a study of four infants three reached normal milestones. The fourth had developmental problems thought not to be related to reboxetine
Sertraline[4,11,23,38,65,72–80]	Undetectable or low. There is one report of an unusually high infant serum level (half maternal serum level). The infant was reported to be 'clinically thriving'.	0.5–3%	Serotonergic overstimulation reported in preterm infant also exposed to sertraline *in utero*. Symptoms included hyperthermia, shivering, myoclonus, tremor, and irritability, high pitched crying, decreased suckling reflex and reactivity. Withdrawal symptoms (agitation, restlessness, insomnia and an enhanced startle reaction) developed in a breastfed neonate, after abrupt withdrawal of maternal sertraline. The neonate was exposed to sertraline *in utero*.	None reported. In a study of 78 infants of mothers taking an SSRI or venlafaxine no difference in weight was noted at 6 months compared with the 'normative' weight.
Trazodone[4,81]	Not assessed.	2.8%	None reported but not assessed.	None reported but not assessed.
Tricyclic Antidepressants (TCAs)[4,14,82–90]	Undetectable or low.	Nortriptyline. Amitriptyline, 1–3%. Clomipramine.	Adverse effects have not been reported in infants exposed to nortriptyline, clomipramine, imipramine, dosulepin and desipramine through breast milk. Severe sedation and poor feeding reported with amitriptyline. Poor suckling, muscle hypotonia, drowsiness and respiratory depression reported with doxepin.	None reported. A study of 15 children did not show a negative outcome in regard to cognitive development in breastfed children 3 to 5 years postpartum.

Table 7.3 (Continued)

Drug	Infant plasma concentrations	Relative infant dose (RID)	Reported acute adverse effects in infant	Reported developmental effects in infant
Venlafaxine,[4,11,23,38,65,91–98]	Undetectable to up to 37% of maternal plasma levels.	6–9%	Lethargy, jitteriness, rapid breathing, poor suckling and dehydration in an infant also exposed *in utero*. Symptoms subsided over a week on breastfeeding. Authors suggested that breastfeeding may have helped manage infant withdrawal symptoms postpartum.	None reported In a study of 78 infants of mothers taking an SSRI or venlafaxine no difference in weight was noted at 6 months compared with the 'normative' weight.
Vortioxetine	No published data available at the time of writing.			

Table 7.4 Antipsychotics in breastfeeding

Drug	Infant plasma concentration	Estimated daily infant dose as proportion of maternal dose (RID)	Acute adverse effects in infant	Developmental effects in infant
Amisulpride[4,94,99–101]	10.5% of the maternal plasma concentration.*	4.7–10.7%	None reported.	None reported.
Aripiprazole[4,102–107]	4% of maternal plasma concentration.*	0.9–8.3%	None reported.	None reported.
Asenapine	No published data available at the time of writing.			
Brexipiprazole	No published data available at the time of writing.			

(Continued)

Table 7.4 (Continued)

Drug	Infant plasma concentration	Estimated daily infant dose as proportion of maternal dose (RID)	Acute adverse effects in infant	Developmental effects in infant
Butyrophenones[4,14,38,82,100,108–111]	Not reported.	Haloperidol = 0.2–12%	One case of hypersomnia, poor feeding, and slowing in motor movements. Mother was also taking risperidone. The effects were noted when haloperidol dose was increased.	Delayed development was noted in three infants exposed to a combination of haloperidol and chlorpromazine in breast milk. Normal development has also been reported.
Cariprazine	No published data available at the time of writing.			
Clozapine[4,14,38,82,109,112–115] NB Avoid	6.5% of maternal plasma concentration.*	1.4%	Sedation, agranulocytosis, decreased sucking reflex, irritability, seizures and cardiovascular instability.	There is one report of delayed speech acquisition. The infant was also exposed to clozapine in utero.
Lurasidone	No published data available at the time of writing.			
Lumateperone tosylate	Published data not available.			
Olanzapine[4,14,38,100,116–128]	Undetectable or low. One case of plasma levels decreasing over 5 months. The authors proposed that infant's capacity to metabolise olanzapine 'developed rapidly' around the age of 4 months.	1.0–1.6%	Somnolence, drowsiness, irritability, tremor, insomnia, lethargy, poor suckling and shaking. One case of jaundice and sedation. Infant was exposed in utero and had cardiomegaly.	One case of lower developmental age than chronological age. Mother was taking additional psychotropic medication. One case of speech delay and one of motor developmental delay. Two cases of failure to gain weight. Normal development has also been reported.

(Continued)

Table 7.4 (Continued)

Drug	Infant plasma concentration	Estimated daily infant dose as proportion of maternal dose (RID)	Acute adverse effects in infant	Developmental effects in infant
Paliperidone	No specific data available. See risperidone.			
Phenothiazines[4,14,82,108–110]	Variable	Chlorpromazine = 0.3%	Lethargy.	Delayed development in three infants exposed to a combination of chlorpromazine and haloperidol.
Pimavanserin	No published data available at the time of writing.			
Quetiapine[4,95,125,129–138]	Undetectable	0.09–0.1%	Excessive sleep. Mother was also taking mirtazapine and a benzodiazepine.	In a small study of quetiapine augmentation of maternal antidepressant there were two cases of mild developmental delays, thought not to be related to quetiapine.
Risperidone[4,111,139–143]	Risperidone undetectable. 9-hydroxyrisperidone – low	Risperidone = 2.8–9.1% 9-hydroxyrisperidone = 3.46–4.7%	One case of hypersomnia, poor feeding, and slowing in motor movements. Mother was also taking haloperidol. The effects were noted when haloperidol dose was increased.	None reported.
Sertindole	No published data available at the time of writing.			
Sulpiride[4,144–148]	Not reported.	2.7–20.7%	None reported.	None reported but not assessed.
Thioxanthenes[4,14,110,149–151]	Not reported.	Zuclopenthixol = 0.4–0.9% Flupentixol = 0.7–1.75%	None reported.	None reported for flupentixol. Not assessed for zuclopenthixol.

(Continued)

Table 7.4 (Continued)

Drug	Infant plasma concentration	Estimated daily infant dose as proportion of maternal dose (RID)	Acute adverse effects in infant	Developmental effects in infant
Ziprasidone[4,22,110,152]	Not reported.	0.07–1.2%	None reported.	None reported.
Iloperidone	No published data available at the time of writing.			

* A proportion of the drug detected may have been due to placental transfer following in utero exposure.

Table 7.5 Mood stabilisers in breastfeeding

Drug	Infant plasma concentration	Estimated daily infant dose as proportion of maternal dose (RID)	Acute adverse effects in infant	Developmental effects in infant
Carbamazepine[4,14,153–163]	Generally low although one report of an infant plasma level within adult therapeutic range.	1.1–7.3%	Adverse effects have not been reported for a number of infants. One case of cholestatic hepatitis, one of transient hepatic dysfunction with hyperbilirubinaemia and elevated GGT. The adverse effects in the first case resolved after discontinuation of breastfeeding and the second resolved despite continued feeding. One case of seizure-like activity, drowsiness, irritability and high-pitched crying. Mother was taking multiple agents.	None reported. A prospective study of children of women with epilepsy found no adverse development at ages 6–36 months. The study assessed outcomes in children exposed to anticonvulsants in utero who were subsequently breastfed compared with those who were not. A study of 199 infants exposed to antiepileptic medications in utero and through breast milk failed to show a difference in IQ between breastfed and non-breastfed infants at the age of 3 years.

(Continued)

Table 7.5 (Continued)

Drug	Infant plasma concentration	Estimated daily infant dose as proportion of maternal dose (RID)	Acute adverse effects in infant	Developmental effects in infant
Carbamazepine (continued)			Poor suckling, poor feeding and 2 cases of hyperexcitability.	A study of 181 children concluded that IQ was not adversely affected by anticonvulsant exposure through breast milk.
Lamotrigine[4,156,161,164–175]	Undetectable to 48% of maternal plasma levels.	9.2–18.3%	No adverse effects have been reported in a number of infants. 7 cases of thrombocytosis One case of a severe cyanotic episode (preceded by mild episodes of apnoea) requiring resuscitation. Neonatal serum concentration was in the upper therapeutic range. Infant exposed in-utero. The mother was taking a high dose (850mg/day). One case of normocytic normochromic anaemia and asymptomatic neutropenia.[176] Three cases of rash. In one case the rash was attributed to eczema, and to soy allergy in another. The third case resolved spontaneously.	No abnormalities reported. A prospective study of children of women with epilepsy found that breastfeeding whilst taking an anticonvulsant was not associated with adverse development of infants at ages 6–36 months. The study assessed outcomes in children exposed to anticonvulsants in utero who were subsequently breastfed compared with those who were not. A study of 199 infants exposed to antiepileptic medications during breast feeding failed to show a difference in IQ between breastfed and non-breastfed infants at the age of 3 years. The infants were exposed to antiepileptic medications in utero. A study of 181 children concluded that IQ was not adversely affected by anticonvulsant exposure through breast milk.

(Continued)

Table 7.5 (*Continued*)

Drug	Infant plasma concentration	Estimated daily infant dose as proportion of maternal dose (RID)	Acute adverse effects in infant	Developmental effects in infant
Lithium[177] NB. Avoid	Undetectable to 57% of maternal plasma levels.	12–30.1%	Early feeding problems, increased urea, raised creatinine, non-specific signs of toxicity. One case of elevated TSH. In utero exposure. One case of cyanosis, lethargy, hypothermia, hypotonia and a heart murmur. In utero exposure. No adverse effects have been reported in others.	None reported.
Topiramate[178,179]	Undetectable to 20% of maternal plasma levels.	3–35%	Diarrhoea	None reported but not assessed.
Valproate[4,14,153–156,161,180,181]	<2% of maternal plasma levels.	1.4–1.7%	Thrombocytopenia and anaemia which reversed on stopping breastfeeding. *In utero* exposure.	A prospective study of children of women with epilepsy found that breastfeeding whilst taking an anticonvulsant was not associated with adverse development of infants at ages 6–36 months. The study assessed outcomes in children exposed to anticonvulsants in utero who were subsequently breastfed compared with those who were not. A study of 199 infants exposed to antiepileptic medications during breast feeding failed to show a difference in IQ between breastfed and non-breastfed infants at the age of 3 years. The infants were exposed to antiepileptic medications *in utero*. A study of 181 children concluded that IQ was not adversely affected by anticonvulsant exposure through breast milk.

(*Continued*)

Table 7.6 Hypnotics in breast-feeding

Drug	Infant plasma concentration	Estimated daily infant dose as proportion of maternal dose (RID)	Acute adverse effects in infant	Developmental effects in infant
Benzodiazepines[4,14,38,182–189]	Not reported	Clonazepam – 2.8% Diazepam – 0.88–7.1% Lorazepam – 2.6–2.9% Oxazepam – 0.28–1%	Sedation, lethargy, weight loss and mild jaundice. One case of persistent apnoea with clonazepam. Restlessness and mild drowsiness with alprazolam. In a telephone survey of 124 women two reported CNS depression in their breastfeeding neonates. One of the children was exposed to benzodiazepines in utero. No adverse effects have been reported in others.	Non reported but not studied.
Promethazine	No published data available at the time of writing.			
Zopiclone, zolpidem and zaleplon[4,190–192]	Not reported.	Zaleplon = 1.5% Zopiclone = 1.5% Zolpidem = 0.02–0.18%	None reported.	None reported but not studied.

Table 7.7 Stimulants in breastfeeding

Drug	Infant plasma concentration	Estimated daily infant dose as proportion of maternal dose (RID)	Acute adverse effects in infant	Developmental effects in infant
Atomoxetine	No published data available at the time of writing			
Dexamfetamine[193]	Undetectable to 14% of maternal plasma level	2.4–10.6%	None reported	None reported but not assessed
Lisdexamfetamine	No published data available at the time of writing			
Methylphenidate[27,194–196]	Undetectable	0.16–0.7%	None reported	None reported
Modafinil[197,198]	Not reported	5.3%	None reported	None reported but not assessed

Report for individual drugs. Table 7.7 does not include this advice (which is often uninformative), but instead uses primary reference sources. It is usually advisable to continue the drug prescribed during pregnancy. Switching drugs postpartum for the purpose of breastfeeding is usually not sensible. Table 7.7 should be used as a guide when initiating treatment postpartum. In each case the previous response (and lack of response) to treatment must be considered.

References

1. Schoretsanitis G, et al. Excretion of antipsychotics into the amniotic fluid, umbilical cord blood, and breast milk: a systematic critical review and combined analysis. *Ther Drug Monit* 2020; 42:245–254.
2. Weissman AM, et al. Pooled analysis of antidepressant levels in lactating mothers, breast milk, and nursing infants. *Am J Psychiatry* 2004; 161:1066–1078.
3. Schmidt FM, et al. Agomelatine in breast milk. *Int J Neuropsychopharmacol* 2013; 16:497–499.
4. Hale TW, et al. *Medications and mothers' milk – 18th edition*. New York, USA: Springer Publishing Company; 2019.
5. Hoffmann E, et al. Brexanolone injection administration to lactating women: breast milk allopregnanolone levels [30J]. *Obstet Gynecol* 2019; 133:115S.
6. Briggs GG, et al. Excretion of bupropion in breast milk. *Ann Pharmacother* 1993; 27:431–433.
7. Chaudron LH, et al. Bupropion and breastfeeding: a case of a possible infant seizure. *J Clin Psychiatry* 2004; 65:881–882.
8. Nonacs RM, et al. Bupropion SR for the treatment of postpartum depression: a pilot study. *Int J Neuropsychopharmacol* 2005; 8:445–449.
9. Haas JS, et al. Bupropion in breast milk: an exposure assessment for potential treatment to prevent post-partum tobacco use. *Tob Control* 2004; 13:52–56.
10. Baab SW, et al. Serum bupropion levels in 2 breastfeeding mother-infant pairs. *J Clin Psychiatry* 2002; 63:910–911.
11. Berle JO, et al. Antidepressant use during breastfeeding. *Curr Womens Health Rev* 2011; 7:28–34.
12. Davis MF, et al. Bupropion levels in breast milk for 4 mother-infant pairs: more answers to lingering questions. *J Clin Psychiatry* 2009; 70:297–298.
13. Neuman G, et al. Bupropion and escitalopram during lactation. *Ann Pharmacother* 2014; 48:928–931.
14. Burt VK, et al. The use of psychotropic medications during breast-feeding. *Am J Psychiatry* 2001; 158:1001–1009.

15. Lee A, et al. Frequency of infant adverse events that are associated with citalopram use during breast-feeding. *Am J Obstet Gynecol* 2004; 190:218–221.

16. Heikkinen T, et al. Citalopram in pregnancy and lactation. *Clin Pharmacol Ther* 2002; 72:184–191.

17. Jensen PN, et al. Citalopram and desmethylcitalopram concentrations in breast milk and in serum of mother and infant. *Ther Drug Monit* 1997; 19:236–239.

18. Spigset O, et al. Excretion of citalopram in breast milk. *Br J Clin Pharmacol* 1997; 44:295–298.

19. Rampono J, et al. Citalopram and demethylcitalopram in human milk; distribution, excretion and effects in breast fed infants. *Br J Clin Pharmacol* 2000; 50:263–268.

20. Schmidt K, et al. Citalopram and breast-feeding: serum concentration and side effects in the infant. *Biol Psychiatry* 2000; 47:164–165.

21. Franssen EJ, et al. Citalopram serum and milk levels in mother and infant during lactation. *Ther Drug Monit* 2006; 28:2–4.

22. Werremeyer A. Ziprasidone and citalopram use in pregnancy and lactation in a woman with psychotic depression. *Am J Psychiatry* 2009; 166:1298.

23. Hendrick V, et al. Weight gain in breastfed infants of mothers taking antidepressant medications. *J Clin Psychiatry* 2003; 64:410–412.

24. Boyce PM, et al. Duloxetine transfer across the placenta during pregnancy and into milk during lactation. *Arch Women's Mental Health* 2011; 14:169–172.

25. Briggs GG, et al. Use of duloxetine in pregnancy and lactation. *Ann Pharmacother* 2009; 43:1898–1902.

26. Lobo ED, et al. Pharmacokinetics of duloxetine in breast milk and plasma of healthy postpartum women. *Clin Pharmacokinet* 2008; 47:103–109.

27. Collin-Lévesque L, et al. Infant exposure to methylphenidate and duloxetine during lactation. *Breastfeed Med* 2018; 13:221–225.

28. Gentile S. Escitalopram late in pregnancy and while breast-feeding (Letter). *Ann Pharmacother* 2006; 40:1696–1697.

29. Castberg I, et al. Excretion of escitalopram in breast milk. *J Clin Psychopharmacol* 2006; 26:536–538.

30. Rampono J, et al. Transfer of escitalopram and its metabolite demethylescitalopram into breastmilk. *Br J Clin Pharmacol* 2006; 62:316–322.

31. Potts AL, et al. Necrotizing enterocolitis associated with in utero and breast milk exposure to the selective serotonin reuptake inhibitor, escitalopram. *J Perinatol* 2007; 27:120–122.

32. Ilett KF, et al. Estimation of infant dose and assessment of breastfeeding safety for escitalopram use in postnatal depression. *Ther Drug Monit* 2005; 27:248.

33. Bellantuono C, et al. The safety of escitalopram during pregnancy and breastfeeding: a comprehensive review. *Hum Psychopharmacol* 2012; 27:534–539.

34. Yoshida K, et al. Fluoxetine in breast-milk and developmental outcome of breast-fed infants. *Br J Psychiatry* 1998; 172:175–178.

35. Lester BM, et al. Possible association between fluoxetine hydrochloride and colic in an infant. *J Am Acad Child Adolesc Psychiatry* 1993; 32:1253–1255.

36. Hendrick V, et al. Fluoxetine and norfluoxetine concentrations in nursing infants and breast milk. *Biol Psychiatry* 2001; 50:775–782.

37. Hale TW, et al. Fluoxetine toxicity in a breastfed infant. *Clin Pediatr* 2001; 40:681–684.

38. Malone K, et al. Antidepressants, antipsychotics, benzodiazepines, and the breastfeeding dyad. *Perspect Psychiatr Care* 2004; 40:73–85.

39. Heikkinen T, et al. Pharmacokinetics of fluoxetine and norfluoxetine in pregnancy and lactation. *Clin Pharmacol Ther* 2003; 73:330–337.

40. Epperson CN, et al. Maternal fluoxetine treatment in the postpartum period: effects on platelet serotonin and plasma drug levels in breast-feeding mother-infant pairs. *Pediatrics* 2003; 112:e425.

41. Taddio A, et al. Excretion of fluoxetine and its metabolite, norfluoxetine, in human breast milk. *J Clin Pharmacol* 1996; 36:42–47.

42. Brent NB, et al. Fluoxetine and carbamazepine concentrations in a nursing mother/infant pair. *Clin Pediatr (Phila)* 1998; 37:41–44.

43. Kristensen JH, et al. Distribution and excretion of fluoxetine and norfluoxetine in human milk. *Br J Clin Pharmacol* 1999; 48:521–527.

44. Burch KJ, et al. Fluoxetine/norfluoxetine concentrations in human milk. *Pediatrics* 1992; 89:676–677.

45. Morris R, et al. Serotonin syndrome in a breast-fed neonate. *BMJ Case Rep* 2015; 2015.

46. Hendrick V, et al. Use of sertraline, paroxetine and fluvoxamine by nursing women. *Br J Psychiatry* 2001; 179:163–166.

47. Piontek CM, et al. Serum fluvoxamine levels in breastfed infants. *J Clin Psychiatry* 2001; 62:111–113.

48. Yoshida K, et al. Fluvoxamine in breast-milk and infant development. *Br J Clin Pharmacol* 1997; 44:210–211.

49. Hagg S, et al. Excretion of fluvoxamine into breast milk. *Br J Clin Pharmacol* 2000; 49:286–288.

50. Arnold LM, et al. Fluvoxamine concentrations in breast milk and in maternal and infant sera. *J Clin Psychopharmacol* 2000; 20:491–492.

51. Kristensen JH, et al. The amount of fluvoxamine in milk is unlikely to be a cause of adverse effects in breastfed infants. *J Hum Lact* 2002; 18:139–143.

52. Wright S, et al. Excretion of fluvoxamine in breast milk. *Br J Clin Pharmacol* 1991; 31:209.

53. Uguz F. Gastrointestinal side effects in the baby of a breastfeeding woman treated with low-dose fluvoxamine. *J Hum Lact* 2015; 31:371–373.

54. Snider DE, Jr., et al. Should women taking antituberculosis drugs breast-feed? *Arch Intern Med* 1984; 144:589–590.

55. Singh N, et al. Transfer of isoniazid from circulation to breast milk in lactating women on chronic therapy for tuberculosis. *Br J Clin Pharmacol* 2008; 65:418–422.

56. Buist A, et al. Mianserin in breast milk (Letter). *Br J Clin Pharmacol* 1993; 36:133–134.

57. Smit M, et al. Mirtazapine in pregnancy and lactation: data from a case series. *J Clin Psychopharmacol* 2015; 35:163–167.

58. Smit M, et al. Mirtazapine in pregnancy and lactation – a systematic review. *Eur Neuropsychopharmacol* 2016; 26:126–135.

59. Buist A, et al. Plasma and human milk concentrations of moclobemide in nursing mothers. *Human Psychopharmacology* 1998; 13:579–582.

CHAPTER 7

60. Pons G, et al. Moclobemide excretion in human breast milk. *Br J Clin Pharmacol* 1990; **29**:27–31.

61. Begg EJ, et al. Paroxetine in human milk. *Br J Clin Pharmacol* 1999; **48**:142–147.

62. Stowe ZN, et al. Paroxetine in human breast milk and nursing infants. *Am J Psychiatry* 2000; **157**:185–189.

63. Misri S, et al. Paroxetine levels in postpartum depressed women, breast milk, and infant serum. *J Clin Psychiatry* 2000; **61**:828–832.

64. Ohman R, et al. Excretion of paroxetine into breast milk. *J Clin Psychiatry* 1999; **60**:519–523.

65. Berle JO, et al. Breastfeeding during maternal antidepressant treatment with serotonin reuptake inhibitors: infant exposure, clinical symptoms, and cytochrome p450 genotypes. *J Clin Psychiatry* 2004; **65**:1228–1234.

66. Merlob P, et al. Paroxetine during breast-feeding: infant weight gain and maternal adherence to counsel. *Eur J Pediatr* 2004; **163**:135–139.

67. Abdul Aziz A, et al. Severe paroxetine induced hyponatremia in a breast fed infant. *J Bahrain Med Soc* 2004; **16**:195–198.

68. Hendrick V, et al. Paroxetine use during breast-feeding. *J Clin Psychopharmacol* 2000; **20**:587–589.

69. Spigset O, et al. Paroxetine level in breast milk. *J Clin Psychiatry* 1996; **57**:39.

70. Uguz F, et al. Short-term safety of paroxetine and sertraline in breastfed infants: a retrospective cohort study from a university hospital. *Breastfeed Med* 2016; **11**:487–489.

71. Hackett LP, et al. Transfer of reboxetine into breastmilk, its plasma concentrations and lack of adverse effects in the breastfed infant. *Eur J Clin Pharmacol* 2006; **62**:633–638.

72. Llewellyn A, et al. Psychotropic medications in lactation. *J Clin Psychiatry* 1998; **59 Suppl 2**:41–52.

73. Mammen OK, et al. Sertraline and norsertraline levels in three breastfed infants. *J Clin Psychiatry* 1997; **58**:100–103.

74. Altshuler LL, et al. Breastfeeding and sertraline: a 24-hour analysis. *J Clin Psychiatry* 1995; **56**:243–245.

75. Dodd S, et al. Sertraline analysis in the plasma of breast-fed infants. *Aust N Z J Psychiatry* 2001; **35**:545–546.

76. Dodd S, et al. Sertraline in paired blood plasma and breast-milk samples from nursing mothers. *Hum Psychopharmacol* 2000; **15**:161–264.

77. Epperson N, et al. Maternal sertraline treatment and serotonin transport in breast-feeding mother-infant pairs. *Am J Psychiatry* 2001; **158**:1631–1637.

78. Stowe ZN, et al. The pharmacokinetics of sertraline excretion into human breast milk: determinants of infant serum concentrations. *J Clin Psychiatry* 2003; **64**:73–80.

79. Muller MJ, et al. Serotonergic overstimulation in a preterm infant after sertraline intake via breastmilk. *Breastfeed Med* 2013; **8**:327–329.

80. Wisner KL, et al. Serum sertraline and N-desmethylsertraline levels in breast-feeding mother-infant pairs. *Am J Psychiatry* 1998; **155**:690–692.

81. Verbeeck RK, et al. Excretion of trazodone in breast milk. *Br J Clin Pharmacol* 1986; **22**:367–370.

82. Yoshida K, et al. Psychotropic drugs in mothers' milk: a comprehensive review of assay methods, pharmacokinetics and of safety of breast-feeding. *J Psychopharmacol* 1999; **13**:64–80.

83. Misri S, et al. Benefits and risks to mother and infant of drug treatment for postnatal depression. *Drug Saf* 2002; **25**:903–911.

84. Yoshida K, et al. Investigation of pharmacokinetics and of possible adverse effects in infants exposed to tricyclic antidepressants in breast-milk. *J Affect Disord* 1997; **43**:225–237.

85. Frey OR, et al. Adverse effects in a newborn infant breast-fed by a mother treated with doxepin. *Ann Pharmacother* 1999; **33**:690–693.

86. Ilett KF, et al. The excretion of dothiepin and its primary metabolites in breast milk. *Br J Clin Pharmacol* 1992; **33**:635–639.

87. Kemp J, et al. Excretion of doxepin and N-desmethyldoxepin in human milk. *Br J Clin Pharmacol* 1985; **20**:497–499.

88. Buist A, et al. Effect of exposure to dothiepin and northiaden in breast milk on child development. *Br J Psychiatry* 1995; **167**:370–373.

89. Khachman D, et al. Clomipramine in breast milk: a case study *J Pharm Clin* 2007; **28**:33–38.

90. Uguz F. Poor feeding and severe sedation in a newborn nursed by a mother on a low dose of amitriptyline. *Breastfeed Med* 2017; **12**:67–68.

91. Koren G, et al. Can venlafaxine in breast milk attenuate the norepinephrine and serotonin reuptake neonatal withdrawal syndrome. *J Obstet Gynaecol Can* 2006; **28**:299–302.

92. Ilett KF, et al. Distribution of venlafaxine and its O-desmethyl metabolite in human milk and their effects in breastfed infants. *Br J Clin Pharmacol* 2002; **53**:17–22.

93. Newport DJ, et al. Venlafaxine in human breast milk and nursing infant plasma: determination of exposure. *J Clin Psychiatry* 2009; **70**:1304–1310.

94. Ilett KF, et al. Assessment of infant dose through milk in a lactating woman taking amisulpride and desvenlafaxine for treatment-resistant depression. *Ther Drug Monit* 2010; **32**:704–707.

95. Misri S, et al. Quetiapine augmentation in lactation: a series of case reports. *J Clin Psychopharmacol* 2006; **26**:508–511.

96. Hendrick V, et al. Venlafaxine and breast-feeding. *Am J Psychiatry* 2001; **158**:2089–2090.

97. Rampono J, et al. Estimation of desvenlafaxine transfer into milk and infant exposure during its use in lactating women with postnatal depression. *Arch Womens Ment Health* 2011; **14**:49–53.

98. Ilett KF, et al. Distribution and excretion of venlafaxine and O-desmethylvenlafaxine in human milk. *Br J Clin Pharmacol* 1998; **45**:459–462.

99. Teoh S, et al. Estimation of rac-amisulpride transfer into milk and of infant dose via milk during its use in a lactating woman with bipolar disorder and schizophrenia. *Breastfeed Med* 2010; **6**:85–88.

100. Uguz F. breastfed infants exposed to combined antipsychotics: two case reports. *Am J Ther* 2016; **23**:e1962–e1964.

101. O'Halloran SJ, et al. A liquid chromatography-tandem mass spectrometry method for quantifying amisulpride in human plasma and breast milk, applied to measuring drug transfer to a fully breast-fed neonate. *Ther Drug Monit* 2016; **38**:493–498.

102. Schlotterbeck P, et al. Aripiprazole in human milk. *Int J Neuropsychopharmacol* 2007; **10**:433.

103. Lutz UC, et al. Aripiprazole in pregnancy and lactation: a case report. *J Clin Psychopharmacol* 2010; **30**:204–205.

104. Watanabe N, et al. Perinatal use of aripiprazole: a case report. *J Clin Psychopharmacol* 2011; **31**:377–379.

105. Mendhekar DN, et al. Aripiprazole use in a pregnant schizoaffective woman. *Bipolar Disorders* 2006; **8**:299–300.

106. Nordeng H, et al. Transfer of aripiprazole to breast milk: a case report. *J Clin Psychopharmacol* 2014; **34**:272–275.

107. Frew JR. Psychopharmacology of bipolar I disorder during lactation: a case report of the use of lithium and aripiprazole in a nursing mother. *Arch Women's Mental Health* 2015; **18**:135–136.

108. Yoshida K, et al. Breast-feeding and psychotropic drugs. *Int Rev Psychiatry (Abingdon, England)* 1996; **8**:117–124.

109. Patton SW, et al. Antipsychotic medication during pregnancy and lactation in women with schizophrenia: evaluating the risk. *Can J Psychiatry* 2002; **47**:959–965.

110. Klinger G, et al. Antipsychotic drugs and breastfeeding. *Pediatr Endocrinol Rev* 2013; **10**:308–317.

111. Uguz F. Adverse events in a breastfed infant exposed to risperidone and haloperidol. *Breastfeed Med* 2019; **14**:683–684.

112. Mendhekar DN. Possible delayed speech acquisition with clozapine therapy during pregnancy and lactation. *J Neuropsychiatry Clin Neurosci* 2007; **19**:196–197.

113. Barnas C, et al. Clozapine concentrations in maternal and fetal plasma, amniotic fluid, and breast milk. *Am J Psychiatry* 1994; **151**:945.

114. Shao P, et al. Effects of clozapine and other atypical antipsychotics on infants development who were exposed to as fetus: a post-hoc analysis. *PLoS One* 2015; **10**:e0123373.

115. Imaz ML, et al. Clozapine use during pregnancy and lactation: a case-series report. *Front Pharmacol* 2018; **9**:264.

116. Goldstein DJ, et al. Olanzapine-exposed pregnancies and lactation: early experience. *J Clin Psychopharmacol* 2000; **20**:399–403.

117. Croke S, et al. Olanzapine excretion in human breast milk: estimation of infant exposure. *Int J Neuropsychopharmacol* 2002; **5**:243–247.

118. Gardiner SJ, et al. Transfer of olanzapine into breast milk, calculation of infant drug dose, and effect on breast-fed infants. *Am J Psychiatry* 2003; **160**:1428–1431.

119. Ambresin G, et al. Olanzapine excretion into breast milk: a case report. *J Clin Psychopharmacol* 2004; **24**:93–95.

120. Lutz UC, et al. Olanzapine treatment during breast feeding: a case report. *Ther Drug Monit* 2008; **30**:399–401.

121. Whitworth A, et al. Olanzapine and breast-feeding: changes of plasma concentrations of olanzapine in a breast-fed infant over a period of 5 months. *J Psychopharmacol* 2010; **24**:121–123.

122. Eli Lilly and Company Limited. Personal correspondence – olanzapine – use in pregnant or nursing women. 2011.

123. Gilad O, et al. Outcome of infants exposed to olanzapine during breastfeeding. *Breastfeed Med* 2010; **6**:55–58.

124. Goldstein DJ, et al. Olanzapine use during breast-feeding. *Schizophr Res* 2002; **53 (Suppl 1)**:185.

125. Aydin B, et al. Olanzapine and quetiapine use during breastfeeding: excretion into breast milk and safe breastfeeding strategy. *J Clin Psychopharmacol* 2015; **35**:206–208.

126. Stiegler A, et al. Olanzapine treatment during pregnancy and breastfeeding: a chance for women with psychotic illness? *Psychopharmacology (Berl)* 2014; **231**:3067–3069.

127. Var L, et al. Management of postpartum manic episode without cessation of breastfeeding: a longitudinal follow up of drug excretion into breast milk. *Eur Neuropsychopharmacol* 2013; **23 (Suppl 1)**:S382.

128. Manouilenko I, et al. Long-acting olanzapine injection during pregnancy and breastfeeding: a case report. *Arch Women's Mental Health* 2018; **21**:587–589.

129. Lee A, et al. Excretion of quetiapine in breast milk. *Am J Psychiatry* 2004; **161**:1715–1716.

130. Gentile S. Quetiapine-fluvoxamine combination during pregnancy and while breastfeeding (Letter). *Arch Women's Mental Health* 2006; **9**:158–159.

131. Seppala J. Quetiapine (Seroquel) is effective and well tolerated in the treatment of psychotic depression during breast feeding. *Eur Neuropsychopharmacol* 2004; **(7 Suppl 1)**: S245.

132. Kruninger U, et al. Pregnancy and lactation under treatment with quetiapine. *Psychiatr Prax* 2007; **34 Suppl 1**:S75–S76.

133. Ritz S. Quetiapine monotherapy in post-partum onset bipolar disorder with a mixed affective state. *Eur Neuropsychopharmacol* 2005; **15 Suppl 3**:S407.

134. Rampono J, et al. Quetiapine and breast feeding. *Ann Pharmacother* 2007; **41**:711–714.

135. Tanoshima R, et al. Quetiapine in human breast milk – population PK analysis of milk levels and simulated infant exposure. *J Popul Ther Clin Pharmacol* 2012; **19**:e259–e298.

136. Yazdani-Brojeni P, et al. Quetiapine in human milk and simulation-based assessment of infant exposure. *Clin Pharmacol Ther* 2010; **87 Suppl 1**:S3–S4.

137. Var L, et al. Management of postpartum manic episode without cessation of breastfeeding: A longitudinal follow up of drug excretion into breast milk. *Eur Neuropsychopharmacol* 2013; **23 Suppl 2**:S382.

138. Van Boekholt AA, et al. Quetiapine concentrations during exclusive breastfeeding and maternal quetiapine use. *Ann Pharmacother* 2015; **49**:743–744.

139. Hill RC, et al. Risperidone distribution and excretion into human milk: case report and estimated infant exposure during breast-feeding. *J Clin Psychopharmacol* 2000; **20**:285–286.

140. Aichhorn W, et al. Risperidone and breast-feeding. *J Psychopharmacol* 2005; **19**:211–213.

141. Ilett KF, et al. Transfer of risperidone and 9-hydroxyrisperidone into human milk. *Ann Pharmacother* 2004; **38**:273–276.

142. Ratnayake T, et al. No complications with risperidone treatment before and throughout pregnancy and during the nursing period. *J Clin Psychiatry* 2002; **63**:76–77.

143. Weggelaar NM, et al. A case report of risperidone distribution and excretion into human milk: how to give good advice if you have not enough data available. *J Clin Psychopharmacol* 2011; **31**:129–131.

144. Ylikorkala O, et al. Treatment of inadequate lactation with oral sulpiride and buccal oxytocin. *Obstet Gynecol* 1984; 63:57–60.

145. Ylikorkala O, et al. Sulpiride improves inadequate lactation. *Br Med J* 1982; 285:249–251.

146. Aono T, et al. Augmentation of puerperal lactation by oral administration of sulpiride. *J Clin Endocrinol Metab* 1970; 48:478–482.

147. Polatti F. Sulpiride isomers and milk secretion in puerperium. *Clin Exp Obstet Gynecol* 1982; 9:144–147.

148. Aono T, et al. Effect of sulpiride on poor puerperal lactation. *Am J Obstet Gynecol* 1982; 143:927–932.

149. Matheson I, et al. Milk concentrations of flupenthixol, nortriptyline and zuclopenthixol and between-breast differences in two patients. *Eur J Clin Pharmacol* 1988; 35:217–220.

150. Kirk L, et al. Concentrations of Cis(Z)-flupentixol in maternal serum, amniotic fluid, umbilical cord serum, and milk. *Psychopharmacology (Berl)* 1980; 72:107–108.

151. Aaes-Jorgensen T, et al. Zuclopenthixol levels in serum and breast milk. *Psychopharmacology (Berl)* 1986; 90:417–418.

152. Schlotterbeck P, et al. Low concentration of ziprasidone in human milk: a case report. *Int J Neuropsychopharmacol* 2009; 12:437–438.

153. Chaudron LH, et al. Mood stabilizers during breastfeeding: a review. *J Clin Psychiatry* 2000; 61:79–90.

154. Wisner KL, et al. Serum levels of valproate and carbamazepine in breastfeeding mother-infant pairs. *J Clin Psychopharmacol* 1998; 18:167–169.

155. Ernst CL, et al. The reproductive safety profile of mood stabilizers, atypical antipsychotics, and broad-spectrum psychotropics. *J Clin Psychiatry* 2002; 63 Suppl 4:42–55.

156. Meador KJ, et al. Effects of breastfeeding in children of women taking antiepileptic drugs. *Neurology* 2010; 75:1954–1960.

157. Zhao M, et al. [A case report of monitoring on carbamazepine in breast feeding woman]. *Beijing Da Xue Xue Bao* 2010; 42:602–603.

158. Froescher W, et al. Carbamazepine levels in breast milk. *Ther Drug Monit* 1984; 6:266–271.

159. Frey B, et al. Transient cholestatic hepatitis in a neonate associated with carbamazepine exposure during pregnancy and breast-feeding. *Eur J Pediatr* 1990; 150:136–138.

160. Merlob P, et al. Transient hepatic dysfunction in an infant of an epileptic mother treated with carbamazepine during pregnancy and breast-feeding. *Ann Pharmacother* 1992; 26:1563–1565.

161. Veiby G, et al. Early child development and exposure to antiepileptic drugs prenatally and through breastfeeding: a prospective cohort study on children of women with epilepsy. *JAMA Neurol* 2013; 70:1367–1374.

162. Pynnonen S, et al. Letter: carbamazepine and mother's milk. *Lancet* 1975; 2:563.

163. Meador KJ, et al. Breastfeeding in children of women taking antiepileptic drugs: cognitive outcomes at age 6 years. *JAMA Pediatrics* 2014; 168:729–736.

164. Ohman I, et al. Lamotrigine in pregnancy: pharmacokinetics during delivery, in the neonate, and during lactation. *Epilepsia* 2000; 41:709–713.

165. Liporace J, et al. Concerns regarding lamotrigine and breast-feeding. *Epilepsy Behav* 2004; 5:102–105.

166. Gentile S. Lamotrigine in pregnancy and lactation (Letter). *Arch Women's Mental Health* 2005; 8:57–58.

167. Page-Sharp M, et al. Transfer of lamotrigine into breast milk (Letter). *Ann Pharmacother* 2006; 40:1470–1471.

168. Rambeck B, et al. Concentrations of lamotrigine in a mother on lamotrigine treatment and her newborn child. *Eur J Clin Pharmacol* 1997; 51:481–484.

169. Tomson T, et al. Lamotrigine in pregnancy and lactation: a case report. *Epilepsia* 1997; 38:1039–1041.

170. Newport DJ, et al. Lamotrigine in breast milk and nursing infants: determination of exposure. *Pediatrics* 2008; 122:e223–e231.

171. Fotopoulou C, et al. Prospectively assessed changes in lamotrigine-concentration in women with epilepsy during pregnancy, lactation and the neonatal period. *Epilepsy Res* 2009; 85:60–64.

172. Nordmo E, et al. Severe apnea in an infant exposed to lamotrigine in breast milk. *Ann Pharmacother* 2009; 43:1893–1897.

173. Wakil L, et al. Neonatal outcomes with the use of lamotrigine for bipolar disorder in pregnancy and breastfeeding: a case series and review of the literature. *Psychopharmacol Bull* 2009; 42:91–98.

174. Birnbaum AK, et al. Antiepileptic drug exposure in infants of breastfeeding mothers with epilepsy. *JAMA Neurol* 2020; 77:441–450.

175. Kacirova I, et al. A short communication: lamotrigine levels in milk, mothers, and breastfed infants during the first postnatal month. *Ther Drug Monit* 2019; 41:401–404.

176. Bedussi F, et al. Normocytic normochromic anaemia and asymptomatic neutropenia in a 40-day-old infant breastfed by an epileptic mother treated with lamotrigine: infant's adverse drug reaction. *J Paediatr Child Health* 2018; 54:104–105.

177. Newmark RL, et al. Risk-benefit assessment of infant exposure to lithium through breast milk: a systematic review of the literature. *Int Rev Psychiatry (Abingdon, England)* 2019; 31:295–304.

178. Westergren T, et al. Probable topiramate-induced diarrhea in a 2-month-old breast-fed child - A case report. *Epilepsy Behav Case Rep* 2014; 2:22–23.

179. Gentile S. Topiramate in pregnancy and breastfeeding. *Clin Drug Investig* 2009; 29:139–141.

180. Piontek CM, et al. Serum valproate levels in 6 breastfeeding mother-infant pairs. *J Clin Psychiatry* 2000; 61:170–172.

181. Bjornsson E. Hepatotoxicity associated with antiepileptic drugs. *Acta Neurol Scand* 2008; 118:281–290.

182. Spigset O, et al. Excretion of psychotropic drugs into breast milk: pharmacokinetic overview and therapeutic implications. *CNS Drugs* 1998; 9:111–134.

183. Hagg S, et al. Anticonvulsant use during lactation. *Drug Saf* 2000; 22:425–440.

184. Iqbal MM, et al. Effects of commonly used benzodiazepines on the fetus, the neonate, and the nursing infant. *Psychiatr Serv* 2002; 53:39–49.

185. Buist A, et al. Breastfeeding and the use of psychotropic medication: a review. *J Affect Disord* 1990; 19:197–206.

186. Fisher JB, et al. Neonatal apnea associated with maternal clonazepam therapy: a case report. *Obstet Gynecol* 1985; 66:34S–35S.

187. Davanzo R, et al. Benzodiazepine e allattamento materno. *Medico E Bambino* 2008; 27:109–114.

188. Kelly LE, et al. Neonatal benzodiazepines exposure during breastfeeding. *J Pediatr* 2012; **161**:448–451.

189. Birnbaum CS, et al. Serum concentrations of antidepressants and benzodiazepines in nursing infants: a case series. *Pediatrics* 1999; **104**:e11.

190. Darwish M, et al. Rapid disappearance of zaleplon from breast milk after oral administration to lactating women. *J Clin Pharmacol* 1999; **39**:670–674.

191. Pons G, et al. Excretion of psychoactive drugs into breast milk. Pharmacokinetic principles and recommendations. *Clin Pharmacokinet* 1994; **27**:270–289.

192. Matheson I, et al. The excretion of zopiclone into breast milk. *Br J Clin Pharmacol* 1990; **30**:267–271.

193. Ilett KF, et al. Transfer of dexamphetamine into breast milk during treatment for attention deficit hyperactivity disorder. *Br J Clin Pharmacol* 2007; **63**:371–375.

194. Hackett LP, et al. Methylphenidate and breast-feeding. *Ann Pharmacother* 2006; **40**:1890–1891.

195. Bolea-Alamanac BM, et al. Methylphenidate use in pregnancy and lactation: a systematic review of evidence. *Br J Clin Pharmacol* 2014; **77**:96–101.

196. Marchese M, et al. Is it safe to breastfeed while taking methylphenidate? *Can Fam Physician* 2015; **61**:765–766.

197. Aurora S, et al. Evaluating transfer of modafinil into human milk during lactation: a case report. *J Clin Sleep Med* 2018; **14**:2087–2089.

198. Calvo-Ferrandiz E, et al. Narcolepsy with cataplexy and pregnancy: a case-control study. *J Sleep Res* 2018; **27**:268–272.

Further reading

National Institute for Health Care and Excellence. Antenatal and postnatal mental health: clinical management and service guidance. Clinical guideline [CG192] 2014 (Last updated February 2020); https://www.nice.org.uk/guidance/cg192

CHAPTER 7

Chapter 8

Hepatic and renal impairment

Hepatic impairment

Patients with hepatic impairment may have:

- **Reduced capacity to metabolise** biological waste products, dietary proteins and foreign substances, such as drugs. Clinical consequences include hepatic encephalopathy and increased dose-related side-effects from drugs.
- **Reduced ability to synthesise** plasma proteins and vitamin K-dependent clotting factors. Clinical consequences include hypoalbuminaemia, leading in extreme cases to ascites. Increased toxicity from highly protein-bound drugs should be anticipated. There is also an increased risk of bleeding from gastro-irritant drugs and perhaps with SSRIs.
- **Reduced hepatic blood flow.** Clinical consequences include oesophageal varices and elevated plasma levels of drugs subject to first-pass metabolism.

General principles

Liver function tests (LFTs) are a poor marker of hepatic metabolising capacity, as the hepatic reserve is large. Note that many patients with chronic liver disease are asymptomatic or have fluctuating clinical symptoms. Always consider the clinical presentation rather than adhere to rigid rules involving LFTs.

There are few clinical studies relating to the use of psychotropic drugs in people with hepatic disease. The following principles should be adhered to:

1. Prescribe as **few drugs** as possible.
2. Use **lower starting doses**, particularly of drugs that are highly protein bound. TCAs, SSRIs (except citalopram), trazodone and antipsychotics may have increased free plasma levels, at least initially. This will not be reflected in measured (total) plasma levels. Use lower doses of drugs known to be subject to extensive first-pass metabolism. Examples include TCAs and haloperidol.

The Maudsley® Prescribing Guidelines in Psychiatry, Fourteenth Edition. David M. Taylor,
Thomas R. E. Barnes and Allan H. Young.
© 2021 David M. Taylor. Published 2021 by John Wiley & Sons Ltd.

3. Be **cautious with drugs that are extensively hepatically metabolised** (mostly psychotropic drugs). Lower doses may be required. Exceptions are sulpiride, amisulpride, lithium and gabapentin, which all undergo no or minimal hepatic metabolism.

4. **Leave longer intervals between dosage increases.** Remember that the half-life of most drugs is prolonged in hepatic impairment, so it will take longer for plasma levels to reach steady state.

5. If albumin is reduced, consider the implications for drugs that are **highly protein bound,** and **if ascites is present consider the increased volume of distribution for water soluble drugs.**

6. **Avoid medicines with a long-half life** or those that require to be metabolised to render them active (**pro-drugs)**

7. Always **monitor carefully for side-effects,** which may be delayed.

8. **Avoid drugs that are very sedative** because of the risk of precipitating hepatic encephalopathy.

9. **Avoid drugs that are very constipating** because of the risk of precipitating hepatic encephalopathy.

10. **Avoid drugs that are known to be hepatotoxic** in their own right (e.g. MAOIs, chlorpromazine).

11. **Choose a low-risk drug** (see Tables below) and **monitor LFTs** weekly, at least initially. If LFTs deteriorate after a new drug is introduced, consider switching to another drug. Note that cross-hepatotoxicity between drugs is possible, especially if they are structurally related.[1]

These rules should always be observed in severe liver disease (low albumin, increased clotting time, ascites, jaundice, encephalopathy, etc.). The information described previously, and on the following pages, should be interpreted in the context of the patient's clinical presentation.

Antipsychotics in hepatic impairment

One-third of patients who are prescribed antipsychotic medication have at least one abnormal LFT, and in 4% at least one LFT is elevated 3 times above the upper limit of normal.[2] Transaminases are most often affected and this generally occurs within 1–6 weeks of treatment initiation.[2] Only rarely does clinically significant hepatic damage result.[2] The development of metabolic syndrome (obesity, insulin resistance) may be linked to the emergence of non-alcoholic fatty liver disease later in treatment.[3,4]

Table 8.1 Antipsychotics in hepatic impairment

Drug	Comments
Amisulpride[5,6]	Predominantly renally excreted, so dosage reduction should not be necessary as long as renal function is normal. Uncommonly associated with rises in transaminases and hepatocellular injury.
Aripiprazole[5-8]	Extensively hepatically metabolised. Limited data that hepatic impairment has minimal effect on pharmacokinetics. SPC states no dosage reduction required in mild-moderate hepatic impairment, but caution required in severe impairment. Small number of reports of hepatotoxicity, increased LFTs, hepatitis and jaundice.[2,9-11]

Table 8.1 (*Continued*)

Drug	Comments
Asenapine[5,6,8]	Hepatically metabolised. SPC recommends avoiding in severe hepatic disease (7-fold increase in asenapine exposure). No dose adjustment required in mild to moderate disease,[12] but be aware of the possibility of increased plasma levels in patients with moderate impairment. Transient, asymptomatic rises in transaminases, AST and ALT are common, especially early in treatment. Single case report of mild cholestatic liver injury resolving on stopping treatment.[13]
Brexpiprazole[6,14]	Little information. Use no more than 3mg/day (schizophrenia) or 2mg/day (depression) in moderate or severe hepatic failure. Long half-life (~90 hours).
Cariprazine[6,15]	Occasional, non-clinically relevant increases in ALT and AST. No dosage adjustment is required in patients with mild or moderate hepatic failure; not recommended in severe hepatic disease (has not been evaluated). Long half-life (~2–4 days). Hepatitis has been reported.
Clozapine[1,5,6,16–18]	Very sedative and constipating. Contraindicated in active liver disease associated with nausea, anorexia or jaundice, progressive liver disease or hepatic failure. In less severe disease, start with 12.5mg and increase slowly, using plasma levels to gauge metabolising capacity and guide dosage adjustment. More frequently associated with changes in liver enzymes than other antipsychotics. Transient elevations in AST, ALT and GGT to over twice the normal range occur in over 10% of physically healthy people, resolving spontaneously in 6–12 weeks.[19] Clozapine-induced hepatitis, jaundice, cholestasis and liver failure have been reported; clozapine should be discontinued if these develop. Successful rechallenge following hepatitis has been described.[20,21] See section on clozapine side effects in Chapter 1.
Flupentixol/ zuclopenthixol[5,6,22,23]	Both are extensively hepatically metabolised. Abnormal liver function tests and (rarely) jaundice have been reported with flupenthixol.[5] Small, transient elevations in transaminases, cholestatic hepatitis and jaundice[5] have been reported in some patients treated with zuclopenthixol. One report of flupentixol-induced hepatitis.[24] No other literature reports of use or harm.[25] Reduce doses by 50% in patients with compromised hepatic function. Depot preparations are best avoided, as altered pharmacokinetics will make dosage adjustment difficult and side effects from dosage accumulation more likely.
Haloperidol[5]	Extensively hepatically metabolised. Halve initial doses. Isolated reports of cholestasis, acute hepatic failure, hepatitis and abnormal liver function tests.[5,6]
Iloperidone[6,8,26]	Hepatically metabolised. Reduce dose in moderate impairment (2-fold increase in active metabolites) and avoid completely in severe hepatic impairment (no studies done). No dose reduction necessary in mild impairment. Infrequent reports of cholelithiasis.
Lumateperone[27,28]	Hepatically metabolised to active metabolites. No dose adjustment required in mild impairment. Increased exposure to lumateperone in moderate and severe impairment – manufacturer recommends avoiding. Increases in transaminases reported in licensing trials.
Lurasidone[5,6,8]	Hepatically metabolised. SPC recommends starting dose of 18.5mg (20mg) in hepatic impairment, maximum dose of 74mg (80mg)/day in moderate hepatic impairment (1.7-fold increase in exposure), and 37mg (40mg) in severe impairment (3-fold increase in exposure). No dose adjustment is required in mild hepatic impairment. Increases in ALT reported infrequently.

(*Continued*)

CHAPTER 8

Table 8.1 (Continued)

Drug	Comments
Olanzapine[1,5,6,8]	Although extensively hepatically metabolised, the pharmacokinetics of olanzapine seem to change little in severe hepatic impairment. It is sedative and anticholinergic (can cause constipation), so caution is advised. Start with 5mg/day in moderate or severe impairment and consider using plasma levels to guide dosage (aim for 20–40μg/L). Dose-related, transient, asymptomatic elevations in ALT and AST are very common in physically healthy adults, particularly early in treatment. People with liver disease or those taking other hepatotoxic drugs may be at increased risk. Rare cases of hepatitis in the literature.
Paliperidone[5,6,8]	Mainly excreted unchanged by the kidneys, so no dosage adjustment required for mild to moderate impairment. However, no data are available with respect to severe hepatic impairment and clinical experience is limited so caution is required. Rises in transaminases and gamma GT reported, some cases of jaundice. May be a good choice for patients with pre-existing hepatic disease.[29–31] One case report of hepatotoxicity with risperidone that did not remit on switching to paliperidone – it is possible that paliperidone may cause hepatotoxicity.[32]
Phenothiazines[5,6]	All cause sedation and constipation. Transient abnormalities in LFTs reported. Associated with cholestasis and some reports of fulminant hepatic cirrhosis. Best avoided completely in hepatic impairment, some phenothiazines are actively contraindicated. Chlorpromazine is particularly hepatotoxic and is also associated with rare cases of immune-mediated obstructive jaundice which may progress to liver disease.
Pimavanserin[6]	Active metabolite has a very long half-life (200 hours) – use not recommended in hepatic impairment. Does not appear to be hepatotoxic.
Quetiapine[5,6,8,33]	Extensively hepatically metabolised but short half-life. Clearance reduced by a mean of 30% in hepatic impairment so start at 25mg/day (IR preparation) or 50mg/day (XL preparation) and increase in 25–50mg/day increments. Can cause sedation and constipation. Transient rises in AST, ALT and GGT reported, rarely jaundice and hepatitis. Several cases of fatal hepatic failure and of hepatocellular damage reported in the literature. A number of studies describe use in patients with alcohol dependence.[34–36]
Risperidone[1,5,6,8]	Extensively hepatically metabolised and highly protein bound. Manufacturers recommend a halved starting dose and slower dose titration. Those with severe impairment should start at 0.5mg bd, and increase by 0.5mg bd at a maximum rate of weekly for doses above 1.5mg bd. Risperidone Consta can be started at 12.5mg fortnightly, or 25mg every two weeks if 2mg daily oral dosing has been tolerated. Transient, asymptomatic elevations in LFTs, cholestatic hepatitis, jaundice, and rare cases of hepatic failure have been reported. Cross-hepatotoxicity with paliperidone has been reported.[32] Steatohepatitis may arise as a result of weight gain.[37]
Sulpiride[5,6]	Almost completely renally excreted with a low potential to cause sedation or constipation. Dosage reduction should not be required. Rises in hepatic enzymes are common. Isolated case reports of cholestatic jaundice and primary biliary cirrhosis.

ALT, alanine aminotransferase; AST, aspartate aminotransferase; bd, bis die (twice a day); GGT, gamma-glutamyl transferase.

Antidepressant medications in hepatic impairment

Of those treated with antidepressants, 0.5–3% develop asymptomatic mild elevation of hepatic transaminases.[38] Onset is normally between several days and six months of treatment initiation and the elderly are more vulnerable.[38] Frank clinically significant liver damage however is rare, mostly idiosyncratic (unpredictable and not related to dose). Cross toxicity within class has been described.[38]

Table 8.2 Antidepressants in hepatic impairment

Drug	Comments
Agomelatine[5,6,38–40]	Liver injury including hepatic failure, liver enzyme increases more than 10× ULN, and hepatitis reported, most commonly in first months of treatment and very occasionally fatal. Contra-indicated in hepatic impairment, including cirrhosis and liver disease. Dose-related increase in transaminases reported; perform LFTs at baseline, 3, 6, 12, 24 weeks during initiation and at each dose increase, and thereafter where clinically indicated. Stop treatment if transaminases rise more than 3× ULN. Use cautiously where other risk factors for hepatic disease are present. Under current monitoring restrictions, risk of liver injury is no higher than for other antidepressants.[41,42]
Brexanolone[6,19]	No dose adjustment required in hepatic impairment. Does not appear to be hepatotoxic, although experience is limited.
Duloxetine[5,6,43–47]	Hepatically metabolised. Clearance markedly reduced even in mild impairment. Reports of hepatocellular injury (liver enzyme increases more than 10× ULN) and, less commonly, jaundice. Hepatic failure, sometimes fatal, has been reported. Contra-indicated in hepatic impairment.
Fluoxetine[5,6,48–52]	Extensively hepatically metabolised with a long half-life (further increased in hepatic insufficiency). Kinetic studies demonstrate accumulation in compensated cirrhosis. Although dosage reduction (of at least 50%) or alternate day dosing are recommended, it would take many weeks to reach steady-state serum levels, making fluoxetine complex to use. Asymptomatic increases in LFTs found in 0.5% of healthy adults. Rare cases of hepatitis reported.
Levomilnacipran, milnacipran[6,19]	No dose adjustment required in hepatic impairment, although the manufacturers of milnacipran recommend avoiding in chronic liver disease, alcohol use or severe dysfunction. Increased liver enzymes have been reported, and hepatitis with milnacipran; discontinue use if jaundice or liver dysfunction occurs.
MAOIs[5,6,53]	Rare cases of fatal hepatic necrosis, hepatotoxicity and jaundice with phenelzine, rarely hepatitis with tranylcypromine and one isolated case of fatal hepatotoxicity with moclobemide. Doses of moclobemide should be reduced to half or one third in hepatic impairment, or the dosing interval increased. Transdermal selegiline has not been associated with liver injury.[54] Non-selective MAOIs are contraindicated in patients with hepatic impairment.
Mirtazapine[5,6,55]	Hepatically metabolised and sedative. 50% dose reduction recommended based on kinetic data, Mild, asymptomatic increases in LFTs seen in healthy adults (ALT >3 times the upper limit of normal in 2%). Few cases of cholestatic and hepatocellular damage reported. Has been used safely in patients with primary biliary cholangitis.[56]
Other SSRIs[5,6,47,52,57–64]	All are hepatically metabolised and accumulate on chronic dosing. Dosage reduction (including reduction of maximum dose by 50%[65] and/or reduced dosing frequency) may be required (see individual SPCs for details). Raised LFTs and rare cases of hepatitis, including chronic active hepatitis, have been reported with paroxetine. Sertraline and fluvoxamine have also been associated with hepatitis. Citalopram, escitalopram and paroxetine have minimal effects on hepatic enzymes and may be the SSRIs of choice although occasional hepatotoxicity has been reported. Paroxetine is used by some specialised liver units with few apparent problems. Sertraline and paroxetine are used in the management of cholestatic pruritus.[66] Be aware of increased risk of bleeding.

(Continued)

CHAPTER 8

Table 8.2 (Continued)

Drug	Comments
Reboxetine[5,6,67]	50% reduction in starting dose recommended. Does not seem to be associated with hepatotoxicity.
Tricyclics[5,6,68]	All are hepatically metabolised, highly protein bound and will accumulate. They vary in their propensity to cause sedation and constipation. All are associated with raised LFTs and rare cases of hepatitis. Sedative TCAs such as trimipramine, imipramine, dothiepin (dosulepin) and amitriptyline are best avoided.
Venlafaxine/ desvenlafaxine[5,6,69,70]	Dosage reduction of 50% advised in mild and moderate hepatic impairment. Rare cases of hepatitis reported.
Vilazodone[6]	No dose adjustment required in hepatic impairment. Does not appear to affect liver enzymes and no cases of hepatotoxicity, but data are limited, and all other SSRIs have been linked to liver toxicity.
Vortioxetine[5,71,72]	Extensively metabolised in the liver. Little experience in hepatic impairment, but pharmacokinetic studies suggest no dose reduction is required. Does not seem to be associated with hepatotoxicity.

ALT, alanine aminotransferase, ULN, upper limit of normal.

Mood stabilisers in hepatic impairment[5,6,73]

Recommendations for the use of mood-stabilising medications in hepatic impairment are summarised in Table 8.3.

Table 8.3 Mood stabilisers in hepatic impairment

Drug	Comments
Carbamazepine[5,6,73]	Extensively hepatically metabolised and potent inducer of CYP450 enzymes (this can cause modest elevations in gamma-GT and alk phos, which in themselves are not an indication for stopping[5]). In chronic stable disease, caution advised. Avoid use in acute liver disease. Reduce starting dose by 50%,[6] and titrate up slowly, using plasma levels to guide dosage. Stop if LFTs deteriorate. Associated with hepatitis, cholangitis, cholestatic and hepatocellular jaundice, and hepatic failure (rare). Adverse hepatic effects are most common in the first 2 months of treatment.[73] Hepatocellular damage is often associated with a poor outcome. Vulnerability to carbamazepine-induced hepatic damage may be genetically determined.[73]
Lamotrigine[19]	Manufacturers recommend 50% reduction in initial dose, dose escalation and maintenance dose in moderate hepatic impairment and 75% in severe hepatic impairment. Discontinue if lamotrigine-induced rash (which can be serious). Extreme caution advised, particularly in women, children, and if co-prescribed with valproate. Elevated LFTs and hepatitis reported.
Lithium[6]	Not metabolised, so dosage reduction not required as long as renal function is normal. Use serum levels to guide dosage and monitor more frequently if ascites status changes (volume of distribution will change). Asymptomatic and transient LFT abnormalities reported in small proportion of patients on long term therapy.[19] One case of ascites and one of hyperbilirubinemia reported over many decades of lithium use worldwide.

(Continued)

Table 8.3 (*Continued*)

Drug	Comments
Valproate[74]	Highly protein bound and hepatically metabolised. Dosage reduction with close monitoring of LFTs in moderate hepatic impairment. Use plasma levels (measure free levels – total concentrations may appear to be normal) to guide dosage. Caution advised. Contraindicated in severe and/or active hepatic impairment, or family history of severe impairment; impairment of usual metabolic pathway can lead to generation of hepatotoxic metabolites via alternative pathway. Risk of liver toxicity is increased in people with hepatic insufficiency if salicylates are used concomitantly. Associated with elevated LFTs and serious hepatotoxicity including fulminant hepatic failure (sometimes fatal). Mitochondrial disease, learning disability, polypharmacy, metabolic disorders and underlying hepatic disease may be risk factors. Particularly hepatotoxic in very young children. The greatest risk is in the first three months of treatment.

Stimulants in hepatic impairment[5,6,75]

Recommendations for the use of stimulant medications in hepatic impairment are outlined in Table 8.4.

Table 8.4 Stimulants in hepatic impairment

Atomoxetine[76]	Reduce initial and target dose by 50% in moderate impairment, and by 75% in severe impairment. Very rare reports of liver toxicity, manifested by elevated hepatic enzymes, and raised bilirubin with jaundice. SPC states 'discontinue in patients with jaundice or laboratory evidence of liver injury, and do not restart'.
Methylphenidate[77]	Rare reports of liver dysfunction and hypersensitivity reactions.
Dexamphetamine/ lisdexamphetamine[78,79]	Little experience in liver disease, manufacturers recommend cautious dose titration. Very rarely associated with abnormal liver function, two case reports of hepatotoxicity.[80,81]

Sedatives in hepatic impairment

Table 8.5 summarises recommended sedatives in hepatic impairment.

Table 8.5 Sedatives in hepatic impairment

Benzodiazepines	Extensively hepatically metabolised. Prolonged duration of effect particularly for drugs with active metabolites (diazepam, midazolam, clonazepam). Lorazepam, oxazepam and temazepam do not have active metabolites and are preferred; lorazepam is considered the best tolerated in advanced liver disease[19] and is commonly used in alcohol withdrawal. Serum enzyme elevations are uncommon and liver injury very rare.[19]
Promethazine[6]	Extensive hepatic metabolism. Manufacturers recommend caution in liver impairment. Jaundice reported with high doses, no reports of LFT abnormalities or toxicity with lower doses.[19]
Z drugs[6,82,83]	Hepatically metabolised, but all have a relatively short half-life (1–7 hours). Reduce initial doses in mild to moderate impairment (use zopiclone 3.75mg, zolpidem 5mg, zaleplon 5mg), avoid in severe impairment. Zaleplon is subject to significant first-pass metabolism and zolpidem plasma concentrations and half-life are significantly increased in hepatic impairment; these agents should be used with caution.[84] Although zopiclone has the longer half-life, this may not be clinically relevant except in severe disease.[83] Zopiclone and zaleplon have not been associated with hepatotoxicity. There are rare reports of abnormal LFTs and a single case of liver injury with zolpidem.[19]

(*Continued*)

CHAPTER 8

Table 8.5 *(Continued)*

Melatonin[6,85]	Complex handling of melatonin in liver impairment: reduced clearance and prolonged half-life contribute to higher circulating levels of endogenous melatonin in daytime hours; negative feedback and accumulation of toxic products results in reduced endogenous production. Relevance to dosing of exogenous melatonin is unclear, although toxicity of melatonin is minimal. Manufacturer recommends avoiding in liver disease. Rarely associated with changes in LFTs.

Other psychotropics in hepatic impairment

Table 8.6 gives a summary of other psychotropics recommended in hepatic impairment.

Table 8.6 Other psychotropics in hepatic impairment

Bremelanotide[6]	No dose adjustment required in mild to moderate hepatic impairment. Use with caution in severe impairment; adverse effects more likely.[27] One case of acute hepatitis reported.
Deutetrabenazine[5,19]	Not studied in hepatic impairment, but based on experience with tetrabenazine, use is contraindicated. Limited information available but clinically relevant hepatotoxicity not reported. Occasional asymptomatic rises in ALT.
Lemborexant[6,27]	No dose adjustment in mild impairment (risk of increased somnolence), starting and maximum dose of 5mg once nightly in moderate impairment, not recommended in severe impairment. Little experience but hepatotoxicity not reported.[86]
Pitolisant[5,27]	Extensively hepatically metabolised. No dose adjustment in mild impairment. In moderate impairment the half-life is doubled; daily dose can be increased two weeks after initiation, daily maximum 18mg. Contraindicated in severe impairment. Hepatic enzyme increases are uncommon.
Solriamfetol[5]	Not metabolised. No known problems in liver impairment, no reports of liver injury.
Valbenazine[6,19]	Hepatically metabolised pro-drug of alpha-dihydrotetrabenazine. Unlike deutetrabenazine, not contra-indicated in liver disease, but maximum dose of 40mg in moderate to severe impairment. Few data, but no reports of clinically relevant liver injury other than a single report of reactivation of pre-existing hepatitis C.

Psychotropics in hepatic impairment

Table 8.7 gives an outline of recommended psychotropics in hepatic impairment.

Table 8.7 Psychotropics in hepatic impairment

Drug group	Recommended drugs
Antipsychotics	**Sulpiride/amisulpride**: no dosage reduction required if renal function is normal **Paliperidone:** if depot required
Antidepressants	**Paroxetine, sertraline, citalopram, or vortioxetine**: start at low dose. Titrate slowly (if required) as above.
Mood-stabilisers	**Lithium**: use plasma levels to guide dosage. Care needed if ascites status changes.
Sedatives	**Lorazepam, oxazepam, temazepam**: as short half-life with no active metabolites Use low doses with caution, as sedative drugs used in severe disease can precipitate hepatic encephalopathy **Zopiclone**: 3.75mg with care in moderate hepatic impairment

Drug-induced hepatic damage

Hy's rule, defined as ALT >3 times the upper limit of normal combined with serum bilirubin >2 times the upper limit of normal, is recommended by the FDA to assess the hepatotoxicity of new drugs.[73]

Drug induced hepatic damage can be due to:

- Direct dose-related hepatotoxicity (Type 1 ADR). A small number of drugs fall into this category, e.g. paracetamol; alcohol.
- Hypersensitivity reactions (Type 2 ADR). These can present with rash, fever and eosinophilia. Almost all drugs have been associated with cases of hepatotoxicity; frequency varies.

Almost any type of liver damage can occur, ranging from mild transient asymptomatic increases in LFTs to fulminant hepatic failure. See tables earlier in this section for details of the hepatotoxic potential of individual drugs.

Risk factors for drug-induced hepatotoxicity include:[87]

- Increasing age
- Female gender
- Alcohol consumption
- Co-prescription of enzyme inducing drugs
- Genetic predisposition
- Obesity
- Pre-existing liver disease (small effect)

When interpreting LFTs, remember that:[88]

- 12% of the healthy adult population have one LFT outside (above or below) the normal reference range.
- Up to 10% of patients with clinically significant hepatic disease have normal LFTs.
- Individual LFTs lack specificity for the liver, but >1 abnormal test greatly increases the likelihood of liver pathology.
- The absolute values of LFTs are a poor indicator of disease severity.

When monitoring LFTs:

- Ideally LFTs should be measured before treatment starts so that 'baseline' values are available.
- LFT elevations of <2 times the upper limit of the normal reference range are rarely clinically significant.
- Most drug related LFT elevations occur early in treatment (first month) and are transient. They may indicate adaptation of the liver to the drug rather than damaged per se. Transient LFT elevations may also occur during periods of weight gain.[89]
- If LFTs are persistently elevated >3-fold, continuing to rise or accompanied by clinical symptoms, the suspected drugs should be withdrawn.
- When tracking change, >20% change in liver enzymes is required to exclude biological or analytical variation.

CHAPTER 8

References

1. Slim M, et al. Hepatic safety of atypical antipsychotics: current evidence and future directions. *Drug Saf* 2016; **39**:925–943.
2. Marwick KF, et al. Antipsychotics and abnormal liver function tests: systematic review. *Clin Neuropharmacol* 2012; **35**:244–253.
3. Morlán-Coarasa MJ, et al. Incidence of non-alcoholic fatty liver disease and metabolic dysfunction in first episode schizophrenia and related psychotic disorders: a 3-year prospective randomized interventional study. *Psychopharmacology (Berl)* 2016; **233**:3947–3952.
4. Baeza I, et al. One-year prospective study of liver function tests in children and adolescents on second-generation antipsychotics: is there a link with metabolic syndrome? *J Child Adolesc Psychopharmacol* 2018; **28**:463–473.
5. Datapharm Communications Ltd. Electronic Medicines Compendium 2020; https://www.medicines.org.uk/emc.
6. IBM Watson Health. IBM Micromedex Solutions 2020; https://www.ibm.com/watson-health/about/micromedex.
7. Mallikaarjun S, et al. Effects of hepatic or renal impairment on the pharmacokinetics of aripiprazole. *Clin Pharmacokinet* 2008; **47**:533–542.
8. Preskorn SH Clinically important differences in the pharmacokinetics of the ten newer "atypical" antipsychotics: part 3. Effects of renal and hepatic impairment. *J Psychiatr Pract* 2012; **18**:430–437.
9. Chico G, et al. Clinical vignettes 482 aripiprazole causes cholelithiasis and hepatitis: a rare finding. *Am J Gastroenterol* 2005; **100**:S164.
10. Kornischka J, et al. Acute drug-induced hepatitis during aripiprazole monotherapy: a case report 2016.
11. Castanheira L, et al. Aripiprazole-induced hepatitis: a case report. *Clin Psychopharmacol Neurosci* (The Official Scientific Journal of the Korean College of Neuropsychopharmacology) 2019; **17**:551–555.
12. Peeters P, et al. Asenapine pharmacokinetics in hepatic and renal impairment. *Clin Pharmacokinet* 2011; **50**:471–481.
13. Schultz K, et al. A case of pseudo-Stauffer's syndrome related to asenapine use. *Schizophr Res* 2015; **169**:500–501.
14. Parikh NB, et al. Clinical role of brexpiprazole in depression and schizophrenia. *Ther Clin Risk Manag* 2017; **13**:299–306.
15. Cutler AJ, et al. Evaluation of the long-term safety and tolerability of cariprazine in patients with schizophrenia: results from a 1-year open-label study. *CNS Spectr* 2018; **23**:39–50.
16. Brown CA, et al. Clozapine toxicity and hepatitis. *J Clin Psychopharmacol* 2013; **33**:570–571.
17. Tucker P Liver toxicity with clozapine. *Aust NZJ Psychiatry* 2013; **47**:975–976.
18. Zarghami M, et al. Concurrent hepatotoxicity and neutropenia induced by clozapine. *Arch Iran Med* 2020; **23**:141–143.
19. LiverTox: Clinical and Research Information on Drug-Induced Liver Injury. Bethesda (MD): National Institute of Diabetes and Digestive and Kidney Diseases 2012; https://www.ncbi.nlm.nih.gov/books/NBK547852.
20. Lally J, et al. Hepatitis, interstitial nephritis, and pancreatitis in association with clozapine treatment: a systematic review of case series and reports. *J Clin Psychopharmacol* 2018; **38**:520–527.
21. Takács A, et al. Clozapine rechallenge in a patient with clozapine-induced hepatitis. *Australas Psychiatry* (Bulletin of Royal Australian and New Zealand College of Psychiatrists) 2019; **27**:535.
22. Amdisen A, et al. Zuclopenthixol acetate in viscoleo – a new drug formulation. An open Nordic multicentre study of zuclopenthixol acetate in Viscoleo in patients with acute psychoses including mania and exacerbation of chronic psychoses. *Acta Psychiatr Scand* 1987; **75**:99–107.
23. Wistedt B, et al. Zuclopenthixol decanoate and haloperidol decanoate in chronic schizophrenia: a double-blind multicentre study. *Acta Psychiatr Scand* 1991; **84**:14–21.
24. Demuth N, et al. [Flupentixol-induced acute hepatitis]. *Gastroenterol Clin Biol* 1999; **23**:152–153.
25. Nolen WA, et al. Disturbances of liver function of long acting neuroleptic drugs. *Pharmakopsychiatr Neuropsychopharmakol* 1978; **11**:199–204.
26. Vanda Pharmaceuticals Inc. FANAPT® (iloperidone) tablets 1mg 2mg 4mg 6mg 8mg 10mg 12mg indication and important safety information 2020; http://www.fanapt.com/product/pi/pdf/fanapt.pdf.
27. U.S. Food & Drug Administration. Drugs@FDA: FDA-approved drugs 2020; https://www.accessdata.fda.gov/scripts/cder/daf.
28. Greenwood J, et al. Lumateperone: a novel antipsychotic for schizophrenia. *Ann Pharmacother* 2020; **55**:98–104.
29. Amatniek J, et al. Safety of paliperidone extended-release in patients with schizophrenia or schizoaffective disorder and hepatic disease. *Clin Schizophr Relat Psychoses* 2014; **8**:8–20.
30. Macaluso M, et al. Pharmacokinetic drug evaluation of paliperidone in the treatment of schizoaffective disorder. *Expert Opin Drug Metab Toxicol* 2017; **13**:871–879.
31. Chang CH, et al. Paliperidone is associated with reduced risk of severe hepatic outcome in patients with schizophrenia and viral hepatitis: a nationwide population-based cohort study. *Psychiatry Res* 2019; **281**:112597.
32. Khorassani F, et al. Risperidone- and paliperidone-induced hepatotoxicity: case report and review of literature. *Am J Health Syst Pharm* 2020; zxaa224.
33. Das A, et al. Liver injury associated with quetiapine: an illustrative case report. *J Clin Psychopharmacol* 2017; **37**:623–625.
34. Monnelly EP, et al. Quetiapine for treatment of alcohol dependence. *J Clin Psychopharmacol* 2004; **24**:532–535.
35. Brown ES, et al. A randomized, double-blind, placebo-controlled trial of quetiapine in patients with bipolar disorder, mixed or depressed phase, and alcohol dependence. *Alcohol Clin Exp Res* 2014; **38**:2113–2118.
36. Vatsalya V, et al. Safety assessment of liver injury with quetiapine fumarate XR management in very heavy drinking alcohol-dependent patients. *Clin Drug Investig* 2016; **36**:935–944.
37. Holtmann M, et al. Risperidone-associated steatohepatitis and excessive weight-gain. *Pharmacopsychiatry* 2003; **36**:206–207.
38. Voican CS, et al. Antidepressant-induced liver injury: a review for clinicians. *Am J Psychiatry* 2014; **171**:404–415.
39. Freiesleben SD, et al. A systematic review of agomelatine-induced liver injury. *J Mol Psychiatry* 2015; **3**:4.

40. Gahr M, et al. Safety and tolerability of agomelatine: focus on hepatotoxicity. *Curr Drug Metab* 2014; **15**:694–702.

41. Billioti de Gage S, et al. Antidepressants and hepatotoxicity: a cohort study among 5 million individuals registered in the French National Health Insurance Database. *CNS Drugs* 2018; **32**:673–684.

42. Pladevall-Vila M, et al. Risk of acute liver injury in agomelatine and other antidepressant users in four European Countries: a cohort and nested case-control study using automated Health Data Sources. *CNS Drugs* 2019; **33**:383–395.

43. Hanje AJ, et al. Case report: fulminant hepatic failure involving duloxetine hydrochloride. *Clin Gastroenterol Hepatol* 2006; **4**:912–917.

44. Vuppalanchi R, et al. Duloxetine hepatotoxicity: a case-series from the drug-induced liver injury network. *Aliment Pharmacol Ther* 2010; **32**:1174–1183.

45. Lin ND, et al. Hepatic outcomes among adults taking duloxetine: a retrospective cohort study in a US health care claims database. *BMC Gastroenterol* 2015; **15**:134.

46. McIntyre RS, et al. The hepatic safety profile of duloxetine: a review. *Expert Opin Drug Metab Toxicol* 2008; **4**:281–285.

47. Bunchorntavakul C, et al. Drug hepatotoxicity: newer agents. *Clin Liver Dis* 2017; **21**:115–134.

48. Schenker S, et al. Fluoxetine disposition and elimination in cirrhosis. *Clin Pharmacol Ther* 1988; **44**:353–359.

49. Cai Q, et al. Acute hepatitis due to fluoxetine therapy. *Mayo Clin Proc* 1999; **74**:692–694.

50. Friedenberg FK, et al. Hepatitis secondary to fluoxetine treatment. *Am J Psychiatry* 1996; **153**:580.

51. Johnston DE, et al. Chronic hepatitis related to use of fluoxetine. *Am J Gastroenterol* 1997; **92**:1225–1226.

52. Hale AS New antidepressants: use in high-risk patients. *J Clin Psychiatry* 1993; **54** Suppl:61–70.

53. Stoeckel K, et al. Absorption and disposition of moclobemide in patients with advanced age or reduced liver or kidney function. *Acta Psychiatr Scand Suppl* 1990; **360**:94–97.

54. Lee KC, et al. Transdermal selegiline for the treatment of major depressive disorder. *Neuropsychiatr Dis Treat* 2007; **3**:527–537.

55. Thomas E, et al. Mirtazapine-induced steatosis. *Int J Clin Pharmacol Ther* 2017; **55**:630–632.

56. Shaheen AA, et al. The impact of depression and antidepressant usage on primary biliary cholangitis clinical outcomes. *PLoS One* 2018; **13**:e0194839.

57. Benbow SJ, et al. Paroxetine and hepatotoxicity. *BMJ* 1997; **314**:1387.

58. Kuhs H, et al. A double-blind study of the comparative antidepressant effect of paroxetine and amitriptyline. *Acta Psychiatr Scand Suppl* 1989; **350**:145–146.

59. de Bree H, et al. Fluvoxamine maleate: disposition in men. *Eur J Drug Metab Pharmacokinet* 1983; **8**:175–179.

60. Green BH Fluvoxamine and hepatic function. *Br J Psychiatry* 1988; **153**:130–131.

61. Milne RJ, et al. Citalopram: a review of its pharmacodynamic and pharmacokinetic properties, and therapeutic potential in depressive illness. *Drugs* 1991; **41**:450–477.

62. Lopez-Torres E, et al. Hepatotoxicity related to citalopram (Letter). *Am J Psychiatry* 2004; **161**:923–924.

63. Colakoglu O, et al. Toxic hepatitis associated with paroxetine. *Int J Clin Pract* 2005; **59**:861–862.

64. Rao N The clinical pharmacokinetics of escitalopram. *Clin Pharmacokinet* 2007; **46**:281–290.

65. Mullish BH, et al. Review article: depression and the use of antidepressants in patients with chronic liver disease or liver transplantation. *Aliment Pharmacol Ther* 2014; **40**:880–892.

66. Düll MM, et al. Treatment of pruritus secondary to liver disease. *Current Gastroenterology Reports* 2019; **21**:48.

67. A T, et al. Pharmacokinetics of reboxetine in volunteers with hepatic impairment. *Clin Drug Investig* 2000; **19**:473–477.

68. Medicines C. Lofepramine (Gamanil) and abnormal blood tests of liver function. *Current Problems* 1988; **23**:2.

69. Archer DF, et al. Cardiovascular, cerebrovascular, and hepatic safety of desvenlafaxine for 1 year in women with vasomotor symptoms associated with menopause. *Menopause* 2013; **20**:47–56.

70. Baird-Bellaire S, et al. An open-label, single-dose, parallel-group study of the effects of chronic hepatic impairment on the safety and pharmacokinetics of desvenlafaxine. *Clin Ther* 2013; **35**:782–794.

71. Ryan PB, et al. Atypical antipsychotics and the risks of acute kidney injury and related outcomes among older adults: a replication analysis and an evaluation of adapted confounding control strategies. *Drugs Aging* 2017; **34**:211–219.

72. Chen G, et al. Vortioxetine: clinical pharmacokinetics and drug interactions. *Clin Pharmacokinet* 2018; **57**:673–686.

73. Bjornsson E Hepatotoxicity associated with antiepileptic drugs. *Acta Neurol Scand* 2008; **118**:281–290.

74. Guo HL, et al. Valproic acid and the liver injury in patients with epilepsy: an update. *Curr Pharm Des* 2019; **25**:343–351.

75. Panei P, et al. Safety of psychotropic drug prescribed for attention-deficit/hyperactivity disorder in Italy. *Adverse Drug Reaction Bulletin* 2010:999–1002.

76. Reed VA, et al. The safety of atomoxetine for the treatment of children and adolescents with attention-deficit/hyperactivity disorder: a comprehensive review of over a decade of research. *CNS Drugs* 2016; **30**:603–628.

77. Tong HY, et al. Liver transplant in a patient under methylphenidate therapy: a case report and review of the literature. *Case Rep Pediatr* 2015; **2015**:437298.

78. Shire Pharmaceuticals Limited. Summary of product characteristics. Elvanse 20mg 30mg 40mg 50mg 60mg 70mg Hard Capsules 2019; https://www.medicines.org.uk/emc/product/2979/smpc.

79. Flynn Pharma Ltd. Summary of product characteristics. Amfexa 5mg 10mg 20mg Tablets 2018; https://www.medicines.org.uk/emc/product/7403/smpc.

80. Vanga RR, et al. Adderall induced acute liver injury: a rare case and review of the literature. *Case Rep Gastrointest Med* 2013; **2013**:902892.

81. Hood B, et al. Eosinophilic hepatitis in an adolescent during lisdexamfetamine dimesylate treatment for ADHD. *Pediatrics* 2010; **125**:e1510–1513.

CHAPTER 8

82. SANOFI. Summary of product characteristics. Stilnoct 5mg 10mg film-coated tablets 2019; https://www.medicines.org.uk/emc/product/4931/smpc.

83. SANOFI. Summary of product characteristics. Zimovane 7.5mg and 3.75mg LS film-coated tablets 2019; https://www.medicines.org.uk/emc/product/2855/smpc.

84. Gunja N The clinical and forensic toxicology of Z-drugs. *J Med Toxicol* 2013; 9:155–162.

85. Flynn Pharma Ltd. Summary of product characteristics. Circadin 2mg prolonged-release tablets 2019; https://www.medicines.org.uk/emc/product/2809/smpc.

86. Kärppä M, et al. Long-term efficacy and tolerability of lemborexant compared with placebo in adults with insomnia disorder: results from the phase 3 randomized clinical trial SUNRISE 2. *Sleep* 2020.

87. Grattagliano I, et al. Biochemical mechanisms in drug-induced liver injury: certainties and doubts. *World J Gastroenterol* 2009; 15:4865–4876.

88. Rosalki SB, et al. Liver function profiles and their interpretation. *Br J Hosp Med* 1994; 51:181–186.

89. Rettenbacher MA, et al. Association between antipsychotic-induced elevation of liver enzymes and weight gain: a prospective study. *J Clin Psychopharmacol* 2006; 26:500–503.

Further reading

Telles-Correia D, et al. Psychotropic drugs and liver disease: A critical review of pharmacokinetics and liver toxicity. *WJGPT*, 2017; 8:26–37.

Renal impairment

Using drugs in patients with renal impairment needs careful consideration. This is partly because some drugs are nephrotoxic but principally because the pharmacokinetics (absorption, distribution, metabolism, excretion) of drugs are altered in renal impairment. In particular, *patients with renal impairment have a reduced capacity to excrete drugs and their metabolites.*

Prescribing in renal impairment – general principles

- *Estimate* **the excretory capacity of the kidney** by calculating the glomerular filtration rate (GFR). GFR is assessed by measurement of:
  - An ideal filtration marker, for example inulin or EDTA (this gives an accurate estimate but expensive and invasive)
  - Serum creatinine – an easy and cheap method but an approximation of function even after necessary adjustments
  - Cystatin C protein – a more expensive test than creatinine but more accurate

- Check **proteinuria** by measuring urinary albumin and calculate albumin/creatinine ratio. This is because proteinuria is a significant risk factor for progression to end-stage renal disease.[1]

- **Use equations which take into account other factors** to improve the precision of GFR determination using serum creatinine and cystatin C (see equations below). Note that these estimates are still less than perfect when compared with directly measured GFR.[2,3] CKD-EPI is more accurate than MDRD and is now preferred:

---

a) Cockroft and Gault equation*

$$CrCl \ (mL/min) = \frac{F \ (140 - age \ (in \ years)) \times ideal \ body \ weight \ (kg))}{Serum \ creatinine \ (\mu mol/L)}$$

F = 1.23 (men) and 1.04 (women)

Ideal body weight should be used for patients at extremes of body weight or else the result of the calculation is a poor estimate.

For men, ideal body weight (kg) = 50kg + 2.3kg per inch over 5 feet

For women, ideal body weight (kg) = 45.5kg + 2.3kg per inch over 5 feet

- Online calculator available at https://www.nuh.nhs.uk/staff-area/antibiotics/creatinine-clearance-calculator.

---

* This equation is not accurate if plasma creatinine is unstable (e.g. acute renal failure), in obesity, in pregnant women, children or in diseases causing production of abnormal amounts of creatinine and has only been validated in White patients. Creatinine clearance is not the same as GFR and is relatively less representative of GFR in severe renal failure.

b) Chronic Kidney Disease Epidemiology Collaboration (CKD-EPI) formula (replaces the previously used Modification of Diet in Renal Disease (MDRD) equation)[2] although some pathology departments still use MDRD.

$$GFR = 141 \times min\ (Scr/\kappa,\ 1)^{\alpha} \times max(Scr/\kappa,\ 1)^{-1.209} \times 0.993^{Age} \times 1.018\ [\text{if female}] \times 1.159\ [\text{if Black}]$$

S_{cr} is serum creatinine in mg/dL,

κ is 0.7 for females and 0.9 for males,

α is –0.329 for females and –0.411 for males,

min indicates the minimum of S_{cr}/κ or 1, and

max indicates the maximum of S_{cr}/κ or 1.

■ Online calculator available at https://www.kidney.org/professionals/kdoqi/gfr_calculator.

■ **Use Cockroft and Gault for drug dose calculation.**

When calculating drug doses use estimated CrCl from the Cockroft and Gault equation.

Do not use the CKD-EPI or MDRD formulae for dose calculation because most current dose recommendations are based on the creatinine clearance estimations from Cockroft and Gault.

Classify the stage of renal impairment[3]

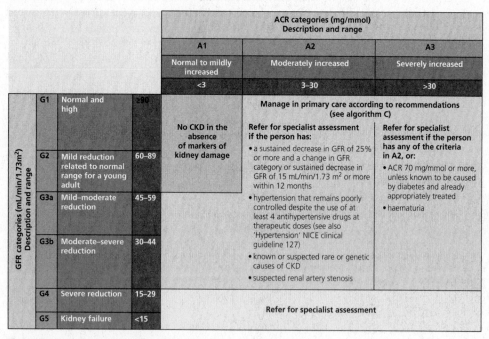

				ACR categories (mg/mmol) Description and range		
				A1	**A2**	**A3**
				Normal to mildly increased	Moderately increased	Severely increased
				<3	3–30	>30
GFR categories (mL/min/1.73m²) Description and range	G1	Normal and high	≥90	No CKD in the absence of markers of kidney damage	Manage in primary care according to recommendations (see algorithm C)	
					Refer for specialist assessment if the person has:	Refer for specialist assessment if the person has any of the criteria in A2, or:
	G2	Mild reduction related to normal range for a young adult	60–89		• a sustained decrease in GFR of 25% or more and a change in GFR category or sustained decrease in GFR of 15 mL/min/1.73 m² or more within 12 months	• ACR 70 mg/mmol or more, unless known to be caused by diabetes and already appropriately treated
	G3a	Mild–moderate reduction	45–59		• hypertension that remains poorly controlled despite the use of at least 4 antihypertensive drugs at therapeutic doses (see also 'Hypertension' NICE clinical guideline 127)	• haematuria
	G3b	Moderate–severe reduction	30–44		• known or suspected rare or genetic causes of CKD	
					• suspected renal artery stenosis	
	G4	Severe reduction	15–29		Refer for specialist assessment	
	G5	Kidney failure	<15			

Figure 8.1 Classification of renal impairment.
Abbreviations: ACR = albumin creatinine ratio; CKD = chronic kidney disease

Notes

- **Monitor decline in renal function over a considerable period** as a 30% change over two years is associated with a 5-fold increase in risk of ESRD. CKD progression is often non-linear.[4]
- **Monitor risk of moving from CKD stages 3–5 (eGFR 10–59) to dialysis/transplantation using Tangri score** at https://qxmd.com/calculate/calculator_125/kidney-failure-risk-equation-8-variable. The four (age, sex, eGFR, urine albumin/creatinine ratio) and eight (as four items plus serum calcium, phosphorus, bicarbonate, albumin) variable equations accurately predict the 2- and 5-year probability of treated kidney failure (dialysis or transplantation) for a potential patient with CKD stages 3–5.[5]
- In general renal function significantly affects overall drug elimination; then the amount of drug excreted unchanged in urine should be 30% or more of the dose.[6]
- **Older adults (>65 years) should be assumed to have at least mild renal impairment.** Their serum creatinine may not be raised because they have a smaller muscle mass.
- **Avoid drugs that are nephrotoxic** (e.g. lithium, NSAIDs) where renal reserve is limited.
- **Be cautious when using drugs that are extensively renally cleared** (e.g. sulpiride, amisulpride, lithium).
- Elimination of drugs metabolised hepatically can be reduced in kidney disease possibly by inhibition of enzymatic activity caused by uraemia.[7]
- **Start at a low dose and increase slowly** because, in renal impairment, the half-life of a drug and the time for it to reach steady state (amount absorbed is the same as cleared when drug is given continuously) are often prolonged. Plasma level monitoring may be useful for some drugs.
- **Try to avoid long-acting drugs** (e.g. depot preparations). Their dose and frequency cannot be easily adjusted should renal function change.
- **Prescribe as few drugs as possible.** Patients with renal failure take many medications requiring regular review. Interactions and side effects can be avoided if fewer drugs are used.
- **Monitor patient for adverse effects.** Patients with renal impairment are more likely to experience side effects and they may take longer to develop than in healthy patients. Adverse effects such as sedation, confusion and postural hypotension can be more common.
- **Be cautious when using drugs with anticholinergic effects,** since they may cause urinary retention.
- There are **few clinical studies** of the use of psychotropic drugs in people with renal impairment. Advice about drug use in renal impairment is often based on knowledge of the drug's pharmacokinetics in healthy patients.
- **The effect of renal replacement therapies (e.g. dialysis) on drugs is difficult to predict.** See Tables 8.4–8.9 that follow. Seek specialist advice.
- **Try to avoid drugs known to prolong QTc interval.** In established renal failure electrolyte changes are common, so probably best to avoid antipsychotics with the greatest risk of QTc prolongation (see section on QTc prolongation).
- **Monitor weight carefully.** Weight gain predisposes to diabetes which can contribute to rhabdomyolysis[8] and renal failure. Psychotropic medications commonly cause weight gain.
- **Be vigilant for serotonin syndrome with antidepressants, dystonias and neuroleptic malignant syndrome (NMS) with antipsychotics.** The resulting rhabdomyolysis can cause renal failure. There are case reports of rhabdomyolysis occurring with antipsychotics without other symptoms of NMS.[9–11]

CHAPTER 8

- **Depression is common in chronic kidney disease** but evidence for effectiveness of antidepressants in this condition is lacking.[12,13] In chronic kidney disease starting some antidepressants at a higher versus lower dose reduces mortality risk.[14] Depression is poorly treated in patients on haemodialysis.[15] Non-drug treatment, for example cognitive behavioural therapy, exercise or relaxation techniques probably reduce depressive symptoms for adults on dialysis.[16] SSRIs are associated with hip fracture in patients on haemodialysis (AOR 1.25; 95% CI 1.17, 1.35).[17]
- **Both schizophrenia and bipolar disorder are associated with an increased risk of chronic kidney disease.**[18,19]
- **Antipsychotics (e.g. olanzapine, quetiapine) may be associated with acute kidney injury**[20] possibly via their effects on blood pressure and urinary retention but studies are conflicting.[21]
- **Mood stabilising anticonvulsants used in bipolar disorder are associated with an increased rate of chronic kidney disease.**[19]

Table 8.8 Antipsychotic medications in renal impairment

Drug	Comments
Amisulpride[22–25]	Primarily renally excreted. 50% excreted unchanged in urine. Limited experience in renal disease. Manufacturer states no data with doses of >50mg but recommends following dosing: 50% of dose if GFR 30–60mL/min; 33% of dose if GFR is 10–30mL/min; no recommendations for GFR <10mL/min so **best avoided in established renal failure**.
Aripiprazole[22,23,25–29]	Less than 1% of unchanged aripiprazole renally excreted. Manufacturer states no dose adjustment required in renal failure as pharmacokinetics are similar in healthy and severely renally diseased patients. There is one case report of safe use of oral aripiprazole 5mg in an 83-year-old man having haemodialysis. Avoid depot formulation where possible although there is a case report of aripiprazole 400mg depot use in a 64-year-old man on haemodialysis.
Asenapine[23,25,30]	Manufacturer states no dose adjustment required for patients with renal impairment but no experience with use if GFR <15mL/min. A 5mg single dose study in renal impairment suggests that no dose adjustment is needed. No dosage adjustment is recommended in patients with mild (eGFR 60–89mL/min/1.73m²), moderate (eGFR 30–59mL/min/1.73m²) or severe (eGFR 15–29mL/min/1.73m²) renal impairment.
Chlorpromazine[22,23,25,31,32]	Less than 1% excreted unchanged in urine. Manufacturer advises avoiding in renal dysfunction. Dosing: GFR 10–50mL/min, dose as in normal renal function; GFR <10mL/min, start with a small dose because of an increased risk of anticholinergic, sedative and hypotensive side effects. Monitor carefully.
Clozapine[23,25,33–37]	Only trace amounts of unchanged clozapine excreted in urine; however, there are rare case reports of interstitial nephritis and acute renal failure. Nocturnal enuresis and urinary retention are common side effects. Contraindicated by manufacturer in severe renal disease. Anticholinergic, sedative and hypotensive side effects occur more frequently in patients with renal disease. Dosing: GFR 10–50mL/min as in normal renal function but with caution; GFR <10mL/min start with a low dose and titrate slowly (based on renal expert opinion). Levels are useful to guide dosing. May cause and aggravate diabetes, a common cause of renal disease. Case reports exist of successful continuation after renal transplantation.[38]

Table 8.8 (Continued)

Drug	Comments
Flupentixol[22,23,25]	Negligible renal excretion of unchanged flupentixol. Dosing: GFR 10–50mL/min dose as in normal renal function; GFR <10mL/min start with ¼ to ½ of normal dose and titrate slowly. May cause hypotension and sedation in renal impairment and can accumulate. Manufacturer recommends caution in renal failure. Avoid depot preparations in renal impairment.
Haloperidol[10,22,23,25,39,40]	Less than 1% excreted unchanged in the urine. Manufacturer advises caution in renal failure. Dosing: GFR 10–50mL/min, dose as in normal renal function; GFR <10mL/min start with a lower dose as can accumulate with repeated dosing. A case report of haloperidol use in renal failure suggests starting at a low dose and increasing slowly. Has been used to treat uraemia associated nausea in renal failure. Avoid depot preparations in renal impairment.
Lumateperone[41,42]	<1% excreted unchanged in urine. Manufacturer advises no dose adjustment needed in renal impairment.
Lurasidone[43]	9% excreted unchanged in the urine. Manufacturer recommends dose adjustment if GFR <50mL/min patients (starting dose is 18.75 (20)mg per day, maximum 74 (80) mg/day) and avoiding if GFR <15mL/min. Renal failure has been reported rarely.
Olanzapine[9,22,23,25,40,44]	57% of olanzapine is excreted mainly as metabolites (7% excreted unchanged) in urine. Dosing: GFR <50mL/min initially 5mg daily and titrate as necessary. Avoid long-acting preparations in renal impairment unless the oral dose is well tolerated and effective. Manufacturer recommends a lower long-acting injection starting dose of 150mg, 4-weekly in patients with renal impairment. May cause and aggravate diabetes, a common cause of renal disease. Hypothermia has been reported when used in renal failure.
Paliperidone[22,23,25]	Paliperidone is also a metabolite of risperidone. 59% excreted unchanged in urine. Dosing: GFR 50–80mL/min, 3mg daily and increase according to response to max of 6mg daily; GFR 10–50mL/min, 3mg alternate days increasing to 3mg daily according to response. Use with caution as clearance is reduced by 71% in severe kidney disease. Manufacturer contraindicates oral form if GFR <10mL/min due to lack of experience and *both* monthly and 3-monthly depot preparations if GFR <50mL/min (reduced loading and maintenance doses if GFR 50 to <80mL/min). There is a single case report of successful paliperidone monthly injection use in a patient with renal failure undergoing haemodialysis.[45]
Pimavanserin[41,46]	<1% excreted unchanged in urine. Manufacturer states no dose adjustment needed in GFR ≥30mL/min but advises to avoid if GFR <30mL/min due to lack of data.
Pimozide[22,23,25]	Less than 1% of pimozide is excreted unchanged in the urine; dose reductions not usually needed in renal impairment. Dosing: GFR 10–50mL/min, dose as in normal renal function; GFR <10mL/min start at a low dose and increase according to response. Manufacturer cautions in renal failure.
Quetiapine[22,23,25,47–49]	Less than 5% of quetiapine excreted unchanged in the urine. Plasma clearance reduced by an average of 25% in patients with a GFR <30mL/min. In patients with GFR of <10–50mL/min start at 25mg/day and increase in daily increments of 25–50mg to an effective dose. Case reports (thrombotic thrombocytopenic purpura, DRESS and non-NMS rhabdomyolysis) resulting in acute renal failure with quetiapine have been published.

(Continued)

Table 8.8 (*Continued*)

Drug	Comments
Risperidone[22,23,25,40,50–53]	Clearance of risperidone and the active metabolite of risperidone (9-OH-) is reduced by 60% in patients with moderate to severe renal disease. Dosing: GFR <50mL/min 0.5mg twice daily for at least 1 week, then increasing by 0.5mg twice daily to 1–2mg bd. The manufacturer advises caution when using risperidone in renal impairment. The long-acting injection should only be used after titration with oral risperidone as described above. If 2mg orally is tolerated, 25mg intramuscularly every 2 weeks can be administered. There are two case reports of successful use of risperidone long-acting injection in haemodialysis at a dose of 50mg 2-weekly in one patient and 37.5mg then 25mg in an older adult. Another describes the successful use of risperidone in a child with steroid-induced psychosis and nephrotic syndrome.
Sulpiride[8,22,23,25,54]	Almost totally renally excreted, with 95% excreted in urine and faeces as unchanged sulpiride. Dosing regimen: GFR 30–60mL/min, give 70% of normal dose; GFR 10–30mL/min give 50% of normal dose; GFR <10mL/min give 34% of normal dose. There is a case report of renal failure with sulpiride due to diabetic coma and rhabdomyolysis. **Probably best avoided in renal impairment.**
Trifluoperazine[25]	Less than 1% excreted unchanged in the urine. Dose GFR <10–50mL/min as for normal renal function – start with a low dose. Very limited data.
Ziprasidone[22,40,55,56]	<1% is renally excreted unchanged. No dose adjustment needed for GFR >10mL/min but care needed with using the injection as it contains a renally eliminated excipient (cyclodextrin sodium). Case report of 80mg twice daily dose used in a patient on haemodialysis who then developed agranulocytosis.[57]
Zuclopenthixol[22,23,25]	10–20% of unchanged drug and metabolites excreted unchanged in urine. Manufacturer cautions use in renal disease as can accumulate. Dosing: 10–50mL/min dose as in normal renal function; GFR <10mL/min start with 50% of the dose and titrate slowly. Avoid both depot preparations (acetate and decanoate) in renal impairment.

Table 8.9 Antidepressants in renal impairment[12]

Drug	Comments
Agomelatine[23]	Negligible renal excretion of unchanged agomelatine. No data on use in renal disease. Manufacturer says pharmacokinetics unchanged in small study of 25mg dose in severe renal impairment but cautions use in moderate or severe renal disease. Nephroprotective effects have been observed in rats.[58,59]
Amitriptyline[22,23,25,32,40,60–64]	<2% excreted unchanged in urine; no dose adjustment needed in renal failure. Dose as in normal renal function but start at a low dose and increase slowly. Monitor patient for urinary retention, confusion, sedation and postural hypotension. Has been used to treat pain in those with renal disease. Plasma level or ECG monitoring may be useful. Associated with acute kidney injury.
Brexanolone[41,65]	Less than 1% excreted unchanged in urine. Manufacturer states no dosage adjustment is recommended in patients with GFR 15–60mL/min; avoid use in patients with GFR <15mL/min because of the potential accumulation of the injection solubilising agent, betadex sulfobutyl ether sodium.

(Continued)

Table 8.9 (Continued)

Drug	Comments
Bupropion[22,23,25,32,40,66–68] (amfebutamone)	0.5% excreted unchanged in the urine. Dosing: GFR <50mL/min, 150mg once daily. A single dose study in haemodialysis patients (stage 5 disease) recommended a dose of 150mg every 3 days. Metabolites may accumulate in renal impairment and clearance is reduced. Elevated levels increase risk of seizures. Has been used to treat sexual dysfunction in mild to moderately depressed patients with chronic kidney disease.
Citalopram[22,23,25,40,69–75]	<13% of citalopram is excreted unchanged in the urine. Single-dose studies in mild and moderate renal impairment show no change in the pharmacokinetics of citalopram. Dosing is as for normal renal function; however, use with caution if GFR <10mL/min due to reduced clearance. The manufacturer does not advise use if GFR <20mL/min. Renal failure has been reported with citalopram overdose. Citalopram can treat depression in chronic renal failure and improve quality of life but use of citalopram (or escitalopram) is associated with a higher risk of sudden cardiac death versus other SSRIs (fluoxetine, fluvoxamine, paroxetine, sertraline) when used in patients on haemodialysis (adjusted hazard ratio, 1.18; 95% CI 1.05, 1.31). A case report of hyponatraemia has been reported in a renal transplant patient on citalopram.
Clomipramine[22,23,25,32,76]	2% of unchanged clomipramine is excreted in the urine. Dosing: GFR 20–50mL/min, dose as for normal renal function; GFR <20mL/min, effects unknown, start at a low dose and monitor patient for urinary retention, confusion, sedation and postural hypotension as accumulation can occur. There is a case report of clomipramine-induced interstitial nephritis and reversible acute renal failure.
Desvenlafaxine[12,22,77,78]	45% of desvenlafaxine is excreted unchanged in the urine. Manufacturer recommends: GFR 30–50mL/min, 50mg per day; GFR <30mL/min, 25mg daily. Half-life is prolonged and desvenlafaxine accumulates as GFR decreases. Urinary retention, delay when starting to pass urine and proteinuria, has been reported as adverse effects.
Dosulepin[22,25,79] (dothiepin)	56% of mainly active metabolites renally excreted. They have a long half-life and may accumulate, resulting in excessive sedation. Dosing: GFR 20–50mL/min, dose as for normal renal function; GFR <20mL/min, start with a small dose and titrate to response. Monitor patient for urinary retention, confusion, sedation and postural hypotension.
Doxepin[22,23,25,32,80]	<1% excreted unchanged in urine. Dosing: GFR 10–50mL/min as in normal renal function but monitor patient for urinary retention, confusion, sedation and postural hypotension; GFR <10mL/min start with a small dose and increase slowly. Manufacturer advises using with caution. Haemolytic anaemia with renal failure has been reported with doxepin. Used topically to treat pruritis in chronic renal failure.
Duloxetine[22,25,81–83]	<1% excreted unchanged in urine. Manufacturer states no dose adjustment is necessary for GFR >30mL/min; however, starting at a low dose and increasing slowly is advised. Duloxetine is contraindicated in patients with a GFR <30mL/min as it can accumulate in chronic kidney disease. Licensed to treat diabetic neuropathic pain and stress incontinence in women. Diabetes is a common cause of renal impairment. Two case reports of acute renal failure with duloxetine have been reported. Serotonin syndrome reported in a patient with chronic kidney disease on trazodone and duloxetine.[84]

(Continued)

Table 8.9 (Continued)

Drug	Comments
Escitalopram[22,25,75,85–87]	8% excreted unchanged in urine. The manufacturer states dosage adjustment is not necessary in patients with mild or moderate renal impairment but caution is advised if GFR <30mL/min, so start with a low dose and increase slowly. A case study of reversible renal tubular defects and another of renal failure have been reported with escitalopram. One study says effective versus placebo in end stage renal disease. Use of escitalopram (or citalopram) is associated with a higher risk of sudden cardiac death versus other SSRIs (fluoxetine, fluvoxamine, paroxetine, sertraline) when used in patients on haemodialysis (adjusted hazard ratio, 1.18; 95% CI 1.05, 1.31).
Fluoxetine[13,22,23,25,32,40,88–91]	2.5–5% of fluoxetine and 10% of the active metabolite norfluoxetine are excreted unchanged in the urine. Dosing: GFR 20–50mL/min dose as normal renal function; GFR <20mL/min use a low dose or on alternate days and increase according to response. Plasma levels after 2 months treatment with 20mg (in patients on dialysis with GFR <10mL/min) are similar to those with normal renal function. Efficacy studies of fluoxetine in depression and renal disease are conflicting. One small placebo controlled study of fluoxetine in patients on chronic dialysis found no significant differences in depression scores between the two groups after 8 weeks of treatment. Another found fluoxetine effective. A case series ($n = 4$) of once-weekly fluoxetine 90mg or 180mg use in depressed patients on haemodialysis describes efficacious use with better tolerability at 90mg dose.
Fluvoxamine[22,25,32,40,63]	2% is excreted unchanged in urine. Little information on its use in renal impairment. Manufacturer cautions in renal impairment. Dosing: GFR 10–50mL/min dose as for normal renal function; GFR <10mL/min dose as for normal renal function but start on a low dose and titrate slowly. Acute renal failure has been reported. Variations in albumin levels might affect serum concentrations of fluvoxamine in haemodialysis.
Imipramine[22,23,25,32,60]	<5% excreted unchanged in the urine. No specific dose adjustment necessary in renal impairment (GFR <10–50mL/min). Monitor patient for urinary retention, confusion, sedation and postural hypotension. Renal impairment with imipramine has been reported and manufacturer advises caution in severe renal impairment. Renal damage reported rarely.
Lofepramine[22,23,25,92]	There is little information about the use of lofepramine in renal impairment. Less than 5% is excreted unchanged in the urine. Dosing: GFR 10–50mL/min dose as in normal renal function; GFR <10mL/min start with a small dose and titrate slowly. Manufacturer contraindicates in severe renal impairment. As with imipramine, desipramine is the major metabolite.
Mirtazapine[22,23,25,93]	75% excreted unchanged in the urine. Clearance is reduced by 30% in patients with a GFR of 11–39mL/min and by 50% in patients with a GFR <10mL/min. Dosing advice: GFR 10–50mL/min dose as for normal renal function; GFR <10mL/min start at a low dose and monitor closely. Mirtazapine has been used to treat pruritis caused by renal failure and appetite loss in patients on dialysis.[94] Rarely associated with kidney calculus formation.
Moclobemide[22,23,25,95,96]	<1% of parent drug excreted unchanged in the urine. However, an active metabolite was found to be raised in patients with renal impairment but was not thought to affect dosing. The manufacturer advises that dose adjustments are not required in renal impairment. Dosing: GFR <10–50mL/min dose as in normal renal function.

(Continued)

Table 8.9 (*Continued*)

Drug	Comments
Nortriptyline[22,25,32,40,60,97]	<5% excreted unchanged in urine. If GFR 10–50mL/min, dose as in normal renal function; if GFR <10mL/min start at a low dose. Plasma level monitoring recommended at doses of >100mg/day, as plasma concentrations of active metabolites are raised in renal impairment. Worsening of GFR in elderly patients has also been reported. Plasma level monitoring can be useful.
Paroxetine[22,23,25,32,98–101]	Less than 2% of oral dose is excreted unchanged in the urine. Single-dose studies show increased plasma concentrations of paroxetine when GFR <30mL/min. Dosing advice differs: GFR 30–50mL/min dose as normal renal function; GFR <10–30mL/min start at 10mg/day (other source says start at 20mg) and increase dose according to response. Paroxetine 10mg daily and psychotherapy have been used successfully to treat depression in patients on chronic haemodialysis. Rarely associated with Fanconi syndrome and acute renal failure.
Phenelzine[22,25]	Approximately 1% excreted unchanged in the urine. No dose adjustment required in renal failure.
Reboxetine[22,23,25,102,103]	Approximately 10% of unchanged drug is excreted unchanged in the urine. Dosing: GFR <20mL/min, 2mg twice daily, adjusting dose according to response. Half-life is prolonged as renal function decreases.
Sertraline[22,23,25,32,104–108]	<0.2% of unchanged sertraline excreted in urine. Pharmacokinetics in renal impairment are unchanged in single dose studies but no published data on multiple dosing. Dosing is as for normal renal function. Sertraline has been used to treat dialysis-associated hypotension[109] and uraemic pruritis; however acute renal failure has been reported so it should be used with caution. Overall, studies of sertraline in patients with depression and chronic kidney disease show lack of efficacy. The CAST study, an RCT of sertraline (median dose 150mg) versus PBO in chronic non-dialysis dependent kidney disease found no significant difference in depressive symptoms.[108] The ASCEND trial of sertraline versus CBT in patients on haemodialysis with depression found no significant differences between sertraline (to 200mg) and CBT in response and remission rates but QIDS-C depression scores at 12 weeks were lower for sertraline than CBT.[110] Another small RCT (ASSertID study) in patients with depression on haemodialysis reported no difference between sertraline and placebo.[111] Has been associated with serotonin syndrome when used in patents on haemodialysis. Case report of neutropenia when used in ESRD.[112] May reduce CRP in patients on haemodialysis with depression[113] and a high CRP may predict response to sertraline (not placebo) in depression with CKD.[114]
Trazodone[22,23,25,115]	<5% excreted unchanged in urine but care needed as approximately 70% of active metabolite also excreted. Dosing: GFR 20–50mL/min, dose as normal renal function; GFR 10–20mL/min, dose as normal renal function but start with small dose and increase gradually; GFR <10mL/min, start with small doses and increase gradually. Serotonin syndrome reported in a patient with chronic kidney disease on trazodone and duloxetine.[84]

(*Continued*)

Table 8.9 (Continued)

Drug	Comments
Trimipramine[22,25,32,60,116,117]	No dose reduction required in renal impairment; however, elevated urea, acute renal failure and interstitial nephritis have been reported. As with all tricyclic antidepressants, monitor patient for urinary retention, confusion, sedation and postural hypotension as patients with renal impairment are at increased risk of having these side-effects.
Venlafaxine[22,23,32,118–120]	1–10% is excreted unchanged in the urine (30% as the active metabolite). Clearance is decreased and half-life prolonged in renal impairment. Dosing advice differs: GFR 30–50mL/min, dose as in normal renal function or reduce by 50%; GFR 10–30mL/min reduce dose by 50% and give tablets once daily; GFR <10mL/min, reduce dose by 50% and give once daily. Rhabdomyolysis and renal failure have been reported rarely with venlafaxine. Has been used to treat peripheral diabetic neuropathy in haemodialysis patients. High doses may cause hypertension.
Vortioxetine[23,121]	Negligible amounts are excreted unchanged in urine. Manufacturer advises that no dose adjustment is needed in renal impairment and end stage disease but advises caution.

Table 8.10 Mood stabilisers in renal impairment

Drug	Comments
Carbamazepine[22,23,25,122–129]	2–3% of the dose is excreted unchanged in urine. Dose reduction not necessary in renal disease, although cases of renal failure, tubular necrosis and tubulointerstitial nephritis have been reported rarely and metabolites may accumulate. Can cause Stevens-Johnson syndrome and toxic epidermal necrolysis which may result in acute renal failure. Maintenance therapy in bipolar disorder is associated with an increased rate of chronic kidney disease.[19]
Lamotrigine[22,23,25,130–134]	<10% of lamotrigine is excreted unchanged in the urine. Single-dose studies in renal failure show pharmacokinetics are little affected: however, inactive metabolites can accumulate (effects unknown) and half-life can be prolonged. Renal failure and interstitial nephritis have also been reported. Dosing: GFR <10–50mL/min, use cautiously, start with a low dose, increase slowly and monitor closely. One source suggests in GFR <10mL/min use 100mg every other day.
Lithium[22,23,25,32,135,136]	Lithium is nephrotoxic and contraindicated in severe renal impairment; 95% is excreted unchanged in the urine. Long-term treatment may result in impaired renal function ('creatinine creep'), permanent changes in kidney histology, microcysts, oncocytoma and collecting duct renal carcinoma, nephrogenic diabetes insipidus, nephrotic syndrome and both reversible and irreversible kidney damage.[137,138] However, shorter studies in younger populations do not show declining GFR[139] or

Table 8.10 (*Continued*)

Drug	Comments
Lithium (continued)	the development of end stage renal disease.[19] These differences may be due to methodology, improved monitoring and targeting recommended maintenance serum levels (0.6–0.8mmol/L in BPAD). Prevent by using once-daily dosing, recommended plasma levels, avoiding intoxication, active monitoring of kidney function and collaboration between psychiatrist, nephrologist and patient in decision making on continuation if CKD occurs.[140] Risk factors for lithium-induced nephrotoxicity include, increasing age, duration of treatment, cumulative dose, lower initial eGFR, female gender, hypertension and diabetes, concomitant nephrotoxic drugs, nephrogenic diabetes insipidus and previous lithium toxicity.[141] If lithium is used in renal impairment, toxicity is more likely and lithium toxicity increases the risk of renal impairment. Renal damage is more likely with chronic toxicity than acute. The manufacturer contraindicates lithium in renal impairment. Dosing: GFR 10–50mL/min, avoid or reduce dose (50–75% of normal dose) and monitor levels; GFR <10mL/min, avoid if possible, however if used it is essential to reduce dose (25–50% of normal dose). There is a case report of successful use in a patient on haemodialysis.[142]
Valproate[22,23,25,143–149]	Approximately 2% excreted unchanged. Dose adjustment usually not required in renal impairment; however, free valproate levels may be increased. Renal impairment, interstitial nephritis, Fanconi syndrome, renal tubular acidosis and renal failure have been reported. Risk factors for renal tubular dysfunction include being bedbound and low serum carnitine and phosphorus levels.[150] Dose as in normal renal function; however, in severe impairment (GFR <10mL/min) it may be necessary to alter doses according to free (unbound) valproate levels. Possibly less likely than lithium to cause chronic kidney disease in patients with bipolar disorder[151] but data are conflicting.[152]

Table 8.11 Anxiolytics and hypnotics in renal impairment

Drug	Comments
Buspirone[22,23,25,32]	Less than 1% is excreted unchanged; however, active metabolite is renally excreted. Dosing advice contradictory, suggest: GFR 10–50mL/min start at a low dose and give twice daily; GFR <10mL/min avoid if possible due to accumulation of active metabolites; if essential, reduce dose by 25–50% if patient is anuric. Manufacturer contraindicates in severe renal impairment.
Chlordiazepoxide[23,25,32]	1–2% excreted unchanged but chlordiazepoxide has a long-acting active metabolite that can accumulate. Dosing: GFR 10–50mL/min, dose as normal renal function; GFR <10mL/min, reduce dose by 50%. Monitor for excessive sedation. Manufacturer cautions in chronic renal disease.
Clomethiazole[22,23,25,153] (chlormethiazole)	0.1–5% of unchanged drug excreted unchanged in urine. Dose as in normal renal function but monitor for excessive sedation. Manufacturer recommends caution in renal disease.
Clonazepam[22,23,25,154]	<0.5% of clonazepam excreted unchanged in urine. Dose adjustment not required in impaired renal function; however, with long-term administration, active metabolites may accumulate, so start at a low doses and increase according to response. Monitor for excessive sedation. Has been used for insomnia in patients on haemodialysis.

(Continued)

Table 8.11 (*Continued*)

Drug	Comments
Diazepam[22,25,32,155]	Less than 0.5% is excreted unchanged. Dosing: GFR 20–50mL/min, dose as in normal renal function; GFR <20mL/min, use small doses and titrate to response. Long-acting, active metabolites accumulate in renal impairment; monitor patients for excessive sedation and encephalopathy. One case of interstitial nephritis with diazepam has been reported in a patient with chronic renal failure.
Eszopiclone[156]	Less than 10% excreted unchanged in the urine. No dose adjustment is needed in renal impairment.
Gabapentin	100% excreted unchanged in urine, clearance is reduced in renal impairment resulting in higher plasma concentrations and longer elimination half-lives.[157] As expected this may result in toxicity in renal impairment if doses are not reduced.[158] Acute renal failure has been reported;[159] myoclonus;[160] altered mental status, fall and fracture when used in patients on haemodialysis for restless legs, itch and neuropathic pain.[161,162] Has been used to treat pruritis, muscle cramps and restless legs syndrome in haemodialysis patients in RCTs.[163–165] Dosing advice differs; GFR 15–60mL/min start low and increase according to response; GFR <15mL/min, 300mg alternate days[32,159] or 100mg at night then increase according to tolerability[25,166] but care toxicity as described above. Manufacturer has table of very specific dosing in renal impairment in SMPC.[159]
Lemborexant[41,167]	<1% excreted unchanged in urine. Manufacturer states no dose adjustment needed in renal impairment but exposure increases during severe renal impairment with a potential increased risk of somnolence.
Lorazepam[22,23,25,32,168–173]	<1% excreted unchanged in urine, dose as in normal renal function but carefully according to response as some may need lower doses. Monitor for excessive sedation. Impaired elimination reported in two patients with severe renal impairment and also reports of propylene glycol in lorazepam injection causing renal impairment and acute tubular necrosis. However, lorazepam injection has been successfully used to treat catatonia in two patients with renal failure.
Nitrazepam[23,25]	Less than 5% excreted unchanged in the urine. Dosing GFR 10–50mL/min as per normal renal function; GFR <10mL/min start with small dose and increase slowly. Manufacturer advises reducing dose in renal impairment. Monitor patient for sedation and unsteadiness.
Pregabalin	Up to 99% excreted unchanged in urine. Acute renal failure reported.[174] Associated with altered mental status and falls when used in patients on haemodialysis,[161] and myoclonus.[175] Case report of seizure on abrupt cessation in patient with CKD.[176] Used to treat uraemic pruritis and neuropathic pain in patients on haemodialysis.[177,178] Dosing advice differs; titrate dosing by tolerability and response for all GFRs; GFR 30–60mL/min, 75mg daily; GFR 15–30mL/min, 25–50mg daily; GFR <15mL/min, 25mg daily. Manufacturer has table of very specific dosing in renal impairment in SMPC.[174]
Oxazepam[22,25,32,179]	Less than 1% excreted unchanged in the urine. Dose adjustment needed in severe renal impairment. Oxazepam may take longer to reach steady state in patients with renal impairment. Dosing: GFR 10–50mL/min, dose as in normal renal function; GFR <10mL/min, start at a low dose and increase according to response. Monitor for excessive sedation.

Table 8.11 (*Continued*)

Drug	Comments
Promethazine[22,23,25,32,180]	Dose reduction usually not necessary; however, promethazine has a long half-life so monitor for excessive sedative effects in patients with renal impairment. Manufacturer advises caution in renal impairment. There is a case report of interstitial nephritis in a patient who was a poor metaboliser of promethazine.
Temazepam[22,23,25,32]	<2% excreted unchanged in urine. In renal impairment the inactive metabolite can accumulate. Monitor for excessive sedative effects. Dosing: GFR 20–50mL/min, dose as normal renal function; GFR <20mL/min, dose as in normal renal function but start with 5mg.
Zolpidem[22,23,25,154,181]	Clearance moderately reduced in renal impairment. No dose adjustment required in renal impairment. Zolpidem 1mg has been used to treat insomnia in patients on haemodialysis. Ongoing RCT of zolpidem to aid sleep in haemodialysis patients with pruritis.[182] Associated with acute pyelonephritis in women.[183]
Zopiclone[22,23,25,184,185]	Less than 5% excreted unchanged in urine. Manufacturer states no accumulation of zopiclone in renal impairment but suggests starting at 3.75mg. Dosing: GFR <10mL/min, start with lower dose. Interstitial nephritis reported rarely.

Table 8.12 Anti-dementia drugs in renal impairment

Drug	Comments
Donepezil[23,25,186–188]	17% excreted unchanged in urine. Dosing is as in normal renal function for GFR <10–50mL/min. Manufacturer states that clearance not affected by renal impairment. Single dose studies find similar pharmacokinetics in moderate and severe renal impairment compared with healthy controls. Has been used at a dose of 3mg/day in an elderly patient with Alzheimer's dementia on dialysis. Single case of rhabdomyolysis causing acute renal failure.[189]
Galantamine[23,25]	18–22% is excreted unchanged in urine. Dose as in normal renal function for GFR 10–50mL/min and at GFR <10mL/min start at a low dose and increase slowly. Manufacturer contraindicates use in GFR <10mL/min. Plasma levels may be increased in patients with moderate and severe renal impairment.
Memantine[22,23,190]	Manufacturers recommend a 10mg dose if GFR 5–29mL/min; 10mg daily for 7 days then increased to 20mg daily if tolerated for GFR >30–49mL/min. Renal tubular acidosis, severe urinary tract infections and alkalisation of urine (e.g. by drastic dietary changes) can increase plasma levels of memantine. Acute renal failure has been reported with memantine.
Rivastigmine[23,25]	0% excreted unchanged in urine. Dosing advice for GFR <50mL/min start at a low dose and gradually increase. Steady state plasma concentrations are not affected by renal function.[191]

Table 8.13 Other psychotropic drugs in renal impairment

Drug	Comments
Bremelanotide[41,192]	64.8% excreted unchanged in urine. Manufacturer states 30–89mL/min no dosage adjustment necessary, caution GFR <30mL/min as increased adverse effects. Exposure is increased in renal impairment. Case report of Melanotan II (bremelanotide is a variation of Melanotan II) and rhabdomyolysis and renal dysfunction.[193]
Deutetrabenazine[194]	No clinical studies in renal impairment. Data limited, no specific dosing advice.
Pitolisant[41,195]	Less than 2% excreted unchanged in urine. Dosing GFR 15–59mL/min, 9mg daily; increase after 7 days to max 18mg once daily;[196] GFR less than 15mL/min not recommended.[196] Peak concentrations and exposure increased in all stages of renal impairment.
Prucalopride[41]	60–65% excreted unchanged in urine. Dosing GFR ≥30mL/min no adjustment necessary; GFR <30mL/min, 1mg daily. Contraindicated by manufacturer in patients requiring dialysis. Exposure increased in moderate and severe renal impairment[197] and raised plasma concentrations in all stages of renal impairment.[198] Case report of acute tubular necrosis and acute renal failure associated with prucalopride use.[199]
Solriamfetol[41,200]	95% excreted unchanged in urine. Dosing advice GFR 60–89mL/min no dose adjustment is required; GFR 30–59mL/min, 37.5mg once daily, increased to maximum of 75mg once daily after 5 days; GFR 15–29mL/min, 5mg once daily; GFR <15mL/min not recommended. In moderate or severe renal impairment risk of increased blood pressure and heart rate because of the prolonged half-life. Increased exposure and $t_{1/2}$ in all stages of renal impairment particularly ESRD.[201]
Valbenazine[41]	<2% excreted unchanged in urine. No adjustment is necessary GFR 30–90mL/min in mild, moderate renal impairment. Manufacturer does not recommend in severe renal impairment GFR <30mL/min.[202] Urinary retention reported as adverse effect in clinical trials.

Summary – recommended psychotropics in renal impairment

Where renal function declines while on existing drug treatment, rule-out existing drugs as a cause of reduced function and continue at a dose suggested in Tables 8.8–8.13. Where new drug treatment is required follow the suggestions below:

Drug group	Recommended drugs
Antipsychotics	■ No agent clearly preferred to another; however, avoid sulpiride and amisulpride ■ avoid highly anticholinergic agents because they can contribute to urinary retention ■ first generation antipsychotic – suggest **haloperidol** 2–6mg a day ■ second generation antipsychotic – suggest **olanzapine** 5mg a day
Antidepressants[203]	■ No agent clearly preferred to another; however, reasonable choices are ■ **Sertraline** but poor efficacy data in renal disease ■ **Citalopram** (care QTc prolonging effects and greater risk of sudden death in those on haemodialysis vs. other SSRIs) ■ **Fluoxetine** but care long half-life and need for alternate day dosing at lower GFRs ■ **CBT** where available
Mood stabilisers	■ No agent clearly preferred to another; however, avoid lithium if possible ■ suggest start one the following at a low dose and increase slowly, monitor for adverse effects: **valproate** or **lamotrigine**
Anxiolytics and hypnotics	■ No agent clearly preferred to another; however, excessive sedation is more likely to occur in patients with renal impairment, so monitor all patients carefully ■ **lorazepam** and **zopiclone** are suggested as reasonable choices
Anti-dementia drugs	■ No agent clearly preferred to another, however, **rivastigmine** is a reasonable choice

References

1. National Institute for Clinical Excellence. 4-year surveillance (2017) – Chronic kidney disease in adults (2014) NICE guideline [CG182]; https://www.nice.org.uk/guidance/cg182/evidence/appendix-a2-cg182-summary-of-new-evidence-from-surveillance-pdf-4429248447.
2. Levey AS, et al. A new equation to estimate glomerular filtration rate. *Ann Intern Med* 2009; **150**:604–612.
3. National Institute for Health and Care Excellence. Chronic kidney disease in adults: assessment and management. Clinical Guidance 182 [CG182] 2015; https://www.nice.org.uk/guidance/cg182.
4. National Institute for Clinical Excellence. Surveillance report 2017 – Chronic kidney disease (stage 4 or 5): management of hyperphosphataemia (2013) NICE Guideline CG157. Chronic kidney disease in adults: assessment and management (2014) NICE guideline CG182 and Chronic kidney disease: managing anaemia (2015) NICE guideline NG8 2017; https://www.nice.org.uk/guidance/cg182/resources/surveillance-report-2017-chronic-kidney-disease-stage-4-or-5-management-of-hyperphosphataemia-2013-nice-guideline-cg157-chronic-kidney-disease-in-adults-assessment-and-management-2014-nice-guideline–pdf-5740305984709.
5. Tangri N, et al. A predictive model for progression of chronic kidney disease to kidney failure. *JAMA* 2011; **305**:1553–1559.
6. Brater DC. Measurement of renal function during drug development. *Br J Clin Pharmacol* 2002; **54**:87–95.
7. Chinnadurai R, et al. Impact of chronic kidney disease on the drugs eliminated predominantly through a non-renal route: a proof of concept study with Citalopram. *Nephrol Dial Transplant* 2019; **34**:gfz103.SP268.
8. Toprak O, et al. New-onset type II diabetes mellitus, hyperosmolar non-ketotic coma, rhabdomyolysis and acute renal failure in a patient treated with sulpiride. *Nephrol Dial Transplant* 2005; **20**:662–663.
9. Baumgart U, et al. Olanzapine-induced acute rhabdomyolysis – a case report. *Pharmacopsychiatry* 2005; **38**:36–37.
10. Marsh SJ, et al. Rhabdomyolysis and acute renal failure during high-dose haloperidol therapy. *Ren Fail* 1995; **17**:475–478.
11. Smith RP, et al. Quetiapine overdose and severe rhabdomyolysis. *J Clin Psychopharmacol* 2004; **24**:343.
12. Nagler EV, et al. Antidepressants for depression in stage 3-5 chronic kidney disease: a systematic review of pharmacokinetics, efficacy and safety with recommendations by European Renal Best Practice (ERBP). *Nephrol Dial Transplant* 2012; **27**:3736–3745.
13. Palmer SC, et al. Antidepressants for treating depression in adults with end-stage kidney disease treated with dialysis. The Cochrane Database of Systematic Reviews 2016:CD004541.
14. Dev V, et al. Higher anti-depressant dose and major adverse outcomes in moderate chronic kidney disease: a retrospective population-based study. *BMC Nephrol* 2014; **15**:79.

15. Guirguis A, et al. Antidepressant usage in haemodialysis patients: evidence of sub-optimal practice patterns. *J Ren Care* 2020; 46:124–132.

16. Natale P, et al. Psychosocial interventions for preventing and treating depression in dialysis patients. Cochrane Database of Systematic Reviews 2019; CD004542.

17. Vangala C, et al. Selective serotonin reuptake inhibitor use and hip fracture risk among patients on hemodialysis. *Am J Kidney Dis* 2020; 75:351–360.

18. Tzeng NS, et al. Is schizophrenia associated with an increased risk of chronic kidney disease? A nationwide matched cohort study. *BMJ Open* 2015; 5:e006777.

19. Kessing LV, et al. Use of lithium and anticonvulsants and the rate of chronic kidney disease: a nationwide population-based study. *JAMA Psychiatry* 2015; 72:1182–1191.

20. Jiang Y, et al. A retrospective cohort study of acute kidney injury risk associated with antipsychotics. *CNS Drugs* 2017; 31:319–326.

21. Ryan PB, et al. Atypical antipsychotics and the risks of acute kidney injury and related outcomes among older adults: a replication analysis and an evaluation of adapted confounding control strategies. *Drugs Aging* 2017; 34:211–219.

22. Truven Health Analytics. Micromedex 2.0. 2017; https://www.micromedexsolutions.com/home/dispatch.

23. Datapharm Ltd. Electronic Medicines Compendium 2020; https://www.medicines.org.uk/emc.

24. Noble S, et al. Amisulpride: a review of its clinical potential in dysthymia. *CNS Drugs* 1999; 12:471–483.

25. Taylor & Francis Group. Renal Drug Database 2020; https://renaldrugdatabase.com.

26. Aragona M. Tolerability and efficacy of aripiprazole in a case of psychotic anorexia nervosa comorbid with epilepsy and chronic renal failure. *Eat Weight Disord* 2007; 12:e54–e57.

27. Mallikaarjun S, et al. Effects of hepatic or renal impairment on the pharmacokinetics of aripiprazole. *Clin Pharmacokinet* 2008; 47:533–542.

28. Tzeng NS, et al. Delusional parasitosis in a patient with brain atrophy and renal failure treated with aripiprazole: case report. *Prog Neuropsychopharmacol Biol Psychiatry* 2010; 34:1148–1149.

29. De Donatis D, et al. Serum aripiprazole concentrations prehemodialysis and posthemodialysis in a schizophrenic patient with chronic renal failure: a case report. *J Clin Psychopharmacol* 2020; 40:200–202.

30. Peeters P, et al. Asenapine pharmacokinetics in hepatic and renal impairment. *Clin Pharmacokinet* 2011; 50:471–481.

31. Fabre J, et al. Influence of renal insufficiency on the excretion of chloroquine, phenobarbital, phenothiazines and methacycline. *Helv Med Acta* 1967; 33:307–316.

32. Aronoff GR, et al. *Drug Prescribing in Renal Failure: Dosing Guidelines for Adults and Children.* 5th edn. Philadelphia: American College of Physicians; 2007.

33. Fraser D, et al. An unexpected and serious complication of treatment with the atypical antipsychotic drug clozapine. *Clin Nephrol* 2000; 54:78–80.

34. Au AF, et al. Clozapine-induced acute interstitial nephritis. *Am J Psychiatry* 2004; 161:1501.

35. Elias TJ, et al. Clozapine-induced acute interstitial nephritis. *Lancet* 1999; 354:1180–1181.

36. Siddiqui BK, et al. Simultaneous allergic interstitial nephritis and cardiomyopathy in a patient on clozapine. *NDT Plus* 2008; 1:55–56.

37. Davis EAK, et al. Clozapine-associated renal failure: a case report and literature review. *Ment Health Clin* 2019; 9:124–127.

38. Lim AM, et al. Clozapine, immunosuppressants and renal transplantation. *Asian J Psychiatr* 2016; 23:118.

39. Lobeck F, et al. Haloperidol concentrations in an elderly patient with moderate chronic renal failure. *J Geriatr Drug Ther* 1986; 1:91–97.

40. Cohen LM, et al. Update on psychotropic medication use in renal disease. *Psychosomatics* 2004; 45:34–48.

41. Lendac Data Systems Ltd. Drugdex Systems 2020; https://www.drugdiscoveryonline.com/doc/drugdex-system-0001.

42. Intra-Cellular Therapies Inc. Highlights of prescribing information. Caplyta (lumateperone) capsules for oral use 2019; https://www.accessdata.fda.gov/drugsatfda_docs/label/2019/209500s000lbl.pdf.

43. Sunovion Pharmaceuticals Europe Ltd. Summary of Product Characteristics. Latuda 18.5mg, 37mg and 74mg film-coated tablets 2020; https://www.medicines.org.uk/emc/medicine/29125.

44. Kansagra A, et al. Prolonged hypothermia due to olanzapine in the setting of renal failure: a case report and review of the literature. *Ther Adv Psychopharmacol* 2013; 3:335–339.

45. Samalin L, et al. Interest of clozapine and paliperidone palmitate plasma concentrations to monitor treatment in schizophrenic patients on chronic hemodialysis. *Schizophr Res* 2015; 166:351–352.

46. ACADIA Pharmaceuticals Inc. Highlights of prescribing information. Nuplazid (pimavanserin) tablets for oral use 2020; https://www.accessdata.fda.gov/drugsatfda_docs/label/2016/207318lbl.pdf.

47. Thyrum PT, et al. Single-dose pharmacokinetics of quetiapine in subjects with renal or hepatic impairment. *Prog Neuropsychopharmacol Biol Psychiatry* 2000; 24:521–533.

48. Huynh M, et al. Thrombotic thrombocytopenic purpura associated with quetiapine. *Ann Pharmacother* 2005; 39:1346–1348.

49. Torroba Sanz B, et al. Permanent renal sequelae secondary to drug reaction with eosinophilia and systemic symptoms (DRESS) syndrome induced by quetiapine. *Eur J Hosp Pharm* 2020:[Epub ahead of print].

50. Snoeck E, et al. Influence of age, renal and liver impairment on the pharmacokinetics of risperidone in man. *Psychopharmacology (Berl)* 1995; 122:223–229.

51. Herguner S, et al. Steroid-induced psychosis in an adolescent: treatment and prophylaxis with risperidone. *Turk J Pediatr* 2006; 48:244–247.

52. Batalla A, et al. Antipsychotic treatment in a patient with schizophrenia undergoing hemodialysis. *J Clin Psychopharmacol* 2010; 30:92–94.

53. Tourtellotte R, et al. Use of therapeutic drug monitoring of risperidone microspheres long-acting injection in hemodialysis: a case report. *Ment Health Clin* 2019; 9:404–407.

54. Bressolle F, et al. Pharmacokinetics of sulpiride after intravenous administration in patients with impaired renal function. *Clin Pharmacokinet* 1989; 17:367–373.

55. Aweeka F, et al. The pharmacokinetics of ziprasidone in subjects with normal and impaired renal function. *Br J Clin Pharmacol* 2000; **49**:27S-33S.

56. Roerig. Highlights of Prescribing Information: GEODON® (ziprasidone HCl) capsules; GEODON® (ziprasidone mesylate) injection for intramuscular use 2020; http://labeling.pfizer.com/ShowLabeling.aspx?id=584.

57. Iskandar JW, et al. Transient agranulocytosis associated with ziprasidone in a 45-year-old man on hemodialysis. *J Clin Psychopharmacol* 2015; **35**:347–348.

58. Basol N, et al. Beneficial effects of agomelatine in experimental model of sepsis-related acute kidney injury. *Ulus Travma Acil Cerrahi Derg* 2016; **22**:121–126.

59. Karaman A, et al. A novel approach to contrast-induced nephrotoxicity: the melatonergic agent agomelatine. *Br J Radiol* 2016; **89**:20150716.

60. Lieberman JA, et al. Tricyclic antidepressant and metabolite levels in chronic renal failure. *Clin Pharmacol Ther* 1985; **37**:301–307.

61. Mitas JA, et al. Diabetic neuropathic pain: control by amitriptyline and fluphenazine in renal insufficiency. *South Med J* 1983; **76**:462–463, 467.

62. Murphy EJ. Acute pain management pharmacology for the patient with concurrent renal or hepatic disease. *Anaesth Intensive Care* 2005; **33**:311–322.

63. Constantino JL, et al. Pharmacokinetics of antidepressants in patients undergoing hemodialysis: a narrative literature review. *Braz J Psychiatry* 2019; **41**:441–446.

64. Chen TY, et al. Amitriptyline-induced acute kidney injury and acute hepatitis: a case report. *Am J Ther* 2021; **28**:e256-e258

65. Sage Therapeutics Inc. Highlights of Prescribing Information. Zulresso (brexanolone) injection for intravenous use [controlled substance schedule pending] 2019; https://www.accessdata.fda.gov/drugsatfda_docs/label/2019/211371lbl.pdf.

66. Turpeinen M, et al. Effect of renal impairment on the pharmacokinetics of bupropion and its metabolites. *Br J Clin Pharmacol* 2007; **64**:165–173.

67. Worrall SP, et al. Pharmacokinetics of bupropion and its metabolites in haemodialysis patients who smoke. A single dose study. *Nephron Clin Pract* 2004; **97**:c83–c89.

68. Ghoreishi A, et al. Bupropion as a treatment for sexual dysfunction among chronic kidney disease patients *Acta Med Iran* 2019; **57**:320–327.

69. Joffe P, et al. Single-dose pharmacokinetics of citalopram in patients with moderate renal insufficiency or hepatic cirrhosis compared with healthy subjects. *Eur J Clin Pharmacol* 1998; **54**:237–242.

70. Kalender B, et al. Antidepressant treatment increases quality of life in patients with chronic renal failure. *Ren Fail* 2007; **29**:817–822.

71. Kelly CA, et al. Adult respiratory distress syndrome and renal failure associated with citalopram overdose. *Hum Exp Toxicol* 2003; **22**:103–105.

72. Spigset O, et al. Citalopram pharmacokinetics in patients with chronic renal failure and the effect of haemodialysis. *Eur J Clin Pharmacol* 2000; **56**:699–703.

73. Hosseini SH, et al. Citalopram versus psychological training for depression and anxiety symptoms in hemodialysis patients. *Iran J Kidney Dis* 2012; **6**:446–451.

74. Sran H, et al. Confusion after starting citalopram in a renal transplant patient. *BMJ Case Rep* 2013; **2013**:bcr2013010511.

75. Assimon MM, et al. Comparative cardiac safety of selective serotonin reuptake inhibitors among individuals receiving maintenance hemodialysis. *J Am Soc Nephrol* 2019; **30**:611–623.

76. Onishi A, et al. Reversible acute renal failure associated with clomipramine-induced interstitial nephritis. *Clin Exp Nephrol* 2007; **11**:241–243.

77. Wyeth Pharmaceuticals Inc. Highlights of Prescribing Information. PRISTIQ® (desvenlafaxine) Extended-Release Tablets, for oral use 2020; http://labeling.pfizer.com/showlabeling.aspx?id=497%20.

78. Nichols AI, et al. The pharmacokinetics and safety of desvenlafaxine in subjects with chronic renal impairment. *Int J Clin Pharmacol Ther* 2011; **49**:3–13.

79. Rees JA. Clinical interpretation of pharmacokinetic data on dothiepin hydrochloride (Dosulepin, Prothiaden). *J Int Med Res* 1981; **9**:98–102.

80. Swarna SS, et al. Pruritus associated with chronic kidney disease: a comprehensive literature review. *Cureus* 2019; **11**:e5256.

81. Lobo ED, et al. Effects of varying degrees of renal impairment on the pharmacokinetics of duloxetine: analysis of a single-dose phase I study and pooled steady-state data from phase II/III trials. *Clin Pharmacokinet* 2010; **49**:311–321.

82. Ho NV, et al. Duloxetine-induced multi-system organ failure: a case report. Poster presented at American Geriatrics Society Annual Meeting, May 11–15, 2011: National Harbor, Maryland; 2011.

83. Nguyen T, et al. Duloxetine uses in patients with kidney disease: different recommendations from the United States versus Europe and Canada. *Am J Ther* 2019; **26**:e516-e519.

84. Uong C, et al. Poster 91 serotonin syndrome in chronic kidney disease patient after given a dose of duloxetine while on trazodone: a case report. *PM&R* 2014; **6** (Suppl): S214–S215.

85. Miriyala K, et al. Renal failure in a depressed adolescent on escitalopram. *J Child Adolesc Psychopharmacol* 2008; **18**:405–408.

86. Adiga GU, et al. Renal tubular defects from antidepressant use in an older adult: an uncommon but reversible adverse drug effect. *Clin Drug Invest* 2006; **26**:607–610.

87. Yazici AE, et al. Efficacy and tolerability of escitalopram in depressed patients with end stage renal disease: an open placebo-controlled study. *Bull Clin Psychopharmacol* 2012; **22**:23–30.

88. Bergstrom RF, et al. The effects of renal and hepatic disease on the pharmacokinetics, renal tolerance, and risk-benefit profile of fluoxetine. *Int Clin Psychopharmacol* 1993; **8**:261–266.

89. Blumenfield M, et al. Fluoxetine in depressed patients on dialysis. *Int J Psychiatry Med* 1997; **27**:71–80.

90. Levy NB, et al. Fluoxetine in depressed patients with renal failure and in depressed patients with normal kidney function. *Gen Hosp Psychiatry* 1996; **18**:8–13.

91. Kauffman KM, et al. Higher dose weekly fluoxetine in hemodialysis patients: a case series report. *Int J Psychiatry Med* 2020; 56: 3–13.

92. Lancaster SG, et al. Lofepramine. A review of its pharmacodynamic and pharmacokinetic properties, and therapeutic efficacy in depressive illness. *Drugs* 1989; 37:123–140.

93. Davis MP, et al. Mirtazapine for pruritus. *J Pain Symptom Manage* 2003; 25:288–291.

94. Shibata K, et al. SP704 The effect of mirtazapine in dialysis patient with appetite loss. *Nephrol Dial Transplant* 2015; 30 (Suppl 3): iii611.

95. Schoerlin MP, et al. Disposition kinetics of moclobemide, a new MAO-A inhibitor, in subjects with impaired renal function. *J Clin Pharmacol* 1990; 30:272–284.

96. Stoeckel K, et al. Absorption and disposition of moclobemide in patients with advanced age or reduced liver or kidney function. *Acta Psychiatr Scand Suppl* 1990; 360:94–97.

97. Pollock BG, et al. Metabolic and physiologic consequences of nortriptyline treatment in the elderly. *Psychopharmacol Bull* 1994; 30:145–150.

98. Doyle GD, et al. The pharmacokinetics of paroxetine in renal impairment. *Acta Psychiatr Scand Suppl* 1989; 350:89–90.

99. Ishii T, et al. A rare case of combined syndrome of inappropriate antidiuretic hormone secretion and Fanconi syndrome in an elderly woman. *Am J Kidney Dis* 2006; 48:155–158.

100. Kaye CM, et al. A review of the metabolism and pharmacokinetics of paroxetine in man. *Acta Psychiatr Scand Suppl* 1989; 350:60–75.

101. Koo JR, et al. Treatment of depression and effect of antidepression treatment on nutritional status in chronic hemodialysis patients. *Am J Med Sci* 2005; 329:1–5.

102. Coulomb F, et al. Pharmacokinetics of single-dose reboxetine in volunteers with renal insufficiency. *J Clin Pharmacol* 2000; 40:482–487.

103. Dostert P, et al. Review of the pharmacokinetics and metabolism of reboxetine, a selective noradrenaline reuptake inhibitor. *Eur Neuropsychopharmacol* 1997; 7 (Suppl 1):S23–S35.

104. Brewster UC, et al. Addition of sertraline to other therapies to reduce dialysis-associated hypotension. *Nephrology (Carlton)* 2003; 8:296–301.

105. Chan KY, et al. Use of sertraline for antihistamine-refractory uremic pruritus in renal palliative care patients. *J Palliat Med* 2013; 16:966–970.

106. Chander WP, et al. Serotonin syndrome in maintenance haemodialysis patients following sertraline treatment for depression. *J Indian Med Assoc* 2011; 109:36–37.

107. Jain N, et al. Rationale and design of the Chronic Kidney Disease Antidepressant Sertraline Trial (CAST). *Contemp Clin Trials* 2013; 34:136–144.

108. Hedayati SS, et al. Effect of sertraline on depressive symptoms in patients with chronic kidney disease without dialysis dependence: the CAST randomized clinical trial. *JAMA* 2017; 318:1876–1890.

109. Razeghi E, et al. A randomized crossover clinical trial of sertraline for intradialytic hypotension. *Iran J Kidney Dis* 2015; 9:323–330.

110. Mehrotra R, et al. Comparative efficacy of therapies for treatment of depression for patients undergoing maintenance hemodialysis: a randomized clinical trial. *Ann Intern Med* 2019; 170:369–379.

111. Friedli K, et al. Sertraline versus placebo in patients with major depressive disorder undergoing hemodialysis: a randomized, controlled feasibility trial. *Clin J Am Soc Nephrol* 2017; 12:280–286.

112. Chien CW, et al. Sertraline-induced neutropenia and fatigue in a patient with end-stage renal disease. *Am J Ther* 2020:[Epub ahead of print].

113. Zahed NS, et al. Impact of sertraline on serum concentration of CRP in hemodialysis patients with depression. *J Renal Inj Prev* 2017; 6:65–69.

114. Gregg LP, et al. Inflammation and response to sertraline treatment in patients with CKD and major depression. *Am J Kidney Dis* 2020; 75:457–460.

115. Catanese B, et al. A comparative study of trazodone serum concentrations in patients with normal or impaired renal function. *Boll Chim Farm* 1978; 117:424–427.

116. Leighton JD, et al. Trimipramine-induced acute renal failure (Letter). *N Z Med J* 1986; 99:248.

117. Simpson GM, et al. A preliminary study of trimipramine in chronic schizophrenia. *Curr Ther Res Clin Exp* 1966; 99:248.

118. Troy SM, et al. The effect of renal disease on the disposition of venlafaxine. *Clin Pharmacol Ther* 1994; 56:14–21.

119. Guldiken S, et al. Complete relief of pain in acute painful diabetic neuropathy of rapid glycaemic control (insulin neuritis) with venlafaxine HCL. *Diabetes Nutr Metab* 2004; 17:247–249.

120. Pascale P, et al. Severe rhabdomyolysis following venlafaxine overdose. *Ther Drug Monit* 2005; 27:562–564.

121. Takeda Pharmaceuticals America Inc. Highlights of Prescribing Information. BRINTELLIX (vortioxetine) tablets 2020; http://www.us.brintellix.com.

122. Hegarty J, et al. Carbamazepine-induced acute granulomatous interstitial nephritis. *Clin Nephrol* 2002; 57:310–313.

123. Hogg RJ, et al. Carbamazepine-induced acute tubulointerstitial nephritis. *J Pediatr* 1981; 98:830–832.

124. Imai H, et al. Carbamazepine-induced granulomatous necrotizing angiitis with acute renal failure. *Nephron* 1989; 51:405–408.

125. Jubert P, et al. Carbamazepine-induced acute renal failure. *Nephron* 1994; 66:121.

126. Nicholls DP, et al. Acute renal failure from carbamazepine (Letter). *Br Med J* 1972; 4:490.

127. Tutor-Crespo MJ, et al. Relative proportions of serum carbamazepine and its pharmacologically active 10,11-epoxy derivative: effect of polytherapy and renal insufficiency. *Ups J Med Sci* 2008; 113:171–180.

128. Verrotti A, et al. Renal tubular function in patients receiving anticonvulsant therapy: a long-term study. *Epilepsia* 2000; 41:1432–1435.

129. Hung CC, et al. Acute renal failure and its risk factors in Stevens-Johnson syndrome and toxic epidermal necrolysis. *Am J Nephrol* 2009; 29:633–638.

130. Fervenza FC, et al. Acute granulomatous interstitial nephritis and colitis in anticonvulsant hypersensitivity syndrome associated with lamotrigine treatment. *Am J Kidney Dis* 2000; 36:1034–1040.

131. Fillastre JP, et al. Pharmacokinetics of lamotrigine in patients with renal impairment: influence of haemodialysis. *Drugs Exp Clin Res* 1993; **19**:25–32.

132. Schaub JE, et al. Multisystem adverse reaction to lamotrigine. *Lancet* 1994; **344**:481.

133. Wootton R, et al. Comparison of the pharmacokinetics of lamotrigine in patients with chronic renal failure and healthy volunteers. *Br J Clin Pharmacol* 1997; **43**:23–27.

134. Bansal AD, et al. Use of antiepileptic drugs in patients with chronic kidney disease and end stage renal disease. *Seminars in Dialysis* 2015; **28**:404–412.

135. Gitlin M. Lithium and the kidney: an updated review. *Drug Saf* 1999; **20**:231–243.

136. Lepkifker E, et al. Renal insufficiency in long-term lithium treatment. *J Clin Psychiatry* 2004; **65**:850–856.

137. McKnight RF, et al. Lithium toxicity profile: a systematic review and meta-analysis. *Lancet* 2012; **379**:721–728.

138. Shine B, et al. Long-term effects of lithium on renal, thyroid, and parathyroid function: a retrospective analysis of laboratory data. *Lancet* 2015; **386**:461–468.

139. Clos S, et al. Long-term effect of lithium maintenance therapy on estimated glomerular filtration rate in patients with affective disorders: a population-based cohort study. *Lancet Psychiatry* 2015; **2**:1075–1083.

140. Schoot TS, et al. Systematic review and practical guideline for the prevention and management of the renal side effects of lithium therapy. *Eur Neuropsychopharmacol* 2020; **31**:16–32.

141. Davis J, et al. Lithium and nephrotoxicity: a literature review of approaches to clinical management and risk stratification. *BMC Nephrol* 2018; **19**:305.

142. Engels N, et al. Successful lithium treatment in a patient on hemodialysis. *Bipolar Disorders* 2019; **21**:285–287.

143. Smith GC, et al. Anticonvulsants as a cause of Fanconi syndrome. *Nephrol Dial Transplant* 1995; **10**:543–545.

144. Fukuda Y, et al. Immunologically mediated chronic tubulo-interstitial nephritis caused by valproate therapy. *Nephron* 1996; **72**:328–329.

145. Watanabe T, et al. Secondary renal Fanconi syndrome caused by valproate therapy. *Pediatr Nephrol* 2005; **20**:814–817.

146. Zaki EL, et al. Renal injury from valproic acid: case report and literature review. *Pediatr Neurol* 2002; **27**:318–319.

147. Tanaka H, et al. Distal type of renal tubular acidosis after anti-epileptic therapy in a girl with infantile spasms. *Clin Exp Nephrol* 1999; **3**:311–313.

148. Knorr M, et al. Fanconi syndrome caused by antiepileptic therapy with valproic acid. *Epilepsia* 2004; **45**:868–871.

149. Rahman MH, et al. Acute hemolysis with acute renal failure in a patient with valproic acid poisoning treated with charcoal hemoperfusion. *Hemodial Int* 2006; **10**:256–259.

150. Koga S, et al. Risk factors for sodium valproate-induced renal tubular dysfunction. *Clin Exp Nephrol* 2018; **22**:420–425.

151. Hayes JF, et al. Adverse renal, endocrine, hepatic, and metabolic events during maintenance mood stabilizer treatment for bipolar disorder: a population-based cohort study. *PLoS Med* 2016; **13**:e1002058.

152. Kessing LV, et al. Continuation of lithium after a diagnosis of chronic kidney disease. *Acta Psychiatr Scand* 2017; **136**:615–622.

153. Pentikainen PJ, et al. Pharmacokinetics of chlormethiazole in healthy volunteers and patients with cirrhosis of the liver. *Eur J Clin Pharmacol* 1980; **17**:275–284.

154. Dashti-Khavidaki S, et al. Comparing effects of clonazepam and zolpidem on sleep quality of patients on maintenance hemodialysis. *Iran J Kidney Dis* 2011; **5**:404–409.

155. Sadjadi SA, et al. Allergic interstitial nephritis due to diazepam. *Arch Intern Med* 1987; **147**:579.

156. Sunovion Pharmaceuticals Inc. Highlights of Prescribing Information. LUNESTA® (eszopiclone) tablets, for oral use 2020; https://www.accessdata.fda.gov/drugsatfda_docs/label/2014/021476s030lbl.pdf.

157. Blum RA, et al. Pharmacokinetics of gabapentin in subjects with various degrees of renal function. *Clin Pharmacol Ther* 1994; **56**:154–159.

158. Miller A, et al. Gabapentin toxicity in renal failure: the importance of dose adjustment. *Pain Med* 2009; **10**:190–192.

159. Upjohn UK Limited. Summary of product characteristics. Neurontin 600mg film-coated tablets 2020; https://www.medicines.org.uk/emc/product/3197/smpc.

160. Yeddi A, et al. Myoclonus and altered mental status induced by single dose of gabapentin in a patient with end-stage renal disease: a case report and literature review. *Am J Ther* 2019; **26**:e768–e770.

161. Ishida JH, et al. Gabapentin and pregabalin use and association with adverse outcomes among hemodialysis patients. *J Am Soc Nephrol* 2018; **29**:1970–1978.

162. Gobo-Oliveira M, et al. Gabapentin versus dexchlorpheniramine as treatment for uremic pruritus: a randomised controlled trial. *Eur J Dermatol* 2018; **28**:488–495.

163. Gunal AI, et al. Gabapentin therapy for pruritus in haemodialysis patients: a randomized, placebo-controlled, double-blind trial. *Nephrol Dial Transplant* 2004; **19**:3137–3139.

164. Beladi Mousavi SS, et al. The effect of gabapentin on muscle cramps during hemodialysis: a double-blind clinical trial. *Saudi J Kidney Dis Transpl* 2015; **26**:1142–1148.

165. Razazian N, et al. Gabapentin versus levodopa-c for the treatment of restless legs syndrome in hemodialysis patients: a randomized clinical trial. *Saudi J Kidney Dis Transpl* 2015; **26**:271–278.

166. Rossi GM, et al. Randomized trial of two after-dialysis gabapentin regimens for severe uremic pruritus in hemodialysis patients. *Intern Emerg Med* 2019; **14**:1341–1346.

167. Eisai Inc. Highlights of Prescribing Information. Dayvigo (lemborexant) tablets for oral use [controlled substance schedule pending] 2019; https://www.accessdata.fda.gov/drugsatfda_docs/label/2019/212028s000lbl.pdf.

168. Huang CE, et al. Intramuscular lorazepam in catatonia in patients with acute renal failure: a report of two cases. *Chang Gung Med J* 2010; **33**:106–109.

169. Reynolds HN, et al. Hyperlactatemia, increased osmolar gap, and renal dysfunction during continuous lorazepam infusion. *Crit Care Med* 2000; 28:1631–1634.

170. Verbeeck RK, et al. Impaired elimination of lorazepam following subchronic administration in two patients with renal failure. *Br J Clin Pharmacol* 1981; 12:749–751.

171. Yaucher NE, et al. Propylene glycol-associated renal toxicity from lorazepam infusion. *Pharmacotherapy* 2003; 23:1094–1099.

172. Zar T, et al. Acute kidney injury, hyperosmolality and metabolic acidosis associated with lorazepam. *Nat Clin Pract Nephrol* 2007; 3:515–520.

173. Hayman M, et al. Acute tubular necrosis associated with propylene glycol from concomitant administration of intravenous lorazepam and trimethoprim-sulfamethoxazole. *Pharmacotherapy* 2003; 23:1190–1194.

174. Upjohn UK Limited. Lyrica 25mg 50mg 75mg 100mg 150mg 200mg 225mg and 300mg hard capsules 2020; https://www.medicines.org.uk/emc/product/10303/smpc.

175. Desai A, et al. Gabapentin or pregabalin induced myoclonus: a case series and literature review. *J Clin Neurosci* 2019; 61:225–234.

176. Du YT, et al. Seizure induced by sudden cessation of pregabalin in a patient with chronic kidney disease. *BMJ Case Rep* 2017; 2017:bcr2016219158.

177. Foroutan N, et al. Comparison of pregabalin with doxepin in the management of uremic pruritus: a randomized single blind clinical trial. *Hemodial Int* 2017; 21:63–71.

178. Otsuki T, et al. Efficacy and safety of pregabalin for the treatment of neuropathic pain in patients undergoing hemodialysis. *Clin Drug Investig* 2017; 37:95–102.

179. Murray TG, et al. Renal disease, age, and oxazepam kinetics. *Clin Pharmacol Ther* 1981; 30:805–809.

180. Leung N, et al. Acute kidney injury in patients with inactive cytochrome P450 polymorphisms. *Ren Fail* 2009; 31:749–752.

181. Drover DR. Comparative pharmacokinetics and pharmacodynamics of short-acting hypnosedatives: zaleplon, zolpidem and zopiclone. *Clin Pharmacokinet* 2004; 43:227–238.

182. Rehman IU, et al. A randomized controlled trial for effectiveness of zolpidem versus acupressure on sleep in hemodialysis patients having chronic kidney disease-associated pruritus. *Medicine (Baltimore)* 2018; 97:e10764.

183. Hsu FG, et al. Use of zolpidem and risk of acute pyelonephritis in women: a population-based case–control study in Taiwan. *J Clin Pharmacol* 2017; 57:376–381.

184. Goa KL, et al. Zopiclone. A review of its pharmacodynamic and pharmacokinetic properties and therapeutic efficacy as an hypnotic. *Drugs* 1986; 32:48–65.

185. Hussain N, et al. Zopiclone-induced acute interstitial nephritis. *Am J Kidney Dis* 2003; 41:E17.

186. Suwata J, et al. New acetylcholinesterase inhibitor (donepezil) treatment for Alzheimer's disease in a chronic dialysis patient. *Nephron* 2002; 91:330–332.

187. Nagy CF, et al. Steady-state pharmacokinetics and safety of donepezil HCl in subjects with moderately impaired renal function. *Br J Clin Pharmacol* 2004; 58 (Suppl 1):18–24.

188. Tiseo PJ, et al. An evaluation of the pharmacokinetics of donepezil HCl in patients with moderately to severely impaired renal function. *Br J Clin Pharmacol* 1998; 46 (Suppl 1):56–60.

189. Sahin OZ, et al. A rare case of acute renal failure secondary to rhabdomyolysis probably induced by donepezil. *Case Rep Nephrol* 2014; 2014:214359.

190. Periclou A, et al. Pharmacokinetic study of memantine in healthy and renally impaired subjects. *Clin Pharmacol Ther* 2006; 79:134–143.

191. Lefevre G, et al. Effects of renal impairment on steady-state plasma concentrations of Rivastigmine: a population pharmacokinetic analysis of capsule and patch formulations in patients with Alzheimer's disease. *Drugs Aging* 2016; 33:725–736.

192. AMAG Pharmaceutical Inc. Highlights of prescribing information. Vyleesi (bremelanotide injection) for subcutaneous use 2019; https://www.accessdata.fda.gov/drugsatfda_docs/label/2019/210557s000lbl.pdf.

193. Nelson ME, et al. Melanotan II injection resulting in systemic toxicity and rhabdomyolysis. *Clin Toxicol (Phila)* 2012; 50:1169–1173.

194. Teva Pharmaceuticals USA Inc. Highlights of prescribing information. Austedo (deutetrabenazine) tablets for oral use 2020; https://www.accessdata.fda.gov/drugsatfda_docs/label/2017/209885lbl.pdf.

195. Lincoln Medical Limited. Wakix 4.5mg/18mg film-coated tablets 2016; https://www.medicines.org.uk/emc/product/7402.

196. Bioprojet Pharma. Highlights of prescribing information. Wakix (pitolisant) tablets for oral use 2019; https://www.accessdata.fda.gov/drugsatfda_docs/label/2019/211150s000lbl.pdf.

197. Smith WB, et al. Effect of renal impairment on the pharmacokinetics of prucalopride: a single-dose open-label Phase I study. *Drug Des Devel Ther* 2012; 6:407–415.

198. Shire Pharmaceuticals Limited. Resolor 1mg and 2mg film-coated tablets 2019; https://www.medicines.org.uk/emc/product/584/smpc.

199. Sivabalasundaram V, et al. Prucalopride-associated acute tubular necrosis. *World J Clin Cases* 2014; 2:380–384.

200. Jazz Pharmaceuticals UK. Sunosi 75mg and 140mg film-coated tablets 2020; https://www.medicines.org.uk/emc/product/11017/smpc.

201. Zomorodi K, et al. Single-dose pharmacokinetics and safety of solriamfetol in participants with normal or impaired renal function and with end-stage renal disease requiring hemodialysis. *J Clin Pharmacol* 2019; 59:1120–1129.

202. Neurocrine Biosciences Inc. Highlights of prescribing information. Ingrezza (valbenazine) capsules for oral use 2020; https://www.accessdata.fda.gov/drugsatfda_docs/label/2017/209241lbl.pdf.

203. Gregg LP, et al. Pharmacologic and psychological interventions for depression treatment in patients with kidney disease. *Curr Opin Nephrol Hypertens* 2020; 29:457–464.

Part 3

Prescribing in specialist conditions

Drug treatment of other psychiatric conditions

Borderline personality disorder (BPD)

Borderline personality disorder (BPD) is common in psychiatric settings, affecting 20% of community psychiatric patients.[1] Common co-morbid conditions affecting patients with BPD include affective disorders (both unipolar and bipolar affective disorder) anxiety spectrum disorders, eating disorders, and drug and alcohol misuse, and the lifetime risk of having at least one co-morbid mental disorder approaches 100%.[2] Co-morbid conditions, such as depression and anxiety, should be managed according to usual guidance for the particular condition, irrespective of any coexisting BPD diagnosis. The suicide rate in BPD is similar to that seen in affective disorders and schizophrenia, affecting about 1-in-10 patients.[3,4]

Although classified as a personality disorder, several aspects of BPD have been assumed to be responsive to drug treatment. These include affective instability, transient or stress-related quasi-psychotic or depressive symptoms, suicidal and self-harming behaviours, and impulsivity.[4] A high proportion of people with BPD are prescribed psychotropic drugs[2,5,6] often in polypharmacy regimes.[7] A survey of prescribing practice in England found that over 90% of patients with BPD had been prescribed psychotropic medication, most commonly antidepressants or antipsychotics, particularly for affective instability.[6] The prevalence of prescribing antipsychotics, antidepressants and mood stabilisers in those with BPD as a sole psychiatric diagnosis is the same as in those with BPD and a clear and documented co-morbid diagnosis of schizophrenia, depression or bipolar disorder, respectively.[6] This suggests that psychotropics are often prescribed for the treatment of BPD per se (for which there is very limited support) rather than for specific co-morbid conditions. No drug is specifically licensed for the treatment of BPD, or indeed any aspect of BPD. Psychological treatments such as DBT are better supported – Cochrane noted 75 randomised controlled trials (RCTs) of psychological treatments in 2020.[8]

In 2009 NICE[9] recommended that:

- Drug treatment should not be used routinely for borderline personality disorder or

The Maudsley® Prescribing Guidelines in Psychiatry, Fourteenth Edition. David M. Taylor, Thomas R. E. Barnes and Allan H. Young.
© 2021 David M. Taylor. Published 2021 by John Wiley & Sons Ltd.

for the individual symptoms or behaviour associated with the disorder (for example, repeated self-harm, marked emotional instability, risk-taking behaviour and transient psychotic symptoms)
- Drug treatment may be considered in the overall treatment of co-morbid conditions
- Short-term use of sedative medication may be considered as part of the overall treatment plan for people with borderline personality disorder in a crisis. The duration of treatment should be agreed with the patient but should be no longer than one week.

NICE guidelines were last reviewed in July 2018, when no changes were recommended.[9] Soon after the initial publication of the NICE guideline for BPD, two further independent systematic reviews were published.[10,11] Essentially the same studies were considered in all three reviews, and where numerical data were combined in meta-analyses the results of these analyses were similar. In addition, all noted that the majority of studies of drug treatment in BPD last for only 6 weeks and that the large number of different outcome measures that were used made it difficult to evaluate and compare studies. NICE considered that the data were not robust enough to be the basis for recommendations to the NHS while the other two reviews concluded that some of the analyses showed promising results and that these were sufficient to inform clinical practice.

A more recent systematic review[12] updated the previous analyses by including 15 studies published between 2010 and 2017. Conclusions were little different from the earlier NICE review – that the body of evidence was insufficient to make clear clinical recommendations. The latest analysis of published, unpublished and ongoing studies[13] concluded not only that no drug treatment has been conclusively shown to be effective in BPD but also that the number of drug trials has declined markedly in the past few years.

Antipsychotics

Open studies, which are admittedly more prone to bias, have found benefit for a number of first- and second-generation antipsychotics over a wide range of symptoms. In contrast, placebo-controlled RCTs generally show more limited benefits for active drug over placebo. The symptoms/symptom clusters that appear to be most responsive to treatment are affect dysregulation, anger, impulsivity and cognitive-perceptual symptoms.[10,11,14,15] Olanzapine may have the best supported effect[12,16,17] but its effect is modest, at best.[12] Open and naturalistic studies report reductions in aggression and self-harming behaviour with clozapine[18-22] and clozapine has been shown to have an anti-aggressive effect in people with schizophrenia.[23] Clozapine seems to reduce the risk of hospital admission in BPD.[22] Quetiapine is perhaps the most widely used antipsychotic in BDP. Its use is supported by a small RCT for which full results were published online in 2020.[24]

Antidepressants

Several open studies have found that selective serotonin reuptake inhibitors (SSRIs) reduce impulsivity and aggression in BPD, but these findings have not been replicated in RCTs. One RCT comparing fluoxetine with DBT showed higher rates of suicide attempts in those given fluoxetine.[25] It can be concluded with reasonable certainty that there is no robust evidence to support the use of antidepressants in treating depressed mood or impulsivity in people with BPD.[10,11]

Mood-stabilisers

Up to a half of people with BPD may be also be diagnosed with a bipolar spectrum disorder[26] (although such diagnoses are rather controversial) and mood-stabilisers are commonly prescribed.[2] There is some evidence that mood stabilisers reduce impulsivity, anger and affect dysregulation in people with BPD.[10,11] **Lithium** is licensed for the control of aggressive behaviour or intentional self-harm.[27] A large RCT of **lamotrigine** found it had no effect on any symptom domain.[28] **Mifepristone** is also ineffective.[29]

Memantine

An RCT of 33 subjects found adjunctive **memantine** 20mg a day to be more effective than placebo[30] and well tolerated. More trials are needed.

Opioid antagonists

Very limited evidence supports the efficacy of **naltrexone** in reducing self-harm and dissociative symptoms,[12,31] but there are no definitive trials supporting the effectiveness of naltrexone in the treatment of patients with BPD.

Management of crisis

Drug treatments are often used during periods of crisis when symptoms can be severe, distressing and potentially life-threatening. In BPD these symptoms can be expected to wax and wane.[3] Consequently, drug therapy may then be required intermittently, and with each episode, the decision to prescribe needs to be informed by a careful consideration of the relative harms and benefits of medication. It is generally easy to see when treatment is required, but much more difficult to decide when modest gains are worthwhile and whether or not continuation is likely to be necessary. The use of psychotropic drugs is not without harm, so treatment should always take the form of a rigorously evaluated short-term trial.

NICE[9] recommend that during periods of crisis, time-limited treatment with a sedative drug may be helpful. Anticipated side effect profile and potential toxicity in overdose should guide choice. For example, benzodiazepines (particularly short-acting drugs) can cause disinhibition in this group of patients,[32] potentially compounding problems. Sedative antipsychotics can cause EPS and/or considerable weight gain, and tricyclic antidepressants are particularly toxic in overdose. A sedative antihistamine such as **promethazine** (25–50mg) is usually well tolerated and may be a helpful short-term treatment when used as part of a coordinated care plan. Its adverse effects (dry mouth, constipation), deleterious effects on sleep architecture and lack of clear anxiolytic effects militate against longer term use.

References

1. Kernberg OF, et al. Borderline personality disorder. *Am J Psychiatry* 2009; 166:505–508.
2. Pascual JC, et al. A naturalistic study of changes in pharmacological prescription for borderline personality disorder in clinical practice: from APA to NICE guidelines. *Int Clin Psychopharmacol* 2010; 25:349–355.
3. Links PS, et al. Prospective follow-up study of borderline personality disorder: prognosis, prediction of outcome, and axis II comorbidity. *Can J Psychiatry* 1998; 43:265–270.
4. Oldham JM. Guideline watch: practice guideline for the treatment of patients with borderline personality disorder. *Focus* 2005; 3:396–400.
5. Baker-Glenn E, et al. Use of psychotropic medication among psychiatric out-patients with personality disorder. *Psychiatrist* 2010; 34:83–86.
6. Paton C. Prescribing for people with emotionally unstable personality disorder under the care of UK mental health services. *J Clin Psychiatry* 2015:e512–e518.
7. Riffer F, et al. Psychopharmacological treatment of patients with borderline personality disorder: comparing data from routine clinical care with recommended guidelines. *Int J Psychiatry Clin Pract* 2019; 23:178–188.
8. Storebø OJ, et al. Psychological therapies for people with borderline personality disorder. *Cochrane Database Syst Rev* 2020; 5:Cd012955.
9. National Institute for Clinical Excellence. Borderline personality disorder: recognition and management. Clinical Guidance 78 [CG78] 2009 (Last checked July 2018); https://www.nice.org.uk/guidance/CG78
10. Lieb K, et al. Pharmacotherapy for borderline personality disorder: Cochrane systematic review of randomised trials. *Br J Psychiatry* 2010; 196:4–12.
11. Ingenhoven T, et al. Effectiveness of pharmacotherapy for severe personality disorders: meta-analyses of randomized controlled trials. *J Clin Psychiatry* 2010; 71:14–25.
12. Hancock-Johnson E, et al. A focused systematic review of pharmacological treatment for borderline personality disorder. *CNS Drugs* 2017; 31:345–356.
13. Stoffers-Winterling J, et al. Pharmacotherapy for borderline personality disorder: an update of published, unpublished and ongoing studies. *Curr Psychiatry Rep* 2020; 22:37.
14. Zanarini MC, et al. A dose comparison of olanzapine for the treatment of borderline personality disorder: a 12-week randomized, double-blind, placebo-controlled study. *J Clin Psychiatry* 2011; 72:1353–1362.
15. Canadian Agency for Drugs and Technologies in Health. Aripiprazole for borderline personality disorder: a review of the clinical effectiveness 2017. https://www.ncbi.nlm.nih.gov/pubmedhealth/PMH0096409.
16. Shafti S, et al. A comparative study on olanzapine and aripiprazole for symptom management in female patients with borderline personality disorder. *Bull Clin Psychopharmacol*, 2015; 25:38–43.
17. Bozzatello P, et al. Efficacy and tolerability of asenapine compared with olanzapine in borderline personality disorder: an open-label randomized controlled trial. *CNS Drugs* 2017; 31:809–819.
18. Benedetti F, et al. Low-dose clozapine in acute and continuation treatment of severe borderline personality disorder. *J Clin Psychiatry* 1998; 59:103–107.
19. Frogley C, et al. A case series of clozapine for borderline personality disorder. *Ann Clin Psychiatry* 2013; 25:125–134.
20. Chengappa KN, et al. Clozapine reduces severe self-mutilation and aggression in psychotic patients with borderline personality disorder. *J Clin Psychiatry* 1999; 60:477–484.
21. Dickens GL, et al. Experiences of women in secure care who have been prescribed clozapine for borderline personality disorder. *Borderline Personal Disord and Emot Dysregul* 2016; 3:12.
22. Rohde C, et al. Real-world effectiveness of clozapine for borderline personality disorder: results from a 2-year mirror-image study. *J Pers Disord* 2017:1–15.
23. Volavka J, et al. Heterogeneity of violence in schizophrenia and implications for long-term treatment. *Int J Clin Pract* 2008; 62:1237–1245.
24. ClinicalTrial.gov. Seroquel extended release (XR) for the management of borderline personality disorder (BPD). ClinicalTrials.gov Identifier: NCT00880919. 2017. https://clinicaltrials.gov/ct2/show/results/NCT00880919?view=results.
25. ClinicalTrial.gov. Treating suicidal behavior and self-mutilation in people with borderline personality disorder. ClinicalTrials.gov Identifier: NCT00533117. 2017. https://clinicaltrials.gov/ct2/show/results/NCT00533117.
26. Deltito J, et al. Do patients with borderline personality disorder belong to the bipolar spectrum? *J Affect Disord* 2001; 67:221–228.
27. Essential Pharma Ltd. Summary of product characteristics. Camcolit 400mg prolonged release Lithium Carbonate. 2020. https://www.medicines.org.uk/emc/product/10829/smpc.
28. Crawford MJ, et al. No effect of lamotrigine in subgroups of patients with borderline personality disorder: response to Smith. *Am J Psychiatry* 2018; 175:1265–1266.
29. ClinicalTrial.gov. Preliminary trial of the effect of Glucocorticoid Receptor Antagonist on borderline personality disorder (BPD). ClinicalTrials.gov Identifier: NCT01212588. 2019. https://clinicaltrials.gov/ct2/show/NCT01212588.
30. Kulkarni J, et al. Effect of the glutamate NMDA receptor antagonist memantine as adjunctive treatment in borderline personality disorder: an exploratory, randomised, double-blind, placebo-controlled trial. *CNS Drugs* 2018; 32:179–187.
31. Moghaddas A, et al. The potential role of naltrexone in borderline personality disorder. *Iran J Psychiatry* 2017; 12:142–146.
32. Gardner DL, et al. Alprazolam-induced dyscontrol in borderline personality disorder. *Am J Psychiatry* 1985; 142:98–100.

Eating disorders

The incidence of eating disorders continues to increase.[1] Lifetime risk of any eating disorder is 8.4% in women and 2.2% in men.[2] Other psychiatric conditions (particularly anxiety, depression and obsessive-compulsive disorder) often coexist with eating disorders, and this may in part explain the benefit sometimes seen with medication. Any medicine prescribed should be accompanied by close monitoring to check for possible adverse reactions.

Anorexia nervosa (AN)

General guidance

Drugs have limited activity in anorexia nervosa (AN), and none is currently licensed for this condition.[3] Prompt weight restoration to a safe weight, family therapy and structured psychotherapy are the main interventions.[4,5] The aim of (physical) treatment is to improve nutritional health through re-feeding with very limited evidence to support the use of any pharmacological interventions other than those prescribed to correct metabolic deficiencies. Medicines may be used to treat co-morbid conditions,[4] but have a very limited role in weight restoration.[6]

Olanzapine is the only drug suggested to have any effect on weight restoration in anorexia nervosa.[7-9] Early data for quetiapine were encouraging[10] but were not replicated in a later RCT.[11] Overall, the body of evidence for pharmacotherapy is said to be 'unsatisfactory'[12] and a meta-analysis found no significant effect over placebo.[13] A network meta-analysis is planned[14] but is yet to be completed. The most recent and largest review of trials and meta-analyses[15] concluded that 'no psychotropic medication has proved efficacious'.

Dronabinol, a synthetic cannabinoid agonist, may induce slight weight gain[16] but is not recommended and adverse effects (dysphoria) are common.[17]

Healthcare professionals should be aware of the risk of medicines that prolong the QT interval. All patients with a diagnosis of anorexia nervosa should have an alert placed in their prescribing record noting that they are at increased risk of arrhythmias secondary to electrolyte disturbances and potential cardiac complications associated with inadequate nutrition. ECG monitoring should be undertaken if the prescription of any medicine that may compromise cardiac functioning is essential.[4]

Physical aspects

Vitamins and minerals

Treatment with a multivitamin/multimineral supplement in oral form is recommended during both inpatient and outpatient weight restoration.[4]

Electrolytes

Electrolyte disturbances (e.g. hypokalaemia) may develop slowly over time and may be asymptomatic and resolve with re-feeding. Hypophosphataemia may also be precipitated by re-feeding. Rapid correction may be hazardous. Oral supplementation is therefore used to prevent serious sequelae rather than simply to restore normal levels. If supplements are used, urea and electrolytes, HCO_3, Ca, P and Mg need to be monitored and an ECG needs to be performed.[18]

Osteoporosis

Bone loss is a serious complication of anorexia with serious consequences. Hormonal treatment using oestrogen or dehydroepiandrosterone (DHEA) does not have a positive impact on bone density and oestrogen is not recommended in children and adolescents due to the risk of premature fusion of the bones.[4] Antipsychotics that raise prolactin levels can further increase the risk of bone loss and osteoporosis. Bisphosphonates are not generally recommended for women with anorexia nervosa due to the lack of data about both the benefits and also safety. They are not licensed for use in premenopausal girls.

Psychiatric aspects

Acute illness: antidepressants

A Cochrane review found no evidence from four placebo-controlled trials that antidepressants improved weight gain, eating disorder or associated psychopathology.[19] It has been suggested that neurochemical abnormalities in starvation may partially explain this non-response.[19] Co-prescribing nutritional supplementation (including tryptophan) with fluoxetine has not been shown to increase efficacy.[20] NICE found little evidence to support the use of antidepressants.[4] Naturalistic studies suggest an important risk of switch to mania.[21] Antidepressants appear to have no role in AN.

Other psychotropic medicines

Antipsychotics (e.g. olanzapine), benzodiazepines or antihistamines (e.g. promethazine) are often used to reduce the high levels of anxiety associated with anorexia nervosa, but they are not usually recommended for the promotion of weight gain.[4] Case reports and retrospective studies have suggested that olanzapine may reduce agitation (and possibly improve weight).[22,23] One RCT[8] showed that 87.5% of patients given olanzapine achieved weight restoration (vs. 55.6% on placebo). Quetiapine may improve psychological symptoms, but there are few data.[10] Only prolactin-sparing antipsychotics should be considered (i.e. avoid risperidone, amisulpride, sulpiride). Pooled effects of antipsychotics on weight are statistically non-existent.[13]

Many other medications[6] have been investigated in small placebo-controlled trials of varying quality and success, these include zinc,[24] naltrexone[25] and cyproheptadine.[26] None is currently widely used in practice. Relamorelin (a ghrelin agonist),[27] oxytocin[28] and testosterone[29] are probably not effective.

Relapse prevention

There is evidence from one small trial that fluoxetine may be useful in improving outcome and preventing relapse of patients with anorexia nervosa after weight restoration.[30] Other studies have found no benefit.[19,31] SSRIs can, albeit very rarely, elevate prolactin.

Co-morbid disorders

Antidepressants are often used to treat co-morbid major depression and obsessive-compulsive disorder. However, caution should be used as these conditions may resolve with weight gain alone.[4] As weight loss is a frequent side effect of bupropion, this antidepressant is contraindicated for the treatment of co-morbid depression in AN.[32] Mania and psychosis occurring in the context of AN are probably best treated with olanzapine, and bipolar depression with olanzapine + fluoxetine.[32]

Bulimia nervosa and binge eating disorder

Psychological interventions should be considered first line for bulimia.[33] Adults with bulimia nervosa and binge eating disorder (BED) may be offered a trial of an antidepressant. SSRIs (specifically fluoxetine[34-36]) are the ADs of first choice. The effective dose of fluoxetine is 60mg daily.[37] Patients should be informed that this can reduce the frequency of binge eating and purging but long-term effects are unknown.[4] Early response (at 3 weeks) is a strong predictor of response overall.[38]

Antidepressants may be used for the treatment of bulimia nervosa in adolescents, but they are not licensed for this age group, and there is little evidence for this practice. They should not be considered as a first line treatment in adolescent bulimia nervosa.[4]

There is some reasonable evidence that topiramate reduces frequency of binge-eating[39] (although it is often poorly tolerated) and rather limited evidence for the usefulness of bupropion,[40] duloxetine,[41] lamotrigine,[42,43] zonisamide,[44,45] acamprosate[46] and sodium oxybate.[47] Systematic reviews[48,49] confirm the modest efficacy of SSRIs and also suggest benefit for lisdexamfetamine (based on a high quality RCT[50]). Lisdexamfetamine is approved for BED in USA.[51] Some limited evidence supports the use of a slow release combination of phentermine and topiramate.[52,53] The noradrenaline/dopamine reuptake inhibitor dasotraline may also be effective[54] but its development ceased in 2020.

Co-morbid depression

Depression is a frequent co-morbidity in BN and BED. Citalopram has been shown to be more effective than fluoxetine for depressive symptoms in BN patients; as weight gain is a frequent side effect of mirtazapine, this antidepressant should be avoided or used with caution for the treatment of co-morbid depression in BED.[32]

Other atypical eating disorders

There have been no useful studies of the use of medicines to treat atypical eating disorders other than anorexia nervosa and BED.[4,55] In the absence of evidence to guide the management of other atypical eating disorders (also known as 'eating disorders not otherwise specified'), it is recommended that the clinician considers following the guidance of the eating disorder that mostly resembles the individual patient's eating disorder.[4]

Summary of NICE guidance on eating disorders[4]

Anorexia nervosa

- Psychological interventions are the treatments of choice and should be accompanied by monitoring of the patient's physical state
- No pharmacological intervention is recommended. A range of medicines may be used in the treatment of co-morbid conditions

Bulimia nervosa

- An evidence-based self-help programme or cognitive behaviour therapy for bulimia nervosa should be the first choice of treatment
- A trial of fluoxetine may be offered as an alternative or additional first step

Binge eating disorder

- An evidence-based self-help programme of cognitive behavioural therapy for binge eating disorder should be the first choice of treatment
- A trial of an SSRI can be considered as an alternative or additional first step
- Lisdexamfetamine is also an option

References

1. Martínez-González L, et al. Incidence of anorexia nervosa in women: a systematic review and meta-analysis. *Int J Environ Res Public Health* 2020; 17:3824.
2. Galmiche M, et al. Prevalence of eating disorders over the 2000–2018 period: a systematic literature review. *Am J Clin Nutr* 2019; 109:1402–1413.
3. Frank GKW. Pharmacotherapeutic strategies for the treatment of anorexia nervosa – too much for one drug? *Expert Opin Pharmacother* 2020; 21:1045–1058.
4. National Institute for Clinical Excellence. Eating disorders: recognition and treatment. NICE guideline [NG69] 2017 (Last update March 2020); https://www.nice.org.uk/guidance/ng69.
5. American Psychiatric Association. Treatment of patients with eating disorders, third edition. *Am J Psychiatry* 2006; 163:4–54.
6. Crow SJ, et al. What potential role is there for medication treatment in anorexia nervosa? *Int J Eat Disord* 2009; 42:1–8.
7. Dunican KC, et al. The role of olanzapine in the treatment of anorexia nervosa. *Ann Pharmacothe* 2007; 41:111–115.
8. Bissada H, et al. Olanzapine in the treatment of low body weight and obsessive thinking in women with anorexia nervosa: a randomized, double-blind, placebo-controlled trial. *Am J Psychiatry* 2008; 165:1281–1288.
9. Leggero C, et al. Low-dose olanzapine monotherapy in girls with anorexia nervosa, restricting subtype: focus on hyperactivity. *J Child Adolesc Psychopharmacol* 2010; 20:127–133.
10. Court A, et al. Investigating the effectiveness, safety and tolerability of quetiapine in the treatment of anorexia nervosa in young people: a pilot study. *J Psychiatr Res* 2010; 44:1027–1034.
11. Powers PS, et al. Double-blind placebo-controlled trial of quetiapine in anorexia nervosa. *Eur Eat Disord Rev* 2012; 20:331–334.
12. Miniati M, et al. Psychopharmacological options for adult patients with anorexia nervosa. *CNS Spectr* 2016; 21:134–142.
13. de Vos J, et al. Meta analysis on the efficacy of pharmacotherapy versus placebo on anorexia nervosa. *J Eat Disord* 2014; 2:27.

14. Wade TD, et al. Comparative efficacy of pharmacological and non-pharmacological interventions for the acute treatment of adult outpatients with anorexia nervosa: study protocol for the systematic review and network meta-analysis of individual data. *J Eat Disord* 2017; 5:24.

15. Blanchet C, et al. Medication in AN: a multidisciplinary overview of meta-analyses and systematic reviews. *J Clin Med* 2019; 8

16. Andries A, et al. Dronabinol in severe, enduring anorexia nervosa: a randomized controlled trial. *Int J Eat Disord* 2014; 47:18–23.

17. Gross H, et al. A double-blind trial of delta 9-tetrahydrocannabinol in primary anorexia nervosa. *J Clin Psychopharmacol* 1983; 3:165–171.

18. Connan F, et al. Biochemical and endocrine complications. *Eur Eat Disord Rev* 2000; 8:144–157.

19. Claudino AM, et al. Antidepressants for anorexia nervosa. *Cochrane Database Syst Rev* 2006:CD004365.

20. Barbarich NC, et al. Use of nutritional supplements to increase the efficacy of fluoxetine in the treatment of anorexia nervosa. *Int J Eat Disord* 2004; 35:10–15.

21. Rossi G, et al. Pharmacological treatment of anorexia nervosa: a retrospective study in preadolescents and adolescents. *Clin Pediatr (Phila)* 2007; 46:806–811.

22. Malina A, et al. Olanzapine treatment of anorexia nervosa: a retrospective study. *Int J Eat Disord* 2003; 33:234–237.

23. La Via MC, et al. Case reports of olanzapine treatment of anorexia nervosa. *Int J Eat Disord* 2000; 27:363–366.

24. Su JC, et al. Zinc supplementation in the treatment of anorexia nervosa. *Eat Weight Disord* 2002; 7:20–22.

25. Marrazzi MA, et al. Naltrexone use in the treatment of anorexia nervosa and bulimia nervosa. *Int Clin Psychopharmacol* 1995; 10:163–172.

26. Halmi KA, et al. Anorexia nervosa. Treatment efficacy of cyproheptadine and amitriptyline *Arch Gen Psychiatry* 1986; 43:177–181.

27. Fazeli PK, et al. Treatment with a ghrelin agonist in outpatient women with anorexia nervosa: a randomized clinical trial. *J Clin Psychiatry* 2018; 79.

28. Russell J, et al. Intranasal oxytocin in the treatment of anorexia nervosa: randomized controlled trial during re-feeding. *Psychoneuroendocrinology* 2018; 87:83–92.

29. Kimball A, et al. A randomized placebo-controlled trial of low-dose testosterone therapy in women with anorexia nervosa. *J Clin Endocrinol Metab* 2019; 104:4347–4355.

30. Kaye WH, et al. Double-blind placebo-controlled administration of fluoxetine in restricting- and restricting-purging-type anorexia nervosa. *Biol Psychiatry* 2001; 49:644–652.

31. Walsh BT, et al. Fluoxetine after weight restoration in anorexia nervosa: a randomized controlled trial. *JAMA* 2006; 295:2605–2612.

32. Himmerich H, et al. Pharmacological treatment of eating disorders, comorbid mental health problems, malnutrition and physical health consequences. *Pharmacol Ther* 2020:107667.

33. Vocks S, et al. Meta-analysis of the effectiveness of psychological and pharmacological treatments for binge eating disorder. *Int J Eat Disord* 2010; 43:205–217.

34. Fluoxetine Bulimia Nervosa Collaborative Study Group. Fluoxetine in the treatment of bulimia nervosa. A multicenter, placebo-controlled, double-blind trial. *Arch Gen Psychiatry* 1992; 49:139–147.

35. Goldstein DJ, et al. Long-term fluoxetine treatment of bulimia nervosa. Fluoxetine Bulimia Nervosa Research Group. *Br J Psychiatry* 1995; 166:660–666.

36. Romano SJ, et al. A placebo-controlled study of fluoxetine in continued treatment of bulimia nervosa after successful acute fluoxetine treatment. *Am J Psychiatry* 2002; 159:96–102.

37. Bacaltchuk J, et al. Antidepressants versus placebo for people with bulimia nervosa. *Cochrane Database Syst Rev* 2003:CD003391.

38. Sysko R, et al. Early response to antidepressant treatment in bulimia nervosa. *Psychol Med* 2010; 40:999–1005.

39. Nourredine M, et al. Efficacy and safety of topiramate in binge eating disorder: a systematic review and meta-analysis. *CNS Spectr* 2020:1–9.

40. White MA, et al. Bupropion for overweight women with binge-eating disorder: a randomized, double-blind, placebo-controlled trial. *J Clin Psychiatry* 2013; 74:400–406.

41. Leombruni P, et al. Duloxetine in obese binge eater outpatients: preliminary results from a 12-week open trial. *Hum Psychopharmacol* 2009; 24:483–488.

42. Guerdjikova AI, et al. Lamotrigine in the treatment of binge-eating disorder with obesity: a randomized, placebo-controlled monotherapy trial. *Int Clin Psychopharmacol* 2009; 24:150–158.

43. Trunko ME, et al. A pilot open series of lamotrigine in DBT-treated eating disorders characterized by significant affective dysregulation and poor impulse control. *Borderline Personality Disord Emot Dysregul* 2017; 4:21.

44. Ricca V, et al. Zonisamide combined with cognitive behavioral therapy in binge eating disorder: a one-year follow-up study. *Psychiatry (Edgmont)* 2009; 6:23–28.

45. Guerdjikova AI, et al. Zonisamide in the treatment of bulimia nervosa: an open-label, pilot, prospective study. *Int J Eat Disord* 2013; 46:747–750.

46. McElroy SL, et al. Acamprosate in the treatment of binge eating disorder: a placebo-controlled trial. *Int J Eat Disord* 2011; 44:81–90.

47. McElroy SL, et al. Sodium oxybate in the treatment of binge eating disorder: an open-label, prospective study. *Int J Eat Disord* 2011; 44:262–268.

48. Hilbert A, et al. Meta-analysis on the long-term effectiveness of psychological and medical treatments for binge-eating disorder. *Int J Eat Disord* 2020; 53:1353–1376.

49. Ghaderi A, et al. Psychological, pharmacological, and combined treatments for binge eating disorder: a systematic review and meta-analysis. *Peer J* 2018; 6:e5113.

50. McElroy SL, et al. Efficacy and safety of lisdexamfetamine for treatment of adults with moderate to severe binge-eating disorder: a randomized clinical trial. *JAMA Psychiatry* 2015; 72:235–246.

51. Citrome L Lisdexamfetamine for binge eating disorder in adults: a systematic review of the efficacy and safety profile for this newly approved indication – what is the number needed to treat, number needed to harm and likelihood to be helped or harmed? *Int J Clin Pract* 2015; 69:410–421.

52. Safer DL, et al. A randomized, placebo-controlled crossover trial of phentermine-topiramate ER in patients with binge-eating disorder and bulimia nervosa. *Int J Eat Disord* 2020; 53:266–277.

53. Guerdjikova AI, et al. Combination phentermine-topiramate extended release for the treatment of binge eating disorder: an open-label, prospective study. *Innov Clin Neurosci* 2018; 15:17–21.

54. Grilo CM, et al. Efficacy and safety of dasotraline in adults with binge-eating disorder: a randomized, placebo-controlled, fixed-dose clinical trial. *CNS Spectr* 2020:1–10.

55. Leombruni P, et al. A 12 to 24 weeks pilot study of sertraline treatment in obese women binge eaters. *Hum Psychopharmacol* 2006; 21:181–188.

Delirium

Delirium is a common neuropsychiatric condition that presents in medical and surgical settings and is known by various names including organic brain syndrome, intensive care psychosis and acute confusional state.[1]

Diagnostic criteria for delirium[2]

- Disturbance of *consciousness* (reduced clarity of awareness of the environment) with reduced ability to focus, sustain or shift attention
- A change in *cognition* (such as memory deficit, disorientation, language disturbance or perceptual disturbance) not better explained by a pre-existing or evolving dementia
- The disturbance develops over a *short period of time* (usually hours to days) and tends to fluctuate over the course of the day
- There is often evidence from the history, physical examination or laboratory findings that the disturbance is due to concomitant medications, a medical condition, substance intoxication or substance withdrawal

Tools for evaluation[3]

A brief cognitive assessment should be included in the examination of patients at risk of delirium. A standardised tool, the Confusion Assessment Method (CAM) is a brief, validated algorithm currently used to diagnose delirium. CAM relies on the presence of acute onset of symptoms, fluctuating course, inattention and either disorganised thinking or an altered level of consciousness.

Clinical subtypes of delirium[4–6]

- **Hyperactive delirium:** Characterised by increased motor activity with agitation, hallucinations and inappropriate behaviour
- **Hypoactive delirium:** Characterised by reduced motor activity and lethargy (has a poorer prognosis)
- **Mixed delirium:** Features of both increased and reduced motor activity

Prevalence

Delirium is present in 10% of hospitalised medical patients and a further 10–30% develop delirium after admission.[4] Postoperative delirium occurs in 15–53% of patients and in 70–87% of those in intensive care.[7]

Risk factors

Delirium is almost invariably multifactorial, and it is often impossible to isolate a single precipitant as the cause.[4] The most important risk factors[4,5,8–10] have consistently emerged as:

- Prior cognitive impairment or dementia
- Older age (>65 years)
- Multiple co-morbidities
- Previous history of delirium, stroke, neurological disease, falls or gait disorder
- Psychoactive drug use
- Polypharmacy (>4 medications)
- Anticholinergic drug use

Outcome

Patients with delirium have an increased length of hospital stay, increased mortality and increased risk of long term institutional placement.[1,5] Hospital mortality rates of patients with delirium range from 6% to 18% and are twice that of matched controls.[5] In older people, the 1-year mortality rate associated with cases of delirium is 35–40%.[7] Up to 60% of individuals suffer persistent cognitive impairment following delirium and these patients are also three times more likely to develop dementia.[1,5]

Management

Preventing delirium is the most effective strategy for reducing its frequency and complications.[7] Delirium is a medical emergency and the identification and treatment of the underlying cause should be the first aim of management.[11]

Non-pharmacological or environmental support strategies should be instituted wherever possible. These include coordinating nursing care, preventing sensory deprivation and disorientation, and maintaining competence.[5,12] Pharmacological treatment should be directed first at the underlying cause (if known) and then at the relief of specific symptoms of delirium.

The common errors in the pharmacological management of delirium are to use antipsychotic medications in excessive doses, give them too late or to overuse benzodiazepines.[4]

General Principles[4,5,13–16]

- Keep the use of sedatives and antipsychotics to a minimum
- Use one drug at a time
- Tailor doses according to age, body size and degree of agitation
- Titrate doses to effect
- Use small doses regularly, rather than large doses less frequently
- Review at least every 24 hours
- Increase scheduled doses if regular 'as needed' doses are required after the initial 24 hours period
- Maintain at an effective dose and discontinue as soon as the clinical situation allows
- Ensure that the diagnosis of delirium is documented both in the patients hospital notes and in their primary health record (include in discharge letter or summary)
- If it has not been possible to discontinue agents prior to discharge, ensure a clear plan for early medication review and follow up in the community is agreed

Choice of drug[17–20]

High quality trials of pharmacological treatments for delirium are lacking, with available studies often small, comprising heterogeneous populations and clinical outcomes, excluding patients with neurologic and psychiatric comorbidities,[21] and producing conflicting results. These problems mean that the results of meta-analyses must be approached with caution; a recent network meta-analysis found a combination of haloperidol and lorazepam to be effective treatment for delirium, but this was based on a single study in cancer patients measuring effect on agitation, not delirium.[22] There is insufficient evidence to recommend any single drug treatment over others. Certain patient populations may derive less benefit from antipsychotic treatment (e.g. those in palliative care may experience worsening of symptoms[23,24]). Treatment choice should therefore be informed by the likelihood of interaction with coexisting medical conditions or other medications (see Table 9.1).

Pharmacological prophylaxis[25–29]

Data around the use of medication to prevent delirium are sparse and conflicting. Most studies use low dose haloperidol in patients deemed at high risk of developing delirium (elderly, post-surgical or ICU patients). Prophylactic low dose haloperidol (around 3mg/day) was thought to reduce the severity and duration of delirium episodes and shorten the length of hospital stay in patients at high risk of developing the condition, but a recent study in older subjects found no effect.[30] Higher doses (>5mg/day) may reduce the incidence in surgical patients,[31] but a large RCT found no benefit to mortality in critically ill patients.[32] Cochrane[25] suggests prophylactic olanzapine may be effective, and a small RCT found some benefit to aripiprazole.[33] Rivastigmine may be effective[34] but Cochrane is dismissive.[25] Data are conflicting for melatonin,[35–37] ramelteon[38–41] and suvorexant[42] but at least these drugs are well tolerated and may reduce sleep disturbance, which contributes to the risk of delirium.[43] Some evidence exists to support non-drug measures to minimise the risk of delirium.[44]

Table 9.1 Drugs used to treat delirium

Drug	Dose	Adverse effects	Notes
First-generation antipsychotics			
Haloperidol[1,5,7,12,30,45–47]	Oral 0.5–1mg bd with additional doses every 4 hourly as needed. (peak effect: 4–6 hours)	EPSE can occur especially at doses above 3mg Prolonged QT interval Increased risk of stroke in patients with dementia	Considered first line agent and is the only licensed treatment in the UK for this indication. No trial data has demonstrated superiority of other antipsychotics over haloperidol; however, care must be taken to monitor for extrapyramidal and cardiac side effects

(Continued)

Table 9.1 (*Continued*)

Drug	Dose	Adverse effects	Notes
Haloperidol (continued)	IM 0.5–1mg, observe for 30–60 minutes and repeat if necessary (peak effect: 20–40 minutes)		Baseline ECG is recommended for all patients, and especially for the elderly or those with a family or personal history of cardiac disease. Low doses (<1mg) are unlikely to cause problems in those with no pre-existing disease[48] Regular monitoring of the ECG and potassium levels should be carried out if there are other conditions present that may prolong the QT interval Avoid in Lewy body dementia and Parkinson's disease Avoid intravenous use where possible. However, in the medical ICU setting, IV is often used with close continuous ECG monitoring

Second-generation antipsychotics

Drug	Dose	Adverse effects	Notes
Amisulpride[12,13,49,50]	Oral 50–300mg od, up to a maximum of 800mg od Doses higher than 300mg should be given in two divided doses	Prolonged QT interval Increased risk of stroke in patients with dementia	Very limited evidence in delirium As amisulpride is almost entirely excreted via the kidneys it is imperative to monitor renal function when used in medically ill or elderly patients
Aripiprazole[12,13,49–51]	Oral 5–15mg/day, up to a maximum of 30mg/day	EPSE less likely than with haloperidol Akathisia or worsening sleep cycle may be problematic Increased risk of stroke in patients with dementia	Very limited evidence Use of the rapid-acting intramuscular preparation has been described[52]
Olanzapine[19,53–57]	Oral 2.5–5mg od, up to a maximum of 20mg/day	EPSE less likely than with haloperidol Sedation is the most commonly reported side effect Increased risk of stroke in patients with dementia	A trial comparing olanzapine, risperidone, haloperidol and quetiapine showed that all were equally efficacious and safe in the treatment of delirium, but the response rate to olanzapine was poorer in the older age group (>75 years)[58] The rapid-acting intramuscular preparations has not been assessed in the treatment of delirium. IV use of the IM preparation has been described[59]

Table 9.1 (*Continued*)

Drug	Dose	Adverse effects	Notes
Risperidone[19,55,56,60–65]	Oral 0.5mg bd with additional doses every 4 hourly as needed Usual maximum 4mg/day	The most commonly reported side effects are hypotension and EPSE Increased risk of stroke in patients with dementia	A trial comparing risperidone with olanzapine showed that both were equally effective in reducing delirium symptoms but the response to risperidone was poorer in the older age group (>70 years)[56]
Quetiapine[19,41,66–72]	Oral 12.5–50mg bd This may be increased every 12 hours to 200mg daily if it is well tolerated	Sedation and postural hypotension are the most common reported side effects Increased risk of stroke in patients with dementia	There are an increasing number of trials demonstrating safety and efficacy of low dose quetiapine compared with haloperidol both in and outside the medical ICU. Now first choice agent in many units
Ziprasidone[73]	IM 10mg every 2 hourly Usual maximum 40mg/day	QT prolongation Increased risk of stroke in patients with dementia	Very limited evidence
Benzodiazepines			
Lorazepam[1,5,7]	Oral/IM 0.25–1mg every 2–4 hourly as needed. Usual maximum 3mg in 24 hours IV use is usually reserved for emergencies	More likely than antipsychotics to cause respiratory depression, over-sedation and paradoxical excitement Associated with prolongation and worsening of delirium symptoms	Used in alcohol or sedative/hypnotic withdrawal, Parkinson's disease and neuroleptic malignant syndrome Otherwise – avoid
Diazepam[74]	Starting oral dose of 5–10mg In the elderly a starting dose of 2mg is recommended	Much longer half-life than lorazepam Associated with prolongation and worsening of delirium symptoms	Used in alcohol or sedative/hypnotic withdrawal, Parkinson's disease and neuroleptic malignant syndrome Otherwise – avoid

(*Continued*)

Table 9.1 (*Continued*)

Drug	Dose	Adverse effects	Notes
Cholinesterase Inhibitors			
Donepezil[75]	Oral 5mg od	Reasonably well tolerated compared with placebo. Nausea, vomiting and diarrhoea are the most common adverse effects reported	Very limited evidence. In the small studies where it has been used, clinical benefits have not been convincing. Not recommended
Rivastigmine[76–78]	Oral 1.5–6mg bd	A study which added rivastigmine to usual care (haloperidol), showed that rivastigmine did not decrease the duration of delirium but in fact was associated with a more severe type of delirium, a longer stay in intensive care and higher mortality compared with placebo	Use of rivastigmine to treat delirium in critically ill patients is not recommended. May have a place in delirium prevention[34]
Other Drugs			
Trazodone[4,7]	25–150mg nocte	Over sedation is problematic	Limited experience – used only in uncontrolled studies. Not recommended
Sodium valproate[79–82]	Oral/IM/IV 250mg bd increased to around 1500mg/day, or 20mg/kg/day. Target plasma levels have not been validated for this indication. Note that physically ill patients may have altered albumin binding of valproate. IV loading doses have also been used in ICU settings	Contraindicated in active liver disease. Monitor for thrombocytopaenia (more common in critically ill patients)	Some case reports of use where antipsychotics and/or benzodiazepines are ineffective; otherwise not recommended

bd, bis die (twice a day); nocte, at night; od, omne in die (once a day)

References

1. van Zyl LT, et al. Delirium concisely: condition is associated with increased morbidity, mortality, and length of hospitalization. *Geriatrics* 2006; **61**:18–21.

2. American Psychiatric Association. *Diagnostic and statistical manual of mental disorders, Fifth Edition (DSM-5)*. Arlington, VA: American Psychiatric Association 2013.

3. Inouye SK, et al. Clarifying confusion: the confusion assessment method. A new method for detection of delirium. *Ann Intern Med* 1990; **113**:941–948.

4. Nayeem K, et al. Delirium. *Clin Med* 2003; **3**:412–415.

5. Potter J, et al. The prevention, diagnosis and management of delirium in older people: concise guidelines. *Clin Med* 2006; **6**:303–308.

6. Fong TG, et al. Delirium in elderly adults: diagnosis, prevention and treatment. *Nat Rev Neurol* 2009; **5**:210–220.

7. Inouye SK. Delirium in older persons. *N Engl J Med* 2006; **354**:1157–1165.

8. Saxena S, et al. Delirium in the elderly: a clinical review. *Postgrad Med J* 2009; **85**:405–413.

9. Naja M, et al. Delirium in geriatric medicine is related to anticholinergic burden. *Eur Geriatr Med* 2013; **4** Suppl 1:S208.

10. Egberts A, et al. Anticholinergic drug burden and delirium: a systematic review. *J Am Med Dir Assoc* 2020:S1525–8610 (1520)30349–30342.

11. Burns A, et al. Delirium. *J Neurol Neurosurg Psychiatry* 2004; **75**:362–367.

12. Schwartz TL, et al. The role of atypical antipsychotics in the treatment of delirium. *Psychosomatics* 2002; **43**:171–174.

13. Seitz DP, et al. Antipsychotics in the treatment of delirium: a systematic review. *J Clin Psychiatry* 2007; **68**:11–21.

14. National Institute for Health and Clinical Excellence. Delirium: diagnosis, prevention and management. [Clinical Guideline 103] 2010 (Last updated March 2019); https://www.nice.org.uk/Guidance/CG103.

15. Donders E, et al. Effect of haloperidol dosing frequencies on the duration and severity of delirium in elderly hip fracture patients. A prospective randomized trial. *Eur Geriatr Med* 2012; **3** Suppl 1:S118–S119.

16. Soiza RL, et al. The Scottish Intercollegiate Guidelines Network (SIGN) 157: guidelines on risk reduction and management of delirium. *Medicina (Kaunas)* 2019; **55**:491.

17. Nikooie R, et al. Antipsychotics for treating delirium in hospitalized adults: a systematic review. *Ann Intern Med* 2019; **171**:485–495.

18. Li Y, et al. Benzodiazepines for treatment of patients with delirium excluding those who are cared for in an intensive care unit. *Cochrane Database Syst Rev* 2020; **2**:Cd012670.

19. Rivière J, et al. Efficacy and tolerability of atypical antipsychotics in the treatment of delirium: a systematic review of the literature. *Psychosomatics* 2019; **60**:18–26.

20. Devlin JW, et al. Clinical practice guidelines for the prevention and management of pain, agitation/sedation, delirium, immobility, and sleep disruption in adult patients in the ICU. *Crit Care Med* 2018; **46**:e825–e873.

21. Martin RC, et al. Assessment of the generalizability of clinical trials of delirium interventions. *JAMA Network Open* 2020; **3**:e2015080.

22. Wu YC, et al. Association of delirium response and safety of pharmacological interventions for the management and prevention of delirium: a network meta-analysis. *JAMA Psychiatry* 2019; **76**:526–535.

23. Finucane AM, et al. Drug therapy for delirium in terminally ill adults. *Cochrane Database Syst Rev* 2020; **1**:Cd004770.

24. Lee KY, et al. Effect of antipsychotics and non-pharmacotherapy for the management of delirium in people receiving palliative care. *J Pain Palliat Care Pharmacother* 2020:1–12.

25. Siddiqi N, et al. Interventions for preventing delirium in hospitalised non-ICU patients. *Cochrane Database Syst Rev* 2016; **3**:Cd005563.

26. Santos E, et al. Effectiveness of haloperidol prophylaxis in critically ill patients with a high risk of delirium: a systematic review. *JBI Database System Rev Implement Rep* 2017; **15**:1440–1472.

27. Fok MC, et al. Do antipsychotics prevent postoperative delirium? A systematic review and meta-analysis. *Int J Geriatr Psychiatry* 2015; **30**:333–344.

28. Schrijver EJ, et al. Efficacy and safety of haloperidol for in-hospital delirium prevention and treatment: A systematic review of current evidence. *Eur J Intern Med* 2016; **27**:14–23.

29. Oh ES, et al. Antipsychotics for preventing delirium in hospitalized adults: a systematic review. *Ann Intern Med* 2019; **171**:474–484.

30. Schrijver E, et al. Haloperidol versus placebo for delirium prevention in acutely hospitalised older at risk patients: a multi-centre double-blind randomised controlled clinical trial. *Age Ageing* 2017; **47**:48–55.

31. Shen YZ, et al. Effects of haloperidol on delirium in adult patients: a systematic review and meta-analysis. *Med Princ Pract* 2018; **27**:250–259.

32. van den Boogaard M, et al. Effect of haloperidol on survival among critically ill adults with a high risk of delirium: the reduce randomized clinical trial. *JAMA* 2018; **319**:680–690.

33. Mokhtari M, et al. Aripiprazole for prevention of delirium in the neurosurgical intensive care unit: a double-blind, randomized, placebo-controlled study. *Eur J Clin Pharmacol* 2020; **76**:491–499.

34. Youn YC, et al. Rivastigmine patch reduces the incidence of postoperative delirium in older patients with cognitive impairment. *Int J Geriatr Psychiatry* 2016; **32**:1079–1084.

35. Asleson DR, et al. Melatonin for delirium prevention in acute medically ill, and perioperative geriatric patients. *Aging Medicine (Milton (NSW))* 2020; **3**:132–137.

36. Campbell AM, et al. Melatonin for the prevention of postoperative delirium in older adults: a systematic review and meta-analysis. *BMC Geriatr* 2019; **19**:272.

37. Ford AH, et al. The healthy heart-mind trial: randomized controlled trial of melatonin for prevention of delirium. *J Am Geriatr Soc* 2020; 68:112–119.

38. Oh ES, et al. Effects of ramelteon on the prevention of postoperative delirium in older patients undergoing orthopedic surgery: the recover randomized controlled trial. *Am J Geriatr Psychiatry* 2021; 29:90–100.

39. Hatta K, et al. Preventive effects of ramelteon on delirium: a randomized placebo-controlled trial. *JAMA Psychiatry* 2014; 71:397–403.

40. Jaiswal SJ, et al. Ramelteon for prevention of postoperative delirium: a randomized controlled trial in patients undergoing elective pulmonary thromboendarterectomy. *Crit Care Med* 2019; 47:1751–1758.

41. Kim MS, et al. Comparative efficacy and acceptability of pharmacological interventions for the treatment and prevention of delirium: A systematic review and network meta-analysis. *J Psychiatr Res* 2020; 125:164–176.

42. Adams AD, et al. The role of suvorexant in the prevention of delirium during acute hospitalization: A systematic review. *J Crit Care* 2020; 59:1–5.

43. Lu Y, et al. Promoting sleep and circadian health may prevent postoperative delirium: A systematic review and meta-analysis of randomized clinical trials. *Sleep Med Rev* 2019; 48:101207.

44. Salvi F, et al. Non-pharmacological approaches in the prevention of delirium. *Eur Geriatr Med* 2020; 11:71–81.

45. Fricchione GL, et al. Postoperative delirium. *Am J Psychiatry* 2008; 165:803–812.

46. Zayed Y, et al. Haloperidol for the management of delirium in adult intensive care unit patients: A systematic review and meta-analysis of randomized controlled trials. *J Crit Care* 2019; 50:280–286.

47. Burry L, et al. Antipsychotics for treatment of delirium in hospitalised non-ICU patients. *Cochrane Database Syst Rev* 2018; 6:Cd005594.

48. Schrijver EJ, et al. Low dose oral haloperidol does not prolong QTc interval in older acutely hospitalised adults: a subanalysis of a randomised double-blind placebo-controlled study. *J Geriatr Cardiol* 2018; 15:401–407.

49. Boettger S, et al. Atypical antipsychotics in the management of delirium: a review of the empirical literature. *Palliat Support Care* 2005; 3:227–237.

50. Leentjens AF, et al. Delirium in elderly people: an update. *Curr Opin Psychiatry* 2005; 18:325–330.

51. Boettger S, et al. Aripiprazole and haloperidol in the treatment of delirium. *Aust NZJ Psychiatry* 2011; 45:477–482.

52. Martinotti G, et al. Psychomotor agitation and hyperactive delirium in COVID-19 patients treated with aripiprazole 9.75mg/1.3 ml immediate release. *Psychopharmacology (Berl)* 2020:1–5.

53. Skrobik YK, et al. Olanzapine vs haloperidol: treating delirium in a critical care setting. *Intensive Care Med* 2004; 30:444–449.

54. Sipahimalani A, et al. Olanzapine in the treatment of delirium. *Psychosomatics* 1998; 39:422–430.

55. Duff G Atypical antipsychotic drugs and stroke – Committee on safety of medicines 2004; https://webarchive.nationalarchives.gov.uk/20141206131857/http://www.mhra.gov.uk/home/groups/pl-p/documents/websiteresources/con019488.pdf.

56. Kim SW, et al. Risperidone versus olanzapine for the treatment of delirium. *Hum Psychopharmacol* 2010; 25:298–302.

57. Grover S, et al. Comparative efficacy study of haloperidol, olanzapine and risperidone in delirium. *J Psychosom Res* 2011; 71:277–281.

58. Yoon HJ, et al. Efficacy and safety of haloperidol versus atypical antipsychotic medications in the treatment of delirium. *BMC Psychiatry* 2013; 13:240.

59. Lorenzo MP, et al. Intravenous olanzapine in a critically ill patient: an evolving route of administration. *Hosp Pharm* 2020; 55:108–111.

60. Bourgeois JA, et al. Prolonged delirium managed with risperidone. *Psychosomatics* 2005; 46:90–91.

61. Gupta N, et al. Effectiveness of risperidone in delirium. *Can J Psychiatry* 2005; 50:75.

62. Liu CY, et al. Efficacy of risperidone in treating the hyperactive symptoms of delirium. *Int Clin Psychopharmacol* 2004; 19:165–168.

63. Horikawa N, et al. Treatment for delirium with risperidone: results of a prospective open trial with 10 patients. *Gen Hosp Psychiatry* 2003; 25:289–292.

64. Han CS, et al. A double-blind trial of risperidone and haloperidol for the treatment of delirium. *Psychosomatics* 2004; 45:297–301.

65. Hakim SM, et al. Early treatment with risperidone for subsyndromal delirium after on-pump cardiac surgery in the elderly: a randomized trial. *Anesthesiology* 2012; 116:987–997.

66. Torres R, et al. Use of quetiapine in delirium: case reports. *Psychosomatics* 2001; 42:347–349.

67. Sasaki Y, et al. A prospective, open-label, flexible-dose study of quetiapine in the treatment of delirium. *J Clin Psychiatry* 2003; 64:1316–1321.

68. Devlin JW, et al. Efficacy and safety of quetiapine in critically ill patients with delirium: a prospective, multicenter, randomized, double-blind, placebo-controlled pilot study. *Crit Care Med* 2010; 38:419–427.

69. Hawkins SB, et al. Quetiapine for the treatment of delirium. *J Hosp Med* 2013; 8:215–220.

70. Tahir TA, et al. A randomized controlled trial of quetiapine versus placebo in the treatment of delirium. *J Psychosom Res* 2010; 69:485–490.

71. Grover S, et al. Comparative effectiveness of quetiapine and haloperidol in delirium: A single blind randomized controlled study. *World J Psychiatry* 2016; 6:365–371.

72. Mangan KC, et al. Evaluating the risk profile of quetiapine in treating delirium in the intensive care adult population: A retrospective review. *J Crit Care* 2018; 47:169–172.

73. Young CC, et al. Intravenous ziprasidone for treatment of delirium in the intensive care unit. *Anesthesiology* 2004; 101:794–795.

74. Chan D, et al. Delirium: making the diagnosis, improving the prognosis. *Geriatrics* 1999; 54:28–42.

75. Sampson EL, et al. A randomized, double-blind, placebo-controlled trial of donepezil hydrochloride (Aricept) for reducing the incidence of postoperative delirium after elective total hip replacement. *Int J Geriatr Psychiatry* 2007; 22:343–349.

76. Dautzenberg PL, et al. Adding rivastigmine to antipsychotics in the treatment of a chronic delirium. *Age Ageing* 2004; 33:516–517.

77. van Eijk MM, et al. Effect of rivastigmine as an adjunct to usual care with haloperidol on duration of delirium and mortality in critically ill patients: a multicentre, double-blind, placebo-controlled randomised trial. *Lancet* 2010; 376:1829–1837.

78. Yu A, et al. Cholinesterase inhibitors for the treatment of delirium in non-ICU settings. *Cochrane Database Syst Rev* 2018; 6:Cd012494.

79. Sher Y, et al. Adjunctive valproic acid in management-refractory hyperactive delirium: a case series and rationale. *J Neuropsychiatry Clin Neurosci* 2015; 27:365–370.

80. Gagnon DJ, et al. Valproate for agitation in critically ill patients: a retrospective study. *J Crit Care* 2017; 37:119–125.

81. Crowley KE, et al. Valproic acid for the management of agitation and delirium in the intensive care setting: a retrospective analysis. *Clin Ther* 2020; 42:e65–e73.

82. Quinn NJ, et al. Prescribing practices of valproic acid for agitation and delirium in the intensive care unit. *Ann Pharmacother* 2021;55:311–317

Drug treatment of psychiatric symptoms occurring in the context of other disorders

General principles of prescribing in HIV

People living with HIV (PLWH) may experience symptoms of mental illness due to a variety of factors (see Box 10.1). In practice, several of these factors may coexist within an individual.

Box 10.1 Factors contributing to the development of psychiatric symptoms in people living with HIV[1]

- Primary (or pre-existing) psychiatric disorders
- Neurobiological changes caused by HIV in the central nervous system (CNS)
- Other infections or CNS tumours
- Antiretroviral drugs and other medical treatments (see Drugs for HIV'in this section)
- Alcohol or substance misuse
- Adverse psychosocial factors (e.g. stigma)
- Awareness of a chronic disease requiring strict adherence to medication

---

When prescribing psychotropics, the following principles should be adhered to:

- Start with a low dose and titrate according to tolerability and response.
- Select the simplest dosing regimen possible. (Remember that the patient's drug regimen is likely to be complex already.)
- Select an agent with the fewest side effects. Drug interactions, medical comorbidities and any ongoing substance misuse must be considered.
- Ensure that management is conducted in close cooperation with the HIV specialists and the rest of the multidisciplinary team.

The Maudsley® Prescribing Guidelines in Psychiatry, Fourteenth Edition. David M. Taylor,
Thomas R. E. Barnes and Allan H. Young.
© 2021 David M. Taylor. Published 2021 by John Wiley & Sons Ltd.

Although most psychotropic agents are thought to be safe in PLWH, definitive data are lacking in many cases, and this group may be more sensitive to higher doses, side effects and interactions.[2] Patients with advanced HIV disease are more likely to suffer exaggerated adverse reactions to psychotropic medication.

Schizophrenia

In general, there is no difference between the pharmacological treatment of schizophrenia in PLWH and the treatment of an uninfected person,[3] but some specific considerations should be kept in mind. PLWH are more susceptible to extrapyramidal side effects (EPSEs)[2] due to HIV invasion into basal ganglia, particularly during advanced illness. Hence, second-generation antipsychotics (SGAs), such as quetiapine, risperidone and aripiprazole have been suggested as first-line choices for the treatment of psychosis unrelated to dementia or delirium.[4] The possible additive metabolic effects of antipsychotics and antiretrovirals require close monitoring. QT interval prolongation can be a complication of HIV progression, co-morbidities, antiretrovirals, as well as antipsychotics.[5] Drug interactions are discussed further in this section.

There are limited published reports of clozapine use for treatment-resistant schizophrenia in PLWH.[6-8] Clozapine can be used in people with refractory schizophrenia and HIV with the aim of achieving control of the viral load. A multidisciplinary approach is required in such cases.[6,8]

However, close monitoring of the white cell count is required since, clozapine, certain antiretroviral therapy (ART), and the HIV virus itself can all have suppressive effects on the bone marrow.[6,8] Clozapine may also be helpful in the treatment of individuals with HIV-associated psychosis with drug-induced parkinsonism.[9]

Delirium

Organic causes should be identified and treated. Short-term symptomatic treatment may include low-dose SGAs (e.g. risperidone[4]). There have been few RCTs in delirious patients with AIDS; earlier studies document the efficacy of typical antipsychotics,[10] and low-dose haloperidol was the agent of choice in one consensus study.[4] However, first-generation antipsychotic (FGAs) should be used cautiously given the increased susceptibility to EPSEs in this patient group.[10] Benzodiazepines should be used cautiously as they may worsen delirium (except when alcohol or benzodiazepine withdrawal is the precipitating factor).[10]

Depression

Depression in PLWH is common, with an estimated prevalence of 20–40%.[11] It may be a consequence of HIV infection or a pre-existing disorder. Studies suggest that depression comorbid with HIV is associated with poor adherence to ART and reduced viral suppression.[12] Antidepressants are more effective than placebo in the treatment of depression in PLWH[12] and may improve adherence to ART,[13] but there is a gap in research comparing antidepressant types in this patient group. Selective serotonin reuptake inhibitors (SSRIs) are preferable as first-line agents. Escitalopram/

citalopram[4,14] have lower risk of pharmacokinetic interactions. Further treatment follows standard protocols for depression. A study of escitalopram found no difference from placebo[15] possibly due to a large placebo response. ECG monitoring is recommended when citalopram/escitalopram is co-administered with ARVs that prolong the QT interval.[5,11] Mirtazapine is effective,[16,17] with relatively low risk of drug interactions,[18] and may be beneficial in coexisting HIV wasting and depression[19] or in reducing methamphetamine use among active users.[20] 'Dual action' antidepressants (duloxetine, venlafaxine) were are equally effective to SSRIs for depressive symptoms in PLWH.[21] Other agents (bupropion,[22] trazodone) are effective but their utility is limited by drug interactions and side effects.

The side-effect burden of TCAs may limit efficacy and compliance, although their use may be appropriate at times. Constipation and dry mouth are frequently reported in PLWH on TCAs.[12] MAOIs are not recommended in PLWH.

Interferon-alpha-induced depression in HIV/HCV co-infected patients

Citalopram has been shown to be an effective and well-tolerated treatment for emergent depression;[23] however, prophylactic use of citalopram (i.e. before depression emerges) cannot be recommended.[24]

Bipolar affective disorder

Mania in PLWH can be primary (pre-existing bipolar affective disorder) or secondary ('HIV mania' associated with late-stage HIV infection). PLWH may be more sensitive to the side effects of mood stabilisers such as neurotoxicity with lithium,[25] especially if they have neurocognitive dysfunction.[25,26] Lithium is renally excreted, and so CYP450 interactions are unlikely. However, it can be problematic in renal impairment, often seen in PLWH. Lithium and tenofovir disoproxil fumarate (TDF) co-therapy was investigated in a randomised placebo controlled trial as both are associated with renal tubular toxicity. The incidence of nephrotoxicity was not increased during the 24 weeks of the trial, but we cannot rule out the risk over long term.[27] Lithium may be used cautiously in PLWH for primary bipolar disorder with close monitoring, but avoided in advanced HIV disease.[28] Carbamazepine should be avoided because of significant drug interactions with and the risk of blood dyscrasias.[28] Valproate can be an alternative in PLWH for bipolar disorder. Monitoring is required due to its risk of hepatotoxicity, blood dyscrasias, pancreatitis and drug interactions. Valproate use is best avoided with other hepatotoxic drugs (e.g. nevirapine, rifampicin).[28] Mood-stabilising antipsychotics such as risperidone, quetiapine and olanzapine are also an option.[4]

Secondary mania ('HIV mania')

Reports of secondary mania, typically occurring in advanced illness in the context of HIV-associated neurocognitive disorders or CNS opportunistic infections,[29] have declined with the widespread use of effective antiretrovirals. The first aim is to identify and treat the potential underlying cause (infections, substance misuse, alcohol withdrawal and metabolic abnormalities). Secondary mania may respond to atypical antipsychotics, quetiapine, olanzapine and aripiprazole (as there is lower risk of EPSEs). A case report describes successful treatment of 'HIV mania' with ziprasidone.[30]

Anxiety disorders

Anxiety disorders are highly prevalent in PLWH. Generalised anxiety, panic disorders and PTSD are commonly reported. SSRIs are first-line options for anxiety and panic disorders treatment in standard guidelines, as well as in PLWH[3] (see 'Depression' in this section for preferred options). Benzodiazepines may have some utility in the acute treatment of anxiety but require caution because of the potential of misuse, possible drug interactions and increased risk of neurocognitive impairment in PLWH.[31]

Lorazepam, oxazepam and temazepam are metabolised by non-CYP450 pathways, hence have lower risk of interactions and may be preferred options for PLWH.[32] Buspirone may also be useful.[33]

HIV-associated neurocognitive disorders

In the current era of effective antiretrovirals, the incidence of severe HIV-associated cerebral disease has declined dramatically; however, more subtle forms of HIV-associated neurocognitive disorders (HAND) remain prevalent.[34,35] Risk factors include comorbidities (e.g. HCV coinfection), HIV infection itself and patient genetic factors. HAND encompasses three sub-disorders, ranging from more common, asymptomatic neurocognitive impairment (ANI), to more severe less common, HIV-associated dementia (HAD) disorders. Screening for cognitive impairment is recommended in PLWH.[11] CogState or the HIV dementia scale have been used though may not identify ANI.[35]

Symptoms include apathy, irritability, inertia, lack of spontaneity, social withdrawal, psychomotor slowing, complaints of diminished attention and concentration, emotional lability, and occasionally, 'HIV mania'.[29]

The main treatment is antiretroviral therapy with high CNS penetration effectiveness (CPE) aiming at reaching good levels in the CNS with minimal drug-related neurotoxicity. Further adjunctive treatments have been studied (minocycline, memantine, selegiline, lithium, valproate, lexipafant, nimodipine, psychostimulants, natalizumab interferons, etc.).[36]

In a recent study paroxetine was associated with neurocognitive improvements (after adjusting for depression),[37] while a trial of rivastigmine patch was negative. Further studies are needed to confirm the effects of these adjunctive treatments for HAND.

Interactions between antiretroviral drugs and psychotropics

Pharmacokinetic interactions between antiretroviral drugs and psychotropics occur frequently and can be clinically significant. Potential interactions should be checked for all patients receiving antiretrovirals and psychotropics concomitantly. Drug history for checking drug interactions should include current prescribed medication, alternative/herbal treatments, recreational drugs and other non-prescribed medicines.[34]

Readers are directed to regularly updated online resources for information about individual pharmacokinetic interactions:

- www.hiv-druginteractions.org (also available as an App)
- www.hivinsite.ucsf.edu

Pharmacodynamic interactions may also occur, usually through overlapping adverse effects.

Potential pharmacodynamic interactions are shown in Table 10.1.

Table 10.1 Potential pharmacodynamic interactions with antiretrovirals.[38]

Potential adverse effect	Implicated antiretroviral drug(s) [32,39,40]	Implications for psychotropic prescribing
Bone marrow suppression	Zidovudine (anaemia, neutropenia)	Concurrent use with certain psychotropics (e.g. clozapine) may increase the risk of myelosuppression/ neutropenia
Bone mineral density reduction	Tenofovir disoproxil fumarate (Tenofovir alafenamide has smaller effect on BMD)	May compound the reductions in bone mineral density possible with prolactin elevating antipsychotics
Creatine kinase (CK) elevations	Dolutegravir, emtricitabine, raltegravir	May be important to acknowledge associated link if diagnosis of NMS is being considered
ECG changes	Atazanavir, darunavir, efavirenz, lopinavir, rilpivirine, ritonavir, saquinavir	May increase risk of arrhythmias associated with certain psychotropic drugs
Cardiovascular effects	Abacavir, darunavir/ritonavir, lopinavir/ ritonavir	Cardiovascular events (e.g. MI) occurred in some cohorts
Renal effects	Tenofovir disoproxil fumarate (if regime includes ritonavir, risk is increased)	Proteinuria, hypophosphatemia, glycosuria, hypokalaemia, renal tubular
Gastrointestinal disturbances	Atazanavir, darunavir, dolutegravir, didanosine, elvitegravir/cobicistat, fosamprenavir, indinavir, lopinavir, nelfinavir, raltegravir, saquinavir, tipranavir, zidovudine	May compound gastrointestinal disturbances associated with certain psychotropics (e.g. SSRIs)
Seizure(s)	Darunavir, efavirenz, maraviroc, ritonavir, saquinavir, zidovudine	May increase seizure risk associated with certain psychotropic drugs
Metabolic abnormalities such as hypertriglyceridaemia, hypercholesterolaemia, insulin resistance, hyperglycaemia and hyperlactataemia	All combination antiretroviral therapy	May compound risk of metabolic adverse effects associated with certain psychotropic drugs (particularly SGAs)

Adverse psychiatric effects of antiretroviral drugs

Psychiatric adverse events have been reported with many antiretroviral drugs, but a causal relationship remains uncertain. Efavirenz has been most commonly implicated, and HIV guidelines suggest avoiding its use in patients with psychiatric illness.[32,34,39]

Table 10.2 summarises the most important psychiatric adverse effects of antiretroviral drugs. Note that this is not an exhaustive list; readers are directed to the SPCs/product labelling for other possible adverse effects. The differential diagnosis of psychiatric side effects is covered elsewhere in the *Guidelines*. Monitoring of people on medicines with psychiatric side effects would be recommended.

Table 10.2 Summary of psychiatric adverse drug reactions (ADRs) with antiretroviral drugs.[32,39-41]

Drug	Adverse psychiatric effects/comment
Nucleoside reverse transcriptase inhibitors	
Abacavir	Depression, anxiety, nightmares, labile mood, mania, psychosis. Very few cases reported; in all reported cases, the patient rapidly returned to baseline after discontinuing drug
Didanosine	Lethargy, nervousness, anxiety, confusion, sleep disturbance, mood disorders, psychosis, mania. Very rare
Emtricitabine	Confusion, irritability, insomnia
Zidovudine	Sleep disturbance, vivid dreams, agitation, mania, depression, psychosis, delirium. Psychiatric ADRs are usually dose-related. The onset varies widely, from <24 hours to 7 months
Non-nucleoside reverse transcriptase inhibitors	
Efavirenz	Somnolence, insomnia, abnormal dreams, impaired concentration, depression, psychosis, and suicidal ideation. Symptoms usually subside or diminish after 2 to 4 weeks. However, subtler, long-term neuropsychiatric effects may occur. Can exacerbate psychiatric symptoms; avoid in patients with a history of psychiatric illness
Etravirine	Sleep disturbance
Nevirapine	Visual hallucinations, persecutory delusions, mood changes, nightmares and vivid dreams, depression. A small handful of cases have been reported. Onset of symptoms was within the first couple of weeks. Symptoms all resolved on discontinuation of nevirapine
Rilpivirine	Depression, suicidality, sleep disturbances. A similar adverse effect profile to efavirenz but a lower incidence of each event. May exacerbate psychiatric symptoms; consider avoiding in patients with a history of psychiatric illness
Integrase strand transfer inhibitors	
Dolutegravir, elvitegravir and raltegravir	Depression and suicidal ideation (symptoms infrequently exacerbated in patients with pre-existing psychiatric conditions)
CCR5 Antagonist	
Maraviroc	Depression, insomnia

References

1. Nanni MG, et al. Depression in HIV infected patients: a review. *Curr Psychiatry Rep* 2015; 17:530.

2. Hill L, et al. Pharmacotherapy considerations in patients with HIV and psychiatric disorders: focus on antidepressants and antipsychotics. *Ann Pharmacother* 2013; 47:75–89.

3. Cohen M, et al. *Comprehensive textbook of AIDS psychiatry: a paradigm for integrated care.* Oxford University Press, Oxford, England; 2017.

4. Freudenreich O, et al. Psychiatric treatment of persons with HIV/AIDS: an HIV-Psychiatry Consensus Survey of Current Practices. *Psychosomatics* 2010; 51:480–488.

5. Liu J, et al. QT prolongation in HIV-positive patients: review article. *Indian Heart J* 2019; 71:434–439.

6. Nejad SH, et al. Clozapine use in HIV-infected schizophrenia patients: a case-based discussion and review. *Psychosomatics* 2009; 50:626–632.

7. Sanz-Cortés S, et al. A case report of schizophrenia and HIV: HAART in association with clozapine. *J Psychiatric Intensive Care* 2009; 5:47–49.

8. Whiskey E, et al. Clozapine, HIV and neutropenia: a case report. *Ther Adv Psychopharmacol* 2018; 8:365–369.

9. Lera G, et al. Pilot study with clozapine in patients with HIV-associated psychosis and drug-induced parkinsonism. *Mov Disord* 1999; 14:128–131.

10. Watkins CC, et al. Cognitive impairment in patients with AIDS - prevalence and severity. *HIV/AIDS (Auckland, NZ)* 2015; 7:35–47.

11. European AIDS Clinical Society. Guidelines Version 10.1 October 2020. 2020; http://www.eacsociety.org/files/guidelines_10.1-english.pdf.

12. Eshun-Wilson I, et al. Antidepressants for depression in adults with HIV infection. *Cochrane Database System Rev* 2018; 1:Cd008525.

13. Gokhale RH, et al. Depression prevalence, antidepressant treatment status, and association with sustained HIV viral suppression among adults living with HIV in care in the United States, 2009-2014. *AIDS Behav* 2019; 23:3452–3459.

14. Currier MB, et al. Citalopram treatment of major depressive disorder in hispanic HIV and AIDS patients: a prospective study. *Psychosomatics* 2004; 45:210–216.

15. Hoare J, et al. Escitalopram treatment of depression in human immunodeficiency virus/acquired immunodeficiency syndrome: a randomized, double-blind, placebo-controlled study. *J Nerv Ment Dis* 2014; 202:133–137.

16. Patel S, et al. Escitalopram and mirtazapine for the treatment of depression in HIV patients: a randomized controlled open label trial. *ASEAN J Psychiatry* 2012; 14.

17. Elliott AJ, et al. Mirtazapine for depression in patients with human immunodeficiency virus. *J Clin Psychopharmacol* 2000; 20:265–267.

18. Adams JL, et al. Treating depression within the HIV 'medical home': a guided algorithm for antidepressant management by HIV clinicians. *AIDS Patient Care STDS* 2012; 26:647–654.

19. Badowski M, et al. Pharmacologic management of human immunodeficiency virus wasting syndrome. *Pharmacotherapy* 2014; 34:868–881.

20. Coffin PO, et al. Effects of mirtazapine for methamphetamine use disorder among cisgender men and transgender women who have sex with men: a placebo-controlled randomized clinical trial. *JAMA Psychiatry* 2020; 77:246–255.

21. Mills JC, et al. Comparative effectiveness of dual-action versus single-action antidepressants for the treatment of depression in people living with HIV/AIDS. *J Affect Disord* 2017; 215:179–186.

22. Currier MB, et al. A prospective trial of sustained-release bupropion for depression in HIV-seropositive and AIDS patients. *Psychosomatics* 2003; 44:120–125.

23. Laguno M, et al. Depressive symptoms after initiation of interferon therapy in human immunodeficiency virus-infected patients with chronic hepatitis C. *Antivir Ther* 2004; 9:905–909.

24. Klein MB, et al. Citalopram for the prevention of depression and its consequences in HIV-hepatitis C coinfected individuals initiating pegylated interferon/ribavirin therapy: a multicenter randomized double-blind placebocontrolled trial. *HIV Clin Trials* 2014; 15:161–175.

25. Ferrando SJ. Psychopharmacologic treatment of patients with HIV/AIDS. *Current psychiatry reports* 2009; 11:235–242.

26. El-Mallakh RS. Mania in AIDS: clinical significance and theoretical considerations. *Int J Psychiatry Med* 1991; 21:383–391.

27. Decloedt EH, et al. Renal safety of lithium in HIV-infected patients established on tenofovir disoproxil fumarate containing antiretroviral therapy: analysis from a randomized placebo-controlled trial. *AIDS Res Ther* 2017; 14:6.

28. Gallego L, et al. Psychopharmacological treatments in HIV patients under antiretroviral therapy. *AIDS Rev* 2012; 14:101–111.

29. Singer EJ, et al. Neurobehavioral Manifestations of Human Immunodeficiency Virus/AIDS: Diagnosis and Treatment. *Neurol Clin* 2016; 34:33–53.

30. Spiegel DR, et al. The successful treatment of mania due to acquired immunodeficiency syndrome using ziprasidone: a case series. *J Neuropsychiatry Clin Neurosci* 2010; 22:111–114.

31. Saloner R, et al. Benzodiazepine use is associated with an increased risk of neurocognitive impairment in people living with HIV. *J Acquir Immune Defic Syndr* 2019; 82:475–482.

32. Panel on Antiretroviral Guidelines for Adults and Adolescents. Guidelines for the use of antiretroviral agents in adults and adolescents living with HIV. Department of Health and Human Services. 2017; https://aidsinfo.nih.gov/contentfiles/lvguidelines/AdultandAdolescentGL.pdf.

33. Brogan K, et al. Management of common psychiatric conditions in the HIV-positive population. *Curr HIV/AIDS Rep* 2009; 6:108–115.

34. Waters L, et al. British HIV Association guidelines for the treatment of HIV-1-positive adults with antiretroviral therapy 2015 (2016 interim update). 2016; http://www.bhiva.org/documents/Guidelines/Treatment/2016/treatment-guidelines-2016-interim-update.pdf.

35. Carroll A, et al. HIV-associated neurocognitive disorders: recent advances in pathogenesis, biomarkers, and treatment. *F1000Res* 2017; 6:312.

36. Ambrosius B, et al. Antineuroinflammatory drugs in HIV-associated neurocognitive disorders as potential therapy. *Neurol Neuroimmunol Neuroinflamm* 2019; 6:e551.

37. Sacktor N, et al. Paroxetine and fluconazole therapy for HIV-associated neurocognitive impairment: results from a double-blind, placebo-controlled trial. *J Neurovirol* 2018; 24:16–27.

38. Panel on Antiretroviral Guidelines for Adults and Adolescents. Guidelines for the Use of Antiretroviral Agents in Adults and Adolescents Living with HIV. Department of Health and Human Services. 2019; https://clinicalinfo.hiv.gov/en.

39. European AIDS Clinical Society. Guidelines Version 9.0 October 2017. http://www.eacsociety.org/files/guidelines_9.0-english.pdf.

40. World Health Organisation. Consolidated guidelines on the use of antiretroviral drugs for treating and preventing HIV infection. Recommendations for a public health approach - Second edition. 2016; http://www.who.int/hiv/pub/arv/arv-2016/en/.

41. Parker C. Psychiatric effects of drugs for other disorders. *Medicine* 2016; 44:768–774.

CHAPTER 10

Epilepsy

Psychiatric comorbidities in epilepsy

People with epilepsy (PWE) have an elevated prevalence of several psychiatric disorders including depression (22.9%), anxiety (20.2%) and psychosis (5.2%).[1,2] Suicide is five-fold higher in PWE compared to the general population[3] and is an important cause of premature mortality.[4] The link between epilepsy and mental illness is bidirectional as patients with depression, anxiety and psychosis have an increased risk of developing new-onset epilepsy.[5,6] Suicide attempts are also associated with the development of epilepsy.[3] This bidirectional relationship might be explained by a common underlying pathology between mental illness and epilepsy. Disturbances in neurotransmission, neuro-inflammation and the HPA axis have all been suggested[7] to be the shared pathology.

Interictal psychiatric disorders (with symptoms occurring independently of seizures) are likely to require treatment with psychotropics.[8–10] When prescribing psychotropics to people with epilepsy, the following general principles[11,12] should be adhered to:

- First, rule out other possible causes of psychiatric symptoms (both peri-ictal and iatrogenic, see Table 10.3).
- Optimise the treatment of epilepsy (ideally before prescribing psychotropics).
- Consider using psychotropics with known antiseizure properties (e.g. antiseizure medications in bipolar disorder).
- Check for interactions with antiseizure medications.
- Start with a low dose and titrate according to tolerability and response (proconvulsive effects are dose-related).
- If seizures do occur, consider changing the psychotropic drug or optimising the antiseizure medication.

Table 10.3 Possible causes of psychiatric symptoms in PWE and their management[5]

Cause of symptoms	Description	Management
Interictal psychiatric disorders	- Symptoms occurring independently of seizures - Although common in PWE, other causes and relatedness to seizures should be ruled out first	- Likely to require treatment with psychotropics - See Table 10.5 for more information about the use of specific psychotropics in PWE
Peri-ictal symptoms	- PWE may experience psychiatric symptoms that are temporally related to seizures	- All peri-ictal psychiatric symptoms (pre-ictal, postictal and ictal) are initially treated by optimising antiseizure medications[11] - Peri-ictal depressive symptoms do not appear to respond to treatment with antidepressants[13,14]
Pre-ictal symptoms	- Typically presents as a dysphoric mood preceding a seizure by a period of 30 minutes to hours to 2 or 3 days	

(Continued)

CHAPTER 10

Table 10.3 *(Continued)*

Cause of symptoms	Description	Management
Post-ictal symptoms	▪ Typically presents between several hours to 7 days following a seizure (depression, anxiety, suicidal ideation and psychosis reported) ▪ PWE and interictal psychiatric disorders may experience worsening of symptoms previously in remission (breakthrough symptoms)	▪ Postictal psychosis can remit spontaneously or respond to treatment with low doses of antipsychotics.[15] Short-term symptomatic treatment with a benzodiazepine or antipsychotic is recommended for up to 3 months[16] Taper off carefully after symptom resolution[14]
Ictal symptoms	▪ May present as ictal fear/panic (most commonly), depressive symptoms, or rarely, psychosis	▪ There is no evidence that psychotropics can prevent ictal symptoms[17]
Para-ictal episodes **'forced normalisation'** *(psychiatric symptoms emerging as a result of a reduction in seizure frequency)*	▪ Psychotic or, less commonly, severe affective symptoms following seizure remission in PWE ▪ Rapid medication titration schedules, rapid seizure control, previously medication-resistant epilepsy, and temporal lobe epilepsy may be risk factors[15]	▪ A decision should be made on how to proceed with antiseizure medications and psychotropics through a process of shared decision-making with carers.[14] Symptomatic treatment with antipsychotics or antidepressants may be indicated
Iatrogenic psychiatric symptoms	▪ Changes in treatments for seizures could result in psychiatric symptoms as a result of: ▪ Starting antiseizure medications with known negative psychotropic properties (particularly in those with a psychiatric history) ▪ Stopping antiseizure medications with beneficial psychotropic properties (e.g. mood stabilisation) ▪ Starting antiseizure medications with enzyme-inducing properties in people stable on psychotropics ▪ Surgery for epilepsy: de novo postsurgical episodes of depression, anxiety and, rarely, psychosis have been reported. Exacerbation of pre-existing conditions more common.	▪ Symptoms are managed by resolving the underlying cause in the first instance ▪ Consider switching antiseizure medications with known negative psychotropic properties to better tolerated antiseizure medications (see Table 10.4) ▪ Antiseizure medications can lower folate levels which may affect mood. Folate levels should be checked and low levels remedied if necessary ▪ If changing antiseizure medications is not suitable, antidepressants can be considered for iatrogenic depressive symptoms[18] ▪ Postsurgical neuropsychiatric symptoms may be treated successfully with psychotropics[17]

Psychiatric side effects of antiseizure medications

Virtually all antiseizure medications are known to have psychotropic effects. These effects can be both helpful and unhelpful. The adverse and beneficial psychiatric side effects of antiseizure medications are summarised in Table 10.4. Readers are directed to the 'Summary of psychiatric side-effects of non-psychotropics' elsewhere in *The Guidelines* for a more detailed summary of psychiatric symptoms associated with antiseizure medications, and for further information about determining causality in any given patient.

Table 10.4 Adverse and beneficial psychiatric side effects of antiseizure medications[5,19,20]

Antiseizure medications	Adverse psychiatric symptoms	Psychiatric benefits
Barbiturates, primidone Benzodiazepines	▪ Behavioural disturbance/ADHD symptoms ▪ Depression, cognitive impairment	▪ Anxiolytic
Carbamazepine, oxcarbazepine	▪ Not reported	▪ Mood stabilising, anti-manic
Ethosuximide	▪ Behavioural disturbance, depression, psychosis	▪ None reported
Felbamate	▪ Anxiety, depression, psychosis	▪ None reported
Gabapentin, pregabalin	▪ Depression and anxiety on cessation	▪ Anxiolytic
Lacosamide	▪ None reported	▪ None reported
Lamotrigine	▪ Anxiogenic in some ▪ Behavioural disturbance in cognitive impairment	▪ Antidepressant ▪ Mood stabilising
Levetiracetam	▪ Anxiety, behavioural disturbance, depression	▪ None confirmed
Perampanel	▪ Behavioural disturbance, depression, psychosis	▪ None reported
Phenytoin	▪ Behavioural disturbance, depression	▪ Anti-manic
Tiagabine	▪ Behavioural disturbance, depression	▪ Anxiolytic
Topiramate	▪ Anxiety, behavioural disturbance, depression	▪ Unclear; possible anti-manic/antipsychotic
Valproate	▪ Behavioural disturbance (at high doses in children)	▪ Mood stabilising, anti-manic ▪ Anti-panic
Vigabatrin	▪ Behavioural disturbance/ADHD symptoms ▪ Depression, psychosis	▪ None reported
Zonisamide	▪ Behavioural disturbance, depression	▪ None confirmed

Interactions[21]

Pharmacokinetic interactions

Important pharmacokinetic interactions exist in both directions between antiseizure medications and psychotropics, primarily mediated through cytochrome P450 enzymes.[8,22] Psychotropics with enzyme-inhibiting effects (e.g. fluoxetine, fluvoxamine, paroxetine, and at higher doses, sertraline) may increase antiseizure medication plasma levels. This is especially relevant to antiseizure medications with a narrow therapeutic index (e.g. carbamazepine and phenytoin). Plasma levels should be monitored, and dosage adjustment may be required. Citalopram and escitalopram are very weak inhibitors of CYP 1A2 and 2D6.

Some antiseizure medications are potent enzyme inducers (e.g. phenytoin, carbamazepine, phenobarbital, primidone) and others are weak inducers (e.g. oxcarbazepine at doses ≥900mg/day, topiramate at doses ≥400mg/day). These drugs can lower plasma levels of multiple psychotropics, possibly leading to treatment failure.

Pharmacodynamic interactions[13]

Adverse effects with antiseizure medications that may overlap with psychotropic adverse effects include:

- Weight gain: Caused by some antiseizure medications (e.g. carbamazepine, gabapentin, pregabalin, valproate)
- Sexual adverse effects: With phenobarbital and primidone but possible with all enzyme-inducing antiseizure medications
- Hyponatraemia: With carbamazepine, oxcarbazepine (note, if severe, it can provoke seizures)
- Osteoporosis and osteopenia: Reported with long-term use of enzyme-inducing antiseizure medications
- Blood dyscrasias: Reported with valproate carbamazepine and especially with felbamate[10]

Psychotropics and the risk of seizures in people with epilepsy

In the general population, the annual incidence of unprovoked seizures is about 50 per 100,000 persons.[23] It is notable that the incidence of unprovoked seizures in the placebo arms of randomised controlled trials of antidepressants and antipsychotics is approximately 15-fold higher, suggesting that both depression and psychosis are risk factors for seizures.[24] A bidirectional relationship between epilepsy and several psychiatric illnesses has been demonstrated, whereby not only do PWE have a higher risk of developing a psychiatric illness, but people with psychiatric illness have a higher risk of developing epilepsy.[5,6] This bidirectional relationship exists for depression, anxiety, psychosis and suicidality.[3,5,6] Thus, the occurrence of seizures may, in some cases, be the expression of the natural progression of a psychiatric illness, unrelated to the use of psychotropics.

Reports of seizures associated with psychotropics must factor in this bidirectional relationship between psychiatric illness and epilepsy. For example, although observational studies have reported an association between antidepressant treatment and seizures,[25] a similar association is also found with non-drug treatments for depression (counselling, for example).[26] These findings are consistent with depression itself being the main risk factor for seizures. In fact, one analysis of controlled studies with psychotropics showed that the incidence of seizures was substantially lower among patients receiving most antidepressants (SSRIs, for example) in comparison with those randomised to placebo.[24] Nonetheless, definitive data are lacking in PWE[27,28] and certain psychotropics have a dose-related risk of seizures within usual dose ranges. Most can cause seizures in overdose. Note also that almost all antidepressants and antipsychotics have been associated with hyponatraemia (see section on hyponatraemia) and seizures may occur if this is severe.[17,29] General guidance on the safety of psychotropics in PWE is summarised in Table 10.5.

Electroconvulsive therapy (ECT) has anticonvulsive properties and is worth considering in the treatment of depression in patients with unstable epilepsy.[8,17,22] ECT does not appear to cause or worsen epilepsy.[17,30]

Table 10.5 Psychotropics in epilepsy

Safety in epilepsy	Drug	Comments
Antidepressants		
Low risk – good choices	SSRIs	Recommended in PWE.[14,18] SSRIs may be anticonvulsant at therapeutic doses[13] but pro-convulsant in overdose.[31] SSRIs with the lowest risk of interactions with antiseizure medications are generally preferred (citalopram/ escitalopram, followed by sertraline).[14,18,32,33] Escitalopram is preferred over citalopram in PWE (lower risk of seizures in overdose).[34] Others have low risk of seizures (e.g. fluoxetine[34]) but drug interactions with antiseizure medications should be considered.[14,18] Fluoxetine may be less likely to provoke seizures in older people than escitalopram or citalopram.[35] Some evidence that sertraline is safe and effective in PWE[36]
	Mirtazapine	Recommended in PWE.[18,37] Not known to be proconvulsive[24]
	Duloxetine	Recommended for PWE.[11,18] Risk of seizures is probably negligible[34,35]
Probably low risk – use with caution (limited evidence)	Agomelatine	Not known to be proconvulsive.[38] Anticonvulsant in animal models[34]
	MAOIs	Not known to be pro-convulsive at therapeutic doses.[34] Low risk of seizures in overdose[17]
	Moclobemide	Not known to be proconvulsive.[34] Anticonvulsant in animal models[34]
	Reboxetine	Small open label study suggests no problems in PWE[39]
	Vortioxetine	Not known to be proconvulsive[34,40] but no experience in PWE[34]
Moderate risk – care required	Lithium	Low risk of seizures.[34] Anticonvulsant in animal models.[34] However, limited data showing increases or decreases in seizures frequency in PWE.[34] For bipolar, consider anticonvulsant mood stabilisers[41]
	Trazodone	Limited data suggest some risk of seizures[34,42]
	Venlafaxine	Effective in PWE[11] and has been recommended[18] but mixed evidence on seizure risk[34]
	Vilazodone	Limited data. Seizure exacerbation in a patient with epilepsy has been reported[34]
Higher risk – avoid (pro-convulsive at therapeutic doses[13])	Amoxapine	Several reports of seizures at therapeutic doses[42]
	Bupropion	Dose-related risk of seizures (particularly with instant-release formulations).[34] Risk is less with slow-release formulations at doses under 300mg/day[34]
	Maprotiline	Several reports of seizures at therapeutic doses[42]
	TCAs	Most TCAs are epileptogenic at higher doses (particularly clomipramine and amitriptyline[10,24,42]). Doxepin possibly lower risk (one small study in PWE).[34] SNRIs are preferred over TCAs in PWE[17]

(Continued)

CHAPTER 10

Table 10.5 (Continued)

Safety in epilepsy	Drug	Comments
Antipsychotics		
Low risk – good choices	Amisulpride/ sulpiride	Considered to be safe in PWE.[43] Renally excreted, so low risk of pharmacokinetic interactions with antiseizure medications. Seizures uncommon in overdose[44]
	Aripiprazole	Rarely lowers seizure threshold.[5] Incidence of seizures similar to placebo in RCTs[24]
	Ziprasidone	
	High potency FGAs	For example, fluphenazine, haloperidol, trifluoperazine, flupentixol. Low risk of lowering the seizure threshold[5]
	Risperidone	Unlikely to lower the seizure threshold.[5] Incidence of seizures similar to placebo in RCTs.[24] Has been recommended for PWE.[32,45] Evidence of safety in a case series of adolescents with epilepsy[46]
Probably low risk – use with caution (limited evidence)	Asenapine	Seizure rate similar to placebo in RCTs.[47] Data and clinical experience of use in PWE is extremely limited
	Brexpiprazole	
	Cariprazine	
	Lurasidone	
Moderate risk – care required	Olanzapine	Olanzapine and quetiapine both associated with seizures in RCTs.[24] However, olanzapine causes more EEG abnormalities.[44] Overall risk of reducing the seizure threshold is considered to be low[5] and olanzapine has been recommended by some for PWE.[32] Data relating to olanzapine are difficult to interpret. EEG changes are seen in some but not all studies[48] and it has been reported to be both anticonvulsant[49] and proconvulsant.[50] Quetiapine has a high risk of drug interaction in PWE[45]
	Quetiapine	
Higher risk – care required	Clozapine	Most epileptogenic antipsychotic.[32] However, has been used successfully in PWE stable on antiseizure medications without worsening seizures[51] and even in treatment-resistant epilepsy.[52] Note, should not be used with carbamazepine (risk of blood dyscrasias and reduced clozapine levels). Valproate or lamotrigine are the antiseizure medications of choice
Higher risk – avoid	Low potency FGAs (e.g. chlorpromazine)	Best avoided in PWE.[31] Doses of chlorpromazine above 1g/day have a 9% incidence of seizures
	Loxapine	Highest rate of seizures amongst the FGAs[53]
	Depot antipsychotics	None of the depot preparations currently available are thought to be epileptogenic, however: ■ The kinetics of depots are complex (seizures may be delayed) ■ If seizures do occur, the offending drug may not be easily withdrawn. Depots should be used with extreme care
	Zotepine	Has established dose-related pro-convulsive effect[44]

(Continued)

Table 10.5 *(Continued)*

Safety in epilepsy	Drug	Comments
Drugs for ADHD		
Low risk	Methylphenidate	Three RCTs support safety and efficacy in children with epilepsy at therapeutic doses (0.3–1mg/kg/day).[10] Two single dose RCTs and one open label extension study demonstrated no effect on seizures in adults.[54,55] A large case control study found an increased rate of seizures after the start of methylphenidate but not in the longer term.[56] This is difficult to interpret but suggests caution would be appropriate
Probably low risk[57,58] – use with caution (limited data)	Amfetamines	Data are limited to one small retrospective study in PWE.[10] No patients who had well controlled epilepsy experienced an increase in seizure frequency.[59] Of note, dexamfetamine was historically used as an adjunctive antiseizure agent[60]
	Atomoxetine	Data are limited to one small retrospective study in PWE.[10] Discontinuation rates were high (though none due to seizure exacerbation[61]). Seizure rate similar to placebo for patients without epilepsy[62]

This table contains information about the pro-convulsive effects of antidepressants and antipsychotics when used in therapeutic doses. See section on psychotropics in overdose for information about supra-therapeutic doses.

Epilepsy and driving

In the United Kingdom, people with epilepsy may not drive a car if they have had a seizure while awake in the previous year. However, they may be eligible to drive if seizures occur only during sleep and this has been an established nocturnal pattern for at least 3 years. The consequences of inducing seizure with antidepressants or antipsychotics can therefore be significant. For further information see "http://www.gov.uk/epilepsy-and-driving" www.gov.uk/epilepsy-and-driving.

References

1. Scott AJ, et al. Anxiety and depressive disorders in people with epilepsy: A meta-analysis. *Epilepsia* 2017; **58**:973–982.
2. Clancy MJ, et al. The prevalence of psychosis in epilepsy; a systematic review and meta-analysis. *BMC Psychiatry* 2014; **14**:75.
3. Hesdorffer DC, et al. Occurrence and recurrence of attempted suicide among people with epilepsy. *JAMA Psychiatry* 2016; **73**:80–86.
4. Thurman DJ, et al. The burden of premature mortality of epilepsy in high-income countries: A systematic review from the mortality task force of the international league against epilepsy. *Epilepsia* 2017; **58**:17–26.
5. Kanner AM. Management of psychiatric and neurological comorbidities in epilepsy. *Nat Rev Neurol* 2016; **12**:106–116.
6. Hesdorffer DC. Comorbidity between neurological illness and psychiatric disorders. *CNS Spectr* 2016; **21**:230–238.
7. Kanner AM. Can neurochemical changes of mood disorders explain the increase risk of epilepsy or its worse seizure control? *Neurochem Res* 2017; **42**:2071–2076.
8. Curran S, et al. Selecting an antidepressant for use in a patient with epilepsy. Safety considerations. *Drug Saf* 1998; **18**:125–133.
9. Blumer D, et al. Treatment of the interictal psychoses. *J Clin Psychiatry* 2000; **61**:110–122.
10. Mula M. The pharmacological management of psychiatric comorbidities in patients with epilepsy. *Pharmacol Res* 2016; **107**:147–153.
11. Elger CE, et al. Diagnosing and treating depression in epilepsy. *Seizure* 2017; **44**:184–193.
12. Anbarasan D. Psychoactive medications and seizures—challenges and pitfalls. *Neurol Rep* 2016; **9**:24–27.

13. Kanner AM. Most antidepressant drugs are safe for patients with epilepsy at therapeutic doses: a review of the evidence. *Epilepsy Behav* 2016; 61:282–286.

14. Kerr MP, et al. International consensus clinical practice statements for the treatment of neuropsychiatric conditions associated with epilepsy. *Epilepsia* 2011; 52:2133–2138.

15. Josephson CB, et al. Psychiatric comorbidities in epilepsy. *Int Rev Psychiatry (Abingdon, England)* 2017; 29:409–424.

16. Maguire M, et al. Epilepsy and psychosis: a practical approach. *Pract Neurol* 2018; 18:106–114.

17. Mula M. *Neuropsychiatric symptoms of epilepsy.* Vol. 1. Basel: Springer International Publishing 2016.

18. Barry JJ, et al. Consensus statement: the evaluation and treatment of people with epilepsy and affective disorders. *Epilepsy Behav* 2008; 13 Suppl 1:S1–29.

19. Schmidt D, et al. Drug treatment of epilepsy in adults. *BMJ* 2014; 348:g254.

20. Piedad J, et al. Beneficial and adverse psychotropic effects of antiepileptic drugs in patients with epilepsy: a summary of prevalence, underlying mechanisms and data limitations. *CNS Drugs* 2012; 26:319–335.

21. Spina E, et al. Clinically significant pharmacokinetic drug interactions of antiepileptic drugs with new antidepressants and new antipsychotics. *Pharmacol Res* 2016; 106:72–86.

22. Harden CL, et al. Mood disorders in patients with epilepsy: epidemiology and management. *CNS Drugs* 2002; 16:291–302.

23. Ngugi AK, et al. Incidence of epilepsy: a systematic review and meta-analysis. *Neurology* 2011; 77:1005–1012.

24. Alper K, et al. Seizure incidence in psychopharmacological clinical trials: an analysis of food and drug administration (FDA) summary basis of approval reports. *Biol Psychiatry* 2007; 62:345–354.

25. Wu CS, et al. Seizure risk associated with antidepressant treatment among patients with depressive disorders: a population-based case-crossover study. *J Clin Psychiatry* 2017; 78:e1226-e1232.

26. Josephson CB, et al. Association of depression and treated depression with epilepsy and seizure outcomes: a multicohort analysis. *JAMA Neurol* 2017; 74:533–539.

27. Farooq S, et al. Interventions for psychotic symptoms concomitant with epilepsy. *Cochrane Database System Rev* 2015:Cd006118.

28. Maguire MJ, et al. Antidepressants for people with epilepsy and depression. *Cochrane Database System Rev* 2014:Cd010682.

29. Maramattom BV. Duloxetine-induced syndrome of inappropriate antidiuretic hormone secretion and seizures. *Neurology* 2006; 66:773–774.

30. Ray AK. Does electroconvulsive therapy cause epilepsy? *JECT* 2013; 29:201–205.

31. Steinert T, et al. [Epileptic seizures during treatment with antidepressants and neuroleptics]. *Fortschr Neurol Psychiatr* 2011; 79:138–143.

32. Mula M. Epilepsy and psychiatric comorbidities: drug selection. *Curr Treat Options Neurol* 2017; 19:44.

33. National Institute for Health and Clinical Excellence. Depression in adults with a chronic physical health problem: treatment and management. Clinical Guidance [CG91]. 2009; http://www.nice.org.uk/CG91.

34. Steinert T, et al. Epileptic seizures under antidepressive drug treatment: systematic review. *Pharmacopsychiatry* 2018; 51:121–135.

35. Finkelstein Y, et al. Second-generation anti-depressants and risk of new-onset seizures in the elderly. *Clin Toxicol (Phila)* 2018; 56:1179–1184.

36. Gilliam FG, et al. A trial of sertraline or cognitive behavior therapy for depression in epilepsy. *Ann Neurol* 2019; 86:552–560.

37. Craig DP, et al. Risk of seizures with antidepressants: what is the evidence? *Drug Ther Bull* 2020; 58:137–140.

38. Servier Laboratories Limited. Summary of product characteristics. Valdoxan. 2020; https://www.medicines.org.uk/emc/medicine/21830.

39. Kuhn KU, et al. Antidepressive treatment in patients with temporal lobe epilepsy and major depression: a prospective study with three different antidepressants. *Epilepsy Behav* 2003; 4:674–679.

40. Lundbeck Limited. Summary of product characteristics. Brintellix (vortioxetine) tablets 5, 10 and 20mg. 2020; https://www.medicines.org.uk/emc/medicine/30904.

41. Knott S, et al. Epilepsy and bipolar disorder. *Epilepsy Behav* 2015; 52:267–274.

42. Johannessen Landmark C, et al. Proconvulsant effects of antidepressants - what is the current evidence? *Epilepsy Behav* 2016; 61:287–291.

43. Elnazer H, et al. Managing aggression in epilepsy. *BJPsych Adv* 2017; 23:253.

44. Steinert T, et al. *Chapter 9 - Seizures A2 - Manu, Peter.* San Diego: Academic Press 2016.

45. Agrawal N, et al. Treatment of psychoses in patients with epilepsy: an update. *Ther Adv Psychopharmacol* 2019; 9:2045125319862968.

46. Gonzalez-Heydrich J, et al. No seizure exacerbation from risperidone in youth with comorbid epilepsy and psychiatric disorders: a case series. *J Child Adolesc Psychopharmacol* 2004; 14:295–310.

47. IBM Watson Health. IBM micromedex solutions. 2020; https://www.ibm.com/watson-health/about/micromedex.

48. Jackson A, et al. EEG changes in patients on antipsychotic therapy: a systematic review. *Epilepsy Behav* 2019; 95:1–9.

49. Qiu X, et al. Antiepileptic effect of olanzapine in epilepsy patients with atypical depressive comorbidity. *Epileptic Disord* 2018; 20:225–231.

50. Mansoor M, et al. Generalised tonic-clonic seizures on the subtherapeutic dose of olanzapine. *BMJ Case Rep* 2019; 12.

51. Langosch JM, et al. Epilepsy, psychosis and clozapine. *Human Psychopharm Clin Experim* 2002; 17:115–119.

52. Jette Pomerleau V, et al. Clozapine safety and efficacy for interictal psychotic disorder in pharmacoresistant epilepsy. *Cogn Behav Neurol* 2017; 30:73–76.

53. Habibi M, et al. The impact of psychoactive drugs on seizures and antiepileptic drugs. *Curr Neurol Neurosci Rep* 2016; 16:71.

54. Adams J, et al. Methylphenidate, cognition, and epilepsy: a 1-month open-label trial. *Epilepsia* 2017; 58:2124–2132.

55. Adams J, et al. Methylphenidate, cognition, and epilepsy: a double-blind, placebo-controlled, single-dose study. *Neurology* 2017; 88:470–476.

56. Man KKC, et al. Association between methylphenidate treatment and risk of seizure: a population-based, self-controlled case-series study. *Lancet Child Adolesc Health* 2020; **4**:435–443.

57. Besag F, et al. Psychiatric and behavioural disorders in children with epilepsy (ILAE Task Force report): epilepsy and ADHD. *Epileptic Disord* 2016; **18**:S8–S15.

58. Besag F, et al. Psychiatric and behavioural disorders in children with epilepsy (ILAE Task Force report): when should pharmacotherapy for psychiatric/behavioural disorders in children with epilepsy be prescribed? *Epileptic Disord* 2016; **18**:S77–S86.

59. Gonzalez-Heydrich J, et al. Comparing stimulant effects in youth with ADHD symptoms and epilepsy. *Epilepsy Behav* 2014; **36**:102–107.

60. Schubert R. Attention deficit disorder and epilepsy. *Pediatr Neurol* 2005; **32**:1–10.

61. Torres A, et al. Tolerability of atomoxetine for treatment of pediatric attention-deficit/hyperactivity disorder in the context of epilepsy. *Epilepsy Behav* 2011; **20**:95–102.

62. Williams AE, et al. Epilepsy and attention-deficit hyperactivity disorder: links, risks, and challenges. *Neuropsychiatr Dis Treat* 2016; **12**:287–296.

Further reading

Kanner AM. Management of psychiatric and neurological comorbidities in epilepsy. *Nat Rev Neurol* 2016; **12**:106–116.

Mula M. Epilepsy and psychiatric comorbidities: drug selection. *Curr Treat Options Neurol* 2017; **19**:44.

22q11.2 deletion syndrome

Clinical features

The commonest autosomal deletion, 22q11.2 Deletion Syndrome (22q11.2DS), is a multisystem disorder with a heterogeneous presentation which varies greatly in severity between affected individuals.[1] Prevalence is estimated to range from 1 per 3000 to 5000 births.[1] The syndrome has been known by many names (including velocardiofacial, DiGeorge or Shprintzen syndrome), in part due to its broad phenotypic range of clinical features (see Box 10.2).

Box 10.2 Clinical features of 22q11.2DS[1]

- Cardiovascular abnormalities including tetralogy of Fallot
- Endocrine abnormalities including hypoparathyroidism
- Genitourinary abnormalities including renal agenesis
- Developmental delays and learning disabilities
- Gastrointestinal abnormalities including constipation

- Immunodeficiency and autoimmune disease
- Palatal abnormalities
- Behavioural phenotypes
- Psychiatric disorders
- Skeletal abnormalities

Psychiatric disorders in people with 22q11.2DS

Around 60% of people with 22q11.2DS are estimated to meet the diagnostic criteria for some type of psychiatric disorder at some point during their lives.[2] Children with 22q11.2DS have an elevated prevalence of anxiety, ADHD and autism spectrum disorders.[1] Anxiety disorders are profoundly increased in adults.[1] Schizophrenia is diagnosed in approximately 25% of individuals with 22q11.2DS.[1]

Few studies have evaluated the safety and efficacy of psychotropics in people with 22q11.2DS. However, standard pharmacological (and non-pharmacological) treatments for ADHD, anxiety, mood disorders and schizophrenia appear to be effective and treatment protocols used in the general population should be followed.[1,3] Although most psychotropics are thought to be safe in people with 22q11.2DS, consideration should be given to medical comorbidities (e.g. cardiovascular disorders), a potentially increased risk of seizures[2] and movement disorders.[1] Endocrine abnormalities (e.g. hypoparathyroidism and hypothyroidism) should be corrected before starting psychotropics because they can mimic psychiatric symptoms and complicate treatment with psychotropics.[2,3] Current evidence and opinion on the treatment of psychiatric disorders in people with 22q11.2DS is summarised in Table 10.6.

Table 10.6 Management of psychiatric disorders in people with 22q11.2DS.[4]

Psychiatric disorder	Treatments
ADHD	■ Although concerns have been raised about the theoretical risk of psychosis with psycho-stimulants in people with 22q11.2DS, standard treatment protocols are advised[2] ■ Two studies support the efficacy of methylphenidate in children with 22q11.2DS.[2] Treatment was generally well tolerated. A comprehensive cardiovascular assessment prior to and during treatment has been recommended
Depression and anxiety	■ **SSRIs**: both depression and anxiety appear to respond favourably to SSRIs.[2,5] Further treatment is per standard protocols ■ S-adenosyl-L-methionine was studied in one small RCT and no significant benefit in depressive (or ADHD) symptoms was detected[2]
Obsessive compulsive disorder	■ One study of four people with OCD and 22q11.2DS found a mean rate of improvement of 35% in symptom score after treatment with fluoxetine (30–60mg/day). Treatment was well tolerated[6]
Schizophrenia	■ Standard treatment protocols are generally recommended.[3,7] People with 22q11.2DS may be more susceptible to seizures and EPSEs with antipsychotics.[4] There is a significantly elevated risk of obesity in 22q11.2DS so metabolic side effects should be closely monitored.[8] Those with cardiac abnormalities have an increased risk of QTc prolongation.[4] Close ECG monitoring is recommended.[4] Antipsychotics with a low effect on the QT interval are preferred.[4] Low starting doses and slow dose titrations are widely recommended.[4] Case reports have described the successful use of aripiprazole, olanzapine, risperidone and quetiapine[5] but treatment-resistance has been demonstrated in many cases.[5] ■ **Clozapine:** found to be effective in one retrospective study of 20 patients with 22q11.2DS.[2] Compared with matched controls, lower doses were needed (a median of 250mg/day for those with 22q11.2DS vs. 450mg/day with matched controls). However, half of the 22q11.2DS group experienced at least one serious adverse effect from clozapine: primarily seizures, but also myocarditis and neutropenia. Several case reports further support the efficacy of clozapine at low doses (median of 200mg/day) for people with 22q11.2DS, while highlighting the risk of seizures (generalised or myoclonic) and thrombocytopenia.[8] Overall, clozapine appears to have demonstrable efficacy at lower than usual doses, but the risk of rare serious adverse events appears to be high.[2] Adjunctive antiseizure medications should be considered.[7,8] ■ **Seizures with other antipsychotics:** investigate low calcium and magnesium levels in all cases and ensure adequate treatment.[7] Consider adjunctive antiseizure medications.[7] ■ **Other agents:** drugs which act directly against catecholamine excess may also be effective. Metyrosine, used as a monotherapy or as an adjunctive agent, was found to be effective 22 of 29 patients recruited to one study.[9] Additional positive case reports have been published.[10] There is single case study where methyldopa was used successfully.[11]

References

1. McDonald-McGinn DM, et al. 22q11.2 deletion syndrome. *Nat Rev Dis Primers* 2015; **1**:15071.

2. Mosheva M, et al. Effectiveness and side effects of psychopharmacotherapy in individuals with 22q11.2 deletion syndrome with comorbid psychiatric disorders: a systematic review. *Eur Child Adolesc Psychiatry* 2020; **29**:1035–1048.

3. Fung WL, et al. Practical guidelines for managing adults with 22q11.2 deletion syndrome. *Genet Med* 2015; **17**:599–609.

4. Baker K, et al. Psychiatric illness. Consensus Document on 22q11 Deletion Syndrome (22q11DS) MaxAppeal 2017; http://www.maxappeal.org.uk/downloads/Consensus_Document_on_22q11_Deletion_Syndrome_Master_2017_(final_draft)_9-end_(1)2018.pdf.

5. Dori N, et al. The effectiveness and safety of antipsychotic and antidepressant medications in individuals with 22q11.2 deletion syndrome. *J Child Adolesc Psychopharmacol* 2017; **27**:83–90.

6. Gothelf D, et al. Obsessive-compulsive disorder in patients with velocardiofacial (22q11 deletion) syndrome. *Am J Med Genet B Neuropsychiatr Genet* 2004; **126b**:99–105.

7. Bassett AS, et al. Practical guidelines for managing patients with 22q11.2 deletion syndrome. *J Pediatr* 2011; **159**:332–339.

8. de Boer J, et al. Adverse effects of antipsychotic medication in patients with 22q11.2 deletion syndrome: A systematic review. *Am J Med Genet A* 2019; **179**:2292–2306.

9. Faedda GL, et al. 4.19 Treatment of velo-cardio-facial syndrome-related psychosis with metyrosine. *J Am Acad Child Adolesc Psychiatry* 2016; **55**:S169.

10. Engebretsen MH, et al. Metyrosine treatment in a woman with chromosome 22q11.2 deletion syndrome and psychosis: a case study. *Int J Dev Disabil* 2017:1–6.

11. O'Hanlon JF, et al. Replacement of antipsychotic and antiepileptic medication by L-alpha-methyldopa in a woman with velocardiofacial syndrome. *Int Clin Psychopharmacol* 2003; **18**:117–119.

Learning disabilities

General considerations[1]

Prescribing psychotropic medications for people with learning disabilities (LD) is a challenging and controversial area of psychiatric practice.[2,3] There are concerns that psychotropic drugs of all kinds (antipsychotics, antidepressants, benzodiazepines (both regular and as required) and antiepileptics as mood stabilisers) are overprescribed with poor review and assessment of their benefit. The learning disabilities field is notable in having only a small therapeutics research base of its own, with particular ethical and practical considerations regarding how emotional and behavioural disturbances are classified and treated. Although prescribing for individuals with mild or borderline intellectual impairment may be undertaken by mainstream mental health services, the assessment and treatment of behavioural and emotional disorders in people with more marked (or, as in the case of autism, atypical) patterns of significant cognitive impairment should be undertaken in the first instance by, or at least in consultation with, specialist clinicians.

The term 'dual diagnosis' in this context refers to the co-occurrence of an identifiable psychiatric disorder (mental illness, personality disorder) and LD. 'Diagnostic overshadowing' is the misattribution of emotional or behavioural problems to LD itself rather than a co-morbid condition. LD is an important risk factor for all psychiatric disorders (including dementia, particularly for individuals with Down syndrome).[4] Where it is possible to diagnose a mental illness using conventional or modified criteria, the drug treatment in the first instance should, in general, be similar to that in the population at large. Most treatment guidelines are increasingly stating their intended applicability to people with LD in this regard.

Mental illness may present in unusual ways in LD, for example, depression as self-injurious behaviour, persecutory ideation as complaints of being 'picked on'. Conversely, behaviours such as self-talk may be normal in some individuals but mistakenly identified as a disorder such as psychosis. In general, diagnosis becomes increasingly complex with increasing severity of disability and associated communication impairment.

Co-morbid autistic spectrum disorder has special assessment considerations and in its own right is an important risk factor for psychiatric disorder, in particular anxiety and depression, bipolar spectrum disorder, severe obsessional behaviour, anger disorders and psychosis-like episodes that may not meet criteria for schizophrenia but nonetheless require treatment. Autistic traits are common amongst patients using LD services. Guidance on the treatment of mental health problems in autism can be found in Chapter 5.

Key practice areas

Capacity and consent: It is uncommon for patients in LD services (who often represent a sub-population of those identified with special educational needs in childhood) to have sufficient understanding of their treatment in order to be able to take truly informed decisions. There is inevitably an increased onus on the clinician to bear the weight of decision-making. The patient's decision-making capacity, depending on the severity of intellectual impairment, may be improved through appropriate verbal and written communication. The involvement of carers in this process is generally essential.

Physical co-morbidity, especially epilepsy: Epilepsy is overrepresented in LD populations, becoming more prevalent as severity increases with approximately one-third of affected individuals developing a seizure disorder by early adulthood. Special consideration is needed when considering the use of medications that may lower seizure threshold or interact with drugs used for epilepsy.

Assessment of care environments: Behavioural and emotional disturbance may sometimes be a reflection of problems or failings in the care environment. Different staff in a care home may have different thresholds of tolerance (or make different attributions) for these difficulties which can lead to varied reports of their significance and impact. Allowing for a period of prospective assessment and using simple assessment tools (e.g. simple ABC or sleep charts) can be very helpful to the clinician in making judgements about recommending medication. If medication is used in a care home, staff may need special education in its use and anticipated side effects and, for 'as required' medications, clear guidelines for its use. This may make it difficult to initiate certain treatments in the community.

Adverse effect sensitivity: It is widely thought that people with LD are especially sensitive to side effects of psychotropics and more at risk of long-term effects such as the metabolic syndrome. However, we only know of one study that has given support to this view. A cohort study extracting information from a large UK primary care database compared the incidence of EPSEs of antipsychotics in adults with LD, with adults without LD. The incidence of EPSE was 30% higher in people with LD than in those without LD.[5] It is good practice to start at lower doses and increase more slowly than might be usual in general psychiatric practice. Notable side effects include worsening of seizures, sedation, extrapyramidal reactions (including with risperidone at normal doses, especially in individuals who already have mobility problems), problems with swallowing (with clozapine and other antipsychotics) and worsening of cognitive function with anticholinergic medications (see section on prescribing in dementia in Chapter 6).

Psychological interventions: In the absence of an identifiable mental illness (including atypical presentations) with clear treatment implications, psychological interventions such as functional behavioural analysis should be considered as first-line intervention for all but the most serious or intractable presentations of behavioural disturbance. In studies where it has been possible to infer severity of challenging behaviour treatment response is generally associated with more severe problems at baseline.

Currently and historically used medications for behaviour disorder

Drug class	Clinical applications	Notes
Antipsychotics[6]	Use in psychosis with LD is justified Used across a broad range of behavioural disturbances[7] May be useful for aggression and irritability	The most widely used[8,9] yet most controversial medication for behavioural problems.[10,11] Although an RCT[12] cast doubt on their efficacy for this indication the study was not without its problems and there is a significant body of other evidence supporting their use including a number of small RCTs in children with LD
		Discontinuation studies in long-term treatment commonly (but not always) show re-emergence of problem behaviours
		NICE suggests considering slow withdrawal of antipsychotics in all those who do not have psychotic symptoms.[13] The UK STOMP programme promotes deprescribing of antipsychotics.[14] It has been successful, but antipsychotics are often replaced by other psychotropics.[15]
		Before the advent of SGAs the best evidence was for **haloperidol**[16] in the context of autism and for zuclopenthixol for behavioural disturbance.[17] Zuclopenthixol may reduce aggression and challenging behaviour.[18]
		Amongst SGAs the best evidence is for **risperidone**[19,20] at low dose (0.5–2mg) for aggression and mood instability, particularly with associated autism though also in non-autistic cases. **Aripiprazole** has an FDA licence for behavioural disturbance in young people with autism.[21,22]
		Some evidence to support **olanzapine**[23] and case reports of **clozapine**[24] for very severe cases of aggression though not widely used and unlikely to be used outside highly specialist (inpatient) settings. In 2015, Cochrane uncovered 38 case reports and chart reviews but found no RCT evidence for the use of clozapine in psychosis in LD.[25]
		Results for **quetiapine** are modest at best.[26]
SSRIs	Helpful for severe anxiety and obsessionality in autistic spectrum disorder. Use here is off-licence unless an additional diagnosis of anxiety disorder or OCD is made Also used as a first-line alternative to antipsychotics for aggression and impulsivity	Commonly used in combination with antipsychotics though limited evidence base for combination treatment. Effectiveness in absence of mood or anxiety-spectrum disorder is unclear, however, and a 2013 Cochrane review was pessimistic[27] about the evidence for their effectiveness for behaviour disorder in autistic children (who may be at heightened risk of adverse effects) though a little more encouraging in adults. Some good evidence for fluoxetine in OCD in LD/autism although dropout rate is high.[28]
		Generally, quality of trials is poor and effects may be exaggerated by use in less severe cases.[29] Caution needed because of the risk of precipitation of hypomania in this population.[30] As with antipsychotics, there are major concerns about overprescribing.[31]
		Venlafaxine is probably not effective.[32]

(Continued)

Drug class	Clinical applications	Notes
Antiseizure medications[33]	Aggression and self-injury	Some uncontrolled studies supporting **sodium valproate**[34] in LD populations though evidence is not strong and research findings contradictory. However, valproate remains best supported of the antiseizure medications for mood lability and aggression partly because of positive studies in non-LD groups.[35]
		Limited studies of **lamotrigine**, mostly in children, suggest no effect, at least in autism and in the absence of affective instability.[26]
		Data for **carbamazepine** also unconvincing, but it is still widely used.[36]
Lithium[37]	Licensed for the treatment of self-injurious behaviour and aggression	Some RCT evidence[38] for LD but no studies in this population for many years[3] although there has been one fairly recent positive RCT for aggression in adolescents without developmental impairment.[39] Experience suggests can be very helpful in individual cases where other treatments have failed and is possibly underused though side effects can be problematic.
		Perhaps best considered where there is a sub-syndromal or nonspecific 'affective component'. Some authorities suggest that, on close examination, challenging behaviour may occur in the context of very rapid cycling bipolar disorder in some individuals with severe and profound learning disability and that the diagnosis is easily missed.
		Some RCT evidence that short term use is reasonably well tolerated (at 6mg/kg).[40]
Methylphenidate	Effective in ADHD associated with LD	NICE[13] conducted a meta-analysis and found clear benefit for methylphenidate (and risperidone and clonidine) in ADHD in the context of LD. Insomnia is common.
Naltrexone[41]	Has been used for severe self-injurious behaviour[42]	Evidence not strong and results are inconsistent. Use may still be an option in severe and intractable cases. One case of successful treatment of kleptomania.[43] Overall, clinical use has declined of late.[44]

References

1. Deb S. The use of medications for the management of problem behaviours in adults who has intellectual [learning] disabilities 2012; http://www.intellectualdisability.info/mental-health/the-use-of-drugs-for-the-treatment-of-behaviour-disorders-in-adults-who-have-learning-intellectual-disabilities.

2. Sheehan R, et al. Psychotropic prescribing in people with intellectual disability and challenging behaviour. *BMJ* 2017; 358:j3896.

3. Ji NY, et al. Pharmacotherapy for mental health problems in people with intellectual disability. *Curr Opin Psychiatry* 2016; 29:103–125.

4. Cooper SA, et al. Mental ill-health in adults with intellectual disabilities: prevalence and associated factors. *Br J Psychiatry* 2007; 190:27–35.

5. Sheehan R, et al. Movement side effects of antipsychotic drugs in adults with and without intellectual disability: UK population-based cohort study. *BMJ Open* 2017; 7:e017406.

6. Antochi R, et al. Psychopharmacological treatments in persons with dual diagnosis of psychiatric disorders and developmental disabilities. *Postgrad Med J* 2003; 79:139–146.

7. Lunsky Y, et al. Antipsychotic use with and without comorbid psychiatric diagnosis among adults with intellectual and developmental disabilities. *Can J Psychiatry* 2017; 63:361–369.

8. Deb S, et al. Characteristics and the trajectory of psychotropic medication use in general and antipsychotics in particular among adults with an intellectual disability who exhibit aggressive behaviour. *J Intellect Disabil Res* 2015; 59:11–25.

9. Sheehan R, et al. Mental illness, challenging behaviour, and psychotropic drug prescribing in people with intellectual disability: UK population based cohort study. *BMJ* 2015; 351:h4326.

10. Deb S, et al. The effectiveness of antipsychotic medication in the management of behaviour problems in adults with intellectual disabilities. *J Intellect Disabil Res* 2007; 51:766–777.

11. Roy D, et al. Pharmacologic management of aggression in adults with intellectual disability. *J Intellect Disabil Res* 2013; 1:28–43.

12. Tyrer P, et al. Risperidone, haloperidol, and placebo in the treatment of aggressive challenging behaviour in patients with intellectual disability: a randomised controlled trial. *Lancet* 2008; 371:57–63.

13. National Institute of Health and Care Excellence. Mental health problems in people with learning disabilities: prevention, assessment and management [NG54] 2016; https://www.nice.org.uk/Guidance/NG54.

14. Shankar R, et al. Stopping, rationalising or optimising antipsychotic drug treatment in people with intellectual disability and/or autism. *Drug Ther Bull* 2019; 57:10–13.

15. Deb S, et al. UK psychiatrists' experience of withdrawal of antipsychotics prescribed for challenging behaviours in adults with intellectual disabilities and/or autism. *BJPsych Open* 2020; 6:e112.

16. Malone RP, et al. The role of antipsychotics in the management of behavioural symptoms in children and adolescents with autism. *Drugs* 2009; 69:535–548.

17. Malt UF, et al. Effectiveness of zuclopenthixol compared with haloperidol in the treatment of behavioural disturbances in learning disabled patients. *Br J Psychiatry* 1995; 166:374–377.

18. Hassler F, et al. Treatment of aggressive behavior problems in boys with intellectual disabilities using zuclopenthixol. *J Child Adolesc Psychopharmacol* 2014; 24:579–581.

19. Nagaraj R, et al. Risperidone in children with autism: randomized, placebo-controlled, double-blind study. *J Child Neurol* 2006; 21:450–455.

20. Pandina GJ, et al. Risperidone improves behavioral symptoms in children with autism in a randomized, double-blind, placebo-controlled trial. *J Autism Dev Disord* 2007; 37:367–373.

21. Owen R, et al. Aripiprazole in the treatment of irritability in children and adolescents with autistic disorder. *Pediatrics* 2009; 124:1533–1540.

22. Marcus RN, et al. A placebo-controlled, fixed-dose study of aripiprazole in children and adolescents with irritability associated with autistic disorder. *J Am Acad Child Adolesc Psychiatry* 2009; 48:1110–1119.

23. Fido A, et al. Olanzapine in the treatment of behavioral problems associated with autism: an open-label trial in Kuwait. *Med Princ Pract* 2008; 17:415–418.

24. Zuddas A, et al. Clinical effects of clozapine on autistic disorder. *Am J Psychiatry* 1996; 153:738.

25. Ayub M, et al. Clozapine for psychotic disorders in adults with intellectual disabilities. *Cochrane Database Syst Rev* 2015:Cd010625.

26. Stigler KA, et al. Pharmacotherapy of irritability in pervasive developmental disorders. *Child Adolesc Psychiatr Clin N Am* 2008; 17:739–752.

27. Williams K, et al. Selective serotonin reuptake inhibitors (SSRIs) for autism spectrum disorders (ASD). *Cochrane Database Syst Rev* 2013; 8:CD004677.

28. Reddihough DS, et al. Effect of fluoxetine on obsessive-compulsive behaviors in children and adolescents with autism spectrum disorders: a randomized clinical trial. *JAMA* 2019; 322:1561–1569.

29. Myers SM. Citalopram not effective for repetitive behaviour in autistic spectrum disorders. *Evid Based Ment Health* 2010; 13:22.

30. Cook EH, Jr., et al. Fluoxetine treatment of children and adults with autistic disorder and mental retardation. *J Am Acad Child Adolesc Psychiatry* 1992; 31:739–745.

31. Oswald DP, et al. Medication use among children with autism spectrum disorders. *J Child Adolesc Psychopharmacol* 2007; 17:348–355.

32. Carminati GG, et al. Using venlafaxine to treat behavioral disorders in patients with autism spectrum disorder. *Prog Neuropsychopharmacol Biol Psychiatry* 2016; 65:85–95.

33. Deb S, et al. The effectiveness of mood stabilizers and antiepileptic medication for the management of behaviour problems in adults with intellectual disability: a systematic review. *J Intellect Disabil Res* 2008; **52**:107–113.

34. Ruedrich S, et al. Effect of divalproex sodium on aggression and self-injurious behaviour in adults with intellectual disability: a retrospective review. *J Intellect Disabil Res* 1999; **43(Pt 2)**:105–111.

35. Donovan SJ, et al. Divalproex treatment for youth with explosive temper and mood lability: a double-blind, placebo-controlled crossover design. *Am J Psychiatry* 2000; **157**:818–820.

36. Unwin GL, et al. Use of medication for the management of behavior problems among adults with intellectual disabilities: a clinicians' consensus survey. *Am J Ment Retard* 2008; **113**:19–31.

37. Pary RJ. Towards defining adequate lithium trials for individuals with mental retardation and mental illness. *Am J Ment Retard* 1991; **95**:681–691.

38. Craft M, et al. Lithium in the treatment of aggression in mentally handicapped patients: a double-blind trial. *Br J Psychiatry* 1987; **150**:685–689.

39. Malone RP, et al. A double-blind placebo-controlled study of lithium in hospitalized aggressive children and adolescents with conduct disorder. *Arch Gen Psychiatry* 2000; **57**:649–654.

40. Yuan J, et al. Lithium treatment is safe in children with intellectual disability. *Front Mol Neurosci* 2018; **11**:425.

41. Campbell M, et al. Naltrexone in autistic children: an acute open dose range tolerance trial. *J Am Acad Child Adolesc Psychiatry* 1989; **28**:200–206.

42. Barrett RP, et al. Effects of naloxone and naltrexone on self-injury: a double-blind, placebo-controlled analysis. *Am J Ment Retard* 1989; **93**:644–651.

43. Mouaffak F, et al. Kleptomania treated with naltrexone in a patient with intellectual disability. *J Psychiatry Neurosci* 2020; **45**:71–72.

44. Sabus A, et al. Management of self-injurious behaviors in children with neurodevelopmental disorders: a pharmacotherapy overview. *Pharmacotherapy* 2019; **39**:645–664.

Huntington's disease – pharmacological treatment

Huntington's disease (HD) is a genetic disease involving slow progressive degeneration of neurones in the striatum with the involvement of the cerebral cortex as the disease progresses.[1] In Western populations HD has a prevalence of 10.6–13.7 individuals per 100,000.[1] The mutant Huntington protein causes neuronal dysfunction and death through several mechanisms, resulting in a triad of motor, cognitive and neuropsychiatric symptoms. There are currently no disease modifying treatments,[1-3] and so, only symptomatic treatment is used, in an attempt to improve quality of life.

Box 10.3 General principles of pharmacological symptom management in Huntington's disease[4,5]

- Tailor management to the needs of the individual patient (treatment is typically initiated when symptoms become bothersome, interfering or socially stigmatising).
- Check whether existing medications are causing or exacerbating symptoms before commencing new treatments.
- Prioritise treatment to target the most troublesome symptoms first, with consideration of comorbid features.
- Balance therapeutic benefit with the potential for adverse effects.
- Start with a low dose and titrate according to tolerability and response (patients are relatively more sensitive to cognitive and motor adverse effects which may also be difficult to distinguish from disease progression).
- Regularly follow up with patients to address changes in treatment (because symptomology evolves with disease progression).

There are few controlled studies to guide practice in this area,[6] though some direction can be drawn from published expert opinion and clinical experience. A summary of the available literature can be found subsequently. Readers are directed to the reports cited for details of dosage regimens and further information about tolerability. Clinicians who treat patients with HD are encouraged to publish reports of both positive and negative outcomes to increase the primary literature base.

Motor symptoms

Motor disturbances follow a biphasic course: an initial hyperkinetic phase with prominent chorea which tends to plateau over time, and a later hypokinetic phase characterised by bradykinesia, dystonia, balance and gait disturbance.[1] With regard to chorea, the goal of treatment is not to obliterate movements but to reduce their severity to achieve better tolerability.[4] Treatment pathways are available to guide management.[7] First-line treatments include tetrabenazine (licensed) or antipsychotics (unlicensed).[7,8] Monotherapy is preferred to prevent an increased risk of adverse effects and complicating the management of non-motor symptoms.[7,8]

CHAPTER 10

Table 10.7 Evidence and experience regarding the pharmacological treatment of motor symptoms in Huntington's disease

Symptoms	Treatments
Chorea	▪ **Tetrabenazine:** Unlike antipsychotics, tetrabenazine's effectiveness is well established.[6,7,9] However, adverse effects including sedation, depression and parkinsonism may limit its clinical benefit. In clinical practice, many prefer to use tetrabenazine first line in patients without depressive symptoms and suicidal behaviour.[7] Compliance with a multiple daily dosing regimen (e.g. TDS) is needed. Deutetrabenazine, licensed in the United States for chorea in HD, has not been directly compared with tetrabenazine but it may offer an improved pharmacokinetic and side effect profile.[9]
	▪ **Antipsychotics:** Considered first-line treatment, particularly in the presence of depression, aggression, psychosis, or when poor drug compliance is suspected[7,8,10] despite a lack of data from RCTs. SGAs such as risperidone or olanzapine are used most commonly.[7] Potentially limiting side effects include dyskinesia, parkinsonism and metabolic syndrome.[4] FGAs have been used successfully but are less popular in clinical practice because of the risk of EPSEs.[10] The Enroll-HD observational database has suggested that risperidone and olanzapine are at least as effective as tetrabenazine[11] but worsen cognition.[12] For severe chorea, antipsychotics and tetrabenazine have been used in combination.[7] Tetrabenazine and deutetrabenazine both have the potential for QT prolongation, as do most antipsychotics.
	▪ **Other agents:** Amantadine, riluzole and nabilone have been recommended as alternatives to tetrabenazine,[13] but the evidence base for beneficial effects with these agents is controversial,[4] and some guidelines recommend against using amantadine and riluzole[7,8] or do not mention at all.[7] Clinical trials with other cannabinoids (nabiximols and cannabidiol) showed no difference from placebo.[14] Clonazepam is sometimes used as an adjunctive therapy in the presence of comorbid features; a small case series reported benefit with high doses.[4,15] Levetiracetam has been used successfully in two small open label studies; somnolence led to a 33% dropout in one study and parkinsonism was also reported.[15] Pridopidine has not been shown to be effective in RCTs so far; further evaluation is required.[16] Other negative studies also include those examining the use of latrepirdine, ethyl-EPA and mavoglurant.[15]
Hypokinetic rigidity	▪ Levodopa may provide partial and temporary relief of symptoms.[7] Note the potential for such drugs to exacerbate behavioural disturbances.[8] Rigidity may be caused/worsened by antipsychotics or tetrabenazine; dose reduction or discontinuation should be considered in the first instance, after weighing any derived benefits against symptoms severity.[7] Positive case reports exist for amantadine and dopamine agonists (though guidelines do not make recommendations on their use).[7]
Myoclonus	▪ Valproate or clonazepam have been suggested, used alone or combination.[7] Levetiracetam is a therapeutic alternative.[7]
Dystonia	▪ Botulinum toxin injections have been suggested for focal dystonia;[7] clonazepam or baclofen has been suggested for non-focal dystonia.[4]

Mental and behavioural symptoms

A wide variety of mental and behavioural symptoms occur in HD, including anxiety, depression, suicidality, preservation, disinhibition, irritability, apathy and, rarely, psychosis.[17] Mental and behavioural symptoms can emerge before motor disturbances and reduce quality of life substantially.[17] In comparison with other HD features, psychiatric

Table 10.8 Evidence and experience regarding the pharmacological treatment of mental and behavioural symptoms in Huntington's disease

Symptoms	Treatments
Anxiety	▪ Reported 16.7–24% lifetime prevalence in HD.[17] There are no RCTs to guide choice; however, olanzapine 5mg/d substantially improved anxiety symptoms in one small open label pilot study.[17] SSRIs and SNRIs have been suggested as first line treatment.[4,7] Some guidelines have recommended considering SGAs (quetiapine,[7] risperidone or olanzapine) for anxiety associated with personality or behavioural disturbances[8] or when other treatments fail.[7] Anxiolytics such as benzodiazepines or buspirone may also be useful.[8]
Depression	▪ Reported 20–56% lifetime prevalence in HD.[17] Treatment is typically required: depression is linked to a lower quality of life in HD and increases the risk of suicide.[17,18] There are no RCTs to guide choice.[19] However, most experts agree that depression in HD responds well to antidepressants. SSRIs are the preferred first-line treatment.[4,7] ▪ **SSRIs:** Two controlled trials examined the effects of fluoxetine and citalopram in non-depressed patients with HD. Despite excluding depressed patients, both showed near significant improvements in depressive symptoms.[19] Note that tetrabenazine is metabolised by CYP2D6; inhibitors of this enzyme (e.g. fluoxetine, paroxetine) may increase levels. ▪ **SNRIs:** Venlafaxine was effective in an uncontrolled study;[19] however, one in five developed side effects, such as nausea and irritability.[17] ▪ **TCAs:** Beneficial effects reported in some cases[20] but generally their use should be avoided or limited. TCAs' anticholinergic properties may worsen hyperkinesias and cognition.[20] Toxicity in overdose may also make them less suitable choices (suicidality is increased in HD[17]). ▪ **Others:** Mirtazapine was used successfully in a case report of severe depression.[4] In a case registry study it was one of the most frequently prescribed treatments for depression in HD.[17] Lithium produced improvements in suicidality in a small case series[19] but experience is very limited, and tolerability may be poor. MAOIs have been used in earlier case studies;[20] a lack of recent experience and important interactions with tetrabenazine make these less suitable. ECT has been suggested in severe cases.[7,21,22]
Obsessive compulsive behaviours or preservation	▪ There are no RCTs.[23] International consensus supports the use of SSRIs first line;[7] use of clomipramine is also supported,[17] but tolerability may be poor. Case studies document the successful use of fluoxetine, paroxetine and sertraline.[4] One study of two patients with preservation and aggression reported beneficial effects with buspirone.[17] For ideational preservation, consensus also supports the use of olanzapine or risperidone (particularly if associated with irritability).[7]
Irritability or agitation[24]	▪ Reported prevalence of 38–73% in HD. Initial management is non-pharmacological (e.g. by addressing possible triggers such as pain or akathisia and using behavioural/psychological approaches). No medications are approved specifically, but expert consensus supports the use of SSRIs as preferred first-line agents with antipsychotics being the next most favoured alternative monotherapy. Clinical features influence treatment choice. For example, SGAs (e.g. olanzapine, risperidone, quetiapine) may be preferred in the presence of chorea, acute irritability, aggression or impulsivity. Benzodiazepines are a popularly used adjunctive therapy. Guidelines have also recommended mirtazapine or mianserin in patients not benefitting from maximum doses of SSRIs, especially in those with a comorbid sleep disorder. In cases nonresponsive to antidepressants and/or antipsychotics, adjunctive mood stabilisers have also been recommended.[7] ▪ **Aggressive behaviours:** A wide variety of psychotropics have been used with reported beneficial effects (e.g. antipsychotics, lithium, valproate, propranolol, medroxyprogesterone, SSRIs, buspirone).[20,25] Antipsychotics have been used most commonly. The evidence base is too limited to make specific treatment recommendations[25] but low-dose antipsychotics can be considered.[4] ECT was helpful in a few case reports agitation refractory to pharmacotherapy.[21]

Table 10.8 *(Continued)*	
Symptoms	**Treatments**
Apathy	■ Common in HD and appears to worsen with disease progression.[17] Some sedative medications (e.g. antipsychotics, benzodiazepines, tetrabenazine) may contribute, so dose reduction or withdrawal should be considered.[7] Bupropion was recently studied in one multicentre RCT and found to be ineffective.[26] Other agents, including methylphenidate, atomoxetine, modafinil, amantadine and bromocriptine have been trialled with little success.[17]
Psychosis	■ One of the least prevalent psychiatric manifestations of HD, perhaps due to the use of antidopaminergics for motor symptoms.[17] There are no RCTs to guide choice; treatment is empirical. Note that antipsychotic drugs may exacerbate any underlying movement disorder. ■ **SGAs:** Olanzapine and risperidone are used most frequently;[17] low starting doses are recommended.[4] Case reports support the efficacy of risperidone, quetiapine, aripiprazole and amisulpride.[20] Clozapine may be considered in refractory cases[5,20] or akinetic forms of HD with debilitating parkinsonian symptoms.[7] ■ **FGAs:** Used less frequently due to the risk of dystonia and parkinsonism; however, haloperidol has been used when chorea is also problematic to the patient.[20]

Table 10.9 Summary of available treatments for mental state and behavioural changes in Huntington's disease[5,7,17]

Symptoms	Most commonly prescribed pharmacological treatments	Alternatives
Anxiety	SSRIs, mirtazapine, pregabalin, venlafaxine	Olanzapine, risperidone, quetiapine benzodiazepines, propranolol, buspirone
Depression or suicidality	SSRIs, mirtazapine, venlafaxine	TCAs; ECT in refractory cases
Obsessive compulsive behaviours	SSRIs	Clomipramine
Irritability or agitation	SSRIs, SGAs (olanzapine, risperidone, sulpiride), tiapride, benzodiazepines	Antiseizure medications (lamotrigine, carbamazepine, valproate), TCAs, buspirone, propranolol; consider trial of an analgesic
Apathy	None	None
Psychosis	Olanzapine, risperidone, haloperidol, sulpiride, tiapride, injectable antipsychotic medication	Clozapine, quetiapine

symptoms are perhaps the most amenable to pharmacotherapy.[5] In general, psychiatric treatment choices are selected as they would be in other conditions,[4] though patients are relatively more sensitive to side effects.[4] The most commonly prescribed psychotropics are summarised in Table 10.8 (mostly based on low quality evidence).[17]

Cognitive symptoms

Cognitive disturbances may emerge many years before motor disturbances;[1] the progression of cognitive decline is gradual[27] and dementia is inevitable in late stages. Although a wide variety of agents have been studied, none has become established treatments and the benefit of most remain unclear.[28] There is insufficient evidence to support the use of acetylcholinesterase inhibitors[29] and no evidence to support any other medications to treat dementia in HD.[30]

References

1. McColgan P, et al. Huntington's disease: a clinical review. *Eur J Neurol* 2018; 25:24–34.
2. Mestre T, et al. Therapeutic interventions for disease progression in Huntington's disease. *Cochrane Database Syst Rev* 2009; 2009:Cd006455.
3. Tabrizi SJ, et al. Huntington disease: new insights into molecular pathogenesis and therapeutic opportunities. *Nat Rev Neurol* 2020; 16:529–546.
4. Killoran A, et al. Current therapeutic options for Huntington's disease: good clinical practice versus evidence-based approaches? *Mov Disord* 2014; 29:1404–1413.
5. Anderson KE, et al. Clinical management of neuropsychiatric symptoms of Huntington disease: expert-based consensus guidelines on agitation, anxiety, apathy, psychosis and sleep disorders. *J Huntington's Dis* 2018; 7:355–366.
6. Mestre T, et al. Therapeutic interventions for symptomatic treatment in Huntington's disease. *Cochrane Database Syst Rev* 2009:CD006456.
7. Bachoud-Lévi AC, et al. International guidelines for the treatment of Huntington's disease. *Front Neurol* 2019; 10:710.
8. Desamericq G, et al. Guidelines for clinical pharmacological practices in Huntington's disease. *Rev Neurol (Paris)* 2016; 172:423–432.
9. Dash D, et al. Therapeutic update on Huntington's disease: symptomatic treatments and emerging disease-modifying therapies. *Neurotherapeutics* 2020:[Epub ahead of print].
10. Unti E, et al. Antipsychotic drugs in Huntington's disease. *Expert Rev Neurother* 2017; 17:227–237.
11. Schultz JL, et al. Comparing risperidone and olanzapine to tetrabenazine for the management of chorea in Huntington disease: an analysis from the Enroll-HD database. *Mov Disord Clin Pract* 2019; 6:132–138.
12. Harris KL, et al. Antidopaminergic treatment is associated with reduced chorea and irritability but impaired cognition in Huntington's disease (Enroll-HD). *J Neurol Neurosurg Psychiatry* 2020; 91:622–630.
13. Armstrong MJ, et al. Evidence-based guideline: pharmacologic treatment of chorea in Huntington disease: report of the guideline development subcommittee of the American Academy of Neurology. *Neurology* 2012; 79:597–603.
14. Dickey AS, et al. Therapy development in Huntington disease: from current strategies to emerging opportunities. *Am J Med Genet A* 2018; 176:842–861.
15. Coppen EM, et al. Current pharmacological approaches to reduce chorea in Huntington's disease. *Drugs* 2017; 77:29–46.
16. Jabłońska M, et al. Pridopidine in the treatment of Huntington's disease. *Rev Neurosci* 2020; 31:441–451.
17. Eddy CM, et al. Changes in mental state and behaviour in Huntington's disease. *Lancet Psychiatry* 2016; 3:1079–1086.
18. Kachian ZR, et al. Suicidal ideation and behavior in Huntington's disease: systematic review and recommendations. *J Affect Disord* 2019; 250:319–329.
19. Moulton CD, et al. Systematic review of pharmacological treatments for depressive symptoms in Huntington's disease. *Mov Disord* 2014; 29:1556–1561.
20. van Duijn E. Medical treatment of behavioral manifestations of Huntington disease. *Handb Clin Neurol* 2017; 144:129–139.
21. Mowafi W, et al. Electroconvulsive therapy for severe depression, psychosis and chorea in a patient with Huntington's disease: case report and review of the literature. *BJPsych Bulletin* 2020:[Epub ahead of print].
22. Adrissi J, et al. Electroconvulsive Therapy (ECT) for refractory psychiatric symptoms in Huntington's disease: a case series and review of the literature. *J Huntington's Dis* 2019; 8:291–300.
23. Oosterloo M, et al. Obsessive-compulsive and perseverative behaviors in Huntington's disease. *J Huntington's Dis* 2019; 8:1–7.
24. Karagas NE, et al. Irritability in Huntington's disease. *J Huntington's Dis* 2020; 9:107–113.
25. Fisher CA, et al. Aggression in Huntington's disease: a systematic review of rates of aggression and treatment methods. *J Huntington's Dis* 2014; 3:319–332.
26. Petersén Å, et al. The psychopharmacology of Huntington disease. *Handb Clin Neurol* 2019; 165:179–189.
27. Ross CA, et al. Huntington disease: natural history, biomarkers and prospects for therapeutics. *Nat Rev Neurol* 2014; 10:204–216.
28. van der Vaart T, et al. Treatment of cognitive deficits in genetic disorders: a systematic review of clinical trials of diet and drug treatments. *JAMA Neurology* 2015; 72:1052–1060.
29. Li Y, et al. Cholinesterase inhibitors for rarer dementias associated with neurological conditions. *Cochrane Database Syst Rev* 2015:Cd009444.
30. O'Brien JT, et al. Clinical practice with anti-dementia drugs: A revised (third) consensus statement from the British Association for Psychopharmacology. *J. Psychopharmacol* 2017; 31:147–168.

Further reading

Bachoud-Lévi AC, et al. International guidelines for the treatment of Huntington's disease. *Frontiers in Neurology* 2019; 10:710.

Multiple sclerosis

Multiple sclerosis (MS) is a common cause of neurological disability affecting approximately 85,000 people in the United Kingdom with the onset usually between 20 and 50 years of age. Individuals with MS experience a variety of psychiatric and neurological disorders such as depression, anxiety, pathological laughter and crying (pseudobulbar affect, PBA), mania and euphoria, psychosis/bipolar disorder, fatigue and cognitive impairment. Psychiatric disorders result from the psychological impact of MS diagnosis and its prognosis, perceived lack of social support or unhelpful coping styles,[1] increased stress,[2] iatrogenic effects of treatments commonly used with MS,[3,4] or damage to neuronal pathways.[3]

Depression

In people with MS, depression is common with a point prevalence of 14–31%[5,6] and lifetime prevalence of up to 50%.[7,8] Suicide rates are 2–7.5 times higher than the general population.[9] Depression is often associated with fatigue and pain, though the relationship direction is unclear. Overlapping symptoms of depression, PBA and MS can complicate diagnosis and so co-operation between neurologists and psychiatrists is essential to ensure optimal treatment for individuals with MS. Depression in MS may result from structural changes in the brain and, as such, it may differ fundamentally from non-MS depression.[10]

The role of interferon-beta in the aetiology of MS depression is unclear, but it is now thought that depression occurs no more frequently in people treated with interferon-beta.[11–13] Standard care for initiation of interferon-beta should include assessment for depression and, for those with a past history of depressive illness, prophylactic treatment with an antidepressant.[3] The same applies to those disease-modifying biological treatments that are associated with depression (daclizumab, alemtuzumab, natalizumab, etc.).[4]

Recommendations for treatment

Depression in MS

Step	Intervention
1	Screen for depression with PHQ-9 HADS/BDI[14]/CES-D.[15] Exclude and treat any organic causes. Consider iatrogenic effects of medications as potential cause of depression. Ensure there is no past history of mania or bipolar disorder. People with mild depression should be considered for cognitive behaviour therapy[16] or self-help.[17]
2	SSRIs should be first-line treatment[3,15,18,19] because of their relatively benign side-effect profile Sertraline was as effective as CBT in one trial,[20] but paroxetine was found to be no more effective than placebo in another study.[21] Fluoxetine was effective in MS-related depression in a small case series.[22] Because of reduced tolerability of side effects in this patient group, medications should be titrated from an initial half dose. Many MS patients are prescribed low-dose TCAs for pain/bladder disturbance and so SSRIs should be used with caution and patients should be observed for serotonin syndrome. For those with co-morbid pain consideration should be given to treating with an SNRI such as duloxetine[23] or venlafaxine.[24] One RCT of desipramine showed it was more effective than placebo, but tricyclics in general are often poorly tolerated.[25] In 2011, Cochrane was not convinced by the studies cited here,[26] but there is little reason to suppose that antidepressants are any less effective in depression associated with physical illness.[27] CBT is the most appropriate psychological intervention with best efficacy in comparison to supportive therapy or usual care, and should be used in conjunction with medication for those who are moderately severely depressed.[20,28,29] Mindfulness training may also help.[30] Omega-3 fatty acids are ineffective.[31]

(Continued)

Step	Intervention

(Continued)

3	If SSRIs are not tolerated or there is no response there are limited data that moclobemide is effective and well tolerated.[32,33] There are no published trials on venlafaxine, duloxetine and mirtazapine but these are used widely. Mirtazapine may worsen fatigue, at least initially.
4	ECT could be considered for people who are actively suicidal or severely depressed and at high risk, but it may trigger an exacerbation of MS symptoms, although some studies suggest that no neurological disturbance occurs.[34]
5	Other treatments that have shown some effect in depression in MS are zinc,[35] vitamin A[36] and co-enzyme Q10.[37] A small trial supports antidepressant effects of fampridine.[38]

Anxiety

Anxiety affects many people with MS, with a point prevalence of up to 50%[39] and lifetime incidence of 35–37%.[40] Elevated rates in comparison with the general population are seen for generalized anxiety disorder, panic disorder, obsessive compulsive disorder[40] and social anxiety. Anxiety appears to be linked to perceived lack of support, increased pain, fatigue, sleep disturbance, depression, alcohol misuse and suicidal ideas. The uncertainty of prognosis in MS is a major cause of anxiety in MS.[41] There are no published trials for the drug treatment of anxiety in MS, but SSRIs can be used and in non-responsive cases, venlafaxine might be an option (based on practice in non MS patients).

Benzodiazepines may be used for acute and severe anxiety but only for a maximum of four weeks and should not be prescribed in the long term. Buspirone and beta-blockers could also be considered although there is no demonstrated efficacy in MS. Pregabalin is also licensed for anxiety and may be useful in this population group especially where pain relief is required.[42,43] People with MS may also respond to CBT. Generally treatment is as for non-MS anxiety disorders (see anxiety section, Chapter 3).

Pseudobulbar affect (PBA)

Up to 10% of individuals with MS experience pathological laughing or crying (PLC) or other incongruence of affect. It is more common in the advanced stages of the disease and is associated with cognitive impairment.[40] There have been a few open label trials recommending the use of small doses of TCAs, for example, amitriptyline or SSRIs, for example, fluoxetine[44,45] in MS. Citalopram,[46] nortriptyline[47] or sertraline[48] have been investigated in people with post-stroke PLC and shown reasonable efficacy and rapid response. Valproic acid may be effective.[49] The combination of dextromethorphan and low-dose quinidine (DMq) is effective.[50] Dextromethorphan plus fluoxetine may show similar effects.[51] In these combinations, dextromethorphan (an analgesic and cough suppressant) is the active ingredient and quinidine/fluoxetine the metabolic inhibitor. DMq is FDA-approved as Nuedexta and once held approval in the EU but is not marketed there.

Bipolar disorder

The incidence of bipolar disorder can be as high as 13% in the MS population[2] compared with 1–6% in the general population. Mania can be induced by drugs such as steroids or baclofen.[52]

Anecdotal evidence suggests that patients presenting with mania/bipolar disorder should be treated with mood stabilisers such as sodium valproate as these are better tolerated than lithium.[53]

Lithium can cause diuresis and thus lead to increased difficulties with tolerance in people with bladder disorder. Mania accompanied by psychosis could be treated with low dose antipsychotics such as risperidone, olanzapine[2] and ziprasidone.[54] Patients requiring psychiatric treatment for steroid-induced mania with psychosis have been known to respond well to olanzapine,[55] further case reports suggest risperidone is also useful. There have been no trials in this area.

Psychosis

Psychosis occurs in 1.1% of the MS population and compared with other psychiatric disorders is relatively uncommon.[54] In a very few cases, psychosis is the presenting complaint of MS.[56] There have been few published trials, but risperidone or clozapine have been recommended because of their low risk of extra pyramidal symptoms.[52] On this basis, olanzapine, aripiprazole and quetiapine might also, in theory at least, be possible options. ECT has been used in refractory cases.[57]

Psychosis may rarely be the presentation of an MS relapse in which case steroids may be beneficial but would need to be given under close supervision. Note also the small risk of psychotic reactions in patients receiving THC-containing formulations.[58,59]

Cognitive impairment

Cognitive impairment occurs in at least 40–65% of people with MS. Some of the medications commonly prescribed can worsen cognition, for example, tizanidine, diazepam, gabapentin.[60] Although there are no published trials, evidence from clinical case studies suggests that the treatment of sleep difficulties, depression and fatigue can enhance cognitive function.[60] There have been two small trials with donepezil for people with mild-moderate cognitive impairment showing moderate efficacy.[61,62] A larger study found no effect.[63] Similarly, data supporting the use of memantine are weak.[64] Overall, no symptomatic treatment has proven worthwhile efficacy[65] and disease modifying agents offer greater promise.[66]

Fatigue

Fatigue is a common symptom in MS with up to 80% of people with MS affected.[67] The aetiology of fatigue is unclear but there have been suggestions that disruption of neuronal networks,[68] depression or psychological reactions,[52] sleep disturbances, inflammation[69] or medication may play a role in its development. Pharmacological and non-pharmacological strategies[67] should be used in a treatment strategy.

Non-pharmacological strategies include reviewing history for any possible contributing factors, assessment and treatment of underlying depression if present, medication, pacing activities and appropriate exercise. One trial suggests that CBT reduces fatigue scores.[70]

Pharmacological strategies include the use of amantadine[71] or modafinil. NICE guidelines suggest no medicine should be used routinely but that amantadine could have a small benefit and should be offered.[72] A Cochrane review of amantadine in people with MS suggested that the quality and outcomes of the amantadine trials are inconsistent and that therefore efficacy remains unclear.[71] A meta-analysis of 11 RCTs found supporting data for amantadine[73] and a later (2020) meta-analysis confirmed its value.[74]

Modafinil has mixed results in clinical trials, but a meta-analysis of five RCTs[75] found clear benefit. Despite doubts over its efficacy modafinil is widely used in MS.[76]

Other pharmacological agents recommended for use in MS fatigue include pemoline, aspirin and Ginseng. A double-blind crossover study of aspirin compared with placebo favoured aspirin but further studies are required.[77] An RCT of pemoline showed double the rate of symptom relief compared with placebo.[78] Data relating to Ginseng are mixed.[79,80]

References

1. Ron MA. Do neurologists provide adequate care for depression in patients with multiple sclerosis? *Nat Clin Pract Neurol* 2006; 2:534–535.

2. Patten SB, et al. Biopsychosocial correlates of lifetime major depression in a multiple sclerosis population. *Mult Scler* 2000; 6:115–120.

3. Servis ME. Psychiatric comorbidity in Parkinson's disease, multiple sclerosis, and seizure disorder. *Continuum* 2006; 12:72–86.

4. Carta MG, et al. Pharmacological management of depression in patients with multiple sclerosis. *Expert Opin Pharmacother* 2018; 19:1533–1540.

5. Gottberg K, et al. A population-based study of depressive symptoms in multiple sclerosis in Stockholm county: association with functioning and sense of coherence. *J Neurol Neurosurg Psychiatry* 2007; 78:60–65.

6. Boeschoten RE, et al. Prevalence of depression and anxiety in multiple sclerosis: A systematic review and meta-analysis. *J Neurol Sci* 2017; 372:331–341.

7. Patten SB, et al. Depression in multiple sclerosis. *Int Rev Psychiatry (Abingdon, England)* 2017:1–10.

8. Kalb R, et al. Depression and suicidality in multiple sclerosis: red flags, management strategies, and ethical considerations. *Curr Neurol Neurosci Rep* 2019; 19:77.

9. Sadovnick AD, et al. Cause of death in patients attending multiple sclerosis clinics. *Neurology* 1991; 41:1193–1196.

10. Corallo F, et al. A complex relation between depression and multiple sclerosis: a descriptive review. *Neurol Sci* 2019; 40:1551–1558.

11. Zephir H, et al. Multiple sclerosis and depression: influence of interferon beta therapy. *Mult Scler* 2003; 9:284–288.

12. Patten SB, et al. Anti-depressant use in association with interferon and glatiramer acetate treatment in multiple sclerosis. *Mult Scler* 2008; 14:406–411.

13. Schippling S, et al. Incidence and course of depression in multiple sclerosis in the multinational beyond trial. *J Neurol* 2016; 263:1418–1426.

14. Moran PJ, et al. The validity of Beck Depression Inventory and Hamilton Rating Scale for Depression items in the assessment of depression among patients with multiple sclerosis. *J Behav Med* 2005; 28:35–41.

15. Pandya R, et al. Predictive value of the CES-D in detecting depression among candidates for disease-modifying multiple sclerosis treatment. *Psychosomatics* 2005; 46:131–134.

16. Minden SL, et al. Evidence-based guideline: assessment and management of psychiatric disorders in individuals with MS: report of the Guideline Development Subcommittee of the American Academy of Neurology. *Neurology* 2014; 82:174–181.

17. Rickards H. Depression in neurological disorders: Parkinson's disease, multiple sclerosis, and stroke. *J Neurol Neurosurg Psychiatry* 2005; 76 Suppl 1:i48-i52.

18. Silveira C, et al. Neuropsychiatric symptoms of multiple sclerosis: state of the art. *Psychiatry Investig* 2019; 16:877–888.

19. Patten SB. Current perspectives on co-morbid depression and multiple sclerosis. *Expert Rev Neurother* 2020; 20:867–874.

20. Mohr DC, et al. Comparative outcomes for individual cognitive-behavior therapy, supportive-expressive group psychotherapy, and sertraline for the treatment of depression in multiple sclerosis. *J Consult Clin Psychol* 2001; 69:942–949.

21. Ehde DM, et al. Efficacy of paroxetine in treating major depressive disorder in persons with multiple sclerosis. *Gen Hosp Psychiatry* 2008; 30:40–48.

22. Flax JW, et al. Effect of fluoxetine on patients with multiple sclerosis. *Am J Psychiatry* 1991; 148:1603.

23. Vollmer TL, et al. A randomized, double-blind, placebo-controlled trial of duloxetine for the treatment of pain in patients with multiple sclerosis. *Pain Practice: The Official Journal of World Institute of Pain* 2014; 14:732–744.

24. Hilty DM, et al. Psychopharmacology for neurologists: principles, algorithms, and other resources. *Continuum* 2006; 12:33–46.

25. Barak Y, et al. Treatment of depression in patients with multiple sclerosis. *Neurologist* 1998; 4:99–104.

26. Koch MW, et al. Pharmacologic treatment of depression in multiple sclerosis. *Cochrane Database Syst Rev* 2011; 2:CD007295.

27. Taylor D, et al. Pharmacological interventions for people with depression and chronic physical health problems: systematic review and meta-analyses of safety and efficacy. *Br J Psychiatry* 2011; 198:179–188.

28. Siegert RJ, et al. Depression in multiple sclerosis: a review. *J Neurol Neurosurg Psychiatry* 2005; 76:469–475.

29. Larcombe NA, et al. An evaluation of cognitive-behaviour therapy for depression in patients with multiple sclerosis. *Br J Psychiatry* 1984; 145:366–371.

30. Grossman P, et al. MS quality of life, depression, and fatigue improve after mindfulness training: a randomized trial. *Neurology* 2010; 75:1141–1149.

31. Shinto L, et al. Omega-3 fatty acids for depression in multiple sclerosis: a randomized pilot study. *PLoS One* 2016; 11:e0147195.

32. Schiffer RB, et al. Antidepressant pharmacotherapy of depression associated with multiple sclerosis. *Am J Psychiatry* 1990; 147:1493–1497.

33. Barak Y, et al. Moclobemide treatment in multiple sclerosis patients with comorbid depression: an open-label safety trial. *J Neuropsychiatry Clin Neurosci* 1999; 11:271–273.

34. Rasmussen KG, et al. Electroconvulsive therapy in patients with multiple sclerosis. *JECT* 2007; 23:179–180.

35. Salari S, et al. Zinc sulphate: A reasonable choice for depression management in patients with multiple sclerosis: A randomized, double-blind, placebo-controlled clinical trial. *Pharmacol Rep* 2015; 67:606–609.

36. Bitarafan S, et al. Effect of vitamin A supplementation on fatigue and depression in multiple sclerosis patients: a double-blind placebo-controlled clinical trial. *Iran J Allergy Asthma Immunol* 2016; 15:13–19.

37. Sanoobar M, et al. Coenzyme Q10 as a treatment for fatigue and depression in multiple sclerosis patients: A double blind randomized clinical trial. *Nutr Neurosci* 2016; 19:138–143.

38. Broicher SD, et al. Positive effects of fampridine on cognition, fatigue and depression in patients with multiple sclerosis over 2 years. *J Neurol* 2018; 265:1016–1025.

39. Jones KH, et al. A large-scale study of anxiety and depression in people with multiple sclerosis: a survey via the web portal of the UK MS Register. *PLoS One* 2012; 7:e41910.

40. Korostil M, et al. Anxiety disorders and their clinical correlates in multiple sclerosis patients. *Mult Scler* 2007; 13:67–72.

41. Butler E, et al. 'It's the unknown' – understanding anxiety: from the perspective of people with multiple sclerosis. *Psychol Health* 2019; 34:368–383.

42. Solaro C, et al. Pregabalin for treating paroxysmal painful symptoms in multiple sclerosis: a pilot study. *J Neurol* 2009; 256:1773–1774.

43. Bittner S, et al. Pregabalin and gabapentin in multiple sclerosis: clinical experiences and therapeutic implications. *Nervenarzt* 2011; 82:1273–1280.

44. Feinstein A, et al. The effects of anxiety on psychiatric morbidity in patients with multiple sclerosis. *Mult Scler* 1999; 5:323–326.

45. Feinstein A, et al. Prevalence and neurobehavioral correlates of pathological laughing and crying in multiple sclerosis. *Arch Neurol* 1997; 54:1116–1121.

46. Andersen G, et al. Citalopram for post-stroke pathological crying. *Lancet* 1993; 342:837–839.

47. Robinson RG, et al. Pathological laughing and crying following stroke: validation of a measurement scale and a double-blind treatment study. *Am J Psychiatry* 1993; 150:286–293.

48. Burns A, et al. Sertraline in stroke-associated lability of mood. *Int J Geriatr Psychiatry* 1999; 14:681–685.

49. Johnson B, et al. Crying and suicidal, but not depressed. Pseudobulbar affect in multiple sclerosis successfully treated with valproic acid: case report and literature review. *Palliative & Supportive Care* 2015; 13:1797–1801.

50. Pioro EP, et al. Dextromethorphan plus ultra low-dose quinidine reduces pseudobulbar affect. *Ann Neurol* 2010; 68:693–702.

51. McGrane I, et al. Treatment of pseudobulbar affect with fluoxetine and dextromethorphan in a woman with multiple sclerosis. *Ann Pharmacother* 2017:1035–1036.

52. Jefferies K. The neuropsychiatry of multiple sclerosis. *Adv Psychiatr Treat* 2006; 12:214–220.

53. Stip E, et al. Valproate in the treatment of mood disorder due to multiple sclerosis. *Can J Psychiatry* 1995; 40:219–220.

54. Davids E, et al. Antipsychotic treatment of psychosis associated with multiple sclerosis. *Prog Neuropsychopharmacol Biol Psychiatry* 2004; 28:743–744.

55. Budur K, et al. Olanzapine for corticosteroid-induced mood disorders. *Psychosomatics* 2003; 44:353.

56. Camara-Lemarroy CR, et al. The varieties of psychosis in multiple sclerosis: A systematic review of cases. *Mult Scler Relat Disord* 2017; 12:9–14.

57. Narita Z, et al. Possible effects of electroconvulsive therapy on refractory psychosis in primary progressive multiple sclerosis: A case report. *Neuropsychopharmacol Rep* 2018; 38:92–94.

58. Aragona M, et al. Psychopathological and cognitive effects of therapeutic cannabinoids in multiple sclerosis: a double-blind, placebo controlled, crossover study. *Clin Neuropharmacol* 2009; 32:41–47.

59. Black N, et al. Cannabinoids for the treatment of mental disorders and symptoms of mental disorders: a systematic review and meta-analysis. *Lancet Psychiatry* 2019; **6**:995–1010.

60. Pierson SH, et al. Treatment of cognitive impairment in multiple sclerosis. *Behav Neurol* 2006; **17**:53–67.

61. Krupp LB, et al. Donepezil improved memory in multiple sclerosis in a randomized clinical trial. *Neurology* 2004; **63**:1579–1585.

62. Greene YM, et al. A 12-week, open trial of donepezil hydrochloride in patients with multiple sclerosis and associated cognitive impairments. *J Clin Psychopharmacol* 2000; **20**:350–356.

63. Krupp LB, et al. Multicenter randomized clinical trial of donepezil for memory impairment in multiple sclerosis. *Neurology* 2011; **76**:1500–1507.

64. Lovera JF, et al. Memantine for cognitive impairment in multiple sclerosis: a randomized placebo-controlled trial. *Mult Scler* 2010; **16**:715–723.

65. Chen MH, et al. Cognitive efficacy of pharmacologic treatments in multiple sclerosis: a systematic review. *CNS Drugs* 2020; **34**:599–628.

66. Patti F. Treatment of cognitive impairment in patients with multiple sclerosis. *Expert Opin Investig Drugs* 2012; **21**:1679–1699.

67. Bakshi R. Fatigue associated with multiple sclerosis: diagnosis, impact and management. *Mult Scler* 2003; **9**:219–227.

68. Sepulcre J, et al. Fatigue in multiple sclerosis is associated with the disruption of frontal and parietal pathways. *Mult Scler* 2009; **15**:337–344.

69. Ormstad H, et al. Chronic fatigue and depression due to multiple sclerosis: immune-inflammatory pathways, tryptophan catabolites and the gut-brain axis as possible shared pathways. *Mult Scler Relat Disord* 2020; **46**:102533.

70. van KK, et al. A randomized controlled trial of cognitive behavior therapy for multiple sclerosis fatigue. *Psychosom Med* 2008; **70**:205–213.

71. Pucci E, et al. Amantadine for fatigue in multiple sclerosis. *Cochrane Database Syst Rev* 2007:CD002818.

72. National Institute for Health and Care Excellence. Multiple sclerosis in adults: management. Clinical Guidance [CG186]. 2014 (last updated November 2019); https://www.nice.org.uk/guidance/cg186.

73. Yang TT, et al. Pharmacological treatments for fatigue in patients with multiple sclerosis: A systematic review and meta-analysis. *J Neurol Sci* 2017; **380**:256–261.

74. Perez DQ, et al. Efficacy and safety of amantadine for the treatment of fatigue in multiple sclerosis: a systematic review and meta-analysis. *Neurodegener Dis Manag* 2020; **10**:383–395.

75. Shangyan H, et al. Meta-analysis of the efficacy of modafinil versus placebo in the treatment of multiple sclerosis fatigue. *Mult Scler Relat Disord* 2018; **19**:85–89.

76. Davies M, et al. Safety profile of modafinil across a range of prescribing indications, including off-label use, in a primary care setting in England: results of a modified prescription-event monitoring study. *Drug Saf* 2013; **36**:237–246.

77. Wingerchuk DM, et al. A randomized controlled crossover trial of aspirin for fatigue in multiple sclerosis. *Neurology* 2005; **64**:1267–1269.

78. Weinshenker BG, et al. A double-blind, randomized, crossover trial of pemoline in fatigue associated with multiple sclerosis. *Neurology* 1992; **42**:1468–1471.

79. Kim E, et al. American ginseng does not improve fatigue in multiple sclerosis: a single center randomized double-blind placebo-controlled crossover pilot study. *Mult Scler* 2011; **17**:1523–1526.

80. Etemadifar M, et al. Ginseng in the treatment of fatigue in multiple sclerosis: a randomized, placebo-controlled, double-blind pilot study. *Int J Neurosci* 2013; **123**:480–486.

Parkinson's disease

Parkinson's disease (PD) is a progressive, degenerative neurological disorder characterised by resting tremor, cogwheel rigidity, bradykinesia and postural instability. The prevalence of co-morbid psychiatric disorders is high. Approximately 25% will suffer from major depression at some point during the course of their illness, a further 25% from milder forms of depression, 25% from anxiety spectrum disorders, 25% from psychosis and up to 80% will develop dementia.[1–3] While depression and anxiety can occur at any time, psychosis, dementia and delirium are more prevalent in the later stages of the illness. Close co-operation between the psychiatrist and neurologist is required to optimise treatment for this group of patients.

Depression in Parkinson's disease

Depression in PD predicts greater cognitive decline, deterioration in functioning and progression of motor symptoms,[4] possibly reflecting more advanced and widespread neurodegeneration involving multiple neurotransmitter pathways.[5] Depression may also occur after the withdrawal of dopamine agonists.[6] Pre-existing dementia is an established risk factor for the development of depression.

Depression in PD – recommendations for treatment	
Step	**Intervention**
1	Exclude/treat organic causes such as hypothyroidism (the prevalence of which is relatively high in PD[4]).
2	**SSRIs** are considered to be first-line treatment although the effect size is modest.[7–9] Some patients may experience a worsening of motor symptoms although the absolute risk is low.[10,11] Care must be taken when combining SSRIs with selegiline, as the risk of serotonin syndrome is increased.[4] The SNRIs venlafaxine[12] and duloxetine[13] also appear to have some effect although venlafaxine may modestly worsen motor symptoms.[12]
	TCAs are generally poorly tolerated because of their anticholinergic (can worsen cognitive problems; constipation) and alpha-blocking effects (can worsen symptoms of autonomic dysfunction). Note though that several meta-analyses[8,9] have reported that low dose TCAs to be more effective than SSRIs,[14–16] although low dose amitriptyline and sertraline seem to be equally effective.[17,18] The most recent network meta-analysis found that SSRIs were the most effective treatments; significantly better than MAOIs and dopamine agonists.[19] Limited evidence supports the safe use of agomelatine.[20,21] Atomoxetine is not effective.[22] CBT should always be considered.[23]
3	Consider augmentation with dopamine agonists/releasers such as pramipexole.[24] Note though that these drugs increase the risk of impulse control disorders.[25,26] They have also rarely been associated with the development of psychosis.[27]
4	Consider **ECT**. Depression and motor symptoms generally respond well,[4] but the risk of inducing delirium is high,[28] particularly in patients with pre-existing cognitive impairment.
5	Follow the algorithm for treatment-resistant depression (see relevant section in Chapter 3) from this point. Be aware of the increased propensity for adverse effects and drug interactions in this patient group.

Psychosis in Parkinson's Disease

Psychosis in PD is often characterised by visual hallucinations.[29] Auditory hallucinations and delusions occur far less frequently,[30] and usually in younger patients.[31] Psychosis and dementia frequently co-exist. Having one predicts the development of the other.[32] Sleep disorders are also an established risk factor for the development of psychosis.[33]

Abnormalities in dopamine, serotonin and acetylcholine neurotransmission have all been implicated, but the exact aetiology of PD psychosis is poorly understood. In the majority of patients, psychotic symptoms are thought to be secondary to dopaminergic medication rather than part of PD itself; psychosis secondary to medication may be determined at least in part through polymorphisms of the ACE gene.[34] From the limited data available, anticholinergics and dopamine agonists seem to be associated with a higher risk of inducing psychosis than levodopa or COMT inhibitors.[30,35] Psychosis is a major contributor to caregiver distress and a risk factor for institutionalisation and early death.[32]

Psychosis in PD – recommendations for treatment	
Step	**Intervention**
1	Exclude organic causes (delirium).
2	Optimise the environment to maximise orientation and minimise problems due to poor caregiver–patient interactions.
3	If the patient has insight and hallucinations are infrequent and not troubling, do not treat.
4	Consider reducing or stopping anticholinergics and dopamine agonists. Monitor for signs of motor deterioration. Be prepared to restart/increase the dose of these drugs again to achieve the best balance between psychosis and mobility.
5	Consider an atypical antipsychotic. The efficacy of clozapine (see below, point 7) is supported by placebo-controlled RCTs.[29] In contrast, there are several negative placebo-controlled trials each for quetiapine and olanzapine.[29] Low-dose quetiapine is the best tolerated, although EPSEs and stereotypical movements can occur. It is probably reasonable to try quetiapine[36] before clozapine but the success rate may be low. Olanzapine, ziprasidone and aripiprazole are likely to all have greater adverse effects on motor function than quetiapine, although one small trial[37] supports the safe use of ziprasidone. Risperidone and typical antipsychotics should be avoided completely. Severe rebound psychosis has been described when antipsychotic drugs (quetiapine or clozapine) are discontinued.
	All antipsychotics may be relatively less effective in managing psychotic symptoms in patients with dementia, and such patients may be more prone to developing motor and cognitive side effects.[38] Antipsychotics have been associated with an increased risk of vascular events in the elderly. In PD all antipsychotics are linked to increased mortality[39] although the effect of clozapine is not known.
6	Consider a **cholinesterase inhibitor**, particularly if the patient has co-morbid dementia[29,40] Cholinesterase inhibitors may also reduce the risk of falls.[41] Early use of donepezil does not prevent or reduce episodes of psychosis although there is some benefit on cognition.[42]

(Continued)

Step	Intervention
	(Continued)
7	Try **clozapine**. Start at 6.25mg – usual dose 25mg–35mg/day.[29,37] Usually safe but NMS has been reported[43]
	Monitor as for clozapine in schizophrenia. Older people are more prone to develop serious blood dyscrasia. A case of aplastic anaemia has been reported.[44]
8	Consider **ECT**.[45] Psychotic and motor symptoms usually respond well,[46] but the risk of inducing delirium is high,[28] particularly in patients with pre-existing cognitive impairment.

Pimavanserin

Pimavanserin is a 5HT2A receptor inverse agonist available in the United States and some other countries. It is effective in PD psychosis but has no dopamine receptor activity and does not worsen PD movement disorder or seem to increase mortality.[47]

Pimavanserin and clozapine are the only drugs recommended for PD psychosis.[48] A recent network meta-analysis suggested only these two drugs had efficacy in PD while having minimal effect on motor function.[49] Other drugs have doubtful efficacy and are poorly tolerated.[49,50]

Cholinesterase inhibitors in PD

Cholinesterase inhibitors have been shown to improve cognition, delusions and hallucinations in patients with Lewy body dementia (which has many similarities to PD). Motor function may deteriorate.[51,52] Improvements in cognitive functioning are modest.[53–55] A Cochrane review and some large RCTs[54,56,57] concluded that there is evidence that cholinesterase inhibitors lead to improvements in global functioning, cognition, behavioural disturbance and activities of daily living in PD. Again, motor function may deteriorate[57,58] with particular increase in tremor.[55] Evidence for memantine is mixed.[59,60] Discontinuation of anticholinergic drugs should improve cognition and psychosis – PD patients often have a very high anticholinergic burden, often unrelated to treatment of PD itself.[61]

Many patients with PD use complementary therapies, some of which may be modestly beneficial – see Zesiewicz et al.[62] Caffeine may offer a protective effect against the development of PD and also modestly improve motor function in established disease.[63]

References

1. Hely MA, et al. The Sydney multicenter study of Parkinson's disease: the inevitability of dementia at 20 years. *Mov Disord* 2008; 23:837–844.

2. Riedel O, et al. Frequency of dementia, depression, and other neuropsychiatric symptoms in 1,449 outpatients with Parkinson's disease. *J Neurol* 2010; 257:1073–1082.

3. Reijnders JS, et al. A systematic review of prevalence studies of depression in Parkinson's disease. *Mov Disord* 2008; 23:183–189.

4. McDonald WM, et al. Prevalence, etiology, and treatment of depression in Parkinson's disease. *Biol Psychiatry* 2003; 54:363–375.

5. Palhagen SE, et al. Depressive illness in Parkinson's disease–indication of a more advanced and widespread neurodegenerative process? *Acta Neurol Scand* 2008; 117:295–304.

6. Rabinak CA, et al. Dopamine agonist withdrawal syndrome in Parkinson disease. *Arch Neurol* 2010; 67:58–63.

7. Rocha FL, et al. Antidepressants for depression in Parkinson's disease: systematic review and meta-analysis. *J Psychopharmacol* 2013; 27:417–423.

8. Liu J, et al. Comparative efficacy and acceptability of antidepressants in Parkinson's disease: a network meta-analysis. *PLoS One* 2013; 8:e76651.

9. Troeung L, et al. A meta-analysis of randomised placebo-controlled treatment trials for depression and anxiety in Parkinson's disease. *PLoS One* 2013; 8:e79510.

10. Gony M, et al. Risk of serious extrapyramidal symptoms in patients with Parkinson's disease receiving antidepressant drugs: a pharmacoepidemiologic study comparing serotonin reuptake inhibitors and other antidepressant drugs. *Clin Neuropharmacol* 2003; 26:142–145.

11. Kulisevsky J, et al. Motor changes during sertraline treatment in depressed patients with Parkinson's disease*. *Eur J Neurol* 2008; 15:953–959.

12. Richard IH, et al. A randomized, double-blind, placebo-controlled trial of antidepressants in Parkinson disease. *Neurology* 2012; 78:1229–1236.

13. Bonuccelli U, et al. A non-comparative assessment of tolerability and efficacy of duloxetine in the treatment of depressed patients with Parkinson's disease. *Expert Opin Pharmacother* 2012; 13:2269–2280.

14. Serrano-Duenas M. A comparison between low doses of amitriptyline and low doses of fluoxetine used in the control of depression in patients suffering from Parkinson's disease. *Rev Neurol* 2002; 35:1010–1014.

15. Menza M, et al. A controlled trial of antidepressants in patients with Parkinson disease and depression. *Neurology* 2009; 72:886–892.

16. Devos D, et al. Comparison of desipramine and citalopram treatments for depression in Parkinson's disease: a double-blind, randomized, placebo-controlled study. *Mov Disord* 2008; 23:850–857.

17. Antonini A, et al. Randomized study of sertraline and low-dose amitriptyline in patients with Parkinson's disease and depression: effect on quality of life. *Mov Disord* 2006; 21:1119–1122.

18. Goodarzi Z, et al. Guidelines for dementia or Parkinson's disease with depression or anxiety: a systematic review. *BMC Neurol* 2016; 16:244.

19. Zhuo C, et al. Efficacy of antidepressive medication for depression in Parkinson disease: a network meta-analysis. *Medicine (Baltimore)* 2017; 96:e6698.

20. Avila A, et al. Agomelatine for depression in Parkinson disease: additional effect on sleep and motor dysfunction. *J Clin Psychopharmacol* 2015; 35:719–723.

21. De Berardis D, et al. Agomelatine treatment of major depressive disorder in Parkinson's disease: a case series. *J Neuropsychiatry Clin Neurosci* 2013; 25:343–345.

22. Weintraub D, et al. Atomoxetine for depression and other neuropsychiatric symptoms in Parkinson disease. *Neurology* 2010; 75:448–455.

23. Dobkin RD, et al. Cognitive-behavioral therapy for depression in Parkinson's disease: a randomized, controlled trial. *Am J Psychiatry* 2011; 168:1066–1074.

24. Barone P, et al. Pramipexole versus sertraline in the treatment of depression in Parkinson's disease: a national multicenter parallel-group randomized study. *J Neurol* 2006; 253:601–607.

25. Antonini A, et al. A reassessment of risks and benefits of dopamine agonists in Parkinson's disease. *Lancet Neurol* 2009; 8:929–937.

26. Weintraub D, et al. Impulse control disorders in Parkinson disease: a cross-sectional study of 3090 patients. *Arch Neurol* 2010; 67:589–595.

27. Li CT, et al. Pramipexole-induced psychosis in Parkinson's disease. *Psychiatry Clin Neurosci* 2008; 62:245.

28. Figiel GS, et al. ECT-induced delirium in depressed patients with Parkinson's disease. *J Neuropsychiatry Clin Neurosci* 1991; 3:405–411.

29. Friedman JH. Parkinson's disease psychosis 2010: a review article. *Parkinsonism Relat Disord* 2010; 16:553–560.

30. Ismail MS, et al. A reality test: how well do we understand psychosis in Parkinson's disease? *J Neuropsychiatry Clin Neurosci* 2004; 16:8–18.

31. Kiziltan G, et al. Relationship between age and subtypes of psychotic symptoms in Parkinson's disease. *J Neurol* 2007; 254:448–452.

32. Factor SA, et al. Longitudinal outcome of Parkinson's disease patients with psychosis. *Neurology* 2003; 60:1756–1761.

33. Reich SG, et al. Ten most commonly asked questions about the psychiatric aspects of Parkinson's disease. *Neurologist* 2003; 9:50–56.

34. Lin JJ, et al. Genetic polymorphism of the angiotensin converting enzyme and L-dopa-induced adverse effects in Parkinson's disease. *J Neurol Sci* 2007; 252:130–134.

35. Stowe RL, et al. Dopamine agonist therapy in early Parkinson's disease. *Cochrane Database of Sys Rev* 2008:Cd006564.

36. Divac N, et al. The efficacy and safety of antipsychotic medications in the treatment of psychosis in patients with Parkinson's disease. *Behav Neurol* 2016; 2016:4938154.

37. Pintor L, et al. Ziprasidone versus clozapine in the treatment of psychotic symptoms in Parkinson disease: a randomized open clinical trial. *Clin Neuro Pharmacol* 2012; 35:61–66.

38. Prohorov T, et al. The effect of quetiapine in psychotic Parkinsonian patients with and without dementia. An open-labeled study utilizing a structured interview. *J Neurol* 2006; 253:171–175.

39. Weintraub D, et al. Association of antipsychotic use with mortality risk in patients with Parkinson disease. *JAMA Neurology* 2016; 73:535–541.

40. Marti M, et al. Dementia in Parkinson's disease. *J Neurol* 2007; **254 Suppl** 1:41–48.

41. Chung KA, et al. Effects of a central cholinesterase inhibitor on reducing falls in Parkinson disease. *Neurology* 2010; 75:1263–1269.

42. Sawada H, et al. Early use of donepezil against psychosis and cognitive decline in Parkinson's disease: a randomised controlled trial for 2 years. *J Neurol Neurosurg Psychiatry* 2018; 89:1332–1340.

43. Mesquita J, et al. Fatal neuroleptic malignant syndrome induced by clozapine in Parkinson's psychosis. *J Neuropsychiatry Clin Neurosci* 2014; 26:E34.

44. Ziegenbein M, et al. Clozapine-induced aplastic anemia in a patient with Parkinson's disease. *Can J Psychiatry* 2003; 48:352.

45. Factor SA, et al. Combined clozapine and electroconvulsive therapy for the treatment of drug-induced psychosis in Parkinson's disease. *J Neuropsychiatry Clin Neurosci* 1995; 7:304–307.

46. Martin BA. ECT for Parkinson's? *CMAJ* 2003; 168:1391–1392.

47. Sarva H, et al. Evidence for the use of pimavanserin in the treatment of Parkinson's disease psychosis. *Ther Adv Neurol Disord* 2016; 9:462–473.

48. Wilby KJ, et al. Evidence-based review of pharmacotherapy used for Parkinson's disease psychosis. *Ann Pharmacother* 2017; 51:682–695.

49. Iketani R, et al. Efficacy and safety of atypical antipsychotics for psychosis in Parkinson's disease: A systematic review and Bayesian network meta-analysis. *Parkinsonism Relat Disord* 2020; 78:82–90.

50. Iketani R, et al. Comparative utility of atypical antipsychotics for the treatment of psychosis in Parkinson's disease: a systematic review and bayesian network meta-analysis. *Biol Pharm Bull* 2017; 40:1976–1982.

51. Richard IH, et al. Rivastigmine-induced worsening of motor function and mood in a patient with Parkinson's disease. *Mov Disord* 2001; **16 Suppl** 1:33–34.

52. McKeith I, et al. Efficacy of rivastigmine in dementia with Lewy bodies: a randomised, double-blind, placebo-controlled international study. *Lancet* 2000; 356:2031–2036.

53. Emre M, et al. Rivastigmine for dementia associated with Parkinson's disease. *N Engl J Med* 2004; 351:2509–2518.

54. Aarsland D, et al. Donepezil for cognitive impairment in Parkinson's disease: a randomised controlled study. *J Neurol Neurosurg Psychiatry* 2002; 72:708–712.

55. Pagano G, et al. Cholinesterase inhibitors for Parkinson's disease: a systematic review and meta-analysis. *J Neurol Neurosurg Psychiatry* 2015; 86:767–773.

56. Rolinski M, et al. Cholinesterase inhibitors for dementia with Lewy bodies, Parkinson's disease dementia and cognitive impairment in Parkinson's disease. *Cochrane Database Syst Rev* 2012; 3:CD006504.

57. Dubois B, et al. Donepezil in Parkinson's disease dementia: a randomized, double-blind efficacy and safety study. *Mov Disord* 2012; 27:1230–1238.

58. Connolly BS, et al. Pharmacological treatment of Parkinson disease: a review. *JAMA* 2014; 311:1670–1683.

59. Emre M, et al. Memantine for patients with Parkinson's disease dementia or dementia with Lewy bodies: a randomised, double-blind, placebo-controlled trial. *Lancet Neurol* 2010; 9:969–977.

60. Seppi K, et al. The movement disorder society evidence-based medicine review update: treatments for the non-motor symptoms of Parkinson's disease. *Mov Disord* 2011; **26 Suppl** 3:S42–S80.

61. Lertxundi U, et al. Anticholinergic burden in Parkinson's disease inpatients. *Eur J Clin Pharmacol* 2015; 71:1271–1277.

62. Zesiewicz TA, et al. Potential influences of complementary therapy on motor and non-motor complications in Parkinson's disease. *CNS Drugs* 2009; 23:817–835.

63. Postuma RB, et al. Caffeine for treatment of Parkinson disease: a randomized controlled trial. *Neurology* 2012; 79:651–658.

Further reading

Assogna F, et al. Drug choices and advancements for managing depression in Parkinson's disease. *Curr Neuropharmacol* 2020; 18:277–287.

Atrial fibrillation – using psychotropics

Atrial fibrillation (AF) is the most common cardiac arrhythmia. It particularly affects older people but may occur in an important proportion of people under 40. Risk factors include anxiety, obesity, diabetes, hypertension, long-standing aerobic exercise and high alcohol consumption.[1-3] AF itself is not usually life-threatening but stasis of blood in the atria during fibrillation predisposes to clot formation and substantially increases the risk of stroke.[4] The use of warfarin or other oral anticoagulants is therefore essential.[3]

AF can be defined as 'lone' or **paroxysmal** (occurring infrequently, and spontaneously reverting to sinus rhythm), **persistent** (repeated and prolonged (> one week) episodes usually, if temporarily, responsive to treatment) or **permanent** (unresponsive). Risk of stroke is increased in all three conditions.[3]

Treatment may involve DC conversion, rhythm control (usually flecainide, propafenone or amiodarone) or rate control (with diltiazem, verapamil or sotalol). With rhythm control the aim is to maintain sinus rhythm, although this is not always achieved. With rate control, AF is allowed to continue but ventricular response is controlled and ventricles are filled passively. Many people with paroxysmal or persistent AF can be effectively cured of the condition by catheter or cryo-ablation of aberrant electrical pathways,[5,6] now a routine and effective procedure.[7]

AF is commonly encountered in psychiatry not least because of the high rates of obesity, diabetes and alcohol misuse seen in mental health patients. When considering the use of psychotropics several factors need to be taken into account:

- Interactions between psychotropics and anticoagulant therapy (see section on SSRIs and bleeding, Chapter 2)
- Arrhythmogenicity of psychotropics prescribed (AF usually results from cardiovascular disease; drugs affecting cardiac ion channels may increase mortality in these patients, especially those with ischaemic disease[8,9])
- Effect on ventricular rate (some drugs induce reflex tachycardia via postural hypotension, others [clozapine, quetiapine] directly increase heart rate)
- Reported association between individual psychotropics and AF (see the subsequent table)
- Risk of interaction with co-prescribed antiarrhythmics or rate-controlling drugs
- Whether AF is paroxysmal (aim to avoid precipitating AF), persistent (aim to avoid prolonging AF) or permanent (aim to avoid increasing ventricular rate)

Recommendations – psychotropics in AF

Condition	Suggested drugs	Drugs to avoid
Schizophrenia/schizoaffective disorder The condition itself may be associated with an increased risk of AF[10] One case–control study suggested antipsychotics increase risk of AF by 17%[11]	In paroxysmal or persistent AF, **cariprazine, brexpiprazole** or **lurasidone** may be appropriate choices In permanent AF with rate control, drug choice is less crucial but probably best to avoid drugs with potent effects on the ECG (ziprasidone, pimozide, sertindole, etc.) and those which increase heart rate	AF reported with clozapine,[12,13] olanzapine[14,15] aripiprazole[16,17] and paliperidone.[18] Causation not clearly established but avoid use in lone, paroxysmal or persistent AF Avoid QT-prolonging drugs in ischaemic heart disease (see section on QT prolongation) Association of antipsychotics with AF[11] may be linked to metabolic disturbance[19] although some studies suggest no link between antipsychotics and AF[20]
Bipolar disorder	**Valproate** **Lithium** **Carbamazepine**	Mood stabilisers appear not to affect risk of AF Valproate may cause A-V conduction block[21] One case of AF following lithium overdose[22] and one in chronic toxicity[23]
Depression Untreated depression predicts recurrence of AF[24] Presence of AF increases risk of depression and anxiety[25]	**SSRIs** but beware interaction with warfarin and other anticoagulants[26] as severe bleeding risk is increased[27] Animal studies suggest an antiarrhythmic effect for SSRIs[28,29] **Paroxetine** improved paroxysmal AF in a series of non-depressed patients[30] **Venlafaxine** does not directly affect atrial conduction[31] and may cardiovert paroxysmal AF[32] AF incidence falls after starting antidepressant treatment[33,34] No evidence that **agomelatine** affects cardiac conduction or clotting	Avoid tricyclics in coronary disease[35] Tricyclics may provoke AF[36,37] but do not increase risk of haemorrhage when combined with warfarin[26] A database study suggests antidepressants in general do not increase risk of AF[38]
Anxiety disorders (anxiety symptoms increase risk of AF)[39]	**Benzodiazepines** **SSRIs** (see previous sections)	Tricyclics (see previous sections) One case of pregabalin-associated AF[40]
Alzheimer's disease	**Acetylcholinesterase inhibitors** (but beware bradycardic effects in patients with paroxysmal 'vagal' AF (paroxysmal AF provoked by low heart rate)) **Rivastigmine** has least interaction potential **Memantine**	Avoid cholinesterase inhibitors in paroxysmal 'vagal' AF

References

1. Chen LY, et al. Epidemiology of atrial fibrillation: a current perspective. *Heart Rhythm* 2007; 4:S1-S6.

2. Tully PJ, et al. Anxiety, depression, and stress as risk factors for atrial fibrillation after cardiac surgery. *Heart Lung* 2011; 40:4–11.

3. National Institute for Health and Care Excellence. Atrial fibrillation: the management of atrial fibrillation. Clinical Guidance 180 2014; http://www.nice.org.uk/guidance/cg180

4. Lakshminarayan K, et al. Clinical epidemiology of atrial fibrillation and related cerebrovascular events in the United States. *Neurologist* 2008; 14:143–150.

5. Rodgers M, et al. Curative catheter ablation in atrial fibrillation and typical atrial flutter: systematic review and economic evaluation. *Health Technol Assess* 2008; 12:iii-198.

6. Latchamsetty R, et al. Catheter ablation of atrial fibrillation. *Cardiol Clin* 2014; 32:551–561.

7. Saglietto A, et al. Impact of atrial fibrillation catheter ablation on mortality, stroke, and heart failure hospitalizations: A meta-analysis. *J Cardiovasc Electrophysiol* 2020; 31:1040–1047.

8. Investigators TCASTI. Effect of the antiarrhythmic agent moricizine on survival after myocardial infarction. *N Engl J Med* 1992; 327:227–233.

9. Epstein AE, et al. Mortality following ventricular arrhythmia suppression by encainide, flecainide, and moricizine after myocardial infarction. The original design concept of the Cardiac Arrhythmia Suppression Trial (CAST). *JAMA* 1993; 270:2451–2455.

10. Emul M, et al. P wave and QT changes among inpatients with schizophrenia after parenteral ziprasidone administration. *Pharmacol Res* 2009; 60:369–372.

11. Chou RH, et al. Antipsychotic treatment is associated with risk of atrial fibrillation: a nationwide nested case-control study. *Int J Cardiol* 2017; 227:134–140.

12. Cam B, et al. [Clozapine and olanzapine associated atrial fibrillation: a case report]. *Turk Psikiyatri Dergisi = Turkish J Psychiatry* 2015; 26:221–226.

13. Low RA, Jr., et al. Clozapine induced atrial fibrillation. *J Clin Psychopharmacol* 1998; 18:170.

14. Waters BM, et al. Olanzapine-associated new-onset atrial fibrillation. *J Clin Psychopharmacol* 2008; 28:354–355.

15. Yaylaci S, et al. Atrial fibrillation due to olanzapine overdose. *Clin Toxicol (Phila)* 2011; 49:440.

16. D'Urso G, et al. Aripiprazole-induced atrial fibrillation in a patient with concomitant risk factors. *Exp Clin Psychopharmacol* 2018; 26:509–513.

17. Stefatos A, et al. Atrial fibrillation and injected aripiprazole: a case report. *Innov Clin Neurosci* 2018; 15:43–45.

18. Schneider RA, et al. Apparent seizure and atrial fibrillation associated with paliperidone. *Am J Health Syst Pharm* 2008; 65:2122–2125.

19. Zeng J, et al. Metabolic disorder caused by antipsychotic treatment may facilitate the development of atrial fibrillation. *Int J Cardiol* 2017; 239:14.

20. Polcwiartek C, et al. Electrocardiogram characteristics and their association with psychotropic drugs among patients with schizophrenia. *Schizophr Bull* 2020; 46:354–362.

21. Davutoglu V, et al. Valproic acid as a cause of transient atrio-ventricular conduction block episodes. *J Atr Fibrillation* 2017; 9:1520.

22. Kalcik MDM, et al. Acute atrial fibrillation as an unusual form of cardiotoxicity in chronic lithium overdose. *J Atr Fibrillation* 2014; 6:1009.

23. Acharya S, et al. Lithium-induced cardiotoxicity: a rare clinical entity. *Cureus* 2020; 12:e7286.

24. Lange HW, et al. Depressive symptoms predict recurrence of atrial fibrillation after cardioversion. *J Psychosom Res* 2007; 63:509–513.

25. Patel D, et al. A systematic review of depression and anxiety in patients with atrial fibrillation: the mind-heart link. *Cardiovasc Psychiatry Neurol* 2013; 2013:159850.

26. Quinn GR, et al. Effect of selective serotonin reuptake inhibitors on bleeding risk in patients with atrial fibrillation taking warfarin. *Am J Cardiol* 2014; 114:583–586.

27. Komen JJ, et al. Concomitant anticoagulant and antidepressant therapy in atrial fibrillation patients and risk of stroke and bleeding. *Clin Pharmacol Ther* 2020; 107:287–294.

28. Pousti A, et al. Effect of sertraline on ouabain-induced arrhythmia in isolated guinea-pig atria. *Depress Anxiety* 2009; 26:E106-E110.

29. Pousti A, et al. Effect of citalopram on ouabain-induced arrhythmia in isolated guinea-pig atria. *Hum Psychopharmacol* 2003; 18:121–124.

30. Shirayama T, et al. Usefulness of paroxetine in depressed men with paroxysmal atrial fibrillation. *Am J Cardiol* 2006; 97:1749–1751.

31. Emul M, et al. The influences of depression and venlafaxine use at therapeutic doses on atrial conduction. *J Psychopharmacol* 2009; 23:163–167.

32. Finch SJ, et al. Cardioversion of persistent atrial arrhythmia after treatment with venlafaxine in successful management of major depression and posttraumatic stress disorder. *Psychosomatics* 2006; 47:533–536.

33. Andrade C. Antidepressants and atrial fibrillation: the importance of resourceful statistical approaches to address confounding by indication. *J Clin Psychiatry* 2019; 80:19f12729.

34. Fenger-Grøn M, et al. Depression, antidepressants, and the risk of non-valvular atrial fibrillation: a nationwide Danish matched cohort study. *Eur J Prev Cardiol* 2019; 26:187–195.

35. Taylor D. Antidepressant drugs and cardiovascular pathology: a clinical overview of effectiveness and safety. *Acta Psychiatr Scand* 2008; 118:434–442.

36. Moorehead CN, et al. Imipramine-induced auricular fibrillation. *Am J Psychiatry* 1965; 122:216–217.

37. Rosen BH. Case report of auricular fibrillation following the use of imipramine (Tofranil). *J Mt Sinai Hosp NY* 1960; 27:609–611.

38. Lapi F, et al. The use of antidepressants and the risk of chronic atrial fibrillation. *J Clin Pharmacol* 2015; 55:423–430.

39. Eaker ED, et al. Tension and anxiety and the prediction of the 10-year incidence of coronary heart disease, atrial fibrillation, and total mortality: the Framingham Offspring Study. *Psychosom Med* 2005; 67:692–696.

40. Chilkoti G, et al. Could pregabalin premedication predispose to perioperative atrial fibrillation in patients with sepsis? *Saudi J Anaesth* 2014; 8:S115–116.

Psychotropics in bariatric surgery

Psychiatric illness is relatively common in patients who have undergone bariatric surgery.[1] Over one-third of those seeking bariatric surgery are prescribed psychotropics.[2] Bariatric surgery can be associated with clinically important changes in drug pharmacokinetics, although it is difficult to predict how psychotropics will be affected because of interindividual differences and limited data. Current research supports the need for close treatment monitoring and the ongoing monitoring of symptoms after bariatric surgery.[3]

Surgical procedures can be classified as:

- **Predominantly restrictive:** sleeve gastrectomy and gastric banding
- **Predominantly malabsorptive:** biliopancreatic diversion and jejunoileal bypass
- **Mixed restrictive/malabsorptive:** Roux-en-Y gastric bypass (RYGB) and gastric reduction duodenal switch (GDRS)

Malabsorptive procedures (including RYGB and GRDS) have a relatively greater potential to alter drug absorption. Most data are derived from studies of patients undergoing RYGB. It is not clear how these data relate to the consequences of other procedures.

Pharmacokinetic changes following bariatric surgery

All procedures may alter the following:

- Tablet disintegration and dissolution times via changes in gastric pH and mixing
- Rate of absorption via changes in the gastric emptying rate
- Drug distribution via loss of adipose tissue (especially lipid soluble drugs) and altered protein binding
- Drug metabolism owing to improvements in hepatic function after weight loss
- Drug excretion via changes in renal function after weight loss

Malabsorptive surgical procedures may further lead to the following:

- Decreased area for drug absorption (reduced functional intestinal length)
- Altered lipophilic drug solubilisation (bypassing proximal small intestine bile salts)
- Reduced intestinal wall drug metabolism via decreased intestinal length

Drug formulations

Any drug formulation that prolongs drug disintegration and dissolution can potentially impair drug absorption following bariatric surgery.[4] Switching to immediate-release formulations before surgery is generally recommended[4,5] (based more on expert consensus rather than any objective data[6]). Orodispersible and liquid preparations do not go through a disintegration phase, and may be preferred if reduced absorption from solid tablets is suspected.[7] Very large tablets (e.g. over 10mm in diameter) should be avoided as passage may be impeded by restrictive procedures.

Drugs

Antidepressants

Table 10.10 Antidepressants in bariatric surgery

Drug	Specific evidence and considerations
SSRIs[8–13]	■ Evidence demonstrates that plasma levels may be significantly reduced following RYGB ■ Malabsorption has been implicated in cases of discontinuation symptoms and loss of efficacy
SNRIs[10,14]	■ Duloxetine levels 42% lower after RYGB compared with matched controls ■ The absorption of venlafaxine MR capsules seems not to be altered by RYGB[15]
Mirtazapine[16,17]	■ Increased appetite and weight gain are possible ■ Has been used successfully for non-mechanical vomiting after RYGB
TCAs[18,19]	■ Single case report suggests therapeutic plasma levels can be achieved within usual dose range after RYGB ■ Plasma levels may be increased after significant weight loss; consider monitoring levels and reducing dose

General summary
- Antidepressants are the best studied psychotropics in the bariatric population. Current evidence suggests that antidepressant absorption is reduced after surgery (though studies are mostly limited to SSRIs after RYGB).
- Signs of reduced absorption may include the rapid development of discontinuation symptoms and later loss of efficacy.
- Patients require close monitoring as those at risk of reduced absorption cannot be reliably predicted.
- The risk of gastric bleeds with bariatric surgery will probably be increased by serotonergic antidepressants

Antipsychotics

Table 10.11 Antipsychotics in bariatric surgery

Drug	Specific evidence and considerations
Asenapine[20]	■ Primarily absorbed via oral mucosa; problems after bariatric surgery are not expected ■ One case report of successful use after RYGB
Cariprazine	■ No data available on absorption after bariatric surgery; follow general recommendations.
Clozapine[21–23]	■ Two case reports of relapse after RYGB[24] ■ Take drug plasma levels before surgery and regularly monitor after ■ Constipation is common after surgery; the manufacturer recommends close monitoring and active treatment ■ Check smoking status (quitting before surgery is encouraged); adjust dose accordingly
Haloperidol[25]	■ Single case report suggests levels after RYGB are similar to those generally reported in the literature

(Continued)

Table 10.11 (*Continued*)

Drug	Specific evidence and considerations
Lurasidone	■ Risk of reduced absorption with reduced/inconsistent calorific intake perioperatively; must be taken with food for absorption (350kcal) ■ One case report of relapse following GRDS; significant reduction in bioavailability and peak serum concentration[26] ■ One case report post-RYGB showed significant reduction in plasma concentration with no worsening of psychotic symptoms[27] ■ Consider switching to alternatives before surgery
Olanzapine[28,29]	■ Evidence of weight gain post-bariatric surgery[26] ■ Conflicting information on site of absorption; follow general recommendations
Quetiapine[7,28]	■ May be absorbed via the stomach and duodenum; monitor mental state ■ Switching to immediate-release preparation and dividing doses ≥300mg has been recommended
Risperidone[30]	■ Consider switching stable patients to an equivalent dose of paliperidone long acting injection ■ Risperidone LAI has been used successfully when oral treatment was not tolerated after bariatric surgery
Ziprasidone[31]	■ Must be taken with food for absorption (500kcal); risk of reduced absorption with reduced/inconsistent calorific intake perioperatively. Consider switching to alternatives before surgery

General summary

■ Antipsychotics are not well studied in bariatric surgery; data are limited to case reports or theoretical concerns
■ Depot antipsychotics avoid the risk of reduced absorption after surgery. Given the limited data on pharmacokinetic changes after surgery and interindividual variability, routinely switching to depot antipsychotics before surgery may not be justified.[7] However, depot preparations remain an option for those stabilised on treatment available as a depot or in patients demonstrating signs of reduced bioavailability after surgery
■ Bariatric surgery may contribute additional cardiac stressors to patients with QT-prolongation;[32] ECG monitoring before surgery is recommended

Mood stabilisers

Table 10.12 Mood stabilisers in bariatric surgery

Drug	Summary of evidence and considerations
Carbamazepine[33]	■ Single case report of agranulocytosis possibly related to increased plasma levels after sleeve gastrectomy
Lamotrigine[28]	■ Possibly absorbed from the stomach and proximal small intestine; monitor for loss of efficacy
Lithium[34–40] (see below)	■ Cases of lithium toxicity following RYGB and sleeve gastrectomy have been reported ■ Switch an equivalent dose of lithium citrate solution ■ In the preoperative period, plasma levels may be affected by prescribed dietary changes ■ In the postoperative period, plasma levels may be affected by malabsorption (mainly absorbed via small intestine), fluid shifts and weight-loss (lithium clearance increased in obesity)

(Continued)

Table 10.12 (*Continued*)

Drug	Summary of evidence and considerations
Valproate[7,34]	▪ Single case report suggests that absorption may be significantly reduced after malabsorptive procedures; no data on restrictive procedures ▪ Dose reductions may be necessary after weight loss (plasma levels related to bodyweight) ▪ Switch to liquid preparation before surgery or if malabsorption suspected on controlled release/enteric coated tablets ▪ Baseline plasma valproate levels, FBC and LFTs with ongoing monitoring recommended ▪ Monitor for clinical signs of poor tolerability, possibly occurring at normal plasma levels

FBC, full blood count; LFT, liver function test; RYGB, Roux-en-Y gastric bypass.

General summary
▪ The literature on mood stabilisers after bariatric surgery is limited to a few case reports; the use of lithium requires particular care owing to its narrow therapeutic index.
▪ The absorption of oral contraceptives may be reduced after bariatric surgery.[41] In patients prescribed teratogenic mood stabilisers, non-oral methods of contraception are recommended.

Lithium around the time of bariatric surgery

The continued use of lithium throughout the perioperative phases of bariatric surgery requires particularly close monitoring. The following guidance is based on available case reports and expert opinion:[40]

▪ Monitor lithium plasma levels weekly in during pre-operative phase and for 6 weeks post-surgery (as fluid intake gradually increases), 2-weekly for 6 months and monthly thereafter. Resume usual lithium monitoring 1 year post-bariatric surgery.
▪ If plasma levels increase by >25% or approach 1.2mmol/L, consider decreasing lithium dose.
▪ Withhold lithium if signs of toxicity are present and review dose.
▪ Monitor mental state periodically, using formal rating scales if possible.
▪ Encourage patient to drink 2.5–3 litres of fluid per day in the pre-operative phase (including liquid meal replacement).

Other drugs

Table 10.13 Miscellaneous agents in bariatric surgery

Drug	Summary of evidence and considerations
Benzodiazepines[42–45]	▪ Bioavailability probably unaffected, shorter time to peak concentration
Methadone[46]	▪ Substantial increase in bioavailability after sleeve gastrectomy in one case report, possibly related increased rate of gastric emptying; consider plasma level and QT monitoring
Methylphenidate[47,48]	▪ Conflicting limited data; one case report of reduced treatment efficacy after RYGB that resolved after switching to transdermal patch suggesting reduced oral bioavailability; another reports signs of toxicity

General recommendations

Box 10.4 General recommendations for prescribing in bariatric surgery[7]

Before surgery	**After surgery (0–6 weeks)**	**After surgery (>6 weeks after)**
■ Do not routinely increase doses; clinically relevant malabsorption cannot be reliably predicted ■ Assess mental state before surgery and consider measuring baseline drug plasma levels ■ Switch modified-release/enteric coated preparations to immediate-release tablets or to liquid preparations	■ Closely monitor for signs of adverse effects and drug malabsorption (symptom re-emergence, discontinuation symptoms) ■ Regularly monitor drug plasma levels if clinically indicated ■ If malabsorption suspected consider the recommended strategies. ■ If medication toxicity suspected withhold and reassess dose	■ Continue regular monitoring for the first year postoperatively, although frequency can be reduced if stable ■ Monitor for an increase in adverse effects, especially if doses were increased in the acute post-operative period ■ Consider returning to presurgical treatment regimen after 1 year (depending on clinical history)

General management strategies for patients demonstrating signs of reduced bioavailability

■ Consider non-oral routes of administration where available (e.g. depots for patients stable on antipsychotics)
■ Dividing doses may improve malabsorption related to a reduced stomach capacity after surgery
■ Switching modified/prolonged/delayed-release to immediate-release formulations
■ Switching solid tablets to liquid or orodispersible preparations to bypass disintegration phase
■ Switching large tablets to smaller ones
■ In cases where doses have been increased to account for reduced bioavailability, monitor for emergent adverse effects as bioavailability may normalise over time.

Psychotropics with a risk of weight gain after bariatric surgery

It is estimated that 10–20% of patients regain a significant amount of weight after bariatric surgery.[49] There is no information on how psychotropics associated with weight gain affect outcomes after surgery, but high-risk drugs should probably be avoided. Patients' individual clinical circumstances should be considered (especially if stable on treatment and at a high risk of relapse) as there is evidence that uncontrolled mental illness is a risk factor for weight regain.[49]

Alcohol[50,51]

Gastric bypass surgery is associated with accelerated alcohol absorption, higher maximum alcohol concentrations and a longer time to elimination. There is also an increased risk of alcohol misuse disorders after gastric bypass. Data are less clear for sleeve gastrectomy and there is no evidence that gastric banding leads to any changes.

Wider considerations[52]

In practice, many patients may not require significant changes to drug treatment after surgery. Relapse of symptoms after surgery may not be related to altered drug pharmacokinetics. Although improvements in mental health are to be anticipated, deterioration can also occur due to a range of factors, including unmet weight-loss expectations, poor tolerability and dissatisfaction after surgical treatment.

References

1. Dawes AJ, et al. Mental health conditions among patients seeking and undergoing bariatric surgery: a meta-analysis. *JAMA* 2016; **315**:150–163.

2. Hawkins M, et al. Psychiatric medication use and weight outcomes one year after bariatric surgery. *Psychosomatics* 2020; **61**:56–63.

3. Gondek W. Psychiatric suitability assessment for bariatric surgery. In S Sockalingam, R Hawa, eds. *Psychiatric care in severe obesity: an interdisciplinary guide to integrated care.* Cham: Springer International Publishing 2017:173–186.

4. Padwal R, et al. A systematic review of drug absorption following bariatric surgery and its theoretical implications. *Obesity Rev Official J Int Assoc Study Obesity* 2010; **11**:41–50.

5. Macgregor AM, et al. Drug distribution in obesity and following bariatric surgery: a literature review. *Obes Surg* 1996; **6**:17–27.

6. Roerig JL, et al. Psychopharmacology and bariatric surgery. *Eur Eating Disord Rev* 2015; **23**:463–469.

7. Bingham KS, et al. Psychopharmacology in bariatric surgery patients. in S Sockalingam, R Hawa, eds. *Psychiatric care in severe obesity: an interdisciplinary guide to integrated care.* Cham: Springer International Publishing 2017:313–333.

8. Faye E, et al. Antidepressant agents in short bowel syndrome. *Clin Ther* 2014; **36**:2029–2033.e2023.

9. Marzinke MA, et al. Decreased escitalopram concentrations post-Roux-en-Y gastric bypass surgery. *Ther Drug Monit* 2015; **37**:408–412.

10. Hamad GG, et al. The effect of gastric bypass on the pharmacokinetics of serotonin reuptake inhibitors. *Am J Psychiatry* 2012; **169**:256–263.

11. Seaman JS, et al. Dissolution of common psychiatric medications in a Roux-en-Y gastric bypass model. *Psychosomatics* 2005; **46**:250–253.

12. Bingham K, et al. SSRI discontinuation syndrome following bariatric surgery: a case report and focused literature review. *Psychosomatics* 2014; **55**:692–697.

13. Roerig JL, et al. Preliminary comparison of sertraline levels in postbariatric surgery patients versus matched nonsurgical cohort. *Surg Obesity Relat Dis Official J Am Soc Bariatric Surgery* 2012; **8**:62–66.

14. Roerig JL, et al. A comparison of duloxetine plasma levels in postbariatric surgery patients versus matched nonsurgical control subjects. *J Clin Psychopharmacol* 2013; **33**:479–484.

15. Krieger CA, et al. Comparison of bioavailability of single-dose extended-release venlafaxine capsules in obese patients before and after gastric bypass surgery. *Pharmacotherapy* 2017; **37**:1374–1382.

16. Teixeira FV, et al. Mirtazapine (Remeron) as treatment for non-mechanical vomiting after gastric bypass. *Obes Surg* 2005; **15**:707–709.

17. Huerta S, et al. Intractable nausea and vomiting following Roux-en-Y gastric bypass: role of mirtazapine. *Obes Surg* 2006; **16**:1399.

18. Broyles JE, et al. Nortriptyline absorption in short bowel syndrome. *JPEN J Parenter Enteral Nutr* 1990; **14**:326–327.

19. Jobson K, et al. Weight loss and a concomitant change in plasma tricyclic levels. *Am J Psychiatry* 1978; **135**:237–238.

20. Tabaac BJ, et al. Pica patient, status post gastric bypass, improves with change in medication regimen. *Ther Adv Psychopharmacol* 2015; **5**:38–42.

21. Kaltsounis J, et al. Intravenous valproate treatment of severe manic symptoms after gastric bypass surgery: a case report. *Psychosomatics* 2000; **41**:454–456.

22. Afshar S, et al. The effects of bariatric procedures on bowel habit. *Obes Surg* 2016; **26**:2348–2354.

23. Mylan Products Ltd. Summary of product characteristics. Clozaril 25mg and 100mg Tablets. 2020; https://www.medicines.org.uk/emc/medicine/32564 .

24. Mahgoub Y, et al. Schizoaffective exacerbation in a Roux-en-Y gastric bypass patient maintained on clozapine. *Prim Care Companion CNS Disord* 2019; **21**:19l02462.

25. Fuller AK, et al. Haloperidol pharmacokinetics following gastric bypass surgery. *J Clin Psychopharmacol* 1986; **6**:376–378.

26. Ward HB, et al. Lurasidone malabsorption following bariatric surgery: a case report. *J Psychiatr Pract* 2019; **25**:313–317.

27. McGrane IR, et al. Roux-en-Y gastric bypass and antipsychotic therapeutic drug monitoring: two cases. *J Pharm Pract* 2020:[Epub ahead of print].

28. Miller AD, et al. Medication and nutrient administration considerations after bariatric surgery. *Am J Health-Syst Pharm AJHP Official J Am Soc Health-Syst Pharm* 2006; **63**:1852–1857.

29. Tran PV, et al. *Olanzapine (Zyprexa): a novel antipsychotic.* Philadelphia: Lippincott Williams & Wilkins 2001.

30. Brietzke E, et al. Long-acting injectable risperidone in a bipolar patient submitted to bariatric surgery and intolerant to conventional mood stabilizers. *Psychiatry Clin Neurosci* 2011; **65**:205–205.

31. Gandelman K, et al. The impact of calories and fat content of meals on oral ziprasidone absorption: a randomized, open-label, crossover trial. *J Clin Psychiatry* 2009; **70**:58–62.

32. Woodard G, et al. Cardiac arrest during laparoscopic Roux-en-Y gastric bypass in a bariatric patient with drug-associated long QT syndrome. *Obes Surg* 2011; **21**:134–137.

33. Koutsavlis I, et al. Dose-dependent carbamazepine-induced agranulocytosis following bariatric surgery (sleeve gastrectomy): a possible mechanism. *Bariatric Surg Pract Patient Care* 2015; **10**:130–134.

34. Dahan A, et al. Lithium toxicity with severe bradycardia post sleeve gastrectomy: a case report and review of the literature. *Obes Surg* 2019; **29**:735–738.

35. Lin YH, et al. Lithium toxicity with prolonged neurologic sequelae following sleeve gastrectomy: a case report and review of literature. *Medicine (Baltimore)* 2020; **99**:e21122.

36. Tripp AC. Lithium toxicity after Roux-en-Y gastric bypass surgery. *J Clin Psychopharmacol* 2011; **31**:261–262.

37. Musfeldt D, et al. Lithium toxicity after Roux-en-Y bariatric surgery. *BMJ Case Rep* 2016; **2016**:bcr2015214056.

38. Walsh K, et al. Lithium toxicity following Roux-en-Y gastric bypass. *Bariatric Surg Pract Patient Care* 2014; **9**:77–80.

39. Alam A, et al. Lithium toxicity following vertical sleeve gastrectomy: a case report. *Clin Psychopharmacol Neurosci* 2016; **14**:318–320.

40. Bingham KS, et al. Perioperative lithium use in bariatric surgery: a case series and literature review. *Psychosomatics* 2016; **57**:638–644.

41. Merhi ZO. Challenging oral contraception after weight loss by bariatric surgery. *Gynecol Obstet Invest* 2007; **64**:100–102.

42. Tandra S, et al. Pharmacokinetic and pharmacodynamic alterations in the Roux-en-Y gastric bypass recipients. *Ann Surg* 2013; **258**:262–269.

43. Chan LN, et al. Proximal Roux-en-Y gastric bypass alters drug absorption pattern but not systemic exposure of CYP3A4 and P-glycoprotein substrates. *Pharmacotherapy* 2015; **35**:361–369.

44. Brill MJ, et al. The Pharmacokinetics of the CYP3A substrate midazolam in morbidly obese patients before and one year after bariatric surgery. *Pharm Res* 2015; **32**:3927–3936.

45. Ochs HR, et al. Diazepam absorption: effects of age, sex, and Billroth gastrectomy. *Dig Dis Sci* 1982; **27**:225–230.

46. Strømmen M, et al. Bioavailability of methadone after sleeve gastrectomy: a planned case observation. *Clin Ther* 2016; **38**:1532–1536.

47. Azran C, et al. Impaired oral absorption of methylphenidate after Roux-en-Y gastric bypass. *Surg Obes Relat Dis* 2017; **13**:1245–1247.

48. Ludvigsson M, et al. Methylphenidate toxicity after Roux-en-Y gastric bypass. *Surg Obesity Relat Dis* 2016; **12**:e55-e57.

49. Karmali S, et al. Weight recidivism post-bariatric surgery: a systematic review. *Obes Surg* 2013; **23**:1922–1933.

50. Ivezaj V, et al. Changes in alcohol use after metabolic and bariatric surgery: predictors and mechanisms. *Curr Psychiatry Rep* 2019; **21**:85.

51. Parikh M, et al. ASMBS position statement on alcohol use before and after bariatric surgery. *Surg Obesity Relat Dis* 2016; **12**:225–230.

52. Stevens T, et al. Your patient and weight-loss surgery. *Adv Psychiatric Treatment* 2012; **18**:418–425.

Prescribing in patients with psychiatric illness at the end of life

Generally, prescribing in patients with psychiatric illness who are approaching end of life should follow the principles of good prescribing practice in palliative care.[1] This includes reviewing the appropriateness of a drug, its dose and potential for its discontinuation. Furthermore, if swallowing becomes impaired, it includes making adjustments, such as the use of liquid preparations or parenteral administration.

There is a lack of specific guidance around long-term psychiatric medications in this setting to support clinicians. This adds to reluctance, particularly by generalists, to adjust or stop such drugs.[2,3] This suggests there is scope for improved liaison between non-psychiatry and psychiatry services.

Physical deterioration may impact on factors (e.g. reducing smoking, drinking less fluid) which in turn alter a drug's pharmacokinetics and/or pharmacodynamics, making ongoing review important. Furthermore, polypharmacy is common, increasing the risk of drug–drug interaction and toxicity, for example, tramadol and SSRI antidepressants leading to serotonin toxicity.

Depression is common[4] but often not recognised at the end of life.[5] This is important, given that antidepressants may be beneficial even when prognosis is short.[6] Mirtazapine and citalopram are most strongly supported for use in this population.[7] Psychostimulants such as modafinil may reduce symptoms of depression in the short term, but there is less evidence for sustained effectiveness.[8]

There is a lack of evidence to guide drug management of anxiety at the end of life.[9,10] Non-drug approaches have a stronger evidence base for effectiveness.[11]

Though commonly used for management of delirium, evidence of effectiveness of antipsychotics is mixed. Nonetheless, national guidelines support their use for very distressed patients or those for whom other approaches have been unsuccessful.[12]

Table 10.14 Examples of drugs prescribed in psychiatry which are also used for symptom management in palliative care[1]

Symptom	Example drugs
Neuropathic pain	Amitriptyline
	Imipramine
	Duloxetine
	Gabapentin/pregabalin
	Clonazepam
Nausea and vomiting	Haloperidol
	Olanzapine
	Lorazepam
Anorexia	Mirtazapine
Skeletal muscle spasm	Diazepam

(*Continued*)

Table 10.14 (Continued)

Symptom	Example drugs
Terminal agitation	Benzodiazepines, for example, midazolam
	Antipsychotics, for example, haloperidol
Overactive bladder symptoms	Amitriptyline
	Duloxetine
Drooling	Amitriptyline
Intractable hiccups	Haloperidol
Pathological laughter or crying	Citalopram
	Sertraline
Sweating	Amitriptyline

References

1. Wilcock A, et al. *PCF7 Palliative Care Formulary*. 7th Edition. Nottingham Palliativedrugs.com Ltd; 2020.
2. Anderson K, et al. Prescriber barriers and enablers to minimising potentially inappropriate medications in adults: a systematic review and thematic synthesis. *BMJ Open* 2014; 4:e006544.
3. Garfinkel D, et al. Inappropriate medication use and polypharmacy in end-stage cancer patients: isn't it the family doctor's role to de-prescribe much earlier? *Int J Clin Pract* 2018; 72:e13061.
4. Rayner L, et al. The clinical epidemiology of depression in palliative care and the predictive value of somatic symptoms: cross-sectional survey with four-week follow-up. *Palliat Med* 2011; 25:229–241.
5. Stiefel F, et al. Depression in palliative care: a pragmatic report from the Expert Working Group of the European Association for Palliative Care. *Support Care Cancer* 2001; 9:477–488.
6. Rayner L, et al. Antidepressants for the treatment of depression in palliative care: systematic review and meta-analysis. *Palliat Med* 2011; 25:36–51.
7. Rayner L, et al. Expert opinion on detecting and treating depression in palliative care: A Delphi study. *BMC Palliat Care* 2011; 10:10.
8. Candy M, et al. Psychostimulants for depression. *Cochrane Database Syst Rev* 2008:Cd006722.
9. Salt S, et al. Drug therapy for symptoms associated with anxiety in adult palliative care patients. *Cochrane Database Syst Rev* 2017; 5:Cd004596.
10. Atkin N, et al. 'Worried to death': the assessment and management of anxiety in patients with advanced life-limiting disease, a national survey of palliative medicine physicians. *BMC Palliat Care* 2017; 16:69.
11. Moorey S, et al. A cluster randomized controlled trial of cognitive behaviour therapy for common mental disorders in patients with advanced cancer. *Psychol Med* 2009; 39:713–723.
12. National Institute for Clinical Excellence. NG31: care of dying adults in the last days of life. 2015; https://www.nice.org.uk/guidance/NG31.

Part 4

Other aspects of psychotropic drug use

Chapter 11

Pharmacokinetics

Plasma level monitoring of psychotropic drugs

Plasma drug concentration or plasma 'level' monitoring is a process often subject to some confusion and misunderstanding. Drug level monitoring, when appropriately used, is of considerable help in optimising treatment and assuring adherence. However, in psychiatry, as in other areas of medicine, plasma level determinations are frequently undertaken without good cause and results acted upon inappropriately.[1] In other instances, therapeutic drug monitoring is underused.

Before taking a blood sample for plasma concentration assay, make sure that the following criteria are satisfied:

- **Is there a clinically useful assay method available?**
  Only a minority of drugs have available assays. The assay must be clinically validated and results available within a clinically useful timescale. Check with your local laboratory.
- **Is the drug at 'steady state'?**
  Plasma levels are usually meaningful only when samples are taken after steady-state levels have been achieved. This takes four to five drug half-lives. A clear exception to this advice is suspected overdose; in such situations attainment of steady state is of no relevance. Another exception is when using blood concentrations to guide titration (e.g. with clozapine).
- **Is the timing of the sample correct?**
  Sampling time is vitally important for many but not all drugs. If the recommended sampling time is, say, 12 hours post-dose, then the sample should be taken 11–13 hours post-dose if possible; 10–14 hours post-dose, if absolutely necessary. A study of clozapine samples taken 1 and 2 hours before and after the 12-hour scheduled sample time showed a mean variation of clozapine blood concentration of less than 10%, but some individuals' levels varied by over 50%.[2] So, if a sample is not taken within 1–2 hours of the required time, it has the potential to

The Maudsley® Prescribing Guidelines in Psychiatry, Fourteenth Edition. David M. Taylor, Thomas R. E. Barnes and Allan H. Young.
© 2021 David M. Taylor. Published 2021 by John Wiley & Sons Ltd.

mislead rather than inform. Always try to take samples as close to the scheduled time as possible. Obviously, if toxicity is suspected, take a sample straightaway, ignoring any scheduled timings.

For trough or 'pre-dose' samples, take the blood sample immediately before the next dose is due. Do not, under any circumstances, withhold the next dose for more than 1 or (possibly) 2 hours until the sample is taken. Withholding for longer than this will inevitably give a misleading result (it will give a lower result than that ever seen in the usual, regular dosing), and this may lead to an inappropriate dose increase. Sampling time is less critical with drugs with a long half-life (e.g. olanzapine, aripiprazole) but, as an absolute minimum, prescribers should always record the time of sampling and time of last dose. This cannot be emphasised enough.

- **Will the level have any inherent meaning?**

  Is there a target range of plasma levels? If so, then plasma levels (from samples taken at the right time) will usefully guide dosing. If there is not an accepted target range, plasma levels can only indicate adherence or potential toxicity. However, if the sample is being used to check compliance, then bear in mind that a plasma level of zero indicates only that the drug has not been taken in the past several days. Plasma levels above zero may indicate erratic compliance, full compliance or even long-standing non-compliance disguised by recent taking of prescribed doses. Note also that target ranges have their limitations: patients may respond to lower levels than the quoted range and tolerate levels above the range; also, ranges quoted by different laboratories vary sometimes widely, often without explanation.

- **Is there a clear reason for plasma level determination?**

  Only the following reasons are valid:
  - to confirm compliance (but see above)
  - if toxicity is suspected
  - if a pharmacokinetic drug interaction is suspected
  - if clinical response is difficult to assess directly (and where a target range of plasma levels has been established)
  - if the drug has a narrow therapeutic index and toxicity concerns are considerable.

Interpreting sample results

The basic rule for sample level interpretation is to act upon assay results only in conjunction with reliable clinical observation (*treat the patient, not the level*). For example, if a patient is responding adequately to a drug but has a plasma level below the accepted target range, then the dose should not normally be increased. If a patient has intolerable adverse effects but a plasma level within the target range, then a dose decrease may be appropriate.

Where a plasma level result is substantially different from previous results, a repeat sample is usually advised. Check dose, timing of dose and recent compliance but ensure, in particular, the correct timing of the sample, or at least that the timing of sampling is known. Many anomalous results are the consequence of changes in sample timing.

A word about target ranges

In psychiatry, target ranges for psychotropic drug concentrations should be treated with some caution. Establishing a range of concentrations associated with response is made difficult by the presence in trials of non-responders (who show no response whatever the blood concentration) and by the presence of placebo responders and spontaneous remitters (who respond at any blood concentration). Establishing a target range based on adverse effects is made difficult by the development of tolerance over time. Thus, most studies aimed at determining target ranges have as much 'noise' as 'signal' and results ultimately represent broad approximations.

Interestingly, drug concentrations associated with response in clinical practice show a fairly close correlation to published target ranges.[3] The lower quartile (25th percentile) of drug concentrations is usually close to the lower end of the target range and the upper quartile (75th percentile) is around the value of, but usually less than, the upper limit. Broadly speaking, this means that around 25% of patients respond below the target range and up to 25% tolerate blood concentrations above the target range (Table 11.1).

Table 11.1 Interpreting sample results for drugs with established target ranges

Drug	Target range	Sample timing	Time to steady state	Comments
Amisulpride	**200–320µg/L** 20–60µg/L (elderly)	Trough	3 days	See text.
Aripiprazole	**150–210µg/L**	Trough	15–16 days	See text.
Carbamazepine[4-6]	**>7mg/L** Bipolar disorder	Trough	2 weeks	Carbamazepine induces its own metabolism. Time to steady state dependent on auto-induction.
Clozapine	**350–600µg/L**	Trough	2–3 days	See text.
Lamotrigine[7-9]	Not established but suggest **2.5–15mg/L**	Trough	5 days Auto-induction is thought to occur, so time to steady state may be longer	Some debate over utility of lamotrigine levels, especially in bipolar disorder. In treatment resistant unipolar depression, plasma levels of above 12.7µmol/L (3.3mg/L) are associated with response.[10,11] Toxicity may be increased above 15mg/L but normally well tolerated.

(Continued)

Table 11.1 (*Continued*)

Drug	Target range	Sample timing	Time to steady state	Comments
Lithium[12–16]	**0.6–1.0mmol/L** (0.4mmol may be sufficient for some patients/indications; >1.0mmol/L required for mania)	12 hours	5 days Post-dose	Well-established target range, albeit derived from ancient data sources. A fairly recent study[17] suggested 0.6mmol/L was the minimum level for a prophylactic effect.
Olanzapine	**20–40µg/L**	12 hours	1 week	See text.
Paliperidone[18]	**20–60µg/L** (9-OH risperidone)	Trough	2–3 days oral 2 months depot	Target range is the same as that established for risperidone.[19] As with risperidone, routine plasma level monitoring is not recommended.
Phenytoin[5]	**10–20mg/L**	Trough	Variable	Follows zero-order kinetics. Free levels may be useful in some circumstances.
Quetiapine	Around **50–100µg/L?**	Trough?	2–3 days oral	Target range poorly defined. Plasma level monitoring not recommended. See text.
Risperidone	**20–60µg/L** (active moiety – risperidone + 9-OH risperidone)	Trough	**2–3 days oral** 6–8 weeks injection	Routine plasma level monitoring is not recommended. See text.
Tricyclics[20]	Nortriptyline **50–150µg/L** Amitriptyline **100–200µg/L**	Trough	2–3 days	Rarely used and of dubious benefit. Use ECG to assess toxicity.
Valproate[4,5,21–23]	**50–100mg/L** Epilepsy and bipolar	Trough	2–3 days	Some doubt over value of levels in epilepsy and in bipolar disorder. Some evidence that, in mania, levels up to 125mg/L are tolerated and more effective than lower concentrations. Valproate plasma levels are linearly related to plasma ammonia.[24]

Amisulpride

Amisulpride plasma levels are closely related to dose with insufficient variation to make routine plasma level monitoring prudent. Higher levels observed in women[25-27] seem to have little significant clinical implication for either therapeutic response or adverse effects. A (trough) threshold for clinical response has been suggested to be approximately 100µg/L[28] and mean levels of 367µg/L[27] have been noted in responders in individual studies. Adverse effects (notably EPS) have been observed at mean levels of 336µg/L,[25] 377µg/L[28] and 395µg/L.[26] A plasma level threshold of below 320µg/L has been found to predict avoidance of EPS.[28] One review[29] has suggested an approximate range of **200–320µg/L** for optimal clinical response and avoidance of adverse effects but a more recent consensus statement[30] suggested a target range of **100–320µg/L**. A dose of 200mg a day is sufficient to give a blood level of 100µg/L[31] so this lower threshold is probably too low for a reliable therapeutic effect. In older patients with psychosis, studies suggest plasma concentrations of **20–60µg/L** may give optimal D_2 occupancy and clinical response.[32,33]

In practice, only a minority of treated patients have 'therapeutic' plasma levels (probably because of poor adherence[34]) so plasma monitoring may be of some benefit. However, amisulpride plasma level monitoring is rarely undertaken and few laboratories offer amisulpride assays. The dose–response relationship is sufficiently robust (in trials, at least) to obviate the need for plasma sampling within the licensed dose range (although note that in older patients doses of 50–100mg a day may be sufficient) and adverse effects are usually well managed by dose adjustment alone. Plasma level monitoring is best reserved for those in whom clinical response is poor, adherence is questioned or in whom drug interactions or physical illness may make adverse effect more likely.

Aripiprazole

Plasma level monitoring of aripiprazole is sometimes undertaken in practice. The dose–response relationship for aripiprazole is well established with a plateau in clinical response and D_2 dopamine occupancy seen in doses above approximately 10mg/day.[35] Plasma levels of aripiprazole, its metabolite, and the total moiety (parent plus metabolite) strongly relate linearly to dose, making it possible to predict, with some certainty, an approximate plasma level for a given dose.[36] Target plasma level ranges for optimal clinical response have been suggested as 146–254µg/L[37] and 150–300µg/L,[38] with adverse effects observed above 210µg/L.[38] Inter-individual variation in aripiprazole plasma levels has been observed but not fully investigated, although gender appears to have little influence.[39,40] Age, metabolic enzyme genotype and interacting medications seem likely causes of variation.[38-41] A putative range between **150µg/L and 210µg/L**[36] has been suggested as a target for patients taking aripiprazole and these are broadly the concentrations seen in patients receiving depot aripiprazole at 300mg and 400mg monthly.[42] Some authorities suggest a lower threshold for clinical effect of 100µg/L[30] – a plasma level usually afforded by an oral dose of 10mg a day.[31,43]

Clozapine

Clozapine plasma levels are broadly related to daily dose,[44] but there is sufficient variation to make impossible any precise prediction of plasma level. Plasma levels are generally lower in younger patients, males,[45] and smokers[46] and higher in Asians.[47] Much lower doses of clozapine are required in East Asians,[48,49] Indians[50] and Bangladeshis.[51] The prevalence of clozapine poor metabolisers is also higher in East Asians.[52,53] A series of algorithms has been developed for the approximate prediction of clozapine levels according to patient factors and these are strongly recommended.[54] Algorithms cannot, however, account for other influences on clozapine plasma levels, such as changes in adherence, inflammation[55] and infection.[56,57]

The plasma level threshold for acute response to clozapine has been suggested to be 200µg/L,[58] 350µg/L,[59–61] 370µg/L,[62] 420 µg/L,[63] 504µg/L[64] and 550µg/L.[65] Limited data suggest a level of at least 200µg/L is required to prevent relapse.[66] Substantial variation in clozapine plasma level may also predict relapse.[67] Changes in an individual's plasma clozapine are common with a tendency for concentrations to slightly decrease over time,[68] although one study suggests a decrease only in norclozapine concentrations.[69]

Despite these somewhat varied estimates of response threshold, plasma levels can be useful in optimising treatment. In those not responding to clozapine, dose should be adjusted to give plasma levels in the range **350–600µg/L** (a range reflecting a consensus of the above findings[30]). Those not tolerating clozapine may benefit from a reduction to a dose giving plasma levels in this range. An upper limit to the clozapine target range has not been defined. Any upper limit must take into account two components: the level above which no therapeutic advantage is gained and the level at which toxicity/tolerability is unacceptable. Plasma levels do seem to predict EEG changes[70,71] and seizures occur more frequently in patients with levels above 1000µg/L,[72] so levels should probably be kept well below this. Other non-neurological clozapine-related adverse effects also seem to be plasma-level related[73] as might be expected. An upper limit has of concentrations around 600–800µg/L has been proposed.[74]

A further consideration is that placing an upper limit on the target range for clozapine levels may discourage potentially worthwhile dose increases within the licensed dose range. Before plasma levels were widely used, clozapine was fairly often given in doses up to 900mg/day, with valproate being added when the dose reached 600mg/day. It remains unclear whether using these high doses can benefit patients with plasma levels already above the accepted threshold. Nonetheless, it is prudent to use an anticonvulsant as prophylaxis against seizures and myoclonus when plasma levels are above 600µg/L (a level based more on repeated recommendation than on a clear evidence-based threshold[74]) and certainly when levels approach 1000µg/L.

Norclozapine is the major metabolite of clozapine. The ratio of clozapine to norclozapine averages 1.25 in populations[75] but may differ for individuals. In chronic dosing, the ratio should remain the same for a given patient. A decrease in ratio may suggest enzyme induction, an increase suggests enzyme inhibition, a non-trough sample or recent missed doses. However, the time of sampling radically alters the clozapine/norclozapine ratio as clozapine is relatively high in early samples and norclozapine is high in late samples.[2] Clozapine metabolism may become saturated at higher doses: the ratio of clozapine to norclozapine increases with increasing plasma levels, suggesting saturation.[76–78] The effect of fluvoxamine also suggests that metabolism via CYP1A2 to norclozapine can be overwhelmed.[79] A recent systematic review concluded that knowledge of clozapine/norclozapine ratio had no clinical utility.[80]

Olanzapine

Plasma levels of olanzapine are linearly related to daily dose,[81] but there is substantial variation,[82] with higher levels seen in women,[64] non-smokers[83] and those on enzyme inhibiting drugs.[83,84] With once-daily dosing, the threshold level for response in schizophrenia has been suggested to be 9.3μg/L (trough sample),[85] 23.2μg/L (12-hour post-dose sample)[64] and 23μg/L at a mean of 13.5 hours post-dose.[86] There is evidence to suggest that levels greater than around 40μg/L (12-hour sampling) produce no further therapeutic benefit than lower levels.[87] Severe toxicity is uncommon but may be associated with levels above 100μg/L, and death is occasionally seen at levels above 160μg/L[88] (albeit when other drugs or physical factors are relevant). A target range for therapeutic use of **20–40μg/L** (12-hour post-dose sample) has been proposed[89] for schizophrenia; the range for mania is probably similar.[90] This target range has recently been widened to **20–80μg/L**[91,92] but the reasons for this are not clear.

Notably, significant weight gain seems most likely to occur in those with plasma levels above 20μg/L.[93] Constipation, dry mouth and tachycardia also seem to be plasma level-related.[94]

In practice, the dose of olanzapine should be largely governed by response and tolerability. However, a survey of UK sample assay results suggested that around 20% of patients on 20mg a day will have sub-therapeutic plasma levels and more than 40% have levels above 40μg/L.[95] Plasma level determinations might then be useful for those suspected of non-adherence, those showing poor tolerability or those not responding to the maximum licensed dose. Where there is poor response and plasma levels are below 20μg/L, dose may then be adjusted to give 12-hour plasma levels of 20–40μg/L, where there is good response and poor tolerability, the dose should be tentatively reduced to give plasma levels below 40μg/L. Changes in dose give proportionate changes in plasma levels.[96] A case might be made to increase the dose to give blood levels in the range 40–80μg/L but only where no other options remain.

Quetiapine

Dose of quetiapine is weakly related to trough plasma samples.[97] Mean levels reported within the dose range 150–800mg/day range from 27μg/L to 387μg/L,[98–103] although the highest and lowest levels are not necessarily found at the lowest and highest doses. Age, gender and co-medication may contribute to the significant inter-individual variance observed in TDM studies, with female gender,[103,104] older age[102,103] and CYP3A4 inhibiting drugs[98,102,103] likely to increase quetiapine concentration. Reports of these effects are conflicting[104] and not sufficient to support the routine use of plasma level monitoring based on these factors alone. Despite the substantial variation in plasma levels at each dose, there is insufficient evidence to suggest a target therapeutic range to aim for (although a target range of 100–500μg/L has been proposed[105]) thus plasma level monitoring is likely to have little value. Moreover, the metabolites of quetiapine have major therapeutic effects and their concentrations are only loosely associated with parent drug levels.[106]

Most current reports of quetiapine concentration associations are derived from analysis of trough samples. Because of the short half-life of quetiapine, trough levels tend to drop to within a relatively small range regardless of dose and previous peak level. Thus peak plasma levels may be more closely related to dose and clinical response,[97] although monitoring of such is not currently justified in the absence of an established peak plasma target range. Interestingly, a study of quetiapine in patients with borderline personality disorder or drug-induced psychosis showed a linear relationship between response and 12-hour plasma level.[104] Peak to trough variation is greater for IR formulations (roughly a maximum of 4000µg/L to zero) than for slow release preparations (roughly a maximum of 3000µg/L to around 100µg/L).[43]

Quetiapine has an established dose–response relationship, and appears to be well tolerated at doses well beyond the licensed dose range.[107] In practice, dose adjustment should be based on patient response and tolerability.

Risperidone

The therapeutic range for risperidone is generally agreed to be **20–60µg/L** of the active moiety (risperidone + 9-OH-risperidone)[91,108,109] although other ranges (25–150µg/L and 25–80µg/L) have been proposed.[110] Plasma levels of 20–60µg/L are usually afforded by oral doses of between 3mg and 6mg a day.[108,111–113] Occupancy of striatal dopamine D_2 receptors has been shown to be around 65% (the minimum required for acute therapeutic effect) at plasma levels of approximately 20µg/L.[109,114]

Risperidone long-acting injection (25mg/2 weeks) appears to afford plasma levels averaging between 4.4µg/L and 22.7µg/L.[112] Dopamine D_2 occupancies at this dose have been variously estimated at between 25% and 71%.[109,115,116] There is considerable inter-individual variation around these mean values with a substantial minority of patients with plasma levels above those shown. Nonetheless, these data do cast doubt on the efficacy of a dose of 25mg/2 weeks,[112] although it is noteworthy that there is some evidence that long-acting antipsychotic preparations are effective despite apparently sub-therapeutic plasma levels and dopamine occupancies.[117] Indeed, evidence continues to grow that sustained high dopamine occupancy is not necessary to prevent recurrence in longer term treatment[118–120] (as opposed to providing acute effects).

Disturbingly, however, a report of assay results for patients receiving RLAI[121] found 50% of patients with levels below 20µg/L and for 10% no risperidone/9-hydroxyrisperidone was detected. Thus therapeutic drug monitoring might be clinically helpful for those on RLAI but this rather defeats the object of a long-acting injection.

Limited data for paliperidone palmitate 1-monthly LAI suggest that standard loading doses give plasma levels of 25–45µg/L; while at steady state, plasma levels ranged from 10–25µg/L for 100mg/month to 15–35µg/L for 150mg/month.[122] Plasma concentrations may gradually rise in the first year of treatment to around 35µg/L (mean dose 138mg/month)[123] and remain stable thereafter.[124] For the 3-monthly injection, steady state plasma concentrations range from 30–55µg/L for 525mg every 3 months, 25–55µg/L for 350mg every 3 months and 20–35µg/L for 263mg every 3 months.[125]

The target ranges listed in Table 11.2 have somewhat dubious usefulness and, in some cases, merely represent the range of values seen in clinical use. Assays for these drugs are likely to be available only in specialist units.

Table 11.2 Target ranges for other psychotropics[30,91]

Antipsychotics	Target range (µg/L)
Asenapine	1–5
Brexpiprazole	40–140
Cariprazine	10–20
Chlorpromazine	30–300
Flupentixol	0.5–5 (*cis*-isomer)
Fluphenazine	1–10
Haloperidol	1–10
Iloperidone	5–10
Lurasidone	15–40
Melperone	30–100
Sulpiride	200–1000
Ziprasidone	50–200
Zuclopenthixol	4–50

Antidepressants	Target range (µg/L)
Agomelatine	7–300
Citalopram	50–110
Desvenlafaxine	100–400
Dosulepin	45–100
Duloxetine	30–120
Escitalopram	15–80
Fluoxetine (+norfluoxetine)	120–500
Fluvoxamine	60–230
Levomilnacipran	80–120
Mianserin	15–70

(*Continued*)

Table 11.2 (Continued)

Antidepressants	Target range (µg/L)
Milnacipran	100–150
Mirtazapine	30–80
Moclobemide	300–1000
Paroxetine	20–65
Reboxetine	60–350
Sertraline	10–150
Trazodone	700–1000
Venlafaxine (+O-desmethylvenlafaxine)	100–400
Vilazodone	30–70
Vortioxetine	15–60

References

1. Mann K, et al. Appropriateness of therapeutic drug monitoring for antidepressants in routine psychiatric inpatient care. *Ther Drug Monit* 2006; 28:83–88.
2. Jakobsen MI, et al. The significance of sampling time in therapeutic drug monitoring of clozapine. *Acta Psychiatr Scand* 2017; 135:159–169.
3. Hiemke C. relationships of psychoactive drugs and the problem to calculate therapeutic reference ranges. *Ther Drug Monit* 2019; 41: 174–179.
4. Taylor D, et al. Doses of carbamazepine and valproate in bipolar affective disorder. *Psychiatric Bulletin* 1997; 21:221–223.
5. Eadie MJ. Anticonvulsant drugs. *Drugs* 1984; 27: 328–363.
6. Chbili C, et al. Relationships between pharmacokinetic parameters of carbamazepine and therapeutic response in patients with bipolar disease. *Ann Biol Clin* (Paris) 2014; 72:453–459.
7. Cohen AF, et al. Lamotrigine, a new anticonvulsant: pharmacokinetics in normal humans. *Clin Pharmacol Ther* 1987; 42:535–541.
8. Kilpatrick ES, et al. Concentration-effect and concentration-toxicity relations with lamotrigine: a prospective study. *Epilepsia* 1996; 37:534–538.
9. Johannessen SI, et al. Therapeutic drug monitoring of the newer antiepileptic drugs. *Ther Drug Monit* 2003; 25:347–363.
10. Kagawa S, et al. Relationship between plasma concentrations of lamotrigine and its early therapeutic effect of lamotrigine augmentation therapy in treatment-resistant depressive disorder. *Ther Drug Monit* 2014; 36:730–733.
11. Nakamura A, et al. Prediction of an optimal dose of lamotrigine for augmentation therapy in treatment-resistant depressive disorder from plasma lamotrigine concentration at week 2. *Ther Drug Monit* 2016; 38:379–382.
12. Schou M. Forty years of lithium treatment. *Arch Gen Psychiatry* 1997; 54: 9–13.
13. Anon. Using lithium safely. *Drug Ther Bull* 1999; 37:22–24.
14. Nicholson J, et al. Monitoring patients on lithium – a good practice guideline. *Psychiatric Bulletin* 2002; 26:348–351.
15. National Institute for Health and Care Excellence. Bipolar disorder: assessment and management: Clinical Guidance [CG185] 2014 (last updated February 2020); https://www.nice.org.uk/guidance/cg185.
16. Severus WE, et al. What is the optimal serum lithium level in the long-term treatment of bipolar disorder–a review? *Bipolar Disorders* 2008; 10:231–237.
17. Nolen WA, et al. The association of the effect of lithium in the maintenance treatment of bipolar disorder with lithium plasma levels: a post hoc analysis of a double-blind study comparing switching to lithium or placebo in patients who responded to quetiapine (Trial 144). *Bipolar Disorders* 2013; 15:100–109.
18. Nazirizadeh Y, et al. Serum concentrations of paliperidone versus risperidone and clinical effects. *Eur J Clin Pharmacol* 2010; 66:797–803.
19. Schoretsanitis G, et al. A systematic review and combined analysis of therapeutic drug monitoring studies for oral paliperidone. *Expert Rev Clin Pharmacol* 2018; 11:625–639.
20. Taylor D, et al. Plasma levels of tricyclics and related antidepressants: are they necessary or useful? *Psychiatric Bulletin* 1995; 19:548–550.

21. Perucca E. Pharmacological and therapeutic properties of valproate. *CNS Drugs* 2002; **16**: 695–714.

22. Allen MH, et al. Linear relationship of valproate serum concentration to response and optimal serum levels for acute mania. *Am J Psychiatry* 2006; **163**:272–275.

23. Bowden CL, et al. Relation of serum valproate concentration to response in mania. *Am J Psychiatry* 1996; **153**:765–770.

24. Vazquez M, et al. Hyperammonemia associated with valproic acid concentrations. *BioMed Research International* 2014; **2014**:217–269.

25. Muller MJ, et al. Amisulpride doses and plasma levels in different age groups of patients with schizophrenia or schizoaffective disorder. *Journal of Psychopharmacology* 2008; **23**:278–286.

26. Muller MJ, et al. Gender aspects in the clinical treatment of schizophrenic inpatients with amisulpride: a therapeutic drug monitoring study. *Pharmacopsychiatry* 2006; **39**:41–46.

27. Bergemann N, et al. Plasma amisulpride levels in schizophrenia or schizoaffective disorder. *Eur Neuropsychopharmacol* 2004; **14**:245–250.

28. Muller MJ, et al. Therapeutic drug monitoring for optimizing amisulpride therapy in patients with schizophrenia. *J Psychiatr Res* 2007; **41**:673–679.

29. Sparshatt A, et al. Amisulpride - dose, plasma concentration, occupancy and response: implications for therapeutic drug monitoring. *Acta Psychiatr Scand* 2009; **120**:416–428.

30. Schoretsanitis G, et al. TDM in psychiatry and neurology: A comprehensive summary of the consensus guidelines for therapeutic drug monitoring in neuropsychopharmacology, update 2017; a tool for clinicians. *World J Biol Psychiatry* 2018; **19**:162–174.

31. Jönsson AK, et al. A compilation of serum concentrations of 12 antipsychotic drugs in a therapeutic drug monitoring setting. *Ther Drug Monit* 2019; **41**:348–356.

32. Reeves S, et al. Therapeutic window of dopamine D2/3 receptor occupancy to treat psychosis in Alzheimer's disease. *Brain* 2017; **140**:1117–1127.

33. Reeves S, et al. Therapeutic D2/3 receptor occupancies and response with low amisulpride blood concentrations in very late-onset schizophrenia-like psychosis (VLOSLP). *Int J Geriatr Psychiatry* 2018; **33**:396–404.

34. Bowskill SV, et al. Plasma amisulpride in relation to prescribed dose, clozapine augmentation, and other factors: data from a therapeutic drug monitoring service, 2002–2010. *Hum Psychopharmacol* 2012; **27**:507–513.

35. Mace S, et al. Aripiprazole: dose–response relationship in schizophrenia and schizoaffective disorder. *CNS Drugs* 2008; **23**:773–780.

36. Sparshatt A, et al. A systematic review of aripiprazole – dose, plasma concentration, receptor occupancy and response: implications for therapeutic drug monitoring. *J Clin Psychiatry* 2010; **71**:1447–1456.

37. Kirschbaum KM, et al. Therapeutic monitoring of aripiprazole by HPLC with column-switching and spectrophotometric detection. *Clin Chem* 2005; **51**:1718–1721.

38. Kirschbaum KM, et al. Serum levels of aripiprazole and dehydroaripiprazole, clinical response and side effects. *World J Biol Psychiatry* 2008; **9**:212–218.

39. Molden E, et al. Pharmacokinetic variability of aripiprazole and the active metabolite dehydroaripiprazole in psychiatric patients. *Ther Drug Monit* 2006; **28**:744–749.

40. Bachmann CJ, et al. Large variability of aripiprazole and dehydroaripiprazole serum concentrations in adolescent patients with schizophrenia. *Ther Drug Monit* 2008; **30**:462–466.

41. Hendset M, et al. Impact of the CYP2D6 genotype on steady-state serum concentrations of aripiprazole and dehydroaripiprazole. *Eur J Clin Pharmacol* 2007; **63**:1147–1151.

42. Mallikaarjun S, et al. Pharmacokinetics, tolerability and safety of aripiprazole once-monthly in adult schizophrenia: an open-label, parallel-arm, multiple-dose study. *Schizophr Res* 2013; **150**:281–288.

43. Korell J, et al. Determination of plasma concentration reference ranges for oral aripiprazole, olanzapine, and quetiapine. *Eur J Clin Pharmacol* 2018; **74**:593–599.

44. Haring C, et al. Influence of patient-related variables on clozapine plasma levels. *Am J Psychiatry* 1990; **147**:1471–1475.

45. Haring C, et al. Dose-related plasma levels of clozapine: influence of smoking behaviour, sex and age. *Psychopharmacology* 1989; **99 Suppl**:S38–S40.

46. Taylor D. Pharmacokinetic interactions involving clozapine. *Br J Psychiatry* 1997; **171**: 109–112.

47. Ng CH, et al. An inter-ethnic comparison study of clozapine dosage, clinical response and plasma levels. *Int Clin Psychopharmacol* 2005; **20**:163–168.

48. Ruan CJ, et al. Clozapine metabolism in East Asians and Caucasians: a pilot exploration of the prevalence of poor metabolizers and a systematic review. *J Clin Psychopharmacol* 2019; **39**:135–144.

49. de Leon J, et al. Do Asian patients require only half of the clozapine dose prescribed for Caucasians? A critical overview. *Indian J Psychol Med* 2020; **42**:4–10.

50. Suhas S, et al. Do Indian patients with schizophrenia need half the recommended clozapine dose to achieve therapeutic serum level? An exploratory study. *Schizophr Res* 2020; **222**:195-201.

51. Bhattacharya R, et al. Clozapine prescribing: comparison of clozapine dosage and plasma levels between White British and Bangladeshi patients. *BJPsych Bulletin* 2021; **45**:22–27.

52. Ruan CJ, et al. Exploring the prevalence of clozapine phenotypic poor metabolizers in 4 Asian samples: they ranged between 2% and 13. *J Clin Psychopharmacol* 2019; **39**:644–648.

53. de Leon J, et al. Using therapeutic drug monitoring to personalize clozapine dosing in Asians. *Asia-Pacific Psychiatry* 2020; **12**:e12384.

54. Rostami-Hodjegan A, et al. Influence of dose, cigarette smoking, age, sex, and metabolic activity on plasma clozapine concentrations: a predictive model and nomograms to aid clozapine dose adjustment and to assess compliance in individual patients. *J Clin Psychopharmacol* 2004; **24**:70–78.

CHAPTER 11

55. Haack MJ, et al. Toxic rise of clozapine plasma concentrations in relation to inflammation. *Eur Neuropsychopharmacol* 2003; 13:381–385.

56. de Leon J, et al. Serious respiratory infections can increase clozapine levels and contribute to side effects: a case report. *Prog Neuropsychopharmacol Biol Psychiatry* 2003; 27:1059–1063.

57. Espnes KA, et al. A puzzling case of increased serum clozapine levels in a patient with inflammation and infection. *Ther Drug Monit* 2012; 34:489–492.

58. VanderZwaag C, et al. Response of patients with treatment-refractory schizophrenia to clozapine within three serum level ranges. *Am J Psychiatry* 1996; 153:1579–1584.

59. Perry PJ, et al. Clozapine and norclozapine plasma concentrations and clinical response of treatment refractory schizophrenic patients. *Am J Psychiatry* 1991; 148:231–235.

60. Miller DD. Effect of phenytoin on plasma clozapine concentrations in two patients. *J Clin Psychiatry* 1991; 52:23–25.

61. Spina E, et al. Relationship between plasma concentrations of clozapine and norclozapine and therapeutic response in patients with schizophrenia resistant to conventional neuroleptics. *Psychopharmacology* 2000; 148:83–89.

62. Hasegawa M, et al. Relationship between clinical efficacy and clozapine concentrations in plasma in schizophrenia: effect of smoking. *J Clin Psychopharmacol* 1993; 13:383–390.

63. Potkin SG, et al. Plasma clozapine concentrations predict clinical response in treatment-resistant schizophrenia. *J Clin Psychiatry* 1994; 55 Suppl B:133–136.

64. Perry PJ. Therapeutic drug monitoring of antipsychotics. *Psychopharmacol Bull* 2001; 35:19–29.

65. Llorca PM, et al. Effectiveness of clozapine in neuroleptic-resistant schizophrenia: clinical response and plasma concentrations. *J Psychiatry Neurosci* 2002; 27:30–37.

66. Xiang YQ, et al. Serum concentrations of clozapine and norclozapine in the prediction of relapse of patients with schizophrenia. *Schizophr Res* 2006; 83:201–210.

67. Stieffenhofer V, et al. Clozapine plasma level monitoring for prediction of rehospitalization schizophrenic outpatients. *Pharmacopsychiatry* 2011; 44:55–59.

68. Lee J, et al. Quantifying intraindividual variations in plasma clozapine levels: a population pharmacokinetic approach. *J Clin Psychiatry* 2016; 77:681–687.

69. Turrion MC, et al. Intra-individual variation of clozapine and norclozapine plasma levels in clinical practice. *Revista De Psiquiatria Y Salud Mental* 2020; 13:31–35.

70. Khan AY, et al. Examining concentration-dependent toxicity of clozapine: role of therapeutic drug monitoring. *J Psychiatr Pract* 2005; 11:289–301.

71. Varma S, et al. Clozapine-related EEG changes and seizures: dose and plasma-level relationships. *Ther Adv Psychopharmacol* 2011; 1:47–66.

72. Greenwood-Smith C, et al. Serum clozapine levels: a review of their clinical utility. *J Psychopharm* 2003; 17:234–238.

73. Yusufi B, et al. Prevalence and nature of side effects during clozapine maintenance treatment and the relationship with clozapine dose and plasma concentration. *Int Clin Psychopharmacol* 2007; 22:238–243.

74. Remington G, et al. Clozapine and therapeutic drug monitoring: is there sufficient evidence for an upper threshold? *Psychopharmacology* 2013; 225:505–518.

75. Couchman L, et al. Plasma clozapine, norclozapine, and the clozapine: norclozapineratio in relation to prescribed dose and other factors: data from a therapeutic drug monitoring service, 1993–2007. *Ther Drug Monit* 2010; 32:438–447.

76. Volpicelli SA, et al. Determination of clozapine, norclozapine, and clozapine-N-oxide in serum by liquid chromatography. *Clin Chem* 1993; 39:1656–1659.

77. Guitton C, et al. Clozapine and metabolite concentrations during treatment of patients with chronic schizophrenia. *J Clin Pharmacol* 1999; 39:721–728.

78. Palego L, et al. Clozapine, norclozapine plasma levels, their sum and ratio in 50 psychotic patients: influence of patient-related variables. *Prog Neuropsychopharmacol Biol Psychiatry* 2002; 26:473–480.

79. Wang CY, et al. The differential effects of steady-state fluvoxamine on the pharmacokinetics of olanzapine and clozapine in healthy volunteers. *J Clin Pharmacol* 2004; 44:785–792.

80. Schoretsanitis G, et al. A comprehensive review of the clinical utility of and a combined analysis of the clozapine/norclozapine ratio in therapeutic drug monitoring for adult patients. *Expert Rev Clin Pharmacol* 2019; 12:603–621.

81. Bishara D, et al. Olanzapine: a systematic review and meta-regression of the relationships between dose, plasma concentration, receptor occupancy, and response. *J Clin Psychopharmacol* 2013; 33:329–335.

82. Aravagiri M, et al. Plasma level monitoring of olanzapine in patients with schizophrenia: determination by high-performance liquid chromatography with electrochemical detection. *Ther Drug Monit* 1997; 19:307–313.

83. Gex-Fabry M, et al. Therapeutic drug monitoring of olanzapine: the combined effect of age, gender, smoking, and comedication. *Ther Drug Monit* 2003; 25:46–53.

84. Bergemann N, et al. Olanzapine plasma concentration, average daily dose, and interaction with co-medication in schizophrenic patients. *Pharmacopsychiatry* 2004; 37:63–68.

85. Perry PJ, et al. Olanzapine plasma concentrations and clinical response in acutely ill schizophrenic patients. *J Clin Psychopharmacol* 1997; 17:472–477.

86. Fellows L, et al. Investigation of target plasma concentration–effect relationships for olanzapine in schizophrenia. *Ther Drug Monit* 2003; 25:682–689.

87. Mauri MC, et al. Clinical outcome and olanzapine plasma levels in acute schizophrenia. *Eur Psychiatry* 2005; 20:55–60.

88. Rao ML, et al. Olanzapine: pharmacology, pharmacokinetics and therapeutic drug monitoring. *Fortschr Neurol Psychiatr* 2001; 69:510–517.

89. Robertson MD, et al. Olanzapine concentrations in clinical serum and postmortem blood specimens–when does therapeutic become toxic? *J Forensic Sci* 2000; 45:418–421.

90. Bech P, et al. Olanzapine plasma level in relation to antimanic effect in the acute therapy of manic states. *Nord J Psychiatry* 2006; 60:181–182.

91. Schoretsanitis G, et al. Blood levels to optimize antipsychotic treatment in clinical practice: a Joint Consensus Statement of the American Society of Clinical Psychopharmacology and the Therapeutic Drug Monitoring Task Force of the Arbeitsgemeinschaft für Neuropsychopharmakologie und Pharmakopsychiatrie. *J Clin Psychiatry* 2020; 81:19cs13169.

92. Noel C. A review of a recently published guidelines' "strong recommendation" for therapeutic drug monitoring of olanzapine, haloperidol, perphenazine, and fluphenazine. *Ment Health Clin* 2019; 9:287–293.

93. Perry PJ, et al. The association of weight gain and olanzapine plasma concentrations. *J Clin Psychopharmacol* 2005; 25:250–254.

94. Kelly DL, et al. Plasma concentrations of high-dose olanzapine in a double-blind crossover study. *Human Psychopharmacol* 2006; 21:393–398.

95. Patel MX, et al. Plasma olanzapine in relation to prescribed dose and other factors: data from a therapeutic drug monitoring service, 1999–2009. *J Clin Psychopharmacol* 2011; 31:411–417.

96. Tsuboi T, et al. Predicting plasma olanzapine concentration following a change in dosage: a population pharmacokinetic study. *Pharmacopsychiatry* 2015; 48:286–291.

97. Sparshatt A, et al. Relationship between daily dose, plasma concentrations, dopamine receptor occupancy, and clinical response to quetiapine: a review. *J Clin Psychiatry* 2011; 72:1108–1123.

98. Hasselstrom J, et al. Quetiapine serum concentrations in psychiatric patients: the influence of comedication. *Ther Drug Monit* 2004; 26:486–491.

99. Winter HR, et al. Steady-state pharmacokinetic, safety, and tolerability profiles of quetiapine, norquetiapine, and other quetiapine metabolites in pediatric and adult patients with psychotic disorders. *J Child Adolesc Psychopharmacol* 2008; 18:81–98.

100. Li KY, et al. Multiple dose pharmacokinetics of quetiapine and some of its metabolites in Chinese suffering from schizophrenia. *Acta Pharmacol Sin* 2004; 25:390–394.

101. McConville BJ, et al. Pharmacokinetics, tolerability, and clinical effectiveness of quetiapine fumarate: an open-label trial in adolescents with psychotic disorders. *J Clin Psychiatry* 2000; 61:252–260.

102. Castberg I, et al. Quetiapine and drug interactions: evidence from a routine therapeutic drug monitoring service. *J Clin Psychiatry* 2007; 68:1540–1545.

103. Aichhorn W, et al. Influence of age, gender, body weight and valproate comedication on quetiapine plasma concentrations. *Int Clin Psychopharmacol* 2006; 21:81–85.

104. Mauri MC, et al. Two weeks' quetiapine treatment for schizophrenia, drug-induced psychosis and borderline personality disorder: a naturalistic study with drug plasma levels. *Expert Opin Pharmacother* 2007; 8:2207–2213.

105. Patteet L, et al. Therapeutic drug monitoring of common antipsychotics. *Ther Drug Monit* 2012; 34:629–651.

106. Fisher DS, et al. Plasma concentrations of quetiapine, N-desalkylquetiapine, o-desalkylquetiapine, 7-hydroxyquetiapine, and quetiapine sulfoxide in relation to quetiapine dose, formulation, and other factors. *Ther Drug Monit* 2012; 34:415–421.

107. Sparshatt A, et al. Quetiapine: dose-response relationship in schizophrenia. *CNS Drugs* 2008; 22:49–68.

108. Olesen OV, et al. Serum concentrations and side effects in psychiatric patients during risperidone therapy. *Ther Drug Monit* 1998; 20:380–384.

109. Remington G, et al. A PET study evaluating dopamine D2 receptor occupancy for long-acting injectable risperidone. *Am J Psychiatry* 2006; 163:396–401.

110. Seto K, et al. Risperidone in schizophrenia: is there a role for therapeutic drug monitoring? *Ther Drug Monit* 2011; 33:275–283.

111. Lane HY, et al. Risperidone in acutely exacerbated schizophrenia: dosing strategies and plasma levels. *J Clin Psychiatry* 2000; 61:209–214.

112. Taylor D. Risperidone long-acting injection in practice - more questions than answers? *Acta Psychiatr Scand* 2006; 114:1–2.

113. Nyberg S, et al. Suggested minimal effective dose of risperidone based on PET-measured D2 and 5-HT2A receptor occupancy in schizophrenic patients. *Am J Psychiatry* 1999; 156:869–875.

114. Uchida H, et al. Predicting dopamine D receptor occupancy from plasma levels of antipsychotic drugs: a systematic review and pooled analysis. *J Clin Psychopharmacol* 2011; 31:318–325.

115. Medori R, et al. Plasma antipsychotic concentration and receptor occupancy, with special focus on risperidone long-acting injectable. *Eur Neuropsychopharmacol* 2006; 16:233–240.

116. Gefvert O, et al. Pharmacokinetics and D2 receptor occupancy of long-acting injectable risperidone (Risperdal Consta™) in patients with schizophrenia. *Int J Neuropsychopharmacol* 2005; 8:27–36.

117. Nyberg S, et al. D2 dopamine receptor occupancy during low-dose treatment with haloperidol decanoate. *Am J Psychiatry* 1995; 152:173–178.

118. Moriguchi S, et al. Estimated dopamine D(2) receptor occupancy and remission in schizophrenia: analysis of the CATIE data. *J Clin Psychopharmacol* 2013; 33:682–685.

119. Tsuboi T, et al. Challenging the need for sustained blockade of dopamine D(2) receptor estimated from antipsychotic plasma levels in the maintenance treatment of schizophrenia: a single-blind, randomized, controlled study. *Schizophr Res* 2015; 164:149–154.

120. Takeuchi H, et al. Dose reduction of risperidone and olanzapine and estimated dopamine D(2) receptor occupancy in stable patients with schizophrenia: findings from an open-label, randomized, controlled study. *J Clin Psychiatry* 2014; 75:1209–1214.

121. Bowskill SV, et al. Risperidone and total 9-hydroxyrisperidone in relation to prescribed dose and other factors: data from a therapeutic drug monitoring service, 2002–2010. *Ther Drug Monit* 2012; 34:349–355.

122. Pandina GJ, et al. A randomized, placebo-controlled study to assess the efficacy and safety of 3 doses of paliperidone palmitate in adults with acutely exacerbated schizophrenia. *J Clin Psychopharmacol* 2010; 30:235–244.

123. Mauri MC, et al. Paliperidone long-acting plasma level monitoring and a new method of evaluation of clinical Stability. *Pharmacopsychiatry* 2017; 50:145–151.

124. Paletta S, et al. Two years of maintenance therapy with paliperidone long-acting in schizophrenia and schizoaffective disorder: a study with plasma levels. *Eur Neuropsychopharmacol* 2016; 26:S556–S557.

125. Berwaerts J, et al. Efficacy and safety of the 3-month formulation of paliperidone palmitate vs placebo for relapse prevention of schizophrenia: A randomized clinical trial. *JAMA Psychiatry* 2015; 72:830–839.

Interpreting postmortem blood concentrations

Much is known about the distribution of drugs in the body during life but relatively little about these same parameters after death. A great many drugs are subject to postmortem distribution changes but, for obvious practical reasons, research into the mechanisms and extent of these effects is very limited. The best that can be said is that a drug *plasma* concentration measured during life may be very different from the concentration measured at some time after death (usually in *whole blood* from the femoral artery).

A number of processes are responsible for these changes. In life, active mechanisms serve to concentrate some drugs in certain organs or tissues. After death, passive diffusion occurs as cell membranes break down and this will mean that postmortem blood samples will, for some drugs, show higher concentrations than were seen during life. (This is known as post mortem redistribution (PMR) and has been described as a 'toxicological nightmare'[1] because of the number of different processes involved.) In addition, central blood vessels surrounding major organs often demonstrate much higher drug concentrations than relatively distant peripheral samples.[2] PMR and other processes are temperature- and time-dependent and so time since death and conditions of storage are important determinants of blood concentration changes.[3] Postmortem redistribution tends to be greater with drugs with a large volume of distribution (i.e. those for which tissue concentrations in life vastly exceed blood concentrations) especially when given over a long period during life.

Other processes of importance[4] include the postmortem synthesis of certain compounds. For example, the body is able to generate gamma-hydroxy butyrate. Trauma may allow the introduction of yeasts that metabolise glucose to alcohol. Another phenomenon is the degradation of drugs by bacteria (e.g. clonazepam and nitrazepam) or fungi. Also, the metabolism of some drugs (cocaine, for example) appears to continue after death (although this may be simple chemical instability of the parent compound).

Table 11.3 lists some of the factors relevant to drug concentration changes after death and the possible consequences of these processes. Generally speaking, an isolated postmortem blood concentration cannot be sensibly interpreted. Even where in-life levels are available, experts agree that, for most drugs in most circumstances, interpretation of blood levels after death is near impossible: high concentrations should certainly not be taken, in the absence of other evidence, to indicate death by overdose, for example. Two valuable reference sources for interpretation of PM sample analysis are the systematic reviews of Ketola and Kriikku[5] and Ketola and Ojanpera.[6] Expert advice should always be sought when considering the role of medication in a death.[7]

Table 11.3 Factors affecting postmortem blood concentrations

Factor	Examples	Consequences
Redistribution of drug from tissues to blood compartment	Most drugs with large volume of distribution, e.g. clozapine,[8,9] olanzapine,[10] methadone,[11] SSRIs,[12] TCAs, mirtazapine,[13] lithium[14]	Postmortem levels up to 10x higher than in-life levels, sometimes higher still[6]
	May not occur to any significant effect with risperidone,[15] aripiprazole[16] or quetiapine[16]	
Uneven distribution of drugs in the blood compartment and in organs (i.e. site of blood collection affects concentration)	Most drugs[5,17], e.g. clozapine, TCAs, SSRIs, duloxetine,[18] benzodiazepines, quetiapine[19]	Concentrations may vary several-fold according to site of collection at postmortem, e.g. femoral blood vs heart blood
Decay of drugs in postmortem tissue (usually by bacterial degradation)	Not widely studied but known to occur with olanzapine, risperidone[20] and some benzodiazepines. Fungi can metabolise amitriptyline, mirtazapine and zolpidem[21,22]	Postmortem levels may be lower than in-life levels
Postmortem metabolism/ degradation	Cocaine metabolised/degraded postmortem. Many other drugs are unstable in postmortem samples. Yeasts may produce ethanol following trauma[4]	Postmortem levels may be lower (cocaine) or higher (alcohol) than in-life levels

References

1. Pounder DJ, et al. Post-mortem drug redistribution–a toxicological nightmare. *Forensic Sci Int* 1990; 45:253–263.
2. Ferner RE. Post-mortem clinical pharmacology. *Br J Clin Pharmacol* 2008; 66:430–443.
3. Flanagan RJ, et al. Analytical toxicology: guidelines for sample collection postmortem. *Toxicol Rev* 2005; 24:63–71.
4. Kennedy MC. Post-mortem drug concentrations. *Intern Med J* 2010; 40:183–187.
5. Ketola RA, et al. Drug concentrations in post-mortem specimens. *Drug Test Anal* 2019; 11:1338–1357.
6. Ketola RA, et al. Summary statistics for drug concentrations in post-mortem femoral blood representing all causes of death. *Drug Test Anal* 2019; 11:1326–1337.
7. Flanagan RJ. Poisoning: fact or fiction? *Med Leg J* 2012; 80:127–148.
8. Flanagan RJ, et al. Effect of post-mortem changes on peripheral and central whole blood and tissue clozapine and norclozapine concentrations in the domestic pig (Sus scrofa). *Forensic SciInt* 2003; 132:9–17.
9. Flanagan RJ, et al. Suspected clozapine poisoning in the UK/Eire, 1992–2003. *Forensic Sci Int* 2005; 155:91–99.
10. Saar E, et al. The time-dependant post-mortem redistribution of antipsychotic drugs. *Forensic Sci Int* 2012; 222:223–227.
11. Caplehorn JR, et al. Methadone dose and post-mortem blood concentration. *Drug Alcohol Rev* 2002; 21:329–333.
12. Lewis RJ, et al. Paroxetine in postmortem fluids and tissues from nine aviation accident victims. *J Anal Toxicol* 2015; 39:637–641.
13. Launiainen T, et al. Drug concentrations in post-mortem femoral blood compared with therapeutic concentrations in plasma. *Drug Test Anal* 2014; 6:308–316.
14. Soderberg C, et al. Reference values of lithium in postmortem femoral blood. *Forensic Sci Int* 2017; 277:207–214.
15. Linnet K, et al. Postmortem femoral blood concentrations of risperidone. *J Anal Toxicol* 2014; 38:57–60.
16. Skov L, et al. Postmortem femoral blood reference concentrations of aripiprazole, chlorprothixene, and quetiapine. *J Anal Toxicol* 2015; 39:41–44.
17. Rodda KE, et al. The redistribution of selected psychiatric drugs in post-mortem cases. *Forensic Sci Int* 2006; 164:235–239.
18. Scanlon KA, et al. Comprehensive duloxetine analysis in a fatal overdose. *J Anal Toxicol* 2016; 40:167–170.
19. Breivik H, et al. Post mortem tissue distribution of quetiapine in forensic autopsies. *Forensic Sci Int* 2020; 315:110413.
20. Butzbach DM, et al. Bacterial degradation of risperidone and paliperidone in decomposing blood. *J Forensic Sci* 2013; 58:90–100.
21. Martinez-Ramirez JA, et al. Search for fungi-specific metabolites of four model drugs in postmortem blood as potential indicators of postmortem fungal metabolism. *Forensic Sci Int* 2016; 262:173–178.
22. Martinez-Ramirez JA, et al. Studies on drug metabolism by fungi colonizing decomposing human cadavers. Part II: biotransformation of five model drugs by fungi isolated from post-mortem material. *Drug Test Anal* 2015; 7:265–279.

Acting on clozapine plasma concentration results

In most developed countries, clozapine blood concentration monitoring is widely used. The table below gives some general advice about actions that should be taken when clozapine levels fall within a certain range. The ranges shown are somewhat arbitrary and convenient – the concentration at which a particular patient might respond cannot be known without a trial of clozapine. Most adverse effects are linearly or exponentially related to dose or plasma level. That is, there is no step-change in risk of seizures, for example, at a particular dose or plasma concentration.[1] As a consequence the Table 11.4 should be considered more an aide to decision-making rather than a rigorous, unbending evidence-based instruction. Note also the effect of tolerance to adverse effects – many patients have a significant adverse effect burden before therapeutic levels are reached,[2] reducing over time as tolerance develops.

CHAPTER 11

Table 11.4 Acting on clozapine plasma concentration results*

Plasma concentration	Response status	Tolerability status	Suggest action
<350µg/L	Poor	Poor	Increase dose very slowly to give level of 350µg/L
	Poor	Good	Increase dose to give level of 350µg/L
	Good	Poor	Maintain dose. Consider cautious dose reduction if tolerability does not improve.
	Good	Good	Continue to monitor. No action required.
350–500µg/L	Poor	Poor	Increase dose slowly, according to tolerability, to give level of >500µg/L. Consider prophylactic anticonvulsant.** If no improvement, consider augmentation.
	Poor	Good	Increase dose slowly, according to tolerability, to give level of >500µg/L. Consider prophylactic anticonvulsant.** If no improvement, consider augmentation.
	Good	Poor	Maintain dose to see if tolerability improves. Consider cautious dose reduction to give plasma level of around 350µg/L.
	Good	Good	Continue to monitor. No action required.
500–1000µg/L	Poor	Poor	Consider use of prophylactic anticonvulsant.** Consider augmentation. Attempt dose reduction if augmentation successful.
	Poor	Good	Consider use of prophylactic anticonvulsant.** Consider augmentation.
	Good	Poor	Attempt slow dose reduction to give plasma level of 350–500µg/L unless there is known non-response at lower level. If this is the case, maintain dose and consider adding anticonvulsant.** Optimise treatment of adverse effects.
	Good	Good	Consider use of prophylactic anticonvulsant.** Maintain dose if good tolerability continues.

(Continued)

Plasma concentration	Response status	Tolerability status	Suggest action
>1000μg/L	Poor	Poor	Add anticonvulsant. Attempt augmentation. Reduce dose to give level of <1000μg/L. Consider abandoning clozapine treatment.
	Poor	Good	Add anticonvulsant. Attempt augmentation. If augmentation successful, reduce dose to give level <1000μg/L. If unsuccessful, consider abandoning clozapine treatment
	Good	Poor	Add anticonvulsant. Attempt slow dose reduction to give plasma level <1000μg/L.
	Good	Good	Add anticonvulsant. Monitor closely; attempt dose reduction only if tolerability declines.

Notes

Poor response	No response or unsatisfactory response to clozapine. For example, not sufficiently well to be discharged.
Good response	Obvious positive changes related to use of clozapine. Patient likely to be suitable for discharge to either supported or unsupported care in the community.
Poor tolerability	Dose constrained by adverse effects such as tachycardia, sedation, hypersalivation, hypotension (see Chapter 1 for suggestions of treatment for adverse effects).
Good tolerability	Patient tolerates treatment well and there are no signs of serious toxicity.
Augmentation	Adding another antipsychotic or mood stabiliser (see Chapter 1).

- In all situations, ensure adequate treatment for clozapine-induced constipation. Constipation is dose-related. Ensure regular bowel movements and record bowel function. Stimulant laxatives such as senna are required (see Chapter 1).
- Seizures are dose- and plasma level-dependent. Suitable anticonvulsants are valproate, lamotrigine, and rarely, topiramate. Use lamotrigine if response poor; valproate if affective symptoms present (see Chapter 2). Note that use of valproate increases risk of neutropenia with clozapine.[3]

* This table applies to results for patients on a stable clozapine dose with confirmed good adherence.

** Anticonvulsants should be used in patients whose plasma level exceeds 600μg/L, unless EEG is normal, and in those with lower plasma levels who suffer clozapine-induced seizures.

References

1. Varma S, et al. Clozapine-related EEG changes and seizures: dose and plasma-level relationships. *Ther Adv Psychopharmacol* 2011; 1:47–66.
2. Yusufi B, et al. Prevalence and nature of side effects during clozapine maintenance treatment and the relationship with clozapine dose and plasma concentration. *Int Clin Psychopharmacol* 2007; 22:238–243.
3. Malik S, et al. Sodium valproate and clozapine induced neutropenia: A case control study using register data. *Schizophr Res* 2018; 195:267–273.

Psychotropics and cytochrome (CYP) function

Information on the effect of drugs on cytochrome function helps predict or confirm suspected interactions which may not have been uncovered in regulatory trials or in clinical use (sometimes called prediction from 'first principles'). Using 'first principles' essentially means understanding and interpreting pharmacokinetic information and anticipating the net effect of combining two or more drugs in vivo.

In addition to the effect of co-administered drugs on CYP function, genetic polymorphism associated with some enzyme pathways (e.g. 2D6, 2C9, 2C19 enzymes) may also account for inter-individual variations in metabolism of certain drugs.

The effects of polymorphism and pharmacokinetic interaction are difficult to predict because some drugs are metabolised by more than one enzyme and an alternative pathway(s) may compensate if other enzyme pathways are inhibited.

The function of CYPs is not the only consideration. P-glycoprotein (P-gp) is a drug transporter protein found in the gut wall. P-gp can eject (active process) drugs that diffuse (passive process) across the gut wall. P-gp is also found in testes and in the blood brain barrier. Drugs that inhibit P-gp are anticipated to increase the uptake of other drugs (that are substrates for P-gp) and drugs that induce P-gp are anticipated to reduce the uptake of drugs (that are substrates for P-gp). Many drugs that are substrates for CYP3A4 have also been found to be substrates for P-gp.

UDP-glucuronosyl transferase (UGT) has been identified as an enzyme that is responsible for phase II (conjugation) reactions. Valproate is a potent inhibitor of UGT, hence its interaction with lamotrigine, a drug which is primarily metabolised by UGT. UGT enzymes are also involved in the metabolism of lumateperone, olanzapine, topiramate and trifluoperazine.

In the table below:
Drugs highlighted in **bold** indicate:

- predominant metabolic enzyme pathway or
- predominant enzyme activity (inhibition or induction)

Drugs annotated with * indicate:

- known to be a minor metabolic enzyme pathway or activity (i.e. not demonstrated to be clinically significant)

Drugs in normal font (not bold and without *) indicate:

- metabolic enzyme pathway(s) or activity where significance is unclear or unknown

NB Information on CYP function derived from individual SPCs and US Labelling (accessed August 2020) and from a recent systematic review.[1]

The tables do not include details of the effects of non-psychotropics on CYP function.

CPY1A2

SUBSTRATES	INHIBITORS	INDUCERS
Agomelatine	**Fluvoxamine**	**'Barbiturates'**
Amitriptyline*	Moclobemide	Carbamazepine
Asenapine	Perphenazine	Modafinil*
Bupropion*		**Phenobarbital**
Caffeine		Phenytoin
Chlorpromazine		
Clomipramine*		
Clozapine		
Duloxetine		
Fluphenazine		
Fluvoxamine		
Imipramine*		
Melatonin		
Mirtazapine*		
Olanzapine		
Perphenazine		
?Pimozide*		
Ramelteon		
Zolpidem*		

CYP2A6

SUBSTRATES	INHIBITORS	INDUCERS
Bupropion*	Tranylcypromine	Phenobarbital
Caffeine		
Nicotine		

CPY2B6

SUBSTRATES	INHIBITORS	INDUCERS
Bupropion	Fluoxetine*	Carbamazepine*
Methadone*	Fluvoxamine	Modafinil*
Nicotine	Memantine	Phenobarbital
Sertraline*	Paroxetine*	Phenytoin
	Sertraline*	

CYP2B7

SUBSTRATES	INHIBITORS	INDUCERS
Buprenorphine*	Not known	Not known

CPY2C8

SUBSTRATES	INHIBITORS	INDUCERS
Zopiclone*	Not known	Not known

CPY2C9

SUBSTRATES	INHIBITORS	INDUCERS
Agomelatine*	Fluoxetine*	Carbamazepine
Amitriptyline	Fluvoxamine	SJW
Bupropion*	Modafinil	
Fluoxetine*	Valproate	
Lamotrigine		
Phenobarbital		
Phenytoin		
Sertraline*		
Valproate		

CPY2C19

SUBSTRATES	INHIBITORS	INDUCERS
Agomelatine*	Escitalopram*	Carbamazepine
Amitriptyline	Fluvoxamine	SJW
Carbamazepine*	Moclobemide	
Citalopram	Modafinil	
Clomipramine*	Topiramate	
Diazepam		
Escitalopram		
Fluoxetine*		
Imipramine*		
?Melatonin		
?Methadone		
Moclobemide		
Phenytoin		
Sertraline*		
Suvorexant		
Trimipramine*		

CPY2D6

SUBSTRATES	INHIBITORS	INDUCERS
Amitriptyline	**Amitriptyline**	Not known
'Amphetamines'	**Asenapine**	
Atomoxetine	**Bupropion**	
Aripiprazole	Chlorpromazine	
Brexpiprazole	Citalopram*	
Cariprazine	Clomipramine	
Chlorpromazine	Clozapine	
Citalopram	**Duloxetine**	
Clomipramine	Escitalopram	
Clozapine*	**Fluoxetine**	
Deutetrabenazine	Fluphenazine	
Donepezil*	Fluvoxamine*	
Duloxetine	Haloperidol	
Escitalopram	Levomepromazine	
Fluoxetine	Methadone*	
Fluvoxamine	Moclobemide	
Fluphenazine	**Paroxetine**	
Galantamine	Perphenazine	
Haloperidol	Reboxetine*	
Iloperidone	Risperidone	
Imipramine	Sertraline	
Methadone*	Venlafaxine*	
Mianserin		
Mirtazapine*		
Moclobemide		
Nortriptyline		
Olanzapine		
Paroxetine		
Perphenazine		
Pimozide*		
Quetiapine*		
Risperidone		
Sertraline		
Trazodone*		
Trimipramine		
Valbenazine		
Venlafaxine		
Vortioxetine		
Zuclopenthixol		

CYP2E1

SUBSTRATES	INHIBITORS	INDUCERS
Bupropion	**Disulfiram**	Ethanol
Ethanol	Paracetamol	

CYP3A4

SUBSTRATES	INHIBITORS	INDUCERS
Alfentanyl	**Fluoxetine**	**Asenapine?**
Alprazolam	Fluvoxamine	**Carbamazepine**
Amitriptyline	**Paroxetine**	**Modafinil**
Aripiprazole	Perphenazine	**Phenobarbital** 'and
Brexpiprazole	Reboxetine*	probably other
Buprenorphine		Barbituates'
Bupropion*		**Phenytoin**
Buspirone		**SJW**
Carbamazepine		Topiramate
Cariprazine		
Chlorpromazine		
Citalopram		
Clomipramine*		
Clonazepam		
Clozapine*		
Diazepam		
Donepezil		
Dosulepin		
Escitalopram*		
Fentanyl		
Fluoxetine*		
Galantamine		
Haloperidol		
Imipramine		
Lemborexant		
Lurasidone		
Methadone		
Midazolam		
Mirtazapine		
Modafinil		
Nitrazepam		
Perphenazine		
Pimavanserin		
Pimozide		
Quetiapine		
Reboxetine		
Risperidone*		
Sertindole		
Sertraline*		
Suvorexant		
Trazodone		
Trimipramine*		
Valbenazine		
Venlafaxine		
Vilazodone		
Zaleplon		
Ziprasidone		
Zolpidem		
Zopiclone		

Reference

1. Schoretsanitis G, et al. TDM in psychiatry and neurology: a comprehensive summary of the consensus guidelines for therapeutic drug monitoring in neuropsychopharmacology, update 2017; a tool for clinicians. *World J Biol Psychiatry* 2018; **19**:162–174.

Smoking and psychotropic drugs

Tobacco smoke contains polycyclic aromatic hydrocarbons that induce certain hepatic enzymes (CYP1A2 in particular).[1] Other enzymes which may be induced by smoking are CYP2C19 and, possibly, CYP3A4 and some variants of UGT (glycosyltransferases).[2] The extent of enzyme induction is determined by the number and type of cigarettes smoked and by the degree of smoke inhalation.[3] For some drugs used in psychiatry smoking significantly reduces drug plasma levels and higher doses are required than in non-smokers. Smoking may also affect alcohol metabolism by inducing CYP2E1.[3]

When people stop smoking, enzyme activity halves roughly every 2 days.[4] (Nicotine replacement or vaping have no effect on this process.) Plasma levels of affected drugs will then rise, sometimes substantially. Dose reduction will usually be necessary. If smoking is re-started, enzyme activity increases, plasma levels fall and dose increases are then required. The process is complicated, and effects are difficult to predict. Of course, few people manage to give up smoking completely, so additional complexity is introduced by intermittent smoking and repeated attempts at stopping completely. Close monitoring of plasma levels (where useful), clinical progress and adverse effect severity are essential.

The table below gives details of psychotropic drugs known to be affected by smoking status.

Drug	Effect of smoking	Action to be taken on stopping smoking	Action to be taken on re-starting
Agomelatine[5]	Plasma levels reduced	Monitor closely Dose may need to be reduced	Consider reintroducing previous smoking dose
Benzodiazepines[3,6]	Plasma levels reduced by 0–50% (depends on drug and smoking status)	Monitor closely Consider reducing dose by up to 25% over one week	Monitor closely Consider re-starting 'normal' smoking dose
Carbamazepine[3]	Unclear, but smoking may reduce carbamazepine plasma levels to a small extent	Monitor for changes in severity of adverse effects	Monitor plasma levels
Chlorpromazine[3,6,7]	Plasma levels reduced. Varied estimates of exact effect	Monitor closely, consider dose reduction	Monitor closely, consider restarting previous smoking dose
Clozapine[8–13]	Reduces plasma levels by up to 50% Plasma level reduction may be greater in those receiving valproate. Effect is reversed by co-administered fluvoxamine[14]	Take plasma level before stopping. On stopping, reduce dose gradually (over a week) until around 75% of original dose reached (i.e. reduce by 25%). Repeat plasma level one week after stopping. Anticipate further dose reductions	Take plasma level before re-starting. Increase dose to previous smoking dose over one week. Repeat plasma level. Deterioration is common if dose increases allow a fall in blood levels[15]

(Continued)

(*Continued*)

Drug	Effect of smoking	Action to be taken on stopping smoking	Action to be taken on re-starting
Doxepin[2,16]	Plasma levels reduced by around 25% (levels of nordoxepin metabolite increased)	Monitor closely Dose may need to be reduced	Consider reintroducing previous dose
Duloxetine[17,18]	Plasma levels may be reduced by up to 50%	Monitor closely Dose may need to be reduced	Consider reintroducing previous smoking dose
Escitalopram[19]	In practice smokers have lower blood levels despite being given higher doses Reduction in levels may be up to 50% (possibly via induction of CYP2C19)	Monitor closely Consider 25% dose reduction	Monitor closely Reinstate smoking dose
Fluphenazine[20]	Reduces plasma levels by up to 50%	On stopping, reduce dose by 25%. Monitor carefully over following 4–8 weeks. Consider further dose reductions	On re-starting, increase dose to previous smoking dose
Fluvoxamine[21]	Plasma levels decreased by around a third	Monitor closely Dose may need to be reduced	Dose may need to be increased to previous level
Haloperidol[22,23]	Reduces plasma levels by around 25–50%	Reduce dose by around 25%. Monitor carefully. Consider further dose reductions	On re-starting, increase dose to previous smoking dose
Loxapine[24] (inhaled)	Half-life reduced from 15.7 hours to 13.6 hours	Monitor	Monitor
Mirtazapine[25]	Unclear, but effect probably minimal	Monitor	Monitor
Olanzapine[13,26–29]	Reduces plasma levels by up to 50%	Take plasma level before stopping. On stopping, reduce dose by 25%. After one week, repeat plasma level. Consider further dose reductions	Take plasma level before restarting. Increase dose to previous smoking dose over one week. Repeat plasma level
Risperidone/ paliperidone[2,30]	Active moiety concentrations probably lower in smokers Minor effect (possibly via induction of CYP3A4)	Monitor closely	Monitor closely

(*Continued*)

(Continued)

Drug	Effect of smoking	Action to be taken on stopping smoking	Action to be taken on re-starting
Trazodone[31]	Around 25% reduction	Monitor for increased sedation. Consider dose reduction	Monitor closely. Consider increasing dose
Tricyclic antidepressants[3,6]	Plasma levels reduced by 25–50%.	Monitor closely. Consider reducing dose by 10–25% over 1 week. Consider further dose reductions	Monitor closely. Consider restarting previous smoking dose
Zuclopenthixol[32,33]	Unclear, but effect probably minimal	Monitor	Monitor

Note: Only cigarette smoking induces hepatic enzymes in the manner described above – nicotine replacement, vaping devices and electronic cigarettes (which do not contain polycyclic aromatic compounds) have no effect on enzyme activity (see Blacker, 2020,[34] for an illustrative case).

References

1. Kroon LA. Drug interactions with smoking. *Am J Health Syst Pharm* 2007; **64**:1917–1921.
2. Scherf-Clavel M, et al. Analysis of smoking behavior on the pharmacokinetics of antidepressants and antipsychotics: evidence for the role of alternative pathways apart from CYP1A2. *Int Clin Psychopharmacol* 2019; **34**:93–100.
3. Desai HD, et al. Smoking in patients receiving psychotropic medications: a pharmacokinetic perspective. *CNS Drugs* 2001; **15**:469–494.
4. Faber MS, et al. Time response of cytochrome P450 1A2 activity on cessation of heavy smoking. *Clin Pharmacol Ther* 2004; **76**:178–184.
5. Servier Laboratories Limited. Summary of Product Characteristics. Valdoxan (Agomelatine) 2020; https://www.medicines.org.uk/emc/medicine/21830.
6. Miller LG. Recent developments in the study of the effects of cigarette smoking on clinical pharmacokinetics and clinical pharmacodynamics. *Clin Pharmacokinet* 1989; **17**:90–108.
7. Goff DC, et al. Cigarette smoking in schizophrenia: relationship to psychopathology and medication side effects. *Am J Psychiatry* 1992; **149**:1189–1194.
8. Haring C, et al. Influence of patient-related variables on clozapine plasma levels. *Am J Psychiatry* 1990; **147**:1471–1475.
9. Haring C, et al. Dose-related plasma levels of clozapine: influence of smoking behaviour, sex and age. *Psychopharmacology* 1989; **99** Suppl:S38–S40.
10. Diaz FJ, et al. Estimating the size of the effects of co-medications on plasma clozapine concentrations using a model that controls for clozapine doses and confounding variables. *Pharmacopsychiatry* 2008; **41**:81–91.
11. Murayama-Sung L, et al. The impact of hospital smoking ban on clozapine and norclozapine levels. *J Clin Psychopharmacol* 2011; **31**:124–126.
12. Cormac I, et al. A retrospective evaluation of the impact of total smoking cessation on psychiatric inpatients taking clozapine. *Acta Psychiatr Scand* 2010; **121**:393–397.
13. Tsuda Y, et al. Meta-analysis: the effects of smoking on the disposition of two commonly used antipsychotic agents, olanzapine and clozapine. *BMJ Open* 2014; **4**:e004216.
14. Augustin M, et al. Effect of fluvoxamine augmentation and smoking on clozapine serum concentrations. *Schizophr Res* 2019; **210**:143–148.
15. Qurashi I, et al. Changes in smoking status, mental state and plasma clozapine concentration: retrospective cohort evaluation. *BJPsych Bulletin* 2019; **43**:271–274.
16. Ereshefsky L, et al. Pharmacokinetic factors affecting antidepressant drug clearance and clinical effect: evaluation of doxepin and imipramine–new data and review. *Clin Chem* 1988; **34**:863–880.
17. Fric M, et al. The influence of smoking on the serum level of duloxetine. *Pharmacopsychiatry* 2008; **41**:151–155.
18. Augustin M, et al. Differences in duloxetine dosing strategies in smoking and nonsmoking patients: therapeutic drug monitoring uncovers the impact on drug metabolism. *J Clin Psychiatry* 2018; **79**:17m12086.

19. Scherf-Clavel M, et al. Smoking is associated with lower dose-corrected serum concentrations of escitalopram. *J Clin Psychopharmacol* 2019; 39:485–488.

20. Ereshefsky L, et al. Effects of smoking on fluphenazine clearance in psychiatric inpatients. *Biol Psychiatry* 1985; 20:329–332.

21. Spigset O, et al. Effect of cigarette smoking on fluvoxamine pharmacokinetics in humans. *Clin Pharmacol Ther* 1995; 58:399–403.

22. Jann MW, et al. Effects of smoking on haloperidol and reduced haloperidol plasma concentrations and haloperidol clearance. *Psychopharmacology* 1986; 90:468–470.

23. Shimoda K, et al. Lower plasma levels of haloperidol in smoking than in nonsmoking schizophrenic patients. *Ther Drug Monit* 1999; 21:293–296.

24. Takahashi LH, et al. Effect of smoking on the pharmacokinetics of inhaled loxapine. *Ther Drug Monit* 2014; 36:618–623.

25. Grasmader K, et al. Population pharmacokinetic analysis of mirtazapine. *Eur J Clin Pharmacol* 2004; 60:473–480.

26. Carrillo JA, et al. Role of the smoking-induced cytochrome P450 (CYP)1A2 and polymorphic CYP2D6 in steady-state concentration of olanzapine. *J Clin Psychopharmacol* 2003; 23:119–127.

27. Gex-Fabry M, et al. Therapeutic drug monitoring of olanzapine: the combined effect of age, gender, smoking, and comedication. *Ther Drug Monit* 2003; 25:46–53.

28. Bigos KL, et al. Sex, race, and smoking impact olanzapine exposure. *J Clin Pharmacol* 2008; 48:157–165.

29. Lowe EJ, et al. Impact of tobacco smoking cessation on stable clozapine or olanzapine treatment. *Ann Pharmacother* 2010; 44:727–732.

30. Schoretsanitis G, et al. Effect of smoking on risperidone pharmacokinetics – a multifactorial approach to better predict the influence on drug metabolism. *Schizophr Res* 2017; 185:51–57.

31. Ishida M, et al. Effects of various factors on steady state plasma concentrations of trazodone and its active metabolite m-chlorophenylpiperazine. *Int Clin Psychopharmacol* 1995; 10:143–146.

32. Jann MW, et al. Clinical pharmacokinetics of the depot antipsychotics. *Clin Pharmacokinet* 1985; 10:315–333.

33. Jorgensen A, et al. Zuclopenthixol decanoate in schizophrenia: serum levels and clinical state. *Psychopharmacology* 1985; 87:364–367.

34. Blacker CJ. Clinical issues to consider for clozapine patients who vape: a case illustration. *Focus (American Psychiatric Publishing)* 2020; 18:55–57.

CHAPTER 11

Drug interactions with alcohol

Drug interactions with alcohol are complex. Many patient-related and drug-related factors need to be considered. It can be difficult to predict outcomes accurately because a number of processes may occur simultaneously or consecutively.

Pharmacokinetic interactions[1–4]

Alcohol (ethanol) is absorbed from the GI tract and distributed in body water. The volume of distribution is smaller in women and the elderly where plasma levels of alcohol will be higher for a given 'dose' of alcohol than in young males. Approximately 10% of ingested alcohol is subjected to first pass metabolism by alcohol dehydrogenase (ADH). A small proportion of alcohol is metabolised by ADH in the stomach. The remainder is metabolised in the liver by ADH and CYP2E1. Women have less capacity to metabolise via ADH than men. CYP2E1 plays a minor role in occasional drinkers but is an important and inducible metabolic route in chronic, heavy drinkers. CYP1A2, CYP3A4 and many other CYP enzymes also play a minor role.[5,6]

CYP2E1 and ADH convert alcohol to acetaldehyde which is both the toxic substance responsible for the unpleasant symptoms of the 'Antabuse reaction' (e.g. flushing, headache, nausea, malaise), and the compound implicated in hepatic damage. It may also have psychotropic effects – ethanol is metabolised to acetaldehyde by CYP2E1 in the brain.[7] The enzyme catalase is also known to metabolise alcohol to acetaldehyde in the brain and elsewhere.[8] Acetaldehyde is further metabolised by aldehyde dehydrogenase to acetic acid and then to carbon dioxide and water.

All of the enzymes involved in the metabolism of alcohol exhibit genetic polymorphism. For example, the majority of people of north Asian origin are poor metabolisers via aldehyde dehydrogenase.[9] Enzyme function can change in response to alcohol. Chronic consumption of alcohol induces CYP2E1 and CYP3A4. The effects of alcohol on other hepatic metabolising enzymes have been poorly studied.

Metabolism of alcohol

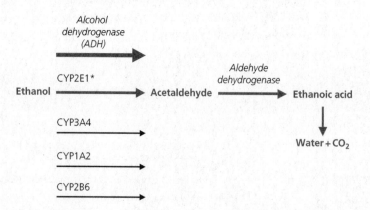

*Minor route in occasional drinkers; major route in misusers and at higher blood alcohol concentration. The ubiquitous enzyme catalase is also able to metabolise ethanol but its overall contribution is not known.

Table 11.5 Drugs that inhibit alcohol dehydrogenase and aldehyde dehydrogenase

Enzyme	Inhibited by	Potential consequences
Alcohol dehydrogenase	Aspirin H$_2$ antagonists	Reduced metabolism of alcohol resulting in higher plasma levels for longer periods of time
Aldehyde dehydrogenase	Chlorpropamide Disulfiram Griseofulvin Isoniazid Isosorbide dinitrate Metronidazole* Nitrofurantoin Sulphamethoxazole Tolbutamide	Reduced ability to metabolise acetaldehyde leading to 'Antabuse' type reaction: facial flushing, headache, tachycardia, nausea and vomiting, arrhythmias and hypotension

*Evidence that metronidazole has any effect on aldehyde dehydrogenase is surprisingly weak.[10–12]

Interactions are difficult to predict in alcohol misusers because two opposing processes may be at work: competition for enzymatic sites during periods of consumption or intoxication (increasing drug plasma levels) and enzyme induction prevailing during periods of sobriety (reducing drug plasma levels[8]). In chronic drinkers, particularly those who binge-drink, serum levels of prescribed drugs may reach toxic levels during periods of intoxication with alcohol and then be sub-therapeutic when the patient is sober. Even in non-intoxicated individuals there is some evidence that co-administered alcohol confers competitive inhibition of CYP3A4, leading to increased exposure to drugs metabolised by this enzyme (Table 11.6).[13] This makes it very difficult to optimise treatment of physical or mental illness.

Table 11.6 Co-administration of alcohol and substrates for CYP2E1 and CYP3A4

	Substrates for enzyme (note: this is not an exhaustive list)	Effects in an intoxicated patient	Effects in a chronic, sober drinker
CYP2E1	Paracetamol Isoniazid Phenobarbitone Warfarin Zopiclone	Competition between alcohol and drug leading to reduced rates of metabolism of both compounds. Increased plasma levels may lead to toxicity	Activity of CYP2E1 is increased up 10-fold Increased metabolism of drugs potentially leading to therapeutic failure

(Continued)

CHAPTER 11

Table 11.6 (Continued)

	Substrates for enzyme (note: this is not an exhaustive list)	Effects in an intoxicated patient	Effects in a chronic, sober drinker
CYP3A4	Alprazolam Aripiprazole Benzodiazepines Carbamazepine Clozapine Donepezil Galantamine Haloperidol Methadone Mirtazapine Quetiapine Risperidone Sildenafil Tricyclics Valproate Venlafaxine 'Z' hypnotics	Competition between alcohol and drug leading to reduced rates of metabolism of both compounds. Increased plasma levels may lead to toxicity	Increased rate of drug metabolism potentially leading to therapeutic failure Enzyme induction can last for several weeks after alcohol consumption ceases

Interactions of uncertain aetiology include increased blood alcohol concentrations in people who take verapamil and decreased metabolism of methylphenidate in people who consume alcohol.

Pharmacodynamic interactions[2–4]

Alcohol enhances inhibitory neurotransmission at $GABA_A$ receptors and reduces excitatory neurotransmission at glutamate NMDA receptors (Table 11.7). It also increases dopamine release in the mesolimbic pathway and may have some effects on serotonin and opiate pathways. Given these actions, alcohol would be expected to cause sedation, amnesia, ataxia and give rise to feelings of pleasure (and/or worsen psychotic symptoms in vulnerable individuals).

Table 11.7 Pharmacodynamic interactions with alcohol

Effect of alcohol	Effect exacerbated by	Potential consequences
Sedation	Other sedative drugs, e.g. Antihistamines Antipsychotics Baclofen Benzodiazepines Lofexidine Opiates Tizanidine Tricyclics Z-hypnotics	Increased CNS depression ranging from increased propensity to be involved in accidents through to respiratory depression and death

(Continued)

Table 11.7 *(Continued)*

Effect of alcohol	Effect exacerbated by	Potential consequences
Amnesia	Other amnesic drugs, e.g. Barbiturates Benzodiazepines Z-hypnotics	Increased amnesic effects ranging from mild memory loss to total amnesia. Usually anterograde amnesia: loss of memory of events after the effects of alcohol begin
Ataxia	ACE inhibitors β-blockers Ca channel blockers Nitrates Adrenergic alpha receptor antagonists, e.g. Clozapine Risperidone Tricyclics	Increased unsteadiness and falls

Alcohol can cause or worsen psychotic symptoms by increasing dopamine release in mesolimbic pathways. The effect of antipsychotic drugs may be competitively antagonised, rendering them less effective (Table 11.8).

Electrolyte disturbances secondary to alcohol-related dehydration can be exacerbated by other drugs that cause electrolyte disturbances such as diuretics.

Note that heavy alcohol consumption can lead to hypoglycaemia in people with diabetes who take insulin or oral hypoglycaemics. Theoretically there is an increased risk of lactic acidosis in patients who take metformin with alcohol. Alcohol can also increase blood pressure.

Chronic drinkers are particularly susceptible to the GI irritant effects of aspirin and NSAIDs.

NB:

In the presence of pharmacokinetic interactions, pharmacodynamic interactions will be more marked. For example, in a chronic heavy drinker who is sober, enzyme induction will increase the metabolism of diazepam which may lead to increased levels of anxiety (treatment failure). If the same patient becomes intoxicated with alcohol, the metabolism of diazepam will be greatly reduced as it will have to compete with alcohol for the metabolic capacity of CYP3A4. Plasma levels of alcohol and diazepam will rise (toxicity). As both alcohol and diazepam are sedative (via $GABA_A$ affinity), loss of consciousness and respiratory depression may occur.

Table 11.8 Psychotropic drugs: choice in patients who continue to drink

	Safest choice	Best avoided
Antipsychotics	**Sulpiride and amisulpride Paliperidone,** if depot required (non-sedative and renally excreted)	**Very sedative antipsychotics** such as chlorpromazine and clozapine
Antidepressants	**SSRI – citalopram, sertraline** Potent inhibitors of CYP3A4 (fluoxetine, paroxetine) may decrease alcohol metabolism in chronic drinkers	**TCAs**, because impairment of metabolism by alcohol (while intoxicated) can lead to increased plasma levels and consequent signs and symptoms of overdose (profound hypotension, seizures, arrhythmias and coma) Cardiac effects can be exacerbated by electrolyte disturbances Combinations of TCAs and alcohol profoundly impair psychomotor skills **Mirtazapine** – often very sedative **MAOIs** as can cause profound hypotension. Also potential interaction with tyramine-containing drinks which can lead to hypertensive crisis
Mood stabilisers	**Valproate Carbamazepine** Note: higher plasma levels achieved during periods of alcohol intoxication may be poorly tolerated	**Lithium**, because it has a narrow therapeutic index and alcohol-related dehydration and electrolyte disturbance can precipitate lithium toxicity

NB. Be aware of the possibility of hepatic failure or reduced hepatic function in chronic alcohol misusers. See section on hepatic impairment in Chapter 8.
Also note risk of hepatic toxicity with some recommended drugs (e.g. valproate).

References

1. Zakhari S. Overview: how is alcohol metabolized by the body? *Alcohol Research & Health: The Journal of the National Institute on Alcohol Abuse and Alcoholism* 2006; **29**:245–254.
2. Tanaka E. Toxicological interactions involving psychiatric drugs and alcohol: an update. *J Clin Pharm Ther* 2003; **28**:81–95.
3. Wan Chih T. Alcohol-related drug interactions. *Pharmacist's Letter/Prescriber's Letter* 2008; **24**:240106.
4. Smith RG. An appraisal of potential drug interactions in cigarette smokers and alcohol drinkers. *J Am Podiatr Med Assoc* 2009; **99**:81–88.
5. Salmela KS, et al. Respective roles of human cytochrome P-4502E1, 1A2, and 3A4 in the hepatic microsomal ethanol oxidizing system. *Alcohol Clin Exp Res* 1998; **22**:2125–2132.
6. Hamitouche S, et al. Ethanol oxidation into acetaldehyde by 16 recombinant human cytochrome P450 isoforms: role of CYP2C isoforms in human liver microsomes. *Toxicol Lett* 2006; **167**:221–230.
7. Koster M, et al. Seizures during antidepressant treatment in psychiatric inpatients–results from the transnational pharmacovigilance project "Arzneimittelsicherheit in der Psychiatrie" (AMSP) 1993–2008. *Psychopharmacology* 2013; **230**:191–201.
8. Cederbaum AI. Alcohol metabolism. *Clin Liver Dis* 2012; **16**:667–685.
9. Wall TL, et al. Biology, genetics, and environment: underlying factors influencing alcohol metabolism. *Alcohol Research: Current Reviews* 2016; **38**:59–68.
10. Williams CS, et al. Do ethanol and metronidazole interact to produce a disulfiram-like reaction? *Ann Pharmacother* 2000; **34**:255–257.
11. Visapää JP, et al. Lack of disulfiram-like reaction with metronidazole and ethanol. *Ann Pharmacother* 2002; **36**:971–974.
12. Mergenhagen KA, et al. Fact versus fiction: a review of the evidence behind alcohol and antibiotic interactions. *Antimicrob Agents Chemother* 2020; **64**:e02167–02119.
13. Huang Z, et al. Influence of ethanol on the metabolism of alprazolam. *Expert Opin Drug Metab Toxicol* 2018; **14**:551–559.

Chapter 12

Other substances

Caffeine

Caffeine is probably the most popular psychoactive substance in the world. Mean daily consumption in the UK is 350–620mg.[1] A quarter of the general population and half of those with psychiatric illness regularly consume over 500mg caffeine/day.[2] Consumption of caffeine should be routinely discussed with an individual to assess its effect on their symptoms and presentation.[3] In particular, caffeine withdrawal can have a marked effect on mental and physical health (Table 12.1).

Chocolate also contains caffeine. Martindale lists over 600 medicines that contain caffeine.[4] Most are available without a prescription and are marketed as analgesics or appetite suppressants.

Table 12.1 Caffeine content of drinks

Drink	Caffeine content
Brewed coffee	100mg/cup
Red Bull	80mg/can (other energy drinks may contain substantially more)
Instant coffee	60mg/cup
Black tea	45mg/cup
Green tea	20–30mg/cup
Soft drinks	25–50mg/can

The Maudsley® Prescribing Guidelines in Psychiatry, Fourteenth Edition. David M. Taylor, Thomas R. E. Barnes and Allan H. Young.
© 2021 David M. Taylor. Published 2021 by John Wiley & Sons Ltd.

Table 12.2 Dose and psychotropic effects of caffeine

Dose	Psychotropic effect
Generally	Central nervous system stimulation Increased catecholamine release, particularly dopamine[5]
Low to moderate dose[2,6]	Elation Impulsivity Peacefulness
Large doses >600mg/day[7] (Sensitive (non-tolerant) individuals may experience effects at lower doses; tolerance develops in long-term users)	Anxiety Insomnia Psychomotor agitation Excitement Rambling speech Delirium Psychosis

General effects of caffeine

- Acute use can increase systolic and diastolic blood pressure (BP) by up to 10mmHg for up to 4 hours.[3] Chronic moderate use probably has little effect on BP.[8]
- May enhance reinforcing effects of nicotine and possibly other drugs of misuse.[4,9]
- Caffeine has *de novo* psychotropic effects (see Table 12.2), may worsen existing psychiatric illness and may interact with psychotropic drugs.
- Caffeine is an antagonist at adenosine A_1 and A_{2A} receptors, thus stimulating dopamine pathways.

Psychotropic effects of caffeine

An established withdrawal syndrome exists. Symptoms include headache, depressed mood, anxiety, fatigue, irritability, nausea, dysphoria and craving.[10]

Pharmacokinetics

- **Absorption**
  - Rapid after oral administration, especially in liquid form.
  - Half-life of 2.5–4.5 hours.
- **Metabolism**
  - Metabolised by CYP1A2, a hepatic cytochrome enzyme that exhibits genetic polymorphism, which may partially account for the large inter-individual differences that are seen in the ability to tolerate caffeine.[11] Note that CYP1A2 is induced by smoking and inhibited by a number of drugs such as fluvoxamine.
  - This metabolic pathway may become saturated at higher doses.[12]
- **Interactions** (Table 12.3)
  - The potential effects of caffeine on the metabolism of other drugs, as well as the potential to induce a caffeine-withdrawal syndrome, should always be considered before substituting caffeine-free drinks.
  - Caffeine competitively inhibits CYP1A2. Plasma levels of some drugs may be reduced if caffeine is withdrawn.

Table 12.3 Interacting substance

Interacting substance	Effect	Comment
CYP1A2 inhibitors: Oestrogens Cimetidine Fluvoxamine (may decrease caffeine clearance by 80%)[13] Disulfiram	Reduce caffeine clearance	Effects of caffeine may be prolonged or increased Adverse effects may be increased May precipitate caffeine toxicity
Cigarette smoke*	CYP1A2 inducer – increasing caffeine metabolism[5]	Smokers may require higher doses of caffeine to gain desired effects[5]
Lithium	High doses of caffeine may reduce lithium levels	Caffeine withdrawal may increase lithium levels[14]
MAOIs	May enhance stimulant CNS effects	
Clozapine	Caffeine may increase clozapine plasma concentrations by up to 60%[15]	Thought to be via competitive inhibition of CYP1A2. Other drugs affected by caffeine-induced inhibition of the enzyme include olanzapine, imipramine and clomipramine
SSRIs	Large doses of caffeine may increase risk of serotonin syndrome[16]	
Benzodiazepines	Caffeine may act as an antagonist	Reduces the efficacy of benzodiazepines[7]

*Vaping has no effect on CYP1A2 function.
CNS, central nervous system; MAOI, monoamine oxidase inhibitor; SSRI, selective serotonin reuptake inhibitor.

Caffeine intoxication

The *Diagnostic and Statistical Manual of Mental Disorders* DSM-V[17] defines caffeine intoxication as the recent consumption of caffeine, usually in excess of 250 mg, accompanied by five or more of the symptoms in Box 12.1.

In caffeine intoxication, these symptoms cause significant distress or impairment in social, occupational or other important areas of functioning and are not due to a general medical condition or better accounted for by another mental disorder (e.g. an anxiety disorder).

Box 12.1 Symptoms of caffeine intoxication

- Restlessness
- Nervousness
- Excitement
- Insomnia
- Flushed face
- Diuresis
- Gastrointestinal disturbance
- Muscle twitching
- Rambling flow of thought and speech
- Tachycardia or cardiac arrhythmia
- Periods of inexhaustibility
- Psychomotor agitation

Caffeine abuse or dependence as a clinical syndrome has been reported[3] and caffeine use disorder and caffeine withdrawal are both DSM-V diagnoses.

Energy drinks

So-called energy drinks contain large amounts of caffeine along with sugar, vitamins and a number of other ingredients such as guarana and taurine. There is some evidence that these drinks can improve attention and short-term memory.[18] Marketing is targeted at adolescents and young adults, some of whom consume large volumes of these drinks, and seem to be particularly vulnerable to developing signs and symptoms of caffeine intoxication. Symptoms of anxiety and depression, frank suicidal behaviour and seizures have been associated with use of these products by young people.[19–21] When combined with alcohol, aggressive behaviour may result.[22] Excessive intake may lead to acute psychosis[23,24] or mania.[25]

Schizophrenia

- Patients with schizophrenia often consume large amounts of caffeine-containing drinks[1] and are twice as likely as controls to consume >200mg caffeine/day.[5]
- Caffeine-containing drinks may be used to relieve dry mouth (as a side effect of some antipsychotic drugs), for the stimulant effects of caffeine (to relieve dysphoria/sedation/negative symptoms)[5] or simply because coffee/tea drinking structures the day or relieves boredom.
- Schizophrenia may increase sensitivity to drug-related cues.[5]
- Moderate caffeine intake may improve cognitive and negative symptoms in schizophrenia, but this is poorly researched.[26]
- Large doses of caffeine can worsen psychotic symptoms[5,27] (in particular, elation and conceptual disorganisation) and result in the prescription of larger doses of antipsychotic drugs.
- The removal of caffeine from the diets of chronically disturbed (challenging behaviour) patients may ultimately lead to decreased levels of hostility, irritability and suspiciousness,[28] although this may not hold true in less disturbed populations.[29]
- Caffeine cessation may be of benefit in clozapine-resistant schizophrenia.[30]

Mood disorders

- Caffeine may elevate mood through increasing noradrenaline release[31] and modest caffeine consumption may protect against depression in those who do not have a pre-existing mood disorder.[32]
- People with mood disorders are more likely to consume caffeine, particularly when depressed.[14,33]
- Depressed patients may be more sensitive to the anxiogenic effects of caffeine.[34,35]
- Excessive consumption of caffeine may precipitate mania.[35,36]
- Caffeine can increase cortisol secretion (gives a false positive in the dexamethasone-suppression test),[37] increase seizure length during electroconvulsive therapy[38] and increase the clearance of lithium by promoting diuresis.[39]

CHAPTER 12

Anxiety disorders

- Caffeine increases vigilance, decreases reaction times, increases sleep latency and worsens sleep quality – effects that may be more marked in poor metabolisers.
- May precipitate or worsen generalised anxiety and panic attacks;[40] vulnerability to these effects may be genetically determined.[9]
- Effects are so marked that caffeine intoxication should always be considered when patients complain of anxiety symptoms or insomnia.
- Symptoms may diminish considerably or even abate completely if caffeine is avoided.[41]
- Patients with panic disorder consume much more caffeine than controls,[42] but the reasons for this are not clear.

Other disorders

Weak evidence supports the benefit of caffeine in attention deficit hyperactivity disorder (ADHD)[43] and that high caffeine consumption may protect against late-life cognitive decline.[44]

Summary

Caffeine:

- is present in high quantities in coffee and some soft drinks, particularly energy drinks.
- may worsen psychosis and anxiety. Young people may be particularly vulnerable.
- inhibits clozapine metabolism.
- may induce intoxication which is characterised by psychomotor agitation and rambling speech.
- may be associated with toxicity when co-administered with CYP1A2 inhibitors such as fluvoxamine.
- can enhance the reinforcing effects of nicotine and possibly other drugs of abuse.

References

1. Rihs M, et al. Caffeine consumption in hospitalized psychiatric patients. Eur Arch Psychiatry Clin Neurosci 1996; 246:83–92.
2. Clementz GL, et al. Psychotropic effects of caffeine. Am Fam Physician 1988; 37:167–172.
3. Ogawa N, et al. Clinical importance of caffeine dependence and abuse. Psychiatry Clin Neurosci 2007; 61:263–268.
4. Pharmaceutical Press. Martindale: the complete drug reference (online). 2020. https://www.medicinescomplete.com/.
5. Adolfo AB, et al. Effects of smoking cues on caffeine urges in heavy smokers and caffeine consumers with and without schizophrenia. Schizophr Res 2009; 107:192–197.
6. Grant JE, et al. Caffeine's influence on gambling behavior and other types of impulsivity. Addict Behav 2018; 76:156–160.
7. Sawynok J. Pharmacological rationale for the clinical use of caffeine. Drugs 1995; 49:37–50.
8. O'Keefe JH, et al. Effects of habitual coffee consumption on cardiometabolic disease, cardiovascular health, and all-cause mortality. JAmCollCardiol 2013; 62:1043–1051.
9. Bergin JE, et al. Common psychiatric disorders and caffeine use, tolerance, and withdrawal: an examination of shared genetic and environmental effects. TwinResHumGenet 2012; 15:473–482.
10. Silverman K, et al. Withdrawal syndrome after the double-blind cessation of caffeine consumption. N Engl J Med 1992; 327:1109–1114.
11. Butler MA, et al. Determination of CYP1A2 and NAT2 phenotypes in human populations by analysis of caffeine urinary metabolites. Pharmacogenetics 1992; 2:116–127.
12. Kaplan GB, et al. Dose-dependent pharmacokinetics and psychomotor effects of caffeine in humans. J Clin Pharmacol 1997; 37:693–703.
13. Medicines Complete. Stockley's drug interactions. 2020. https://www.medicinescomplete.com/.
14. Baethge C, et al. Coffee and cigarette use: association with suicidal acts in 352 Sardinian bipolar disorder patients. Bipolar Disorders 2009; 11:494–503.

15. Carrillo JA, et al. Effects of caffeine withdrawal from the diet on the metabolism of clozapine in schizophrenic patients. J Clin Psychopharmacol 1998; **18**:311–316.

16. Shioda K, et al. Possible serotonin syndrome arising from an interaction between caffeine and serotonergic antidepressants. Human Psychopharmacology 2004; **19**:353–354.

17. American Psychiatric Association. Diagnostic and Statistical Manual of Mental Disorders, Fifth Edition (DSM-5). Arlington, VA: American Psychiatric Association 2013.

18. Wesnes KA, et al. An evaluation of the cognitive and mood effects of an energy shot over a 6h period in volunteers: a randomized, double-blind, placebo controlled, cross-over study. Appetite 2013; **67**:105–113.

19. Szpak A, et al. A case of acute suicidality following excessive caffeine intake. J Psychopharmacol 2012; **26**:1502–1510.

20. Trapp GS, et al. Energy drink consumption among young Australian adults: associations with alcohol and illicit drug use. Drug Alcohol Depend 2014; **134**:30–37.

21. Pennington N, et al. Energy drinks: a new health hazard for adolescents. J Sch Nurs 2010; **26**:352–359.

22. Sheehan BE, et al. Caffeinated and non-caffeinated alcohol use and indirect aggression: the impact of self-regulation. Addict Behav 2016; **58**:53–59.

23. Görgülü Y, et al. A case of acute psychosis following energy drink consumption. Noro Psikiyatri Arsivi 2014; **51**:79–81.

24. Kelsey D, et al. A case of psychosis and renal failure associated with excessive energy drink consumption. Case Reports in Psychiatry 2019; **2019**:3954161.

25. Quadri S, et al. An energy drink-induced manic episode in an adolescent. Prim Care Companion CNS Disord 2018; **20**: 18l02318

26. Topyurek M, et al. Caffeine effects and schizophrenia: is there a need for more research? Schizophr Res 2019; **211**:34–35.

27. Wang HR, et al. Caffeine-induced psychiatric manifestations: a review. Int Clin Psychopharmacol 2015; **30**:179–182.

28. De Freitas B, et al. Effects of caffeine in chronic psychiatric patients. Am J Psychiatry 1979; **136**:1337–1338.

29. Koczapski A, et al. Effects of caffeine on behavior of schizophrenic inpatients. Schizophr Bull 1989; **15**:339–344.

30. Dratcu L, et al. Clozapine-resistant psychosis, smoking, and caffeine: managing the neglected effects of substances that our patients consume every day. Am J Ther 2007; **14**:314–318.

31. Achor MB, et al. Diet aids, mania, and affective illness. Am J Psychiatry 1981; **138**:392.

32. Wang L, et al. Coffee and caffeine consumption and depression: A meta-analysis of observational studies. Aust N Z J Psychiatry 2016; **50**:228–242.

33. Maremmani I, et al. Are "social drugs" (tobacco, coffee and chocolate) related to the bipolar spectrum? J AffectDisord 2011; **133**:227–233.

34. Lee MA, et al. Anxiogenic effects of caffeine on panic and depressed patients. Am J Psychiatry 1988; **145**:632–635.

35. Rizkallah E, et al. Could the use of energy drinks induce manic or depressive relapse among abstinent substance use disorder patients with comorbid bipolar spectrum disorder? BipolarDisord 2011; **13**:578–580.

36. Machado-Vieira R, et al. Mania associated with an energy drink: the possible role of caffeine, taurine, and inositol. Can J Psychiatry 2001; **46**:454–455.

37. Uhde TW, et al. Caffeine-induced escape from dexamethasone suppression. Arch Gen Psychiatry 1985; **42**:737–738.

38. Cantu TG, et al. Caffeine in electroconvulsive therapy. Ann Pharmacother 1991; **25**:1079–1080.

39. Mester R, et al. Caffeine withdrawal increases lithium blood levels. Biol Psychiatry 1995; **37**:348–350.

40. Bruce MS. The anxiogenic effects of caffeine. Postgrad Med J 1990; **66 Suppl 2**:S18–S24.

41. Bruce MS, et al. Caffeine abstention in the management of anxiety disorders. Psychol Med 1989; **19**:211–214.

42. Santos VA, et al. Panic disorder and chronic caffeine use: a case-control study. Clin Pract Epidemiol Ment Health 2019; **15**:120–125.

43. Ioannidis K, et al. Ostracising caffeine from the pharmacological arsenal for attention-deficit hyperactivity disorder–was this a correct decision? A literature review. Journal of Psychopharmacology (Oxford, England) 2014; **28**:830–836.

44. Panza F, et al. Coffee, tea, and caffeine consumption and prevention of late-life cognitive decline and dementia: a systematic review. J Nutr Health Aging 2015; **19**:313–328.

CHAPTER 12

Nicotine

Nicotine is consumed by vaping or tobacco smoking. Less than a quarter of the general population, 40–50% of those with depression[1] and 70–80% of those with schizophrenia, use nicotine.[2] Nicotine causes peripheral vasoconstriction, tachycardia and increased blood pressure.[3] People with schizophrenia who smoke are more likely to develop the metabolic syndrome, compared with those who do not smoke.[4] As well as nicotine, cigarettes also contain tar (a complex mixture of organic molecules, many carcinogenic), a cause of cancers of the respiratory tract, chronic bronchitis and emphysema.[5] Electronic cigarettes contain only nicotine (alongside some necessary excipients), which has very limited toxicity and is not thought to be carcinogenic. Vaping is thus preferred for all smokers, albeit with some reservations in regard to quality control of content and the so-called re-normalisation of smoking. Vaping is probably not without risk, but this is a complex area beyond the scope of this book.

Nicotine is highly addictive: an effect which may be at least partially genetically determined.[6] People with mental illness are 2–3 times more likely than the general population to develop and maintain nicotine addiction.[1] Chronic smoking contributes to the increased morbidity and mortality from respiratory and cardiovascular disease that is seen in this patient group. Nicotine also has psychotropic effects. Smoking can affect the metabolism (and therefore the efficacy and toxicity) of drugs prescribed to treat psychiatric illness.[7] See section on 'Smoking and psychotropic drugs' in Chapter 11. Nicotine use may be a gateway drug to experimenting with other psychoactive substances.

Psychotropic effects

Nicotine is highly lipid-soluble and rapidly enters the brain after inhalation. Nicotine receptors are found on dopaminergic cell bodies and stimulation of these receptors leads to dopamine release.[1] Dopamine release in the limbic system is associated with pleasure: dopamine is the brain's 'reward' neurotransmitter. Nicotine may be used by people with mental health problems as a form of 'self-medication' (e.g. to alleviate the negative symptoms of schizophrenia or antipsychotic-induced dysphoria or for its anxiolytic effect[8]). Drugs that increase the release of dopamine reduce the craving for nicotine. They may also worsen psychotic illness (see under smoking cessation below).

Nicotine improves concentration and vigilance,[1] probably by enhancing the effects of glutamate, acetylcholine and serotonin.[8]

Schizophrenia

Seventy to eighty per cent of people with schizophrenia regularly smoke cigarettes[2] (with increasing numbers switching to vaping[9,10]) and this increased tendency to smoke predates the onset of psychiatric symptoms.[11] Smoking might actually be a cause of schizophrenia.[12] Possible explanations for higher rates of nicotine use are as follows:[13] smoking causes dopamine release, leading to feelings of well-being and a reduction in negative symptoms;[8] smoking alleviates some of the side effects of antipsychotics such as drowsiness and extrapyramidal symptoms (EPS)[1] and cognitive slowing;[14,15] smoking

CHAPTER 12

serves as a means of structuring the day (a behavioural filler); smoking arises as a result of a familial vulnerability[16] or smoking may be used as a means of alleviating the deficit in auditory gaiting that is found in schizophrenia.[17] Nicotine may also improve working memory and attentional deficits.[18–20] Nicotinic receptor agonists may have beneficial effects on neurocognition,[21,22] although none is licensed for this purpose. Note though that cholinergic drugs may exacerbate nicotine dependence.[23] A single-photon emission computed tomography (SPECT) study has shown that the greater the occupancy of striatal D_2 receptors by antipsychotic drugs, the more likely the patient is to smoke.[24] This may partly explain the clinical observation that smoking cessation may be more achievable when clozapine (a weak dopamine antagonist) is prescribed in place of a conventional antipsychotic. It has been suggested that people with schizophrenia find it particularly difficult to tolerate nicotine withdrawal symptoms[7] (although some certainly can quit[25]). Switching to nicotine replacement therapy or vaping may thus be a preferred option.[26,27] A switch to vaping has been shown to be well tolerated even in severe mental illness.[28]

Depression and anxiety

In 'normal' individuals a moderate consumption of nicotine is associated with pleasure and a decrease in anxiety and feelings of anger.[29] The mechanism of this anxiolytic effect is not understood. People who suffer from anxiety and/or depression are more likely to smoke[30,31] and find it more difficult to stop.[29,32] Nicotine itself might have antidepressant activity.[33] Nicotine withdrawal can precipitate or exacerbate depression in those with a history of the illness,[29] and cigarette smoking may directly increase the risk of symptoms of depression.[34] In contrast, some studies suggest that stopping smoking actually improves depression and anxiety.[35,36] These contradictory findings might be explained by the fact that early withdrawal worsens depression whereas successful cessation improves depression in the longer term. A Cochrane review[37] suggests smoking cessation is achievable in depressed smokers, but a recent twin study found that depression made smoking cessation much less likely.[38]

Patients with depression are at increased risk of cardiovascular disease. By directly causing tachycardia and hypertension,[3] nicotine may, in theory, exacerbate this problem. More importantly, smoking is a well-known independent risk factor for cardiovascular disease, probably because it hastens atherosclerosis. Vaping, while not carcinogenic, probably does increase risk of cardiovascular disease.[39] A recent study suggests nicotine addiction and depression severity are independently linked.[40]

Movement disorders and Parkinson's disease

By increasing dopaminergic neurotransmission, nicotine provides a protective effect against both drug-induced EPS and idiopathic Parkinson's disease. Smokers are less likely to suffer from antipsychotic-induced movement disorders than non-smokers[1] and use anticholinergics less often.[7] Parkinson's disease occurs less frequently in smokers than in non-smokers and the onset of clinical symptoms is delayed.[1,41] This may reflect the inverse association between Parkinson's disease and sensation-seeking behavioural traits, rather than a direct effect of nicotine.[42]

Drug interactions

Polycyclic hydrocarbons in tobacco smoke are known to stimulate the hepatic microsomal enzyme system, particularly P4501A2,[8] the enzyme responsible for the metabolism of many psychotropic drugs. Smoking can lower the blood levels of some drugs by up to 50%.[8] This can affect both efficacy and side effects and needs to be taken into account when making clinical decisions. The drugs most likely to be affected are clozapine,[43] fluphenazine, haloperidol, chlorpromazine, olanzapine, many tricyclic antidepressants, mirtazapine, fluvoxamine and propranolol. Vaping has no effect on hepatic enzyme function. See section on 'Smoking and psychotropic drugs' in Chapter 11.

Withdrawal symptoms[7]

Withdrawal symptoms occur within 6–12 hours of stopping smoking and include intense craving, depressed mood, insomnia, anxiety, restlessness, irritability, difficulty concentrating and increased appetite. Nicotine withdrawal can be confused with depression, anxiety, sleep disorders and mania. Withdrawal can also exacerbate the symptoms of schizophrenia.

Smoking cessation

See section on 'Nicotine and smoking cessation' in Chapter 4 – Addictions and substance misuse.

References

1. Goff DC et al. Cigarette smoking in schizophrenia: relationship to psychopathology and medication side effects. Am J Psychiatry 1992; **149**:1189–1194.
2. Winterer G. Why do patients with schizophrenia smoke? Curr Opin Psychiatry 2010; **23**:112–119.
3. Benowitz NL et al. Cardiovascular effects of nasal and transdermal nicotine and cigarette smoking. Hypertension 2002; **39**:1107–1112.
4. Yevtushenko OO et al. Influence of 5-HT2 C receptor and leptin gene polymorphisms, smoking and drug treatment on metabolic disturbances in patients with schizophrenia. Br J Psychiatry 2008; **192**:424–428.
5. Anderson JE et al. Treating tobacco use and dependence: an evidence-based clinical practice guideline for tobacco cessation. Chest 2002; **121**:932–941.
6. Berrettini W. Nicotine addiction. Am J Psychiatry 2008; **165**:1089–1092.
7. Ziedonis DM et al. Schizophrenia and nicotine use: report of a pilot smoking cessation program and review of neurobiological and clinical issues. Schizophr Bull 1997; **23**:247–254.
8. Lyon ER. A review of the effects of nicotine on schizophrenia and antipsychotic medications. Psychiatr Serv 1999; **50**:1346–1350.
9. Sharma R et al. Motivations and limitations associated with vaping among people with mental illness: a qualitative analysis of reddit discussions. Int J Environ Res Public Health 2016; **14**:7.
10. Bianco CL. Rates of electronic cigarette use among adults with a chronic mental illness. Addict Behav 2019; **89**:1–4.
11. Weiser M et al. Higher rates of cigarette smoking in male adolescents before the onset of schizophrenia: a historical-prospective cohort study. Am J Psychiatry 2004; **161**:1219–1223.
12. Hunter A et al. The effects of tobacco smoking, and prenatal tobacco smoke exposure, on risk of schizophrenia: a systematic review and meta-analysis. Nicotine Tobacco Res 2020; **22**:3–10.
13. Caponnetto P et al. Tobacco smoking, related harm and motivation to quit smoking in people with schizophrenia spectrum disorders. Health Psychol Res 2020; **8**:9042.
14. Harris JG et al. Effects of nicotine on cognitive deficits in schizophrenia. Neuropsychopharmacology 2004; **29**:1378–1385.
15. Gupta T et al. Nicotine usage is associated with elevated processing speed, spatial working memory, and visual learning performance in youth at ultrahigh-risk for psychosis. Psychiatry Res 2014; **220**:687–690.
16. Ferchiou A et al. Exploring the relationships between tobacco smoking and schizophrenia in first-degree relatives. Psychiatry Res 2012; **200**:674–678.
17. McEvoy JP et al. Smoking and therapeutic response to clozapine in patients with schizophrenia. Biol Psychiatry 1999; **46**:125–129.

CHAPTER 12

18. Jacobsen LK et al. Nicotine effects on brain function and functional connectivity in schizophrenia. Biol Psychiatry 2004; 55:850–858.

19. Sacco KA et al. Effects of cigarette smoking on spatial working memory and attentional deficits in schizophrenia: involvement of nicotinic receptor mechanisms. Arch Gen Psychiatry 2005; 62:649–659.

20. Smith RC et al. Effects of nicotine nasal spray on cognitive function in schizophrenia. Neuropsychopharmacology 2006; 31:637–643.

21. Olincy A et al. Proof-of-concept trial of an alpha7 nicotinic agonist in schizophrenia. Arch Gen Psychiatry 2006; 63:630–638.

22. Lieberman JA et al. Cholinergic agonists as novel treatments for schizophrenia: the promise of rational drug development for psychiatry. Am J Psychiatry 2008; 165:931–936.

23. Kelly DL et al. Lack of beneficial galantamine effect for smoking behavior: a double-blind randomized trial in people with schizophrenia. Schizophr Res 2008; 103:161–168.

24. de Haan L et al. Occupancy of dopamine D2 receptors by antipsychotic drugs is related to nicotine addiction in young patients with schizophrenia. Psychopharmacology (Berl) 2006; 183:500–505.

25. Gilbody S et al. Smoking cessation for people with severe mental illness (SCIMITAR+): a pragmatic randomised controlled trial. Lancet Psychiatry 2019; 6:379–390.

26. Caponnetto P et al. Impact of an electronic cigarette on smoking reduction and cessation in schizophrenic smokers: a prospective 12-month pilot study. Int J Environ Res Public Health 2013; 10:446–461.

27. Kozak K et al. Pharmacotherapy for smoking cessation in schizophrenia: a systematic review. Expert Opin Pharmacother 2020; 21:581–590.

28. Hickling LM et al. A pre-post pilot study of electronic cigarettes to reduce smoking in people with severe mental illness. Psychol Med 2019; 49:1033–1040.

29. Glassman AH. Cigarette smoking: implications for psychiatric illness. Am J Psychiatry 1993; 150:546–553.

30. Nunes SO et al. The shared role of oxidative stress and inflammation in major depressive disorder and nicotine dependence. Neurosci Biobehav Rev 2013; 37:1336–1345.

31. Tsuang MT et al. Genetics of smoking and depression. Hum Genet 2012; 131:905–915.

32. Wilhelm K et al. Clinical aspects of nicotine dependence and depression. Med Today 2004; 5:40–47.

33. Gandelman JA et al. Transdermal nicotine for the treatment of mood and cognitive symptoms in nonsmokers with late-life depression. J Clin Psychiatry 2018; 79:18m12137.

34. Boden JM et al. Cigarette smoking and depression: tests of causal linkages using a longitudinal birth cohort. Br J Psychiatry 2010; 196:440–446.

35. Taylor G et al. Change in mental health after smoking cessation: systematic review and meta-analysis. BMJ 2014; 348:g1151.

36. Cather C et al. Improved depressive symptoms in adults with schizophrenia during a smoking cessation attempt with varenicline and behavioral therapy. J Dual Diagn 2017; 13:168–178.

37. van der Meer RM et al. Smoking cessation interventions for smokers with current or past depression. Cochrane Database Syst Rev 2013; 8:CD006102.

38. Ranjit A et al. Depressive symptoms predict smoking cessation in a 20-year longitudinal study of adult twins. Addict Behav 2020; 108:106427.

39. Schweitzer RJ et al. E-cigarette use and indicators of cardiovascular disease risk. Curr Epidemiol Rep 2017; 4:248–257.

40. Bainter T et al. A key indicator of nicotine dependence is associated with greater depression symptoms, after accounting for smoking behavior. PLoS One 2020; 15:e0233656.

41. Scott WK et al. Family-based case-control study of cigarette smoking and Parkinson disease. Neurology 2005; 64:442–447.

42. Evans AH et al. Relationship between impulsive sensation seeking traits, smoking, alcohol and caffeine intake, and Parkinson's disease. J Neurol Neurosurg Psychiatry 2006; 77:317–321.

43. Derenne JL et al. Clozapine toxicity associated with smoking cessation: case report. Am J Ther 2005; 12:469–471.

Psychotropic drugs in special conditions

Psychotropics in overdose

Suicide attempts and suicidal gestures are frequently encountered in psychiatric and general practice, and psychotropic drugs are often taken in overdose (Table 13.1). This section gives brief details of the toxicity in overdose of commonly used psychotropics. It is intended to help guide drug choice in those thought to be at risk of suicide, to give some indication of safe quantities to prescribe and to help identify symptoms of overdose. This section gives no information on the treatment of psychotropic overdose and readers are directed to specialist poisons centres. In all cases of suspected overdose, urgent referral to acute medical facilities is, of course, strongly advised.

Table 13.1 Psychotropic drugs in overdose

Drug or drug group	Toxicity in overdose	Smallest dose likely to cause death	Signs and symptoms of overdose
Antidepressants			
Agomelatine[1,2]	Low	No deaths reported. In early trials, 800mg was maximum tolerated dose. EU SPC reports no serious effects from 2.45g overdose. A mixed overdose of 7.5g caused only drowsiness and mild tachycardia.	Sedation, agitation, stomach pains, dizziness.

(Continued)

The Maudsley® Prescribing Guidelines in Psychiatry, Fourteenth Edition. David M. Taylor, Thomas R. E. Barnes and Allan H. Young.

Table 13.1 (*Continued*)

Drug or drug group	Toxicity in overdose	Smallest dose likely to cause death	Signs and symptoms of overdose
Bupropion[3–6]	Moderate	Around 4.5g, although largest overdose of 13.5g was not fatal.[7]	Tachycardia, seizures, QRS prolongation, QT prolongation, arrhythmia. Agitation and toxic psychosis also reported. Fatal serotonin syndrome may occur if taken with venlafaxine.[8]
Duloxetine[9–12]	Low	Unclear – no deaths from single overdose reported but involved in numerous mixed overdose deaths.	Drowsiness, bradycardia, hypotension. May be asymptomatic.
Lofepramine[13,14]	Low	Unclear. Fatality unlikely if lofepramine taken alone.	Sedation, coma, tachycardia, hypotension.
MAOIs[13,15–17] (not moclobemide)	High	Phenelzine – 400mg Tranylcypromine – 200mg	Tremor, weakness, confusion, sweating, tachycardia, hypertension.
Mianserin[18–20]	Low	Unclear but probably more than 1000mg. Fatality unlikely if mianserin taken alone.	Sedation, coma, hypotension, hypertension, tachycardia, possible QT prolongation.
Mirtazapine[3,21–24]	Low	Fatality unlikely in overdose of mirtazapine alone. One death reported following overdose with 990mg.[25]	Sedation; even large overdose may be asymptomatic. Tachycardia/hypertension sometimes seen. Agitation.
Moclobemide[26,27]	Low	Unclear, but probably more than 8g. Fatality unlikely if moclobemide taken alone.	Vomiting, sedation, disorientation.
Reboxetine[3,28]	Low	Not known. Fatality unlikely in overdose of reboxetine alone.	Sweating, tachycardia, changes in blood pressure.
SSRIs[14,29–32]	Low	Unclear. Probably above 1–2g. Fatality unlikely if SSRI taken alone.	Vomiting, tremor, drowsiness, tachycardia, ST depression. Seizures and QT prolongation possible. Citalopram most toxic of SSRIs in overdose[24,33] (coma, seizures, arrhythmia); escitalopram is less toxic.[34,35]
Trazodone[10,36–39]	Low	Unclear but probably more than 10g. Fatality unlikely in overdose of trazodone alone. Mortality rate about 1 in 10,000 exposures.[24]	Drowsiness, nausea, hypotension, dizziness. Rarely QT prolongation, arrhythmia.
Tricyclics[13,15,16,40] (not lofepramine)	High	Around 500mg. Doses over 50mg/kg usually fatal.	Sedation, coma, tachycardia, arrhythmia (QRS, QT prolongation), hypotension, seizures.

Table 13.1 (Continued)

Drug or drug group	Toxicity in overdose	Smallest dose likely to cause death	Signs and symptoms of overdose
Venlafaxine[3,41–43] (desvenlafaxine causes similar effects but may be less toxic[44])	Moderate	Probably above 5g, but seizures may occur after ingestion of 1g.	Vomiting, sedation, tachycardia, hypertension, seizures, acidosis. Rarely QT prolongation, arrhythmia, rhabdomyolysis. Very rarely cardiac arrest/MI, heart failure.
Vilazodone[45,46]	Low	Doses below 300mg are not fatal. No fatalities recorded in 714 exposures.[24]	Drowsiness, agitation, vomiting, seizures.
Vortioxetine[47]	Low	Unclear. An overdose of 250mg caused no symptoms.	Nausea, somnolence, diarrhoea, pruritis.

Antipsychotics

Drug or drug group	Toxicity in overdose	Smallest dose likely to cause death	Signs and symptoms of overdose
Amisulpride[48–50]	Moderate	Around 16g.	QT prolongation, arrhythmia, cardiac arrest.
Aripiprazole[51–53]	Low	Unclear. Fatality unlikely when taken alone.	Sedation, lethargy, GI disturbance, drooling.
Asenapine[54]	Probably low	Unclear. No deaths from overdose reported. Oral absorption very limited.	Sedation, confusion, facial dystonia, benign ECG changes.
Brexpiprazole[55]	Probably low	No information available.	Presumably agitation and nausea?
Butyrophenones[56–58] (e.g. haloperidol)	Moderate	Haloperidol – probably above 500mg. Arrhythmia may occur at 300mg.	Sedation, coma, dystonia, NMS, QT prolongation, arrhythmia.
Cariprazine[59]	Low	EU SPC reports one overdose of 48mg.	Sedation, low blood pressure.
Clozapine[60,61]	Moderate	Around 2g; much lower in those not tolerant to its effects.[62]	Lethargy, coma, tachycardia, hypotension, hypersalivation, pneumonia, seizures.
Iloperidone[63–65]	Probably moderate	Unclear but probably more than 500mg.	Potent effect on QT interval. Sedation, tachycardia, respiratory depression, hypotension likely.
Lumateperone[66]	Probably low	No overdoses reported.	Presumably sedation and dizziness?
Lurasidone[67]	Low	Unclear. An overdose of 1360mg was not fatal.[68] One study reported no deaths in 821 exposures.[24]	Very limited information. Minimal effect on QT interval.
Olanzapine[60,69–71]	Moderate	Unclear. Probably substantially more than 200mg.	Lethargy, confusion, myoclonus, myopathy, hypotension, tachycardia, delirium. Possibly QT prolongation.

(Continued)

CHAPTER 13

Table 13.1 (*Continued*)

Drug or drug group	Toxicity in overdose	Smallest dose likely to cause death	Signs and symptoms of overdose
Phenothiazines[56,72-74] (e.g. chlorpromazine, fluphenazine)	Moderate	Chlorpromazine 5–10g.	Sedation, coma, tachycardia, arrhythmia, pulmonary oedema, hypotension, QT prolongation, seizures, dystonia, NMS.
Pimavanserin[75]	Not known	No overdoses reported but pimavanserin prolongs QT interval in clinical doses.	Probably QT prolongation and arrhythmia. ? Nausea, vomiting, confusion.[76]
Quetiapine[24,60,77-80]	Moderate	Unclear. Probably more than 5g. Fatalities can occur in single substance overdose.	Lethargy, delirium, tachycardia, QT prolongation, respiratory depression, hypotension, rhabdomyolysis, NMS.
Risperidone[60,81,82] (assume the same for paliperidone)	Low	Unclear. Fatality rare in those taking risperidone or paliperidone alone.	Lethargy, dystonia, tachycardia, changes in blood pressure, QT prolongation. Renal failure with paliperidone.
Ziprasidone[83-88]	Low	Around 10g. Fatality unlikely when taken alone.	Drowsiness, lethargy. QT prolongation, torsades de pointes.

Mood stabilisers

Drug or drug group	Toxicity in overdose	Smallest dose likely to cause death	Signs and symptoms of overdose
Carbamazepine[89,90]	Moderate	Around 20g, but seizures may occur at around 5g.	Somnolence, coma, respiratory depression, ataxia, seizures, tachycardia, arrhythmia, electrolyte disturbance.
Lamotrigine[91,92]	Low	At least 4g. Two deaths reported – one after 4g, the other after 7.5g, but overdoses of >40g have not proved fatal.	Drowsiness, vomiting, ataxia, seizures, tachycardia, dyskinesia, QT prolongation.
Lithium[93-95]	Moderate	Chronic toxicity probably more dangerous but single overdose is occasionally fatal. Six acute overdose deaths recorded in UK 2005–2012.[96]	Nausea, diarrhoea, tremor, confusion, weakness, lethargy, seizures, coma, cardiovascular collapse, bradycardia, arrhythmia, heart block, renal failure.
Valproate[97-101]	Moderate	Unclear but probably more than 20g. Doses over 400mg/kg cause severe toxicity.	Somnolence, coma, cerebral oedema, respiratory depression, blood dyscrasia, hypotension, hypothermia, seizures, electrolyte disturbance (hyperammonaemia).

Others

Drug or drug group	Toxicity in overdose	Smallest dose likely to cause death	Signs and symptoms of overdose
Benzodiazepines[102,103]	Low	Probably more than 100mg diazepam equivalents. Fatality unusual if taken alone. Alprazolam is most toxic.	Drowsiness, ataxia, nystagmus, respiratory dysarthria, depression, coma.
Buspirone[24]	Low	Limited data. Deaths not reported.	Not known.

Table 13.1 (*Continued*)

Drug or drug group	Toxicity in overdose	Smallest dose likely to cause death	Signs and symptoms of overdose
Methadone[104,105]	High	20–50mg may be fatal in non-users. Co-ingestion of benzodiazepines increases toxicity.	Drowsiness, nausea, hypotension, respiratory depression, coma, rhabdomyolysis.
Modafinil[106–108]	Low	Unclear, but no fatalities reported. Overdoses of >6g have not caused death.	Tachycardia, insomnia, agitation, anxiety, nausea, hypertension, dystonia.
Pregabalin[109,110]	Low	No deaths reported. One overdose of 8.4g caused unconsciousness and coma.	May be asymptomatic. Sedation and coma may occur.
Suvorexant[108]	Low	Unclear. No deaths reported.	Sedation, vomiting.
Zolpidem[111,112]	Low	Unclear. Probably >200mg. Fatality rare in those taking zolpidem alone.	Drowsiness, agitation, respiratory depression, tachycardia, coma.
Zopiclone[102,113,114]	Low	Unclear. Probably >100mg. Fatality rare in those taking zopiclone alone.	Ataxia, nausea, diplopia, drowsiness, coma.

ECG, electrocardiogram; GI, gastrointestinal; MAOI, monoamine oxidase inhibitor; MI, myocardial infarction; NMS, neuroleptic malignant syndrome; SPC, summary of product characteristics; SSRI, selective serotonin reuptake inhibitor.

High = Less than 1 week's supply likely to cause serious toxicity or death.
Moderate = 1–4 weeks' supply likely to cause serious toxicity or death.
Low = Death or serious toxicity unlikely even if more than 1 month's supply taken.

CHAPTER 13

References

1. Howland RH Critical appraisal and update on the clinical utility of agomelatine, a melatonergic agonist, for the treatment of major depressive disease in adults. *Neuropsychiatr Dis Treat* 2009; 5:563–576.
2. Wong A, et al. Agomelatine overdose and related toxicity. *Toxicology Communications* 2018; 2:62–65.
3. Buckley NA, et al. 'Atypical' antidepressants in overdose: clinical considerations with respect to safety. *Drug Saf* 2003; 26:539–551.
4. Mercerolle M, et al. A fatal case of bupropion (Zyban) overdose. *J Anal Toxicol* 2008; 32:192–196.
5. Murray B, et al. Single-agent bupropion exposures: clinical characteristics and an atypical cause of serotonin toxicity. *J Med Toxicol* 2020; 16:12–16.
6. Overberg A, et al. Toxicity of bupropion overdose compared with selective serotonin reuptake inhibitors. *Pediatrics* 2019; 144:e20183295.
7. Zhu Y, et al. Atypical findings in massive bupropion overdose: a case report and discussion of psychopharmacologic issues. *J Psychiatr Pract* 2016; 22:405–409.
8. Alibegović A, et al. Fatal overdose with a combination of SNRIs venlafaxine and duloxetine. *Forensic Sci Med Pathol* 2019; 15:258–261.
9. Menchetti M, et al. Non-fatal overdose of duloxetine in combination with other antidepressants and benzodiazepines. *World J Biol Psychiatry* 2009; 10:385–389.
10. White N, et al. Suicidal antidepressant overdoses: a comparative analysis by antidepressant type. *J Med Toxicol* 2008; 4:238–250.
11. Darracq MA, et al. A retrospective review of isolated duloxetine-exposure cases. *ClinToxicol(Phila)* 2013; 51:106–110.
12. Scanlon KA, et al. Comprehensive duloxetine analysis in a fatal overdose. *J Anal Toxicol* 2016; 40:167–170.
13. Cassidy S, et al. Fatal toxicity of antidepressant drugs in overdose. *Br Med J* 1987; 295:1021–1024.
14. Henry JA, et al. Relative mortality from overdose of antidepressants. *BMJ* 1995; 310:221–224.
15. Crome P. Antidepressant overdosage. *Drugs* 1982; 23:431–461.
16. Henry JA. Epidemiology and relative toxicity of antidepressant drugs in overdose. *Drug Saf* 1997; 16:374–390.

17. Waring WS, et al. Acute myocarditis after massive phenelzine overdose. *Eur J Clin Pharmacol* 2007; **63**:1007–1009.

18. Chand S, et al. One hundred cases of acute intoxication with minaserin hydrochloride. *Pharmacopsychiatry* 1981; **14**:15–17.

19. Scherer D, et al. Inhibition of cardiac hERG potassium channels by tetracyclic antidepressant mianserin. *Naunyn Schmiedebergs Arch Pharmacol* 2008; **378**:73–83.

20. Koseoglu Z, et al. Bradycardia and hypotension in mianserin intoxication. *Hum Exp Toxicol* 2010; **29**:887–888.

21. Bremner JD, et al. Safety of mirtazapine in overdose. *J Clin Psychiatry* 1998; **59**:233–235.

22. LoVecchio F, et al. Outcomes after isolated mirtazapine (Remeron) supratherapeutic ingestions. *J Emerg Med* 2008; **34**:77–78.

23. Berling I, et al. Mirtazapine overdose is unlikely to cause major toxicity. *ClinToxicol(Phila)* 2014; **52**:20–24.

24. Nelson JC, et al. Morbidity and mortality associated with medications used in the treatment of depression: an analysis of cases reported to u.s. poison control centers, 2000-2014. *Am J Psychiatry* 2017; **174**:438–450.

25. Vignali C, et al. Mirtazapine fatal poisoning. *Forensic Sci Int* 2017; **276**:e8-e12.

26. Hetzel W. Safety of moclobemide taken in overdose for attempted suicide. *Psychopharmacology (Berl)* 1992; **106** Suppl: S127-S129.

27. Myrenfors PG, et al. Moclobemide overdose. *J Intern Med* 1993; **233**:113–115.

28. Baldwin DS, et al. Tolerability and safety of reboxetine. *Rev Contemp Pharmacother* 2000; **11**:321–330.

29. Cheeta S, et al. Antidepressant-related deaths and antidepressant prescriptions in England and Wales, 1998-2000. *Br J Psychiatry* 2004; **184**:41–47.

30. Barbey JT, et al. SSRI safety in overdose. *J Clin Psychiatry* 1998; **59** Suppl 15:42–48.

31. Jimmink A, et al. Clinical toxicology of citalopram after acute intoxication with the sole drug or in combination with other drugs: overview of 26 cases. *Ther Drug Monit* 2008; **30**:365–371.

32. Tarabar AF, et al. Citalopram overdose: late presentation of torsades de pointes (TdP) with cardiac arrest. *J Med Toxicol* 2008; **4**:101–105.

33. Kraai EP, et al. Citalopram overdose: a fatal case. *J Med Toxicol* 2015; **11**:232–236.

34. Yilmaz Z, et al. Escitalopram causes fewer seizures in human overdose than citalopram. *Clin Toxicol (Phila)* 2010; **48**:207–212.

35. van GF, et al. Clinical and ECG effects of escitalopram overdose. *Ann Emerg Med* 2009; **54**:404–408.

36. Gamble DE, et al. Trazodone overdose: four years of experience from voluntary reports. *J Clin Psychiatry* 1986; **47**:544–546.

37. Martinez MA, et al. Investigation of a fatality due to trazodone poisoning: case report and literature review. *J Anal Toxicol* 2005; **29**:262–268.

38. Dattilo PB, et al. Prolonged QT associated with an overdose of trazodone. *J Clin Psychiatry* 2007; **68**:1309–1310.

39. Service JA, et al. QT prolongation and delayed atrioventricular conduction caused by acute ingestion of trazodone. *Clin Toxicol (Phila)* 2008; **46**:71–73.

40. Caksen H, et al. Acute amitriptyline intoxication: an analysis of 44 children. *Hum Exp Toxicol* 2006; **25**:107–110.

41. Howell C, et al. Cardiovascular toxicity due to venlafaxine poisoning in adults: a review of 235 consecutive cases. *Br J Clin Pharmacol* 2007; **64**:192–197.

42. Hojer J, et al. Fatal cardiotoxicity induced by venlafaxine overdosage. *Clin Toxicol (Phila)* 2008; **46**:336–337.

43. Taylor D. Venlafaxine and cardiovascular toxicity. *BMJ* 2010; **340**:327.

44. Cooper JM, et al. Desvenlafaxine overdose and the occurrence of serotonin toxicity, seizures and cardiovascular effects. *Clin Toxicol (Phila)* 2017; **55**:18–24.

45. Russell JL, et al. Pediatric ingestion of vilazodone compared to other selective serotonin reuptake inhibitor medications. *Clin Toxicol (Phila)* 2017; **55**:352–356.

46. Allergan USA I. Highlights of prescribing information: VIIBRYD (vilazodone hydrochloride) tablets. 2020; https://www.allergan.com/assets/pdf/viibryd_pi.

47. Mazza MG, et al. Vortioxetine overdose in a suicidal attempt: A case report. *Medicine (Baltimore)* 2018; **97**:e10788.

48. Isbister GK, et al. Amisulpride deliberate self-poisoning causing severe cardiac toxicity including QT prolongation and torsades de pointes. *Med J Aust* 2006; **184**:354–356.

49. Ward DI. Two cases of amisulpride overdose: A cause for prolonged QT syndrome. *Emerg Med Australas* 2005; **17**:274–276.

50. Isbister GK, et al. Amisulpride overdose is frequently associated with QT prolongation and torsades de pointes. *J Clin Psychopharmacol* 2010; **30**:391–395.

51. Lofton AL, et al. Atypical experience: a case series of pediatric aripiprazole exposures. *Clin Toxicol (Phila)* 2005; **43**:151–153.

52. Carstairs SD, et al. Overdose of aripiprazole, a new type of antipsychotic. *J Emerg Med* 2005; **28**:311–313.

53. Forrester MB. Aripiprazole exposures reported to Texas poison control centers during 2002-2004. *J Toxicol Environ Health A* 2006; **69**:1719–1726.

54. Taylor JE, et al. A case of intentional asenapine overdose. *PrimCare CompanionCNSDisord* 2013; **15**:PCC.13l01547.

55. U.S. Food & Drug Administration. Drugs@FDA: FDA-approved drugs. 2020; https://www.accessdata.fda.gov/scripts/cder/daf/.

56. Haddad PM, et al. Antipsychotic-related QTc prolongation, torsade de pointes and sudden death. *Drugs* 2002; **62**:1649–1671.

57. Levine BS, et al. Two fatalities involving haloperidol. *J Anal Toxicol* 1991; **15**:282–284.

58. Henderson RA, et al. Life-threatening ventricular arrhythmia (torsades de pointes) after haloperidol overdose. *Hum Exp Toxicol* 1991; **10**:59–62.

59. Recordati Pharmaceuticals Limited. Summary of product characteristics. Reagila 1.5 mg, 3mg, 4.5mg, and 6mg hard capsules. 2020; https://www.medicines.org.uk/emc/product/9401/smpc.

60. Trenton A, et al. Fatalities associated with therapeutic use and overdose of atypical antipsychotics. *CNS Drugs* 2003; **17**:307–324.

61. Flanagan RJ, et al. Suspected clozapine poisoning in the UK/Eire, 1992-2003. *Forensic Sci Int* 2005; **155**:91–99.

62. Shigeev SV, et al. Clozapine intoxication: theoretical aspects and forensic-medical examination. *Sud Med Ekspert* 2013; **56**:41–46.

63. Vigneault P, et al. Iloperidone (Fanapt(R)), a novel atypical antipsychotic, is a potent HERG blocker and delays cardiac ventricular repolarization at clinically relevant concentration. *Pharmacol Res* 2012; **66**:60–65.

64. Vanda Pharmaceuticals Inc. Highlights of prescribing information: FANAPT® (iloperidone) tablets. 2020; https://www.fanapt.com/product/pi/pdf/fanapt.pdf.

65. Amon J, et al. A case of iloperidone overdose in a 27-year-old man with cocaine abuse. *SAGE Open Medical Case Reports* 2016; 4:2050313x16660485.

66. Vyas P, et al. An evaluation of lumateperone tosylate for the treatment of schizophrenia. *Expert Opin Pharmacother* 2020; **21**:139–145.

67. Sunovion Pharmaceuticals Europe Ltd. Summary of Product Characteristics. Latuda 18.5mg, 37mg and 74mg film-coated tablets 2020; https://www.medicines.org.uk/emc/medicine/29125.

68. Molnar GP, et al. Acute lurasidone overdose. *J Clin Psychopharmacol* 2014; **34**:768–770.

69. Chue P, et al. A review of olanzapine-associated toxicity and fatality in overdose. *J Psychiatry Neurosci* 2003; **28**:253–261.

70. Waring WS, et al. Olanzapine overdose is associated with acute muscle toxicity. *Hum Exp Toxicol* 2006; **25**:735–740.

71. Morissette P, et al. Olanzapine prolongs cardiac repolarization by blocking the rapid component of the delayed rectifier potassium current. *Journal of Psychopharmacology (Oxford, England)* 2007; **21**:735–741.

72. Buckley NA, et al. Cardiotoxicity more common in thioridazine overdose than with other neuroleptics. *J Toxicol Clin Toxicol* 1995; **33**:199–204.

73. Li C, et al. Acute pulmonary edema induced by overdosage of phenothiazines. *Chest* 1992; **101**:102–104.

74. Flanagan RJ. Fatal toxicity of drugs used in psychiatry. *Human Psychopharmacology* 2008; **23 Suppl 1**:43–51.

75. Sahli ZT, et al. Pimavanserin: novel pharmacotherapy for Parkinson's disease psychosis. *Expert Opinion on Drug Discovery* 2018; 13:103–110.

76. Vanover KE, et al. Pharmacokinetics, tolerability, and safety of ACP-103 following single or multiple oral dose administration in healthy volunteers. *J Clin Pharmacol* 2007; **47**:704–714.

77. Langman LJ, et al. Fatal overdoses associated with quetiapine. *J Anal Toxicol* 2004; **28**:520–525.

78. Hunfeld NG, et al. Quetiapine in overdosage: a clinical and pharmacokinetic analysis of 14 cases. *Ther Drug Monit* 2006; **28**:185–189.

79. Strachan PM, et al. Mental status change, myoclonus, electrocardiographic changes, and acute respiratory distress syndrome induced by quetiapine overdose. *Pharmacotherapy* 2006; **26**:578–582.

80. Ngo A, et al. Acute quetiapine overdose in adults: a 5-Year retrospective case series. *Ann Emerg Med* 2008; **52**:541–547.

81. Liang CS, et al. Acute renal failure after paliperidone overdose: a case report. *J Clin Psychopharmacol* 2012; **32**:128.

82. Lapid MI, et al. Acute dystonia associated with paliperidone overdose. *Psychosomatics* 2011; **52**:291–294.

83. Gomez-Criado MS, et al. Ziprasidone overdose: cases recorded in the database of Pfizer-Spain and literature review. *Pharmacotherapy* 2005; **25**:1660–1665.

84. Arbuck DM. 12,800-mg ziprasidone overdose without significant ECG changes. *Gen Hosp Psychiatry* 2005; **27**:222–223.

85. Insa Gomez FJ, et al. Ziprasidone overdose: cardiac safety. *Actas Esp Psiquiatr* 2005; **33**:398–400.

86. Klein-Schwartz W, et al. Prospective observational multi-poison center study of ziprasidone exposures. *Clin Toxicol (Phila)* 2007; **45**:782–786.

87. Tan HH, et al. A systematic review of cardiovascular effects after atypical antipsychotic medication overdose. *Am J Emerg Med* 2009; **27**:607–616.

88. Alipour A, et al. Torsade de pointes after ziprasidone overdose with coingestants. *J Clin Psychopharmacol* 2010; **30**:76–77.

89. Spiller HA. Management of carbamazepine overdose. *Pediatr Emerg Care* 2001; **17**:452–456.

90. Schmidt S, et al. Signs and symptoms of carbamazepine overdose. *J Neurol* 1995; **242**:169–173.

91. Alabi A, et al. Safety profile of lamotrigine in overdose. *Ther Adv Psychopharmacol* 2016; **6**:369–381.

92. Alyahya B, et al. Acute lamotrigine overdose: a systematic review of published adult and pediatric cases. *Clin Toxicol (Phila)* 2018; **56**:81–89.

93. Tuohy K, et al. Acute lithium intoxication. *Dial Transplant* 2003; **32**:478–481.

94. Chen KP, et al. Implication of serum concentration monitoring in patients with lithium intoxication. *Psychiatry Clin Neurosci* 2004; **58**:25–29.

95. Offerman SR, et al. Hospitalized lithium overdose cases reported to the California poison control system. *Clin Toxicol (Phila)* 2010; **48**:443–448.

96. Ferrey AE, et al. Relative toxicity of mood stabilisers and antipsychotics: case fatality and fatal toxicity associated with self-poisoning. *BMC Psychiatry* 2018; **18**:399.

97. Isbister GK, et al. Valproate overdose: a comparative cohort study of self poisonings. *Br J Clin Pharmacol* 2003; **55**:398–404.

98. Spiller HA, et al. Multicenter case series of valproic acid ingestion: serum concentrations and toxicity. *J Toxicol Clin Toxicol* 2000; **38**:755–760.

99. Sztajnkrycer MD. Valproic acid toxicity: overview and management. *J Toxicol Clin Toxicol* 2002; **40**:789–801.

100. Eyer F, et al. Acute valproate poisoning: pharmacokinetics, alteration in fatty acid metabolism, and changes during therapy. *J Clin Psychopharmacol* 2005; **25**:376–380.

101. Robinson P, et al. Severe hypothermia in association with sodium valproate overdose. *N Z Med J* 2005; **118**:U1681.

102. Reith DM, et al. Comparison of the fatal toxicity index of zopiclone with benzodiazepines. *J Toxicol Clin Toxicol* 2003; **41**:975–980.

103. Isbister GK, et al. Alprazolam is relatively more toxic than other benzodiazepines in overdose. *Br J Clin Pharmacol* 2004; **58**:88–95.

104. Gable RS. Comparison of acute lethal toxicity of commonly abused psychoactive substances. *Addiction* 2004; **99**:686–696.

105. Caplehorn JR, et al. Fatal methadone toxicity: signs and circumstances, and the role of benzodiazepines. *Aust N Z J Public Health* 2002; 26:358–362.

106. Spiller HA, et al. Toxicity from modafinil ingestion. *Clin Toxicol (Phila)* 2009; 47:153–156.

107. Carstairs SD, et al. A retrospective review of supratherapeutic modafinil exposures. *J Med Toxicol* 2010; 6:307–310.

108. Russell J, et al. Retrospective assessment of toxicity following exposure to Orexin pathway modulators modafinil and suvorexant. *Toxicology Communications* 2019; 3:33–36.

109. Miljevic C, et al. A case of pregabalin intoxication. *Psychiatrike = Psychiatriki* 2012; 23:162–165.

110. Wood DM, et al. Significant pregabalin toxicity managed with supportive care alone. *J Med Toxicol* 2010; 6:435–437.

111. Gock SB, et al. Acute zolpidem overdose–report of two cases. *J Anal Toxicol* 1999; 23:559–562.

112. Garnier R, et al. Acute zolpidem poisoning–analysis of 344 cases. *J Toxicol Clin Toxicol* 1994; 32:391–404.

113. Pounder D, et al. Zopiclone poisoning. *J Anal Toxicol* 1996; 20:273–274.

114. Bramness JG, et al. Fatal overdose of zopiclone in an elderly woman with bronchogenic carcinoma. *J Forensic Sci* 2001; 46:1247–1249.

Driving and psychotropic medicines

Everyone has a duty to drive reasonably, and in almost all countries drivers are legally responsible for accidents they cause whether or not under the influence of drugs and alcohol.[1]

Many factors have been shown to affect driving performance. These include age, gender, personality, physical and mental state and being under the influence of alcohol, prescribed medicines, street drugs or over-the-counter medicines.[2,3] Studying the effects of any of these individual factors in isolation is extremely difficult. Some studies have attempted to categorise medicinal drugs according to how they affect driving performance,[4] and some have assessed the effect of medication on tests such as response-time and attention,[5] but these tests do not directly measure ability to drive.

As many as 10% of people killed or injured in road traffic accidents (RTAs) are taking psychotropic medication (Table 13.2).[5] Patients with personality disorders and alcoholism have the highest rates of motoring offences and are more likely to be involved in accidents.[5] In most countries people whose driving ability may be impaired through their illness or prescribed medication are required to inform their motor insurer. Failure to do so is considered to be 'withholding a material fact' and may render the insurance policy void.

Effects of mental illness

In the UK, severe mental disorder is a prescribed disability for the purposes of the Road Traffic Act 1988.[6] Regulations define mental disorder as including mental illness, arrested or incomplete development of the mind, psychopathic disorder or severe impairment of intelligence or social functioning. There is an assessing fitness to drive guide at www.gov.uk. Amongst physical conditions commonly seen in mental illness licence restrictions may also apply to people with diabetes, particularly if treated with insulin or if there are established micro- or macro-vascular complications. In the USA, regulations related to driving and mental health disorders vary somewhat from state to state (see Department of Motor Vehicles website for each state).

Many people with early dementia are capable of driving safely.[7,8] In the UK, all drivers with new diagnoses of Alzheimer's disease and other dementias must notify the Driver and Vehicle Licensing Agency (DVLA).[7] The doctor may need to make an immediate decision on safety to drive and ensure that the licensing agency is notified.[9] There are no data to support ongoing driving assessments as a way of maintaining driving ability or improving road safety of drivers with dementia.[10] In the USA, some states mandate doctors to report a diagnosis of dementia, but in others the issue may only arise on licence renewal.

Psychiatric medicines, driving and UK law

Most countries prohibit the use of a range of illicit substances when driving. In the UK, drug-driving law gives threshold blood concentration for eight drugs associated with illicit use (zero tolerance approach – threshold set to reveal any recent use) and eight medicinal drugs.[11] For the latter group, Table 13.3 gives the legal limit and expected plasma concentrations in clinical use.

CHAPTER 13

Table 13.2 Psychotropics and driving

Drug	Effect
Alcohol	Alcohol causes sedation and impaired coordination, vision, attention and information-processing. Alcohol-dependent drivers are twice as likely to be involved in traffic accidents and offences than licensed drivers as a whole,[5] and a third of all fatal RTAs involve alcohol-dependent drivers.[5] Young drivers who use alcohol in combination with illicit drugs are particularly at high risk.[12,13]
Antiseizure medication	Initial, dose-related side effects may affect driving ability (e.g. blurred vision, ataxia and sedation). There are strict rules regarding epilepsy and driving. Lamotrigine may have limited effects on driving ability.[14]
Antidepressants	People who are prescribed an antidepressant have an increased risk of being involved in a RTA particularly at treatment initiation. SSRIs may have some advantages over TCAs, but driving ability is still diminished compared with healthy individuals,[15] suggesting that depression itself may make a major contribution.[16,17] SSRIs tend not to impair driving in healthy volunteers.[18–20] In remitted patients on SSRIs, driving performance may likewise not be impaired.[21] Initiation effects caused by mirtazapine diminish to an extent when it is given as a single dose at night, but many people experience substantial hangover which can impair driving.[22] Effects may disappear in chronic treatment.[23] Trazodone also appears to impair driving ability.[24] Agomelatine and venlafaxine may actually improve driving performance.[25] Vortioxetine has no effect.[23] Intranasal esketamine seems to have no effect on driving ability 8 hours post dose.[26]
Antipsychotics	Sedation and EPS can impair coordination and response time.[2] A high proportion of patients treated with antipsychotics may have an impaired ability to drive.[27,28] One study found that patients with schizophrenia taking atypical antipsychotics or clozapine performed better in tests of skills related to car-driving ability than patients with schizophrenia taking first-generation antipsychotics,[29] but 25% of all patients were severely impaired with respect to driving skills.
Hypnotics and Anxiolytics	Benzodiazepines cause sedation and impaired attention, information processing, memory and motor coordination, and along with opiates are the medicines most frequently implicated in RTAs.[30,31] When used as anxiolytics and hypnotics, benzodiazepines, zopiclone and zolpidem are associated with an increased risk of RTAs.[30] There is some gender variation in the pharmacokinetics of zolpidem with females having higher drug plasma concentrations than males for any given dose; the driving ability of females may therefore be particularly impaired.[3] Zolpidem may additionally be associated with automatism and 'sleep driving'.[32] Zaleplon and the newer hypnotics acting at melatonin or serotonin receptors have not been found to have any negative residual effects on driving ability.[33] Orexin receptor antagonists (suvorexant and lemborexant), available in some countries, appear not to impair driving the day after being taken.[34,35]
Lithium	Lithium may impair visual adaptation to the dark,[2] but the implications for driving safety are unknown. Many patients treated with lithium can be shown to be unfit to drive,[14] although the exact contribution of lithium is difficult to determine. Elderly people who take lithium may be at increased risk of being involved in an injurious motor vehicle crash.[36]
Methylphenidate	Some studies have demonstrated that reaction time is longer in patients with ADHD which may in turn be associated with increased driving risks.[37] Other studies have found that methylphenidate improved driving performance in adults with ADHD,[38] again suggesting that illness may make a bigger contribution to fitness to drive than the specific pharmacology of the treatment.[38]
Opioids	Opioids have major adverse effect on the risk of RTA.[39] Buprenorphine and methadone reduce driving ability at low doses in non addicts.[40]

ADHD, attention deficit hyperactivity disorder; EPS, extrapyramidal symptoms; RTA, road traffic accident; SSRI, selective serotonin reuptake inhibitor; TCA, tricyclic antidepressant.

Table 13.3 Benzodiazepines concentration in normal dosing and the legal limit

Drug/daily dose	Range of concentrations reported (legal limit)
Clonazepam 0.5–6.0mg[41,42]	5–80µg/L (50)
Diazepam 5–30mg[43]	50–1000µg/L (550)
Flunitrazepam 0.5–2.0mg[44,45]	10–20µg/L (300)
Lorazepam 1–4mg[46,47]	10–70µg/L (100)
Oxazepam 15–30mg[48]	250–600µg/L (300)
Temazepam 10–20mg[49]	200–900µg/L (1000)

In regards to methadone, doses of up to 80mg a day generally give plasma levels below the UK legal limit.[50] The legal limits listed here apply only to those who are lawfully prescribed the drug in question – the driver may be subject to prosecution if it can be proved the drugs were taken illicitly.

Other medicines

Many psychotropics can impair alertness, concentration and driving performance. Medicines that block H_1, α_1-adrenergic or cholinergic receptors may be particularly problematic. Effects are particularly marked at the start of treatment and after increasing the dose. Drivers must be made aware of any potential for impairment and are advised to evaluate their driving performance at these times. They must stop driving if adversely affected.[51] The use of alcohol will further increase any impairment.

Some antipsychotics and antidepressants lower the seizure threshold. In the UK, the DVLA advises this is taken into consideration when prescribing for a driver. Further information about the effects of psychotropics on driving can be found in Table 13.2.

Medication-induced sedation

Many psychotropics are sedating. The more sedating a medicine is, the more likely it is to impair driving ability. Other medicines, either prescribed or bought over the counter, may also be sedative and/or affect driving ability (e.g. antihistamines[5]). One study found that 89% of patients taking other psychotropics in addition to antidepressants failed a battery of 'fitness to drive' tests.[52] Since the degree of sedation any individual will experience is very difficult to predict, patients prescribed sedating medicines should be advised not to drive if they feel sedated. In the UK, it is the responsibility of the driver to ensure they are fit to drive.

DVLA – duty of the driver

In the UK, it is the legal responsibility of the licence holder or applicant to notify the DVLA of any medical condition which may affect safe driving. A list of relevant medical conditions can be found in the DVLA assessing fitness-to-drive guide.[53]

DVLA – duty of the prescriber

Make sure the patient understands that their condition may impair their ability to drive. If the patient is incapable of understanding, notify the DVLA immediately. Explain to the patient that they have a legal duty to inform the DVLA.

Note: The DVLA guidance specifies that patients under S17 of the Mental Health Act must be able to satisfy the standards of fitness for their respective conditions and be free from any effects of medication which would affect driving adversely, before resuming driving. Very few patients will fulfil these criteria.

General Medical Council guidelines for prescribers[54]

- Patients who disagree with the diagnosis or the effect of the condition on their ability to drive should seek a second opinion and refrain from driving until this has been obtained.
- If the patient continues to drive while unfit, you should make every reasonable effect to persuade them to stop. This may include telling their next of kin if they agree you may do the driving.
- If they continue to drive, inform the DVLA. Tell the patient you are going to do this and write to the patient to confirm you have done so. Document the advice given clearly in the patient's notes.

References

1. Annas GJ. Doctors, drugs, and driving – tort liability for patient-caused accidents. *N Engl J Med* 2008; **395**:521–525.
2. Metzner JL, et al. Impairment in driving and psychiatric illness. *J Neuropsychiatry Clin Neurosci* 1993; **5**:211–220.
3. Farkas RH, et al. Zolpidem and driving impairment – identifying persons at risk. *N Engl J Med* 2013; **369**:689–691.
4. Alvarez J, et al. ICADTS Working Group: Categorization system for medicinal drugs affecting driving performance. 2007; http://www.icadts.nl/medicinal.html.
5. Noyes R, Jr. Motor vehicle accidents related to psychiatric impairment. *Psychosomatics* 1985; **26**:569–580.
6. The National Archives. Road Traffic Act 1991. 1991; http://www.legislation.gov.uk/ukpga/1991/40/contents.
7. Driver and Vehicle Licensing Agency. Assessing fitness to drive – a guide for medical professionals. 2016 (last updated 2018); www.gov.uk/dvla/fitnesstodrive.
8. Piersma D, et al. Prediction of fitness to drive in patients with Alzheimer's dementia. *PLoS One* 2016; **11**:e0149566.
9. Breen DA, et al. Driving and dementia. *BMJ* 2007; **334**:1365–1369.
10. Martin AJ, et al. Driving assessment for maintaining mobility and safety in drivers with dementia. *Cochrane Database Syst Rev* 2013; **8**:CD006222.
11. Department for Transport. Changes to drug driving law. 2013 (last updated August 2017); https://www.gov.uk/government/collections/drug-driving.
12. Biecheler MB, et al. SAM survey on "drugs and fatal accidents": search of substances consumed and comparison between drivers involved under the influence of alcohol or cannabis. *Traffic Inj Prev* 2008; **9**:11–21.
13. Oyefeso A, et al. Fatal injuries while under the influence of psychoactive drugs: a cross-sectional exploratory study in England. *BMC Public Health* 2006; **6**:148.
14. Segmiller FM, et al. Driving ability according to German guidelines in stabilized bipolar I and II outpatients receiving lithium or lamotrigine. *J Clin Pharmacol* 2013; **53**:459–462.

15. Brunnauer A, et al. The effects of most commonly prescribed second generation antidepressants on driving ability: a systematic review : 70th Birthday Prof. Riederer. *J Neural Transm* 2013; **120**:225–232.

16. Bramness JG, et al. Minor increase in risk of road traffic accidents after prescriptions of antidepressants: a study of population registry data in Norway. *J Clin Psychiatry* 2008; **69**:1099–1103.

17. Verster JC, et al. Psychoactive medication and traffic safety. *Int J Environ Res Public Health* 2009; **6**:1041–1054.

18. Iwamoto K, et al. The effects of acute treatment with paroxetine, amitriptyline, and placebo on driving performance and cognitive function in healthy Japanese subjects: a double-blind crossover trial. *Human Psychopharmacol* 2008; **23**:399–407.

19. Ridout F, et al. A placebo controlled investigation into the effects of paroxetine and mirtazapine on measures related to car driving performance. *Human Psychopharmacol* 2003; **18**:261–269.

20. Wingen M, et al. Actual driving performance and psychomotor function in healthy subjects after acute and subchronic treatment with escitalopram, mirtazapine, and placebo: a crossover trial. *J Clin Psychiatry* 2005; **66**:436–443.

21. Miyata A, et al. Driving performance of stable outpatients with depression undergoing real-world treatment. *Psychiatry Clin Neurosci* 2018; **72**:399–408.

22. Verster JC, et al. Mirtazapine as positive control drug in studies examining the effects of antidepressants on driving ability. *Eur J Pharmacol* 2015; **753**:252–256.

23. Theunissen EL, et al. A randomized trial on the acute and steady-state effects of a new antidepressant, vortioxetine (Lu AA21004), on actual driving and cognition. *Clin Pharmacol Ther* 2013; **93**:493–501.

24. Ip EJ, et al. The effect of trazodone on standardized field sobriety tests. *Pharmacotherapy* 2013; **33**:369–374.

25. Brunnauer A, et al. Driving performance and psychomotor function in depressed patients treated with agomelatine or venlafaxine. *Pharmacopsychiatry* 2015; **48**:65–71.

26. van de Loo A, et al. The effects of intranasal esketamine (84 mg) and oral mirtazapine (30 mg) on on-road driving performance: a double-blind, placebo-controlled study. *Psychopharmacology (Berl)* 2017; **234**:3175–3183.

27. Grabe HJ, et al. The influence of clozapine and typical neuroleptics on information processing of the central nervous system under clinical conditions in schizophrenic disorders: implications for fitness to drive. *Neuropsychobiology* 1999; **40**:196–201.

28. Wylie KR, et al. Effects of depot neuroleptics on driving performance in chronic schizophrenic patients. *J Neurol Neurosurg Psychiatry* 1993; **56**:910–913.

29. Brunnauer A, et al. The impact of antipsychotics on psychomotor performance with regards to car driving skills. *J Clin Psychopharmacol* 2004; **24**:155–160.

30. Dassanayake T, et al. Effects of benzodiazepines, antidepressants and opioids on driving: a systematic review and meta-analysis of epidemiological and experimental evidence. *Drug Saf* 2011; **34**:125–156.

31. Rudisill TM, et al. Medication use and the risk of motor vehicle collisions among licensed drivers: a systematic review. *Accid Anal Prev* 2016; **96**:255–270.

32. Poceta JS. Zolpidem ingestion, automatisms, and sleep driving: a clinical and legal case series. *J Clin Sleep Med* 2011; **7**:632–638.

33. Verster JC, et al. Hypnotics and driving safety: meta-analyses of randomized controlled trials applying the on-the-road driving test. *Current Drug Safety* 2006; **1**:63–71.

34. Vermeeren A, et al. On-the-road driving performance the morning after bedtime administration of lemborexant in healthy adult and elderly volunteers. *Sleep* 2019; **42**:zsy260.

35. Vermeeren A, et al. On-the-road driving performance the morning after bedtime use of suvorexant 15 and 30 mg in healthy elderly. *Psychopharmacology (Berl)* 2016; **233**:3341–3351.

36. Etminan M, et al. Use of lithium and the risk of injurious motor vehicle crash in elderly adults: case-control study nested within a cohort. *BMJ* 2004; **328**:558–559.

37. Hashemian F, et al. A comparison of the effects of reboxetine and placebo on reaction time in adults with Attention Deficit-Hyperactivity Disorder (ADHD). *Daru* 2011; **19**:231–235.

38. Classen S, et al. Evidence-based review on interventions and determinants of driving performance in teens with attention deficit hyperactivity disorder or autism spectrum disorder. *Traffic Inj Prev* 2013; **14**:188–193.

39. Hetland A, et al. Medications and impaired driving. *Ann Pharmacother* 2014; **48**:494–506.

40. Strand MC, et al. Pharmacokinetics of single doses of methadone and buprenorphine in blood and oral fluid in healthy volunteers and correlation with effects on psychomotor and cognitive functions. *J Clin Psychopharmacol* 2019; **39**:489–493.

41. Sjo O, et al. Pharmacokinetics and side-effects of clonazepam and its 7-amino-metabolite in man. *Eur J Clin Pharmacol* 1975; **8**:249–254.

42. Berlin A, et al. Pharmacokinetics of the anticonvulsant drug clonazepam evaluated from single oral and intravenous doses and by repeated oral administration. *Eur J Clin Pharmacol* 1975; **9**:155–159.

43. Rutherford DM, et al. Plasma concentrations of diazepam and desmethyldiazepam during chronic diazepam therapy. *Br J Clin Pharmacol* 1978; **6**:69–73.

44. Wickstrom E, et al. Pharmacokinetic and clinical observations on prolonged administration of flunitrazepam. *Eur J Clin Pharmacol* 1980; **17**:189–196.

45. Mattila MA, et al. Flunitrazepam: a review of its pharmacological properties and therapeutic use. *Drugs* 1980; **20**:353–374.

46. Greenblatt DJ, et al. Single- and multiple-dose kinetics of oral lorazepam in humans: the predictability of accumulation. *J Pharmacokinet Biopharm* 1979; **7**:159–179.

47. Greenblatt DJ, et al. Pharmacokinetic comparison of sublingual lorazepam with intravenous, intramuscular, and oral lorazepam. *J Pharm Sci* 1982; **71**:248–252.

CHAPTER 13

48. Smink BE, et al. The concentration of oxazepam and oxazepam glucuronide in oral fluid, blood and serum after controlled administration of 15 and 30 mg oxazepam. *Br J Clin Pharmacol* 2008; **66**:556–560.

49. Greenblatt DJ, et al. Clinical pharmacokinetics of the newer benzodiazepines. *Clin Pharmacokinet* 1983; **8**:233–252.

50. Ferrari A, et al. Methadone – metabolism, pharmacokinetics and interactions. *Pharmacol Res* 2004; **50**:551–559.

51. Department of Transport. Medication and Road Safety: A Scoping Study. Road Safety Research Report No. 116. 2010; https://webarchive.nationalarchives.gov.uk/20101007211118/http://www.dft.gov.uk/pgr/roadsafety/research/rsrr/theme3/report16findings.pdf

52. Grabe HJ, et al. The influence of polypharmacological antidepressive treatment on central nervous information processing of depressed patients: implications for fitness to drive. *Neuropsychobiology* 1998; **37**:200–204.

53. Driver and Vehicle Licensing Agency. At a glance guide to the current medical standards of fitness to drive. 2013 (last updated March 2020); https://www.gov.uk/government/publications/at-a-glance.

54. General Medical Council. Good practice in prescribing and managing medicines and devices. 2013; https://www.gmc-uk.org/guidance/ethical_guidance/14316.asp.

Psychotropics and surgery

There are few studies of the effects of non-anaesthetic drugs on surgery and the anaesthetic process.[1,2] Practice is largely based on theoretical considerations, case reports, clinical experience and personal opinion. Any guidance given in this area is therefore somewhat speculative. The decision as to whether or not to continue a drug during surgery and the perioperative period should take into account a number of interacting factors. Some general considerations include the following:

- Patients are at risk of aspirating their stomach contents during general anaesthesia. For this reason they are usually prevented from eating for at least 6 hours before surgery. However, clear fluids leave the stomach within 2 hours of ingestion and so fluids that enable a patient to take routine medication may be allowed up to 2 hours before surgery.[3]
- There are some interactions between drugs used during surgery and routine medication that constitute an absolute contra-indication. This is usually managed by the anaesthetist through their choice of anaesthetic drugs, but may involve temporary cessation of regular medication. Significant interactions between medicines used during surgery and psychotropics include the following:
  - Enflurane may precipitate seizures in patients taking tricyclic antidepressants.[4-6]
  - Pethidine and other serotonergic opioids may precipitate fatal 'excitatory' reactions in patients taking MAOIs and may cause serotonin syndrome in patients taking SSRIs.[4-7]
  - Volatile anaesthetics (halothane, enflurane, etc.) prolong QTc[8] and should usually not be given to patients on QT-prolonging drugs who have ECG evidence of QT prolongation.

In addition:
- Major surgical procedures induce profound physiological changes, which include electrolyte disturbances and the release of cortisol and catecholamines.
- Postoperatively, surgical stress and some agents used in anaesthesia may lead to gastric or gastrointestinal stasis. Oral absorption of drugs is therefore likely to be compromised.

To continue or not to continue?

For the most part, psychotropic drugs should be continued during the perioperative period, assuming agreement of the anaesthetist/anaesthesiologist concerned. Table 13.4 provides some discussion of the merits or otherwise of continuing individual psychotropics during surgery.

Psychotropic and other drugs are frequently (albeit accidentally and/or unthinkingly) withheld from preoperative patients simply because they are 'nil by mouth'.[1] Patients may be labelled 'nil by mouth' for several reasons, including pre-operative preparation, unconsciousness, to rest the gut postoperatively or as a result of the surgery itself. Patients may also develop an intolerance to oral medicines at any time during a stay in hospital, often because of nausea and vomiting. When it is decided to continue a psychotropic, this decision needs to be explicitly outlined to medical and nursing staff so that treatment is not unintentionally withheld.

Table 13.4 Psychotropic and surgery

Drug or drug group	Considerations	Safe in surgery?	Alternative formulations
Antiseizure medications[4,9–11]	▪ CNS depressant activity may reduce anaesthetic requirements ▪ Drug level monitoring may be required ▪ Reduced dose of propofol may be required ▪ Has been used pre-operatively and has analgesic properties	Probably, usually continued for people with epilepsy	Carbamazepine liquid or suppositories are available in most countries: 100mg tablet = 125mg suppository. Maximum by rectum 1g daily in four divided doses. Phenytoin is available IV or liquid: IV dose = oral dose Sodium valproate is available IV or liquid: IV dose = oral dose. Before crushing tablets and mixing with water, confirm stability with either local guidelines or the drug company. Liquid and dispersible tablets fairly widely available.
Antidepressants – MAOIs[3,4,12–16]	▪ Dangerous, potentially fatal interaction with pethidine and dextromethorphan (serotonin syndrome or coma/respiratory depression may occur) ▪ Action of inhaled anaesthetics and neuromuscular blockers is reduced ▪ Sympathomimetic agents may result in hypertensive crisis (avoid ketamine, ephedrine, pancuronium)[17] ▪ Phenylephrine, epinephrine and norepinephrine give exaggerated response ▪ MAO inhibition lasts for up to 2 weeks: early withdrawal is required ▪ Switching to moclobemide 2 weeks before surgery allows continued treatment up until day of surgery (do not give moclobemide on the day of surgery)	Probably not, but careful selection of anaesthetic agents may reduce risks if continuation is essential	None

Table 13.4 *(Continued)*

Drug or drug group	Considerations	Safe in surgery?	Alternative formulations
Antidepressants – SSRIs[4–7,15,18–20]	▪ Danger of serotonin syndrome if administered with pethidine, fentanyl, pentazocine or tramadol ▪ Occasional seizures reported ▪ Cessation may result in withdrawal syndrome and increased risk of relapse ▪ Rule-out hyponatraemia in all surgical patients[21] ▪ Various interactions with drugs used in surgery including blocking conversion of pro-drugs such as codeine and oxycodone ▪ Venlafaxine may provoke opioid-induced rigidity ▪ Increases risk of perioperative bleeding	Probably, but avoid other serotonergic agents	Liquid escitalopram, fluoxetine and paroxetine are available in most countries. Oral disintegrating tablets of mirtazapine have been used perioperatively (for nausea).[22]
Antidepressants – tricyclics[4–6,15,18,20,23]	▪ α_1 blockade may lead to hypotension and interfere with effects of epinephrine and norepinephrine ▪ Care needed with activities that increase sympathetic stimulation (e.g. intubation)[17] ▪ Danger of serotonin syndrome (clomipramine; amitriptyline) if administered with pethidine, pentazocine or tramadol ▪ Many drugs prolong QT interval so arrhythmia more likely ▪ Most drugs lower seizure threshold ▪ May lessen core hypothermia ▪ Sympathomimetic agents may give exaggerated response ▪ Effects persist for several days after cessation so will need to be stopped some time before surgery ▪ Clomipramine, amitriptyline may increase bleeding risk ▪ Analgesic effect may decrease opiate requirements	Unclear, but anaesthetic agents need to be carefully chosen Some authorities recommend slow discontinuation before surgery	Liquid amitriptyline is available. It is acidic and may interact with enteral feeds. Dosulepin capsules can be opened and mixed with water before flushing well. This is preferred to crushing tablets. Most tricyclics have potent local anaesthetic effects – oral delivery in liquid form is likely to cause local anaesthesia.

(Continued)

Table 13.4 (Continued)

Drug or drug group	Considerations	Safe in surgery?	Alternative formulations
Antipsychotics[4,15,24–28]	▪ Some antipsychotics widely used in anaesthetic practice ▪ Increased risk of arrhythmia with most drugs ▪ α_1 blockade may lead to hypotension and interfere with effects of epinephrine and norepinephrine ▪ Most drugs lower seizure threshold ▪ May enhance interoperative core hypothermia ▪ Some evidence of safe use in surgery[29] ▪ Clozapine may delay recovery from anaesthesia ▪ Gaseous anaesthetics may affect dopamine metabolism ▪ Preoperative olanzapine reduces risk of delirium[30] as may preoperative aripiprazole[31] ▪ Use of SGAs may reduce postoperative nausea[32]	Probably, usually continued to avoid relapse[33]	Liquid preparations of some antipsychotics are available. Some 'specials' liquids can be made for NG delivery. Before crushing tablets and mixing with water, confirm stability with either local guidelines or the drug manufacturer.
Benzodiazepines[4,9]	▪ Reduced requirements for induction and maintenance anaesthetics ▪ Many have prolonged action (days or weeks), so early withdrawal is necessary ▪ Withdrawal symptoms possible	Probably; usually continued	Liquid, IM, IV and rectal diazepam are available (do not use IM route). Buccal liquid available for midazolam Sublingual (use normal tablets), IM, IV and lorazepam are available.
Lithium[3,4,12,15]	▪ Prolongs the action of both depolarising and non-depolarising muscle relaxants ▪ Surgery-related electrolyte disturbance and reduced renal function may precipitate lithium toxicity. Avoid dehydration and NSAIDs ▪ Possible increased risk of arrhythmia	Probably safe in minor surgery but usually discontinued before major procedures and re-started once electrolytes normalise Slow discontinuation is essential – anaesthetists may not appreciate this[34]	The bioavailability of lithium varies between brands. Care is needed with equivalent doses of salts: lithium carbonate 200mg = lithium citrate 509mg. Liquid lithium citrate is available and is usually administered twice daily.

(Continued)

Table 13.4 (*Continued*)

Drug or drug group	Considerations	Safe in surgery?	Alternative formulations
Methadone [3,9]	▪ May reduce opiate requirements ▪ Naloxone may induce withdrawal ▪ Methadone prolongs QT interval ▪ When using opiates, use only full agonists (avoid buprenorphine)	Probably, usually continued	IM dose = oral dose
Modafinil[35,36]	▪ Limited data suggest no interference with anaesthesia ▪ Improves recovery after anaesthesia	Probably, data limited	None
Pregabalin[37]	▪ Preoperative pregabalin reduces post-op nausea	Yes	None

CNS, central nervous system; IM, intramuscular; IV, intravenous; MAOI, monoamine oxidase inhibitor; NSAID, non-steroidal anti-inflammatory drug; SSRI, selective serotonin reuptake inhibitor; TCA, tricyclic antidepressant.

Smoking

For many patients undergoing surgery and recovery in a hospital there will be little or no opportunity to smoke. Abrupt cessation of smoking is likely to affect mental state and may also result in drug toxicity if psychotropics are continued (see section on 'Smoking and psychotropic drugs', Chapter 11 – Pharmacokinetics).

Changing formulation

Alternative routes and formulations may be sought for a variety of reasons related to surgery. When changing the route or formulation, bioavailability may also change and so care should be taken to ensure the appropriate dose and frequency is prescribed. Oral preparations may sometimes be administered via a nasogastric (NG), percutaneous endoscopic gastrostomy (PEG) or jejunostomy tube, either in liquid formulations or as crushed tablets. Bioavailability issues may arise because of adsorption of drugs to the delivery tube material.

Risks associated with discontinuing psychotropics

▪ Relapse (especially if treatment ceased for more than a few days)[38]
▪ Worsening of condition. For example, abrupt cessation of lithium worsens outcome in bipolar affective disorder,[39] as does abrupt stopping of antidepressants[40] and antipsychotics[41]
▪ Suicide. Cessation of antidepressants may increase risk of suicide[42]
▪ Withdrawal symptoms. These may complicate diagnosis in the perioperative period
▪ Delirium. Common in those discontinuing antipsychotics[43] and antidepressants[6]

Risks associated with continuing psychotropics

- Potential for interactions (pharmacokinetic and pharmacodynamics) with anaesthetic and perioperative drugs
- Increased likelihood of bleeding (e.g. with SSRIs)[44]
- Hypo/hypertension (depending on psychotropic)[23,24]
- Effects on core body temperature (e.g. with phenothiazines)

References

1. Noble DW, et al. Interrupting drug therapy in the perioperative period. *Drug Saf* 2002; 25:489–495.
2. Noble DW, et al. Risks of interrupting drug treatment before surgery. *BMJ* 2000; 321:719–720.
3. Anon. Drugs in the peri-operative period: 1–stopping or continuing drugs around surgery. *Drug Ther Bull* 1999; 37:62–64.
4. Smith MS, et al. Perioperative management of drug therapy, clinical considerations. *Drugs* 1996; 51:238–259.
5. Chui PT, et al. Medications to withhold or continue in the preoperative consultation. *Curr Anaesth Crit Care* 1998; 9:302–306.
6. Kudoh A, et al. Antidepressant treatment for chronic depressed patients should not be discontinued prior to anesthesia. *Can J Anaesth* 2002; 49:132–136.
7. Spivey KM, et al. Perioperative seizures and fluvoxamine. *Br J Anaesth* 1993; 71:321.
8. Schmeling WT, et al. Prolongation of the QT interval by enflurane, isoflurane, and halothane in humans. *Anesth Analg* 1991; 72:137–144.
9. Morrow JI, et al. Essential drugs in the perioperative period. *Curr Pract Surg* 1990; 90:106–109.
10. Bloor M, et al. Antiepileptic drugs and anesthesia. *Paediatr Anaesth* 2017; 27:248–250.
11. Bhosale UA, et al. Comparative pre-emptive analgesic efficacy study of novel antiepileptic agents gabapentin, lamotrigine and topiramate in patients undergoing major surgeries at a tertiary care hospital: a randomized double blind clinical trial. *J Basic Clin Physiol Pharmacol* 2017; 28:59–66.
12. Rahman MH, et al. Medication in the peri-operative period. *Pharm J* 2004; 272:287–289.
13. Blom-Peters L, et al. Monoamine oxidase inhibitors and anesthesia: an updated literature review. *Acta Anaesthesiol Belg* 1993; 44:57–60.
14. Hill S, et al. MAOIs to RIMAs in anaesthesia–a literature review. *Psychopharmacology (Berl)* 1992; 106 Suppl:S43-S45.
15. Huyse FJ, et al. Psychotropic drugs and the perioperative period: a proposal for a guideline in elective surgery. *Psychosomatics* 2006; 47:8–22.
16. Bajwa SJ, et al. Psychiatric diseases: need for an increased awareness among the anesthesiologists. *JAnaesthesiolClinPharmacol* 2011; 27:440–446.
17. Aroke EN, et al. Perioperative considerations for patients with major depressive disorder undergoing surgery. *J Perianesth Nurs* 2020; 35:112–119.
18. Takakura K, et al. Refractory hypotension during combined general and epidural anaesthesia in a patient on tricyclic antidepressants. *Anaesth Intensive Care* 2008; 34:111–114.
19. Roy S, et al. Fentanyl-induced rigidity during emergence from general anesthesia potentiated by venlafexine. *Can J Anaesth* 2003; 50:32–35.
20. Mahdanian AA, et al. Serotonergic antidepressants and perioperative bleeding risk: a systematic review. *ExpertOpinDrug Saf* 2014; 13:695–704.
21. Levine SM, et al. Selective serotonin reuptake inhibitor-induced hyponatremia and the plastic surgery patient. *Plast Reconstr Surg* 2017; 139:1481–1488.
22. Chang FL, et al. Efficacy of mirtazapine in preventing intrathecal morphine-induced nausea and vomiting after orthopaedic surgery*. *Anaesthesia* 2010; 65:1206–1211.
23. Kudoh A, et al. Chronic treatment with antidepressants decreases intraoperative core hypothermia. *Anesth Analg* 2003; 97:275–279.
24. Kudoh A, et al. Chronic treatment with antipsychotics enhances intraoperative core hypothermia. *Anesth Analg* 2004; 98:111–115.
25. Doherty J, et al. Implications for anaesthesia in a patient established on clozapine treatment. *Int J Obstet Anesth* 2006; 15:59–62.
26. Geeraerts T, et al. Delayed recovery after short-duration, general anesthesia in a patient chronically treated with clozapine. *Anesth Analg* 2006; 103:1618.
27. Adachi YU, et al. Isoflurane anesthesia inhibits clozapine- and risperidone-induced dopamine release and anesthesia-induced changes in dopamine metabolism was modified by fluoxetine in the rat striatum: an in vivo microdialysis study. *Neurochem Int* 2008; 52:384–391.
28. Parlow JL, et al. Single-dose haloperidol for the prophylaxis of postoperative nausea and vomiting after intrathecal morphine. *Anesth Analg* 2004; 98:1072–1076.
29. Kim DH, et al. Adverse events associated with antipsychotic use in hospitalized older adults after cardiac surgery. *J Am Geriatr Soc* 2017; 65:1229–1237.
30. Larsen KA, et al. Administration of olanzapine to prevent postoperative delirium in elderly joint-replacement patients: a randomized, controlled trial. *Psychosomatics* 2010; 51:409–418.
31. Mokhtari M, et al. Aripiprazole for prevention of delirium in the neurosurgical intensive care unit: a double-blind, randomized, placebo-controlled study. *Eur J Clin Pharmacol* 2020; 76:491–499.

32. Jabaley CS, et al. Chronic atypical antipsychotic use is associated with reduced need for postoperative nausea and vomiting rescue in the postanesthesia care unit: a propensity-matched retrospective observational study. *Anesth Analg* 2020; **130**:141–150.

33. Kaye AD, et al. Perioperative implications of common and newer psychotropic medications used in clinical practice. *Best Pract Res Clin Anaesthesiol* 2018; **32**:187–202.

34. Attri JP, et al. Psychiatric patient and anaesthesia. *Indian JAnaesth* 2012; **56**:8–13.

35. Larijani GE, et al. Modafinil improves recovery after general anesthesia. *Anesth Analg* 2004; **98**:976–981.

36. Doyle A, et al. Day case general anaesthesia in a patient with narcolepsy. *Anaesthesia* 2008; **63**:880–882.

37. Grant MC, et al. The effect of preoperative pregabalin on postoperative nausea and vomiting: a meta-analysis. *Anesth Analg* 2016; **123**:1100–1107.

38. De Baerdemaeker L, et al. Anaesthesia for patients with mood disorders. *Curr Opin Anaesthesiol* 2005; **18**:333–338.

39. Faedda GL, et al. Outcome after rapid vs gradual discontinuation of lithium treatment in bipolar disorders. *Arch Gen Psychiatry* 1993; **50**:448–455.

40. Baldessarini RJ, et al. Illness risk following rapid versus gradual discontinuation of antidepressants. *Am J Psychiatry* 2010; **167**:934–941.

41. Horowitz MA, et al. Tapering of SSRI treatment to mitigate withdrawal symptoms. *Lancet Psychiatry* 2019; **6**:538–546.

42. Yerevanian BI, et al. Antidepressants and suicidal behaviour in unipolar depression. *Acta Psychiatr Scand* 2004; **110**:452–458.

43. Copeland LA, et al. Postoperative complications in the seriously mentally ill: a systematic review of the literature. *Ann Surg* 2008; **248**:31–38.

44. Paton C, et al. SSRIs and gastrointestinal bleeding. *BMJ* 2005; **331**:529–530.

CHAPTER 13

Chapter 14

Miscellany

Enhancing medication adherence

The World Health Organisation (WHO) has defined adherence to long-term therapy, as 'the extent to which a person's behaviour – taking medication, following a diet, and/or executing lifestyle changes, corresponds with agreed recommendations from a health-care provider'.[1] Subsequently, in the UK, National Institute for Health and Care Excellence (NICE) guidance also defined adherence as 'the extent to which patient's action matches the agreed recommendation'. Adherence to medication demands collaboration and agreement between the patient and the prescriber. NICE recommended that, as long as the patient has capacity to consent, their right not to take medication should be respected.[2] If the prescriber considers that this decision may lead to an adverse outcome, the reasons for the patient's decision and the prescriber's concerns should be recorded. In fact, in its guidelines for treatment of schizophrenia, NICE emphasised the need for increased research into the effectiveness of psychosocial interventions in the absence of prescribed antipsychotics.[3] However, a meta-analysis[4] and systematic review[5] of such psychodynamic interventions, which included studies in unmedicated patients, confirmed the superiority of treatment with antipsychotics. The most recent systematic review of psychosocial interventions for psychotic patients (with no or low-dose antipsychotic) found the effect of such interventions to be equal to treatment with antipsychotics.[6]

Medication adherence is directly related to better clinical outcome. A 20-year follow-up study of 62,250 patients with schizophrenia reported a significantly lower suicide mortality during antipsychotic use compared with non-use and when all-cause mortality was considered, the most beneficial outcome was associated with clozapine intake.[7] Unsurprisingly, the WHO states, 'increasing the effectiveness of adherence interventions may have far greater impact on the health of the population than any improvements in specific medical treatments'.[1] This is a long way of saying that we don't need better drugs, we need better adherence.

The Maudsley® Prescribing Guidelines in Psychiatry, Fourteenth Edition. David M. Taylor,
Thomas R. E. Barnes and Allan H. Young.
© 2021 David M. Taylor. Published 2021 by John Wiley & Sons Ltd.

Adherence is a complex behaviour which is influenced by malleable underlining factors. Consequently, determinants of non-adherence can be modified through patient-specific and factor-focused interventions. Most adherence-enhancing interventions have been criticised for not being based on a sound theoretical framework and for lack methodological rigour.[8] Low-quality studies and their outcomes are often not duplicated in different settings. This phenomenon was also highlighted by the most recent Cochrane review of adherence interventions when they reported that only 11 studies out of 182 included papers had the lowest risk of bias.[9]

Rate of non-adherence to medication

Reviews of adherence generally conclude that approximately 50% of people do not take their medication as prescribed, and that this proportion is similar across chronic physical and mental disorders.[9] This, however, may be an over-simplification in that it is probable that only a very small proportion of patients are fully adherent, the majority are partially adherent to varying degrees, and a few never take any medication at all of their own volition.[10]

There is some variation in adherence rates both over time and across settings. For example, 10 days after discharge from hospital, up to 25% of patients with schizophrenia are partially or completely non-adherent and this figure rises to 50% at one year and 75% by two years.[11] Other studies have reported 25.8% complete discontinuation of medication within one-year of discharge from hospital.[12] In some mental healthcare settings the rate of non-adherence may be up to 90%.[13] A great deal of poor adherence occurs without the knowledge of the prescriber. In one study,[14] prescribers identified only half of those who were non-adherent. In another, 35% of patients referred for treatment of refractory schizophrenia had sub-therapeutic plasma concentrations and many of them had plasma levels of zero.[15]

Impact of non-adherence

Poor adherence to medication is a major risk factor for worse outcomes including relapse in people with schizophrenia,[16–18] bipolar disorder[19] and depression.[20,21] Wider health benefits are also lost. For example, compared with depressed patients who take an antidepressant, those who do not have a 20% increased risk of an incident myocardial infarction.[21] Non-adherence to medication may have serious consequences which are preventable by implementing routine monitoring. Indeed, analyses of data collected as part of the national confidential inquiry into suicide and homicide by people with mental illness revealed that healthcare providers that had a policy in place regarding how to manage patients who are not taking their medication as prescribed had 20% fewer suicides than providers that did not have such a policy.[22] Of course, a major contributor to worsened outcomes in poorly adherent individuals is the nature in which the medication is stopped – often abruptly and without monitoring. Abrupt cessation of almost all psychotropic drugs has been shown to worsen prognosis (see sections on de-prescribing).

Strategies for improving adherence

Systematic reviews suggest that patient-specific interventions are more likely to enhance adherence in patients with serious mental disorders.[23] In addition, NICE has reviewed the evidence for adherence over a range of health conditions. They conclude that no specific intervention can be recommended for all patients.

Note that few studies in this area specifically recruited non-adherent patients (the refusal rate in such patients is likely to be high) and the specific barriers to adherence are rarely identified. The small effect size seen in many studies may simply be a consequence of this unfocused approach. Intervention Mapping (IM) framework[24] provides a clear path for recognising determinants of non-adherence and to choose the evidence-based methods in order to change the underlining factors. IM provides a foundation for targeted, patient-centred, and implementable interventions.

Mapping out interventions

Stage 1 – Recognising facilitators of non-adherence.[25,26] Some common factors are listed here under each category.

Determinants of medication non-adherence

Intentional non-adherence

Illness-related factors	Treatment-related factors	Clinician- and organisational-related factors	Patient-related factors	Environment-related factors	Unintentional non-adherence
Lack of motivation	Side effects	Therapeutic alliance	Denial	Family's beliefs	Forgetfulness
Poor insight	Dysfunctional beliefs	Lack of follow-ups	Insight	Cultural beliefs	Disorganised lifestyle
Grandiose		Limited consultation time	Co-morbidity	Religious beliefs	
Delusions			Physical impairments/ barriers		
Cognitive deficit					
Thought disorder					

Stage 2 – Linking determinants of non-adherence to evidence-based interventions[27]

Adherence-enhancing interventions

Intentional non-adherence	Unintentional non-adherence
Psychoeducation is the foundation for all adherence interventions, but without behaviour changing components it is not overwhelmingly effective. Provides both verbal and written information. **Motivational interview** for goal-setting.	Simplifying dose regimen Pharmacy interventions – Medication-taking aids

(Continued)

CHAPTER 14

(Continued)

Adherence-enhancing interventions

Intentional non-adherence	Unintentional non-adherence
Adherence therapy for exploring dysfunctional beliefs about medication or the illness, providing information and goal setting. It requires more time and multiple sessions. **Cognitive behavioural therapy** to eradicate or control the residual symptoms that prevent adherence. To address dysfunctional beliefs about treatment. **Cognitive remediation** to help with cognitive deficit in psychotic patients and thought disorder. **Mindfulness** to help with symptoms. **Monitor side effects** regularly and periodically. **Therapeutic alliance** – patients tend to please their clinicians. Non-judgemental attitude and openness on clinician's part allow patients to communicate their dysfunctional thoughts and behaviour. **Family intervention**; psychoeducation and family therapy.	Pairing-up medication – taking with a daily activity. e.g. having breakfast, brushing teeth or before bedtime. Use technology: messaging service, email and telephone. **Pharmacy interventions** for those with physical impairment (e.g. opening bottles).

Stage 3 – Assessing medication adherence[28,29]

Assessments methods	Variables measured	Advantages	Disadvantages
Direct (Objective)			
Blood test	Drug/metabolite plasma levels	Accurate	Invasive
			Costly
			Interpersonal variations: fast or slow metabolisers
			Not reliable for all drugs (see discussion in accompanying text)
			Only a result of zero can be definitively interpreted
Indirect (Subjective)			
Pill count	Number of missing tablets	Simple to use (useful in clinical trials)	Labour-intensive in clinical practice
			Substantial evidence that pill counts grossly underestimate levels of adherence[14]
Electronic database-clinical/pharmacy records	History of non-adherence Pharmacy dispensing and collection records (e.g. Medication Possession Ratio – MPR)	Readily accessible Easy to identify non-adherent patients Inexpensive Non-invasive	Not reliable evidence for medication being ingested; only shows collection and possession

(Continued)

Assessments methods	Variables measured	Advantages	Disadvantages
Self-reported	Validated assessment scales (questionnaires) (e.g. Medication Adherence Rating Scale – MARS)	Easy to use Inexpensive	Subject to reporting bias Tendency to please clinicians Massively overestimates adherence Subjective
Electronic monitoring devices (e.g. Medication Event Monitoring System – MEMS)[14]	Number of times medication container has been opened and (assumed) percentage of doses removed	Amongst the most accurate methods Objective Provides additional information on medication-taking behaviour	Expensive Bulky containers Not evidence for ingestion of medication – only of container opening Patients feel under surveillance

Note that blood tests can provide an accurate plasma level of some drugs or their metabolites at the time of sampling, but they do not provide any information about the patterns of medication-taking behaviour, levels of adherence or factors that may change adherence.[29]

For some antipsychotics such as clozapine, olanzapine and risperidone, blood tests can be useful to directly assess plasma levels. It is important to note that plasma levels of these drugs achieved with a fixed dose vary somewhat and it is not possible to accurately determine partial non-adherence (i.e. total non-adherence will be readily revealed but partial and full adherence may be difficult to tell apart).

Monitoring adherence and assessing attitudes to medication

Psychiatrists generally prefer to use direct questioning over the use of more intrusive/objective methods of assessing adherence and so partial or non-adherence may go undetected.[30] NICE recommends that the patient should be asked in a non-judgemental way if they have missed any doses over a specific time period such as the previous week.[2]

A number of rating scales and checklists are available that help to guide and structure discussion around attitudes to medication. The most widely used is the Drug Attitude Inventory (DAI)[31] which consists of a mix of positive and negative statements about medication; 30 statements in its full form and 10 in its abbreviated form. It is designed to be completed by the patient who simply agrees or disagrees with each statement. The total score is an indicator of the patient's overall perception of the balance between the benefits and harms associated with taking medication, and therefore likely adherence. Attitudes to medication as measured using the DAI have been shown to be a useful predictor of compliance over time.[32] Other available checklists include the Rating of Medication Influences Scale (ROMI),[33] the Beliefs about Medicines Questionnaire[34] and the Medication Adherence Rating Scale (MARS).[18]

CHAPTER 14

Medication-taking aids

'Compliance aids' that contain compartments that accommodate up to four doses of multiple medicines each day may be helpful in patients who are clearly motivated to take medication but find this difficult because of disorganisation or cognitive deficits. It should be noted that only 10% of non-adherent patients say that they simply forgot to take medication[35] and that medication-taking aids are not a substitute for lack of insight or lack of motivation to take medication. Some medicines are unstable when removed from blister packaging and placed in a compliance aid. These include oro-dispersible formulations which are often prescribed for non-adherent patients. In addition, medication-taking aids are labour-intensive (expensive) to fill, it can be difficult to change prescriptions at short notice and the process of filling of these devices is particularly error-prone.[36]

Depot/long-acting antipsychotics

Meta-analyses of clinical trials have shown that the relative and absolute risks of relapse with depot maintenance treatment were 30% and 10% lower, respectively, than with oral treatment.[37,38] NICE recommends that depots are an option in patients who are known to be non-adherent to oral treatment and/or those who prefer this method of administration.[3] However, it is worthy of mentioning that switching a non-adherent patient from oral antipsychotics to a long-acting injectable formulation does not address the determinants of non-adherence in that person. This has been highlighted by a recent systematic review which reported a rate of discontinuation of above 50% in those who had been prescribed second-generation depots.[39] The prescribing of long-acting antipsychotics does not 'cure' non-adherence, but it does prevent sudden cessation of medication and its consequences (all depots provide a slow decline in plasma levels) and it provides certainty about the level of adherence (the injection is either given or it is not).

Depots are probably underused, for example, an US study found that depot preparations were prescribed for fewer than one in five patients with a recent episode of non-adherence.[40]

An alternative to depots is the use of long-acting oral antipsychotics such as penfluridol, which can be given weekly.[41] Supervised administration obviates the need for injections but does not provide the same level of certainty over compliance given the facility patients sometimes show for disguising the taking of oral medication.

In the USA Abilify MyCite is approved for use. This is a version of aripiprazole with a transmitting sensor embedded in the formulation which is able to confirm that a tablet has been taken. Evidence for its effectiveness is slim.[42]

Financial incentives

There is evidence from controlled trials in a number of disease areas supporting the potential of financial incentives to enhance medication adherence. Paying people to take their medication is extremely controversial, though some clinicians have found this strategy to be effective in improving adherence. The effect could not be maintained in an RCT at 6- and 24-month follow-up after payments were stopped and complete adherence was achieved in only 28% of patients receiving the incentives.[43] Other RCTs also have demonstrated a significant increase in adherence during the trial and a decline at follow-up when payments had stopped.[44] Offering financial incentives did not reduce patients' motivation for treatment.[45] A systematic review of acceptability of financial incentives for health-related behaviours has raised concerns about the validity and reliability of these interventions given their methodological limitations.[46]

References

1. World Health Organisation. Adherence to long-term therapies: evidence for action. 2003. https://apps.who.int/iris/bitstream/handle/10665/42682/9241545992.pdf.

2. National Institute for Health and Care Excellence. Medicines adherence: involving patients in decisions about prescribed medicines and supporting adherence. Clinical Guideline [CG76]. 2009 (last checked March 2019); https://www.nice.org.uk/guidance/cg76/chapter/introduction.

3. National Institute for Health and Care Excellence. Psychosis and schizophrenia in adults: prevention and management Clinical Guidance [CG178]. 2014 (last checked March 2019); https://www.nice.org.uk/guidance/cg178.

4. Malmberg L et al. Individual psychodynamic psychotherapy and psychoanalysis for schizophrenia and severe mental illness. *Cochrane Database Syst Rev* 2001:Cd001360.

5. Mueser KT et al. Psychodynamic treatment of schizophrenia: is there a future? *Psychol Med* 1990; **20**:253–262.

6. Cooper RE et al. Psychosocial interventions for people with schizophrenia or psychosis on minimal or no antipsychotic medication: a systematic review. *Schizophr Res* 2019; **225**: 15–30.

7. Taipale H et al. 20-year follow-up study of physical morbidity and mortality in relationship to antipsychotic treatment in a nationwide cohort of 62,250 patients with schizophrenia (FIN20). *World Psychiatry* 2020; **19**:61–68.

8. Zullig LL et al. Moving from the trial to the real world: improving medication adherence using insights of implementation science. *Annu Rev Pharmacol Toxicol* 2019; **59**:423–445.

9. Nieuwlaat R et al. Interventions for enhancing medication adherence. *Cochrane Database Syst Rev* 2014:Cd000011.

10. Masand PS et al. Partial adherence to antipsychotic medication impacts the course of illness in patients with schizophrenia: a review. *Prim Care Companion J Clin Psychiatry* 2009; **11**:147–154.

11. Leucht S et al. Epidemiology, clinical consequences, and psychosocial treatment of nonadherence in schizophrenia. *J Clin Psychiatry* 2006; **67** Suppl 5:3–8.

12. Zhou Y et al. Factors associated with complete discontinuation of medication among patients with schizophrenia in the year after hospital discharge. *Psychiatry Res* 2017; **250**:129–135.

13. Cramer JA et al. Compliance with medication regimens for mental and physical disorders. *Psychiatr Serv* 1998; **49**:196–201.

14. Remington G et al. The use of electronic monitoring (MEMS) to evaluate antipsychotic compliance in outpatients with schizophrenia. *Schizophr Res* 2007; **90**:229–237.

15. McCutcheon R et al. Antipsychotic plasma levels in the assessment of poor treatment response in schizophrenia. *Acta Psychiatr Scand* 2018; **137**:39–46.

16. Morken G et al. Non-adherence to antipsychotic medication, relapse and rehospitalisation in recent-onset schizophrenia. *BMC Psychiatry* 2008; **8**:32.

17. Knapp M et al. Non-adherence to antipsychotic medication regimens: associations with resource use and costs. *Br J Psychiatry* 2004; **184**:509–516.

18. Jaeger S et al. Adherence styles of schizophrenia patients identified by a latent class analysis of the Medication Adherence Rating Scale (MARS): a six-month follow-up study. *Psychiatry Res* 2012; **200**:83–88.

19. Lang K et al. Predictors of medication nonadherence and hospitalization in Medicaid patients with bipolar I disorder given long-acting or oral antipsychotics. *J Med Econ* 2011; **14**:217–226.

20. Mitchell AJ et al. Why don't patients take their medicine? Reasons and solutions in psychiatry. *Adv Psychiatr Treat* 2007; **13**:336–346.

21. Scherrer JF et al. Antidepressant drug compliance: reduced risk of MI and mortality in depressed patients. *Am J Med* 2011; **124**:318–324.

22. Appleby L et al. National confidential inquiry into suicide and homicide by people with mental illness. 2013; http://www.bbmh.manchester.ac.uk/cmhr/research/centreforsuicideprevention/nci/.

23. Nosè M et al. Systemic review of clinical interventions for reducing treatment non-adherence in psychosis. *Epidemiol Psichiatr Soc* 2003; **12**:272–286.

24. Kok G et al. A taxonomy of behaviour change methods: an intervention mapping approach. *Health Psychol Rev* 2016; **10**:297–312.

25. Pedley R et al. Qualitative systematic review of barriers and facilitators to patient-involved antipsychotic prescribing. *Br J Psych Open* 2018; **4**:5–14.

26. Semahegn A et al. Psychotropic medication non-adherence and its associated factors among patients with major psychiatric disorders: a systematic review and meta-analysis. *Syst Rev* 2020; **9**:17.

27. Hartung D et al. Interventions to improve pharmacological adherence among adults with psychotic spectrum disorders and bipolar disorder: a systematic review. *Psychosomatics* 2017; **58**:101–112.

CHAPTER 14

28. Forbes CA et al. A systematic literature review comparing methods for the measurement of patient persistence and adherence. *Curr Med Res Opin* 2018; **34**:1613–1625.

29. Anghel LA et al. An overview of the common methods used to measure treatment adherence. *Med Pharm Rep* 2019; **92**:117–122.

30. Vieta E et al. Psychiatrists' perceptions of potential reasons for non- and partial adherence to medication: results of a survey in bipolar disorder from eight European countries. *J Affect Disord* 2012; **143**:125–130.

31. Hogan TP et al. A self-report scale predictive of drug compliance in schizophrenics: reliability and discriminative validity. *Psychol Med* 1983; **13**:177–183.

32. O'Donnell C et al. Compliance therapy: a randomised controlled trial in schizophrenia. *BMJ* 2003; **327**:834.

33. Weiden P et al. Rating of medication influences (ROMI) scale in schizophrenia. *Schizophr Bull* 1994; **20**:297–310.

34. Horne R et al. The beliefs about medicines questionnaire: the development and evaluation of a new method for assessing the cognitive representation of medication. *Psychology and Health* 1999; **14**:1–24.

35. Perkins DO. Predictors of noncompliance in patients with schizophrenia. *J Clin Psychiatry* 2002; **63**:1121–1128.

36. Barber ND et al. Care homes' use of medicines study: prevalence, causes and potential harm of medication errors in care homes for older people. *Qual Saf Health Care* 2009; **18**:341–346.

37. Leucht C et al. Oral versus depot antipsychotic drugs for schizophrenia–a critical systematic review and meta-analysis of randomised long-term trials. *Schizophr Res* 2011; **127**:83–92.

38. Leucht S et al. Antipsychotic drugs versus placebo for relapse prevention in schizophrenia: a systematic review and meta-analysis. *Lancet* 2012; **379**:2063–2071.

39. Gentile S. Discontinuation rates during long-term, second-generation antipsychotic long-acting injection treatment: a systematic review. *Psychiatry Clin Neurosci* 2019; **73**:216–230.

40. West JC et al. Use of depot antipsychotic medications for medication nonadherence in schizophrenia. *Schizophr Bull* 2008; **34**:995–1001.

41. Soares BG et al. Penfluridol for schizophrenia. *Cochrane Database Syst Rev* 2006:Cd002923.

42. Cosgrove L et al. Digital aripiprazole or digital evergreening? A systematic review of the evidence and its dissemination in the scientific literature and in the media. *BMJ Evid Based Med* 2019; **24**:231–238.

43. Priebe S et al. Financial incentives to improve adherence to antipsychotic maintenance medication in non-adherent patients: a cluster randomised controlled trial. *Health Technol Assess* 2016; **20**:1–122.

44. Noordraven EL et al. Financial incentives for improving adherence to maintenance treatment in patients with psychotic disorders (money for medication): a multicentre, open-label, randomised controlled trial. *Lancet Psychiatry* 2017; **4**:199–207.

45. Noordraven EL et al. The effect of financial incentives on patients' motivation for treatment: results of 'Money for Medication', a randomised controlled trial. *BMC Psychiatry* 2018; **18**:144.

46. Hoskins K et al. Acceptability of financial incentives for health-related behavior change: an updated systematic review. *Prev Med* 2019; **126**:105762.

Re-starting psychotropic medications after a period of non-compliance

A common scenario when a patient is admitted to hospital is that they have been non-compliant with their medications for some time before admission. The clinical question of whether to re-start the medication and at which dose is a complex one. The risk of withdrawal symptoms and relapse must be balanced against the risk of adverse drug reactions when medications are re-introduced too quickly. There is little published evidence on this area, with most guidance (of undeclared provenance) coming from manufacturers, so the below guidance should be followed with caution.

Summary of Product Characteristics (SPCs) and other formal regulatory documents tend not to deal with this clinical scenario, but official Patient Information Leaflets often do. These leaflets are unanimous in advising that on no account should a double dose be given to make up for a missed dose. The vast majority advise only on what to do if a single dose has been missed. In this case, some leaflets advise taking the missed dose later (providing it is not too close to the next dose), whereas others recommend skipping the missed dose altogether and starting again with the next dose.

In the event that more than one dose has been missed, the first question is whether or not this is the appropriate drug for a patient to be taking. Poor compliance often indicates some dissatisfaction on the part of the patient. If it is a drug with a short half-life or one that requires lengthy re-titration, it may not be appropriate to re-start prescribing for a patient who is frequently non-compliant. Similarly, if a patient is intoxicated with alcohol or drugs, it may not be sensible to restart medication at that time. Find out if there are any particular reasons for non-compliance. In schizophrenia and schizoaffective disorder consider the appropriateness of a long-acting injection.

Regarding the question as to whether to re-start the drug at the same dose or whether to re-titrate from a lower dose, clearly the time since the last dose is vitally important. If more than a week or two has passed, then all drugs will probably need to be restarted as if new treatment (although for many drugs that do not require titration this will mean starting back on the same dose as before). The only exceptions are long-acting depot formulations and oral drugs with long half-lives such as aripiprazole, cariprazine and penfluridol.

Table 14.1 summarises our recommendations. The drugs in the first column have specific safety issues that mean they require re-titration after the specified length of time. The drugs in the middle column are thought to be safe because the maximum dose is usually no higher than the highest recommended starting dose. Drugs in the right column are thought to be safe to restart at the prior dose because a similar drug appears in the middle column, because clinical experience suggests they are safe or because the risks associated with giving un-titrated high doses are thought to be low.

Lamotrigine

Lamotrigine has been associated with life-threatening cutaneous reactions, especially with high initial doses. The manufacturer's product information therefore advises that if five half-lives have elapsed since the last lamotrigine dose was given, lamotrigine should be titrated as if for the first time. The half-life in healthy subjects on no other medication is around 33 hours. This is affected by other medications and is approximately 14 hours when given with glucuronidation-inducing drugs such as carbamazepine or phenytoin. The half-life is increased to approximately 70 hours when given with valproate. This means that the time before complete re-titration is necessary therefore varies between 3 and 7 days, depending on the other drugs prescribed.[1]

Table 14.1 Restarting medication up to two weeks after stopping oral treatment (data obtained from EU regulatory documents (SPCs)[2])

Drugs that require re-titration			Drugs that are usually safe for restarting at the previous dose	Drugs that are probably safe for restarting at the previous dose
Drug	**Time after which re-titration must be performed**	**Further guidance**		
Clozapine	48 hours	See 'Re-starting clozapine after after a break in treatment' in Chapter 1	Acamprosate	Antipsychotics (except clozapine, quetiapine and risperidone)
			Asenapine	
			Fluoxetine	Carbamazepine
			Haloperidol	Cholinesterase inhibitors
			Isocarboxazid	CNS stimulants
			Lofepramine	
Lamotrigine	3–7 days	See discussion in the text	Methylphenidate	Disulfiram
			Phenelzine	Lithium (titration advised if renal function has changed)
			Sulpiride	
Methadone	3 days	See 'Opioid dependence' in Chapter 4	Tranylcypromine	MAOIs
Buprenorphine	3 days		Valproate	Memantine
				Naltrexone
				Other antidepressants (but beware loss of tolerance to sedative effects)
Paliperidone long-acting injection	Depends on formulation	See 'Paliperidone palmitate long-acting injection' in Chapter 1		Pregabalin
				SSRIs
				TCAs (but beware loss of tolerance to sedative and hypotensive effects)
Aripiprazole long-acting injection	>5 weeks if 2nd or 3rd dose missed	See 'Aripiprazole long-acting injection' in Chapter 1		
	>6 weeks in chronic treatment			

CNS, central nervous system; MAOI, monoamine oxidase inhibitor; SSRI, selective serotonin reuptake inhibitor; TCA, tricyclic antidepressant.

References

1. Aurobindo Pharma – Milpharm Ltd. Summary of Product Characteristics. Lamotrigine 25mg Tablets. 2019; https://www.medicines.org.uk/emc/product/4736/smpc.
2. EMC. https://www.medicines.org.uk/emc/; accessed June 2020.

Biochemical and haematological effects of psychotropics

Almost all psychotropics have haematology or biochemistry-related adverse effects that may be detected using routine blood tests. While many of these changes are idiosyncratic and not clinically significant, others, such as the agranulocytosis associated with agents such as clozapine, will require regular monitoring of the full blood count. In general, where an agent has a high incidence of biochemical/haematological side-effects or a rare but potentially fatal effect, regular monitoring is required as discussed in other sections.

For other agents, laboratory-related side effects are comparatively rare (prevalence usually less than 1%), are often reversible upon cessation of the putative offending agent and not always clinically significant. It should further be noted that medical co-morbidity, polypharmacy and the effects of non-prescribed agents including substances of abuse and alcohol may also influence biochemical and haematological parameters. In some cases, where a clear temporal association between starting the agent and the onset of laboratory changes is unclear, then withdrawal and re-challenge with the agent in question may be considered. Where there is doubt as to the aetiology and significance of the effect, the appropriate source of expert advice should always be consulted.

Tables 14.2 and 14.3 summarise those agents with identified biochemical and haematological effects, with information compiled from various sources.[1-9] In many cases the evidence for these various effects is limited, with information obtained mostly from case reports, case series and information supplied by manufacturers. For further details about each individual agent, the reader is encouraged to consult the appropriate section of the Guidelines as well as other specialist sources, particularly product literature relating to individual drugs.

Table 14.2 Summary of biochemical changes associated with psychotropics

Parameter	Reference range[10]	Agents reported to raise levels	Agents reported to lower levels
Alanine aminotransferase (ALT)	Females: ≤34U/L Males: ≤45U/L (may be higher in obese subjects)	**Antipsychotics:** asenapine, benperidol, cariprazine, clozapine, haloperidol, loxapine, olanzapine, phenothiazines, quetiapine, risperidone/paliperidone **Antidepressants:** agomelatine, bupropion, MAOIs, mianserin, mirtazapine, SNRIs, SSRIs (especially paroxetine and sertraline), TCAs, trazodone, vortioxetine **Anxiolytics/hypnotics:** barbiturates, benzodiazepines, buspirone, clomethiazole, promethazine, suvorexant, tasimelteon, zolpidem **Mood stabilisers:** carbamazepine, lamotrigine, valproate **Other:** alcohol, atomoxetine, beta-blockers, caffeine, cocaine, disulfiram, naltrexone, opioids, stimulants (abused)	Vigabatrin

(Continued)

Table 14.2 (*Continued*)

Parameter	Reference range[10]	Agents reported to raise levels	Agents reported to lower levels
Albumin	35–50g/L (gradually decreases after age 40)	Microalbuminuria may be a feature of metabolic syndrome secondary to psychotropic use (especially phenothiazines, clozapine, olanzapine and possibly quetiapine)	Chronic use of amfetamine or cocaine
Alkaline phosphatase	50–120U/L	Baclofen, beta-blockers, benzodiazepines, caffeine (excess/chronic use), carbamazepine, citalopram, clozapine, disulfiram, duloxetine, galantamine, haloperidol, loxapine, memantine, modafinil, nortriptyline, olanzapine, phenytoin, sertraline, topiramate, trazodone, valbenazine, valproate; also associated with agents causing NMS	Buprenorphine, fluoxetine (in children), zolpidem (rarely)
Ammonia	11–32μmol/L (increased following meals and exercise)	Barbiturates, carbamazepine, tobacco smoking, topiramate, valproate (may present with signs of encephalopathy)	None known
Amylase	28–100U/L	Alcohol (acute), donepezil, opioids, pregabalin, rivastigmine, SSRIs (rarely) **Agents associated with pancreatitis:** alcohol, carbamazepine, clozapine, olanzapine, valproate	None known
Aspartate aminotransferase (AST)	Females: ≤34U/L Males: ≤45U/L	As for Alanine Transferase; baclofen. Note: ALT is preferred as an indicator of liver damage.	Trifluoperazine, vigabatrin
Bicarbonate	22–29mmol/L	Laxative abuse	Agents associated with SIADH: all antidepressants, antipsychotics (clozapine, haloperidol, olanzapine, phenothiazines, pimozide, risperidone/paliperidone, quetiapine); carbamazepine; also associated with agents causing metabolic acidosis (alcohol, cocaine, topiramate, zonisamide)

Table 14.2 (*Continued*)

Parameter	Reference range[10]	Agents reported to raise levels	Agents reported to lower levels
Bilirubin	≤21µmol/L (total)	Amitriptyline, atomoxetine, benzodiazepines, carbamazepine, chlordiazepoxide, chlorpromazine, citalopram, clomethiazole, clozapine, disulfiram, imipramine, fluphenazine, lamotrigine, meprobamate, milnacipran, olanzapine, phenothiazines, phenytoin, promethazine, sertraline, valbenazine, valproate; also associated with agents causing cholestasis/hepatic damage	Barbiturates
C-reactive protein	<10mg/L	Buprenorphine (rare); also associated with agents causing myocarditis (clozapine)	None known
Calcium	2.20–2.60mmol/L (total, adjusted) 1.15–1.34mmol/L (ionised)	Lithium (rare)	Barbiturates, carbamazepine, haloperidol, valproate
Carbohydrate-deficient transferrin (CDT)	≤1.5%	Alcohol (CDT levels of 1.6–1.9% suggest high intake; levels ≥ 2% suggest excessive intake)	None known
Chloride	95–108mmol/L	Agents causing hyperchloremic metabolic acidosis: topiramate, zonisamide	Medications associated with SIADH: all antidepressants, antipsychotics (clozapine, haloperidol, olanzapine, phenothiazines, pimozide, risperidone/paliperidone, quetiapine); carbamazepine, laxative abuse
Cholesterol (total)	≤5.2mmol/L (usually compared to recommended action limits rather than reference ranges)	Antipsychotics, especially those implicated in the metabolic syndrome (phenothiazines, clozapine, olanzapine and quetiapine). Rarely: aripiprazole, beta-blockers (additive effects with clozapine), carbamazepine, disulfiram, duloxetine, memantine, mirtazapine, modafinil, phenytoin, rivastigmine, sertraline, venlafaxine	Prazosin, thyroid agents

CHAPTER 14

(*Continued*)

Table 14.2 (*Continued*)

Parameter	Reference range[10]	Agents reported to raise levels	Agents reported to lower levels
Creatine Kinase	Females: 25–200U/L Males: 40–320U/L (range for Caucasians; may be higher in other ethnic groups)	Bremelanotide, brexpiprazole, cariprazine, clonidine, clozapine (when associated with seizures), cocaine, dexamfetamine, donepezil, olanzapine, pregabalin; also associated with agents causing NMS and SIADH; agents administered intramuscularly	None known
Creatinine	Females: 55–100µmol/L Males: 60–120µmol/L	Clozapine, lithium, lurasidone, thioridazine, valproate, medications associated with rhabdomyolysis (benzodiazepines, dexamfetamine, pregabalin, thioridazine); also associated with agents causing renal impairment, NMS and SIADH	None known
Ferritin	Females: 15–150µg/L Males: 30–400µg/L (increases with age)	Alcohol (acutely and in alcoholic liver disease)	None known
Gamma-glutamyl transferase (GGT)	Females: ≤38 U/L Males: ≤55 U/L (limits two-fold higher in persons of African ancestry)	**Antidepressants:** mirtazapine, SSRIs (paroxetine and sertraline implicated), TCAs, trazodone, venlafaxine **Antiseizure medications/mood stabilisers:** carbamazepine, lamotrigine, phenytoin, phenobarbitone, valproate **Antipsychotics:** benperidol, chlorpromazine, clozapine, fluphenazine, haloperidol, olanzapine, quetiapine **Other:** alcohol, barbiturates, clomethiazole, dexamfetamine, modafinil, tobacco smoking	None known
Glucose	Fasting: 2.8–6.1mmol/L Random: <11.1mmol/L	**Antidepressants:** MAOIs*, SSRIs/ SNRIs*, TCAs* **Antipsychotics:** chlorpromazine, clozapine, haloperidol*, olanzapine*, quetiapine and others **Substances of abuse:** amfetamine, methadone, opioids **Other:** Baclofen, beta-blockers*, bupropion*, caffeine* (in diabetics), clonidine, donepezil, gabapentin, galantamine, lithium*, nicotine, sympathomimetics, thyroid agents, valbenazine	Alcohol; rarely with duloxetine, haloperidol, pregabalin, TCAs Medications associated with metabolic syndrome may result in raised or decreased glucose levels
HbA1c	20–39mmol/mol		Lithium, MAOIs, SSRIs

CHAPTER 14

Table 14.2 (Continued)

Parameter	Reference range[10]	Agents reported to raise levels	Agents reported to lower levels
Lactate dehydrogenase	90–200U/L (levels rise gradually with age)	Benzodiazepines, clozapine, methadone, TCAs (especially imipramine), valproate, also associated with agents causing NMS	None known
Lipoproteins: HDL	>1.2mmol/L	Carbamazepine, nicotine, phenobarbital, phenytoin	Beta-blockers, olanzapine, phenothiazines, valproate
Lipoproteins: LDL	<3.5mmol/L	Beta-blockers, caffeine (controversial), carbamazepine, chlorpromazine, clozapine, iloperidone, memantine, mirtazapine, modafinil, olanzapine, phenothiazines, quetiapine, risperidone/paliperidone, rivastigmine, venlafaxine	Prazosin
Phosphate	0.8–1.5mmol/L	Dexamfetamine; also associated with agents causing NMS	Carbamazepine, lithium, mianserin, topiramate
Potassium	3.5–5.3mmol/L	Beta-blockers, lithium	Alcohol, disulfiram, caffeine, cocaine, haloperidol, lithium, mianserin, pregabalin, reboxetine, rivastigmine, sodium oxybate, sympathomimetics, topiramate, zonisamide; may also be a feature of delirium tremens
Prolactin	Normal: <350mU/L Abnormal: >600mU/L	**Antidepressants:** especially amoxapine, MAOIs and TCAs; SSRIs and venlafaxine also implicated **Antipsychotics:** amisulpride, haloperidol, pimozide, risperidone/paliperidone, sulpiride and others (aripiprazole[†], asenapine, brexpiprazole, cariprazine, clozapine, lurasidone, olanzapine, quetiapine and ziprasidone have minimal effects on prolactin levels) **Other:** benzodiazepines, buspirone, deutetrabenazine, opioids, ramelteon, tetrabenazine, valbenazine	Aripiprazole, dopamine agonists, pirenzepine
Protein (total)	60–80g/L	None known	Olanzapine (rarely)

(Continued)

CHAPTER 14

Table 14.2 (Continued)

Parameter	Reference range[10]	Agents reported to raise levels	Agents reported to lower levels
Sodium	133–146mmol/L	Lithium (in overdose)	**Antidepressants:** especially SSRIs/SNRIs; others also implicated **Antipsychotics:** all (via SIADH) **Mood stabilisers:** carbamazepine, lithium, valproate **Other:** benzodiazepines, clonidine, donepezil, memantine, rivastigmine Hyponatraemia should be considered in any patient on an antidepressant who develops confusion, convulsions or drowsiness
Testosterone	Males: 9.9–27.8nmol/L Females: 0.22– 2.9nmol/L	Diazepam	Opioids, ramelteon
Thyroid-stimulating hormone	0.3–4.0mU/L	Aripiprazole, carbamazepine, lithium, quetiapine, rivastigmine, sertraline, valproate (slightly)	Moclobemide, thyroid agents
Thyroxine	Free: 9–26pmol/L Total: 60–150nmol/L	Rarely; amfetamine (heavy abuse), moclobemide, propranolol	Barbiturates, carbamazepine, liothyronine, lithium (causes decreased T4 secretion), opioids, phenytoin, valproate. Rarely implicated: aripiprazole, clozapine, quetiapine, rivastigmine, sertraline
Triglycerides			None known
Triiodothyronine	Free 3.0–6.8pmol/L; total 1.2–2.9nmol/L	Heroin, methadone	Free T3: valproate; total T3: carbamazepine, lithium, propranolol
Urate (uric acid)	Females: 0.16–0.36mmol/L Males: 0.21–0.43mmol/L (increases with age)	Alcohol (acute), caffeine (false positive), clozapine, levodopa, olanzapine, pindolol, prazosin, topiramate, zonisamide	Sertraline (slightly)
Urea	2.5–7.8mmol/L (increases with age)	Carbamazepine, levodopa; rarely with agents associated with anticonvulsant hypersensitivity syndrome and rhabdomyolysis	None known

*May also be associated with hypoglycaemia.
† May also be associated with subnormal prolactin levels.

Table 14.3 Summary of haematological changes associated with psychotropics

Parameter	Reference range	Agents reported to raise levels	Agents reported to lower levels
Activated partial thromboplastin time	23–33 seconds	Phenothiazines (especially chlorpromazine)	Modafinil (rare)
Basophils	0.0–0.1 × 10⁹/L	Clozapine, TCAs (especially desipramine)	None known
Eosinophils	0.04–0.40 × 10⁹/L	Amoxapine, beta-blockers, bupropion, buspirone, carbamazepine, chloral hydrate, chlorpromazine, clonazepam, clozapine, donepezil, fluphenazine, haloperidol, loxapine, meprobamate, maprotiline, methylphenidate (IV abuse only), modafinil, naltrexone (parenterally administered), olanzapine, promethazine, quetiapine, risperidone/paliperidone, SSRIs, TCAs, tetrazepam, tryptophan*, valproate, venlafaxine; may also be a feature of agents causing a hypersensitivity syndrome	None known
Erythrocyte sedimentation rate	Females: 1–12mm/h Males: 1–10mm/h (increases with age)	Clozapine, dexamfetamine, levomepromazine, maprotiline, SSRIs	Buprenorphine
Haemoglobin	Females: 115–165g/L Males: 130–180g/L	Clozapine, testosterone, tobacco smoking	Aripiprazole, barbiturates, buprenorphine, bupropion, carbamazepine, chlordiazepoxide, chlorpromazine, donepezil, duloxetine, galantamine, MAOIs, memantine, meprobamate, mianserin, phenytoin, promethazine, rivastigmine, tramadol, trifluoperazine, vigabatrin
Lymphocytes	1.5–4.5 × 10⁹/L	Naltrexone, opioids, tobacco smoking, valproate; may also be a feature of drugs causing hypersensitivity syndrome	Alcohol (chronic), chloral hydrate, clozapine, lithium, mirtazapine (rarely)

(Continued)

CHAPTER 14

Table 14.3 (*Continued*)

Parameter	Reference range	Agents reported to raise levels	Agents reported to lower levels
Mean cell haemoglobin	27–32pg	Medications associated with megaloblastic anaemia e.g. all antiseizure medications, nitrous oxide	None known
Mean cell haemoglobin concentration	320–360g/L		
Mean cell volume	80–100fL	Alcohol	
Monocytes	0.2–0.8 × 10⁹/L	Haloperidol	None known
Neutrophils	2.0–7.5 × 10⁹/L (may be lower in people of African descent due to benign ethnic neutropenia)	Bupropion, carbamazepine†, citalopram, chlorpromazine, clozapine†, duloxetine, fluoxetine, fluphenazine, haloperidol, lamotrigine, lithium, maprotiline, olanzapine, quetiapine, risperidone/paliperidone, rivastigmine, tiotixene, trazodone, venlafaxine	**Agents associated with agranulocytosis:** amoxapine, aripiprazole, barbiturates, carbamazepine, chlordiazepoxide, chlorpromazine, clozapine‡, cocaine (adulterated), diazepam, fluphenazine, haloperidol, meprobamate, mianserin, mirtazapine, olanzapine, pirenzepine, promethazine, risperidone/paliperidone, TCAs (especially imipramine), tranylcypromine, valproate **Agents associated with leucopoenia:** amitriptyline, amoxapine, asenapine, bupropion, carbamazepine, cariprazine, chlorpromazine, citalopram, clomipramine, clonazepam, clozapine, duloxetine, fluoxetine, fluphenazine, galantamine, haloperidol, lamotrigine, lorazepam, lumateperone, lurasidone, memantine, meprobamate, mianserin, mirtazapine, modafinil, nitrous oxide, olanzapine, oxazepam, phenelzine, pregabalin, promethazine, quetiapine, tranylcypromine, valproate, venlafaxine, ziprasidone **Agents associated with neutropenia:** sertraline, trazodone, valproate
Packed cell volume	Females: 0.37–0.47L/L Males: 0.40–0.52L/L	Clozapine (rare), testosterone	Benzodiazepines (rare), buprenorphine, naltrexone, vigabatrin

Table 14.3 (*Continued*)

Parameter	Reference range	Agents reported to raise levels	Agents reported to lower levels
Platelets	150–450 × 10⁹/L	Lamotrigine, lithium†	Alcohol, barbiturates, beta-blockers, benzodiazepines, bupropion, buspirone, carbamazepine, chlordiazepoxide, chlorpromazine, clonazepam, clonidine, clozapine†, cocaine, diazepam, donepezil, duloxetine, fluoxetine, fluphenazine, lamotrigine, meprobamate, methadone, methylphenidate, mirtazapine, naltrexone, nitrous oxide, olanzapine, pirenzepine, promethazine, quetiapine, risperidone/paliperidone, rivastigmine, sertraline, TCAs, tranylcypromine, trazodone, trifluoperazine, valproate, venlafaxine, ziprasidone; may also be a feature of drugs causing hypersensitivity syndrome **Agents associated with impaired platelet aggregation:** chlordiazepoxide, citalopram, diazepam, fluoxetine, fluvoxamine, paroxetine, piracetam, sertraline, valproate
Prothrombin time (PT)/international normalised ratio (INR)	PT: 10–13 seconds INR: 0.8–1.2	Chloral hydrate, disulfiram, fluoxetine, fluvoxamine, mirtazapine, valproate; also agents interacting with warfarin	Barbiturates, carbamazepine, phenytoin, tiotixene
Red blood count	Males: 4.5–6.5 × 10¹²/L Females: 3.8–5.8 × 10¹²/L	Lithium, testosterone	Buprenorphine, carbamazepine, chlordiazepoxide, chlorpromazine, donepezil, haloperidol, meprobamate, phenytoin, quetiapine, trifluoperazine

(*Continued*)

Table 14.3 (*Continued*)

Parameter	Reference range	Agents reported to raise levels	Agents reported to lower levels
Red cell distribution width	11.5–14.5%	Agents associated with anaemia e.g.: carbamazepine, chlordiazepoxide, citalopram, clonazepam, diazepam, lamotrigine, memantine, mirtazapine, sertraline, tranylcypromine, trazodone, valproate, venlafaxine	None known
Reticulocyte count	0.5–2.5% (or 50–100 × 10⁹/L)	None known	Carbamazepine, chlordiazepoxide, chlorpromazine, meprobamate, phenytoin, trifluoperazine **Agents associated with pure red cell aplasia:** carbamazepine, clozapine, valproate

*Previous reports of eosinophilia-myalgia syndrome may have been due to a contaminant from a single manufacturer.

†May raise or lower levels.

‡Note that in rare cases clozapine has been associated with a 'morning pseudo-neutropenia' with lower levels of circulating neutrophil levels. As neutrophil counts may show circadian rhythms, repeating the FBC at a later time of day may be instructive.

References

1. BMJ Group and Pharmaceutical Press. British National Formulary 2020; https://www.medicinescomplete.com.
2. Aronson J. *Meyler Side Effects of Drugs: the International Encyclopedia of Adverse Drug Reactions and Interactions*. Elsevier Science; 2015.
3. Foster R. *Clinical Laboratory Investigation and Psychiatry. A Practical Handbook*. New York: Informa 2008.
4. Oyesanmi O, et al. Hematologic side effects of psychotropics. *Psychosomatics* 1999; 40: 414–421.
5. Stubner S, et al. Blood dyscrasias induced by psychotropic drugs. *Pharmacopsychiatry* 2004; 37 Suppl 1:S70-S78.
6. Pharmaceutical Press. Martindale: the Complete Drug Reference (online) 2020; https://www.medicinescomplete.com.
7. LiverTox: clinical and Research Information on Drug-Induced Liver Injury. Bethesda (MD): National Institute of Diabetes and Digestive and Kidney Diseases 2012; https://www.ncbi.nlm.nih.gov/books/NBK547852.
8. Medicines Complete. AHFS Drug Information 2020; https://www.medicinescomplete.com/mc/ahfs/current.
9. U.S. Food & Drug Administration. Drugs@FDA: FDA-Approved Drugs 2020; https://www.accessdata.fda.gov/scripts/cder/daf.
10. Association for Clinical Biochemistry and Laboratory Medicine. Analyte Monographs Alongside the National Library of Medicine Catalogue 2020; http://www.acb.org.uk/whatwedo/science/amalc.aspx.

Summary of psychiatric side effects of non-psychotropics

It is increasingly recognised that non-psychotropic medications can induce a wide range of psychiatric symptoms.[1] Up to two-thirds of all drugs have potential psychiatric side effects listed in their product labelling,[2] although in most cases the evidence supporting a causal link is limited. Psychiatric side effects are poorly characterised in drug clinical trials, often only becoming apparent during post-marketing surveillance.[3] Given this level of uncertainty, suspected psychiatric side effects should be diagnosed and managed on a case-by-case basis. As a general guide, the psychiatric side effects of non-psychotropics are shown in Table 14.4. For individual drugs and agents not listed below, additional sources of information and the product literature should be consulted. Note that psychiatric side effects of drugs used in psychiatry and drugs for HIV and epilepsy are summarised elsewhere in the *Guidelines*.

Table 14.4 Summary of psychiatric adverse drug reactions (ADRs) with non-psychotropics[4–7]

Drug	Psychiatric side effect	Comment
ACE inhibitors		
E.g. Captopril, lisinopril	Fatigue, hallucinations, delirium, mood disturbances	Captopril most strongly associated with mood effects. Overall limited psychiatric ADRs
Analgesics		
Opioids	Sedation, dysphoria, confusion, mood changes including euphoria, sleep disturbances, hallucinations, psychosis, delirium, dependence	Psychiatric ADRs are relatively common with opioids. Psychosis during opioid withdrawal has also been reported rarely[8]
$5HT_1$ agonists (e.g. sumatriptan)	Fatigue, anxiety, panic attacks	
Antibiotics		
Cephalosporins, penicillins, quinolones (including fluoroquinolones), tetracyclines	Sleep disturbances (insomnia and somnolence, abnormal dreams, nightmares), anxiety, delirium and confusional states, depression and agitation, psychotic symptoms (e.g. hallucinations, suicidal ideation)	All antibiotics can cause delirium. Patients with underlying medical conditions can be at higher risk of developing psychiatric ADRs. Of the quinolones, ciprofloxacin causes the most psychiatric ADRs, including mood disturbances, agitation and confusion. Onset of psychiatric ADRs can be fast, e.g. after one dose

(Continued)

Table 14.4 (*Continued*)

Drug	Psychiatric side effect	Comment
Antimalarials		
Chloroquine, mefloquine	Psychosis including hallucinations, panic attacks, suicidal ideation and attempts, anxiety, depression, restlessness, confusion. Abnormal dreams/nightmares are common with mefloquine	Symptoms begin early in treatment. Patients should be advised to stop treatment if these develop and seek medical advice. Psychiatric ADRs are more common with mefloquine than chloroquine. Reactions can even occur after discontinuation of the drug. Mefloquine should not be prescribed for patients with an active or a history of a psychiatric diagnosis
Antiparkinsonian treatments		
Levodopa	Visual hallucinations, depression, hypomania, sleep disturbances, abnormal dreams, cognitive impairment, agitation, psychosis, delirium	
Dopamine agonists	Sedation, psychomotor agitation, anxiety, akathisia, sleep disturbances, psychosis, cognitive impairment, delirium, visual hallucinations	These are associated with more psychiatric adverse effects than levodopa
Amantadine	Decreased concentration, sleep disturbances, visual hallucinations, irritability, anxiety, depression, euphoria, fatigue, psychosis, delirium	
Selegiline (MAO-B inhibitor)	Sleep disturbances, agitation, psychosis	Primary metabolites include levamfetamines
Entacapone (COMT inhibitor)	Sleep disturbances, hallucinations, delirium	
Cardiovascular agents		
β-Blockers	Fatigue, sedation, sleep disturbances and nightmares, cognitive impairment, depression, hallucinations, psychosis, delirium	Disturbances more common with lipophilic β-blockers (e.g. propranolol, metoprolol) than with hydrophilic β-blockers (e.g. atenolol, sotalol, nadolol). Propranolol most commonly associated with depressive symptoms, but even with this drug, causality has not clearly been established. Reports of psychiatric ADRs from numerous clinical trials are equivocal.

Table 14.4 (*Continued*)

Drug	Psychiatric side effect	Comment
Calcium channel blockers (e.g. diltiazem, amlodipine)	Mood changes, lethargy, dysphoria, mania, psychosis, delirium, akathisia	Causal association not clearly demonstrated
Statins[9–11] (e.g. simvastatin, atorvastatin)	Cognitive impairment, memory impairment, depression, emotional lability, irritability, sleep disturbance	Causal associations between statins and changes in mood, sleep and cognition have not established in systematic reviews of RCTs. Statins penetrate the blood-brain barrier; simvastatin has the highest permeability. Switching to hydrophilic statins (e.g. pravastatin, rosuvastatin) has been suggested in suspected cases of moderate-severe psychiatric ADRs
Corticosteroids		
Glucocorticoids (e.g. betamethasone, prednisolone, prednisone)	Mood disorders, suicidal ideation, euphoria, agitation, sleep disturbances, psychosis and delirium, dementia, cognitive impairment	Clear causal association. Onset of psychiatric ADRs are often very sudden, and within the first 1–2 week of starting treatment. Symptoms generally respond to dose decreases and have been reported in association with several routes of administration (including oral, parenteral and inhaled), although are probably less common with inhalation. Symptoms usually resolve on gradual discontinuation, although duration of symptoms varies considerably
Other agents		
Chemotherapeutic agents (e.g. 5-fluorouracil, asparaginase, bortezomib, ifosfamide, vincristine)	More commonly: cognitive impairment, delirium, psychosis Less commonly: depression, anxiety, suicidal ideation	Almost all chemotherapeutic agents are associated with significant psychiatric ADRs which may be multifactorial in origin (i.e. secondary to the disease process, ADRs and psychological distress). Cancer therapy-associated cognitive changes include difficulty in executive functions, multitasking, short-term memory recall and attention. Cognitive changes seem to be dose dependent, and certain drugs (methotrexate, fludarabine, cytarabine, 5-fluorouracil, cisplatin), are associated with worse cognitive effects
Cimetidine	Cognitive impairment, delirium	

(Continued)

CHAPTER 14

Table 14.4 (*Continued*)

Drug	Psychiatric side effect	Comment
Interferon-α and interferon-β	Depression, loss of efficacy of previously effective antidepressants, suicidal ideation, delirium, non-specific psychiatric symptoms. Rare case reports of psychosis and mania with interferon-α	Psychiatric ADRs are relatively unlikely with interferon-β but much more widely reported with interferon-α. Interferon-α-associated depression responds to antidepressants, use of which can be preventive. Novel diagnostic biomarkers have been investigated to predict which patients are likely to develop interferon-α-associated psychiatric ADRs
Isotretinoin[12]	Depression, suicidal ideation, psychosis	Sporadic reports of psychiatric ADRs but a causal link between isotretinoin therapy and depression, anxiety, mood changes, or suicidal ideation/ suicide has not been established. Moreover, a recent systematic review found that the treatment of acne improves depressive symptoms.[13] Rare, idiosyncratic reactions cannot be ruled out; if they occur the drug should be discontinued. Risk is no higher in those with prior suicide attempts and is not dose or treatment duration related

Differential diagnosis of psychiatric side effects

A wide range of confounding factors complicate the diagnosis (and perhaps also the recognition) of psychiatric side effects. For example, physical illness, co-prescribed medication, non-prescribed agents, pre-existing mental illness may all influence the clinical presentation and outcome. Factors determining the probability of a causal relationship between drugs and psychiatric side-effects are shown in Box 14.1. To further support clinical decision-making, the Naranjo scale can be used to assess the likelihood of any adverse reaction being drug-related (Table 14.5). Although cessation of the implicated non-psychotropic might be indicated in some cases; such decisions require individual considerations beyond the scope of this book.

Table 14.5 Adapted Naranjo adverse drug reactions (ADR) probability scale criteria[14]

Questions	Yes	No	NA/unknown
1. Are there previous *conclusive* reports on this reaction?	+1	0	0
2. Did the ADR appear after the suspected drug was administered?	+2	−1	0
3. Did the ADR improve when the drug was discontinued?	+1	0	0
4. Did the ADR appear with re-challenge?	+2	−1	0
5. Are there alternative causes for the ADR?	−1	+2	0
6. Did the reaction appear when placebo was given?	−1	+1	0
7. Was the drug detected in the blood at toxic levels?	+1	0	0
8. Was the ADR more severe when the dose was increased, or less severe when the dose was decreased?	+1	0	0
9. Did the patient have a similar reaction to the same or similar drugs in *any* previous exposure?	+1	0	0
10. Was the ADR confirmed by any objective evidence?	+1	0	0

Probability score: ≥9 = definite; 5–8 = probable; 1–4 = possible; ≤0 = doubtful

Box 14.1 Factors determining the probability of a causal relationship between drugs and psychiatric side effects[4,15]

- Temporal relationship between the drug exposure and the psychiatric side effect
- Evidence of the specific psychiatric side effects occurring with the suspected drug
- Plausible pharmacological mechanism for the psychiatric side effect (e.g. dopamine agonists and psychosis)
- Presence of alternative explanations for symptoms (e.g. pre-existing mental illness, de novo psychiatric illness, other drugs)
- Response of symptoms to the withdrawal of the drug
- Effect of re-challenge with the same drug

References

1. Rudorfer MV, et al. Assessing Psychiatric Adverse Effects during Clinical Drug Development. *Pharmaceut Med* 2012; 26:363–394.
2. Smith DA. Psychiatric side effects of non-psychiatric drugs. *S DJ Med* 1991; 44:291–292.
3. Holvey C, et al. Psychiatric side effects of non-psychiatric drugs. *Br J Hosp Med (Lond)* 2010; 71:432–436.
4. Gupta A, et al. Adverse psychiatric effects of non-psychotropic medications. *BJ Psych Advances* 2016; 22:325–334.
5. Huffman JC, et al. Neuropsychiatric consequences of cardiovascular medications. *Dialogues Clin Neurosci* 2007; 9:29–45.
6. Munjampalli SK, et al. Medicinal-Induced Behavior Disorders. *Neurol Clin* 2016; 34:133–169.
7. Parker C. Psychiatric effects of drugs for other disorders. *Medicine* 2016; 44:768–774.
8. Maremmani AG, et al. Substance abuse and psychosis. *The Strange Case of Opioids. Eur Rev Med Pharmacol Sci* 2014; 18:287–302.
9. Ott BR, et al. Do statins impair cognition? A systematic review and meta-analysis of randomized controlled trials. *J Gen Intern Med* 2015; 30:348–358.
10. Swiger KJ, et al. Statins, mood, sleep, and physical function: a systematic review. *Eur J Clin Pharmacol* 2014; 70:1413–1422.
11. Tuccori M, et al. Neuropsychiatric adverse events associated with statins: epidemiology, pathophysiology, prevention and management. *CNS Drugs* 2014; 28:249–272.
12. Liu M, et al. Neurological and Neuropsychiatric Adverse Effects of Dermatologic Medications. *CNS Drugs* 2016; 30:1149–1168.
13. Huang YC, et al. Isotretinoin treatment for acne and risk of depression: A systematic review and meta-analysis. *J Am Acad Dermatol* 2017; 76:1068-1076.e1069.
14. Naranjo CA, et al. A method for estimating the probability of adverse drug reactions. *Clin Pharmacol Ther* 1981; 30:239–245.
15. World Health Organisation and Uppsala Monitoring Centre. The use of the WHO-UMC system for standardised case causality assessment. 2004; http://www.who.int/medicines/areas/quality_safety/safety_efficacy/WHOcausality_assessment.pdf.

Further reading

Bangert MK, et al. Neurological and psychiatric adverse effects of antimicrobials. CNS Drugs 2019; 33:727–753.

Prescribing drugs outside their licensed indications ('off-label' prescribing or unapproved use of approved drugs)

A Product Licence (PL) is granted when regulatory authorities are satisfied that the drug in question has proven efficacy in the treatment of a specified disorder, along with an acceptable side-effect profile, relative to the severity of the disorder being treated and other available treatments. Licensed indications are preparation-specific, outlined in the Summary of Product Characteristics (SPC), and may be different for branded and generic formulations of the same drug.[1] In the US, product 'labelling' has a similar legal status to EU licensing.

The decision of a manufacturer to seek a PL for a given indication is essentially a commercial one; potential sales are balanced against the cost of conducting the necessary clinical trials. It therefore follows that drugs may be effective outside their licensed indications for different disease states, age ranges, doses and durations. The absence of a formal PL or labelling may simply reflect the absence of controlled trials supporting the drug's efficacy in these areas. In other cases (e.g. sertraline or quetiapine in GAD) there is sufficient evidence but a licence has not been sought by the manufacturer. Importantly, however, it is also possible that trials have been conducted but given negative or equivocal results. Clinicians often assume that drugs with a similar mode of action will be similarly effective for a given indication, and in many cases this may be true. For example, the efficacy of aripiprazole, olanzapine, quetiapine and risperidone in reducing behavioural and psychological symptoms (BPSD) in people with dementia is similar,[2] yet in the EU, only risperidone is licensed for this indication.

Prescribing a drug within its licence or labelling does not guarantee that the patient will come to no harm. Likewise, prescribing outside a licence does not mean that the risk-benefit ratio is automatically adverse. In the BPSD example given above, risperidone is not clearly better tolerated than other antipsychotics.[2] Prescribing outside a licence, usually called 'off-label', does confer extra responsibilities on prescribers, who will be expected to be able to show that they acted in accordance with a respected body of medical opinion (the Bolam test)[3] and that their action was capable of withstanding logical analysis (the Bolitho test).[4] Both have effectively been superseded, or at least clarified, by the Montgomery vs Lanarkshire Health Board appeal case decision[5] which stated:

An adult person of sound mind is entitled to decide which, if any, of the available forms of treatment to undergo, and her consent must be obtained before treatment interfering with her bodily integrity is undertaken. The doctor is therefore under a duty to take reasonable care to ensure that the patient is aware of any material risks involved in any recommended treatment, and of any reasonable alternative or variant treatments. The test of materiality is whether, in the circumstances of the particular case, a reasonable person in the patient's position would be likely to attach significant to the risk, or the doctor is or should reasonable be aware that the particular patient would be likely to attach significance to it.

Thus, in the UK at least, the prescriber has a duty to make a patient aware of any material risks associated with the prescribing of any medicines and to outline alternatives.

CHAPTER 14

The General Medical Council allows doctors to prescribe off-label but only where the prescriber is satisfied that there is enough evidence or experience to support efficacy and safety.[6]

In the USA, it is lawful to prescribe off label 'within a legitimate health care practitioner-patient relationship'.[7] Marketing of off-label use is forbidden but information may be provided following an unsolicited request.[8] Off-label prescribing has been estimated to represent 13% of all prescribing in mental health conditions in the USA.[9]

It has been suggested that off-label prescribing in psychiatry is less likely to be supported by a strong evidence base than off-label prescribing in other areas of medicine.[10] In psychiatry, small (underpowered) studies (with wide confidence intervals) often influence practice, particularly with respect to treatment resistant illness (a great many examples can be found in this publication). When these small studies are combined in the form of a meta-analysis, considerable heterogeneity is often found suggesting publication bias (that is, that some negative studies are not published). Treatments may therefore become incorporated into 'routine custom and practice' in the absence of any evidence supporting efficacy and/or tolerability, and these treatments may sometimes continue to be used despite the findings of later, larger, and more definitive negative studies and meta-analyses. The use of omega-3 fatty acids in schizophrenia is a good example of this. An example of widespread off-label prescribing of a psychotropic in non-mental health conditions is amitriptyline – 93% of UK primary care prescriptions are off-label.[11]

The psychopharmacology special interest group at the Royal College of Psychiatrists published a consensus statement on the use of licensed medicines for unlicensed uses[12] which was updated in 2017.[13] They note that unlicensed use is common in general adult psychiatry with cross-sectional studies showing that up to 50% of patients are prescribed at least one drug outside the terms of its licence. They also note that the prevalence of this type of prescribing is likely to be higher in patients under the age of 18 or over 65, in those with a learning disability, in women who are pregnant or lactating and in those patients who are cared for in forensic psychiatry settings. The main recommendations in the consensus statement are summarised below.

Before prescribing 'off-label':

- Exclude licensed alternatives (e.g. they have proved ineffective or poorly tolerated).
- Ensure familiarity with the evidence base for the intended unlicensed use. If unsure, seek advice from another clinician (and possibly a specialist pharmacist).
- Consider and document the potential risks and benefits of the proposed treatment. Share this risk assessment with the patient, and carers if applicable. Document the discussion and the patient's consent or lack of capacity to consent.
- If prescribing responsibility is to be shared with primary care, ensure that the risk assessment and consent issues are shared with the GP.
- Monitor for efficacy and side effects; start a low dose and increase slowly.
- Consider publishing the case to add to the body of knowledge.
- Withdraw any treatment that is ineffective or where emergent risks outweigh the benefits.

The more experimental the unlicensed use is, the more important it is to adhere to the above guidance.

Examples of acceptable use of drugs outside their product licences/labels

Table 14.6 gives examples of common unlicensed uses of drugs in psychiatric practice. These examples would all fulfil the Bolam and Bolitho criteria in principle. An exhaustive list of unlicensed uses is impossible to prepare as: the evidence base is constantly changing and because the expertise and experience of prescribers varies. A particular strategy may be justified in the hands of a specialist in psychopharmacology based on a tertiary referral centre but be much more difficult to justify if initiated by someone with a special interest in psychotherapy who rarely prescribes.

Table 14.6 Examples of common unlicensed uses of drugs in psychiatric practice

Drug/drug group	Unlicensed use(s)	Further information
Second generation antipsychotics	Psychotic illness other than schizophrenia	Licensed indications vary markedly, and in most cases are unlikely to reflect real differences in efficacy between drugs
Clozapine	Bipolar disorder	Substantial evidence to support efficacy when standard treatments have failed to control symptoms
Cyproheptadine	Akathisia	Some evidence to support efficacy in this distressing and difficult to treat adverse effect of antipsychotics
Fluoxetine/Sertraline	Generalised anxiety disorder	Substantial supporting evidence
Ketamine (racemate)	Refractory depression	Substantial evidence with both racemate and S-isomer
Melatonin (circadin)	Insomnia in children	Licence covers adults >55 years only. Probably preferable to unlicensed formulations of melatonin
Methylphenidate	ADHD in children under 6	Established clinical practice
Naltrexone	Self-injurious behaviour in people with learning disabilities	Limited evidence base Acceptable in specialist hands
Sodium valproate	Treatment and prophylaxis of bipolar disorder	Established clinical practice Evidence from other valproate preparations

CHAPTER 14

Note that some drugs do not have a UK licence for any indication. Two commonly prescribed examples in psychiatric practice are immediate release formulations of melatonin (used to treat insomnia in children and adolescents) and pirenzepine (used to treat clozapine-induced hypersalivation). Awareness of the evidence base and documentation of potential benefits, side effects and patient consent are especially important here.

References

1. Datapharm Communications Ltd. Summary of product characteristics. Electronic Medicines Compendium 2020; http://www.medicines.org.uk/emc.
2. Maher AR, et al. Efficacy and comparative effectiveness of atypical antipsychotic medications for off-label uses in adults: a systematic review and meta-analysis. *JAMA* 2011; **306**:1359–1369.
3. Bolam v Friern Barnet Hospital Management Committee. *The Weekly Law Reports* 1957; **1**:582.
4. Bolitho v City and Hackney Health Authority. *The Weekly Law Reports* 1997; **3**:1151.

5. British and Irish Legal Information Institute. Montgomery (Appellant) v Lanarkshire Health Board (Respondent) (Scotland) 2015; http://www.bailii.org/uk/cases/UKSC/2015/11.html.

6. General Medical Council. Good practice in prescribing and managing medicines and devices 2013; https://www.gmc-uk.org/guidance/ethical_guidance/14316.asp.

7. Buckman Co. v. Plaintiffs' Legal Comm. 531 U.S. 341 2001; https://www.law.cornell.edu/supct/html/98-1768.ZO.html.

8. FindLaw. Off-label use promotion is protected free speech 2012; https://blogs.findlaw.com/second_circuit/2012/12/off-label-use-promotion-is-protected-free-speech.html.

9. Vijay A, et al. Patterns and predictors of off-label prescription of psychiatric drugs. *PLoS One* 2018; 13:e0198363.

10. Epstein RS, et al. The many sides of off-label prescribing. *ClinPharmacolTher* 2012; 91:755–758.

11. Wong J, et al. Off-label indications for antidepressants in primary care: descriptive study of prescriptions from an indication based electronic prescribing system. *BMJ* 2017; 356:j603.

12. Royal College of Psychiatrists. College Report 142. Use of licensed medicines for unlicensed applications in psychiatric practice 2007; http://www.rcpsych.ac.uk/publications/collegereports/cr/cr142.aspx.

13. Royal College of Psychiatrists Psychopharmacology Committee. Use of licensed medicines for unlicensed applications in psychiatric practice. 2nd edition. College Report CR210 2017; http://www.rcpsych.ac.uk/files/pdfversion/CR210.pdf.

Further reading

Frank B, et al. Psychotropic medications and informed consent: a review. *Ann Clin Psychiatry* 2008; 20:87–95. General Medical Council. Good practice in prescribing and managing medicines and devices. 2013. http://www.gmc-uk.org/guidance/ethical_guidance/14316.asp.

Sharma, et al. BAP position statement: off-label prescribing of psychotropic medication to children and adolescents. *J Psychopharmacol* 2016; 30:416–421.

CHAPTER 14

The Mental Health Act in England and Wales

The 1983 Mental Health Act (MHA) as amended by the 2007 MHA is the legislation within England and Wales that provides the framework for detaining and treating people with mental disorder in hospital. It also allows for the supervision of people in the community.

The guidance here provides a quick summary of the sections that prescribers are likely to come across in their day to day work. It is not an exhaustive list. The Act has a statutory Code of Practice for practitioners and Chapter 25 of the Code provides detailed guidance on the treatment rules of the Act.[1] The MHA may be accessed at www.legislation.gov.uk.

Civil and forensic detention sections

Section 2	Admission for assessment which lasts for up to 28 days
Section 3	Admission for treatment which may last up to 6 months and is renewable
Section 36	Remand to hospital for treatment
Section 37	Hospital Order made by the courts (runs like a S3)
Notional 37	Treat as if subject to S37. This term is used informally under a number of different circumstances. One example is where a patient previously detained under S47/49 and their restriction order expires
Section 38	Interim Hospital Order
Section 41	Restriction Order an order made by the Crown Court restricting discharge. Accompanies S37 and is written as S37/41
Section 47	Transfer to hospital of prisoners
Section 49	A restriction order which usually accompanies S47 (Written as S47/49)
Section 48	Applies to un-sentenced prisoners in need of urgent treatment and is accompanied by S49 (Written as S48/49)
Section 58	**Treatment requiring consent or a second opinion** Please note **in law it is the Responsible Clinician (RC) who is accountable for the operation of S58**

It is important to note that the power to treat under Section 58 is only for treatment of mental disorder. Physical treatment (generally) is governed by the normal rules of consent or, if the person lacks capacity, the authority of the Mental Capacity Act.

The RC is usually the patient's consultant.

For the first three months of detention the RC may give medication (with or without consent) to a person under one of the detention sections named above for the treatment of their mental disorder. Thereafter the patient's consent or a second opinion must be sought. The three months countdown starts when medication for mental disorder is first administered whilst the patient is detained. Be aware that this includes a patient detained under S2 who is then without a break, changed to and detained under S3. For practical purposes the three month rule is usually calculated from the date of first detention.

If a patient consents to treatment, the RC completes a form **T2**.

If a patient has not given consent or has not got the capacity to consent a second opinion appointed doctor (SOAD) is called. The SOAD then completes a form **T3**.

A copy of the forms T2 and T3 should be kept with the patient's medication chart as recommended in paragraph 25.75 of the Code of Practice.[1]

Completion of forms T2 and T3

The following should be stated on the forms:

- The name of the drug **or** the class of drug
- If the class of drug is stated, the number of drugs allowed at any one time
- The route of administration
- The maximum dosage with reference to BNF guidance

For example, antipsychotic, second generation × 1 (oral) within BNF maximum dose limits.

For a patient who has capacity and is consenting to treatment and is only willing to take a particular drug it is appropriate for the RC to write the name of the drug instead of the name of the class of drug on the T2.

For example, olanzapine tablets only (oral) within BNF maximum dose limits.

Psychotropics not found in the BNF may be written on a T2 or T3 with its indication.

For example, melperone tablets (oral) up to a maximum of 25mg daily for the treatment of schizophrenia.

Non-psychotropics used for the treatment of mental disorder should be included on the T2 and T3, for example omega-3 fatty acids (fish oils) in schizophrenia. Antimuscarinics used to treat hypersalivation and the extrapyramidal adverse effects of antipsychotics should be included too.

Arranging and preparing for SOAD visits

The Code at paragraph 25.51 states: Clinicians should consider seeking a review by a specialist mental health pharmacist before seeking a SOAD certificate, particularly if the patient's medication regime is complex or unusual.

Statutory consultees

SOADs should consult with two people before issuing a T3. One must be a nurse. The other must not be a nurse or a doctor. Both must have been involved with the patient's treatment. These two people are known as statutory consultees. Mental health pharmacists can perform this role where they have been involved in any recent review of a patient's medication.

The Code of Practice 25.56 states:

Statutory consultees may expect to have a private discussion with the SOAD and to be listened to with consideration. Issues that the consultees may be asked about include, but are not limited to:

- the proposed treatment and the patient's ability to consent to it;
- their understanding of the past and present views and wishes of the patient;
- other treatment options and the way in which the decision on the treatment proposal was arrived at;
- the patient's progress and the views of the patient's carers; and
- where relevant, the implications of imposing treatment on a patient who does not want it and the reasons why the patient is refusing treatment.

What is consent?

The Code of 24.34 defines consent as:

... the voluntary and continuing permission of a patient to be given a particular treatment, based on a sufficient knowledge of the purpose, nature, likely effects and risks of that treatment, including the likelihood of its success and any alternatives to it. Permission given under any unfair or undue pressure is not consent.

For a patient to consent formally they must have the 'capacity' to make a decision.

What is capacity?

The Mental Capacity Act 2005 states that

- people must be assumed to have capacity unless it is established that they lack capacity;
- people are not to be treated as unable to make a decision unless all practicable steps to help them do so have been taken without success; and
- people are not to be treated as unable to make a decision merely because they make an unwise decision

A patient is deemed to lack capacity if they cannot:

- understand relevant information about the decision to be made
  or
- retain that information in their mind
  or
- use or weigh that information as part of the decision making process
  or
- communicate their decision (by talking, using sign language or any other means).

CHAPTER 14

The patient needs to fail on only one of the four points above to be deemed not to have capacity. Capacity may change over time so reassessment is important. A person may lack capacity about one decision but not about another.

Section 62 urgent treatment

If after three months medication is needed urgently to treat a patient's mental disorder and it is not covered by a T2 or T3, S62 may be applied.

The Code of Practice 25.38 states

> This applies only if the treatment in question is immediately necessary to:
>
> - save the patient's life;
> - prevent a serious deterioration of the patient's condition, and the treatment does not have unfavourable physical or psychological consequences which cannot be reversed;
> - alleviate serious suffering by the patient, and the treatment does not have unfavourable physical or psychological consequences which cannot be reversed and does not entail significant physical hazard; or
> - prevent patients behaving violently or being a danger to themselves or others, and the treatment represents the minimum interference necessary for that purpose, does not have unfavourable physical or psychological consequences which cannot be reversed and does not entail significant physical hazard.

Each Trust should design a form for the clinician in charge of treatment (usually the consultant) to state what the treatment is, why it is immediately necessary and the length of treatment.

Section 132 duty of managers of hospitals to give information to detained patients

With regards to S132 and consent to treatment the code of practice 4.20 states

> Patients must be told what the Act says about treatment for their mental disorder. In particular they must be told:
>
> - the circumstances (if any) in which they can be treated without their consent – and the circumstances in which they have the right to refuse treatment;
> - the role of second opinion appointed doctors (SOADs) and the circumstances in which they may be involved; and
> - (where relevant) the rules on electro-convulsive therapy (ECT) and medication administered as part of ECT.

Electro-convulsive therapy ECT

Section 58a deals with ECT. Treatment for ECT is authorised on forms:

T4	For consenting adults 18 and over, may be written by the RC or SOAD
T5	For consenting patients under 18, to be written by a SOAD only
T6	For patients who lack capacity. To be written by a SOAD only

All patients under the age of 18 who are to receive ECT, whether or not they are detained under the MHA, must have treatment authorised on a T5 or T6.

Patients who have the capacity to consent must not receive ECT unless they do consent (in emergencies this can however be overridden under Section 62 of the Act). There is no three-month rule with regards to ECT and this also applies to medication given as part of ECT. Hence a form for ECT must always be in place regardless of the first date of detention. The forms should indicate the maximum number of treatments the patient is to receive (Code of Practice paragraph 25.23).

Community patients

Patients on a Community Treatment Order (CTO) should have treatment authorised on one of the following forms:

| CTO11 | Written by a SOAD, after one month on a CTO, when the patient lacks capacity |
| CTO12 | Written by the RC when the patient has capacity and is consenting to treatment, after one month on a CTO |

There is no legal authority to give patients medication in the community if they refuse it.

Reference

1. Department of Health. Code of practice: mental Health Act 1983. Updated 31 October 2017. https://www.gov.uk/government/publications/code-of-practice-mental-health-act-1983#history.

CHAPTER 14

Site of administration of intramuscular injections

Table 14.7 gives the sites of administration formally indicated in the individual product's EU licence. Other routes and sites may be possible, but pharmacokinetic analysis of administration via these sites is generally not available.

Table 14.7 Site of administration of intramuscular injections

Antipsychotic generic name and formulation	Site(s) of administration
Typical antipsychotic (FGA) depots	
Bromperidol decanoate (available in Belgium, Germany, Italy and the Netherlands[1]) (in sesame oil)	Deep intramuscular injection into the gluteal muscle. SPC in some countries recommend to alternate injections into the left and right sides to prevent pain at the injection site.[2]
Clopentixol decanoate (in Viscoleo® thin vegetable oil)	Deep intramuscular injection into the **gluteal region**.[3,4]
Flupentixol decanoate (in thin vegetable oil derived from coconuts)	Deep intramuscular injection into the **upper outer buttock** (dorsogluteal) or **lateral thigh** (vastus lateralis).[5]
Fluphenazine decanoate (in sesame oil)	Deep intramuscular injection into the **gluteal region**.[5] Can also be administered into the **lateral surface of the thigh muscle** but this is **unlicensed use**. Administration into the deltoid is not recommended by manufacturer.[6]
Fluspirilene (available in some EU countries, Canada, Argentina and Israel[7]) (in vegetable oil[8])	Deep intramuscular injection into the **gluteus muscle** (intragluteal). Because of its microcrystalline form, irritation and inflammation symptoms may occur at the injection site. Manufacturer recommends to alternate between left and right gluteal muscle.[2,9]
Haloperidol decanoate (in sesame oil)	Deep intramuscular injection into the **gluteal region** using an appropriate needle, preferably 2–2.5 inches long, of at least 21 gauge.[5] Can also be administered into the **deltoid muscle** according to the manufacturer.[10] **Although** this is an **unlicensed use** one trial suggests it is safe and effective.[11]
Perphenazine decanoate (in clinical use in the Nordic countries, Belgium, Portugal and the Netherlands[12]) (in sesame oil)	Deep intramuscular injection.[12,13] No other information available.
Perphenazine enanthate (in clinical use in the Nordic countries, Belgium, Portugal and the Netherlands[12]) (in sesame oil)	Deep intramuscular injection into the **gluteal** region.[12,14]

Table 14.7 (*Continued*)

Antipsychotic generic name and formulation	Site(s) of administration
Pipotiazine palmitate (in sesame oil)	Deep intramuscular injection into the muscle in **the thigh** or **bottom.**[15]
Zuclopenthixol decanoate (in thin vegetable oil derived from coconuts)	Deep intramuscular injection into the **upper outer buttock** (dorsogluteal) or **lateral thigh** (vastus lateralis).[5]

Atypical antipsychotic (SGA) depots

Antipsychotic generic name and formulation	Site of administration
Aripiprazole Powder and vehicle for prolonged release suspension	*Gluteal muscle* administration[5] The recommended needle for gluteal administration is a 38mm (1.5inch), 22 gauge hypodermic safety needle; for obese patients (body mass index >28kg/m²), a 50mm (2inch), 21 gauge hypodermic safety needle should be used. Gluteal injections should be alternated between the two gluteal muscles. *Deltoid muscle* administration[5] The recommended needle for deltoid administration is a 25mm (1inch), 23 gauge hypodermic safety needle; for obese patients, a 38mm (1.5inch), 22 gauge hypodermic safety needle should be used. Deltoid injections should be alternated between the two deltoid muscles. The powder and vehicle vials and the pre-filled syringe are for single-use only.[5]
Aripiprazole lauroxil	Intramuscular administration into the **deltoid** or **gluteal** muscle.[16]
Olanzapine pamoate monohydrate Powder and vehicle for prolonged release suspension	Olanzapine pamoate monohydrate should only be administered by deep intramuscular **gluteal** injection by a healthcare professional trained in the appropriate injection technique and in locations where post-injection observation and access to appropriate medical care in the case of overdose can be assured.[17]
Paliperidone palmitate Prolonged release suspension for injection	Injected slowly, deep into the **deltoid or dorsogluteal muscle** (the two initial loading doses should be administered in the deltoid muscle so as to attain therapeutic concentrations rapidly).[5,18] Administration should be in a single injection. The dose should not be given in divided injections.[18]

(*Continued*)

CHAPTER 14

Table 14.7 (Continued)

Antipsychotic generic name and formulation	Site(s) of administration
Paliperidone palmitate Prolonged release suspension for injection every 3 months	***Deltoid muscle** administration*[19] The specified needle for administration of Trevicta into the deltoid muscle is determined by the patient's weight. • For those ≥90kg, the thin wall 1½inch, 22 gauge (0.72mm × 38.1mm) needle should be used. • For those <90kg, the thin wall 1inch, 22 gauge (0.72mm × 25.4mm) needle should be used. It should be administered into the centre of the deltoid muscle. Deltoid injections should be alternated between the two deltoid muscles. ***Gluteal muscle** administration*[19] The needle to be used for administration of TREVICTA into the gluteal muscle is the thin wall 1½inch, 22 gauge (0.72mm × 38.1mm) needle regardless of body weight. It should be administered into the upper-outer quadrant of the gluteal muscle. Gluteal injections should be alternated between the two gluteal muscles.
Risperidone microspheres Powder and vehicle for prolonged-release suspension	Deep intramuscular **deltoid or gluteal** injection using the appropriate safety needle. For deltoid administration, use the 1-inch needle alternating injections between the two arms. For gluteal administration, use the 2-inch needle alternating injections between the two buttocks.[20]

Intramuscular injections for rapid tranquilisation

Antipsychotic generic name and Formulation	Site of administration
Aripiprazole Solution for injection	To enhance absorption and minimise variability, injection into the **deltoid or deep within the gluteus maximus muscle**, avoiding adipose regions, is recommended.[21]
Haloperidol Solution for injection	Intramuscular administration.[22] Preferably, **gluteal muscle** is selected when the dosage volume is high. **Deltoid muscle** is preferred for low doses of the injection. However, there is no information on the dosage limit for these specific muscle groups. Choice of site is at the discretion of the prescriber, according to the manufacturer.[23]
Lorazepam Solution for injection	Intramuscular administration. Can be administered into the **gluteal, deltoid or frontal thigh area** according to the manufacturer.[24] A 1:1 dilution of Ativan Injection with normal saline or Sterile Water for Injection BP is recommended in order to facilitate intramuscular administration and absorption.[25]

Table 14.7 (Continued)

Antipsychotic generic name and formulation	Site(s) of administration
Olanzapine Powder for solution for injection	Inject slowly, deep into the muscle mass. The exact site of administration is not specified and choice of muscle site should be a clinical decision, according to the manufacturer.[26] Dissolve the contents of the vial using 2.1mL of Sterile Water for Injection to provide a solution containing approximately 5mg/mL of olanzapine. The resulting solution should appear clear and yellow. Use immediately (within 1 hour) after reconstitution. *Discard any unused portion.*[27]
Promethazine hydrochloride Solution for injection	By deep intramuscular injection. Can be administered into the **thigh, upper arm** or **gluteal region**. Ensure muscle mass is sufficient for the volume being injected.[6]
Other Intramuscular injections	
Clotiapine 40mg/4mL injection (available in Argentina, Belgium, Israel, Italy, Luxemburg, South Africa, Spain, Switzerland and Taiwan[28])	By intramuscular injection.[28] No other information available.
Clozapine intramuscular injection 25mg/mL (unlicensed)[29,30]	Only for deep intramuscular administration into the **gluteal** muscle. 25mg IM clozapine = 50mg oral. The maximum volume that can be injected into each site is 4mL (100mg). For doses greater than 100mg daily, the dose may be divided and administered into two sites. (Injection sites should be rotated as per usual IM practice.)

CHAPTER 14

References

1. Purgato M et al. Bromperidol decanoate (depot) for schizophrenia. *Cochrane Database Syst Rev* 2012; 11:Cd001719.
2. Eumedica. Medical information department – written communication, 2020.
3. Aaes-Jørgensen T et al. Serum concentrations of the isomers of clopenthixol and a metabolite in patients given cis(Z)-clopenthixol decanoate in viscoleo. *Psychopharmacology (Berl)* 1983; **81**:68–72.
4. Chakravarti SK et al. Zuclopenthixol acetate (5% in 'Viscoleo'): single-dose treatment for acutely disturbed psychotic patients. *Curr Med Res Opin* 1990; **12**:58–65.
5. Janssen UK. Guidance on the administration to adults of oil-based depot and other long-acting intramuscular antipsychotic injections. 2016. http://www2.hull.ac.uk/fhsc/pdf/SOP%20IM%20Injection%205th%20Edition%20SOP%20FINAL.pdf.
6. Sanofi. Medical information department – verbal and written communication, 2017.
7. Abhijnhan A et al. Depot fluspirilene for schizophrenia. *Cochrane Database Syst Rev* 2007; **2007**:Cd001718.
8. Spanarello S et al. The pharmacokinetics of long-acting antipsychotic medications. *Curr Clin Pharmacol* 2014; **9**:310–317.
9. iMedikament.de. IMAP. 2015. https://imedikament.de/imap.
10. Janssen. Medical information department – verbal and written communication, 2017.
11. McEvoy JP et al. Effectiveness of paliperidone palmitate vs haloperidol decanoate for maintenance treatment of schizophrenia: a randomized clinical trial. *JAMA* 2014; **311**:1978–1987.
12. Quraishi S et al. Depot perphenazine decanoate and enanthate for schizophrenia. *Cochrane Database Syst Rev* 2000:Cd001717.
13. Laakeinfo.fi. Peratsin Dekanoaatii injektioneste, liuos 108mg/ml. 2019. https://laakeinfo.fi/Medicine.aspx?m=2333.
14. Starmark JE et al. Abscesses following prolonged intramuscular administration of perphenazine enantate. *Acta Psychiatr Scand* 1980; **62**:154–157.

15. South London and Maudsley NHS Foundation Trust. Pipotiazine palmitate. 2015. https://www.slam.nhs.uk/media/12994/pipotiazine-palmitate.pdf.

16. Turncliff R et al. Relative bioavailability and safety of aripiprazole lauroxil, a novel once-monthly, long-acting injectable atypical antipsychotic, following deltoid and gluteal administration in adult subjects with schizophrenia. *Schizophr Res* 2014; 159:404–410.

17. Eli Lily and Company Limited. Summary of product characteristics. Zypadhera 210mg powder and solvent for prolonged release suspension for injection. 2020. https://www.medicines.org.uk/emc/product/6429/smpc.

18. Janssen-Cilag Ltd. Summary of product characteristics. Xeplion 25mg, 50mg, 75mg, 100mg, and 150mg prolonged-release suspension for injection. 2018. https://www.medicines.org.uk/emc/medicine/31329.

19. Janssen-Cilag Ltd. Summary of product characteristics. TREVICTA 175mg, 263mg, 350mg, 525mg prolonged release suspension for injection. 2019. https://www.medicines.org.uk/emc/medicine/32050.

20. Janssen-Cilag Limited. Summary of product characteristics. RISPERDAL CONSTA 25mg powder and solvent for prolonged-release suspension for intramuscular injection. 2018. https://www.medicines.org.uk/emc/medicine/9939.

21. Otsuka Pharmaceutical (UK) Ltd. Abilify 7.5mg/ml solution for injection (intramuscular). 2020. https://www.medicines.org.uk/emc/product/6239/smpc.

22. ADVANZ Pharma. Haloperidol injection BP 5mg/ml. 2017. https://www.medicines.org.uk/emc/product/514.

23. Concordia International. Medical information department – verbal and written communication, 2017.

24. Pfizer. Medical information department – verbal and written communication, 2017.

25. Pfizer Limited. Ativan 4mg/ml solution for injection. 2019. https://www.medicines.org.uk/emc/product/5473/smpc.

26. Lilly UK. Medical information department – verbal and written communication, 2017.

27. Eli Lilly and Company (NZ) Limited. Zyprexa IM inj New Zealand datasheet. 2019. https://medsafe.govt.nz/Profs/Datasheet/z/ZyprexaIMinj.pdf.

28. Carpenter S et al. Clotiapine for acute psychotic illnesses. *Cochrane Database Syst Rev* 2004:Cd002304.

29. Henry R et al. Evaluation of the effectiveness and acceptability of intramuscular clozapine injection: illustrative case series. *Br J Psych Bull* 2020:1–5. 44:239–243

30. Casetta C et al. A retrospective study of intramuscular clozapine prescription for treatment initiation and maintenance in treatment-resistant psychosis. *Br J Psychiatry* 2020: 217:506–513

CHAPTER 14

Intravenous formulations in psychiatry

The intravenous (IV) route is one of the main parenteral routes for drug administration outside psychiatry (see Table 14.8). Advantages include rapid onset of action, precise titration, patient-specific dosing and bypass of liver metabolism. Hypersensitivity reactions, prevalence of adverse effects, infection risk and a higher overall cost some of its most debated downsides. Unlike other areas of medicine, IV has been significantly under-utilised in psychiatry. A testament to this is the audit undertaken by the Prescribing for Mental Health Observatory in 2013 in the UK – from the recorded 2,172 episodes of acute disturbance, use of IV medication was limited to only two instances.[1]

While the main focus of delivering psychotropic medication through the IV route has been the management of acutely disturbed behaviour, its indications include a wide range of diagnoses, including affective and anxiety disorder, among others. Given the special care and expertise needed for the safe administration of IV formulations, they are most commonly considered when standard options fail to produce the desirable effect and in special clinical settings where trained staff, optimal monitoring, resuscitation equipment and ventilators are all at hand, such as the general hospital.[2] Some drugs may only be given by the IV route (brexanolone for example).

Table 14.8 Intravenous medication in psychiatry

Medication	Indication	Class	Dose[a]	Adverse Effects[b]	Comments
Biperiden[3]	Akathisia	Peripheral anticholinergic	5mg	None of note	Weak evidence
Brexanolone[4,5] (allopregnanolone)	Postnatal Depression	GABA – A positive allosteric modulator	Weight-based dosing, with a recommended maximal dose of 90µg/kg/hour	Sleepiness, dry mouth, loss of consciousness, and hot flushes	The intravenous infusion takes about 60 hours (2½ days) to complete
Citalopram	Depression[6,7]	SSRI	10–20mg	Fatigue, insomnia, anxiety, headaches	No serious adverse events reported
	Treatment-resistant OCD[8]		20–80mg		
Clomipramine[8–11]	Treatment-resistant OCD	TCA	150–250mg	Nausea, hypotension, bradycardia	Significant improvement sometimes noted
Dexmedetomidine[12–17]	Acute disturbance	Highly selective α_2-adrenergic receptor agonist	0.2–1.4µg/kg/hour	Bradycardia, hypotension	Only appropriate for in an ICU setting
Diazepam[18]	Acute disturbance	Benzodiazepine	5–20mg	Respiratory depression	Widely used, despite the dearth of available evidence

(Continued)

CHAPTER 14

Table 14.8 (*Continued*)

Medication	Indication	Class	Dose[a]	Adverse Effects[b]	Comments
Droperidol[19–24]	Acute disturbance	Butyrophenone (D2 antagonist)	5–10mg	Historical concerns over QT prolongation have been contested in subsequent reviews and trials	Combination with midazolam is more effective than either IV droperidol is superior to lorazepam
Haloperidol	Acute disturbance[24–27]	Butyrophenone (D2 antagonist)	5–10mg	Dystonia, hypoxia	Lack of robust recent evidence ECG essential
	Delirium[28–30]		2–2.5mg every 4–8 hours Up to 10mg slow bolus	Over sedation hypokinesia	Most recent evidence showed effect not superior to placebo in ICU delirium ECG essential
Ketamine	Acute disturbance[31–34]	NMDA antagonist	1–5mg/kg	No effect on respiratory drive. May increase heart rate and blood pressure	Supported by the Royal College of Emergency Medicine
	Depression[35–43]		0.5mg/kg, diluted in 0.9% saline, over a 40-minute period (absolute dose 26–60mg)	No serious adverse events. Dissociation was common. Transient blood pressure elevation	Most recent evidence supports weekly infusions and is more positive than previous Cochrane review (2015)[44]
	Bipolar depression[44,45]		0.5mg/kg	Well tolerated	Cochrane (2015)[44] suggests evidence is limited, though a 2018 study found it safe and effective
	Fatigue[46]		0.5mg/kg	Mild and transient	Apparently safe and effective
Lorazepam	Acute disturbance[23]	Benzodiazepine		No significant side effects reported	Inferior to IV droperidol
	Delirium[29]		3mg of lorazepam in 25mL of 0.9% normal saline solution	Difficult to say as was given in combination with haloperidol	Combination with haloperidol more effective than haloperidol
Midazolam[20,21,47,48]	Acute disturbance	Benzodiazepine	2.5–15mg	Safe but respiratory depression is a possibility, especially in higher doses	High dose protocols are not more effective but have higher adverse events incidence. Combination with droperidol more effective

Table 14.8 (Continued)

Medication	Indication	Class	Dose[a]	Adverse Effects[b]	Comments
Nitroprusside[49]	Schizophrenia	Vasodilator	0.5μg/kg/hour	Well tolerated	Probably not efficacious
Olanzapine[20–22,50–52]	Acute disturbance	Atypical antipsychotic	1.25–20mg	Hypoxia, respiratory depression, bradycardia	Safe with appropriate monitoring
Scopolamine[53] (hyoscine)	Depression	Anticholinergic	4μg/kg	No serious adverse events. Drowsiness, blurred vision, dry mouth, light-headedness and reduced blood pressure were reported	Effective
Trazodone[54]	Depression	SARI	25–100mg in 250mL of saline	No serious adverse events. Sedation, rash, dizziness	No difference compared with IV Clomipramine
Valproate	Acute disturbance[55]	Mood stabiliser	20mg/kg	Sedation	As effective as Haloperidol with less severe side effects
	Acute mania[56]		500mg		Possibly faster-acting than haloperidol

[a]The range of doses as described in the included studies.
[b]As reported in studies, though not exclusively.

References

1. POMH-UK. Topic 16a. Rapid tranquillisation in the context of the pharmacological management of acutely-disturbed behaviour. Royal College of Psychiatrists, 2017.
2. Patel MX, et al. Joint BAP NAPICU evidence-based consensus guidelines for the clinical management of acute disturbance: de-escalation and rapid tranquillisation. *Journal of Psychopharmacology* 2018; 32:601–640.
3. Hirose S, et al. Intravenous Biperiden in Akathisia: an open pilot study. *The International Journal of Psychiatry in Medicine* 2000; 30:185–194.
4. Meltzer-Brody S, et al. Brexanolone injection in post-partum depression: two multicentre, double-blind, randomised, placebo-controlled, phase 3 trials. *The Lancet* 2018; 392:1058–1070.
5. Kanes S, et al. Brexanolone (SAGE-547 injection) in post-partum depression: a randomised controlled trial. *The Lancet* 2017; 390:480–489.
6. Pompili M, et al. Response to intravenous antidepressant treatment by suicidal vs. *Nonsuicidal Depressed Patients. J Affect Disord* 2010; 122:154–158.
7. Altamura AC, et al. Intravenous augmentative citalopram versus clomipramine in partial/nonresponder depressed patients: a short-term, low dose, randomized, placebo-controlled study. *Journal of Clinical Psychopharmacology* 2008; 28:406–410.
8. Pallanti S, et al. Citalopram intravenous infusion in resistant obsessive-compulsive disorder: an open trial. *J Clin Psychiatry* 2002; 63:796–801.
9. Koran LM, et al. Rapid benefit of intravenous pulse loading of clomipramine in obsessive-compulsive disorder. *Am J Psychiatry* 1997; 154:396–401.
10. Fallon BA, et al. Intravenous clomipramine for obsessive-compulsive disorder refractory to oral clomipramine: a placebo-controlled study. *Arch Gen Psychiatry* 1998; 55:918–924.
11. Karameh WK, et al. Intravenous clomipramine for treatment-resistant obsessive-compulsive disorder. *Int J Neuropsychopharmacol* 2015; 19.
12. Jakob SM, et al. Dexmedetomidine vs midazolam or propofol for sedation during prolonged mechanical ventilation: two randomized controlled trials. *Jama* 2012; 307:1151–1160.

CHAPTER 14

13. Calver L, et al. Dexmedetomidine in the emergency department: assessing safety and effectiveness in difficult-to-sedate acute behavioural disturbance. *Emergency Medicine Journal: EMJ* 2012; **29**:915–918.

14. Ahmed S, et al. *Dexmedetomidine Use in the ICU: Are We There Yet? Critical Care (London, England)* 2013; **17**:320.

15. Pasin L, et al. Dexmedetomidine reduces the risk of delirium, agitation and confusion in critically Ill patients: a meta-analysis of randomized controlled trials. *Journal of Cardiothoracic and Vascular Anesthesia* 2014; **28**:1459–1466.

16. Riker RR, et al. Dexmedetomidine vs midazolam for sedation of critically ill patients: a randomized trial. *Jama* 2009; **301**:489–499.

17. Bielka K, et al. Addition of dexmedetomidine to benzodiazepines for patients with alcohol withdrawal syndrome in the intensive care unit: a randomized controlled study. *Annals of Intensive Care* 2015; **5**:33.

18. Lerner Y, et al. Acute high-dose parenteral haloperidol treatment of psychosis. *Am J Psychiatry* 1979; **136**:1061–1064. 1010.1176/ajp.1136.1068.1061.

19. Knott JC, et al. Randomized clinical trial comparing intravenous midazolam and droperidol for sedation of the acutely agitated patient in the emergency department. *Annals of Emergency Medicine* 2006; **47**:61–67.

20. Chan EW, et al. Intravenous droperidol or olanzapine as an adjunct to midazolam for the acutely agitated patient: a multicenter, randomized, double-blind, placebo-controlled clinical trial. *Annals of Emergency Medicine* 2013; **61**:72–81.

21. Yap CYL, et al. Intravenous midazolam-droperidol combination, droperidol or olanzapine monotherapy for methamphetamine-related acute agitation: subgroup analysis of a randomized controlled trial. *Addiction* 2017; **112**:1262–1269.

22. Taylor DM, et al. Midazolam-droperidol, droperidol, or olanzapine for acute agitation: a randomized clinical trial. *Annals of Emergency Medicine* 2017; **69**:318–326.e311.

23. Richards JR, et al. Chemical restraint for the agitated patient in the emergency department: lorazepam versus droperidol. *The Journal of Emergency Medicine* 1998; **16**:567–573.

24. Thomas H, Jr., et al. Droperidol versus haloperidol for chemical restraint of agitated and combative patients. *Annals of Emergency Medicine* 1992; **21**:407–413.

25. Möller HJ, et al. Efficacy and side effects of haloperidol in psychotic patients: oral versus intravenous administration. *Am J Psychiatry* 1982; **139**:1571–1575.

26. Nielssen O, et al. Intravenous sedation of involuntary psychiatric patients in New South Wales. *Aust N Z J Psychiatry* 1997; **31**:273–278.

27. MacNeal JJ, et al. Use of haloperidol in PCP-intoxicated individuals. *Clinical Toxicology (Philadelphia, Pa)* 2012; **50**:851–853.

28. Page VJ, et al. Effect of intravenous haloperidol on the duration of delirium and coma in critically ill patients (Hope-ICU): a randomised, double-blind, placebo-controlled trial. *The Lancet Respiratory Medicine* 2013; **1**:515–523.

29. Hui D, et al. Effect of Lorazepam With Haloperidol vs Haloperidol Alone on Agitated Delirium in Patients With Advanced Cancer Receiving Palliative Care: A Randomized Clinical Trial. *JAMA* 2017; **318**:1047–1056.

30. Girard TD, et al. Haloperidol and Ziprasidone for treatment of delirium in critical illness. *N Engl J Med* 2018; **379**:2506–2516.

31. The Royal College of Emergency Medicine Guidelines for the Management of Excited Delirium/Acute Behavioural Disturbance (ABD). in M Gillings JG, M Aw-Yong, eds., 2016.

32. Isbister GK, et al. Ketamine as rescue treatment for difficult-to-sedate severe acute behavioral disturbance in the emergency department. *Ann Emerg Med* 2016; **67**:581–587.e581.

33. Le Cong M, et al. Ketamine sedation for patients with acute agitation and psychiatric illness requiring aeromedical retrieval. *Emergency Medicine Journal: EMJ* 2012; **29**:335–337.

34. Riddell J, et al. Ketamine as a first-line treatment for severely agitated emergency department patients. *Am J Emerg Med* 2017; **35**:1000–1004.

35. Caddy C, et al. Ketamine and other glutamate receptor modulators for depression in adults. *The Cochrane Database of Systematic Reviews* 2015:Cd011612.

36. Phillips JL, et al. Single, Repeated, and Maintenance Ketamine Infusions for Treatment-Resistant Depression: A Randomized Controlled Trial. *Am J Psychiatry* 2019; **176**:401–409.

37. McGirr A, et al. A systematic review and meta-analysis of randomized, double-blind, placebo-controlled trials of ketamine in the rapid treatment of major depressive episodes. *Psychological Medicine* 2015; **45**:693–704.

38. Fava M, et al. Double-blind, placebo-controlled, dose-ranging trial of intravenous ketamine as adjunctive therapy in treatment-resistant depression (TRD). *Molecular Psychiatry* 2020; **25**:1592–1603.

39. Singh JB, et al. A Double-Blind, Randomized, Placebo-Controlled, Dose-Frequency Study of Intravenous Ketamine in Patients With Treatment-Resistant Depression. *Am J Psychiatry* 2016; **173**:816–826.

40. Rodrigues NB, et al. Safety and tolerability of IV Ketamine in adults with major depressive or bipolar disorder: results from the Canadian rapid treatment center of excellence. *Expert Opinion on Drug Safety* 2020:1–10.

41. Salloum NC, et al. Efficacy of intravenous ketamine treatment in anxious versus nonanxious unipolar treatment-resistant depression. *Depress Anxiety* 2019; **36**:235–243.

42. Finnegan M, et al. Ketamine versus midazolam for depression relapse prevention following successful electroconvulsive therapy: a randomized controlled pilot trial. *J Ect* 2019; **35**:115–121.

43. Grunebaum MF, et al. Ketamine for rapid reduction of suicidal thoughts in major depression: a midazolam-controlled randomized clinical trial. *Am J Psychiatry* 2018; **175**:327–335.

44. McCloud TL, et al. Ketamine and other glutamate receptor modulators for depression in bipolar disorder in adults. Cochrane Database of Systematic Reviews 2015; CD011611.

45. Zheng W, et al. Rapid and longer-term antidepressant effects of repeated-dose intravenous ketamine for patients with unipolar and bipolar depression. *J Psychiatr Res* 2018; **106**:61–68.

46. Fitzgerald K, et al. Pilot randomized active-placebo controlled double-blind trial of low dose ketamine for the treatment of multiple sclerosis-related fatigue (1642). *Neurology* 2020; **94**:1642.

47. TREC G. Rapid tranquillisation for agitated patients in emergency psychiatric rooms: a randomised trial of midazolam versus haloperidol plus promethazine. *Bmj* 2003; **327**:708–713.

48. Spain D, et al. Safety and effectiveness of high-dose midazolam for severe behavioural disturbance in an emergency department with suspected psychostimulant-affected patients. *Emergency Medicine Australasia: EMA* 2008; **20**:112–120.

49. Brown HE, et al. Efficacy and Tolerability of Adjunctive Intravenous Sodium Nitroprusside Treatment for Outpatients With Schizophrenia: A Randomized Clinical Trial. *JAMA Psychiatry* 2019; **76**:691–699.

50. Martel ML, et al. A Large Retrospective Cohort of Patients Receiving Intravenous Olanzapine in the Emergency Department. *Acad Emerg Med* 2016; **23**:29–35.

51. Cole JB, et al. A Prospective Observational Study of Patients Receiving Intravenous and Intramuscular Olanzapine in the Emergency Department. *Ann Emerg Med* 2017; **69**:327–336.e322.

52. Sud P, et al. Intravenous droperidol or olanzapine as an adjunct to midazolam for the acutely agitated patient: a multicenter, randomized, double-blind, placebo-controlled clinical trial. *Annals of Emergency Medicine* 2013; **61**:597–598.

53. Drevets WC, et al. Replication of scopolamine's antidepressant efficacy in major depressive disorder: a randomized, placebo-controlled clinical trial. *Biol Psychiatry* 2010; **67**:432–438.

54. Buoli M, et al. Is trazodone more effective than clomipramine in major depressed outpatients? A single-blind study with intravenous and oral administration. *CNS Spectrums* 2019; **24**:258–264.

55. Asadollahi S, et al. Efficacy and safety of valproic acid versus haloperidol in patients with acute agitation: results of a randomized, double-blind, parallel-group trial. *International Clinical Psychopharmacology* 2015; **30**:142–150.

56. Sekhar S, et al. Efficacy of sodium valproate and haloperidol in the management of acute mania: a randomized open-label comparative study. *J Clin Pharmacol* 2010; **50**:688–692.

CHAPTER 14

Index

The Maudsley® Prescribing Guidelines in Psychiatry, Fourteenth Edition. David M. Taylor,
Thomas R. E. Barnes and Allan H. Young.
© 2021 David M. Taylor. Published 2021 by John Wiley & Sons Ltd.